Principles and Practice of

Pediatric Cardiology

Incorporating Care of Fetal Life, Newborn, Infant, Children and Adolescents

Volume 2

Principles and Practice of
Pediatric Cardiology

Incorporating Care of Fetal Life, Newborn, Infant, Children and Adolescents

Volume 2

KC Verma
MBBS, DCH, MD, DM (Cardiology), FICP (USA), FRST M&H (Lond), FCSI (India)
Senior Consulting Heart Specialist and
Formerly Professor in Cardiovascular and Thoracic Unit
Govt. Medical College, Jammu (J&K)

CBS

CBS Publishers & Distributors Pvt Ltd

New Delhi • Bengaluru • Chennai • Kochi • Kolkata • Mumbai
Hyderabad • Nagpur • Patna • Pune • Vijayawada

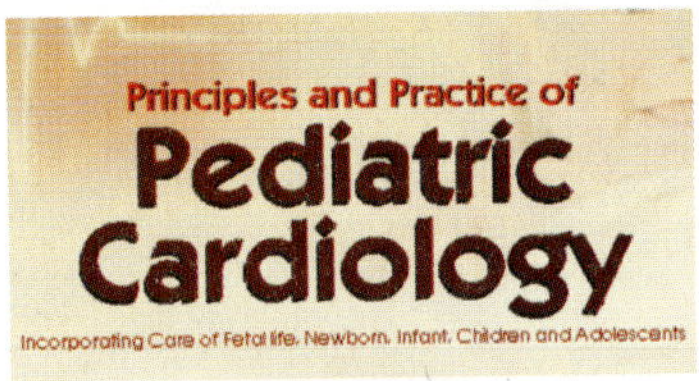

Volume 2

ISBN: 978-81-239-2926-2

First Edition: 2016

Published by Satish Kumar Jain and produced by Varun Jain for
CBS Publishers & Distributors Pvt Ltd
4819/XI Prahlad Street, 24 Ansari Road, Daryaganj, New Delhi 110 002, India.
Ph: 23289259, 23266861, 23266867   Fax: 011-23243014   Website: www.cbspd.com
e-mail: delhi@cbspd.com; cbspubs@airtelmail.in.

Corporate Office: 204 FIE, Industrial Area, Patparganj, Delhi 110 092
Ph: 4934 4934   Fax: 4934 4935   e-mail: publishing@cbspd.com; publicity@cbspd.com

Branches

- **Bengaluru:** Seema House 2975, 17th Cross, K.R. Road, Banasankari 2nd Stage, Bengaluru 560 070, Karnataka
  Ph: +91-80-26771678/79   Fax: +91-80-26771680   e-mail: bangalore@cbspd.com
- **Chennai:** No. 7, Subbaraya Street, Shenoy Nagar, Chennai 600 030, Tamil Nadu
  Ph: +91-44-26680620, 26681266   Fax: +91-44-42032115   e-mail: chennai@cbspd.com
- **Kochi:** Ashana House, 39/1904, AM Thomas Road, Valanjambalam, Ernakulam 682 016, Kochi, Kerala
  Ph: +91-484-4059061-65,67   Fax: +91-484-4059065   e-mail: kochi@cbspd.com
- **Kolkata:** No. 6/B, Ground Floor, Rameswar Shaw Road, Kolkata-700014 (West Bengal), India
  Ph: +91-33-2289-1126, 2289-1127, 2289-1128   e-mail: kolkata@cbspd.com
- **Mumbai:** 83-C, Dr E Moses Road, Worli, Mumbai-400018, Maharashtra
  Ph: +91-22-24902340/41   Fax: +91-22-24902342   e-mail: mumbai@cbspd.com

Representatives

- **Hyderabad** 0-9885175004
- **Nagpur** 0-9021734563
- **Patna** 0-9334159340
- **Pune** 0-9623451994
- **Vijayawada** 0-9000660880

Printed at RP Printers

to

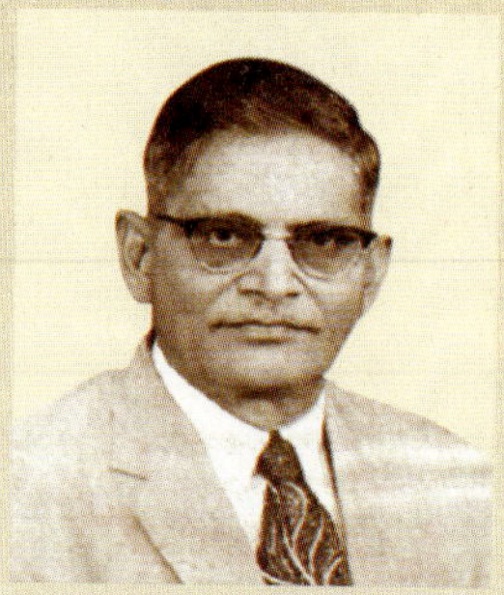

ST Achar MD, FRCP **(1902–1968)**

Dr ST Achar was born on the 11th september 1902 and he retired from service on the 10th september 1965. He entered Madras Medical College Services in 1928 after a brilliant academic career (MBBS First class and first rank 1927; first in the competitive examination for entry into service 1928). In 1948, he was selected to organize the Pediatric of the Madras Medical College occupying the first chair in pediatric in India. Under his chairmanship, this department was upgraded into a full-fledged All India Institute of Pediatrics in 1957 with Dr Achar as its first Director. His main scientific published work had been on pediatric nutritional problems on childhood cirrhosis and on diarrhoeal disorders and had earned for him nation-wide recognition and international reputation. By his hard work and dedication, he gained international fame. He was visiting Lecturer in USA in 1959 and was delegate to the World International Pediatric Congress in 1950 (Zurich) and read his resereach papers in various conferences in 1956 (Copenhagen), 1959 (Montreal), 1965 (Tokyo). He had laid down his office in September 1965 after 37 years of official service. In recognition to his scientific contributions and abilities, the Indian Council of Medical Research had selected him as Emeritus Medical Scientist to do research work in any institution of his choice for five years—an honour conferred for the first time by the council on retired persons unfortunately, he could not complete this mission as he passed away in june 1968.

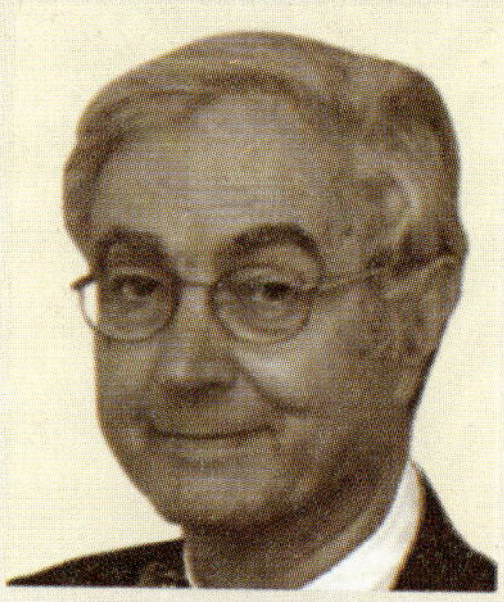

Alexander Nadas (1913–2000)

Dr Alexander Sandor Nadas of Harvard was described as the Father of Paediatric Cardiology. Dr Alexander Sandor Nadas, who trained generations of pediatric cardiologists at Children's Hospital in Boston and at Harvard Medical School, died on Tuesday at his home in Needham, Mass. He was 86.

Dr Nadas, a long-time former resident of Wellesley, Mass, retired in 1982 as chairman emeritus of the hospital's department of cardiology and in 1984 as professor emeritus of pediatrics at the medical school. He had been associated with Children's Hospital since 1949 and was credited with helping build the department's national and international renown for the care of children with heart disease. Harvard Medical School and Children's Hospital honored Dr. Nadas in 1989 by establishing a professorship in his name. And, just days before he died, the American Heart Association gave him its Paul Dudley White Award for his work as a pediatric cardiologist.

Dr Nadas's research centered on cardiovascular physiology and the physiology of congenital heart disease in children. He was the author of hundreds of clinical research papers, and wrote four editions of a textbook for medical students, Pediatric Cardiology, first published in 1957 by WB Saunders.

Preface

This book in its general section deals with brief account of **Anatomy and physiology** including **foetal circulation** of the cardiovascular system.

Examination of heart patient, with physical techniques of history taking, recording of symptoms and signs of heart disease along with thorough bodily examination of a patient has been lucidly detailed in this book.

As this book progresses in its chapters, it discusses the **latest innovations in both non-invasive and invasive techniques** such as cardiovascular imaging, stress testing, CMRI and cardiac CT, Holter study, nuclear evaluation of cardiac functions, echocardiography (transthoracic, transesophageal and intracardiac), cardiac catheterization and angiography.

Subject of **Cardiac arrhythmia** in children which is difficult to understand by both the postgraduates of general medicine and cardiac fellows has been made easy to grasp its fundamentals of diagnosis and treatment with both invasive and minimally invasive techniques.

A brief description of diagnosis and management of **rheumatic fever**, acute and chronic rheumatic valvular dysfunctions, infective endocarditis, pericardial diseases and cardiac tumors, emerging problems of metabolic syndrome, juvenile atherosclerosis, thyroid hormone disorders, mitral valve prolapse, sudden death syndrome and common cardio-pulmonary emergencies has been included skilfully.

This manuscript deals with **congenital heart diseases in younger age group of patients**, which carry maximum burden in cardiology and the author has been able to review its chapter with utmost care and construct its format in such a way that it could be understood with ease and comprehension by the readers of pediatric cardiology.

Heart failure remains as one of the leading causes of deaths in children and is often found to be the terminal event of various congenital and acquired heart ailments, particularly in malnourished patients in tropical and subtropical regions of the world including Indian subcontinent. This chapter has been written with simple text describing both types of systolic and diastolic heart failures supported with self-explanatory illustrations.

With the progress in the field of **interventional cardiology**, most of cardiac defects are being managed with the application of percutaneous catheter techniques in the closure of congenital intracardiac defects with occluders, ablation of foci of cardiac arrhythmias, AV and semilunar valve placement and percutaneous coronary interventions. The author has been able to mention a brief account of this technology.

Currently **medical genomics and stem cell technolgy** have revolutionized the management of various cardiovascular diseases by regenerating the damaged myocardium due to blocked blood supply of coronary vessels and peripheral arteries by advanced atherosclerosis. With the help of genetic engineering and genomic formulations, the scientists have been able to manufacture almost all the damaged tissues of the body. The author has been able to describe a brief review in this context and certainly this will evoke a healthy response among both the geneticists and medical workers, particularly with the recent introduction of **leadless pacemaker** and genetically prepared **pacing cellular system** in the management of cardiac arrhythmias.

Since large number of young adults are taking parts in different **sports** activities, it is therefore important for a specialised doctor in sport medicine to conduct a thorough examination before their selection into a particular sport. Some of them may be having congenital or acquired cardiovascular disorders and are therefore not fit for such exercising activities. The author, therefore, has made a comprehensive review guiding sports doctors in their final selection.

Robotic cardiac surgery in the management of various congenital and acquired cardiac defects and ***in utero* interventions** with minimal invasion, lesser operative time and least discomfort are becoming the popular techniques of the present time and author of this book, therefore has been able to attach a brief review of the subject in separate chapters.

Since we are living in a tropical country and systemic invasion by various viral and bacterial infections and parasitic infestations lead to high morbidity and mortality with cardiorespiratory failure particularly among the malnourished children. The author, therefore, thought it proper to add a brief review of **tropical cardiology.**

Many patients live at distance places from their consulting cardiologist and only way to approach them in hour of emergency, is through the mode of telecommunication, i.e. **"Telemedicine"**. Therefore, a brief review in this subject has been attached for the benefit of the pediatric patients.

This book in its present format and contents is considered as a treasure house of knowledge of cardiology and would certainly act as a ready reckoner to the budding cardiologist, cardiac fellows, junior and senior residents of general medicine for their understanding of the anatomical and physiological basis of cardiovascular system.and various newer non-invasive and invasive methodologies employed in the assessment and management of different cardiovascular disorders.

KC Verma

Acknowledgements

I am very grateful to my wife Dr Mrs Urmil Kanta Verma, Formerly Professor in Department of Blood Transfusion Medicine and Pathology for providing me a perfect congenial atmosphere and all material and moral support needed for writing such a specialised book on Pediatric Cardiology. I also appreciate the support of my grand daughter, Adwita Verma by posing as a physical model in chapter "Yogic exercises in children and adolescents".

Under the perfect guidance of Production manager, Vice-President and CMD of CBSP&D, New Delhi, contributions and hard work rendered by various individuals with respect to its perfect designing, typesetting, preparation of thousands of figures and line diagrams, which itself was a big challenging task, is joyfully acknowledged.

KC Verma

Contents

26 Diagnosis and Management of Cardiac Tumors

Cardiac tumours are benign or malignant neoplasms arising primarily in the inner lining, muscle layer, or the surrounding pericardium of the heart. They can be primary or metastatic. Primary cardiac tumours are rare in paediatric practice. In contrast, the incidence of cardiac tumours during foetal life has been reported to be approximately 0.14%. The vast majority of primary cardiac tumours in children are benign, whilst approximately 10% are malignant. Secondary malignant tumours are 10–20 times more prevalent than primary malignant tumours. Rhabdomyoma is the most common cardiac tumour during foetal life and childhood. It accounts for more than 60% of all primary cardiac tumours. The frequency and type of cardiac tumours in adults differ from those in children with 75% being benign and 25% being malignant. Myxomas are the most common primary tumours in adults constituting 40% of benign tumours. Sarcomas make up 75% of malignant cardiac masses. Echocardiography, computing tomography (CT) and magnetic resonance imaging (MRI) of the heart are the main noninvasive diagnostic tools. Cardiac catheterisation is seldom necessary. Tumour biopsy with histological assessment remains the gold standard for confirmation of the diagnosis. Surgical resection of primary cardiac tumours should be considered to relieve symptoms and mechanical obstruction to blood flow. The outcome of surgical resection in symptomatic, nonmyxomatous benign cardiac tumours is favourable. Patients with primary cardiac malignancies may benefit from palliative surgery but this approach should not be recommended for patients with metastatic cardiac tumours. Surgery, chemotherapy and radiotherapy may prolong survival. The prognosis for malignant primary cardiac tumours is generally extremely poor (Fig. 26.6 and Table 26.1).

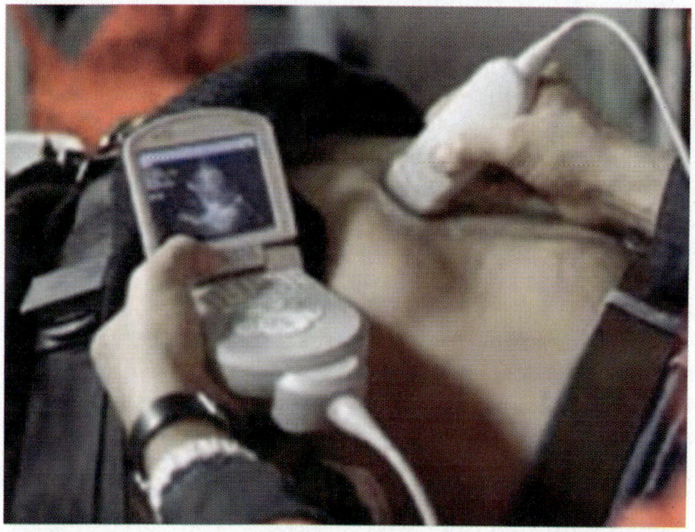

Fig. 26.1: *Hand held echocardiography is a useful tool for investigating a child with cardiac mass*

DIAGNOSIS OF CARDIAC TUMORS

Rhabdomyoma is the most common cardiac tumour during fetal life and childhood. This is usually followed by teratoma, fibroma and haemangioma. Myxoma is exceedingly rare in foetuses and neonates. Likewise, fibroma and intracardiac teratoma are exceptionally rare in adults but more commonly seen in the first year of life during childhood. Rhabdomyoma and pericardial teratoma make up more than 70% of the primary tumours of the heart in foetuses, neonates, and infants (Figs 26.2, 26.31 and 26.32).

Cardiac tumours may present in foetal or postnatal life. The presenting features depend on the size and location of the mass. In the foetus, a tumour can be noted on a routine antenatal anomaly scan as an intracardiac mass. The manifestations of a cardiac tumour in foetal life include arrhythmia, congestive heart failure, hydrops, and not infrequently stillbirth. In postnatal life, cardiac tumours may affect the integrity and function of the adjacent cardiac structures leading to severely compromised blood flow due to inflow or outflow tract obstruction, cyanosis, murmur, respiratory distress, myocardial dysfunction, valvular insufficiency, arrhythmias and sudden death.

Table 26.1: *Frequency distribution of cardiac tumours*

Types of tumors	*Frequency (%)*
Primary benign	
Rhabdomyoma	40–60
Teratoma	15–19
Fibroma	12–16
Myxoma	2–4
Haemangioma	5
Lymphangioma	
Haemangiopericytoma	Very rare
Oncocytic tumours	Rare
Primary malignant	
Rabdomyosarcomas	2
Fibrosarcoma	2
Secondary metastatic tumours	
Neuroblastoma	Rare
Leukaemia	Very rare
Lymphoma	Rare
Melanoma	Rare

Source: Uzun et al. orphanet journal of rare Diseases, 2007 2:11

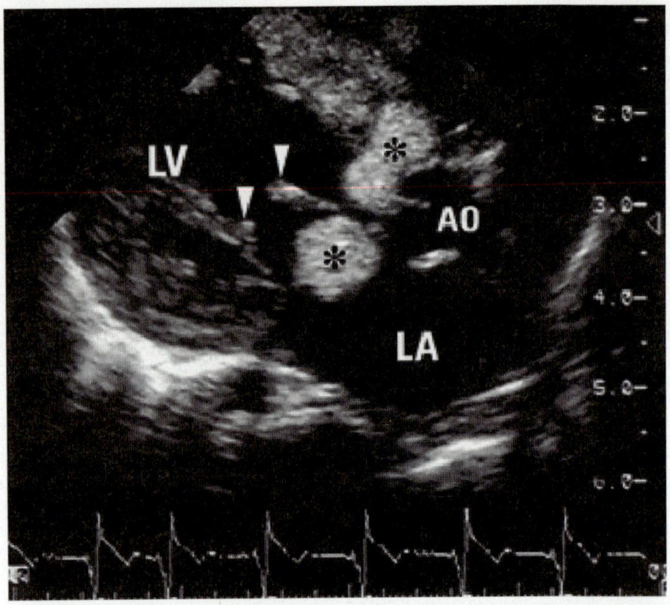

Fig. 26.2: *Multiple rhabdomyomas in tuberous sclerosis. Parasternal long-axis echocardiogram demonstrates two well-defined echogenic lesions (*) consistent with rhabdomyomas. One of these causes obstruction to left ventricle (LV) inflow with associated thickening of mitral valve leaflets (arrow heads) which narrows LV outflow tract. AO, aorta; LA, left atrium*

The diagnosis of cardiac tumours can be established in symptomatic patients, but in rare cases sudden death is the presenting feature. Echocardiography or magnetic resonance imaging (MRI) is usually adequate to facilitate the diagnosis of cardiac tumours. Cardiac catheterisation is rarely necessary. Tumour biopsy, with histological assessment, remains as the gold standard for confirmation of the diagnosis (Fig. 26.1).

Due to the progressive nature of pregnancy, fetal cardiac tumours are expected to grow antenatally and it is not unusual for cardiac lesions to be missed at an early obstetric scan. Some tumours can be detected from 20 weeks onwards but the majority will develop later in the course of the pregnancy. Most fetal cardiac tumours will be readily detectable in the late second or third trimester.

BENIGN CARDIAC TUMOURS

Rhabdomyoma

The most common primary cardiac tumour in infants and children is rhabdomyoma. It accounts for more than 60% of all primary cardiac tumours. Rhabdomyomas are usually located within the ventricles but not infrequently they may also originate in the atriums. Their location in the atrioventricular junction may have a rather peculiar effect where tumour may act like an accessory pathway with resultant pre-excitation on twelve lead electrocardiogram (ECG) (Figs 26.16 to 26.18).

Fetal diagnosis of cardiac rhabdomyoma is most commonly made on a 20-week anomaly scan after incidental detection of multiple intracardiac masses. Occasionally, cardiac rhabdomyoma may be noted coincidentally during evaluation for fetal cardiac arrhythmia.

Although the association of multiple cardiac rhabdomyomas with tuberous sclerosis has long been recognised, the association with a single rhabdomyoma is not clear. However, in case of a solitary tumour a careful examination of cardiac chambers should be made in order not to miss smaller lesions elsewhere. Multiple cardiac rhabdomyomas in fetal life may herald the diagnosis of tuberous sclerosis well before the other features of the disease, such as skin signs or seizures, emerge in infancy. The incidence of tuberous sclerosis in patients with cardiac rhabdomyoma has been reported to be between 60% and 80%.

Equally in patients with the diagnosis of tuberous sclerosis, cardiac rhabdomyoma can be detected between 43% and 72% of cases and their presence may assist in making a definitive diagnosis of the condition. However, the diagnosis of tuberous sclerosis must only be made on the basis of strict criteria, and the presence of multiple cardiac rhabdomyomas, whilst raising strong suspicions, is not by itself sufficient evidence to establish the diagnosis. Nevertheless, detection of multiple cardiac tumours should raise a strong suspicion of rhabdomyoma, hence tuberous sclerosis. In such patients, a detailed family history should be obtained and genetic counselling should be offered.

Clinical examination may reveal a murmur, reduced peripheral pulses or cyanosis. Arrhythmias are not a rare event and have been reported to occur in 16–47% of cases with cardiac rhabdomyoma. Atrial or ventricular arrhythmias frequently occur but a higher incidence of Wolff-Parkinson-White syndrome has been noted in patients with tuberous sclerosis (1.5%) compared to the general population (0.15%). This may be explained by the fact that the tumour cells may create continuity at the atrioventricular junction between the atrial and the ventricular myocardium. Since the tumour cells are structurally similar to Purkinje cells they can function like accessory pathways. As the tumour regresses, the associated arrhythmias also undergo spontaneous resolution and loss of the delta wave is frequently encountered (Figs 26.16 to 26.18).

Macroscopically rhabdomyomas appear uniform, round and solid, and are brighter than the neighbouring healthy myocardium. Their predominant location is the ventricular myocardium, but they can also be seen in the atrial wall. Rhabdomyomas are most commonly multiple and intracavitary extensions are found in up to 50% of patients. Echocardiography is diagnostic and shows multiple bright intramural masses with luminal extensions.

Microscopically each tumour shows pathognomonic spider cells with centrally placed cytoplasm containing the nucleus and myofibrils radiating to the cell wall. Rhabdomyomas are not considered to be true tumours and many authors would describe them as hamartomas of striated muscular fibres occurring solely in the heart. Rhabdomyomas exhibit immunoreactivity with the muscle markers desmin, actin, myoglobin, vimentin, and also with hamartin and tuberin. Immunohistochemical studies showed that the spider cells exhibit immunoreactivity with ubiquitin. The ubiquitin pathway is associated with the degradation of myoflaments, progression of cytoplasmic vacuolisation with the formation of spider cells, enlargement of glycogen vacuoles, apoptosis, myxoid degeneration and regression of the rhabdomyomas. These above events may provide plausible explanation for the spontaneous regression of rhabdomyomas. The outcome of antenatally detected cardiac rhabdomyomas is favourable. Once foetal somatic growth is completed, hamartomas lose their mitotic potential and undergo apoptosis. The majority of tumours will regress towards the end of the third trimester although rarely some may continue to grow larger. Despite the expected shrinkage of these tumours, unexpected foetal loss may occur due to arrhythmias or obstruction of blood flow.

After birth, rhabdomyoma cells lose their ability to divide and regression of the tumour in infancy is an expected outcome, regardless of size of the tumour. Hence, following birth, tumour regression is a rule rather than an exception. Complete resolution of more than 80% of the tumours may occur during early childhood.

Thus, due to high rate of spontaneous regression after birth these tumours can be managed conservatively with echocardiography and ECG monitoring. Surgical intervention should be preserved only for sick patients with symptoms of severe obstruction with haemodynamic compromise or haemodynamically significant and intractable arrhythmias that are unresponsive to antiarrhythmic drugs.

Fibroma (Figs 26.3 and 26.4)

Fibromas are solitary tumours that are mainly located in the ventricular septum. Fibromas are derived from connective tissue fibroblasts. They are primarily seen in childhood and the size may vary from 1–10 cm. Fibroma may invade the ventricular muscle, replace the working myocardium and may result in intractable congestive heart failure or cyanosis. Not infrequently, a fibroma may extend into the ventricular conduction system and can cause ventricular arrhythmias.

Macroscopically, a fibroma is clearly demarcated from the myocardium, but interdigitations with the surrounding myocardium can be seen on microscopy. Calcification of the central portion of the tumour is pathognomonic for fibroma reflecting poor blood supply to the mass.

Cardiac fibromas usually remain dormant and spontaneous regression rarely occurs, therefore total surgical resection is normally recommended. Large tumours can be resected subtotally. If progressive loss of working myocardial fibres continues and cardiac failure does not resolve following tumour resection, heart transplantation may be considered.

Teratoma (Figs 26.5, 26.9, 26.26 and and 26.28)

Cardiac teratoma is a rare tumour of the heart and pericardium. Teratomas are the second most common tumour in the fetus and neonate after rhabdomyoma. Most commonly, these tumours are detected in the pericardial cavity attached to the pulmonary artery and aorta. The tumour size within the heart varies from 2 to 9 cm in diameter, and intrapericardial tumours as large as 15 cm have been reported. Intracardiac tumours arise from the atrial or ventricular wall as nodular masses protruding into the cardiac chambers. Cardiac and pericardial teratomas are easily detected in the fetus and neonate by two

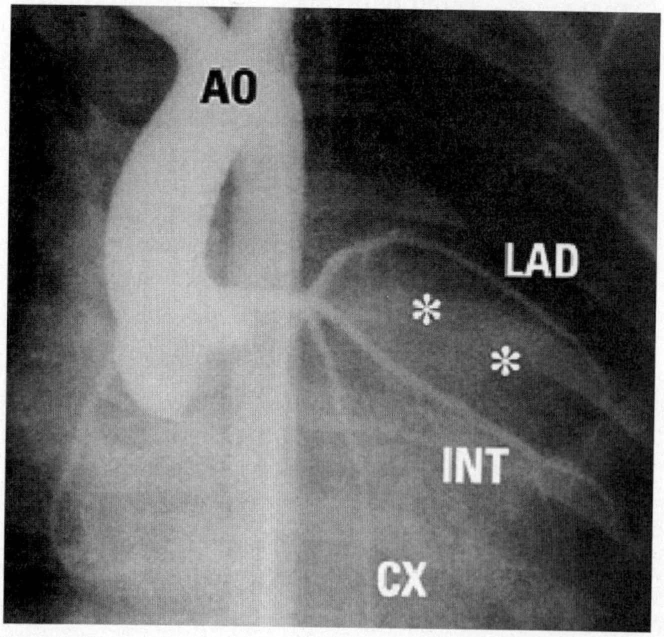

Fig. 26.3: *Coronary angiogram in septal fibroma. Retrograde aortic root injection in frontal projection demonstrates filling of both coronary arteries. Left anterior descending artery (LAD) is displaced cranially by tumor mass (*), whereas intermediate artery (INT) is displaced posteroinferiorly. Main tumor mass is in anterior interventricular and anterior left ventricle free wall. AO, aorta; CX, circumflex*

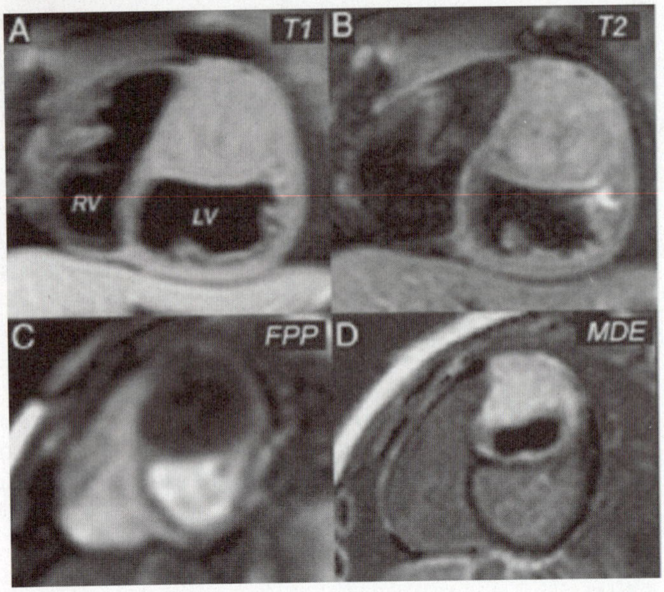

Fig. 26.4: *LV fibroma typical large fibroma involving the anterior wall of the left ventricle (LV). (A) Isointense signal on T1-TSE; (B) slightly hyperintense on T2-TSE; (C) strongly hypointense on FPP; and (D) strongly hyperintense on myocardial delayed enhancement (MDE) with a central dark core. RV, right ventricle*

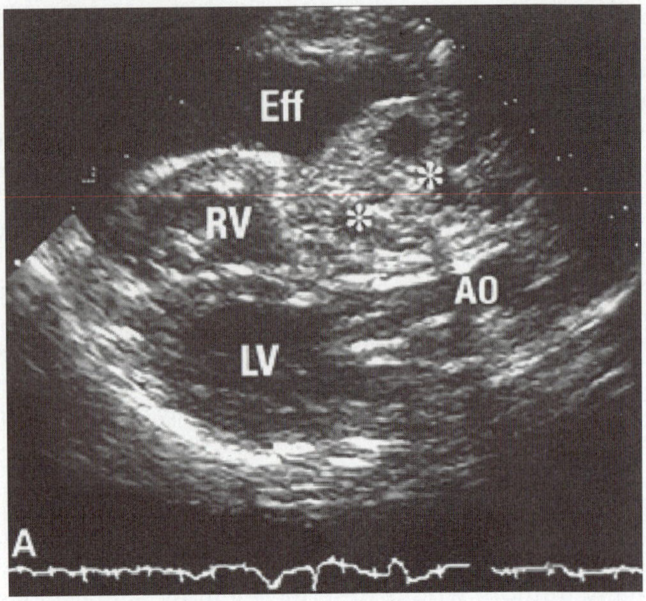

Fig. 26.5: *Pericardial teratoma. (A) Modified parasternal long-axis view of echocardiogram demonstrates intrapericardial tumor (*) displacing aorta posteriorly. Note pericardial effusion. At surgery, tumor was easily shelled out of pericardial space and on sectioning had both cystic and solid elements. AO, aorta; Eff, effusion; L, left; LV, left ventricle; R, right; RV, right ventricle*

dimensional echocardiography as heterogeneous and encapsulated cystic masses.

The main clinical findings in the foetus or neonate relate to the mass effect of the tumour and to the accumulation of fluid in the pericardial space. Fetal hydrops and stillbirth may occur. Respiratory distress, cyanosis and congestive heart failure are predominant signs in the neonate. Pericardial effusion may lead to cardiac compression and tamponade. The pericardial effusion is usually serous and contains small numbers of mesothelial cells.

Macroscopically teratomas have a typical cystic and multilobulated appearance.

Teratomas histologically contain multiple immature elements including epithelium, neuroglial tissue, thyroid, pancreas, smooth and skeletal muscle, cartilage and bone Although teratomas have been considered to be benign, tumour recurrence after resection or malignant differentiation has been reported. Most intrapericardial teratomas can be easily dissected off from the great vessels; on the contrary, surgical removal of intracardiac ones is technically more difficult.

Myxoma (Fig. 26.7)

Myxoma is the most common primary cardiac tumour in adults (65%) with particular predilection to females. The left atrium is the most common location (90%) but they can be seen on the right atrium as well. In 90% of cases, the myxoma is solitary. Myxomas usually do not cause cardiac murmurs, but more often they present with breathlessness, syncope, embolus, congestive heart failure, arrhythmias and constitutional symptoms. As the presenting symptoms may not suggest a cardiac cause, myxomas may present late in the disease and at this stage cardiac signs may then also ensue. On occasions, left-sided myxomas may cause diastolic murmurs or added sounds ("diastolic plop") due to inflow obstruction. Right-sided myxomas are rare and they may lead to tricuspid or pulmonary artery obstruction or pulmonary embolism.

Familial occurrence of myxomas has been reported, usually seen in younger patients. These myxomas are associated with multiple endocrine syndromes including LAMB (lentigines, atrial myxoma, mucocutaneous myxoma, and blue naevi) and NAME (naevi, atrial myxoma, myxoid neurofibromata and ephelides). Familial tumours are predominantly multiple but the sporadic cases are mostly solitary. Screening of first-degree relatives cases of multiple myxomas should therefore be considered.

Macroscopically, myxomas are pedunculated with a short, broad-based attachment to the atrial wall. They are gelatinous in consistency. The echocardiographic appearance of a myxoma is highly suggestive of the diagnosis: it has a pedicle, with irregular, nonhomogenous small lucencies or calcifications on it and the location is characteristically to the atrial septum, around foramen ovale. In contrast, an intracardiac thrombus is usually homogenous in appearance.

The treatment of choice is complete surgical excision of the myxoma with removal of substantial portion of healthy adjacent endocardial tissue. If the surrounding tissue along with the myxoma is not resected completely, the tumour is likely to recur. Prognosis following surgery is quite good, albeit with a recurrence rate of up to a 5% if there has been inadequate resection, intraoperative implantation, tumour embolisation, or unrecognised multiple lesions. Survival after surgery has been reported to be excellent with no late

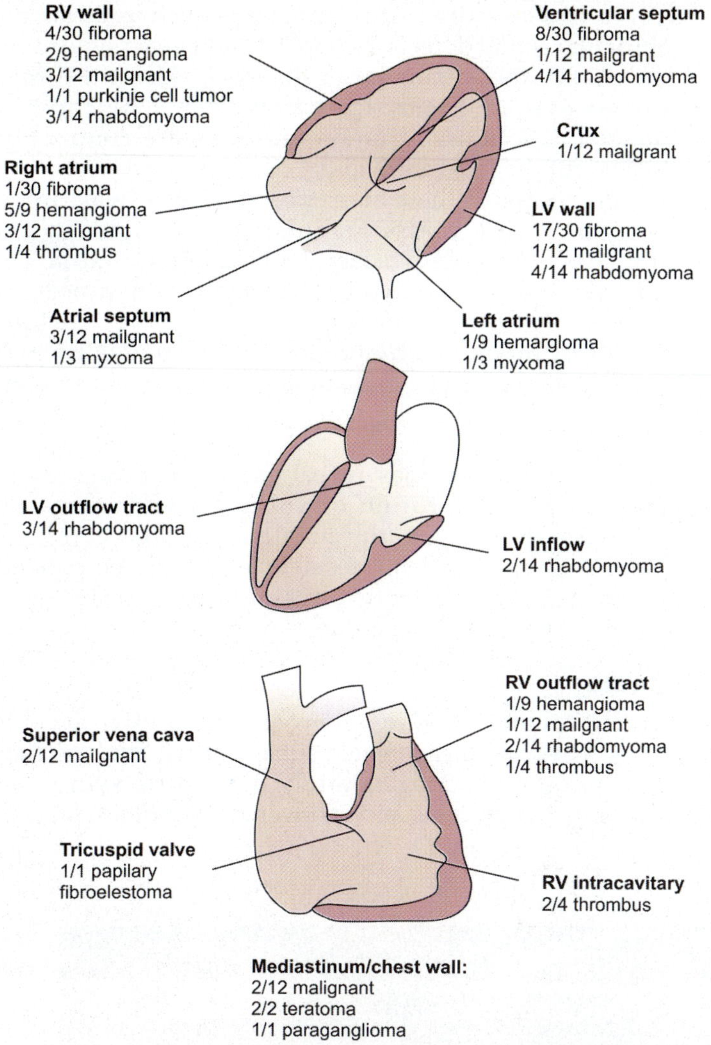

Fig. 26.6: *Locations of cardiac tumors schematic depiction of locations of cardiac tumors. Ratios refer to number of cases of each tumor type in this location divided by the total number of cases with same tumor type. Note that 1 tumor might involve several locations. LV, left ventricle; RV, right ventricle*

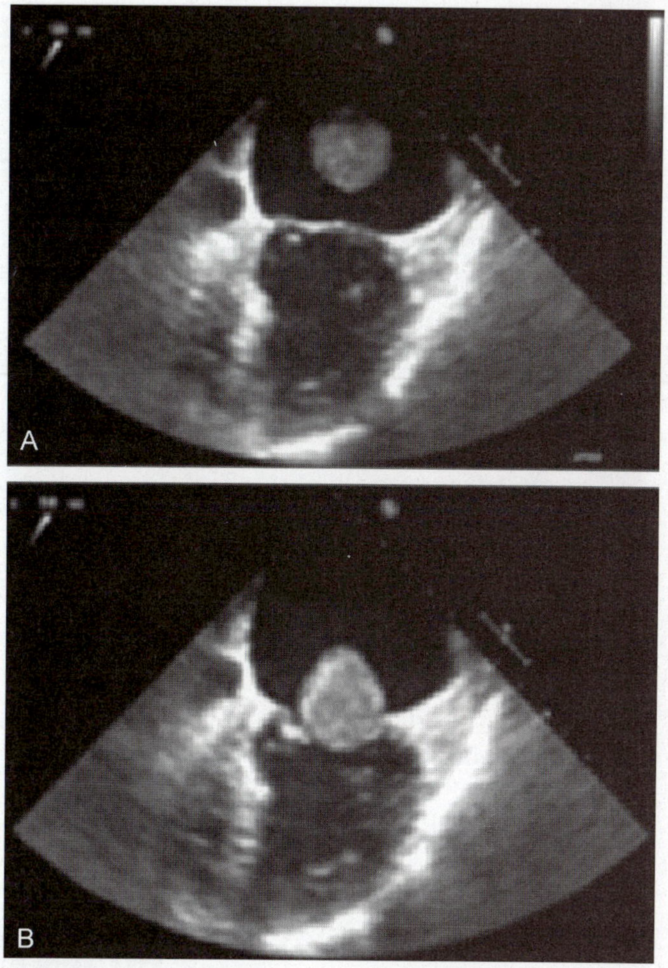

Fig. 26.7: *Intraoperative transesophageal echocardiogram showing the free-floating myxoma in the left atrium (A) and the myxoma obstructing the mitral valve orifice at end-diastole (B)*

deaths attributable to surgery or to myxoma recurrence during 16 years of follow-up.

Haemangioma (Fig. 26.7)

Haemangioma is an exceedingly rare tumour and can be located anywhere within the cardiac layers with slight predilection to the ventricular septum and right atrium. Macroscopically, haemangiomas are subendocardial nodules measuring 2–4 cm in diameter. Microscopically, they may have capillary, cavernous, intramuscular or haemangioendotheliomatous features. The presence of multiple haemangiomas in the skin should raise suspicion of a cardiac haemangioma in the neonate.

Haemangiomas are benign tumours and undergo spontaneous regression with a good prognosis. However, their clinical course may be unfavourable in infants due to high-output cardiac failure, haemorrhage from ruptured vessels and thrombocytopaenia. Ventricular tachycardia and cardiac tamponade are not uncommon. Complete surgical excision may be difficult because of the vascular nature of the tumour.

Histiocytoid nodule–oncocytic cardiomyopathy–Purkinje cell tumour.

These hamartomatous masses differ distinctly from rhabdomyomas. They are mostly found in infants and young children presenting with refractory arrhythmias or sudden unexpected death. They have a predilection to the female sex. These masses have been described with a variety of names such as infantile histiocytic cardiomyopathy, oncocytic cardiomyopathy, histiocytoid cardiomyopathy, Purkinje cell tumour, focal lipid cardiomyopathy, and idiopathic infantile cardiomyopathy.

The most common clinical presentation is refractory arrhythmias such as ventricular fibrillation, ventricular tachycardia, and junctional tachycardia. Premature ventricular contractions, supraventricular tachycardia, and partial or complete atrioventricular block can also be seen. Oncocytic cardiomyopathy is an important cause of sudden unexpected death in infancy.

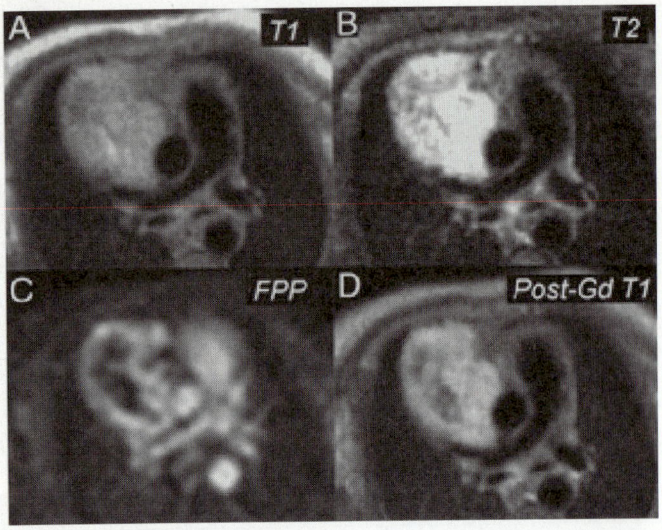

Fig. 26.8: *Right atrial hemangioma. (A) Iso- to slightly hyperintense signal on T1-TSE; (B) strongly hyperintense signal on T2-TSE; (C) inhomogeneous, strongly hyperintense signal on FPP with avid perfusion of the tumor; and (D) hyperintense signal on post-contrast T1-TSE*

Macroscopically, these masses present as focal yellowish nodules or yellow areas of discoloration composed of vacuolated histiocyte-like cells within the myocardium. In up to one-third of patients the tumours may be associated with cardiac or extracardiac anomalies such as atrial and ventricular septal defects, hypoplastic left heart syndrome, cleft palate, and anomalies of the eyes, skin and central nervous system. Their size varies from 1 to 2 mm in diameter. The most common locations are conduction system and the left ventricle.

Microscopically, these masses contain large oval cardiac myocytes with a coarse granular pale cytoplasm. The cytoplasm is filled with bizarre looking mitochondria. The term oncocytic cardiomyopathy describes the process of the granules (mitochondria) replacing the working myofibrils. Infants with oncocytic cardiomyopathy may show similar oncocytic cells in other organs including the trachea, adrenal, thyroid, anterior pituitary and salivary glands.

Echocardiography may reveal nodular deposits on the ventricular endocardium or valves. If left untreated, oncocytic cardiomyopathy may have a fatal course in infants with multiple unresectable lesions. Some patients may benefit from electrophysiological studies with mapping and surgical excision.

Lipoma

Cardiac lipomas are rare lesions and occur exclusively in adults. They are encapsulated subepicardial masses. They are commonly silent but rarely may cause symptoms including arrhythmias and atrioventricular block.

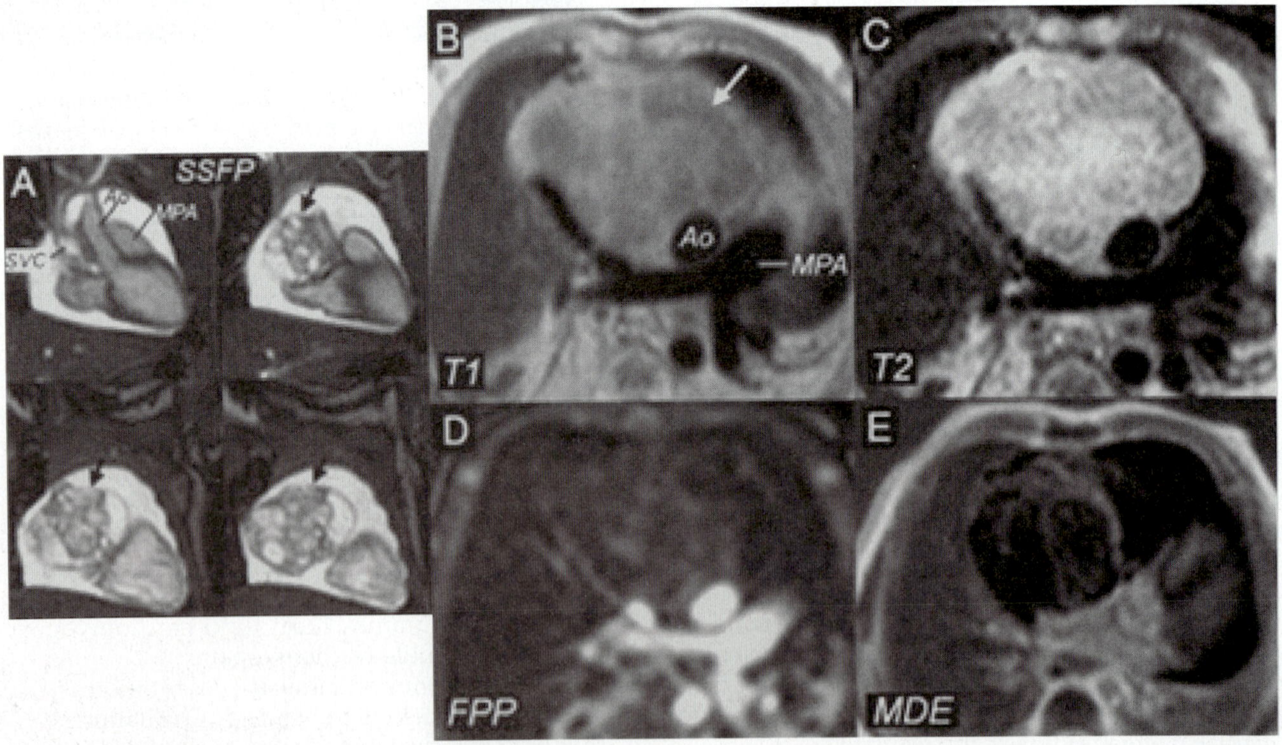

Fig. 26.9: *Intrapericardial teratoma (A) Cine steady-state free precession (SSFP) cine in the coronal plane showing a large multicystic tumor (arrow); (B) axial plane T1-TSE showing inhomogeneous isointense signal; (C) hyperintense signal on T2-TSE; (D) strongly hypointense signal on FPP; and (E) hypointense signal on myocardial delayed enhancement (MDE) imaging. MPA, main pulmonary artery; SVC, superior vena cava*

MALIGNANT CARDIAC TUMOURS

Primary Malignant Cardiac Tumours

Up to a quarter of all cardiac tumours may exhibit some features of malignancy. Ninety five percent of these primary malignancies are sarcomas, the other 5% are lymphomas. Sarcomas are more common in adults and most commonly located in the right atrium. These mesenchymal tumours show various morphologies. The clinical course is usually aggressive with extensive local infiltration, intracavity obstruction and death.

Angiosarcoma

Angiosarcomas are the most common primary cardiac malignancy and more common in male sex. Eighty percent of these tumours originate in the right atrium or pericardium. Echocardiography shows a broad based atrial mass close to the inferior vena cava with frequent epicardial, endocardial or intracavity extensions. Local pulmonary, pleural and mediastinal metastases are frequent. Clinical findings include right-sided heart failure, pericardial disease, pleuritic chest pain, dyspnoea, and pericardial effusion. Some patients (10%) may present with nonspecific symptoms such as fever, weight loss, and malaise. The outlook is poor, and most patients die shortly after the onset of symptoms.

Rhabdomyosarcoma

Rhabdomyosarcomas are the second most common primary malignancy of the heart. Their origin is of striated muscle. These malignancies are most common in adult males and can occur in any heart chamber. The most common presenting symptoms are nonspecific including fever, anorexia, malaise and weight loss. The symptoms associated with pericardial disease, pleural effusion, and embolic phenomena are also common. As compared to angio-

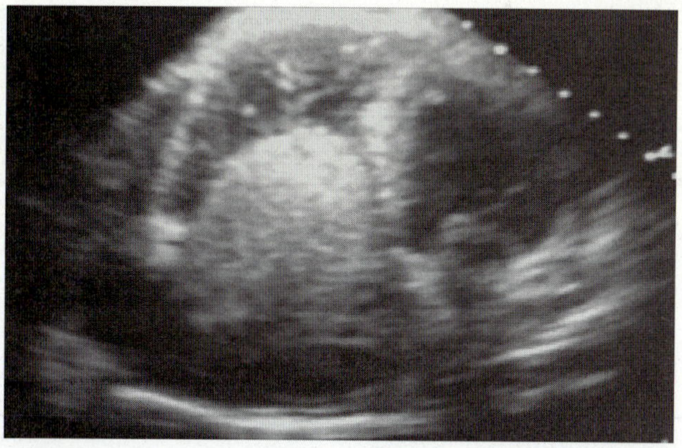

Fig. 26.11: *Two dimensional echocardiograph in apical four chamber view (A4C) shows a right atrial, single, mobile, homogenous, large 7 × 10 cm mass, without satellite lesions, and causing dynamic obstruction to the right ventricular inflow and outflow tract*

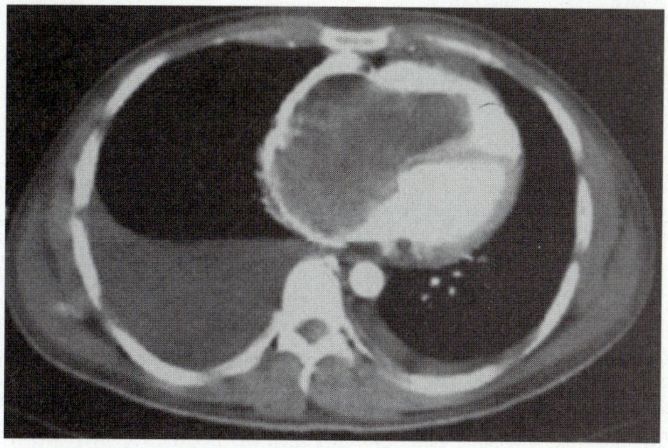

Fig. 26.12: *Computerized tomography with contrast shows a single and large contrast non-enhancing intracardiac mass occupying right atrium and right ventricle with right ventricular outflow tract and inferior vena cava extension. This typical description is consistent with intracardiac thrombus*

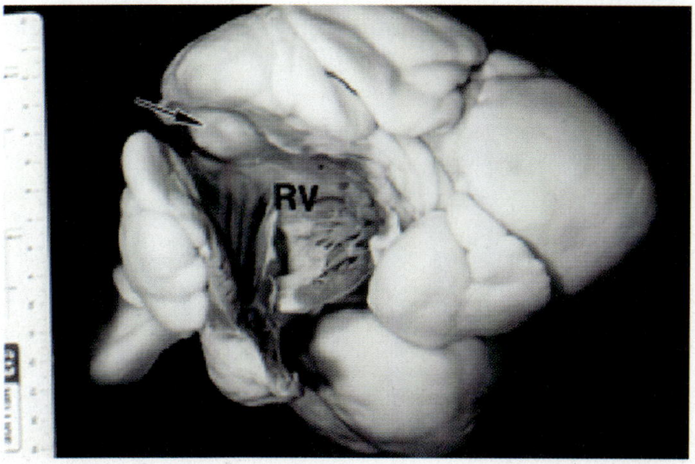

Fig. 26.10: *The anterior aspect of the heart. There are multiple, confluent subepicardial lipomas that originate from all four cardiac chambers and protrude into the pericardial cavity. An extensive fatty deposition (arrow) within the ventricular septum bulged into the right ventricular infundibulum. Abbreviation: RV, right ventricle*

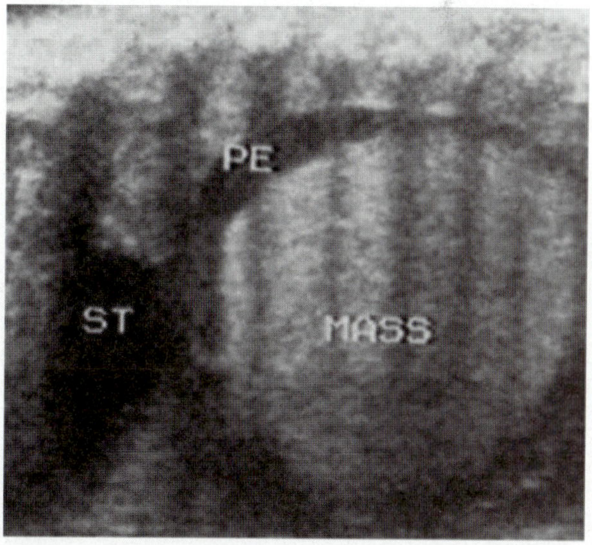

Fig. 26.13: *Left longitudinal view of fetal heart. A large echodense mass, outlined by a pleural effusion (PE), fills the large chest. The stomach (ST) is noted just below the diaphragm*

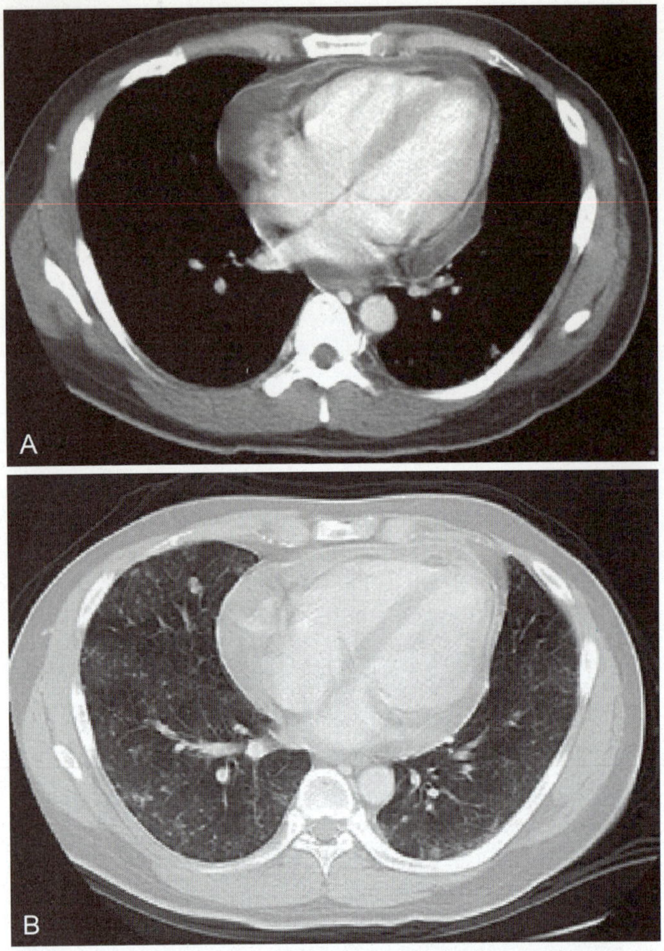

Fig. 26.14: *Patient with chest pain, hemoptysis, and right atrial mass. (A) Axial CT section through the chest after intravenous contrast, mediastinal window shows a filling defect in the right atrial lumen that extends across the adjacent wall of the right atrium into the epicardial fat. There is also a moderate-sized pericardial effusion. (B) Axial CT section through the chest, lung window demonstrates multiple bilateral small pulmonary nodules*

sarcoma, diffuse pericardial involvement is not common and the tumour rarely invades beyond the parietal pericardium. The prognosis is poor.

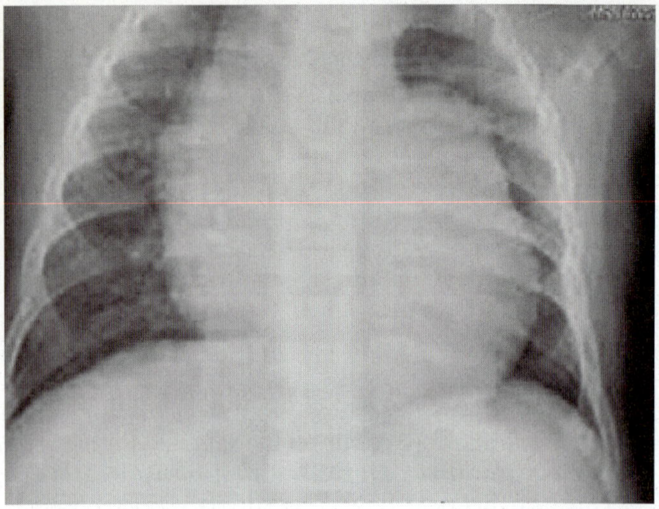

Fig. 26.15: *Plain film showing cardiomegaly with evidence of both left atrium and left ventricle enlargement in a patient with intracardiac mass*

Fibrosarcoma

Fibrosarcomas are mesenchymal tumours with fibroblastic origin. These tumours can be seen within the left or right heart chambers. At postmortem, they are usually found in multiple intracardiac sites as firm, greyish-white small nodules. The clinical findings include heart murmurs, nonspecific ECG changes, chest pain, fever and malaise. They may spread to surrounding structures. The outlook is poor with death ensuing within a year of diagnosis (Figs 26.16 to 26.18).

Lymphoma (Fig. 26.20)

Primary lymphoma of the heart is rare and involves only the heart or the pericardium. These tumours man be seen in various cardiac sites without any specific predilection. They may present with congestive heart failure, cardiomegaly, or pericardial effusion and may be seen as part of the acquired immunodeficiency syndrome. Surgical resection and radiotherapy offer limited success.

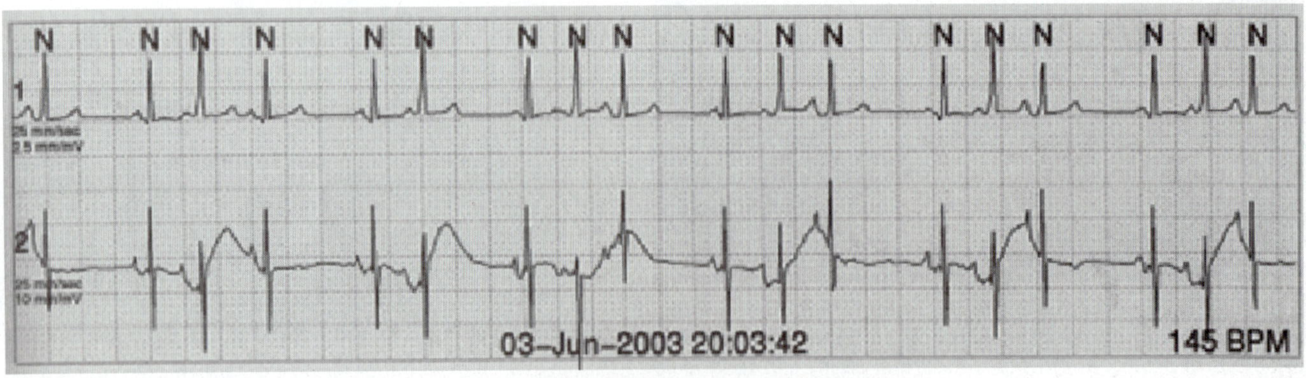

Fig. 26.16: *A 24-hour Holter on a child, a month after birth shows pre-excitation and premature atrial beats in one of the patients with cardiac tumor*

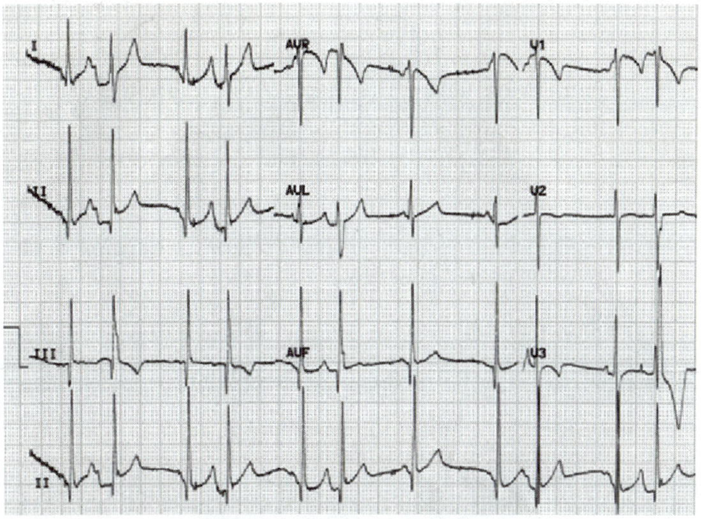

Fig. 26.17: *In 3-years-old child with intracardiac neoplasm, 12-lead ECG reveals ongoing premature atrial complexes*

Intrapericardial Phaeochromocytoma

These tumours are soft, vascular and originate from autonomic paraganglia. They may be found within the atrium, in the atrial septum, in coronary, pulmonary, or aortic locations. If the tumour can be resected, the prognosis is favourable.

Secondary Malignant (Metastatic) Cardiac Tumours

The incidence of cardiac metastases with malignant tumours is estimated to be approximately 1% and 20 times higher than primary malignancies of the heart. The most common cardiac metastases originate from lung tumours in men and breast tumours in women. Metastatic tumours are mostly located in the epicardial surface of the heart.

Macroscopically, carcinomatous metastatic tumours are multiple small, discrete and firm nodules. Carcinomas are more frequent than sarcomatous infiltrations.

Melanoma shows a special affinity to spread to heart with equal distribution to all four chambers. Leukemias and lymphomas may cause intramyocardial infiltration, haemorrhagic pericardial effusion, but occasionally they can remain asymptomatic.

The majority of metastatic tumours remain silent but some may present with arrhythmias, cardiac failure, or pericardial effusion.

Diagnostic Techniques (Figs 26.1, 26.2, 26.5, 26.7, 26.11, 26.13, 26.19–26.21, 26.23, 26.33)

Echocardiography, computing tomography (CT) and MRI of the heart are the main noninvasive diagnostic tools. Open surgical or endomyocardial biopsy is only utilised to reveal the histology of the lesion before surgical resection. A thorough metastatic check should be carried out with CT or MRI imaging before removal of malignant cardiac tumours. A bone marrow biopsy or bone scan may be necessary (Figs 26.4, 26.8, 26.9, 26.12, 26.14).

Surgical Intervention

Resection

Myxomas should be excised completely along with a small rim of surrounding healthy myocardium. In view of their potential for embolisation or valvular obstruction, early resection of myxomas is recommended.

Surgical resection of primary cardiac tumours should only be considered to relieve symptoms and mechanical obstruction to blood flow. The outcome of surgical resection in symptomatic, nonmyxomatous benign cardiac tumours is favourable.

Primary cardiac malignancies may benefit from palliative surgery but this approach cannot be recommended for patients with metastatic cardiac tumours. Surgery, chemotherapy and radiotherapy may prolong survival. The prognosis for malignant primary cardiac tumours is generally extremely poor.

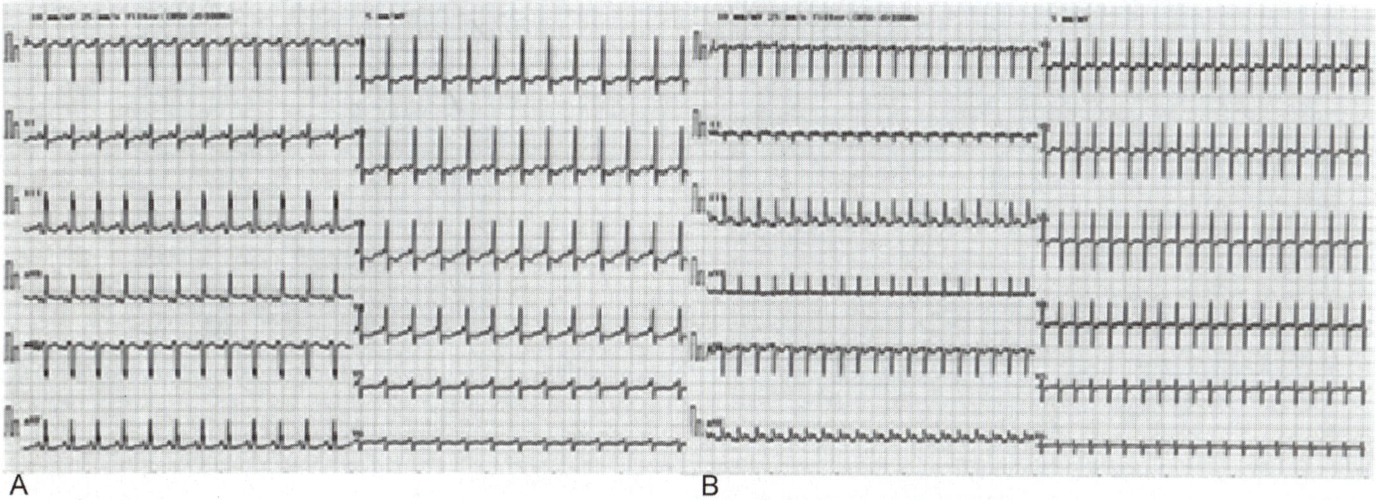

A B

Fig. 26.18: *Electrocardiogram of the sinus rhythm showed pre-excitation (A) and supraventricular tachycardia (B) in a child with cardiac tumor*

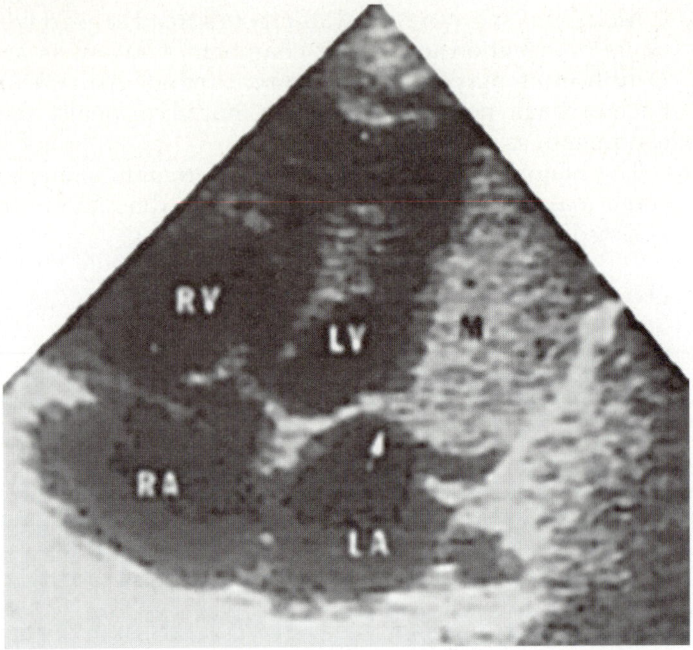

Fig. 26.19: *Two dimensional echocardiogram of the heart in the four chamber view demonstrates a large echogenic mass (M) abutting the left ventricle (LV) and the left atrium (LA). The possibility of invasion of the mitral valve (arrow) could not be excluded. The left ventricular wall could not be demonstrated to be free of the lesion. (RA, right atrium; RV, right ventricle)*

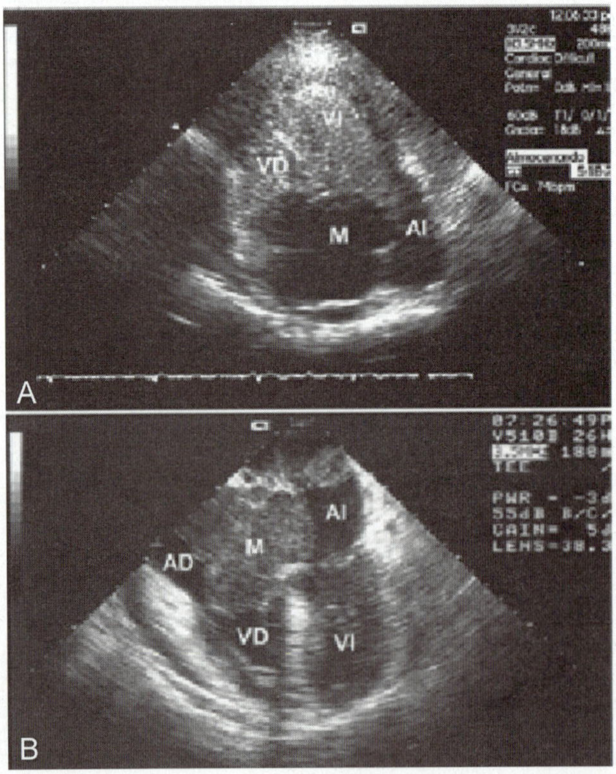

Fig. 26.20: *Primary cardiac lymphoma (A) Transthoracic echocardiogram, apical four chamber view after intravenous contrast injection. (B) Transesophageal echocardiogram, four chamber view without contrast. RA, right atrium; LA, left atrium; M, mass; LV, left ventricle; RV, right ventricle*

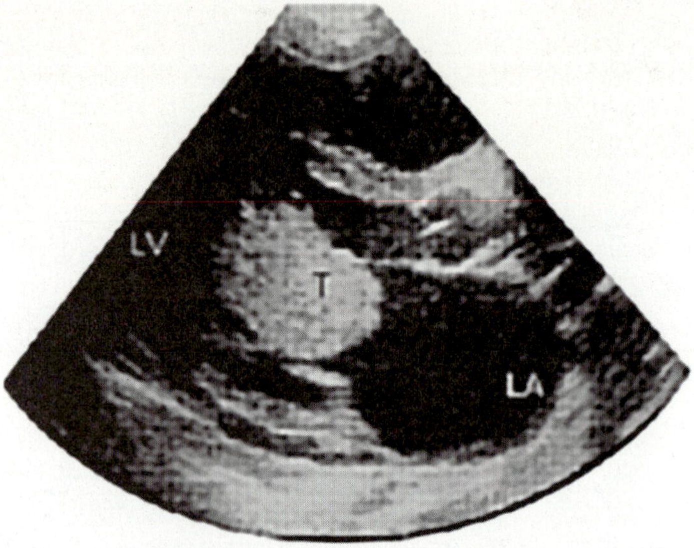

Fig. 26.21: *Transthoracic echocardiogram of the patient, demonstrating a large mass (T) in the left atrium (LA), intermittently prolapsing into the left ventricle (LV)*

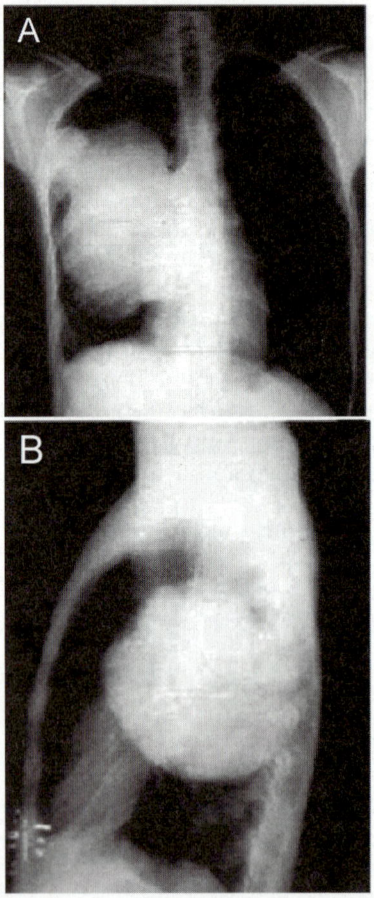

Fig. 26.22: *Skiagram chest showing anteroposterior (A) and lateral right (B) chest X-ray showing the large right pulmonary mass with clear hilar involvement*

Transplantation

If the resection of the tumour is not achievable in severely symptomatic patients, orthotopic cardiac transplantation

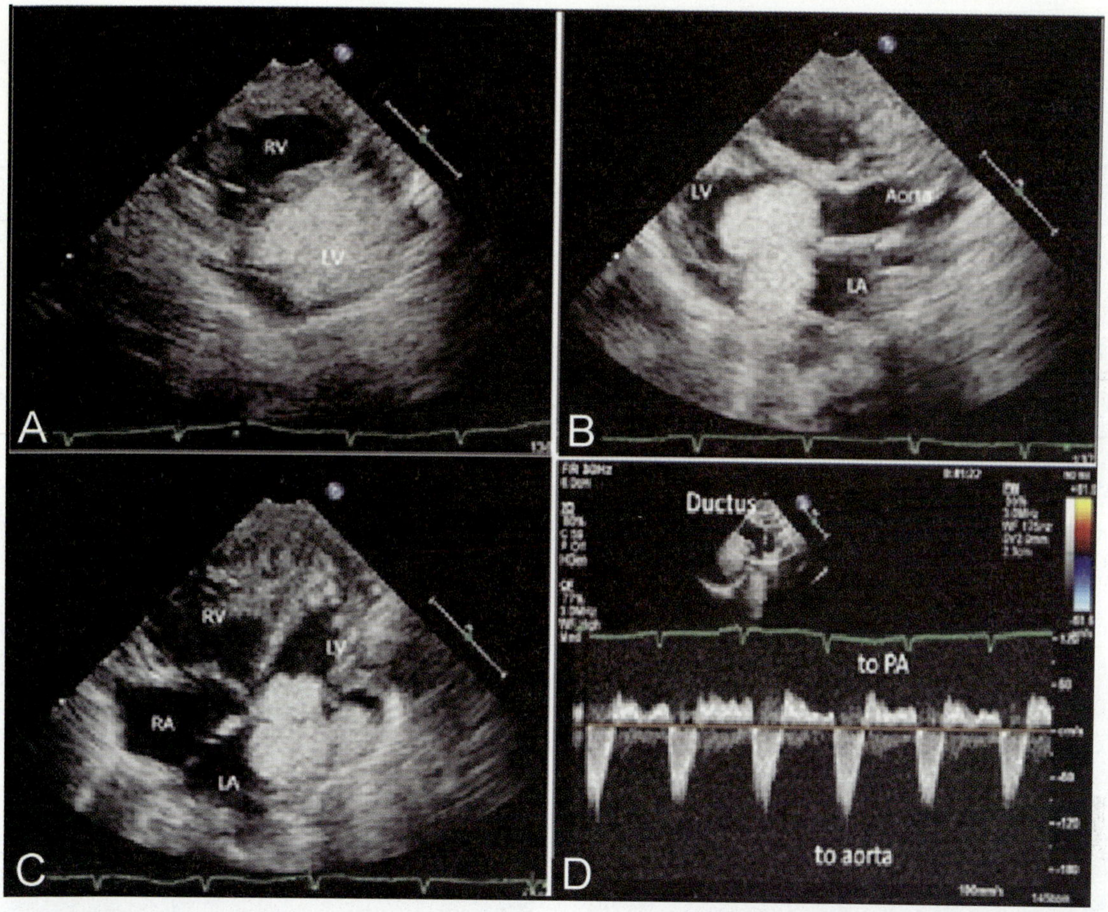

Fig. 26.23: *Echocardiography shows a large tumor widely extended from the left atrium (LA) through mitral valve to the left ventricle (LV) in the short (A), parasternal; (B), and four-chamber; (C) views. Doppler ultrasound showed reversed ductus flow from pulmonary artery to aorta which dominant to ductus flow from aorta to pulmonary artery; (D). RA, right atrium, RV, right ventricle, LA, left atrium, LV, left ventricle, PA, pulmonary artery*

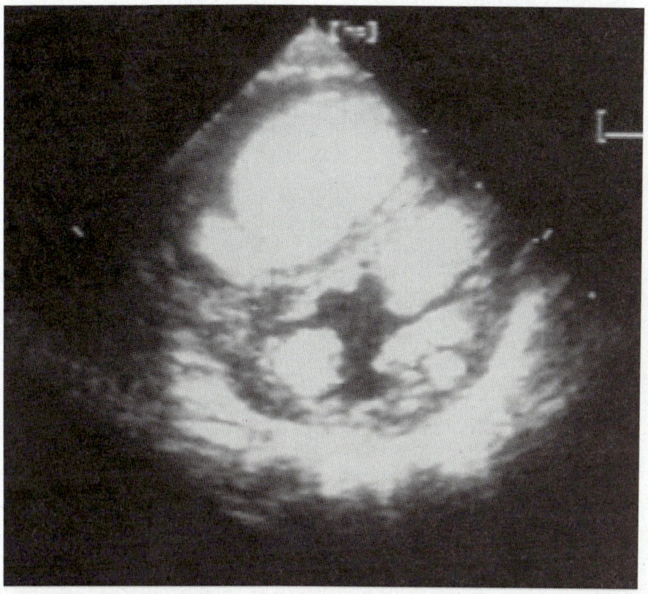

Fig. 26.24: *Echocardiography on a newborn child shows multiple rhabdomyomas in both ventricles. In this child, the diagnosis of tuberous sclerosis was confirmed*

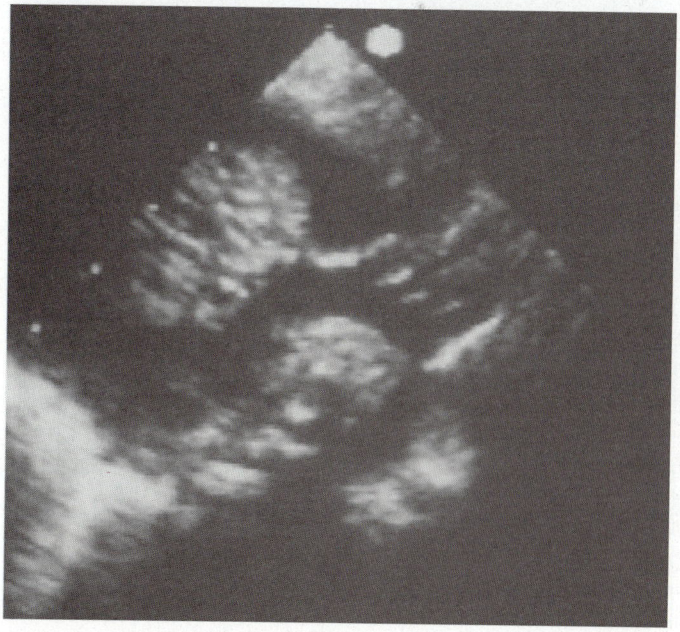

Fig. 26.25: *Echocardiogram demonstrating a cystic teratoma attached to the aortic root (Ao)*

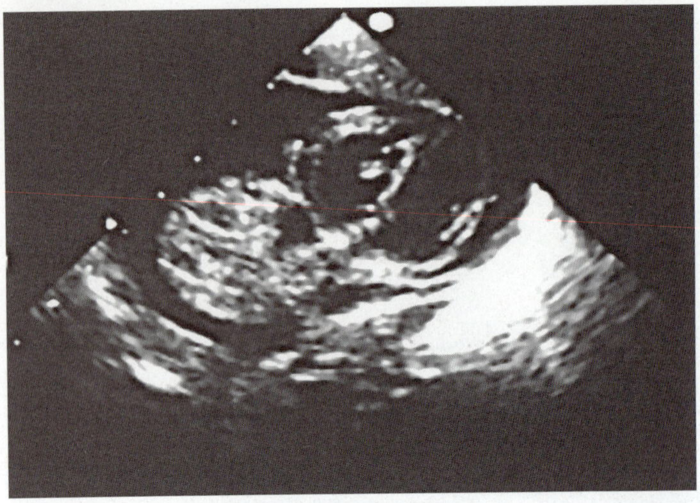

Fig. 26.26: *Echocardiogram demonstrating pericardial effusion (*) and cystic teratoma in a child*

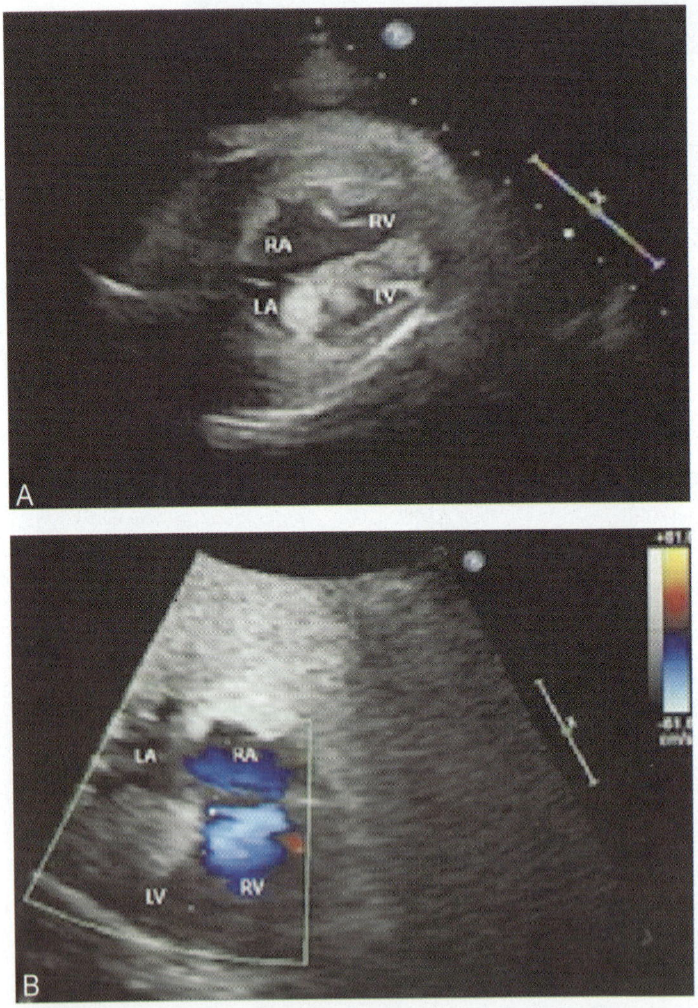

Fig. 26.27: *Fetal echocardiography at 35 weeks of gestation showed a giant tumor involving mitral valve which extended from the left atrium to the left ventricle (A) Color Doppler ultrasound showed severely reduced left ventricular inflow flow (B) and antegrade aortic flow*

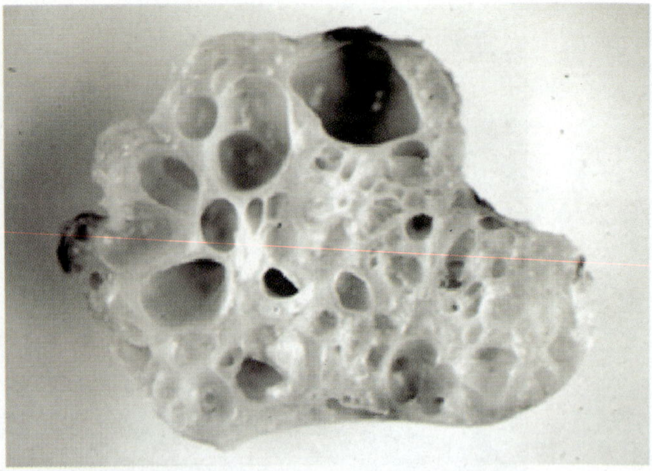

Fig. 26.28: *Morbid anatomy of a mass typical cystic and multi-lobular appearance of a teratoma excised from heart*

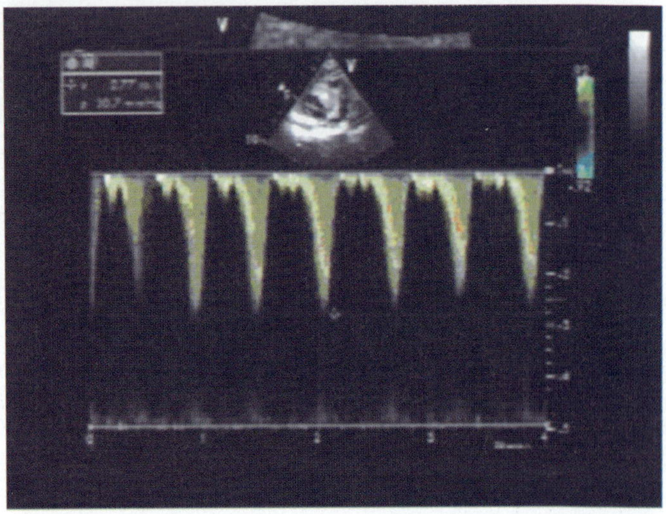

Fig. 26.29: *Doppler echostudy showing right ventricular (RV) tumour in a 2-year-old child resulting in RV outflow tract obstruction. The Doppler velocity is 2.77 m/sec*

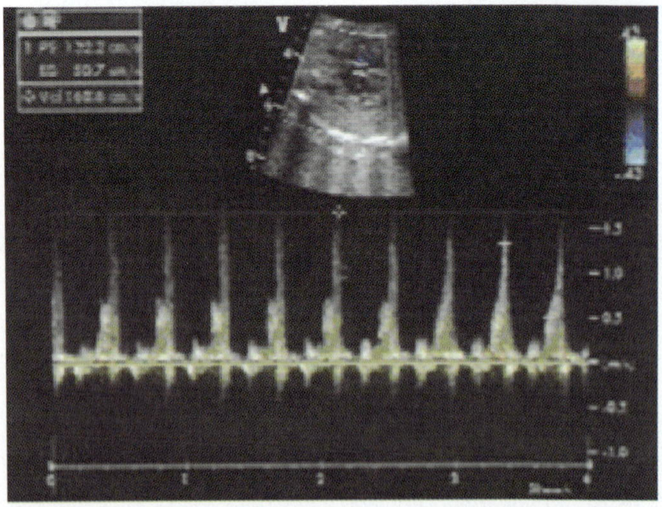

Fig. 26.30: *Doppler echo study showing a foetal tumour in the left ventricular (LV) cavity causing LV outflow tract obstruction*

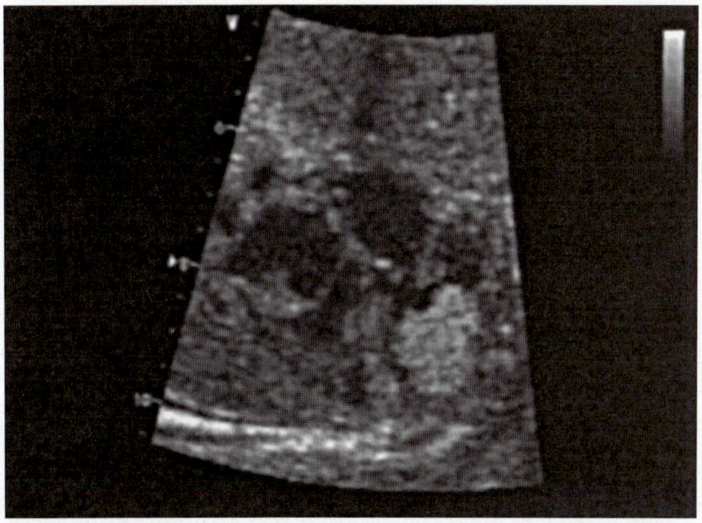

Fig. 26.31: *Multiple rhabdomyomas are found on a foetal ultrasound at 20 weeks of gestation. Rhabdomyomas appears brighter than the surrounding myocardium*

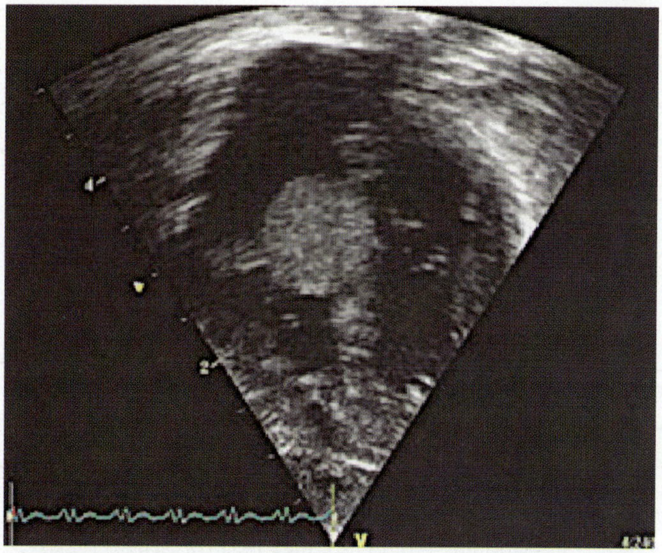

Fig. 26.32: *Apical four chamber view showing rhabdomyoma on the tricuspid valve with some inflow obstruction*

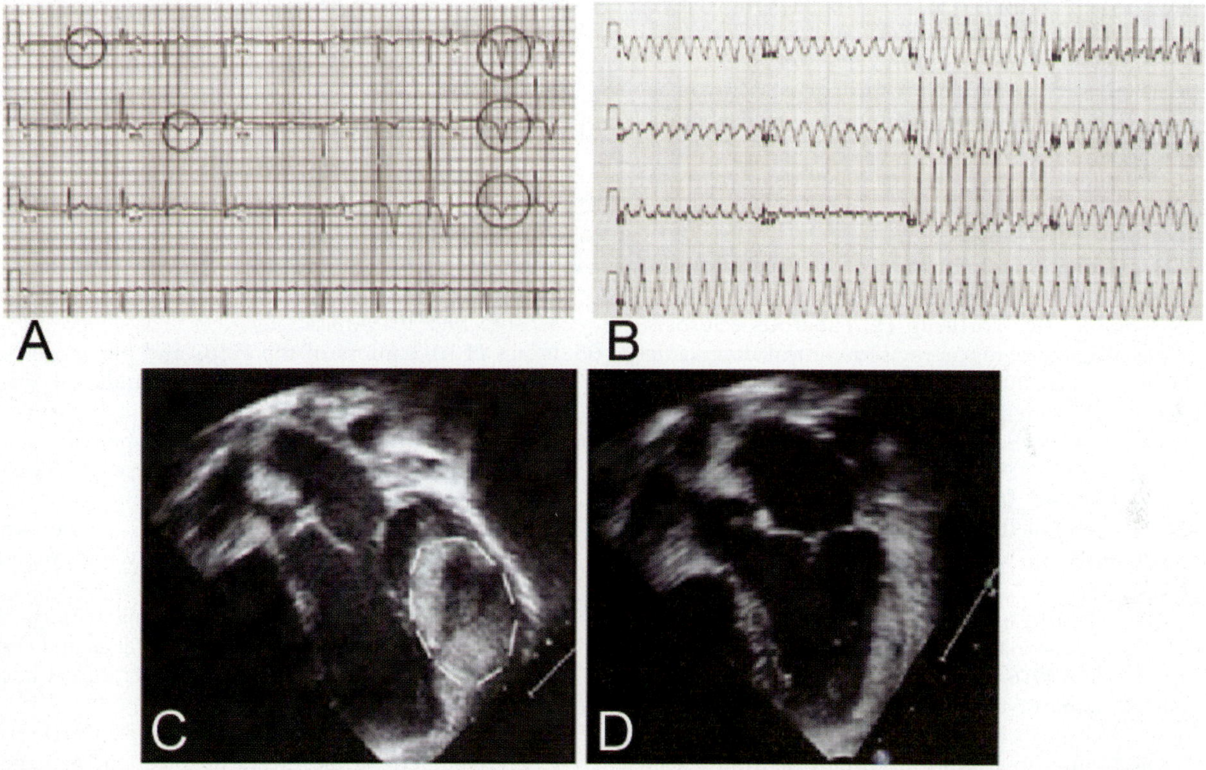

Fig. 26.33: *Patient with a left ventricular fibroma. (A) Common electrocardiographic changes in this patient and a majority of patients with left ventricular fibromas demonstrating T-wave inversions in left lateral leads, (B) electrocardiogram of this patient in ventricular tachycardia, and (C) preoperative and postoperative echocardiographic images of the same patient after surgical resection of a large left lateral ventricular fibroma*

may be considered. This treatment modality is only an option for patients with unresectable cardiac tumours with no evidence of metastatic involvement of the heart.

BIBLIOGRAPHY

1. McAllister HA Jr: Primary tumours of the heart and pericardium. Pathol Annu 1979, 14:325–355.
2. Nadas AS, Ellison RC: Cardiac tumors in infancy. Am J Cardiol 1968, 21:363–366.

3. Holley DG, Martin GR, Brenner JI: Diagnosis and management of fetal cardiac tumors: a multicenter experience and review of published reports. J Am Coll Cardiol 1995, 26:516–520.
4. Lam KY, Dickens P, Chan AC: Tumors of the heart. A 20-year experience with a review of 12,485 consecutive autopsies. Arch Pathol Lab Med 1993, 117:1027–1031.
5. Bulkley BH, Hutchins GM: Atrial myxomas: a fifty year review. Am Heart J 1979, 97:639–643.
6. Chan HS, Sonley MJ, Moes CA, Daneman A, Smith CR, Martin DJ: Primary and secondary tumours of childhood involving the heart, pericardium, and great vessels. A report of 75 cases and review of the literature. Cancer 1985, 56:825–836.
7. Beghetti M, Gow RM, Haney I, Mawson J, Williams WG, Freedom RM: Pediatric primary benign cardiac tumours: a 15-year review. Am Heart J 1997, 134:1107–1114.
8. Groves AM, Fagg NL, Cook AC, Allan LD: Cardiac tumours in intrauterine life. Arch Dis Child 1992, 67:1189–1192.
9. Simcha A, Wells BG, Tynan MJ, Waterston DJ: Primary cardiac tumours in childhood. Arch Dis Child 1971, 46:508–514.
10. Nir A, Tajik AJ, Freeman WK, Seward JB, Offord KP, Edwards WD, Mair DD, Gomez MR: Tuberous sclerosis and cardiac rhabdomyoma. Am J Cardiol 1995, 76:419–421.
11. Webb DW, Thomas RD, Osborne JP: Cardiac rhabdomyomas and their association with tuberous sclerosis. Arch Dis Child 1993, 68:367–370.
12. Harding CO, Pagon RA: Incidence of tuberous sclerosis in patients with cardiac rhabdomyoma. Am J Med Genet 1990, 37(4):443–446.
13. Watson GH: Cardiac rhabdomyoma in tuberous sclerosis. Ann NY Acad Sci 1991, 61:50–57.
14. Roach ES, Gomez MR, Northrup H: Tuberous sclerosis complex consensus conference: revised clinical diagnostic criteria. J Child Neurol 1998, 13(12):624–628.
15. Mas C, Penny DJ, Menahem S: Pre-excitation syndrome secondary to cardiac rhabdomyomas in tuberous sclerosis. J Paediatr Child Health 2000, 36(1):84–86.
16. Callaghan FJ, Clarke AC, Joffe H, Keeton B, Martin R, Salmon A, Thomas RD, Osborne JP: Tuberous sclerosis complex and Wolff-Parkinson-White syndrome. Arch Dis Child 1998, 78:159–162.
17. Fenoglio JJ, McAllister HA, Ferrans VJ: Cardiac rhabdomyoma: a clinicopathologic and electron microscopic study. Am J Cardiol 1976, 38(2):241–251.
18. Krymskaya VP: Tumour suppressors hamartin and tuberin: intracellular signalling. Cell Signal 2003, 15(8):729–739.
19. Satge D, De Geeter B: Rhabdomyomes cardiaques et apoptose: les régressions sont-elles controlées par l'organisme? Arch Mal Coeur Vaiss 1992, 85:603–608.
20. Smythe JF, Dyck JD, Smallhorn JF, Freedom RM: Natural history of cardiac rhabdomyoma in infancy and childhood. Am J Cardiol 1990, 66:1247–1249.
21. Uzun O, McGawley G, Wharton GA: Multiple cardiac rhabdomyomas: tuberous sclerosis or not? Heart 1997, 77:388.
22. Paladini D, Palmieri S, Russo MG, Pacileo G: Cardiac multiple rhabdomyomatosis: prenatal diagnosis and natural history. Ultrasound Obstet Gynecol 1996, 7:84–85.
23. Bosi G, Linthermans JP, Pellegrino PA, Svaluto-Moreolo G, Vliers A: The natural history of cardiac rhabdomyoma with and without tuberous sclerosis. Acta Paediatr 1996, 85:928–931
24. Corno A, de Simone G, Catena G, Marcelletti C: Cardiac rhabdomyoma: surgical treatment in the neonate. J Thorac Cardiovasc Surg 1984, 87:725–731.
25. Black MD, Kadletz M, Smallhorn JF, Freedom RM: Cardiac rhabdomyomas and onstructive left heart disease: histologically but not functionally benign. Ann Thorac Surg 1998, 65:1388–1390.
26. Isaacs H Jr: Fetal and Neonatal Cardiac Tumors. Pediatr Cardiol 2004, 25:252–273.
27. Becker AE: Primary heart tumors in the pediatric age group: a review of salient pathologic features relevant for clinicians. Pediatr Cardiol 2000, 21:317–332.
28. Marin-Garcia J, Fitch CW, Shenefelt RE: Primary right ventricular tumor (fibroma) simulating cyanotic heart disease in a newborn. J Am Coll Cardiol 1984, 3:868–871.
29. Soler-Soler J, Romero-Gonzalez R: Calcified intramural fibroma of the left ventricle. Eur J Cardiol 1975, 3:71–73.
30. Burke AP, Rosado-de-Christensen M, Templeton PA, Virmani R: Cardiac fibroma: clinicopathologic correlates and surgical treatment. J Thorac Cardiovasc Surg 1994, 108:862–867.
31. Geha AS, Weidman WH, Soule EH, McGoon DC: Intramural ventricular cardiac fibroma. Successful removal in two cases and review of the literature. Circulation 1967, 36:427–440.
32. Ali SZ, Susin M, Kahn E, Hajdu SI: Intracardiac teratoma in a child simulating an atrioventricular nodal tumour. Pediatr Pathol 1994, 14:913–917.
33. Fyler DC: Report of the New England Regional Infant Cardiac Program. Pediatrics 1980, 65(suppl):376.
34. Isaacs H Jr: Tumors. In Potter's Pathology of the Fetus and Infant. Volume 2. Edited by Gilbert-Barness E. St Louis: Mosby; 1997:1319–1323.
35. Isaacs H Jr: Tumors of the Fetus and Newborn. In Major Problems in Pathology. Volume 35. Saunders, Philadelphia: Saunder; 1997:330–343.
36. Becker AE: Primary heart tumors in the pediatric age group: a review of salient pathologic features relevant for clinicians. Pediatr Cardiol 2000, 21:317–332.
37. Uzun O, Dickinson DF, Watterson KG: Acute tamponade due to massive cystic teratoma in a newborn infant. Heart 1996, 76(2):188.
38. Carter D, Bibro MC, Touloukian RJ: Benign clinical behavior of immature mediastinal teratoma in infancy and childhood: report of two cases and review of the literature. Cancer 1982, 49:398–402.
39. Benatar A, Vaughan J, Nicolini U, Trotter S, Corrin B, Lincoln C: Prenatal pericardiocentesis: its role in the management of intrapericardial teratoma. Obstet Gynecol 1992, 79:856–859.
40. Takach TJ, Reul GJ, Ott DA, Cooley DA: Primary cardiac tumours in infants and children: immediate and long-term operative results. Ann Thorac Surg 1996, 62:559–564.
41. Reynen K: Cardiac myxomas. N Engl J Med 1995, 33:1610–1617.
42. Carney JA, Hruska LS, Beauchamp GD, Gordon H: Dominant inheritance of the complex of myxomas, spotty pigmentation, and endocrine overactivity. Mayo Clin Proc 1986, 61:165–172.
43. Obeid AI, Marvasti M, Parker F, Rosenberg J: Comparison of transthoracic and transesophageal echocardiography in

diagnosis of left atrial myxomas. Am J Cardiol 1989, 63:1006–1008.
44. Cohen MV: Left atrial myxoma: echocardiographic identification. J Med Soc NJ 1979, 76:213–215.
45. Berning J, Egeblad H, Lauridsen P, Wennevold A: The diagnostic challenge of left atrial myxoma. Acta Med Scand 1979, 206:115–121.
46. Sellke FW, Lemmer JH Jr, Vandenberg BF, Ehrenhaft JL: Surgical treatment of cardiac myxomas: long-term results. Ann Thorac Surg 1990, 50:557–561.
47. Kabbani SS, Jokhadar M, Meada R, Jamil H, Abdun F, Sandouk A, Nabhani F: Atrial myxoma: report of 24 operations using the biatrial approach. Ann Thorac Surg 1994, 58:483–488.
48. Lijoi A, Scoti P, Faveto C, Canale C, Parodi E, Passerone GC, Dottori V, Venere G: Surgical management of intracardiac myxomas a 16-year experience. Tex Heart Inst J 1993, 20:231–234.
49. Burke A, Johns JP, Virmani R: Hemangiomas of the heart. A clinicopathologic study of ten cases. Am J Cardiovasc Pathol 1990, 3:283–290.
50. Tseng JJ, Chou MM, Lee YH, Ho ES: In utero diagnosis of cardiac hemangioma. Ultrasound Obset Gynecol 1999, 13:363–365
51. Cartagena AM, Levin TL, Issenberg H, Goldman HS: Pericardial effusion and cardiac hemangioma in the neonate. Pediatr Radiol 1993, 23:384–385.
52. Ilbawi M, DeLeon S, Riggs T, Hernandez R: Primary vascular tumours of the heart in infancy. Report of a case with successful surgical management. Chest 1982, 81:511–512.
53. Baillie T, Chan YF, Koelmeyer TD, Cluroe AD: Test and teach. Ill-defined subendocardial nodules in an infant. Histiocytoid cardiomyopathy. Pathology 2001, 33:230–234.
54. Bird LM, Krous HF, Eichenfield LF, Swalwell CI, Jones MC: Female infant with oncocytic cardiomyopathy and microphthalmia with linear skin defects (MLS): a clue to the pathogenesis of oncocytic cardiomyopathy? Am J Med Genet 1994, 53:141–148.
55. Bove KE, Schwartz DC: Focal lipid cardiomyopathy in an infant with paroxysmal atrial tachycardia. Arch Pathol 1973, 95:26–36.
56. Gelb AB, Van Meter SH, Billingham ME, Berry GJ, Rouse RV: Infantile histiocytoid cardiomyopathy–myocardial or conduction system hamartoma: what is the cell type involved? Hum Pathol 1993, 24:1226–1231.
57. Kearney DL, Titus JL, Hawkins EP, Ott DA, Garson A Jr: Pathologic features of myocardial hamartomas causing childhood tachyarrhythmias. Circulation 1987, 75:705–710.
58. Keller BB, Mehta AV, Shamszadeh M, Marino TA, Sanchez GR, Huff DS, Dunn JM: Oncocytic cardiomyopathy of infancy with Wolff-Parkinson-White syndrome and ectopic foci causing tachydysrhythmias in children. Am Heart J 1987, 114:782–792.
59. Malhotra V, Ferrans VJ, Virmani R: Infantile histiocytoid cardiomyopathy: three cases and literature review. Am Heart J 1994, 128:1009–1021.
60. Franciosi RA, Singh A: Oncocytic cardiomyopathy syndrome. Hum Pathol 1988, 19:1361–1362.
61. Silver MM, Burns JE, Sethi RK, Rowe RD: Oncocytic cardiomyopathy in an infant with oncocytosis in exocrine and endocrine glands. Hum Pathol 1980, 11:598–605.
62. Marx GR, Bierman FZ, Matthews E, Williams R: Two-dimensional echocardiographic diagnosis of intracardiac masses in infancy. JAm Coll Cardiol 1984, 3:827–832.
63. Murphy MC, Sweeney MS, Putnam JB Jr, Walker WE, Frazier OH, Ott DA, Cooley DA: Surgical treatment of cardiac tumours: a 25-year experience. Ann Thorac Surg 1990, 49:612–617.
64. Val-Bernal JF, Villoria F, Fernández FA: Polypoid (pedunculated) subepicardial lipoma: a cardiac lesion resembling the epiploic appendage. Cardiovasc Pathol 2000, 9:55–57.
65. Ashar K, van Hoeven KH: Fatal lipoma of the heart.Am J Cardiovasc Pathol 1992, 4:85–90.
66. Roberts WC: Primary and secondary neoplasms of the heart. Am J Cardiol 1997, 80:671–682.
67. Herrmann MA, Shankerman RA, Edwards WD, Shub C, Schaff HV: Primary cardiac angiosarcoma: a clinicopathologic study of six cases. J Thorac Cardiovasc Surg 1992, 103:655–664.
68. Lazarus KH, D'Orsogna DE, Bloom KR, Rouse RG: Primary pericardial sarcoma in a neonate. Am J Pediatr Hematol Oncol 1989, 11:343–347.
69. Shapiro LM: Cardiac tumours: diagnosis and management. Heart 2001, 85:218–222.
70. Roberts WC, Glancy DL, De Vita VT: Heart in malignant lymphoma (Hodgkin's disease, lymphosarcoma, reticulum cell sarcoma and mycosis fungoides). A study of 196 autopsy cases. Am J Cardiol 1968, 22:85–107.
71. Holladay AO, Siegel RJ, Schwartz DA: Cardiac malignant lymphoma in acquired immune deficiency syndrome. Cancer 1992, 70(8):2203–2207.
72. Aravot DJ, Banner NR, Cantor AM, Theodoropoulos S, Yacoub MH: Location, localisation and surgical treatment of cardiac phaeochromocytoma. Am J Cardiol 1992, 69(3):283–285.
73. Jeevanandam V, Oz MC, Shapiro B, Barr ML, Marboe C, Rose EA: Surgical management of cardiac phaeochromocytoma. Resection versus transplantation. Ann Surg 1995, 221:415–419.
74. Abraham KP, Reddy V, Gattuso P: Neoplasms metastatic to the heart: review of 3314 consecutive autopsies. Am J Cardiovasc Pathol 1990, 3:195–198.
75. Gibbs P, Cebon JS, Calafiore P, Robinson WA: Cardiac metastases from malignant melanoma. Cancer 1999, 85:78–84.
76. Thurber DL, Eduards JE, Achor RWR: Secondary malignant tumors of the pericardium. Circulation 1962, 26:228.
77. Dein JR, Frist WH, Stinson EB, Miller DC, Baldwin JC, Oyer PE, Jamieson S, Mitchell RS, Shumway NE: Primary cardiac neoplasms: early and late results of surgical treatment in 42 patients. J Thorac Cardiovasc Surg 1987, 93:502–511.
78. Larrieu AJ, Jamieson WR, Tyers GF, Burr LH, Munro AI, Miyagishima RT, Gerein AN, Allen P: Primary cardiac tumours: experience with 25 cases. J Thorac Cardiovasc Surg 1982, 83:339–348.

27 Mitral Valve Prolapse (MVP) in Children and Adolescents

Mitral valve prolapse (MVP) is one of the most common causes of atypical chest pain in school going young girls. The physicians advice is seeked when the patient presents with precordial pain or frequent palpitation.

Mitral valve prolapse (MVP), the most common anomaly of the mitral valve apparatus, occurs when one or both mitral valve leaflets excessively billows into the left atrium toward the end of systole. Mitral regurgitation (MR) develops in some patients with MVP, particularly those with more significant prolapse, when the valve edges fail to coapt. An extreme form of prolapse could include chordal rupture, in which the prolapsed mitral valve is flail. Mitral valves excised from patients with severe MR secondary to MVP have large leaflets and show various histologic alterations.

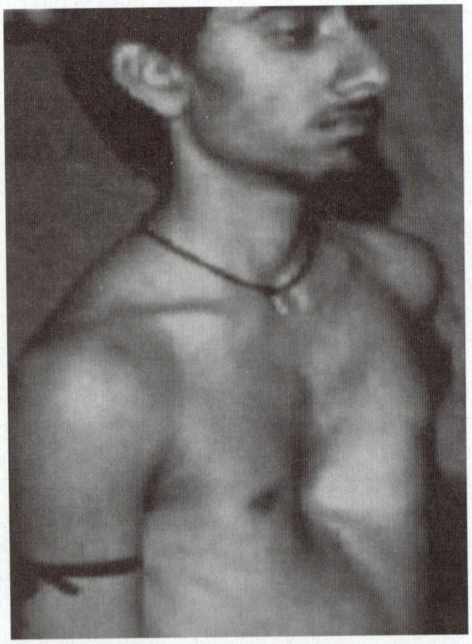

Fig. 27.1: *A young male showing pectus excavatum type of chest deformity with mitral valve prolapse and PDA*

Besides the symptoms attributable to the MR, various neuroendocrine and autonomic disturbances occur in some patients with MVP. In these patients, prolapse may be an epiphenomenon of the underlying autonomic or neurohumoral illness. The term MVP syndrome is often used to refer to the collection of these manifestations. However, in a significant proportion of patients, the mitral valve prolapse is trivial, and no such associated manifestations are present. In these patients, MVP constitutes an essentially benign condition.

Physicians were aware of MVP syndrome as early as 1916, when Sir James MacKenzie described the soldier's heart in spare, thin young men with great vasomotor instability, easy fatigability, breathlessness, and pain over the region of the heart. Kerley first described the syndrome in 1920, and Lincoln described the syndrome in 1928. In 1963,

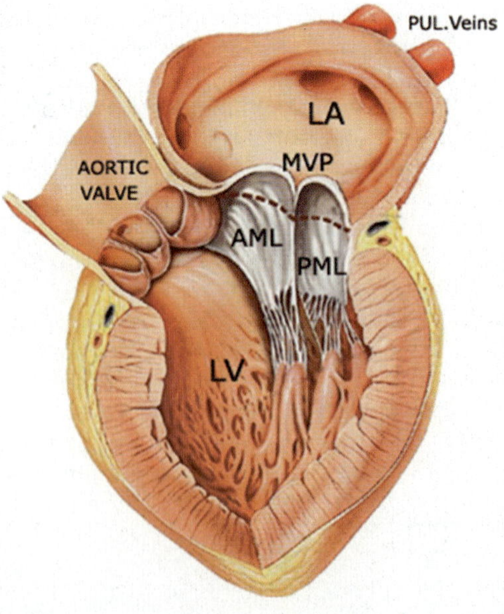

Fig. 27.2: *Shows a normal demarkating line between LA and LV with mitral valve that separates the left atrium from the left ventricle It also shows mitral valve prolapsing into the LA*

Barlow and colleagues made the first clinical diagnosis of the syndrome as it is known today. The advent of echocardiography led to further advances and formed the basis of current knowledge. Idiopathic MVP may be congenital in some patients, but recognition may be delayed until adolescence or adulthood. Associated complicating issues include cardiac arrhythmia, heart failure secondary to severe MR (rare), and, occasionally, thromboembolic events. Familial cases are known and occur in an autosomal dominant pattern with variable penetrance and expression (familial MVP).

Pathophysiology

MVP is a heterogeneous disorder and may originate from various underlying causes affecting one or more portions of the mitral valve leaflets, chordae tendineae, papillary muscle, and/or valve annulus. The syndrome may occur in isolation or in association with generalized connective tissue abnormalities, such as Marfan and Ehlers-Danlos syndromes, in which specific enzymatic defects are found. MVP may occur in the context of inflammatory disease such as rheumatic fever or endocarditis (Figs 27.3 and 27.4).

Table 27.1: *Conditions associated with mitral valve proplase*

1. Ostium secundum atrial septal defect, VSD, coarctation of aorta
2. Martan's syndrome
3. Rheumatic heart disease
4. Ischemic heart disease
5. Hypertrophic cardiomyopathy
6. Periarteritis nodosa/aorto-arteritis
7. Wolff-Parkinson-White syndrome
8. Ebstein's anomaly of the tricuspid valve
9. Ehlers-Danlos syndrome
10. Trauma

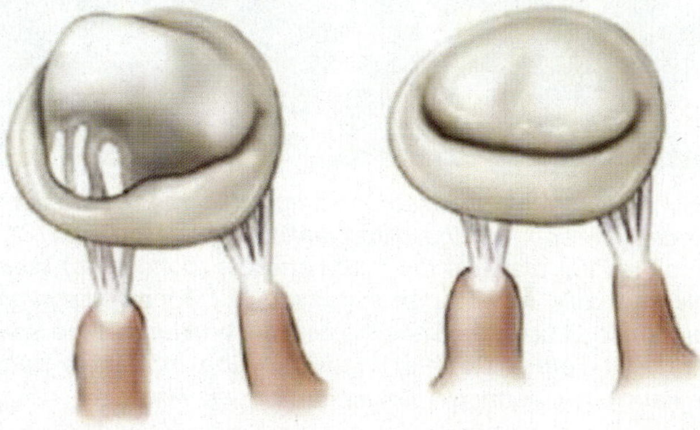

Fig. 27.3: *Anatomical features of normal (left) and prolased (right) MV in MVP*

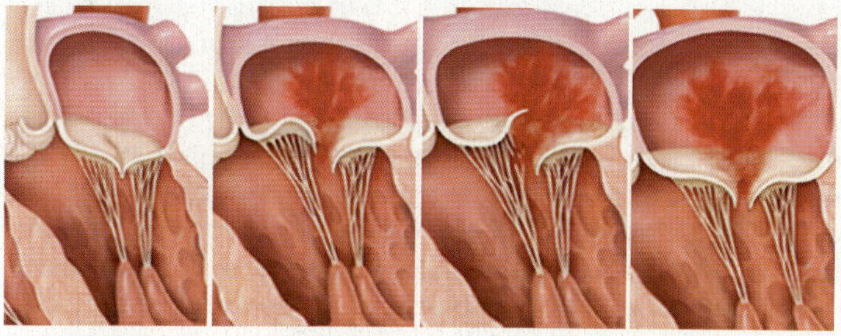

Fig. 27.4: *Valvular positions in normal MV and comparing with mitral regurgitation of MVP and other common causes of MR*

MVP may be secondary to rupture or dysfunction of the papillary muscles following myocardial infarction or ischemia, rupture of chordae tendineae due to infective endocarditis, or abnormal left ventricular wall motion in the setting of myocardial ischemia and/or primary myocardial disease. In these patients, the posterior leaflet in the floppy valve tends to have a significantly longer basal free-edge length and more frequent chordal rupture compared with patients with postinflammatory disease. A connective tissue abnormality, possibly related to collagen metabolism, may underlie the idiopathic disorder. Abnormalities of collagen and elastic fibers have been documented in floppy mitral valves (FMV). Urokinase-plasminogen activator (PLAU), which is suggested in the pathogenesis of elastin and collagen degradation in arterial aneurysm, has also been implicated in MVP (PLAU T4065C TC genotype). A locus for autosomal dominant MVP has also been described on chromosome 11p15.4. Electron microscopy of the affected valve leaflets shows a haphazard arrangement, disruption, and fragmentation of collagen fibrils. Myxomatous proliferation of the mitral valve, in which the middle spongiosa layer is predominantly involved, leads to the presence of unusually large amounts of myxomatous material and acid mucopolysaccharide. Degeneration of collagen within the central core of the chordae tendineae may lead to chordal rupture. MVP can also follow rheumatic fever and myocardial infarction, in which case the prolapse is secondary to inflammatory or ischemic chordal rupture, respectively.

Metabolic and neuroendocrine abnormalities also occur in MVP and may separately result in prolapse unrelated to a connective tissue disorder. In such patients, increased norepinephrine and epinephrine may be found.

Abnormalities in autonomic and neuroendocrine regulation have been demonstrated including hyper-response to adrenergic stimulation, parasympathetic abnormalities (vagal withdrawal), altered baroreflex activity, renin-aldosterone regulation abnormalities, decreased intravascular volume, decreased left ventricular volume in upright posture, and atrial natriuretic factor secretion abnormalities (Figs 27.2 and 27.3).

Incidence

MVP is the most prevalent cardiac valve disorder. MVP is a common finding in otherwise healthy teenagers and young adults, particularly those patients who present with palpitations, chest pain, or dizziness. More than one-third of cases in younger children are associated with other congenital heart defects. Reports vary, but 3–5% of pediatric patients likely have clinically significant MVP.

Global Occurrence

Prevalence rates are 1–2% in children and 5–15% in adolescents and young adults. In a series of 278 surgically removed mitral valves with pure regurgitation, MVP was present in 43%.

Mortality/morbidity: When present, coexistent abnormalities dictate the risk. Presence of significant MR and prolonged QT interval on ECG may also influence outcome.

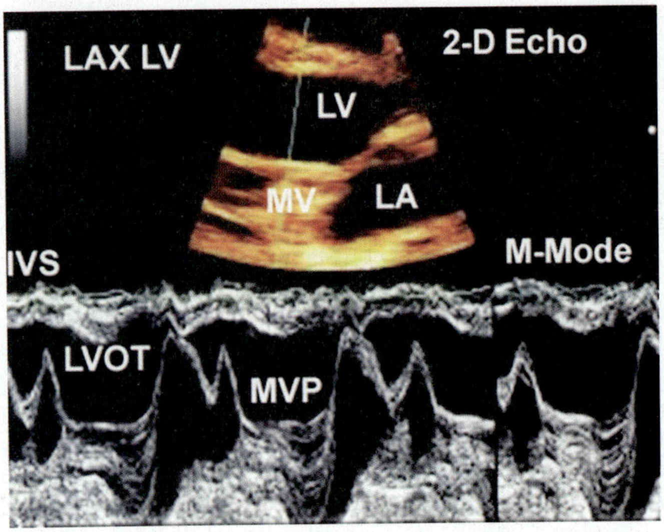

Fig. 27.5: *Two dimensional (top) and M-mode echocardiography (bottom) showing significant prolapse of anterior*

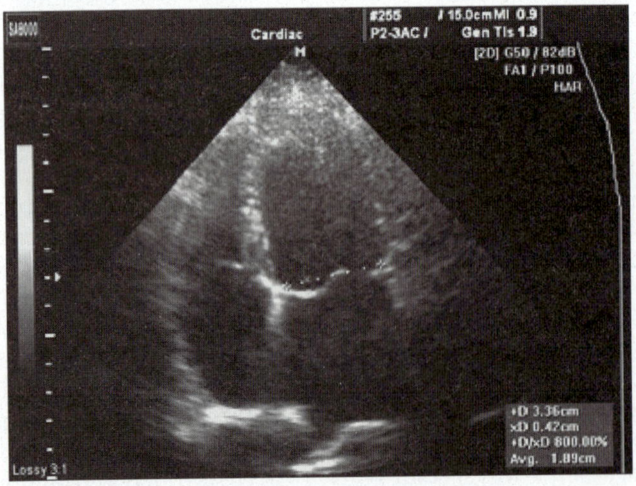

Fig. 27.6: *Apical four chamber view showing typical prolapse of anterior mitral leaflet into left atrium from the imaginary line across the mitral annulus*

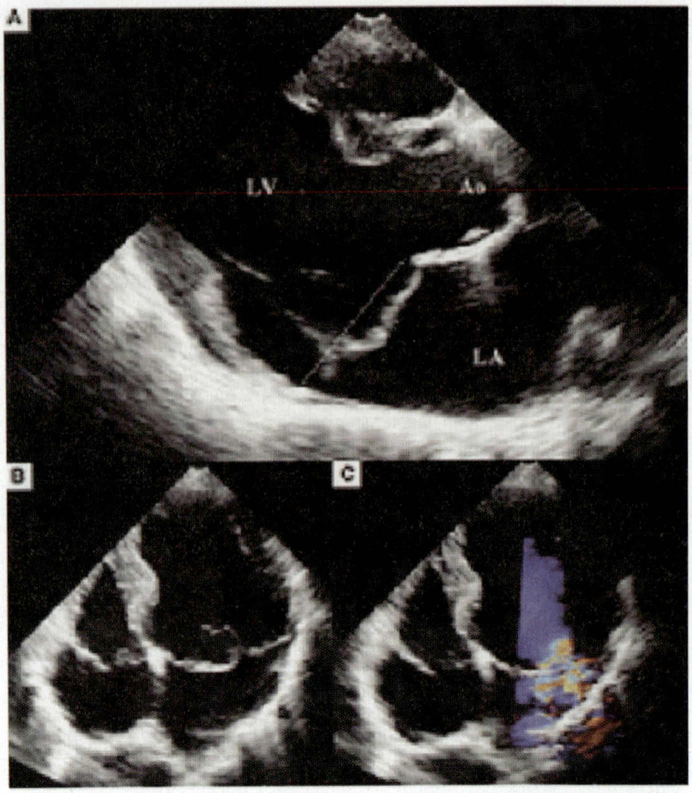

Fig. 27.7: *Mitral valve prolapse. (A) Echocardiographic parasternal long-axis view showing the mitral leaflets prolapsing more than 2 mm above the plane of the mitral annulus (dotted line) during systole in a child with Marfan syndrome. (B) Echocardiographic apical four chamber view showing bileaflet prolapse in the same patient. (C) Colour Doppler view showing moderate mitral regurgitation. Ao, aorta; LA, left atrium; LV, left ventricle*

QT prolongation is slightly more prevalent among patients with MVP and may be associated with repolarization abnormalities and arrhythmia vulnerability. When severe, MR can lead to heart failure.

Mortality is rare in children. Sudden death is also rare and occurs more often in young women with a history of recurrent syncope, sustained supraventricular tachycardia, or complex ventricular tachycardia. Family history of cardiac sudden death often is a risk-stratifying indicator. Development of MR and the progression of mild or moderate MR to severe MR are important determinants to morbidity. One study showed that the prevalence of MR increased from 29% of patients to 43% of patients during 4.3 years of follow-up. Other possible complications include congestive cardiac failure, rupture of chordae tendineae, infective endocarditis (in 0.1–0.3 cases per 100 patient years), thromboembolic phenomena including cerebrovascular accidents, and sudden death. Cardiac arrhythmias such as ventricular tachycardia and fibrillation are more common in MVP.

Sex Distribution

Some studies show MVP is twice as frequent in females as in males.

Age Distribution

Although findings are more frequent in older children and adults, the defect is believed to be present at birth.

Clinical examination: Most patients are asymptomatic and mitral valve prolapse (MVP) is an incidental auscultatory finding. Beta-blockers may markedly attenuate or abolish the symptoms, a fact that is important to remember while evaluating a patient who is receiving these agents. Findings are more marked when patients are examined in the outpatient department rather than in the inpatient setting, reflecting the contributory role of adrenergic state (Fig. 27.1).

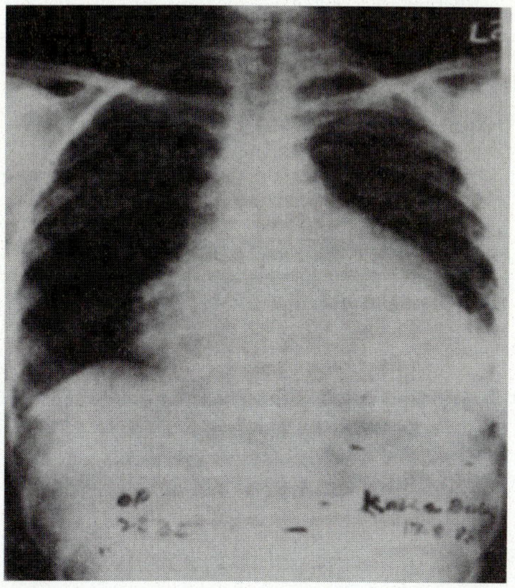

Fig. 27.8: *X-ray chest (PA view) shows cardomegaly (LV type) in mitral valve prolapse with MR*

Chest pain occurs in 10% of patients diagnosed with MVP and may be caused by any of the following fact.

Excessive stretching of the chordae tendineae, leading to traction on papillary muscles.

Coronary microembolism from platelet aggregates and fibrin deposits in the angle between the left atrium and the posterior mitral leaflet. Inappropriate tachycardia and excessive postural changes and physical and emotional stresses hyperadrenergic state, which increases myocardial oxygen demand.

Coronary Artery Spasm

Palpitations

Palpitations are present in 7.4% of patients.

Occurrence may be related to cardiac arrhythmia, although this has not been conclusively proven.

Fatigability and dyspnea: These often develop upon exertion.

The cause may be alterations in centrally modulated breathing cycle control.

Neuropsychiatric

Panic attacks may occur.

Nervousness, presyncope, and syncope occur in 0.9% of patients.

Thromboembolism, arrhythmia, or vasodepressor-vasovagal problems may be involved.

Pulse

Findings are usually normal.

Pulse is occasionally irregular in the presence of premature contractions.

Exaggerated tachycardia (high-volume in severe MR) following exertion is not unusual.

Skeletal abnormalities are observed in two-thirds of patients. These do not fit into any of the recognized connective tissue disorders although an occasional patient may have Marfan or other related syndromes. Common findings are as follows:

- Hypomastia
- Thin children
- Height-to-weight ratio greater than normal
- Arm span greater than height (dolichostenomelia)
- Arachnodactyly
- Scoliosis
- Narrow anteroposterior chest diameter (straight back)
- Pectus excavatum or pectus carinatum (Fig. 20.4)
- Cathedral palate
- Crowding of teeth
- Joint hypermobility.

Auscultation: Apical midsystolic nonejection click and late systolic murmur are the hallmarks, but either may occur alone. Heart sounds are usually normal, but the first heart sound (S1) may be accentuated when prolapse occurs early in systole because of the summation of S1 and mitral click. Multiple clicks occur when prolapse of different leaflets occurs at different times during the systole and may resemble pericardial friction rub.

In patients with redundant floppy mitral valves and significant MR, the murmur may be holosystolic and the click may be absent.

In cases in which the posterior mitral valve leaflet is prolapsing, the murmur may radiate along the left sternal border to the aortic area, thus mimicking left ventricular outflow tract murmur. If the anterior leaflet prolapses, the murmur radiates to the axilla and the spine.

Dynamic auscultation: In the sitting or standing position in late systole, the click may appear earlier and the murmur may be more prominent. The systolic click moves toward S1 upon standing, often merging with S1 if marked postural tachycardia occurs, and new clicks may appear. If an exaggerated heart rate response occurs, the murmur becomes longer and often louder to holosystolic. Occasionally (Fig. 27.9), the murmur is present only in the upright posture.

When squatting from standing position, the click and murmur may move back to late systole. Continuous auscultation while the patient is standing from squatting position, reveals the click and murmur moving back to early systole on a beat-to-beat basis as the heart rate accelerates. A systolic precordial honk or whooping sound may occasionally be heard with the murmur. Often these are heard only in the sitting or standing position and may be

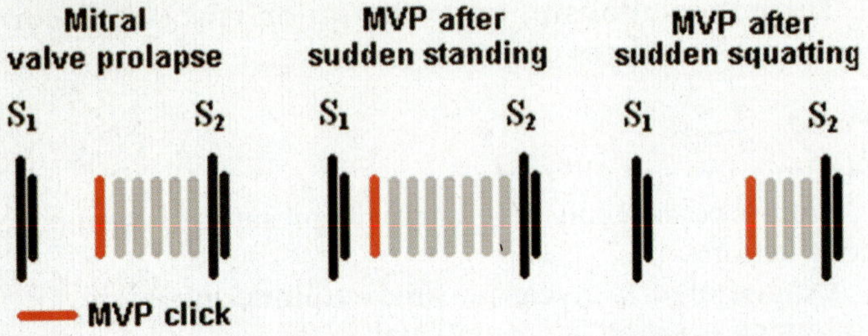

Fig. 27.9: *Mitral valve prolapse response to dynamic auscultation. MVP click and murmur varies after sudden standing and sudden squatting as demonstrated in this illustration. It therefore helps in differentiating others conditions with click and murmur*

limited to a few beats immediately after standing.

Dynamic auscultatory changes reflect alterations in the timing of the MVP, the timing and extent of the MR, the expected changes in left ventricular volume, myocardial contractility, and heart rate. In the upright posture, venous return decreases, as does the left ventricular volume. The reflex tachycardia that occurs in the upright position further reduces left ventricular volume. Timing and degree of the prolapse are determined by the position of the mitral leaflets at end diastole, which, in turn, is dependent on the distance from the mitral valve annulus to the attachment of the chordae to papillary muscles. Low left ventricular end-diastolic volume shortens the mitral annular papillary muscle distance, allowing the leaflets to prolapse earlier in systole.

Prompt squatting from standing position increases venous return and left ventricular volume; thus, the systolic click and murmur may become late systolic. Squatting, however, may also be associated with an increase in peripheral vascular resistance, which, in turn, increases the tension on the mitral valve apparatus, preferentially directing blood flow into the left atrium, rather than to the peripheral circulation. The late systolic click and murmur then become accentuated in the squatting position.

Other maneuvers are possible as follows, but none is as practical and helpful as a systematically performed postural dynamic auscultation.

- Leg elevation
- Isometric hand grip exercise
- Valsalva maneuver
- Application of tourniquets to the extremities
- Lower body negative pressure or amyl nitrate inhalation causes
- Heritable disorders of connective tissue
- Marfan syndrome
- Ehlers-Danlos syndrome types I, II, IV
- Stickler syndrome
- Polycystic kidney disease, adult type
- Osteogenesis imperfecta
- Fragile X syndrome
- Martin-Bell syndrome
- Pseudoxanthoma elasticum
- Periarteritis nodosa
- Skeletal abnormalities
- Asthenic habitus
- Straight back syndrome
- Pectus excavatum (Fig. 27.1)
- Pectus carinatum
- Cardiac abnormalities
- Atrial septal defect (ostium secundum) including atrial septal aneurysm, tricuspid valve prolapse, aortic valve prolapse, and Ebstein anomaly of tricuspid valve
- Holt-Oram syndrome
- Accessory atrioventricular pathways
- Coronary artery anomalies
- Hypertrophic cardiomyopathy.

Other disease

- Graves disease
- Thyroiditis
- Sickle cell disease
- Muscular dystrophy
- Myotonic dystrophy
- Von Willebrand disease
- Several reports suggest magnesium deficiency underlies the disease in some patients.

Laboratory Studies

Perform blood and other laboratory tests as dictated by the condition of the patient.

Imaging Studies

Radiography

Chest radiography findings are normal. Cardiac size and pulmonary venous congestion appear when MR is severe. Skeletal surveys reveal any abnormalities (Fig. 27.8).

Echo-Doppler Studies

This is an essential tool to identify the presence and magnitude of mitral valve prolapse (MVP), the thickness of mitral valve leaflets, mitral annulus size, chordae tendineae length, and left ventricular and left atrial size and function. The test also reveals any associated heart diseases. Multiple views of the mitral valve annulus are essential, and the echo-Doppler findings have to be correlated with clinical details (Figs 27.5 to 27.7, 27.10).

Two dimensional, real-time echocardiographic pictures from parasternal long-axis window show the mitral valve leaflets coming together in systole and billowing into the left atrium beyond the atrioventricular junction. The medial aspect of the anterior leaflet and middle scallop of the posterior leaflet are visualized from this view. The lateral scallop of posterior leaflet can be seen only from the apical four chamber window, and, at times, MVP can be focal. The echocardiographic description of the MVP should include structural changes, such as leaflet thickening, redundancy, annular dilatation and chordal elongation. A varying degree of noncoaptation of the leaflets is present, and MR can be identified by Doppler-color, pulse wave, and continuous wave. The MR jet can be defined, and its magnitude and direction estimated. The size of the left atrium and left ventricle are increased in the presence of moderate-to-severe MR (Fig. 27.7).

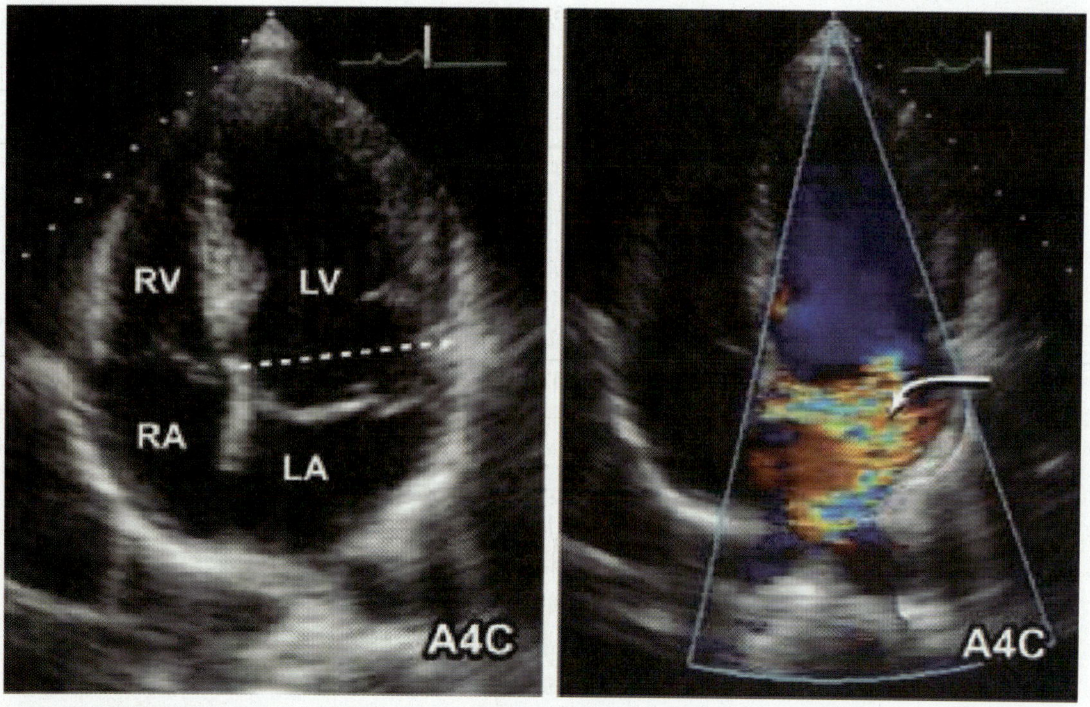

Fig. 27.10: *Bileaflet prolapse is easily visualized in the apical four chamber (A4C) view. However, the mitral valve profile is normally exaggerated in this view and may lead to overdiagnosis of mitral valve prolapse (left panel). Severe mitral regurgitation was present (right panel)*

Three dimensional echocardiography is reportedly very helpful in delineating the prolapse and associated regurgitation. It has also been reported to provide information that helps in surgical repair.

Transesophageal echocardiography has also improved the identification of leaflet morphology, assisting surgical repair (Fig. 27.13).

M-mode echocardiography shows a characteristic posterior movement of the posterior mitral leaflet during mid or late systole or pansystolic prolapse of both anterior and posterior mitral leaflets toward the left atrium. With the availability of two dimensional and Doppler studies, MVP should no longer be diagnosed solely on M-mode Echo Scans. These studies, particularly transesophageal echocardiography, also help to identify potential embolic sources in patients with focal neurologic symptoms or signs. Findings are always interpreted in the context of the clinical evaluation by dynamic auscultation. The diagnostic accuracy improves by use of a constellation of findings, which include structural and functional changes. Patients with echocardiographic criteria for MVP without evidence of thickened redundant leaflets or significant MR, require careful review before MVP is diagnosed. Mere sagging of anterior leaflet in the four chamber view does not indicate MVP. Patients with typical auscultatory findings may be diagnosed even with questionable echocardiographic findings.

Rarely, patients with MVP may have typical echocardiographic findings but no abnormality on auscultation. Patients with suggestive symptoms and no auscultatory findings, who have nonspecific echocardiographic changes, present a real challenge and may require periodic reevaluation before a firm diagnosis can be made. Family history could be of help in some of these patients. Stress **scintigraphy**: myocardial perfusion scintigraphy (e.g. using thallium-201) during exercise may help to identify the rare patient with MVP and myocardial ischemia (Figs 27.9 and 27.10).

Other Tests

Electrocardiography (Fig. 27.11)

Results are usually normal; however, in about one half of children and adolescents, the findings may reveal inverted or biphasic T waves, especially in leads II, III, aVF, and/or V5-6. The T-wave abnormalities may vary at different times in the same patient and may improve with exercise or with beta-blocker therapy.

Arrhythmias described at rest or during exercise include premature atrial (23.6%) or ventricular (27.3%) contractions, supraventricular tachycardia, and conduction abnormalities. Patients with MVP demonstrate a higher frequency of left-sided accessory pathways. More serious findings include ventricular tachycardia and fibrillation.

A higher incidence of arrhythmia may be due to a prolonged QT interval. Diastolic depolarization of muscle fibers in the anterior mitral leaflet in response to stretch may also have a role.

Slow response action potentials originating in the atrial-like muscle fibers in the mitral valve leaflets can lead to sustained rhythmic action that penetrates the cardiac chambers.

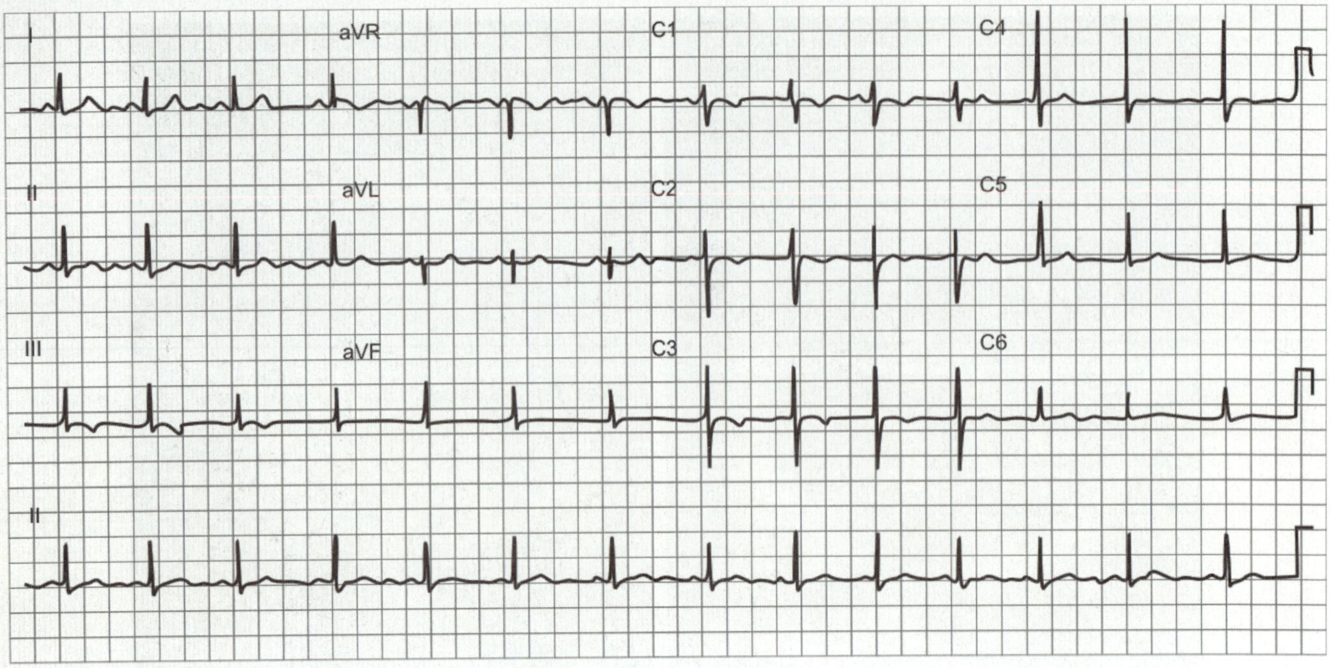

Fig. 27.11: *12-electrocardiogram of a child with mitral valve prolapse (MVP) showing T-wave inversion in leads III and aVF*

Phonocardiography: This was previously used as an adjunct to confirm the auscultatory findings.

Invasive and noninvasive Procedures

Ambulatory 24-hour Electrocardiogram

A Holter monitor may help to identify the nature and frequency of arrhythmic activity. Premature ventricular beats (38%), multiform couplets, and tachyarrhythmias (8%) are usual findings (Fig. 27.12).

Exercise testing: This is useful in patients with palpitations and exercise-related symptoms.

Premature ventricular beats (16%), ventricular tachycardia (4%), and supraventricular ecotopy are common findings. Ventricular fibrillation is a rare finding.

Cardiac Catheterization and Angiography

These tests are generally restricted to patients with MVP and severe MR who may require valve repair or replacement.

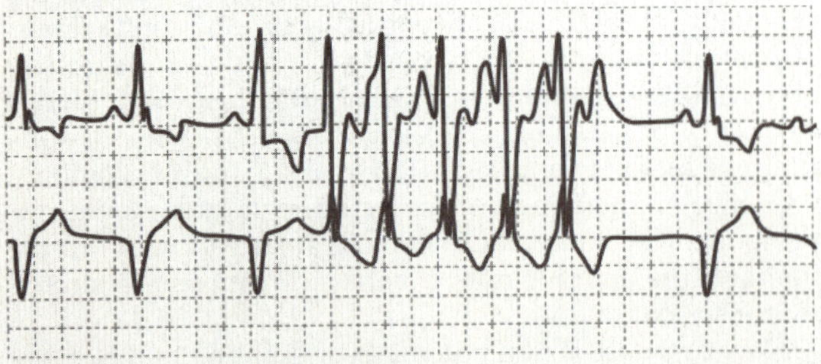

Fig. 27.12: *Two channel Holte recording strips with 5 beats run of ventricular tachycardia in patient with mitral valve prolapse with mitral regurgitation*

Associated coronary artery disease can also be confirmed or excluded. A left ventricular angiogram, taken in the right anterior oblique view, best shows the posterior leaflet. A left anterior oblique projection shows the anterior leaflet (Fig. 27.14).

Other abnormalities that may be revealed include dilatation, decreased systolic contraction, calcification of the mitral annulus, and poor contraction of the basal portion of the left ventricle.

Electrophysiology

Indications for electrophysiology (EPS) are similar to those in general clinical practice.

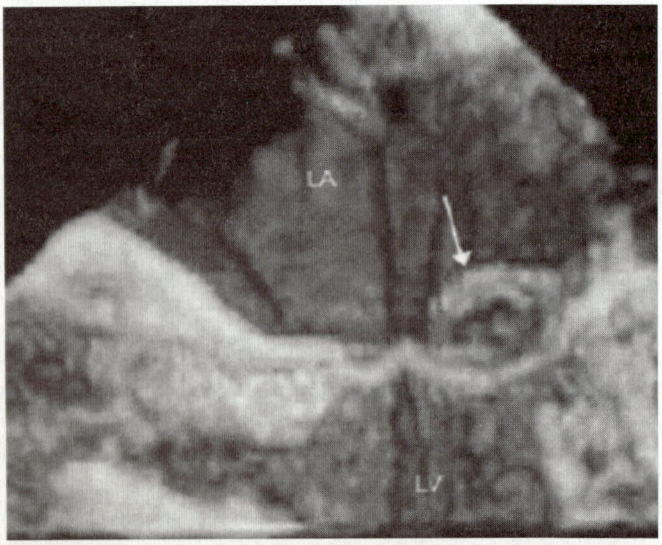

Fig. 27.13: *Three dimensional reconstruction obtained from the TEE in a patient with prolapse posterior mitral valve leaflet (arrow)*

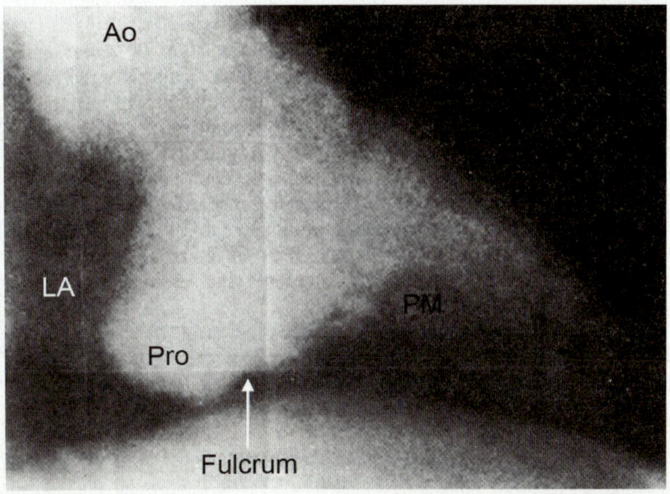

Fig. 27.14: *Left ventricular angiogram during systole demonstrating prolapse of mitral valve (Pro). The posteromedial commissural scallop of the posterior mitral leaflet extends posteriorly and inferiorly to the fulcrum (arrow)*

EPS is useful in the presence of supraventricular tachycardia because accessory atrioventricular pathways are common in patients with MVP. In this subset of patients, EPS is important because radiofrequency ablation can be performed during the same procedure, with a very high curative success rate.

Tilt test: Upright tilt studies with blood pressure and cardiac rhythm monitoring may be valuable in patients with light-headedness or syncope when vasodepressor-vasovagal reaction is suspected and confirmation of clinical symptoms is desired.

Histologic Findings

Mitral valves excised from patients with severe MR secondary to MVP have large leaflets and show various alterations. The most specific, fundamental, and characteristic histologic changes are (1) collagen dissolution and disruption in the pars fibrosa of the mitral valve leaflet and (2) replacement of the dense collagenous fibrosa by loose myxomatous connective tissue with high acid mucopolysaccharide content.

Similar histologic abnormalities are observed in chordae tendineae. Scanning electron photomicrographs demonstrate surface folds and focal loss of endothelial cells on mitral valve leaflets obtained from patients with severe MVP and significant MR. These surface abnormalities may predispose to thromboembolic complications and/or infectious endocarditis. Continuous pressure and stress on the leaflets and chordae tendineae during left ventricular systole contribute to gradual progression of these histologic changes.

Medical treatment: In childhood, the condition is not progressive, and specific therapy is not indicated for the vast majority. Asymptomatic patients with isolated mitral systolic clicks need only counseling and reassurance. Avoid excessive use of caffeine, cigarettes, alcohol, and prescription or over-the-counter drugs that contain stimulants such as epinephrine or ephedrine to minimize catecholamine and cyclic adenosine monophosphate (AMP) stimulation. Prevention of volume depletion before, during, and immediately after exercise may help. Subacute bacterial endocarditis antibiotic prophylaxis coverage for at-risk procedures is indicated in patients with mitral valve prolapse (MVP) and MR.

Additional dental care recommended for patients at risk for infective endocarditis includes the following:
- Regular toothbrushing after eating no cookies, sweets, or sweet drinks between meals
- Regular dental checks every 6 months
- Fluoride supplements in locations where the fluoride in drinking water is less than 0.3 ppm for children younger than 2 years or less than 0.7 ppm for children younger than 2 years
- Dental treatments (more than 2) scheduled at an interval of 14 days or longer.

Surgical intervention: Recent advances have made reconstructive mitral valve surgery feasible in patients with congestive heart failure, severe MR secondary to MVP, or both. For details of surgical intervention, results, postoperative care, and complications of MR.

Robotic Mitral Valve Repair (Figs 27.15 and 27.16)

Robotic mitral valve repair allows complete anatomic correction of all categories of leaflet prolapse using techniques identical to open approaches. Robotic repair effectively corrects mitral regurgitation, offers excellent freedom from adverse events, and facilitates rapid weaning from ventilation, translating into earlier hospital dismissal. Safety and efficacy after both open and robotic mitral valve repair are higher than recently reported in the EVEREST II trial and establish a benchmark against which nonsurgical therapies should be evaluated.

Group consultations: A multidisciplinary approach is preferable with a team from the following specialties:
- Pediatrics
- Pediatric cardiology

Radiology
- Genetics
- Cardiothoracics
- Physiotherapy
- Family medicine
- Orthopedics.

Advice for physical activity: A gradual return to exercise may be tolerated. In the absence of studies on the effect of exercise on the progression of MVP, the best approach at present is based on common sense and good clinical judgment.
- Patients with symptoms of syncope, presyncope, or palpitations upon exertion should undergo thorough evaluations and avoid competitive sports for at least 6 months after the last significant episode.
- In the presence of significant MR, limitations apply as for any other cause of MR.

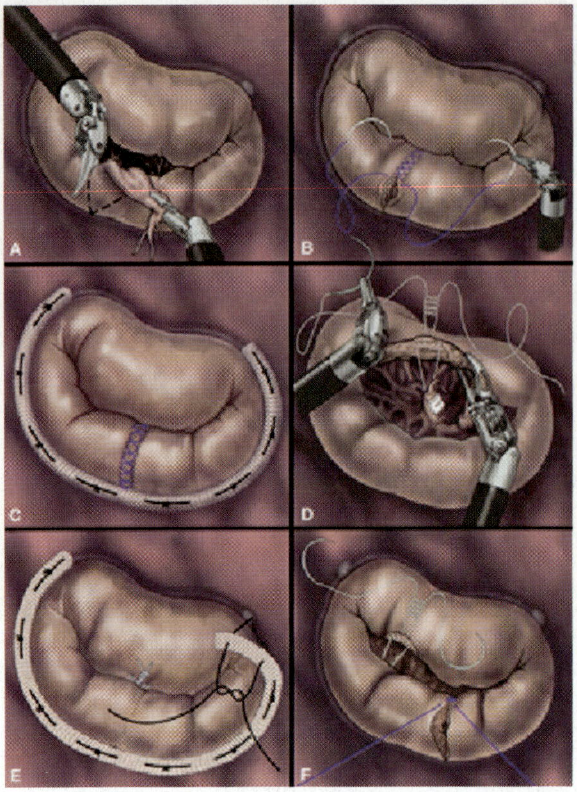

Fig. 27.15: *Robotic mitral valve repair for all prolapse subsets using techniques identical to open valvuloplasty: Standard Mayo Clinic mitral valve repair techniques using robotic instrumentation. (A) The extent of posterior leaflet prolapse is determined and a triangular-shaped resection performed to eliminate redundancy predominating at the leading edge, restoring the position of the coapting margin to the annular plane and decreasing leaflet height. (B) The remaining leaflet edges are reapposed using a 2-layer prolene stitch, restoring normal leaflet coaptation. (C) After posterior leaflet correction, a standard-length 63-mm flexible posterior annuloplasty band is inserted using interrupted Ethibond sutures from right to left fibrous trigones. (D) Anterior leaflet prolapse is corrected by placing two 5-0 Gore-Tex (WL Gore & Associates, Inc, Flagstaff, Ariz) neochords between the subtending papillary muscle to the unsupported leaflet edge using a double-armed Gore-Tex pledget-backed mattress stitch. E, After anterior leaflet correction, a 63 mm flexible posterior annuloplasty band is inserted using interrupted Ethibond sutures from right to left fibrous trigones. (F) Bileaflet repair is performed using a combination of posterior leaflet resection/reconstruction, anterior leaflet neochord resuspension, and standard-length 63-mm flexible posterior annuloplasty band*

- Coexisting aortic root dilatation and aortic regurgitation can further limit activity.
- Patients with cardiac arrhythmia should have periodic exercise tests performed and ambulatory ECG recordings obtained while doing the type of exercise they are likely to undertake.
- Sudden death is extremely uncommon in MVP.

Pharmacotherapy in Mitral Valve Prolapse

Anticongestive heart failure therapy: Antibiotic prophylaxis during surgery, dental, and genitourinary procedures. Only necessary if associated mitral regurgitation.

Antiarrhythmic therapy: It may be indicated in patients with documented and/or symptomatic arrhythmia, dependent on findings of noninvasive and/or invasive electrophysiologic testing.

Beta-blockers: It may be beneficial for symptom prevention, reduction in ectopy, treatment of vasodepressor syncope, panic attacks, or antiarrhythmic therapy.

Antiplatelet therapy: It used in patients with thromboembolic episodes.

ACE inhibitors: It used in patients with significant MR. Low-dose aspirin and/or anticoagulant therapy. Considered in patients with thromboembolic episodes.

Beta-adrenergic blocking agents: These agents block the beta-adrenergic receptor and are modulators of the autonomic system. They inhibit chronotropic, inotropic and vasodilatory responses to beta-adrenergic stimulation.

Propranolol (Inderal)

Description: Inhibits beta1 and beta 2-adrenergic receptors. Class II antiarrhythmic, nonselective, beta-adrenergic receptor blocker with membrane-stabilizing activity that decreases automaticity of contractions.

Pediatric dose: 1–4 mg/kg/d PO divided bid/qid.

Antiplatelet Agents

These drugs are used for secondary prevention of thrombotic cerebrovascular or cardiac disease.

Aspirin: Anacin, bayer, empirin.

Description: Inhibits prostaglandin synthesis, which prevents formation of platelet-aggregating thromboxane A2.

Pediatric dose: 5–10 mg/kg/d PO; not to exceed 100 mg/d.

Diuretics: These drugs are used to release retained fluid and lower preload.

Furosemide (Lasix)

Description: Inhibits reabsorption of fluid from ascending limb of the Henle loop in renal tubule. Administered IV. It has venodilation action; thus, also lowers preload even before diuresis effect. It is useful in acute heart failure and exacerbations of chronic heart failure.

Pediatric dose: 1–4 mg/kg PO qd or bid; or 1–4 mg/kg IV q 8 h.

ACE inhibitors: These agents reduce afterload and decrease myocardial remodeling, which worsens chronic heart failure.

Captopril (Capoten)

Description: Accepted as essential part of heart failure therapy. Not only gives symptomatic improvement but also prolongs survival.

Adult dose: 6.25–25 mg PO tid.

Pediatric dose: 0.1–1 mg/kg PO tid; initiate at lower dosage range and titrate upward.

Table 27.2: *Antibiotic recommendation to prevent bacterial endocarditis in mitral valve prolapse*

Dental or respiratory-tract procedures	*Genitourinary or gastrointestinal surgery or instrumentation*
1. Penicilin V, 2 gm orally 1 hour before the procedure and 1 gm 6 hour later	1. Ampicilin 2 g, IM or IV, puls gentamicin, 1.5 mg/kg, IM or IV, ½ to 1 hour before the procedure and repeated 8 hour later.
2. If unable to take medications by mouth, 2 million units penicillin G, IV or IM, 30–60 min before the procedure and 1 million units 6 hours later.	2. If allergic to penicillin; vancomycin, 1 gm IV slowly over 1 hour, puls gentamicin, 1.5 mg/kg, IM or IV, 1 hour before the procedure. These doses are repeated once 8–12 hour later.
3. If allergic to penicillin, either erythromycin, 1 gm orally, 1 hour before the procedure and 500 mg 6 hour later; or vancomycin, 1 gm slowly IV for 1 hour before the procedure.	3. For minor or repetitive procedures in low-risk patients, amoxicillin, 3 gm orally 1 hour before the procedure and 1.5 gm 6 hours later unless renal function is compromised.
4. In high-risk patients with prosthetic heart valves, ampicillin 1–2 gm, IM or IV, puls gentamicin, 1.5 mg/kg IV, 30 min before teh procedure; and either the same medication 8 hour later or penicillin V, 1 gm orally, 6 hours later.	

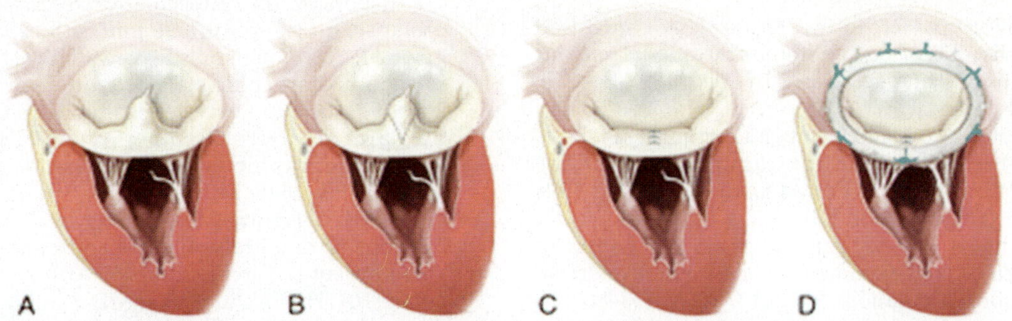

Fig. 27.16: *Triangular resection and ring annuloplasty. (A) Fibroelastic deficiency with P2 (posterior middle scallop) prolapse. (B) Dashed lines represent area of leaflet to be excised. (C) Reconstructed leaflet after triangular resection. (D) Completed repair after ring annuloplasty*

Digoxin (Lanoxin)

Description: It improves myocardial contractility, reduces heart rate, and lowers sympathetic stimulation in chronic heart failure.

Pediatric dose: Maintenance dose: preterm infant: 5–7.5 mcg/kg/d PO. Term infant: 6–10 mcg/kg/d PO. 1 month to 2 years: 10–15 mcg/kg/d PO. 2–5 years: 7.5–10 mcg/kg/d PO. 5–10 years: 5–10 mcg/kg/d. PO > 10 years: 2.5–5 mcg/kg/d PO. Daily dose typically divided bid for.

Medical/Legal Aspects in MVP

- Failure to make the diagnosis
- Failure to fully investigate patients who are symptomatic
- Failure to restrict exercise in patients who are symptomatic
- Failure to recognize the higher risk of arrhythmia during anesthesia and the perioperative period
- Patients with mitral valve prolapse (MVP) syndrome require a careful history and thorough physical examination because of the possibility of misinterpreting history, physical findings, borderline laboratory test results, and nonspecific ECG or echocardiography changes.

Over diagnosis: Any unexplained symptoms should be viewed with due concern and investigated.

Special concerns: Diagnosis should include the type of prolapse (late systolic, holosystolic, anterior, or posterior leaflet), thickness of MV leaflets, size of mitral annulus, and the left ventricular and left atrial size and function. The diagnosis should also include presence, severity, and timing of MR; define jet direction and magnitude; and clearly list associated abnormalities. Patients with orthostatic syncope secondary to dehydration should take excess salt and water during and following sport activities and competition.

Patients are more sensitive to volume depletion; hence chronic diuretic therapy should be avoided.

BIBLIOGRAPHY

1. Alpert MA, Mukerji V, Sabeti M, et al: Mitral valve prolapse, panic disorder, and chest pain. Med Clin North Am 1991 Sep; 75(5): 1119–33.
2. American College of Cardiology/American Heart Association: ACC/AHA guidelines for the management of patients with valvular heart disease. A report of the American College of Cardiology/American Heart Association. Task Force on Practice Guidelines (Committee

on Management of Patients with Valvular Heart Disease. J Am Coll Cardiol 1998 Nov; 32(5): 1486–588.
3. American College of Cardiology/American Heart Association: ACC/AHA 2006 guidelines for the management of patients with valvular heart disease. A report of the American College of Cardiology/American Heart Association Task Force on Practice Guidelines (writing committee to revise the 1998 guidelines for the Manag. J Am Coll Cardiol 2006; 48:1–148.
4. Aviernos JF, Gersh BJ, Melton LJ, et al: Natural history of asymptomatic mitral valve prolapse in the community. Circulation 2002; 106: 1355–1361.
5. Barnett HJ, Boughner DR, Taylor DW, et al: Further evidence relating mitral-valve prolapse to cerebral ischemic events. N Engl J Med 1980 Jan 17; 302(3): 139–44.
6. Bryhn M, Persson S: The prevalence of mitral valve prolapse in healthy men and women in Sweden. An echocardiographic study. Acta Med Scand 1984; 215(2): 157–60.
7. Ciancamerla F, Paglia I, Catuzzo B, et al: Sudden death in mitral valve prolapse and severe mitral regurgitation. Is chordal rupture an indication to early surgery?. J Cardiovasc Surg (Torino) 2003 Apr; 44(2): 283–6.
8. Clemens JD, Horwitz RI, Jaffe CC, et al: A controlled evaluation of the risk of bacterial endocarditis in persons with mitral-valve prolapse. N Engl J Med 1982 Sep 23; 307(13): 776–81.
9. Cohn LH, Couper GS, Aranki SF, et al: Long-term results of mitral valve reconstruction for regurgitation of the myxomatous mitral valve. J Thorac Cardiovasc Surg 1994 Jan; 107(1): 143–50; discussion 150–1.
10. Dajani AS, Taubert KA, Wilson W, et al: Prevention of bacterial endocarditis. Recommendations by the American Heart Association. Circulation 1997 Jul 1; 96(1): 358–66.
11. David TE, Omran A, Armstrong S, et al: Long-term results of mitral valve repair for myxomatous disease with and without chordal replacement with expanded polytetrafluoroethylene sutures. J Thorac Cardiovasc Surg 1998 Jun; 115(6): 1279–85.
12. Davidsen B, Egeblad H, Pietersen A: Thromboembolism in patients with advanced mitral valve prolapse. J Intern Med 1989 Dec; 226(6): 433–6.
13. Devereux RB, Kramer-Fox R, Shear MK, et al: Diagnosis and classification of severity of mitral valve prolapse: methodologic, biologic, and prognostic considerations. Am Heart J 1987 May; 113(5): 1265–80.
14. Devereux RB, Kramer-Fox R, Brown WT, et al: Relation between clinical features of the mitral prolapse syndrome and echocardiographically documented mitral valve prolapse. J Am Coll Cardiol 1986 Oct; 8(4): 763–72.
15. Devereux RB, Hawkins I, Kramer-Fox R, et al: Complications of mitral valve prolapse. Disproportionate occurrence in men and older patients. Am J Med 1986 Nov; 81(5): 751–8.
16. Devereux RB: Recent developments in the diagnosis and management of mitral valve prolapse. Curr Opin Cardiol 1995 Mar; 10(2): 107–16.
17. Devlin WH, Starling MR: Outcome of valvular heart disease with vasodilator therapy. Compr Ther 1994; 20(10): 569–74.
18. Freed LA, Levy D, Levine RA, et al: Prevalence and clinical outcome of mitral-valve prolapse. N Engl J Med 1999 Jul 1; 341(1): 1–7.
19. Freed LA, Benjamin EJ, Levy D, et al: Mitral valve prolapse in the general population: the benign nature of echocardiographic features in the Framingham Heart Study. J Am Coll Cardiol 2002 Oct 2; 40(7): 1298–304.
20. Gilon D, Buonanno FS, Joffe MM, et al: Lack of evidence of an association between mitral-valve prolapse and stroke in young patients. N Engl J Med 1999 Jul 1; 341(1): 8–13.
21. Glesby MJ, Pyeritz RE: Association of mitral valve prolapse and systemic abnormalities of connective tissue. A phenotypic continuum. JAMA 1989 Jul 28; 262(4): 523–8.
22. Grayburn PA: Vasodilator therapy for chronic aortic and mitral regurgitation. Am J Med Sci 2000 Sep; 320(3): 202–8.
23. Grigioni F, Enriquez-Sarano M, Ling LH, et al: Sudden death in mitral regurgitation due to flail leaflet. J Am Coll Cardiol 1999 Dec; 34(7): 2078–85.
24. Kligfield P, Hochreiter C, Kramer H, et al: Complex arrhythmias in mitral regurgitation with and without mitral valve prolapse: contrast to arrhythmias in mitral valve prolapse without mitral regurgitation. Am J Cardiol 1985 Jun 1; 55(13 Pt 1): 1545–9.
25. Kostuk WJ, Boughner DR, Barnett HJ, Silver MD: Strokes: A complication of mitral–leaflet prolapse?. Lancet 1977 Aug 13; 2(8033): 313–6.
26. Kramer HM, Kligfield P, Devereux RB, et al: Arrhythmias in mitral valve prolapse. Effect of selection bias. Arch Intern Med 1984 Dec; 144(12): 2360–4.
27. Kulan K, Komsuoglu B, Tuncer C, Kulan C: Significance of QT dispersion on ventricular arrhythmias in mitral valve prolapse. Int J Cardiol 1996 Jun; 54(3): 251–7.
28. Levine RA, Stathogiannis E, Newell JB, et al: Reconsideration of echocardiographic standards for mitral valve prolapse: lack of association between leaflet displacement isolated to the apical four chamber view and independent echocardiographic evidence of abnormality. J Am Coll Cardiol 1988 May; 11(5): 1010–9.
29. Levine RA, Triulzi MO, Harrigan P, Weyman AE: The relationship of mitral annular shape to the diagnosis of mitral valve prolapse. Circulation 1987 Apr; 75(4): 756–67.
30. Levine RA, Handschumacher MD, Sanfilippo AJ, et al: Three-dimensional echocardiographic reconstruction of the mitral valve, with implications for the diagnosis of mitral valve prolapse. Circulation 1989 Sep; 80(3): 589–98.
31. Levine RA, Stathogiannis E, Newell JB, et al: Reconsideration of echocardiographic standards for mitral valve prolapse: lack of association between leaflet displacement isolated to the apical four chamber view and independent echocardiographic evidence of abnormality. J Am Coll Cardiol 1988 May; 11(5): 1010–9.
32. Levy D, Savage D: Prevalence and clinical features of mitral valve prolapse. Am Heart J 1987 May; 113(5): 1281–90.
33. Ling LH, Enriquez-Sarano M, Seward JB, et al: Early surgery in patients with mitral regurgitation due to flail leaflets: a long-term outcome study. Circulation 1997 Sep 16; 96(6): 1819–25.
34. MacMahon SW, Roberts JK, Kramer-Fox R, et al: Mitral valve prolapse and infective endocarditis. Am Heart J 1987 May; 113(5): 1291–8.
35. MacMahon SW, Hickey AJ, Wilcken DE, et al: Risk of infective endocarditis in mitral valve prolapse with and without precordial systolic murmurs. Am J Cardiol 1987 Jan 1; 59(1): 105–8.
36. Markiewicz W, Stoner J, London E, et al: Mitral valve prolapse in one hundred presumably healthy young females. Circulation 1976 Mar; 53(3): 464–73.
37. Marks AR, Choong CY, Sanfilippo AJ, et al: Identification of high-risk and low-risk subgroups of patients with mitral-valve prolapse. N Engl J Med 1989 Apr 20; 320(16): 1031–6.
38. Martinez-Rubio A, Schwammenthal Y, Schwammenthal E, et al: Patients with valvular heart disease presenting with sustained ventricular tachyarrhythmias or syncope: results of programmed ventricular stimulation and long-term follow-up. Circulation 1997 Jul 15; 96(2): 500–8.

39. Mylonakis E, Calderwood SB: Infective endocarditis in adults. N Engl J Med 2001 Nov 1; 345(18): 1318–30.
40. Nidorf SM, Weyman AE, Hennessey R: The relationship between mitral valve morphology and prognosis in patients with mitral valve prolapse: a prospective echocardiographic study of 568 patients. J Am Soc Echocardiogr 1993; 6: 58.
41. Cheunsuchon P, Chuangsuwanich T, Samanthai N, Warnnissorn M, Leksrisakul P, Thongcharoen P. Surgical pathology and etiology of 278 surgically removed mitral valves with pure regurgitation in Thailand. Cardiovasc Pathol. Mar-Apr 2007;16(2):104–10.
42. Deng YB, Takenaka K, Sakamoto T, et al. Follow-up in mitral valve prolapse by phonocardiography, M-mode and two-dimensional echocardiography and Doppler echocardiography. Am J Cardiol. Feb 1 1990;65(5):349–54.
43. AAP. Mitral valve prolapse and athletic participation in children and adolescents. Pediatrics. May 1995;95(5):789–90.
44. American College of Cardiology/American Heart Association Task Force on Practice Guidelines; Society of Cardiovascular Anesthesiologists; Society for Cardiovascular Angiography and Interventions; Society of Thoracic Surgeons, et al. ACC/AHA 2006 guidelines for the management of patients with valvular heart disease: a report of the American College of Cardiology/American Heart Association Task Force on Practice Guidelines (writing committee to revise the 1998 Guidelines for the Management of Patients With Valvular Heart Disease): developed in collaboration with the Society of Cardiovascular Anesthesiologists: endorsed by the Society for Cardiovascular Angiography and Interventions and the Society of Thoracic Surgeons. Circulation. Aug 1 2006;114(5):e84–231.
45. Bassili A, Mokhtar SA, Dabous NI, et al. Congenital heart disease among school children in Alexandria, Egypt: an overview on prevalence and relative frequencies. J Trop Pediatr. Dec 2000;46(6):357–62.
46. Beroukhim RS, Reed JH, Schaffer MS, Yetman AT. Surgical correction of mitral valve prolapse : a cure for recurrent ventricular tachycardia in Marfan syndrome?. Pediatr Cardiol. Nov-Dec 2006;27(6):755–8.
47. Bisset GS, Schwartz DC, Meyer RA, et al. Clinical spectrum and long-term follow-up of isolated mitral valve prolapse in 119 children. Circulation. Aug 1980;62(2):423–9.
48. Blum A, Shapira Y, Yeganh S, Rabinkov M. Mitral valve prolapse and thromboembolic events. Isr Med Assoc J. Apr 2001;3(4):282–3.
49. Bonow RO, Carabello BA, Kanu C, et al. ACC/AHA 2006 Guidelines for the Management of Patients with Valvular Heart Disease: A Report of the American College of Cardiology/American Heart Association Task Force on Practice Guidelines. Circulation. Aug 1 2006;114(5):e84–231.
50. Carolei A, Marini C, Ferranti E, et al. A prospective study of cerebral ischemia in the young. Analysis of pathogenic determinants. The National Research Council Study Group. Stroke. Mar 1993;24(3):362–7.
51. Chauvaud S. Congenital mitral valve surgery: techniques and results. Curr Opin Cardiol. Mar 2006;21(2):95–9.
52. Cheng TO. Heart rate variability and QT dispersion in mitral valve prolapse. J Electrocardiol. Jan 2001;34(1):89.
53. Cheng TO, Wang XF, Zheng LH. Three-dimensional transesophageal echocardiography in the diagnosis of mitral valve prolapse. Am Heart J. Dec 1994;128(6 Pt 1):1218–24.
54. Chou HT, Chen YT, Shi YR, Tsai FJ. Association between angiotensin I-converting enzyme gene insertion/deletion polymorphism and mitral valve prolapse syndrome. Am Heart J. Jan 2003;145(1):169–73.
55. Chou HT, Hung JS, Chen YT, et al. Association between angiotensinogen gene M235T polymorphism and mitral valve prolapse syndrome in Taiwan Chinese. J Heart Valve Dis. Nov 2002;11(6):830–6.
56. Chou HT, Shi YR, Hsu Y, Tsai FJ. Association between fibrillin-1 gene exon 15 and 27 polymorphisms and risk of mitral valve prolapse. J Heart Valve Dis. Jul 2003;12(4):475–81.
57. Colomina MJ, Puig L, Godet C, et al. Prevalence of asymptomatic cardiac valve anomalies in idiopathic scoliosis. Pediatr Cardiol. Jul–Aug 2002;23(4):426–9.
58. Cooke RA, Chambers JB. Anorexia nervosa and the heart. Br J Hosp Med. Oct 4–17 1995;54(7):313–7.
59. Corrado D, Basso C, Nava A, et al. Sudden death in young people with apparently isolated mitral valve prolapse. G Ital Cardiol. Nov 1997;27(11):1097–105.
60. Corrado D, Thiene G, Nava A, et al. Sudden death in young competitive athletes: clinicopathologic correlations in 22 cases. Am J Med. Nov 1990;89(5):588–96.
61. Corrao S, Scaglione R, Arnone S, Licata G. Left ventricular diastolic filling alterations in subjects with mitral valve prolapse: a Doppler echocardiographic study. Eur Heart J. Mar 1993;14(3):369–72.
62. David TE, Omran A, Armstrong S, et al. Long-term results of mitral valve repair for myxomatous disease with and without chordal replacement with expanded polytetrafluoroethylene sutures. J Thorac Cardiovasc Surg. Jun 1998;115(6):1279–85; discussion 1285–6.
63. Dreyfus GD, Corbi P, Rubin S, Aubert S. Posterior leaflet preservation in mitral valve prolapse: a new approach to mitral repair. J Heart Valve Dis. Jul 2006;15(4):528–30.
64. Freed LA, Acierno JS, Dai D, et al. A locus for autosomal dominant mitral valve prolapse on chromosome 11p15.4. Am J Hum Genet. Jun 2003;72(6):1551–9.
65. Fuzellier JF, Chauvaud SM, Fornes P, et al. Surgical management of mitral regurgitation associated with Marfan's syndrome. Ann Thorac Surg. Jul 1998;66(1):68–72.
66. Glesby MJ, Pyeritz RE. Association of mitral valve prolapse and systemic abnormalities of connective tissue. A phenotypic continuum. JAMA. Jul 28 1989;262(4):523–8.
67. Gorgulu S, Eren M, Norgaz T, Tezel T. Comparison of echocardiographic methods in assessing severity of mitral regurgitation in patients with mitral valve prolapse. J Heart Valve Dis. Jan 2004;13(1):38–45.
68. Hamada T, Koshino Y, Misawa T, et al. Mitral valve prolapse and autonomic function in panic disorder. Acta Psychiatr Scand. Feb 1998;97(2):139–43.
69. Henneke KH, Pongratz G, Feistel H, et al. Assessment of cardiac adrenergic supply in mitral valve prolapse using m–[123I]iodobenzylguanidine scintigraphy. Int J Cardiol. Dec 1992;37(3):389–94.
70. Ismajli J, Shabani X, Manaj R, Emini M, Bajraktari G. Mitral valve prolapse, atrial flutter, and syncope in a young female patient. Med Sci Monit. 2006;12:110–3.
71. James PA, Aftimos S, Skinner JR. Familial mitral valve prolapse associated with short stature, characteristic face, and sudden death. Am J Med Genet A. May 15 2003;119(1):32–6.
72. Kaminer SJ, Hixon RL, Strong WB. Evaluation and recommendations for participation in athletics for children with heart disease. Curr Opin Pediatr. Oct 1995;7(5):595–600.
73. Karakurum B, Topçu S, Yildirim T, Karatas M, Turan I, Tan M. Silent cerebral infarct in patients with mitral valve prolapse. Int J Neurosci. Nov 2005;115(11):1527–37.

28 Cardiomyopathies in Children and Adolescents

With the pediatric population, cardiomyopathy occurs in approximately 12 children out of every million with about 1,000–5,000 new cases diagnosed each year. The majority of diagnosed children are infants under the age of 12 months with fewer cases between the ages of 1–12 years. When cardiomyopathy is diagnosed in children before puberty, it is considered extremely unusual and it may not have the same causes, manifestations or disease progression as cardiomyopathy in adults. There is a vast amount of literature on adult cardiomyopathy but not all of the information is relevant to children diagnosed with the disease. Unfortunately, there has been little research and focus on pediatric cardiomyopathy over the years. Consequently, the causes are not well understood. According to the Pediatric Cardiomyopathy Registry, less than 25% of all patients have an identified cause despite

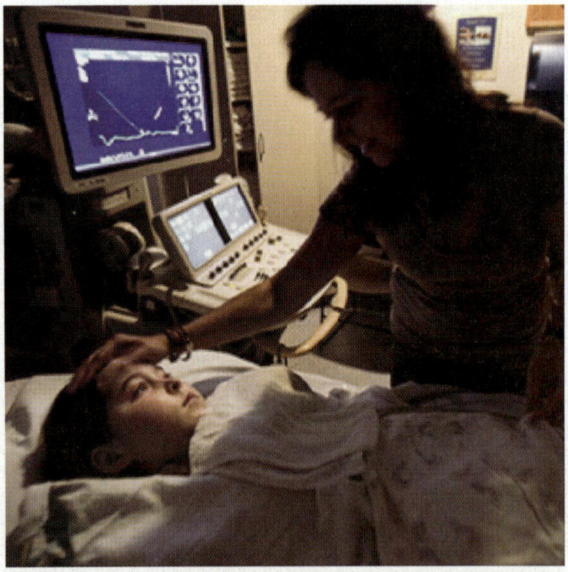

Fig. 28.1: *Mother is sitting at the bedside of the young child suffering with DCM in intensive care unit*

Table 28.1: *Etiological classification of cardiomyopathy*

Dilated cardiomyopathy (Fig. 28.2)
Idiopathic cardiomyopathy
Familial cardiomyopathy
Noncompacted myocardium
Postpartum cardiomyopathy
hemachromatosis
Infectious
Postviral myocarditis
Human immunodeficiency virus related
Legionella infection
Sepsis (gram negative)
Toxic cardiomyopathy
Adriamycin
Alcohol
Carbon monoxide poisoning
Other chemotherapy
High-output cardiomyopathy
Tachycardia-mediated cardiomyopathy thyrotoxicosis
Nutritional (beriberi, thiamine deficiency)
Peripheral left to right shunt lesions
Anemia
Hypertrophic cardiomyopathy
Asymmetric septal hypertrohy (idiopathic hypertrophic cardiomyopathy)
Obstructive vs. nonobstructive
Concentric hypertrophic cardiomyopathy
Isolated apical hypetrophic cardiomyopathy
Atypical hypertrophic cardiomyopathy
Restrictive cardiomyopathy
Idiopathic
Infiltrative
Amyloidosis
Glycogen storage diseases
Hemachromatosis
Postradiation therapy
Endocardial fibroelastosis
Other
Friedreich ataxia
Muscular dystrophies

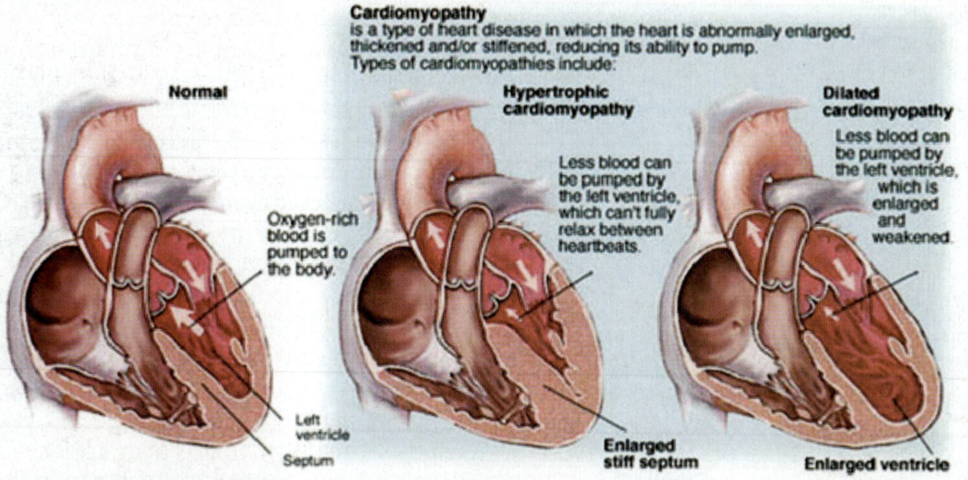

Fig. 28.2: *Comparative description of normal heart functioning with two common types of cardiomyopathies*

rigorous, standardized evaluation. What is known is that the underlying causes of cardiomyopathy in infants and children may be considerably different from that diagnosed in adolescents and adults with similar symptoms. Pediatric cardiomyopathy is more likely to be due to genetic factors while lifestyle or environmental factors play a greater role in adult cardiomyopathy.

In rare cases, pediatric cardiomyopathy may be a symptom of a larger genetic disorder that may not be immediately detected. For example, when an infant or young child is diagnosed with dilated cardiomyopathy, a rare genetic heart disease called Barth Syndrome or a mitochondrial defect (i.e. Kearns-Sayre syndrome) may be the cause. Similarly, a child with severe hypertrophic cardiomyopathy may actually have Noonan Syndrome, Pompe disease (type II glycogen storage disease), a fatty acid oxidation disorder, or mitochondrial HCM. It is therefore important for any diagnosed child to be properly evaluated for other suspected genetic disorders. A thorough evaluation remains a complicated and expensive process due to the large number of rare genetic causes, the broad range of symptoms and the existence of many specialized biochemical, enzymatic and genetic tests. Verifying a diagnosis may require getting additional blood, urine or tissue tests and consulting other specialists such as a neurologist and geneticist.

Cardiomyopathy in children may also present differently from diagnosed teenagers or adult. It is considered unusual when an infant or a child is diagnosed with symptoms at such a young age. Typically, symptoms are not apparent until the late teens or adult years when most patients are diagnosed. With hypertrophic cardiomyopathy, the disease commonly develops in association with growth and is detected when a child progresses through puberty. Even in genetically affected family members, a child that carries the muted gene from birth may appear to have a normal heart and be asymptomatic until puberty.

A diagnosis at a young age usually, but not always, signifies a serious heart condition that requires aggressive treatment. The concern lies in the uncertainty of how the heart muscle will respond with each additional growth spurt. With some older children, the condition may stabilize over time with the aid of certain medications or surgery. In severe cases, small children may experience progressive symptoms quickly leading to heart failure. This presentation contrasts with most diagnosed adults who may only have minor symptoms without serious limitations or major problems for years.

Aside from differences in the cause and manifestation, cardiomyopathy may also progress differently in children than adults. When children are diagnosed at an early age, the prognosis may be poor depending on the form of cardiomyopathy and the stage of the disease. For example, dilated cardiomyopathy can progress quite rapidly when diagnosed in young children. Up to 40% of diagnosed children with dilated cardiomyopathy fail medical management within the first year of diagnosis and of those that survive many have permanently impaired heart function. Children diagnosed with hypertrophic

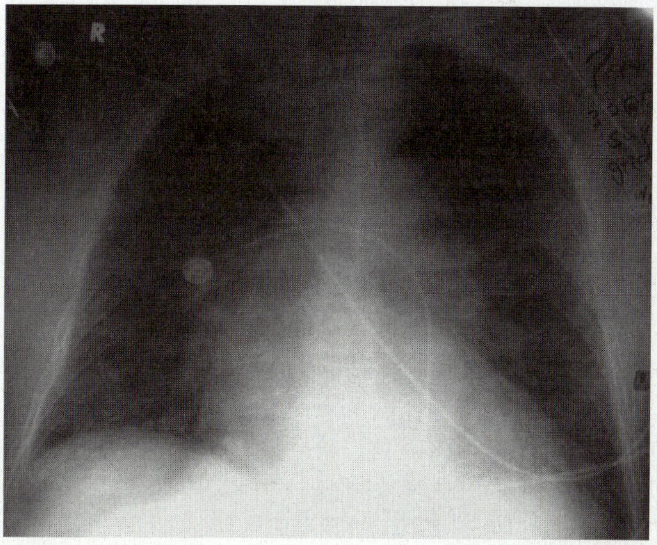

Fig. 28.3: *Chest X-ray showing gross cardiomegaly with bilateral congestion due to congestive heart failure in DCM*

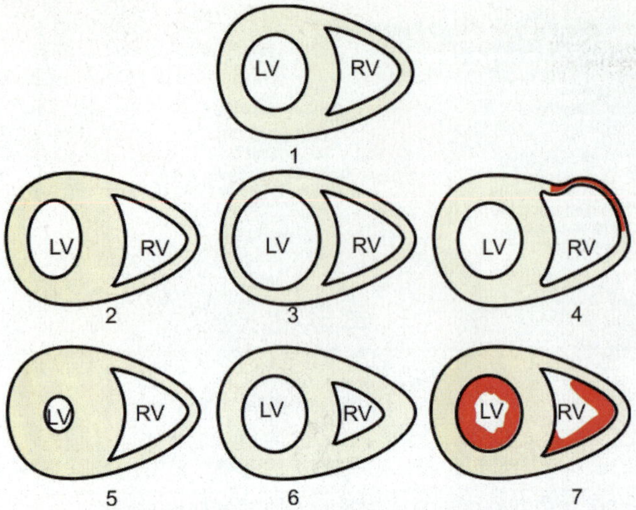

Fig. 28.4: *Diagrammatic representation of different types of cardiomyopathies at short-axis views and right and left ventricles at mid-septal levels. 1. Normal; 2. HCM, nonobstructive hypertrophic cardiomyopathy; 3. DCM, dilated cardiomyopathy; 4. ARVD, arrhythmogenic right ventricular dysplasia; 5. HOCM, hypertrophic obstructive cardiomyopathy; 6. RCM, restrictive cardiomyopathy; 7. EMF, endomyocardial fibrosis or obliterative cardiomyopathy*

cardiomyopathy seem to fare better but the outcome is highly variable. Mortality and heart transplant rates of childhood cardiomyopathies are much higher than in adults due to the rarity and uncertainty of the disease. Less than optimal outcomes may be attributed to the more fragile state of infants and young children or it may be a function of the disease's advanced progression associated with another genetic disorder. Another unfortunate reason is that cardiomyopathy is not usually detected until the end stage when obvious symptoms of heart failure are apparent. Cardiomyopathy can be easily missed in routine check-ups when there are no obvious symptoms (i.e. heart murmur) or when there is no reason for diagnostic testing (i.e. no family history of the disease).

TYPES OF CARDIOMYOPATHIES (Table 28.1)

- Common types
  a. Dilated cardiomyopathy (DCM)
  b. Hypertrophic cardiomyopathy (HOCM)
  c. Restrictive cardiomyopathy (RCM)
- Less common types
  a. Arrhythmogenic RV cardiomyopathy
  b. Noncompaction cardiomyopathy (NCC)
  c. Takotsubo cardiomyopathy.

A. Dilated Cardiomyopathy

Dilated or congestive cardiomyopathy (DCM) is diagnosed when the heart is enlarged (dilated) and the pumping chambers contract poorly (usually left side worse than right).

This condition is the most common form of cardiomyopathy and accounts for approximately 55–60% of all childhood cardiomyopathies. According to the pediatric cardiomyopathy registry database, this form of myopathy is detected in roughly one per 200,000 children with roughly one new case per 160,000 children reported each year in the United States. It can have both genetic and infectious/environmental causes.

It is more commonly diagnosed in younger children with the average age at diagnosis being 2 years. Dilated cardiomyopathy can be familial (genetic), and it is estimated that 20–30% of children with DCM have a relative with the disease although they may not have been diagnosed or have symptoms.

Signs and Symptoms of DCM

Dilated cardiomyopathy can appear along a spectrum of no symptoms, subtle symptoms, or in the more severe cases, congestive heart failure (CHF), which occurs when the heart is unable to pump blood well enough to meet the body tissue needs for oxygen and nutrients.

When only subtle symptoms exist, infants and young children are sometimes diagnosed with a viral upper respiratory tract infection or recurrent "pneumonia" without realizing that a heart problem is the basis for these symptoms.

Older children and adolescents are less likely to be diagnosed with viral syndromes and more likely to present with decreased exercise capacity or easy fatigability. With CHF, babies and young children will usually have more noticeable clinical changes such as irritability, failure to thrive (poor gain weight), increased sweating especially with activities, pale color, faster breathing and/or wheezing.

In older children, congestive heart failure can manifest as difficulty breathing and/or coughing, pale color, decreased urine output and swelling, excessive sweating,

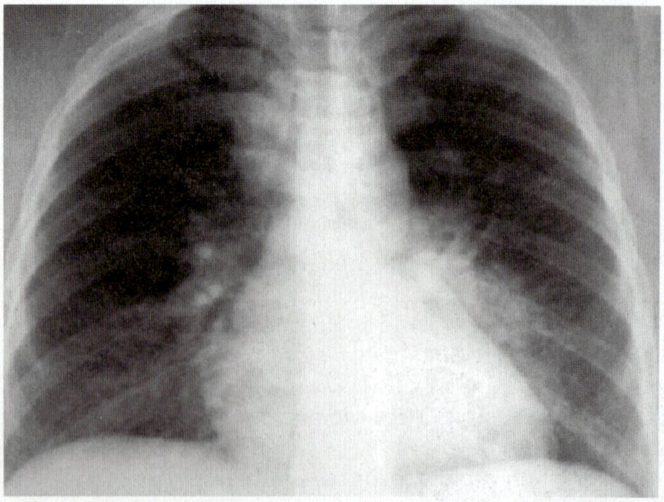

Fig. 28.5: *Chest radiograph in a patient presenting with heart failure, which was subsequently found to be the result of dilated cardiomyopathy. Although cardiac size is at the upper limit of normal, left ventricular function is poor, causing severe pulmonary edema with bilateral alveolar edema and marked dilatation of the superior vena cava*

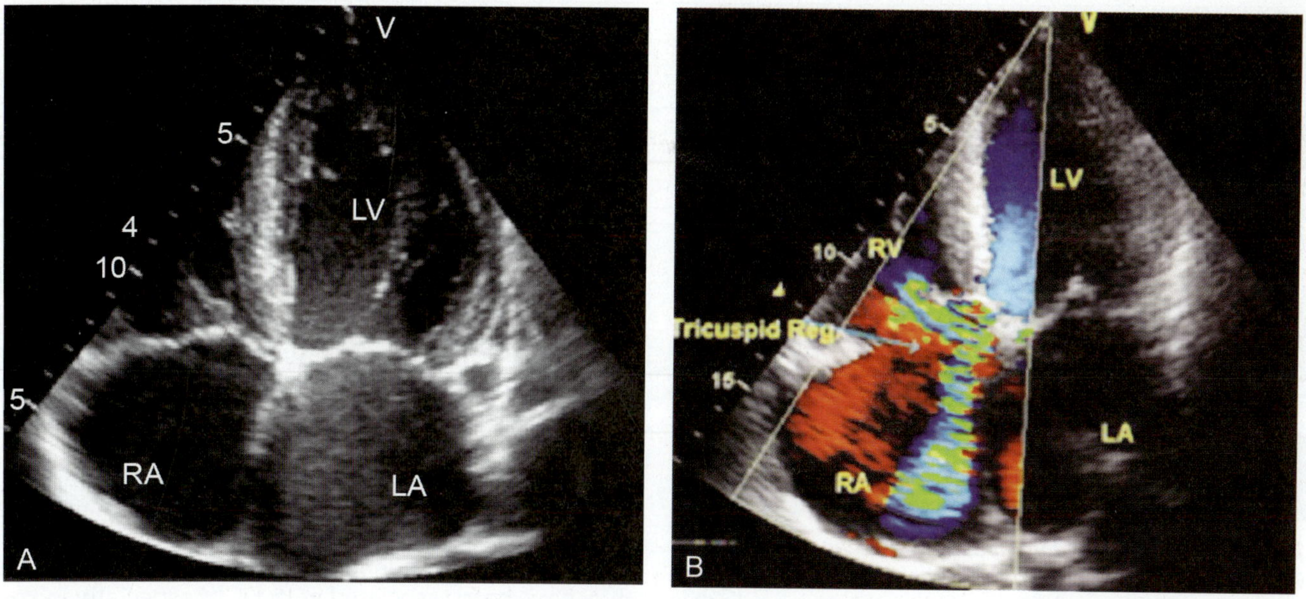

Fig. 28.6: *Dilated cardiomyopathy in a 20-year-old adolescent with AIDS. (A) Apical four chamber echocardiographic view shows marked enlargement of all four chambers, as well as spontaneous echo contrast ("smoke") in the left-sided chambers because of a very low ejection fraction and sluggish flow. (B) Apical fourc hamber view obtained with color Doppler flow imaging shows an eccentric jet of severe regurgitation through the tricuspid valve. LA, left atrium, LV, left ventricle, RA, right atrium, RV, right*

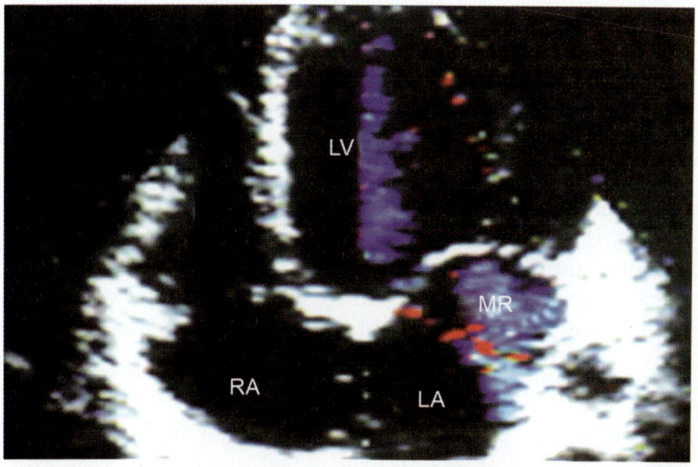

Fig. 28.7: *Apical two dimensional echocardiogram with color Doppler display (systolic image) in a patient with dilated cardiomyopathy shows a jet of mitral regurgitation (MR) into a large left atrium (LA) (Doppler-encoded blue). Note the dilatation of the left ventricle (LV) compared with the right ventricle*

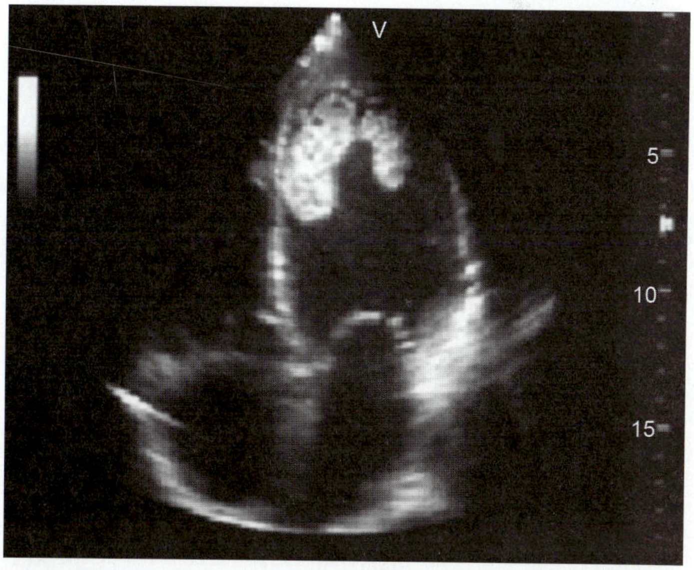

Fig. 28.8: *Peripartum cardiomyopathy with left ventricular thrombus*

and fatigue with minimal activities. Until the diagnosis is made in many children, chronic coughing and wheezing, particularly during activities, can be misinterpreted as asthma.

Some patients with DCM caused by viral myocarditis (weakened, enlarged heart muscle usually due to a viral infection) can have a rapid increase in the number and severity of CHF symptoms such that within 24–48 hours the child can become very ill requiring emergency hospitalization, and occasionally, advanced life support.

Symptoms due to heart rhythm problems (or arrhythmias, which means irregular, fast or slow heart rates) can also be either the first symptom or a symptom that appears after other symptoms have led to a diagnosis of DCM. Symptoms of rhythm problems include palpitations (feeling of funny or fast heart beats), syncope (fainting), seizures (convulsions), or even sudden cardiac arrest (heart stops beating effectively requiring resuscitation). These symptoms can occur at any age and with any stage of cardiomyopathy, even if other more

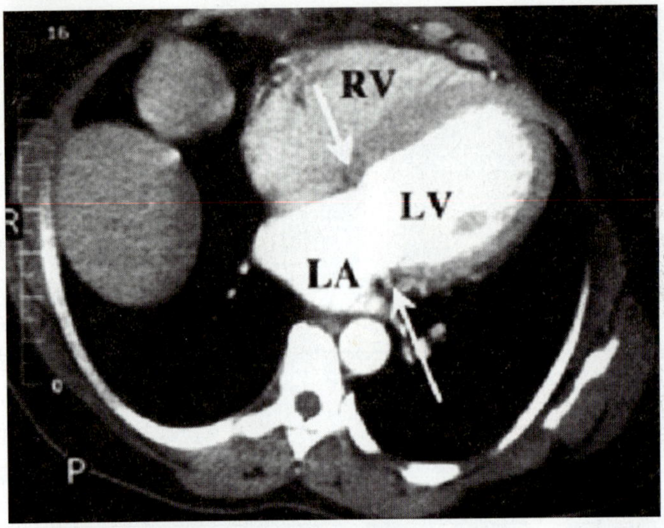

Fig. 28.9: *Spiral computed tomography (CT) scan obtained with intravenous contrast enhancement at the level of the center of the mitral valve (between arrows) and tricuspid valve in a patient with dilated cardiomyopathy. Left ventricle (LV) is dilated compared with the right ventricle (RV)*

severe symptoms of congestive heart failure have not yet appeared.

Diagnosis of DCM

Once there is clinical suspicion based on the patient history and physical examination, the diagnosis of DCM is primarily based on echocardiography. With this test, your physician will be using ultrasound beams to evaluate the heart looking for dilated chambers and decreased pump function. Along with the echocardiogram, there are other tests that will likely be done to confirm the diagnosis or provide clues as to the cause.

A chest X-ray will show the heart size and can be used as a reference to follow increases in heart size that may occur over time.

An electrocardiogram, or EKG, records the electrical conduction through the heart and is used to look for evidence of thickened or enlarged chambers as well as abnormal heart beats that can occur in children with this diagnosis. To more completely evaluate for the presence or absence of these abnormal heart rhythms, which may effect treatment, your doctor may also order a Holter monitor which records heart beats over a 24–48 hour period. (Figs 28.10, 28.12 and 28.16).

A treadmill test can also be useful in some children (beyond age 5–7 years) who can cooperate with this study. This exercise test is used to assess the energy reserve of your child's heart and, in cases when children do not respond adequately to medicines, this test may also help to predict the need for heart transplantation.

Depending on your child's age, a battery of blood tests may be done in order to identify treatable causes for the cardiomyopathy. This may include testing for certain viral infections such as adenovirus and the coxsackie viruses as they have been associated with DCM especially in younger children. In many cases, no cause is discovered, and the cardiomyopathy may be referred to as "idiopathic" (cause unknown). Many heart failure specialists believe this "idiopathic" form of the cardiomyopathy is genetic. While genetic screening has not yet become a standard procedure, some physicians may send blood to molecular testing labs located in a few centers around the country so that limited genetic testing can be performed looking for possible mutations currently known to cause dilated cardiomyopathy. If your physicians believe the cause is genetic (especially common in older children and adolescents), evaluation, usually with echo, of other family members is recommended to rule out presence of this disease in other close relatives (parents, siblings).

Finally, in more advanced cases of DCM, cardiac catheterization may be performed. During this procedure, a catheter (thin plastic tube) will be slowly advanced through an artery or vein into the heart (while watching its

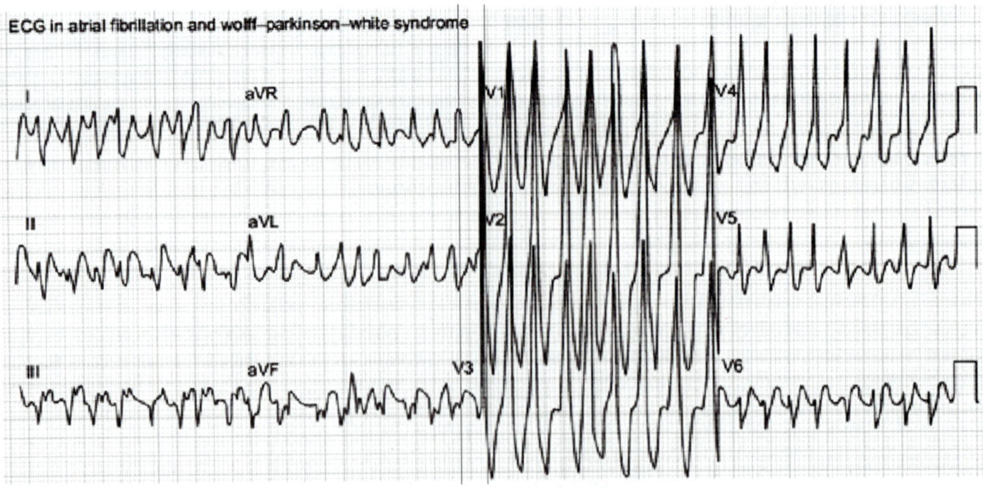

Fig. 28.10: *This ECG shows preexcited atrial fibrillation. The shortest RR Interval is 200 milliseconds; intervals < 260 milliseconds are associated with a risk of sudden death in patient with DCM*

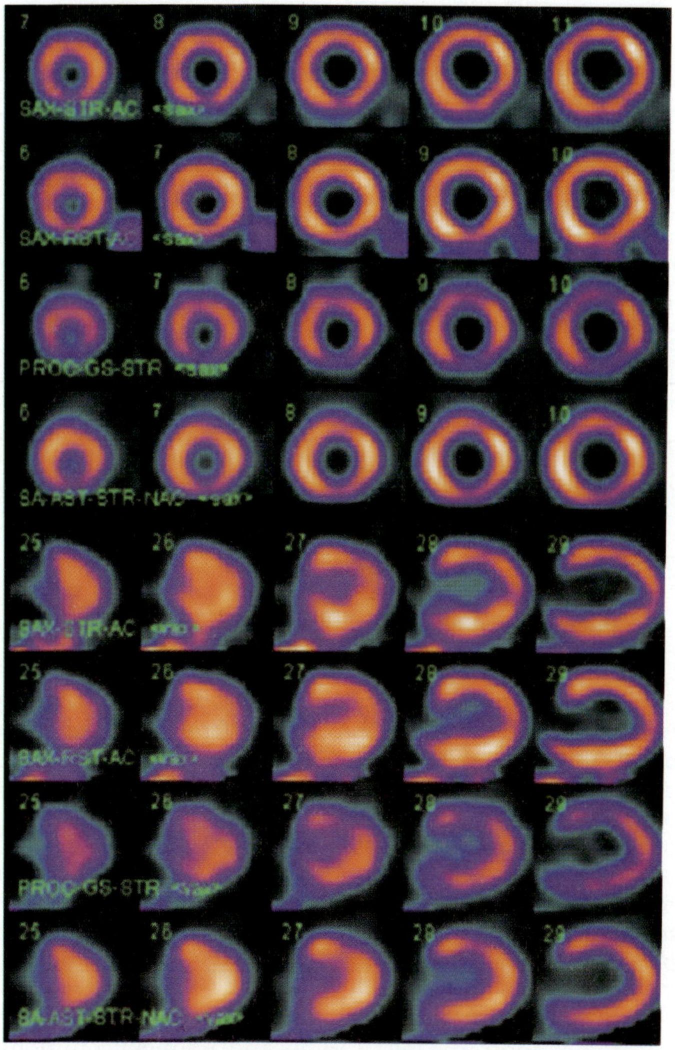

Fig. 28.11: *Tec99 Sestamibi cardiac perfusion study demonstrates dilated left ventricular cavity*

course on a TV monitor) so that pressures within the heart chambers can be measured.

A cardiac biopsy, which involves removing tiny pieces of heart muscle for inspection under the microscope, may be performed to help distinguish between infectious and genetic causes. The information provided during the catheterization may also be helpful if transplantation is being considered as one of the treatment options for your child.

Etiological Factors in DCM

While other causes of DCM have been identified and are briefly discussed in other sections of this brochure, mounting scientific evidence is beginning to suggest that individual genetic "mutations" may be among the more common causes of DCM in children. For a greater understanding of the basics of human inheritance patterns and a more detailed discussion of the potential genetic causes of DCM, the reader is encouraged to read separate sections entitled "Overview of Inheritance" and "Genetics of Cardiomyopathies" printed elsewhere in this brochure.

Current Treatment

Currently, there are no therapies that can "cure" DCM; however, many treatments are available that can improve symptoms and decrease risk in children with DCM. The choice of a specific therapy depends on the clinical condition of the child, the risk of dangerous events and the ability of the child to tolerate the therapy. In the following sections, current medical and nonmedical therapies for DCM are summarized.

Medical Therapy

The majority of children with DCM have signs and symptoms of heart failure. The most common types of medications used to treat heart failure include diuretics,

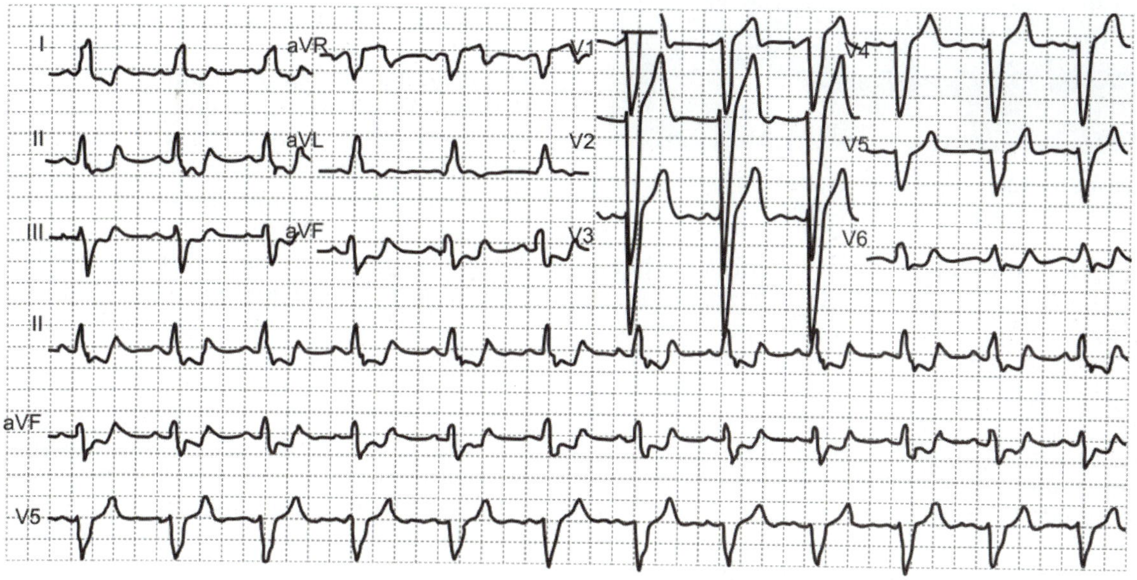

Fig. 28.12: *LBBB in dialated cardiomyopathy*

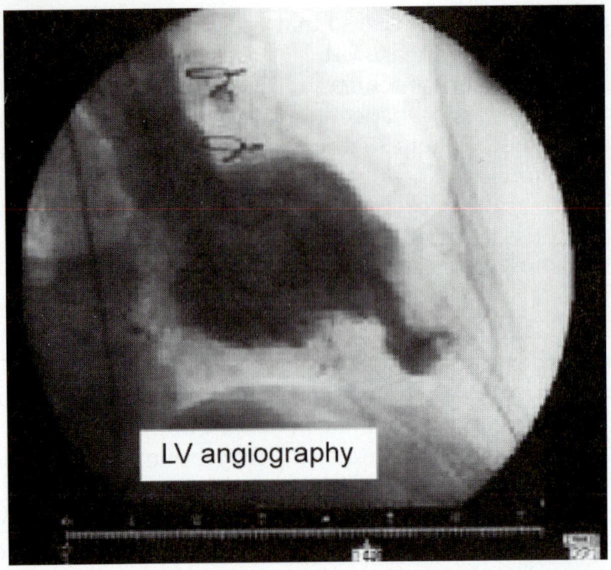

Fig. 28.13: *LV angiography showing apical left ventricular dyskinesis (ventricular aneurysm) presenting as a dilated cardiomyopathy*

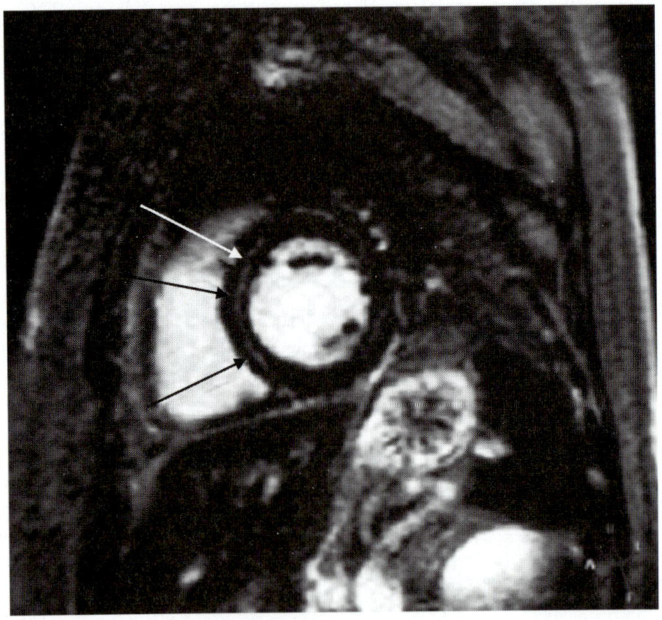

Fig. 28.14: *Typical mid-septal rim of nonischemc hyperenhancement in a patient with dilated cardiomyopathy*

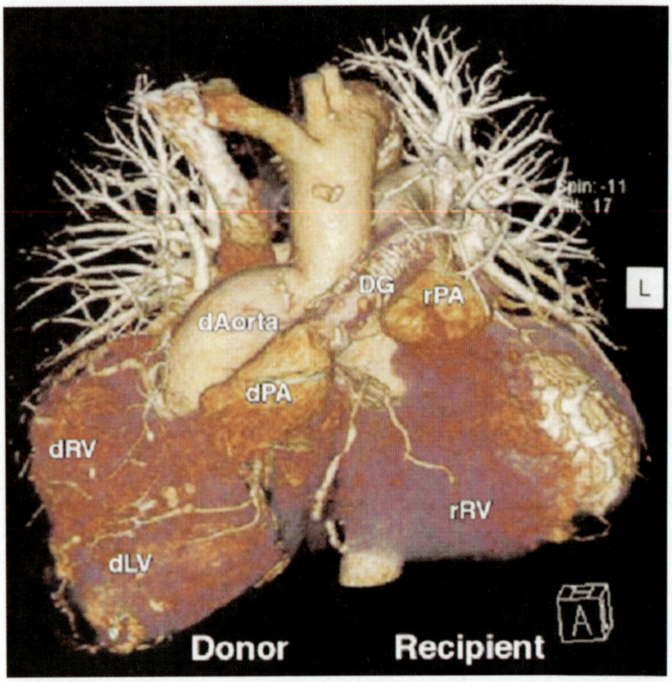

Fig. 28.15: *An adolescent with dilated cardiomyopathy. Heterotopic heart transplantation was performed 6 years earlier. dAorta, aorta of donor heart; dPA, main pulmonary arteries of donor heart; dRV, right ventricle of donor heart; dLV, left ventricle of donor heart; dRA, right atrium of donor heart; rRA, right atrium of recipient heart; rRV, right ventricle of recipient heart; DG, polyester textile fiber (Dacron, DuPont) tube graft. Heterotopic heart transplant is shown by 3D volume rendering (VR) reconstructed by cardiac CT. VR image shows relationship between donor and recipient hearts*

inotropic agents, afterload reducing agents and beta-blockers.

Diuretics, sometimes called "water pills", reduce excess fluid in the lungs or other organs by increasing urine production. The loss of excess fluid reduces the workload of the heart, reduces swelling and helps children breathe more easily. Diuretics can be given either orally or intravenously. Common diuretics include furosemide, spironolactone, bumetanide and metolazone. Common side effects of diuretics include dehydration and abnormalities in the blood chemistries (particularly potassium loss).

Inotropic agents are used to help the heart contract more effectively. Inotropic medications and are most commonly used intravenously to support children who have severe heart failure and are not stable enough to be home. Common types of inotropic medications include:

- ***Digoxin*** (taken by mouth): It improves the contraction of the heart. Side effects include low heart rate, and, with high blood levels, vomiting and abnormal heart rhythm.
- ***Dobutamine***, dopamine, epinephrine, norepinephrine (intravenous medications given in the hospital) medications that increase blood pressure and the strength of heart contractions. Side effects include increased heart rate, arrhythmias and for some, constriction of the arteries.
- ***Vasopressin*** (intravenous medication): It increases blood pressure and improves blood flow to kidneys. Side effects include excessive constriction of the arteries and low sodium.
- ***Milrinone*** (intravenous medication): It improves heart contraction and decreases the work of the heart by relaxing the arteries. Side effects include low blood pressure, arrhythmias and headaches.

Afterload reducing agents reduce the work of the heart by relaxing the arteries and allowing the blood to flow more easily to the body. Common afterload reducing medications include:

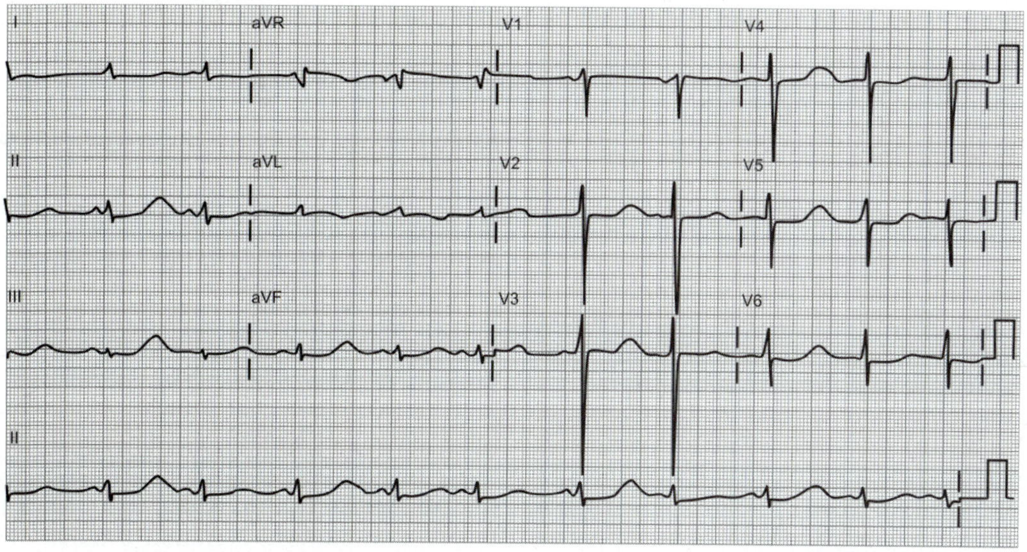

Fig. 28.16: *ECG morphology of an ischemic cardiomyopathy with prolonged Qt interval*

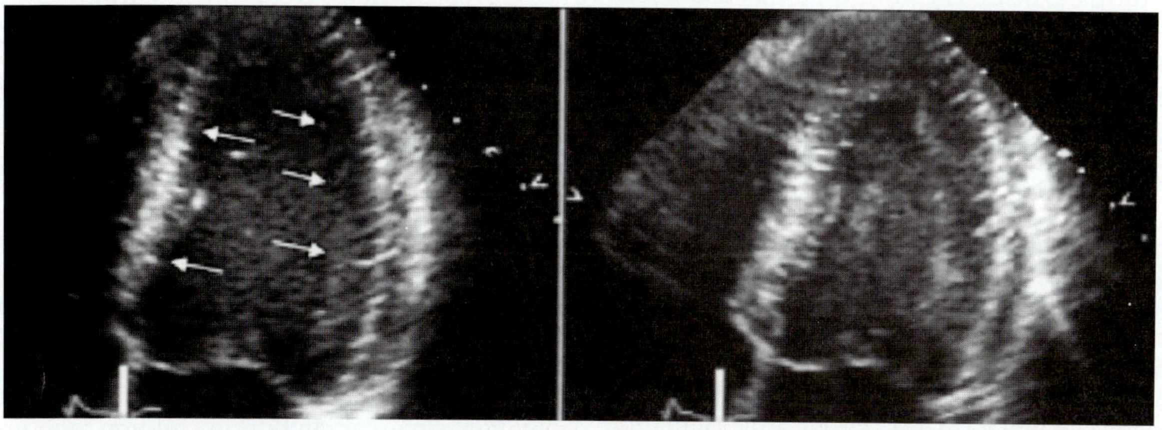

Fig. 28.17: *Transthoracic two dimensional echocardiogram (apical four chamber view, end systolic) at rest (left panel) and during infusion of low dose dobutamine (right panel) in a patient with ischaemic cardiomyopathy and severe hypokinesia of the septum and lateral wall. During low dose dobutamine, improved contraction of the dysfunctional segments indicates myocardial viability*

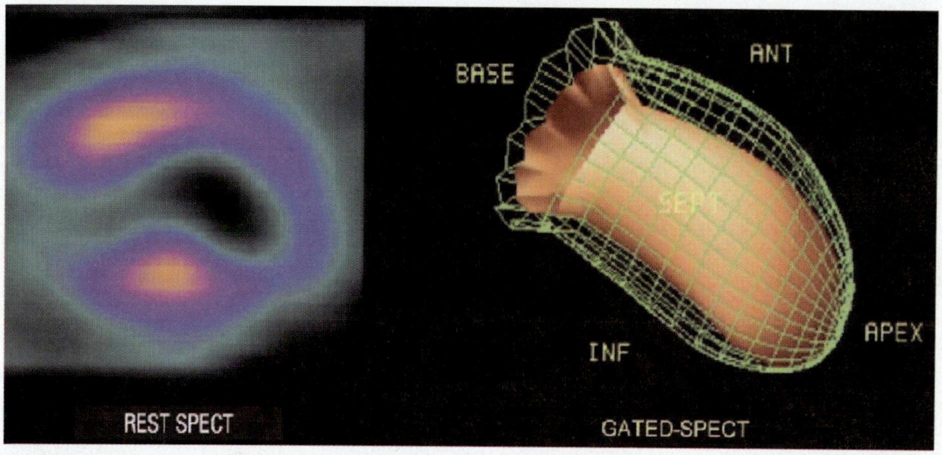

Fig. 28.18: *Left: divergent left ventricular pattern (transversal diameter at the apical level > transversal diameter at the basal level in vertical long-axis view) and absence of anteroapical uptake in myocardial perfusion SPECT at rest in a patient with anterior infarction. These criteria are highly specific for myocardial nonviability. Right: gated-SPECT of the same patient in whom anterior akinesia and septal and apical dyskinesia can be observed. End-diastolic volume, 248 mL; end-systolic volume, 203 mL; ejection fraction, 18%. Ant, anterior; Inf, inferior; SPECT, Single-Photon Emission Computed Tomography*

- ***Angiotensin converting enzyme inhibitors (ACE inhibitors):*** Captopril, enalapril, lisinopril, monopril (taken by mouth). Side effects include low blood pressure, low white blood cell count, high potassium levels and kidney or liver abnormalities.
- ***Angiotensin I blocker:*** Losartan (taken by mouth), side effects include diarrhea, muscle cramps and dizziness.
- ***Milrinone*** is an inotropic agent that also relaxes the arteries.

Beta-blockers slow the heartbeat and reduce the work needed for contraction of the heart muscle. Slowing down the heart rate can help to keep a weakened heart from overworking. In some cases, beta-blockers allow an enlarged heart to become more normal in size. Common beta-blockers (taken by mouth) include carvedilol, metoprolol, propanolol and atenolol. Side effects include dizziness, low heart rate, low blood pressure, and, in some cases, fluid retention, fatigue, impaired school performance and depression. In addition to improving the symptoms of heart failure, ACE inhibitors and beta-blockers have been shown to return the heart size toward normal and lessen the number of deaths and hospitalizations in adult patients with dilated cardiomyopathy without symptoms. An ACE inhibitor is recommended in children with dilated cardiomyopathy even in the absence of symptoms. Currently, no firm recommendations are available for beta-blockers in children.

Anticoagulation Medications

In children with a heart that does not contract well, there is a risk of blood clots forming inside the heart possibly leading to a stroke. Anticoagulation medications, also known as blood thinners are often used in these situations. The choice of anticoagulation drug depends on how likely it is that a blood clot will form. Less strong anticoagulation medications include aspirin and dipyridamole. Stronger anticoagulation drugs are warfarin, heparin, and enoxaparin; these drugs require careful monitoring with regular blood testing. While variable, common side effects of anticoagulants include excessive bruising or bleeding from otherwise minor skin injuries, interaction with other medications and, for warfarin, fluctuations in anti-coagulation blood levels caused by changes in daily dietary intake. Information regarding which food groups can significantly affect warfarin levels can be obtained from your cardiologist.

Antiarrhythmia Medications

In some DCM patients, especially those with very dilated and poorly contractile ventricles, there may be a higher risk of an abnormal, life-threatening heart rhythm (ventricular tachycardia), and medications are used to prevent or control this abnormal rhythm which then keeps the heart beating in a regular pattern. Common antiarrhythmia medications include: amiodarone, procainamide and lidocaine. General side effects may include slower heart rate, lower blood pressure, GI upset (nausea/constipation), headache, depressed mood, difficulties concentrating, dizziness, and skin rash among others. Consult your cardiologist for drug-specific side effects once a particular antiarrhythmic medicine has been prescribed.

Pacing Therapies for DCM

Pacemakers

Pacemakers are small, battery-operated devices that are placed under the skin of the chest or abdomen and attached to electrical wires (leads) which are threaded to the heart. Depending on which type of pacemaker is used, these leads are attached to muscle tissue either on the inside or outside of the heart. The devices monitor the heartbeat and help to maintain a regular rhythm in children who are prone to have abnormal heartbeats.

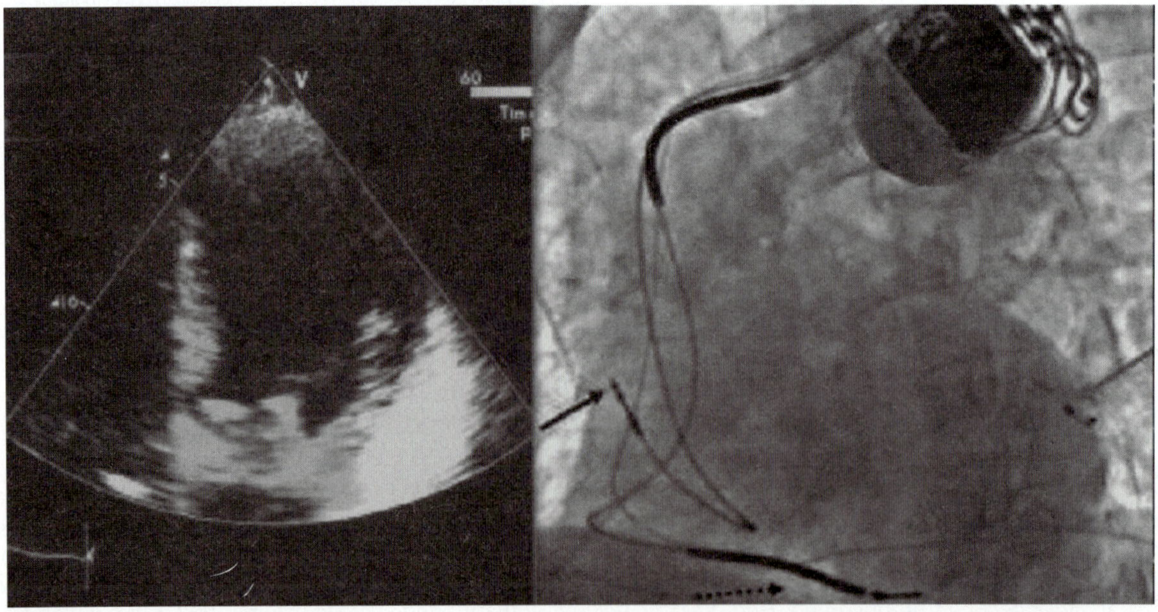

Fig. 28.19: *(Left) echocardiography showing diastolic wall motion defect in cardiac failure. Right shows CRT in dilated cardiomyopathy*

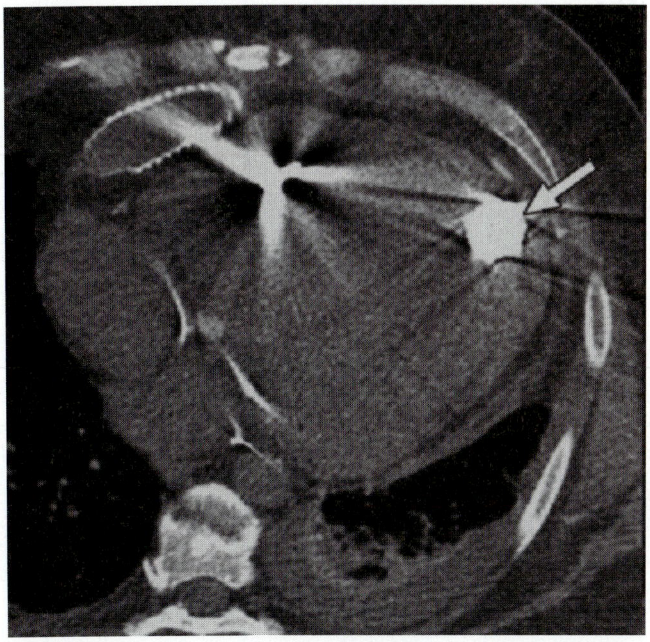

Fig. 28.20: *A young person with HeartMate II (Thoratec) that was implanted for ischemic cardiomyopathy and ejection fraction of 10%*

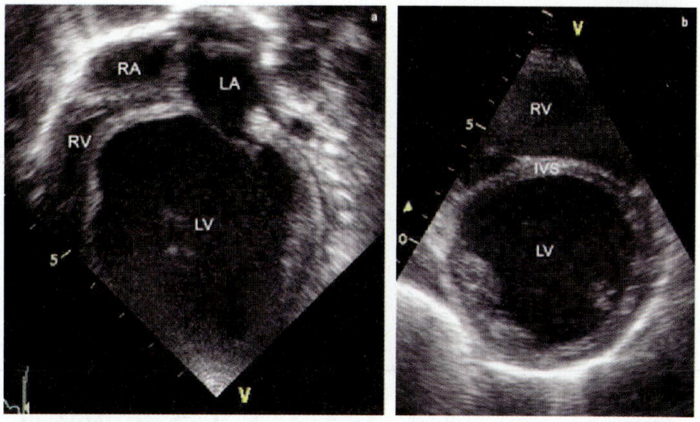

Fig. 28.21: *Dilated cardiomyopathy. (A) A four-chamber echocardiogram showing a hugely dilated left ventricle that is squashing the right ventricle. (B) Short-axis view. The myocardium is thinned*

In some patients with DCM, the heart rate can become too slow either due to abnormally slow conduction of impulses through the heart or as a side effect of medications. In those instances, a "back-up" pacemaker can be implanted to help maintain an appropriate heart rate. Conversely, as mentioned above, patients with DCM can develop abnormally fast, life-threatening arrhythmias (ventricular tachycardia and/or fibrillation). Implantable cardioverter defibrillators (ICDs) can be used in those children to convert these arrhythmias to a normal rhythm (Fig. 28.20).

Finally, a biventricular pacing system has recently become part of the standard therapy in adults with end-stage heart failure associated with DCM, and this treatment modality is currently being evaluated in children.

Implantable Cardioverter Defibrillator (ICD)

ICDs are designed to prevent sudden death from a serious arrhythmia known as ventricular tachycardia or fibrillation. An ICD constantly monitors heart rate, and when ventricular tachycardia or fibrillation is detected, the ICD delivers a shock to the heart that restores normal rhythm. ICDs are used in patients with hypertrophic cardiomyopathy who are felt to be at high risk for a sudden death and in children with dilated cardiomyopathy who have serious ventricular arrhythmias. Biventricular pacemaker.

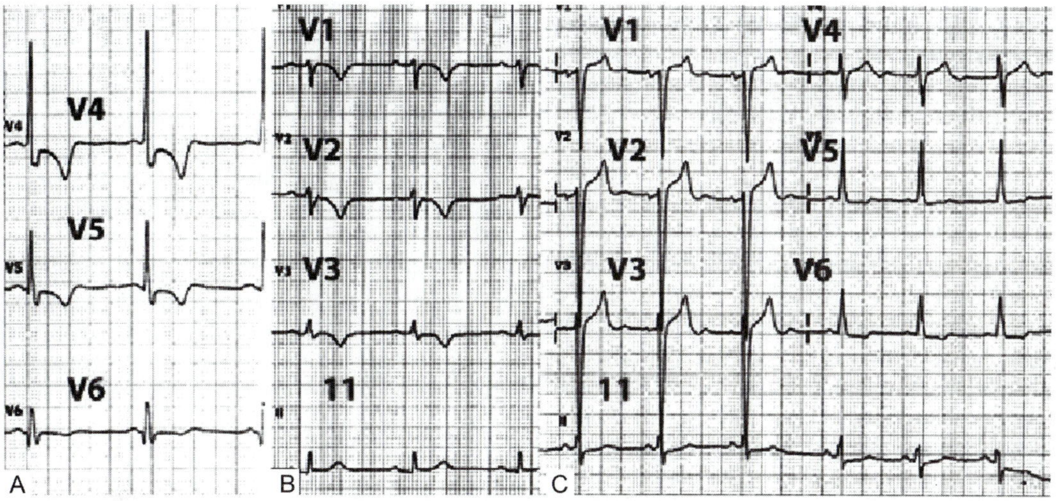

Fig. 28.22: *A young patient with inherited cardiomyopathy. (A) Lateral precordial leads of a patient with hypertrophic cardiomyopathy showing Q wave (V6), ST depression, and T wave inversion associated with large voltage QRS complexes. (B) Right precordial leads of a patient with arrhythmogenic right ventricular cardiomyopathy showing epsilon wave (V2), QRS prolongation, and T wave inversion. (C) Precordial leads of a patient with dilated cardiomyopathy showing incomplete left bundle-branch block and electrocardiographic left atrial enlargement*

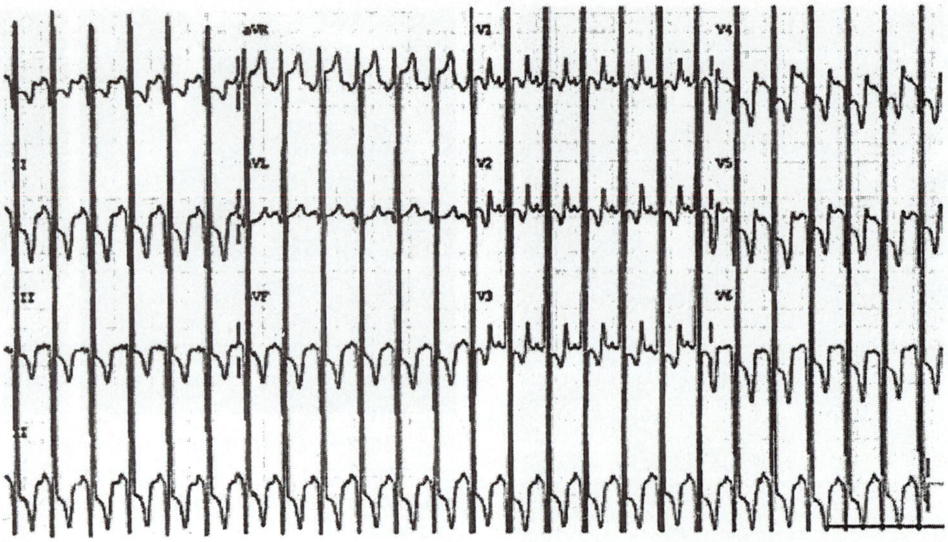

Fig. 28.23: *ECG showing sinus tachycardia, giant T wave inversion and generalised increased QRS voltage with LVH in an adolescent with hypertrophic cardiomyopathy*

In recent promising studies in adult patients with dilated cardiomyopathy, a special pacemaker that can pace both the right and left ventricles has been designed. This system, which has to be specially timed, allows the two ventricles to contract together and improves the synchrony of contraction between the walls of the left ventricle. Study results have shown that, when added to other medical treatments, this mode of pacing has helped some patients live longer with fewer hospitalizations and, in some cases, has decreased the need for transplantation. At the time of this publication, use of biventricular pacing in children is in the early stages of development. It is not yet known which children may benefit most from this form of pacing or the best way to implant the system. Nonetheless, this approach is considered an adjunctive therapy to medicines that patients are already receiving and should not be thought of as a medicine replacement. Over the next few years, study results in children in whom biventricular pacing is being used may help cardiologists better understand which patients may benefit most from this therapy and under what circumstances.

Surgical Options for DCM

No surgery has been effective in improving the heart function in dilated cardiomyopathy. In a few patients with a severely dilated left ventricle and a very leaky (regurgitant) mitral valve, surgery to repair or replace the mitral valve may help the heart function improve temporarily. Heart transplantation is the only effective surgery offered for patients with DCM who have severe heart failure that does not respond to medications or other treatments.

Cardiac Assist Devices (Mechanical Hearts)

Cardiac assist devices are machines that do the work of the heart using a mechanical pump to deliver blood to the body. Cardiac assist devices are implanted when all other therapies have failed and the heart failure is severe. They improve blood flow to the body and allow other organs to recover from the stress of heart failure. These devices are typically used as bridges to transplantation. That is, they are used to support a child either until the heart function has recovered enough to effectively circulate blood through the body or until a suitable donor organ can be found. In pediatric patients, they are designed as a temporary means of support and cannot be used as a permanent alternative to the child's own heart or a transplanted heart. Potential complications of cardiac assist devices include infection, blood clots, stroke and mechanical problems with the devices themselves. There are a variety of cardiac assist devices available. The type of cardiac assist device that is used for an individual child depends on body size and also the type of assist support needed (Fig. 28.20).

Heart Transplantation

Dilated cardiomyopathy is one of the leading reasons for heart transplantation in children. Heart transplant is only considered in children who have such serious heart disease that there are no other medications or support devices available to sustain the child. A heart transplant offers the child with DCM the chance to return to a normal lifestyle. While a donor heart can cure the symptoms of heart failure and greatly improve survival, it is a major operation with considerable risks and long-term complications. Once a transplant is done, other concerns arise, such as infection, organ rejection, coronary artery disease, and the side effects of medications (Fig. 28.15).

Prognosis

Many children with DCM are able to lead relatively normal lives once the diagnosis has been established and appropriate therapies have been started. The long-term prognosis varies depending on the cause, severity and degree of functional impairment. Children with DCM

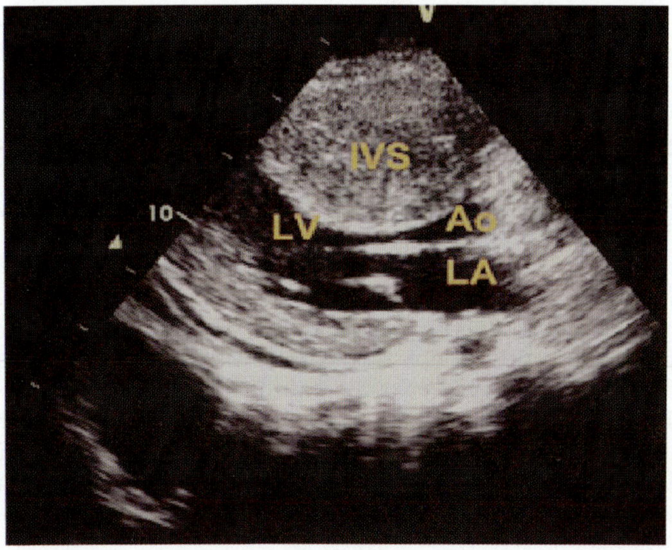

Fig. 28.24: *Diffuse hypertrophy variant of hypertrophic cardiomyopathy (HCM). This pattern of hypertrophy is classically seen in younger patients. Ao, aorta; IVS, interventricular septum; LA, left atrium; LV, left ventricle*

should be watched closely for the development of heart failure, abnormal heart rhythms, blood clots inside the heart and other signs that the heart is not able to maintain normal blood flow. Once signs of heart failure or significantly abnormal rhythms appear, aggressive therapy is begun with close monitoring for signs of worsening blood flow to the vital organs. If other organs show signs of damage or the heart failure does not respond to medications, a cardiac assist device and/or transplant is considered early, as the waiting time for a donor heart can be unpredictable. It is important that a child with cardiomyopathy be closely monitored at a center with expertise in pediatric heart failure, arrhythmias, cardiac assist devices and transplantation in order to ensure rapid response to any worsening of his or her condition. In children with DCM, approximately 35% recover completely, 35% stabilize and the remaining may progressively worsen. Children with DCM are more prone to congestive heart failure and have a higher rate of heart transplantation compared with other forms of cardiomyopathy. However, improved medical therapy may eventually change this scenario.

Current average 5-year survival rates for children with DCM are 40–50%. If the cause of DCM is myocarditis, children are more likely to improve and have a better outcome than children with other causes of DCM.

Living with DCM

The diagnosis of DCM affects many areas of a child's life. The following sections outline the general approaches to living with this disease. It is important that specific recommendations are developed by the team caring for the child.

Physical Activity

Children with DCM are not allowed to play competitive sports because of the possibility of a sudden collapse or increased heart failure. A competitive sport is an organized team activity for which training is required.

A child with dilated cardiomyopathy and no heart failure symptoms can be allowed to perform recreational athletic activities, also known as low-dynamic or low-static sports, in a noncompetitive situation. In milder cases, the child may even participate in gym class after careful discussions between the child, teacher, and parents to ensure that the

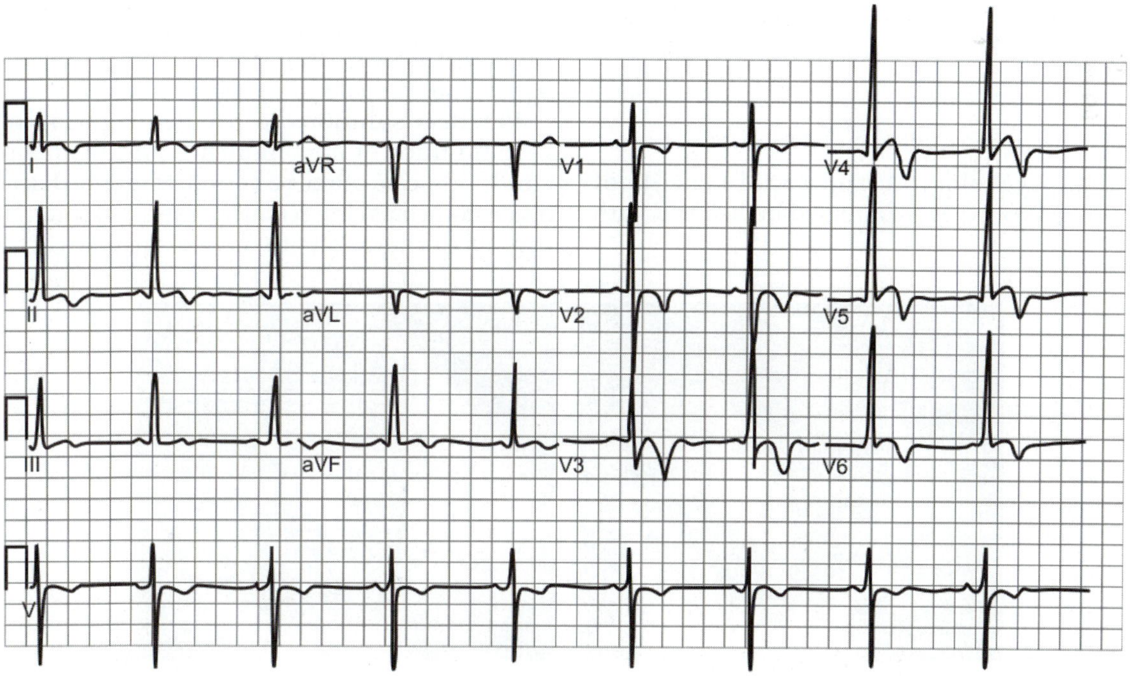

Fig. 28.25: *ECG from a 13-year-old boy with apical hypertrophic cardiomyopathy. Note elevated QRS voltages associated with left ventricular hypertrophy and inverted T waves in all precordial leads*

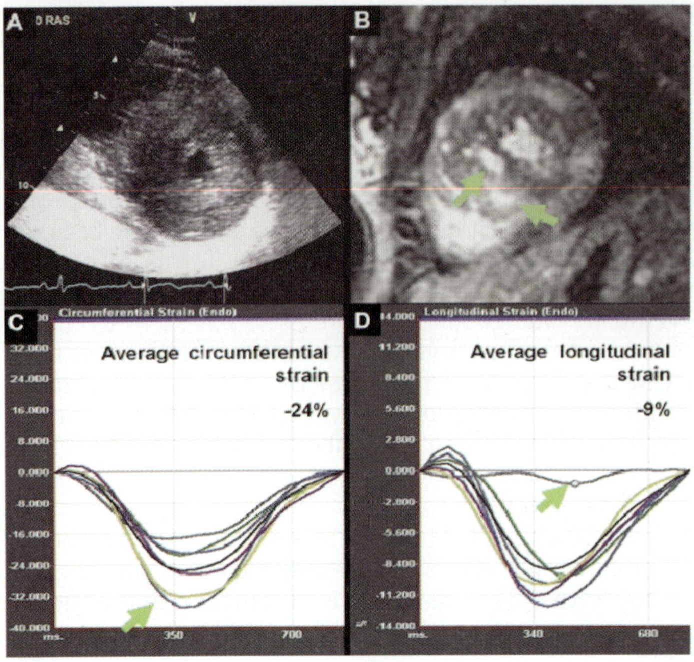

Fig. 28.26: *Myocardial mechanics in a 21-year-old female patient with hypertrophic cardiomyopathy. Panels A and B show the cross-sectional view of the left ventricle obtained from 2D echocardiography and MRI, respectively. Note the localized and spotty enhancement seen on delayed enhanced MRI (green arrows). Panels C and D show the disparate patterns of shortening mechanics (2D Cardiac Performance Analysis; TomTec, Munich, Germany). Midinferior segments (C) (green arrow) show preserved circumferential strains, whereas the same segment shows marked attenuation of longitudinal strain (D) (green arrow)*

level of activity does not cause overexertion (breathlessness, chest pain, excessive sweating). Specific activity recommendations should be individualized by the treating cardiologist.

Attending School by the Child

The intellectual, psychological, and social benefits of attending school cannot be overestimated in the child with DCM.

Adjusting medication schedules so they do not interfere with school activities, discussing safe activity levels with school personnel, and providing tutoring to maintain academic performance are important interventions that can help a child to stay in school and keep up with their peers. Often close communication between the parents, medical care team, and the school nurse can help to keep a child up to date in school.

Mixing with Friends

Every effort should be made to allow a child with DCM to spend time with friends. The child should also be allowed to participate in recreational activities whenever possible. However, an effort should be made to avoid contact with those who are acutely ill with fever, even though many children with this disease are able to tolerate upper respiratory tract illnesses (common colds) well.

Psychological Issues and Councelling

Adjusting to having a chronic illness is stressful not only for the child but for the entire family as well. The child's reaction to having DCM often depends on the stage of the child's development. Discussions about the disease should be tailored to the specific concerns of the child. Child-life professionals and pediatric psychiatrists are important resources to help children cope, and their services are often available through the treating center.

Acceptance of DCM Child by Family Members

The impact of a diagnosis of DCM is felt throughout the child's immediate and extended family. It is important for parents and other caregivers to realize that they are not alone in feeling the weight of responsibility that comes with taking care of a child with a chronic illness. Anticipating and/or preventing the stress imposed by an illness is an important part of caring for the child and family, and personnel at the treating medical center can help to identify issues that can lead to increased stress.

Practical solutions to problems giving medications, keeping track of appointments, and maintaining normal family life can often be found through discussions with nurse clinicians, the social worker, psychiatrist, and other parents of children with dilated cardiomyopathy.

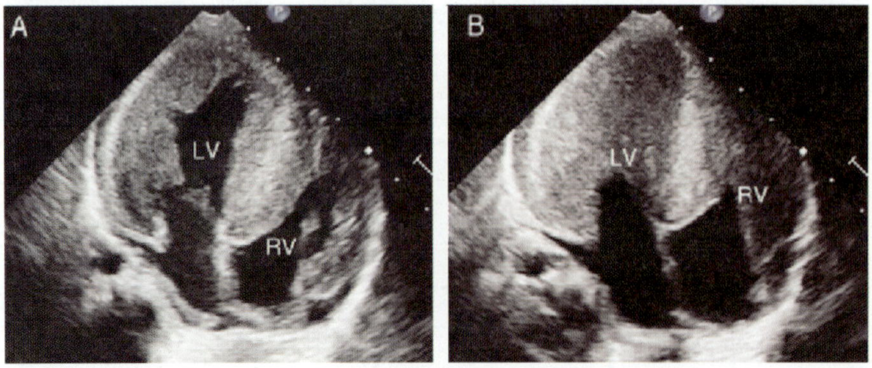

Fig. 28.27: *Echocardiograms taken in apical four chamber view showing gross thickening of the left ventricular myocardium in a young patient with hypertrophic cardiomyopathy. (A) diastole, (B) systole views*

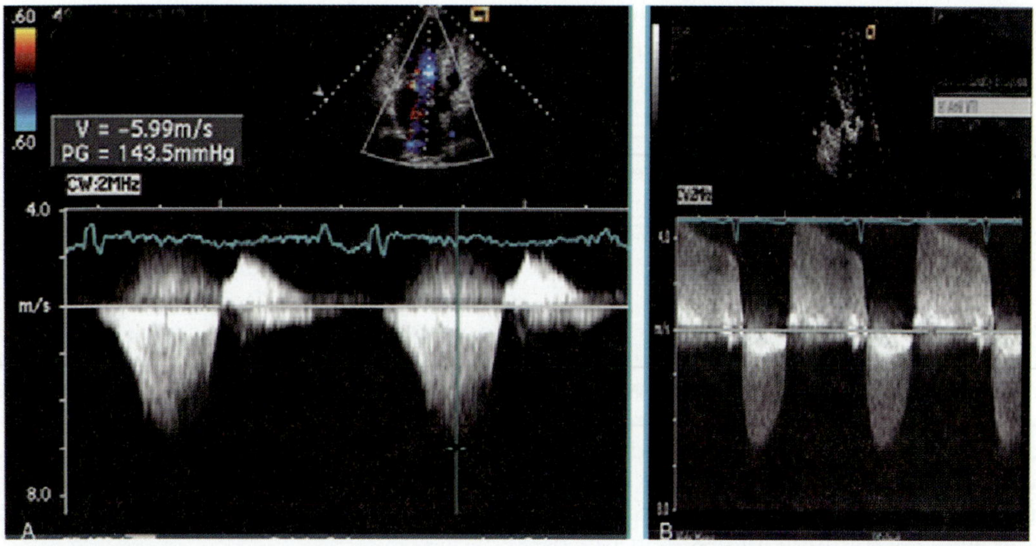

Fig. 28.28: *Comparison of Doppler profiles of hypertrophic cardiomyopathy (HCM) (A) and aortic stenosis (B). Because aortic stenosis is a fixed obstruction, a contour of the aortic valve gradient can be seen. In contrast, the Doppler profile of HCM is seen as the classic dagger shape, reflecting the dynamic obstruction*

Healthy Diet

All children with DCM should follow a healthy diet. The recommendations published in 2005 by the United States Department of Agriculture (USDA) can be found at the following website address: http://www.mypyramid.gov. Certain types of DCM are associated with an inability to digest certain types of food, and in these cases, a special diet is developed in consultation with metabolic specialists. In children with dilated cardiomyopathy and heart failure, a low salt diet is recommended to avoid fluid retention.

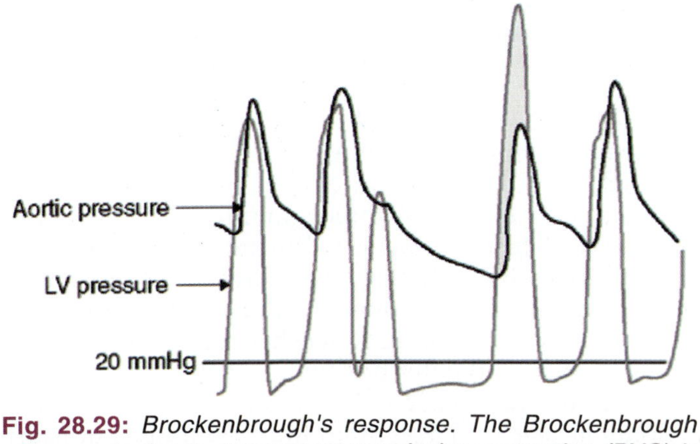

Fig. 28.29: *Brockenbrough's response. The Brockenbrough response in the postpremature ventricular contraction (PVC) is classic for hypertrophic cardiomyopathy (HCM). Post-PVC, there is increased preload secondary to a compensatory pause. The increased contractility associated with the post-PVC beat results in increased left ventricular outflow tract (LVOT) obstruction in HCM patients and a subsequent increase in the left ventricular-aortic gradient and decreased aortic pulse pressure during the post-PVC beat. In contrast, in subjects with no LVOT obstruction, a PVC results in increased cardiac contractility, but there is no left ventricle-aortic gradient, either at rest or in the post-PVC beat. The aortic pulse pressure in the post-PVC beat usually increases because of the increased contractility. LV, left ventricular*

Some children with heart failure may not grow well. In these cases, a diet that increases calories is recommended.

Children who are taking some medications may have low levels of magnesium or potassium and a diet that has a higher amount of one or both of these two electrolytes may be recommended. Some children with severe heart failure can retain extra body fluid, and it may be necessary to limit the amount that a child can drink to prevent fluid from accumulating in the lungs.

Health Maintenance for Children with DCM

Routine pediatric care is important for children with DCM. Regular well child visits and standard childhood immunizations should be performed. The influenza vaccine should be administered on a yearly basis. Children under age 2 year should receive Synagis for protection against respiratory syncytial virus (RSV).

A medical alert bracelet is an important safety measure for children with DCM. In the event of an emergency, these bracelets allow medical personnel to know details about a child's illness, especially if a family member is not available.

Future Research in DCM

Much progress has been made in our ability to diagnose DCM in both the clinical and molecular arenas. However, much additional research is needed in this field. Areas of research to be highlighted over the next decade include:

1. Better understanding of DCM as a disease process and the characteristics of the disease as they relate to outcome, which will lead to better management strategies.
2. Increased clinical trials which will lead to new drug development and more effective therapies.
3. Molecular identification of novel genetic mutations as well as more precise diagnostic genetic testing/screening which will result in more accurate diagnosis.

It is the expectation of the medical community that the data derived from exploring these avenues of scientific research will translate into a clinician's ability to tailor medical therapy based on a given child's precise diagnosis. Achieving this goal over the next couple of decades will represent a large milestone in the field of pediatric cardiomyopathy research and will, hopefully, improve the ongoing care and prognosis of children afflicted with this heart muscle disease.

B. Hypertrophic Cardiomyopathy (HCM)

Most often diagnosed during infancy or adolescence, hypertrophic cardiomyopathy (HCM) is the second most common form of heart muscle disease, is usually genetically transmitted, and comprises about 35–40% of cardiomyopathies in children.

HCM affects up to 500,000 people in the United States with children under age 12 accounting for less than 10% of all cases. According to the Pediatric Cardiomyopathy Registry, HCM occurs at a rate of 5 per 1 million children. "Hypertrophic" refers to an abnormal growth of muscle fibers in the heart. In HCM, the thick heart muscle is stiff, making it difficult for the heart to relax and for blood to fill the heart chambers. While the heart squeezes normally, the limited filling prevents the heart from pumping enough blood, especially during exercise.

Although HCM can involve both lower chambers, it usually affects the main pumping chamber (left ventricle) with thickening of the septum (wall separating the pumping chambers), posterior wall or both. With hypertrophic obstructive cardiomyopathy (HOCM), the muscle thickening restricts the flow of blood out of the heart.

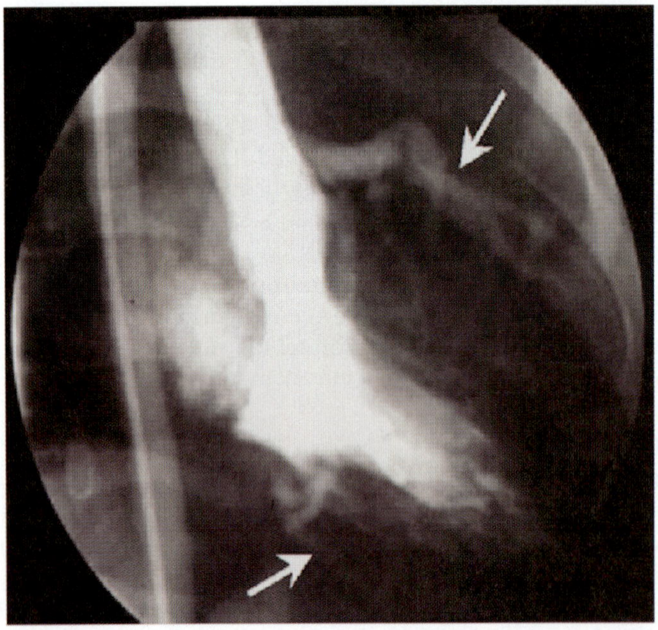

Fig. 28.30: *Cardiomyopathy, hypertrophic. Conventional end-systolic right anterior oblique left ventriculogram acquired during cardiac catheterization study, shows a small left-ventricular cavity with mild mitral regurgitation (M). Note the increased distance between the ventricular cavity and the coronary arteries (arrows), which define the epicardial surface of the heart as the myocardium becomes thickened in systole*

Often, leakage of the mitral valve causes the blood in the lower chamber (left ventricle) to leak back into the upper chamber (left atrium). In less than 10% of patients, the disease may progress to a point where the heart muscle thins and the left ventricle dilates resulting in reduced heart function similar to that seen in DCM.

HCM is most often diagnosed during infancy or adolescence. Gene defects can be familial, and it is estimated that 50–60% of children with HCM have a relative with the disease, although they may not have been diagnosed or have symptoms.

Signs and Symptoms of HCM

There is tremendous variation in how HCM presents and progresses. While some children have no or mild symptoms, others may have more severe symptoms including heart failure. Some patients develop abnormal heart rhythms (arrhythmias) that may put them at increased risk for sudden cardiac death. Children under 1 year of age often have symptoms of congestive heart failure whereas older children may be symptom free and, therefore, may be unaware that HCM is present. Onset of symptoms often coincides with the rapid growth and development of late childhood and early adolescence. The strenuous exercise of competitive sports has also been known to make symptoms of HCM more apparent.

Disease severity and symptoms are related to the extent and location of the hypertrophy and whether there is obstruction to blood leaving the heart or valve leakage from the left-sided pumping chamber back into the left atrium above. The first sign of HCM may be a murmur, although this is usually absent in the nonobstructive form of HCM. Symptoms in children with HCM can include dyspnea (shortness of breath during exercise), angina (chest pain), presyncope (light-headedness or dizziness), syncope (fainting), exercise intolerance or palpitations/arrhythmias (irregular heartbeats). Symptoms in infants may be more difficult to detect but include difficulty breathing, poor growth, excessive sweating (diaphoresis) or crying and agitation during feeding thought to be due to chest pain.

Children with severe HCM may have symptoms of heart failure such as difficulty breathing, swelling around the eyes and legs (edema), tiredness or weakness, coughing, abdominal pain and vomiting. Mild symptoms of heart failure can also resemble asthma. Children with HCM may also develop an abnormal heartbeat (arrhythmia), either beating too fast (tachycardia) or too slow (bradycardia). Symptoms resulting from rhythm problems can appear without a child having congestive heart failure or other more obvious symptoms of HCM. The risk of sudden death from arrhythmia is higher with this form of cardiomyopathy compared with other forms of pediatric myopathy especially among adolescent patients. Finally, in some cases of HCM (especially those with extreme wall thickness), the disease evolves towards progressive wall

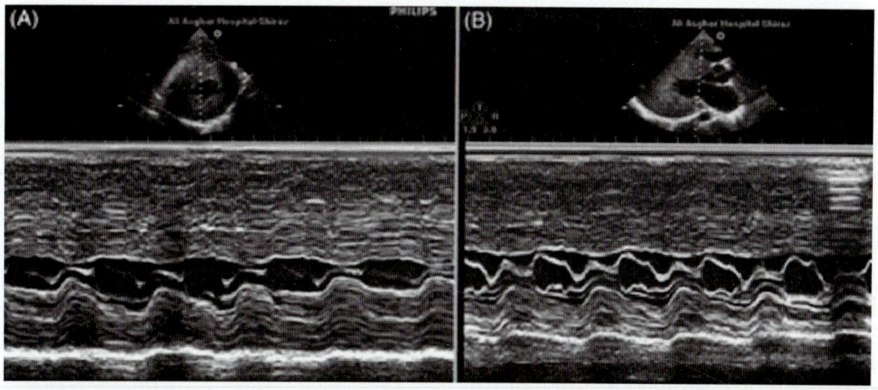

Fig. 28.31: *M-mode echocardiography in parasternal window of a patient presented with recurrent episodes of syncope. (A) Short-axis view of the left ventricle at the level of papillary muscle which shows severe hypertrophy of the left ventricle more prominently in the septum. (B) M-mode echocardiography of the mitral valve in long-axis view demonstrates systolic anterior motion of the mitral valve leaflets*

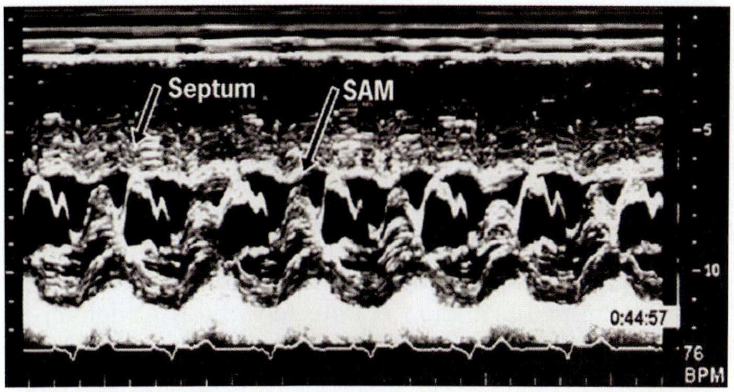

Fig. 28.32: *M-mode echocardiogram in obstructive hypertrophic cardiomyopathy showing systolic anterior motion of the mitral valve (SAM) (arrows indicating septum and mitral valve leaflet contact)*

thinning and LV chamber dilation until the heart appears to have all the features of DCM. In these cases, a family history of HCM, a prior echocardiogram that showed HCM or a cardiac biopsy may help to differentiate between the two.

Diagnosis of HCM (Figs 28.23–28.32)

Once suspected, the diagnosis of hypertrophic cardiomyopathy is established with an echocardiogram (or ultrasound of the heart) looking for abnormally thick walls predominantly in the left pumping chamber (left ventricle). In addition, the extent of obstruction or muscular narrowing through the outlet of the left ventricle to the aorta (main vessel which carries blood to the body) will be assessed. This diagnosis can only be made after other potential causes of abnormal wall thickening (i.e. aortic valve stenosis,

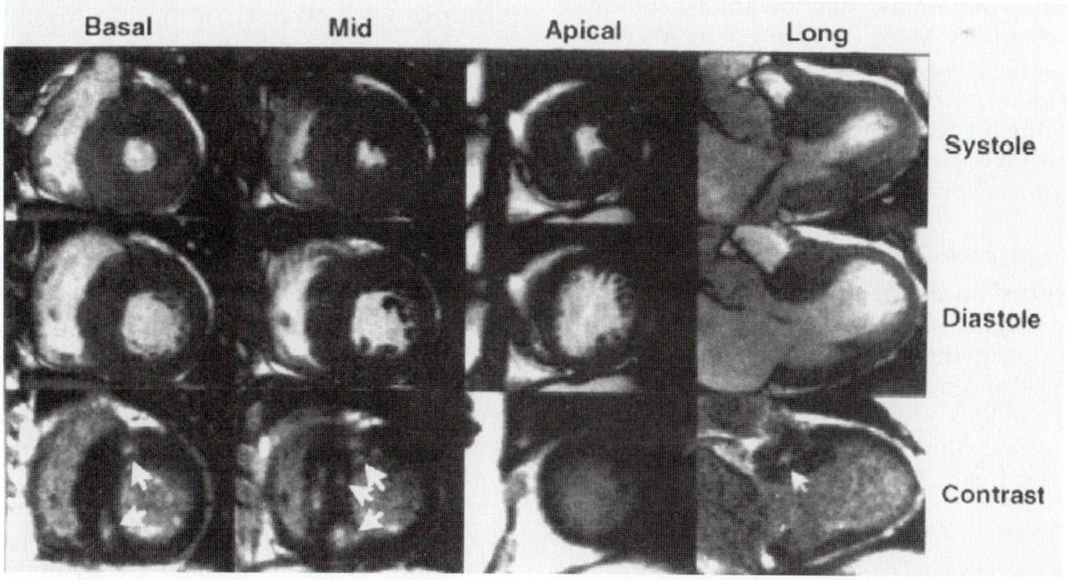

Fig. 28.33: *Scans showing hypertrophy (maximum wall thickness, 27 mm) and scarring. There are multiple foci of scar tissue, which are located predominantly in the mid-myocardial region (Mid) and are not present in the lateral free wall. The long-axis (long) cine images demonstrate systolic anterior motion of the mitral valve, systolic flow turbulence in the left ventricular outflow tract, and mitral regurgitation in patient with myocardial scarring in asymptomatic or mildly symptomatic hypertrophic cardiomyopathy*

coarctation of the aorta, high blood pressure, etc.) are eliminated either by physical examination echocardiogram.

An electrocardiogram, or EKG, which records the electrical impulses sent through the heart, may show evidence of thickened pumping chambers. Many cardiologists will order a Holter monitor to record your child's heartbeats over a 24–48 hour period. This will allow your physician to check for abnormal, and sometimes life-threatening, heart rhythms, which can occur more often in children with HCM. To further estimate your child's risk for developing these abnormal heart rhythms, some cardiologists may ask, in children old enough to cooperate, to perform an exercise treadmill test. Since the cause of this form of cardiomyopathy varies and depends on your child's age, additional laboratory testing may be requested. In some cases, an accumulation of abnormal proteins or sugars (glycogen) may occur in the heart causing the increased wall thicknesses. In others, genetic mutations or abnormalities in the mitochondria (powerhouses of the cells) produce this effect. Blood testing and, in some cases, a muscle biopsy from the leg or arm can help to identify the cause or help your doctor formulate a prognosis.

Genetic testing is available for some but not all forms of HCM. In the next decade, as more genetic bases for HCM are identified, genetic testing may become a routine part of the HCM evaluation.

Finally, because most patients with this diagnosis have inherited the disease, once confirmed in your child, your cardiologist will likely recommend screening (usually with echocardiogram) of the child's parents, siblings and perhaps other close relatives to discover whether this disease is present in any other family members.

Etiological Factors in HCM

Mounting scientific evidence is beginning to suggest that individual genetic "mutations" may be among the more common causes of HCM in children. For a greater understanding of the basics of human inheritance patterns and a more detailed discussion of the potential genetic causes of HCM, the reader is encouraged to read separate sections entitled "Overview of Inheritance" and "Genetics of Cardiomyopathies" printed elsewhere in this brochure.

Current Treatment for HCM

Currently, there are no therapies that can "cure" HCM; however, many treatments are available that can improve symptoms and potentially decrease risk in children with HCM. The choice of a specific therapy depends on the clinical condition of the child, the risk of dangerous events and the ability of the child to tolerate the therapy. In the following sections, treatments for HCM are summarized.

Medical Therapies

Medications are used to treat children with HCM who have symptoms such as difficulty breathing, chest pain, decreased activity tolerance or fatigue and generally include beta-blocking and calcium channel-blocking medicines.

Beta-blocking

Medications are used to slow the heartbeat and allow the heart to fill more completely when the thick muscle in the ventricular septum narrows the outflow of blood from the heart. These medications can cause excessive slowing of the heart rate, low blood pressure, dizziness, and in some cases, fluid retention, fatigue, impaired school performance and depression. Calcium channel blockers improve the filling of the heart by reducing the stiffness of the heart muscle, and are used in patients with chest pain or breathlessness. Side effects can include excessive slowing of the heart rate and lower blood pressure. Common calcium channel blockers are verapamil and diltiazem. Diuretics, which must be used with caution in this disease, are used to decrease fluid accumulation (when present) from the lungs in children with severe hypertrophic cardiomyopathy. In the case of HCM which has progressed into a myopathy with DCM features (occurs relatively infrequently as a later stage of HCM—see previous discussion of HCM), therapies used to treat HCM will no longer be effective, and standard medicines for the treatment of DCM will be substituted.

Pacing Therapies for HCM

Implantable Cardioverter Defibrillator (ICD)

ICDs are designed to prevent sudden death from a serious arrhythmia known as ventricular tachycardia or fibrillation. An ICD constantly monitors heart rate, and when ventricular tachycardia or fibrillation is detected, the ICD delivers a shock to the heart that restores normal rhythm. ICDs are used in patients with hypertrophic cardiomyopathy who are felt to be at high risk for a sudden death or have documented serious ventricular arrhythmias (Fig. 28.35).

Surgery for HCM

Septal myomectomy is a surgery that is performed in patients with hypertrophic cardiomyopathy when symptoms of heart failure have developed because the thickened muscle of the septum (the wall dividing the two sides of the heart) has narrowed (obstructed) the blood flow out of the heart, and medical therapy has not been effective. The surgery involves removing the muscle that has obstructed the blood flow. While septal myomectomy is effective in controlling symptoms, it does not stop hypertrophy from progressing, nor does it treat the life-threatening abnormal rhythms associated with HCM.

Heart Transplantation

Currently, transplantation for HCM is not routinely performed. Two exceptions include medically refractory ventricular arrhythmias, and HCM which has developed features of DCM not responsive to standard DCM therapy. A heart transplant will offer that child the chance to return to a normal lifestyle. While a donor heart can cure the symptoms of heart failure and greatly improve survival, it is a major operation with considerable risks and long-term complications. Once a transplant is done, other concerns arise, such as infection, organ rejection, coronary artery disease, and the side effects of medications.

Prognosis

Many children with HCM can lead relatively normal lives once the diagnosis has been established and appropriate therapies have been started. The long-term prognosis varies depending on the cause, severity and degree of functional impairment. Children with HCM should be watched closely for increasing symptoms of activity intolerance and the development of DCM features with heart failure and symptoms of palpitations or syncope which might suggest abnormal heart rhythms that require more thorough investigation. It is important that a child with HCM be closely monitored at a center with expertise in pediatric cardiomyopathy, arrhythmias and transplantation in order to ensure rapid response to any worsening of his or her condition.

The outcome of HCM is highly variable with some patients remaining asymptomatic, some developing symptoms and possibly progressive heart failure, and all remaining at risk for sudden death. Heart transplant is performed uncommonly and is primarily reserved for patients with severe, uncontrollable heart failure. Average 10-year survival rates for older children with HCM are > 90% although infants with HCM typically do far more poorly.

Living with HCM

The diagnosis of HCM affects many areas of a child's life. The following sections outline the general approaches to living with this disease. It is important that specific recommendations are developed by the team caring for the child.

Physical Activity

Children with HCM are not allowed to play competitive sports because of the possibility of a sudden collapse or increased heart failure. A competitive sport is an organized team activity for which training is required.

A child with hypertrophic cardiomyopathy may be allowed to perform low-impact activities based on their clinical status, degree of potential outflow obstruction and relative risk of arrhythmias. However, specific activity recommendations should be individualized by the treating cardiologist.

Attending School by the Child

The intellectual, psychological and social benefits of attending school cannot be overestimated in the child with HCM. Adjusting medication schedules so they do not interfere with school activities, discussing safe activity levels with school personnel, and providing tutoring to maintain academic performance are important interventions that can help a child to stay in school and keep up with their peers. Often close communication between the parents, medical care team, and the school nurse can help to keep a child up to date in school.

Mixing with Friends

Every effort should be made to allow a child with HCM to spend time with friends. Depending on the specific recommendations of the treating cardiologist, the child may be allowed to participate in light activities when possible. However, an effort should be made to avoid contact with those who are acutely ill with fever, even though many children with this disease are able to tolerate upper respiratory tract illnesses (common colds) well.

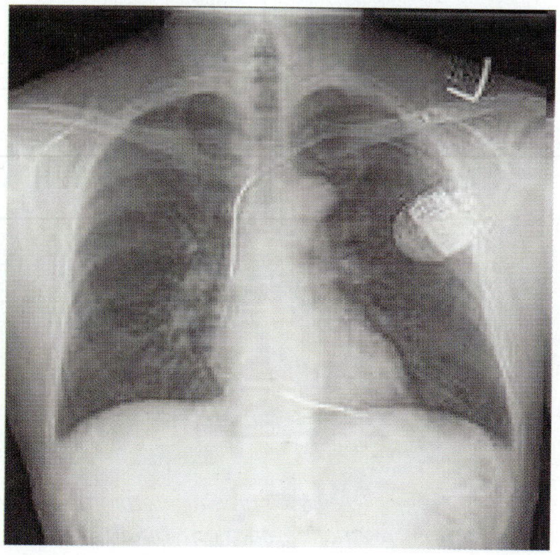

Fig. 28.34: *Chest X-ray showing an implantable cardioverter-defibrillator in patient with hypertrophic obstructive cardiomyopathy*

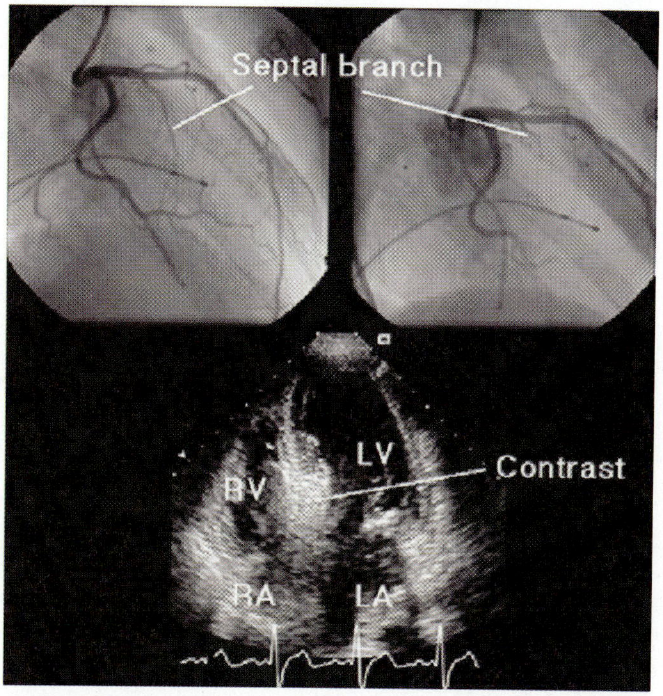

Fig. 28.35: *The septal branch of the left anterior descending coronary artery in a patient with hypertrophic obstructive cardiomyopathy (top panels). Estimation of the size of the septal vascular territory with myocardial contrast echocardiography (lower panel). LA, left atrium; RA, right atrium; LV, left ventricle; RV, right ventricle*

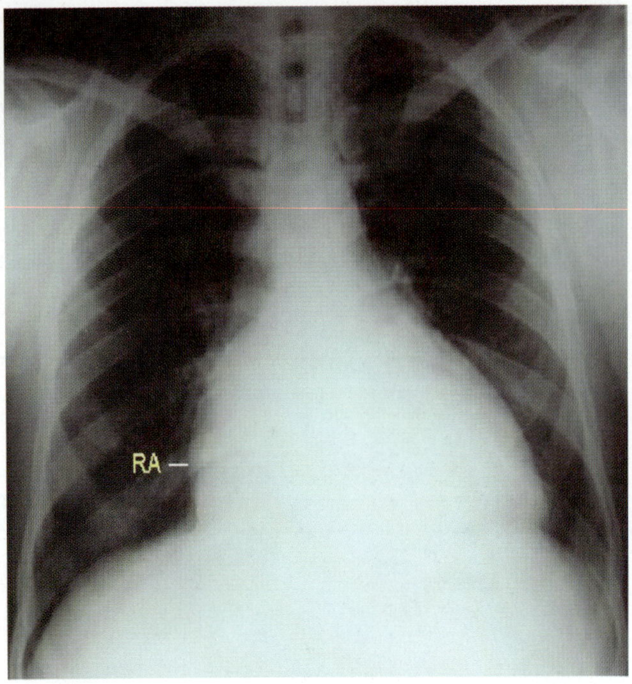

Fig. 28.36: *X-ray chest PA view showing cardiomegaly with right atrial enlargement in restrictive cardiomyopathy*

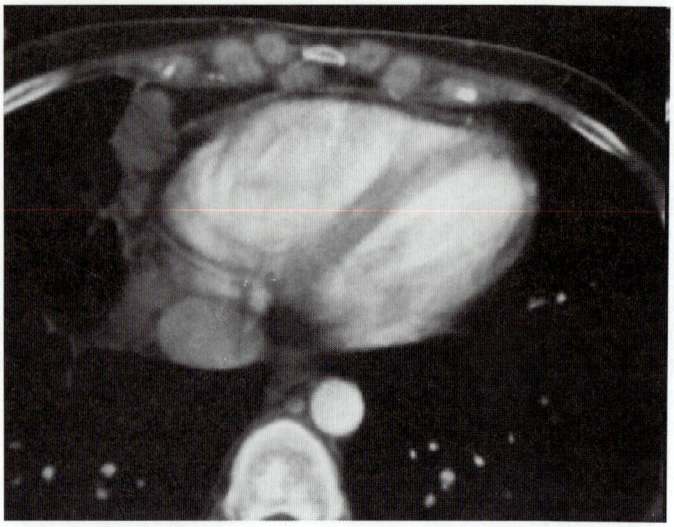

Fig. 28.37: *Restrictive cardiomyopathy. Axial contrast-enhanced CT image through the heart shows a thin pericardium without calcification. Note the cardiophrenic and internal mammary lymph nodes. The patient had extensive mediastinal and hilar adenopathy, as well as interstitial lung changes*

Psychological Issues and Councelling

Adjusting to having a chronic illness is stressful not only for the child but for the entire family as well. The child's reaction to having HCM often depends on the stage of the child's development. Discussions about the disease should be tailored to the specific concerns of the child. Child-life professionals and pediatric psychiatrists are important resources to help children cope, and their services are often available through the treating center.

Family

The impact of a diagnosis of HCM is felt throughout the child's immediate and extended family. It is important for

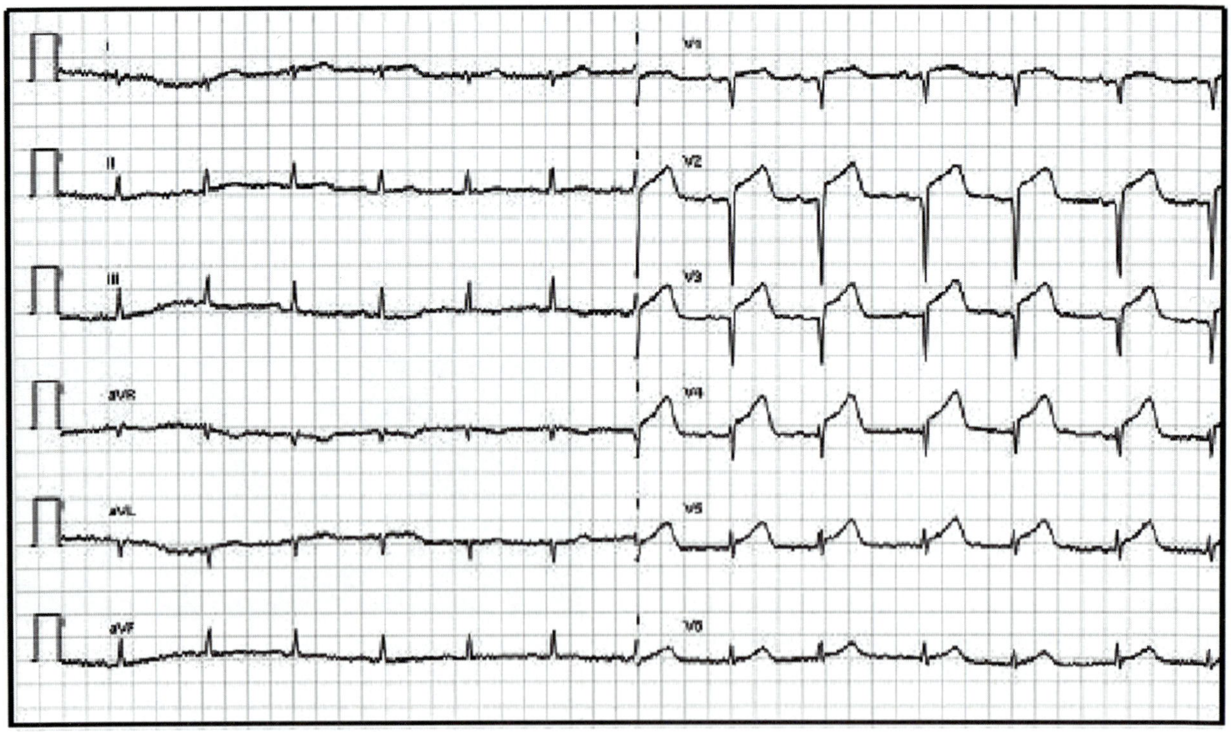

Fig. 28.38: *Mixed constrictive-restrictive cardiomyopathy ECG shows sinus rhythm (79/min) with absent progression of R-wave (V1-V4) and omozonal ST elevation*

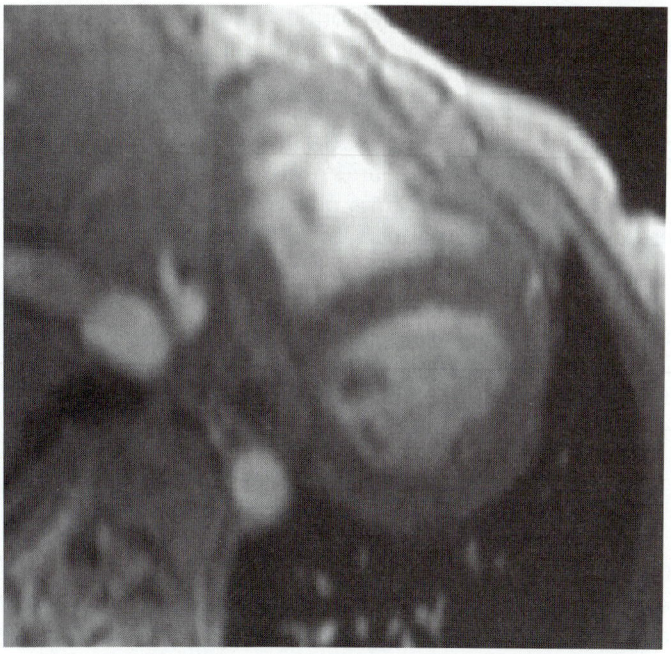

Fig. 28.39: *Restrictive cardiomyopathy. Axial double inversion-recovery MRI of the heart in a 20-year-old adolescent with sarcoid demonstrates a normal pericardium*

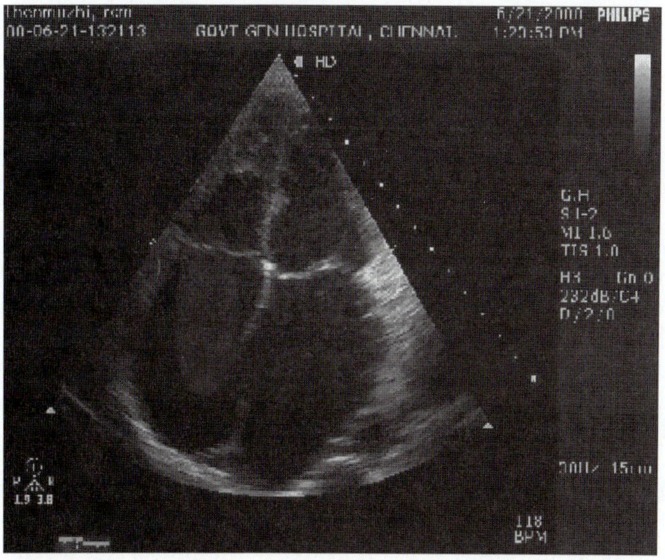

Fig. 28.40: *A classical restrictive cardiomyopathy. Both atria balloon out as they face stiff resistance from the ventricles*

parents and other caregivers to realize that they are not alone in feeling the weight of responsibility that comes with taking care of a child with a chronic illness. Anticipating and/or preventing the stress imposed by an illness is an important part of caring for the child and family, and personnel at the treating medical center can help identify issues that can lead to increased stress.

Practical solutions to problems giving medications, keeping track of appointments, and maintaining normal family life can often be found through discussions with nurse clinicians, the social worker, psychiatrist, and other parents of children with hypertrophic cardiomyopathy.

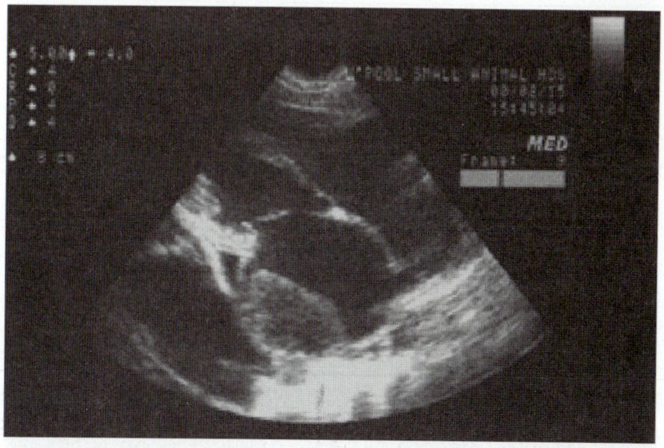

Fig. 28.41: *Real-time ultrasound from a 5-year-old boy with restrictive cardiomyopathy showing pleural effusion and a thrombus in the left atrium*

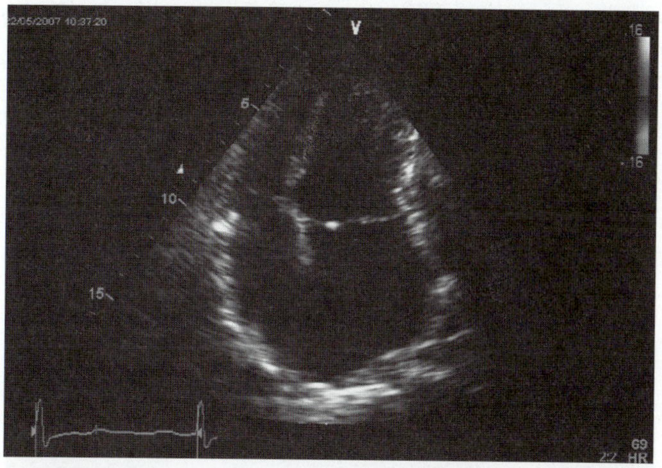

Fig. 28.42: *Two dimensional apical four chamber image showing moderate to severe biatrial enlargement in a patient with restrictive cardiomyopathy*

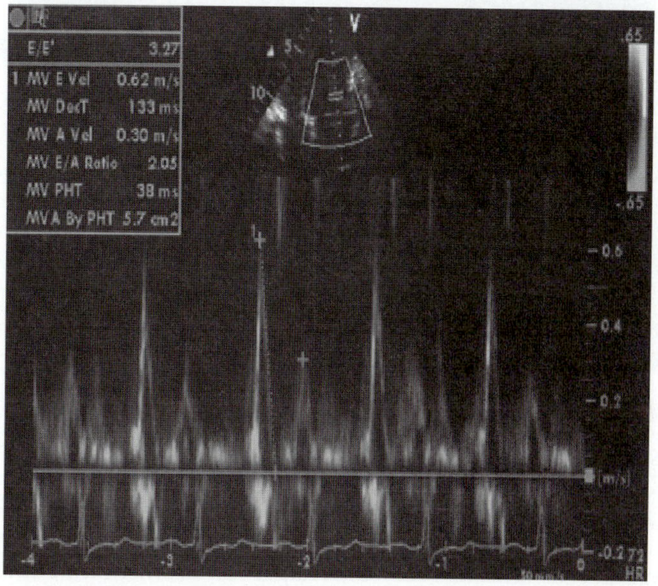

Fig. 28.43: *Pulsed wave Doppler of transmitral flow; mitral valve E and A velocity measured 0.74 and 0.36 m/s, respectively in restrictive cardiomyopathy*

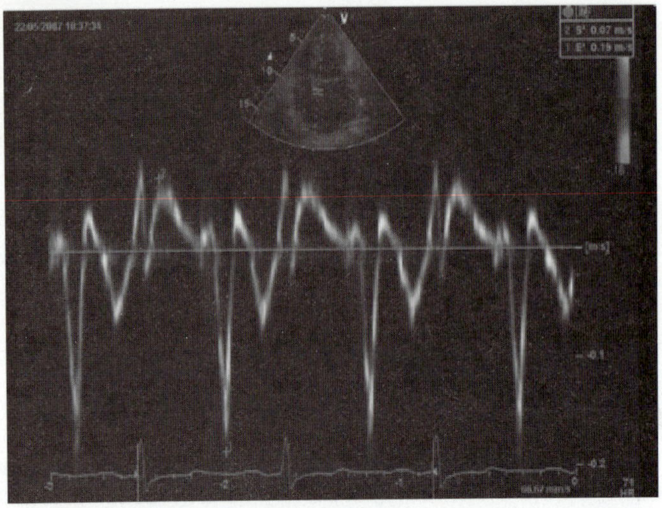

Fig. 28.44: *Tissue Doppler imaging; E and S measured 19 and 7 cm/s, respectively, E/E ratio was 3 in case of a restrictive cardiomyopathy*

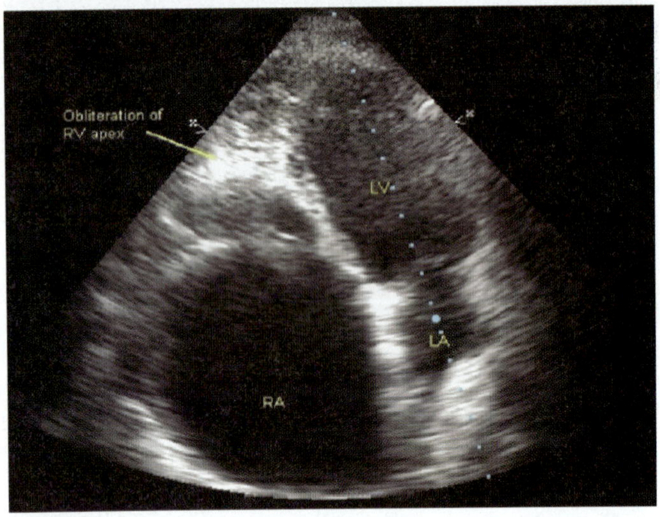

Fig. 28.45: *Echocardiogram in right ventricular endomyocardial fibrosis*

Healthy Diet

All children with HCM should follow a healthy diet. The recommendations published in 2005 by the United States Department of Agriculture (USDA) can be found at the following website address: http://www.mypyramid.gov.

Certain types of HCM may require alteration of dietary intake, and in these cases, a special diet may be developed in consultation with metabolic specialists.

Health Maintenance for Children with HCM

Routine pediatric care is important for children with HCM. Regular well child visits and standard childhood immunizations should be performed. The influenza vaccine should be administered on a yearly basis. Children under age 2 year should receive Synagis for protection against respiratory syncytial virus (RSV).

A medical alert bracelet is an important safety measure for children with HCM. In the event of an emergency, these bracelets allow medical personnel to know details about a child's illness, especially if a family member is not available.

Future Research in HCM?

Much progress has been made in our ability to diagnose HCM in both the clinical and molecular arenas. However, much additional research is needed in this field. Areas of research to be highlighted over the next decade include:

1. Better understanding of HCM as a disease process and the characteristics of the disease as they relate to outcome, which will lead to better management strategies (Fig. 28.36).
2. Increased clinical trials which will lead to new drug development and more effective therapies.
3. Molecular identification of novel genetic mutations as well as more precise diagnostic genetic testing/screening which will result in more accurate diagnosis.

It is the expectation of the medical community that the data derived from exploring these avenues of scientific research will translate into a clinician's ability to tailor medical therapy based on a given child's precise diagnosis. Achieving this goal over the next couple of decades will represent a large milestone in the field of pediatric cardiomyopathy research and will, hopefully, improve the ongoing care and prognosis of children afflicted with this heart muscle disease.

C. Restrictive Cardiomyopathy

Restrictive cardiomyopathy (RCM) is a rare form of heart muscle disease that is characterized by restrictive filling of the ventricles. In this disease, the contractile function (squeeze) of the heart and wall thicknesses are usually normal, but the relaxation or filling phase of the heart is very abnormal. This occurs because the heart muscle is stiff and poorly compliant and does not allow the ventricular chambers to fill with blood normally. This inability to relax and fill with blood results in a "back up" of blood into the atria (top chambers of the heart), lungs and body causing the symptoms and signs of heart failure.

Within the broad category of cardiomyopathy, RCM is the least common in children, accounting for 2.5–5% of the diagnosed cardiomyopathies (occurs in less than 1 per million children). The average age at diagnosis is 5–6 years. RCM appears to affect girls somewhat more often than boys. There is a family history of cardiomyopathy in approximately 30% of cases. In most cases, the cause of the disease is unknown (idiopathic) although a genetic cause is suspected in most cases of pediatric RCM.

Diagnosis of RCM (Figs 28.36–28.45)

In children, the first symptoms of RCM often seem related to problems other than the heart. The most common symptoms at first may appear to be lung related. Children with RCM frequently have a history of "repeated lung infections" or "asthma". In these cases, referral to a cardiologist eventually occurs when a large heart is seen on chest X-ray. The second most common reason for referral is an abnormal physical finding during a doctor's examination. Children who have ascites (fluid in the abdomen), hepatomegaly (enlarged liver) and edema (fluid causing puffy looking feet, legs, hands or face) are often sent to see a gastroenterologist first. Referral to a cardiologist is made when additional cardiac signs or symptoms occur, a chest X-ray is found to be abnormal or no specific gastrointestinal cause is found for the edema or enlarged liver. When the first sign of the disease is an abnormal heart sound, or signs of heart failure are recognized, then earlier referral to a cardiologist occurs. In approximately 10% of cases, fainting is the first symptom causing concern. Unfortunately, sudden death has been the initial presentation in some patients. Diagnosis of RCM Restrictive cardiomyopathy is among the rarest of childhood cardiomyopathies. Its diagnosis is difficult to establish early in the clinical course due to the lack of symptoms. Therefore, in many cases, this diagnosis is made only after presentation with symptoms such as decreased exercise tolerance, new heart sound (gallop), syncope (passing out) or chest pain with exercise.

Once suspected, there are certain tests that can help to confirm this diagnosis.

An electrocardiogram, or EKG, which records the electrical conduction through the heart, can be very helpful. This can show abnormally large electrical forces from enlargement of the atria (upper chambers) of the heart.

An echocardiogram, or ultrasound of the heart, can provide additional clues to help to make this diagnosis. Generally, in children with RCM, the echocardiogram shows marked enlargement of the atria (upper chambers), normal sized ventricles (lower chambers) and normal heart function. In more advanced disease states, pulmonary artery pressure (blood pressure in the lungs) will be increased and can often be estimated during the echocardiogram.

Cardiac catheterization is usually the next procedure done to confirm the diagnosis. During this procedure, a catheter (thin plastic tube) will be slowly advanced through an artery or vein into the heart (while watching its course on a TV monitor) so that pressures within the heart chambers can be measured. These measurements often show significantly elevated pressures during the relaxation period of the heart (when it fills with blood before the next beat) and varying degrees of increased pulmonary artery

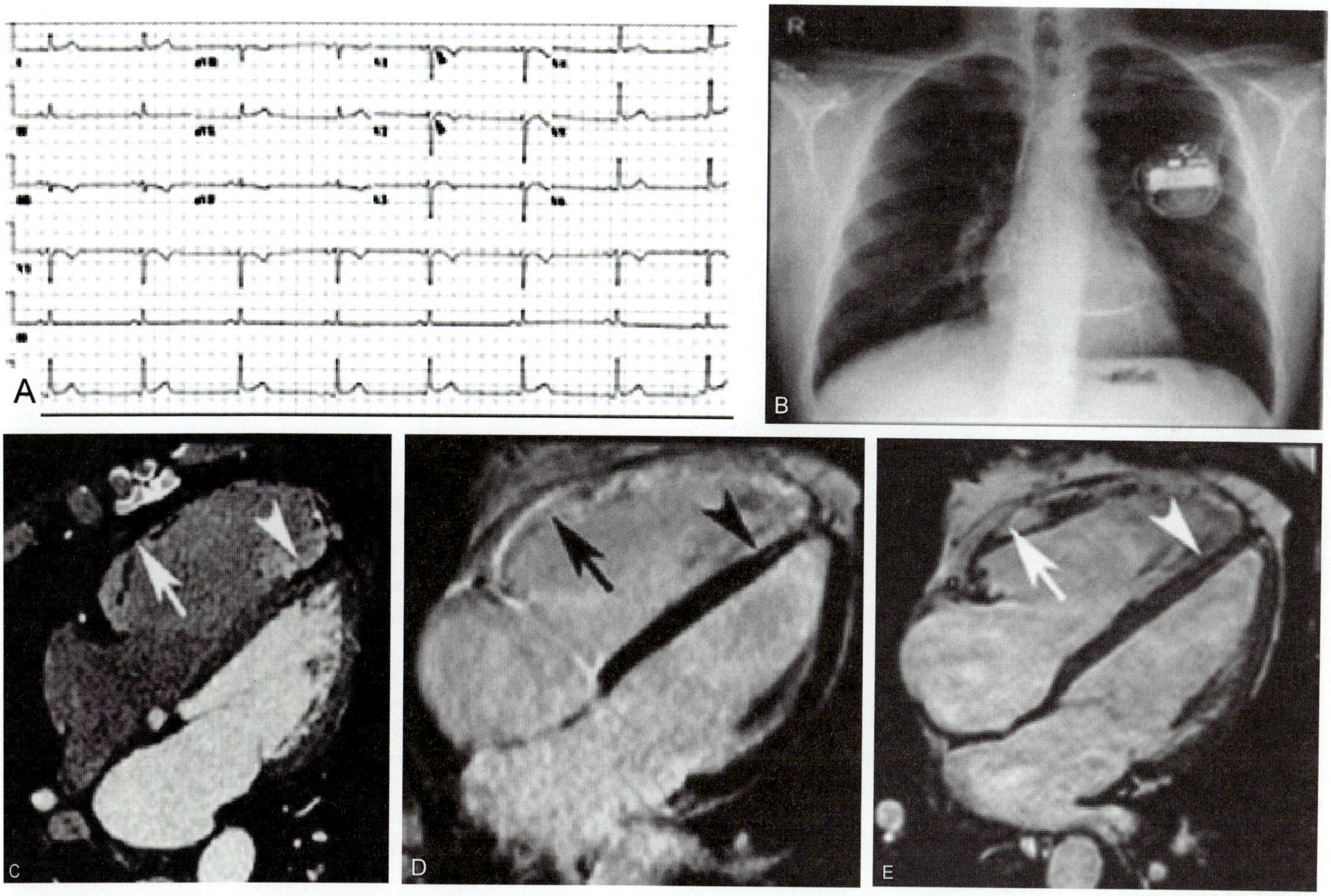

Fig. 28.46: *(A) ECG with typical signs for ARVC; negative T waves and Epsilon waves in the precordial leads (arrow). (B) Chest X-ray after ICD implantation. Both the atrial and ventricular leads are visible. (C through E) Signal attenuation in RV septum on MDCT (C), increased signal intensity on delayed enhancement images (D), and decreased signal intensity on steady-state free precession images (E)*

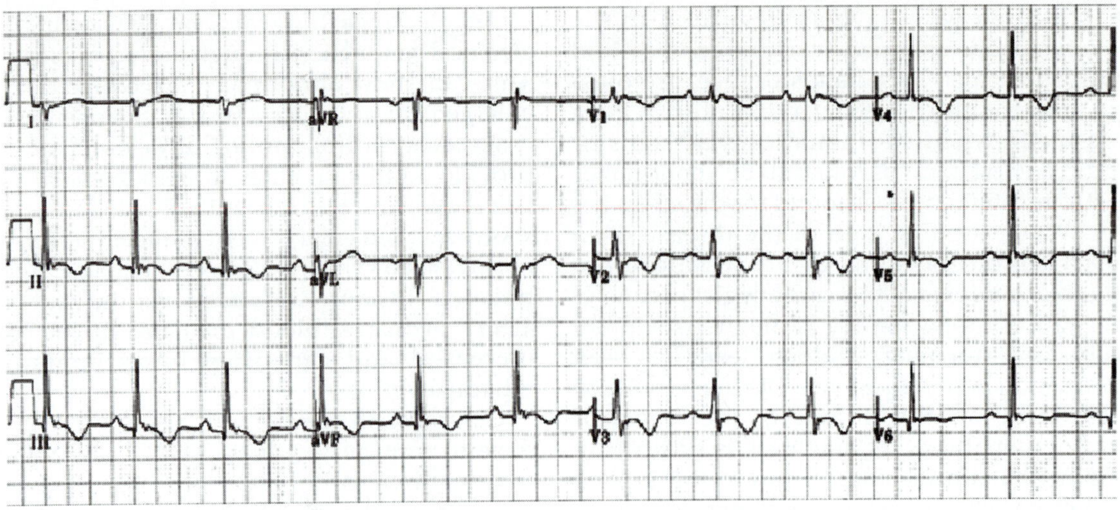

Fig. 28.47: *Right ventricular hypertrophy in a patient with arrhythmogenic right ventricular cardiomyopathy: Right axis deviation. R/S ratio in V1 > 1 right ventricular strain pattern with T-wave inversion and ST depression in the right precordial (V1-3) and inferior (II, III, aVF) leads*

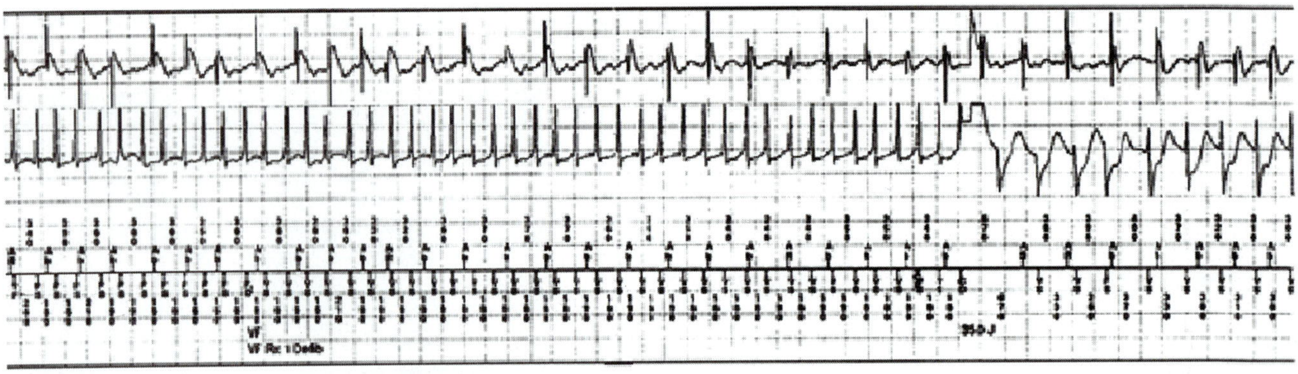

Fig. 28.48: *Electrophysiological study: it showed caffeine-induced malignant ventricular arrhythmia in a young patient with arrhythmogenic cardiomyopathy. At electrophysiological study, long runs of self-terminating atrial and ventricular tachycardia were inducible from the right-ventricular upper lateral regions of RV*

pressure (which can confirm the echo estimates) in the absence of any other structural heart disease. In very rare cases, based on clinical symptoms and prior laboratory evaluation, a cardiac biopsy may be performed. This involves removing tiny pieces of heart muscle for inspection under the microscope to search for potential causes of this condition (such as amyloidosis or sarcoidosis, which are common causes of RCM in adults but rarely in pediatric patients).

Finally, since childhood RCM is often genetic and in many cases will be inherited, once this diagnosis is established, your doctor will likely request that parents, siblings of the patient and sometimes other close relatives be screened with an echocardiogram to rule out the presence of this disease in other family members.

Etiological Factors in RCM

Although the cause of RCM is not known in most pediatric cases, there is some scientific evidence suggesting that individual genetic "mutations" may be a cause in some cases of RCM in children. For a greater understanding of the basics of human inheritance patterns and a more detailed discussion of the potential genetic causes of RCM.

Current Treatment

Currently, there are no therapies that can "cure" RCM; however, some treatments are available that can improve symptoms in children with RCM. The choice of a specific therapy depends on the clinical condition of the child, the risk of dangerous events and the ability of the child to tolerate the therapy. Medical Therapies to Treat RCM and Associated Heart Failure Some children with RCM have signs and symptoms of heart failure due to the abnormal relaxation properties of the heart muscle. The most common types of medications used to treat heart failure under these circumstances include diuretics, beta-blockers and occasionally afterload reducing agents.

Diuretics, sometimes called "water pills", reduce excess fluid in the lungs or other organs by increasing urine production.

Diuretics can be given either orally or intravenously. Common diuretics include furosemide, spironolactone, bumetanide and metolazone. Common side effects of diuretics include dehydration and abnormalities in the blood chemistries (particularly potassium loss). In patients with RCM, diuretics must be used very carefully and given only in doses to treat extra lung and abdominal fluid without inducing excessive fluid loss as this may cause symptomatically low blood pressure.

Beta-blockers slow the heartbeat and increase the relaxation time of the heart. This may allow the heart to fill better with blood before each heart beat and decrease some of the symptoms created by the stiff pumping chambers. Common beta-blockers (taken by mouth) include carvedilol, metoprolol, propanolol and atenolol. Side effects include dizziness, low heart rate, low blood pressure, and, in some cases, fluid retention, fatigue, impaired school performance and depression.

Anticoagulation Medications

In children with a heart that does not relax well, there is a risk of blood clots forming inside the heart possibly leading to a stroke. Anticoagulation medications, also known as blood thinners, are often used in these situations. The choice of anticoagulation drug depends on how likely it is that a blood clot will form. Less strong anticoagulation medications include aspirin and dipyridamole. Stronger anticoagulation drugs are warfarin, heparin, and enoxaparin; these drugs require careful monitoring with regular blood testing. While variable, common side effects of anticoagulants include excessive bruising or bleeding from otherwise minor skin injuries, interaction with other medications and, for warfarin, fluctuations in anticoagulation blood levels caused by changes in daily dietary intake. Information regarding which food groups can significantly affect warfarin levels can be obtained from your cardiologist.

Surgical Intervention in Restrictive Cardiomyopathy

No surgery has been effective in improving the heart function in restrictive cardiomyopathy. Heart transplantation is the only effective surgery offered for patients with RCM, particularly those who already have symptoms at the time of diagnosis or in whom reactive pulmonary hypertension exists.

Heart Transplantation

Since there are no proven effective therapies for children with RCM, transplantation is the only known intervention for this disease. This is especially true in cases where evaluation has demonstrated the presence of pulmonary hypertension, which can be fatal if not treated. For children with RCM, heart transplantation can address both the abnormal heart function as well as associated pulmonary hypertension. A heart transplant offers the child with RCM the chance to return to a normal lifestyle. While a donor heart can cure the symptoms of heart failure and greatly improve survival, it is a major operation with considerable risks and long-term complications. Once a transplant is done, other concerns arise, such as infection, organ rejection, coronary artery disease, and the side effects of medications.

Prognosis

The long-term prognosis for children with RCM varies depending on the symptoms at the time of diagnosis and the presence of pulmonary hypertension. Children with RCM should be watched closely for the development of excess fluid retention, abnormal heart rhythms, blood clots inside the heart or evidence of progressive pulmonary hypertension.

As discussed previously, RCM is rare, and there is limited information on this disease in children. Once diagnosed, approximately 20% develop thrombotic or embolic events (blood clots). The average 2-year survival rate for children with RCM is 45–70% including those treated with heart transplantation. Survival increases significantly for children who are transplanted. Irreversible pulmonary hypertension (high blood pressure in the lung vessels) has been the only major risk factor associated with poor outcome among these patients. Therefore, it is important that transplant be considered sooner than later to optimize long-term survival, as the waiting time for a donor heart can be unpredictable. Finally, a child with RCM should be closely monitored at a center with expertise in pediatric heart failure, cardiomyopathy, arrhythmias and transplantation in order to ensure rapid response to any worsening of his or her condition.

Living with RCM

The diagnosis of RCM affects many areas of a child's life. The following sections outline the general approaches to living with RCM. It is important that specific recommendations are developed by the team caring for the child with restrictive cardiomyopathy.

Physical Activity and Sports

Children with RCM are not allowed to play competitive sports because of the possibility of a sudden collapse or increased heart failure. A competitive sport is an organized team activity for which training is required.

A child with restrictive cardiomyopathy and no heart failure symptoms can be allowed to perform recreational athletic activities, also known as low-dynamic or low-static sports, in a noncompetitive situation. Specific activity recommendations should be individualized by the treating cardiologist.

Attending School

The intellectual, psychological and social benefits of attending school cannot be overestimated in the child with RCM.

Adjusting medication schedules so they do not interfere with school activities, discussing safe activity levels with school personnel, and providing tutoring to maintain academic performance are important interventions that can help a child to stay in school and keep up with their peers. Often close communication between the parents, medical care team, and the school nurse can help to keep a child up to date in school.

Mixing with Friends

Every effort should be made to allow a child with RCM to spend time with friends. The child should also be allowed to participate in recreational activities whenever possible. However, an effort should be made to avoid contact with those who are acutely ill with fever, even though many children with RCM are able to tolerate upper respiratory tract illnesses (common colds) well.

Psychological Issues

Adjusting to having a chronic illness is stressful for the child and the family. The child's reaction to having RCM often depends on the stage of the child's development. Discussions about the disease should be tailored to the specific concerns of the child. Child-life professionals and pediatric psychiatrists are important resources to help children cope, and their services are often available through the treating center.

Acceptance of RCM Child by Family Members

The impact of a diagnosis of RCM is felt throughout the child's immediate and extended family. It is important for parents and other caregivers to realize that they are not alone in feeling the weight of responsibility that comes with taking care of a child with a chronic illness. Anticipating and/or preventing the stress imposed by an illness is an important part of caring for the child and family and personnel at the cardiomyopathy center can help to identify issues that can lead to increased stress.

Practical solutions to problems giving medications, keeping track of appointments, and maintaining normal family life can often be found through discussions with nurse clinicians, the social worker, psychiatrist, and other parents of children with RCM.

Healthy Diet

All children with RCM should follow a healthy diet. In children with RCM and extra lung and abdominal fluid, a low-salt diet is recommended to avoid excessive fluid retention. Some children with heart failure may not grow well. In these cases, a diet that increases calories is recommended.

Children who are taking some medications may have low levels of magnesium or potassium and a diet that has a higher amount of one or both of these two electrolytes may be recommended. Some children with severe heart failure can retain extra body fluid, and it may be necessary to limit the amount that a child can drink to prevent fluid from accumulating in the lungs.

Health Maintenance with Regular Medical Check Up

Routine pediatric care is important for children with RCM. Regular well child visits and standard childhood immunizations should be performed. The influenza vaccine should be administered on a yearly basis. Children under age 2 year should receive Synagis for protection against respiratory syncytial virus.

A medical alert bracelet is an important safety measure for children with RCM. In the event of an emergency, these bracelets allow medical personnel to know details about a child's illness, especially if a family member is not available.

Futuristic Goals in RCM

Slowly, progress is being made in our ability to diagnose RCM in both the clinical and molecular arenas. However, much additional research is needed in this field. Areas of research to be highlighted over the next decade include:

1. Better understanding of RCM as a disease process and the characteristics of the disease as they relate to outcome, which will lead to better management strategies.
2. Increased clinical trials which will lead to new drug development and more effective therapies.
3. Molecular identification of novel genetic mutations as well as more precise diagnostic genetic testing/screening which will result in more accurate diagnosis.

It is the expectation of the medical community that the data derived from exploring these avenues of scientific research will translate into a clinician's ability to tailor medical therapy based on a given child's precise diagnosis. Achieving this goal over the next couple of decades will represent a large milestone in the field of pediatric cardiomyopathy and will, hopefully, improve the ongoing care and prognosis of children afflicted with these heart muscle diseases.

D. Arrhythmogenic Right Ventricular Dysplasia (ARVD)

There are other forms of cardiomyopathy which comprise only a very small percentage of the total (~2–3%) number of cardiomyopathies in children. These cardiomyopathies may have overlapping features with any of the previous types described and include arrhythmogenic right ventricular dysplasia (ARVD), mitochondrial and left ventricular noncompaction cardiomyopathies (LVNC).

Patients with ARVD have dilated, poorly functioning right ventricles which have fatty deposits within the walls and are at risk for abnormally fast, life-threatening heart rhythms (ventricular tachycardia). This myopathy can be diagnosed (usually due to the abnormal rhythms) either in early infancy or later in adolescence/adulthood by echocardiogram or MRI, and its prognosis depends, in part, on the age at presentation (Figs 28.46 and 28.51). Mitochondrial myopathies are rare and often present early in life. Hearts in the affected patients are often thick-walled (hypertrophic) although dilated hearts with poor function can also occur with this type of myopathy. This cardiomyopathy is caused by abnormalities in the mitochondria of the cells, which are small structures within each cell responsible for generating the energy the cell uses for its normal activities. These cardiomyopathies are often associated with other muscle, liver, neurologic and/or developmental abnormalities and are usually genetically passed from an affected mother to her children (Fig. 28.49).

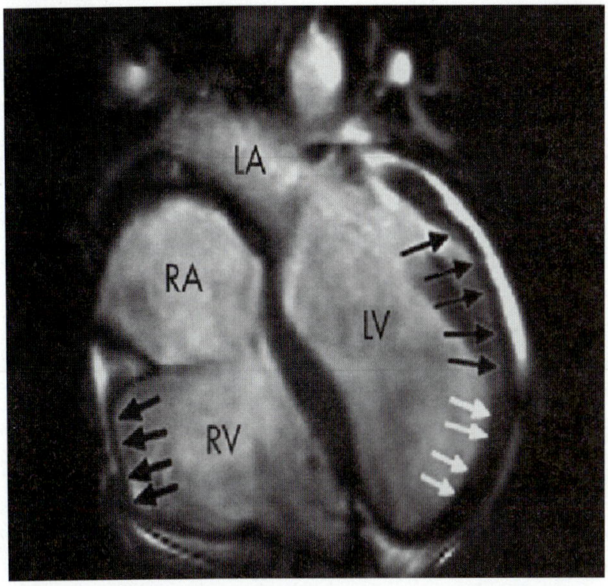

Fig. 28.49: *ARVC Four chamber view shows severe global enlargement of the right ventricle (RV) with localised dilation at the inflow tract (black arrows). The left ventricle (LV) is also moderately dilated. Regional thinning of the posterolateral LV wall is observed (black arrows). Normal LV wall thickness is highlighted by white arrows for comparison. LA, left atrium; RA, right atrium*

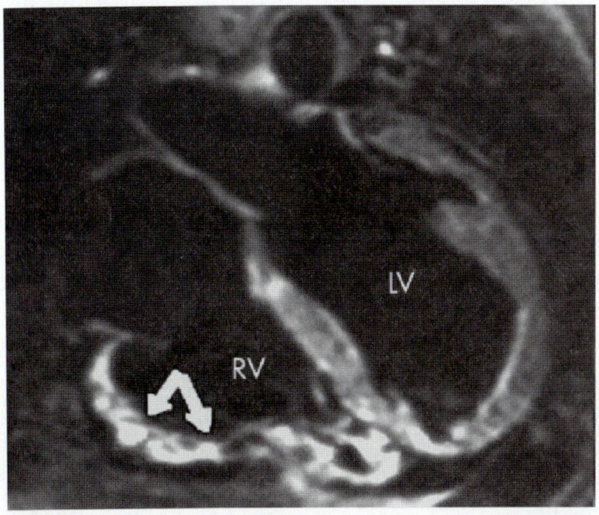

Fig. 28.50: *T2 weighted spin echo image in the four chamber view with fat suppression. The bright areas within the grey myocardium (white arrows) are likely to represent oedema, suggesting the presence of patchy inflammatory infiltrates as seen in ARVC*

Finally, left ventricular noncompaction (LVNC) cardiomyopathy is characterized by deep trabeculations (or crevices) within muscle of the left ventricular walls. These hearts may have features of both dilated and/or hypertrophic cardiomyopathy. Conditions associated with LVNC include mitochondrial and metabolic disorders as well as systemic (whole body) processes such as Barth syndrome. Barth syndrome has a constellation of abnormalities including cyclic neutropenia or periodic

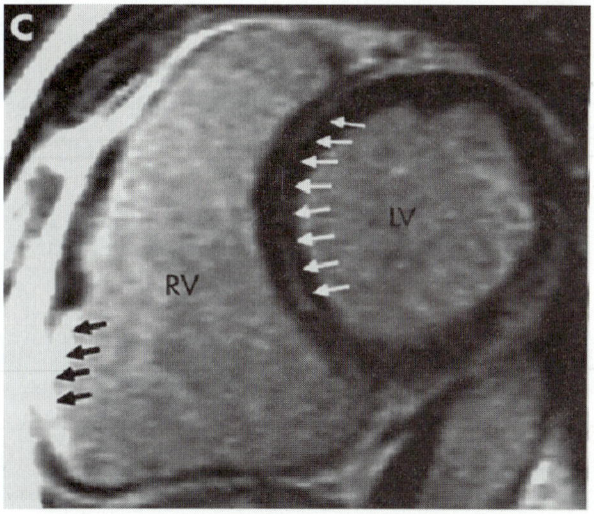

Fig. 28.51: *Following intravenous administration of gadolinium-DTPA, late enhancement was observed in both the right ventricle (RV) (black arrows) and the septum (white arrows). Since fat was absent from these regions on corresponding T1 weighted turbospin images, the appearances are consistent with myocardial fibrosis. The mid-myocardial distribution is typical of fibrosis secondary to ARVC.*

fluctuations in the white blood cell count (which may not be apparent in early infancy), hypotonia (weak muscles) and LVNC cardiomyopathy. Barth syndrome has recently been linked to an abnormality in the X-chromosome and is passed from mother to son.

Symptoms of ARVD, Mitochondrial and LVNC Cardiomyopathies

Symptoms (the problems noted by the child and/or family) and signs (the problems detected by your physician) of cardiomyopathy in children are dependent on several factors including the type, cause and severity of the specific cardiomyopathy, the age when the problems started, and the effects of treatment. Since patients with ARVD generally have symptoms consistent with DCM, and patients with mitochondrial or LVNC cardiomyopathies can have symptoms seen with either HCM or DCM.

Diagnosis of ARVD, mitochondrial and LVNC cardiomyopathies as with presenting symptoms, the clinical diagnosis of these rare forms of cardiomyopathy will depend on the features of the specific cardiomyopathy. That is, the diagnostic criteria in a child with ARVD will generally follow that of DCM while the mitochondrial and LVNC myopathies will follow that of either DCM or HCM depending on the clinical manifestations of the myopathy.

The diagnosis of ARVD can be difficult especially in children given its low incidence. However, opposed to the usual form of DCM, which involves the left ventricle to a greater extent, ARVD typically involves the right ventricle preferentially and often times, the clinical suspicion for ARVD can be further explored with MRI which, in many cases, can differentiate fatty deposits from muscle tissue within the wall of the right ventricle that are commonly

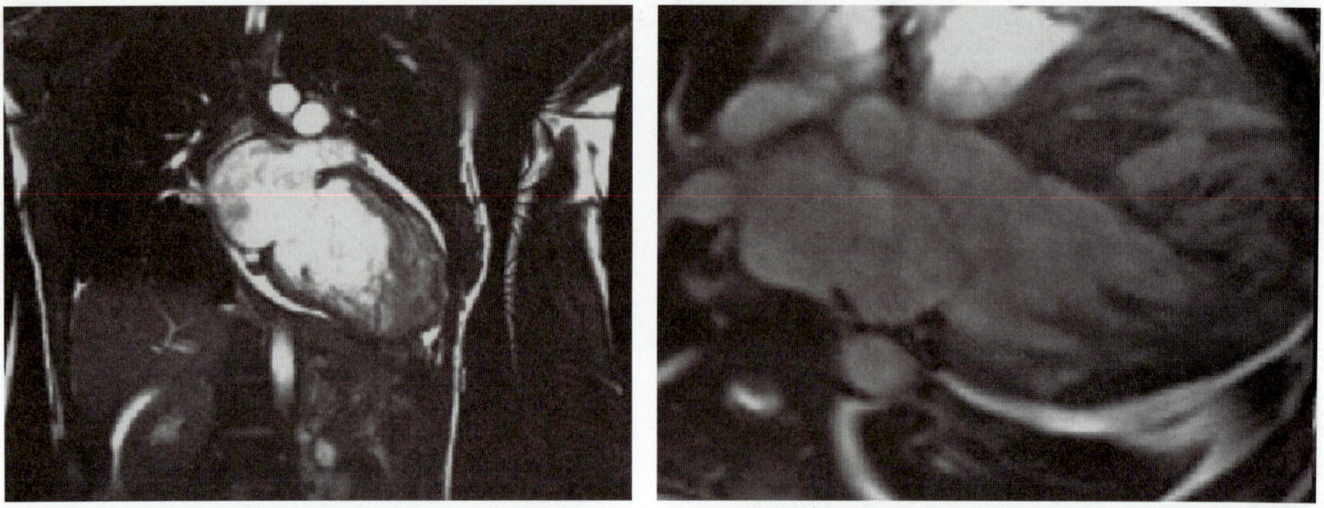

Fig. 28.52: *Images from cardiac MRI showing a markedly dilated left ventricle and left atrium. The left ventricle shows prominent trabeculation particularly along the apex. A small pericardial effusion and a small pleural effusion are also noted in a case with non-compacted cardiomyopathy*

seen with this disease. The diagnosis can usually be confirmed with visualization of significant fatty deposition within the right ventricular walls (where muscle should be) from biopsy specimens obtained during cardiac catheterization.

Patients with mitochondrial cardiomyopathy often have other associated medical problems such as hearing or vision problems, skeletal muscle weakness in the arm and leg muscles and/or central nervous system issues including learning problems, developmental delay or loss of developmental milestones. Once suspected, in addition to the cardiac assessment (for DCM or HCM) outlined elsewhere in this brochure, a muscle biopsy performed to evaluate both structure and function of the mitochondria can help to verify this diagnosis. A cardiac biopsy is generally not useful because the volume of muscle tissue necessary to perform the mitochondrial analyses can only be safely obtained from arm or leg muscles.

The diagnosis of LVNC can often by strongly suspected when deep crevices or trabeculations are noted with the walls of the left ventricle during an echocardiogram. Very few other cardiac diagnoses have these specific findings. Genetic testing may become more available in the near future to assess identified causes of LVNC especially among male children and those suspected of having Barth syndrome (see following discussion on the G4.5 mutation testing).

Causes of the Miscellaneous Cardiomyopathies

Currently, the cause of these "rare" cardiomyopathies in most children is incompletely understood, but in a subset of children it is clear that the cause is an error or mistake in a gene. For a greater understanding of the basics of human inheritance patterns and a more detailed discussion of the potential genetic causes of the "rare" cardiomyopathies.

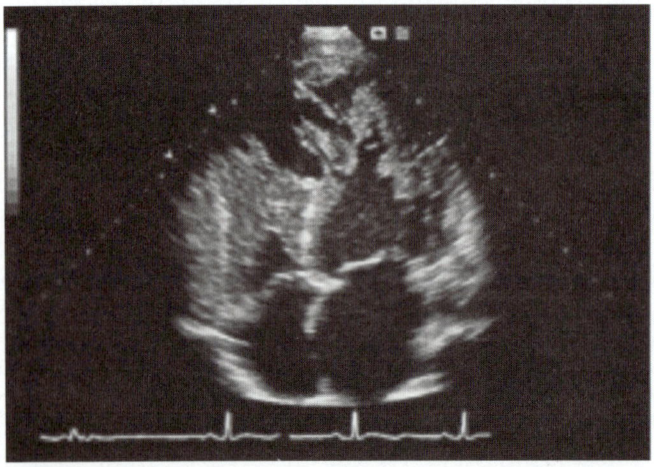

Fig. 28.53: *Apical four chamber view on transthoracic echocardiogram (apex up) revealing a left ventricle with a thick spongy endocardial surface that is severely trabeculated at the apex characteristic of left ventricular noncompaction*

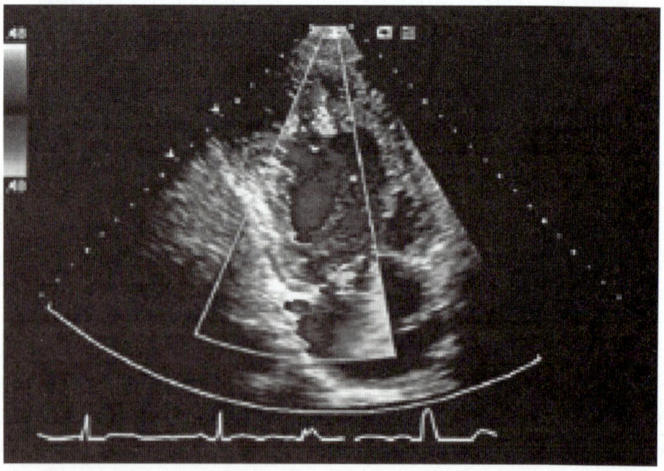

Fig. 28.54: *Apical two chamber view on transthoracic echocardiogram (apex up) with low-scale color Doppler showing multiple large recesses in the left ventricular apex being perfused from the left ventricular cavity in LV type of noncompaction cardiomyopathy*

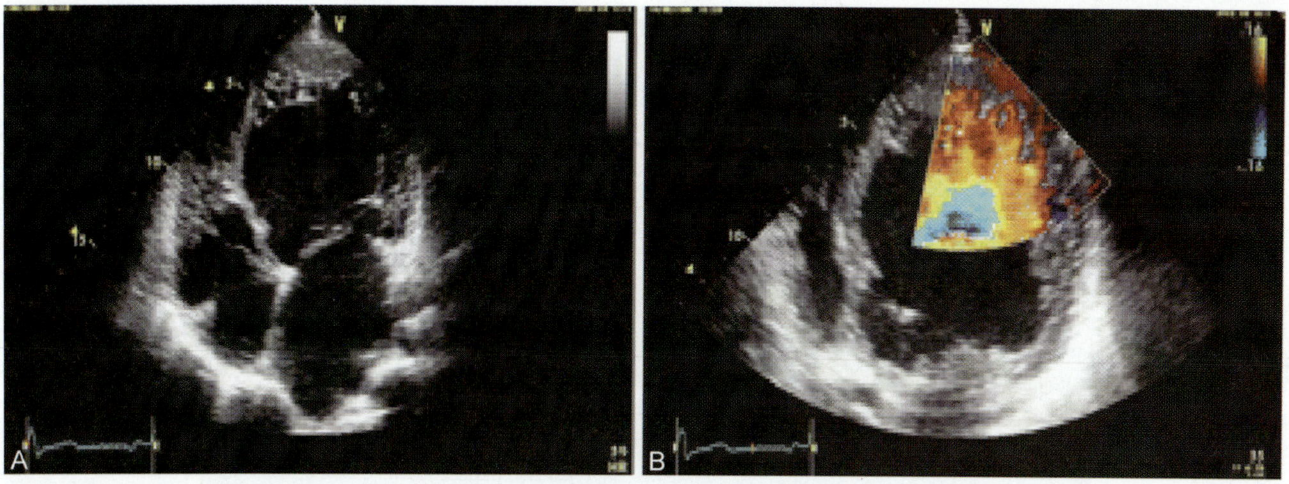

Fig. 28.55: *Left ventricular noncompaction. (A) There is marked LV dilatation and dysfunction, thinning of the septum and hypertrophy, excessive trabeculation of the lateral wall and apex. (B) Colour flow mapping shows flow within deep recesses, extending to the epicardium at the apex*

Current Management

Currently, there are no therapies that can "cure" cardiomyopathy; however, many treatments are available that can improve symptoms and decrease risk in children with cardiomyopathy. The choice of a specific therapy depends on the type of cardiomyopathy, the clinical condition of the child, the risk of dangerous events and the ability of the child to tolerate the therapy. To review detailed therapies for both the dilated and hypertrophic forms of cardiomyopathy that apply to ARVD, mitochondrial myopathy or LVNC, the reader is directed to the pertient sections on treatment written for DCM and HCM elsewhere in this brochure.

Prognosis

Many children with cardiomyopathy are able to lead relatively normal lives once the diagnosis has been established and appropriate therapies have been started. The long-term prognosis varies depending on the type of cardiomyopathy and the degree of functional impairment. Children with cardiomyopathy should be watched closely for the development of heart failure, abnormal heart rhythms, blood clots inside the heart and other signs that the heart is not able to maintain normal blood flow. Once signs of heart failure or significantly abnormal rhythms appear, aggressive therapy is begun with close monitoring for signs of worsening blood flow to the vital organs. If other organs show signs of damage or the heart failure does not respond to medications, a cardiac assist device and/or transplant is considered early, as the waiting time for a donor heart can be unpredictable. It is important that a child with cardiomyopathy be closely monitored at a center with expertise in pediatric heart failure, cardiomyopathy, arrhythmias, cardiac assist devices and transplantation in order to ensure rapid response to any worsening of his or her condition.

In children with DCM, approximately 35% recover completely, 35% stabilize and the remaining may progressively worsen. Children with DCM are more prone to congestive heart failure and have a higher rate of heart transplantation compared with other forms of cardiomyopathy. However, improved medical therapy may eventually change this scenario.

Current average 5-year survival rates for children with typical DCM are 40–50%. Survival rates for ARVD, LVNC and mitochondrial myopathies are much less well established.

The outcome of hypertrophic cardiomyopathy is highly variable with some patients remaining asymptomatic, some developing symptoms and possibly progressive heart failure, and all remaining at risk for sudden death. Heart transplant is performed uncommonly and is primarily reserved for patients with severe, uncontrollable heart

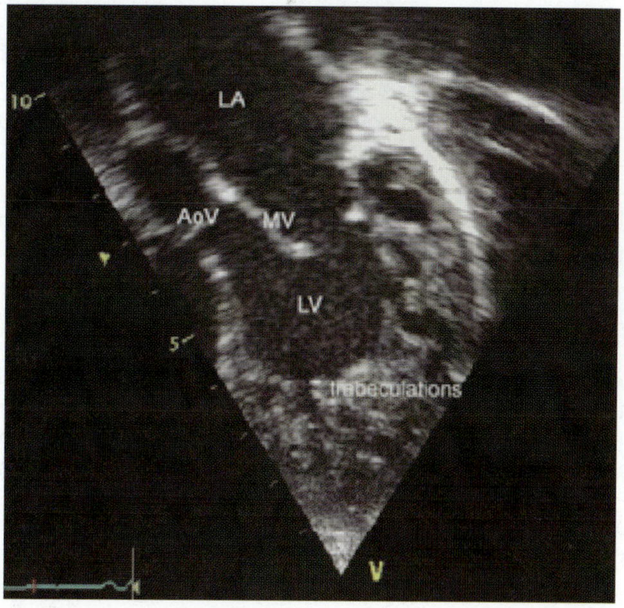

Fig. 28.56: *Echocardiogram showing the left heart structures and left ventricular noncompaction. The apex of the left ventricle is normally smooth but in this case heavily trabeculated*

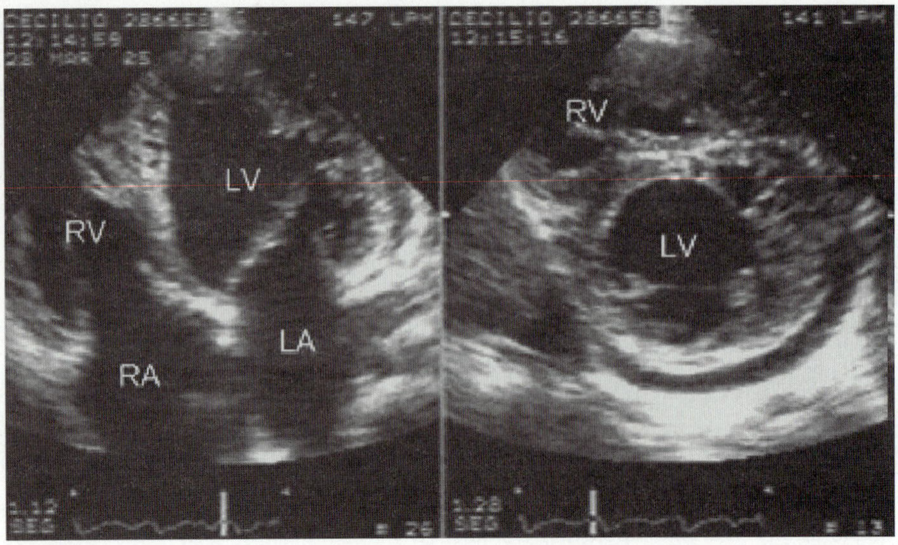

Fig. 28.57: *Two dimensional apical four chamber and parasternal short-axis images at the level of the ventricles show dilatation of both ventricles, multiple trabeculae and intertrabecular recesses in inferior, lateral, anterior walls, middle and apical portions of the septum and apex of the left ventricle in a case with noncompacted cardiomyopathy*

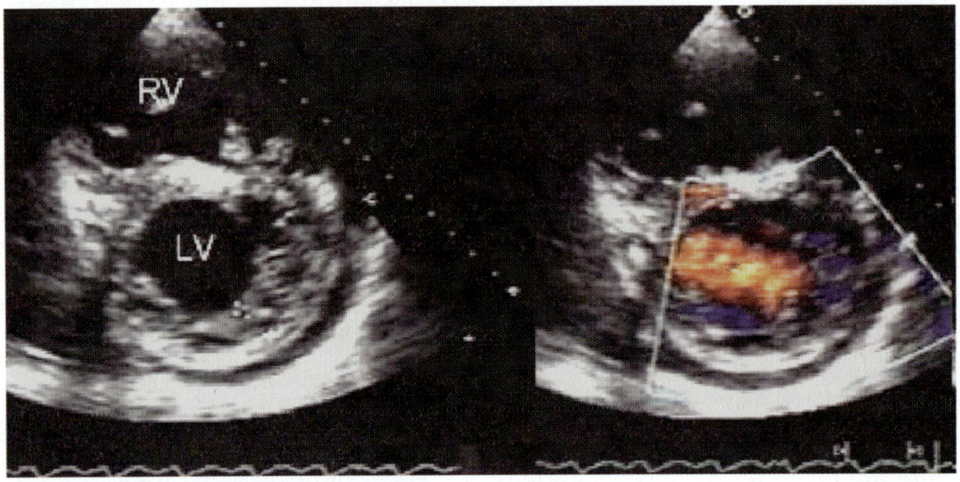

Fig. 28.58: *Short axis two dimensional parasternal and color Doppler images at the level of both ventricles show the noncompacted: compacted wall ratio and how the color enters the intertrabecular recesses in a case with noncompacted cardiomyopathy*

failure. Average 10-year survival rates for older children with HCM are > 90% although infants with HCM typically do far more poorly.

Living with Cardiomyopathy

The diagnosis of cardiomyopathy affects many areas of a child's life. The following sections outline the general approaches to living with cardiomyopathy. It is important that specific recommendations are developed by the team caring for the child with cardiomyopathy.

Physical Activity and Sports

Children with cardiomyopathy are not allowed to play competitive sports because of the possibility of a sudden collapse or increased heart failure. A competitive sport is an organized team activity for which training is required.

A child with the dilated subtype of rare cardiomyopathy (LVNC and ARVD) and no heart failure symptoms can be allowed to perform recreational athletic activities, also known as low-dynamic or low-static sports, in a non-competitive situation.

In milder cases of cardiomyopathy, the child may even participate in gym class after careful discussions between the child, teacher, and parents to ensure that the level of activity does not cause overexertion (breathlessness, chest pain, excessive sweating). Children with the hypertrophic subtype of cardiomyopathy (i.e. mitochondrial) are prohibited from serious recreational sports because of the possibility of a sudden collapse and death. Specific activity recommendations should be individualized by the treating cardiologist.

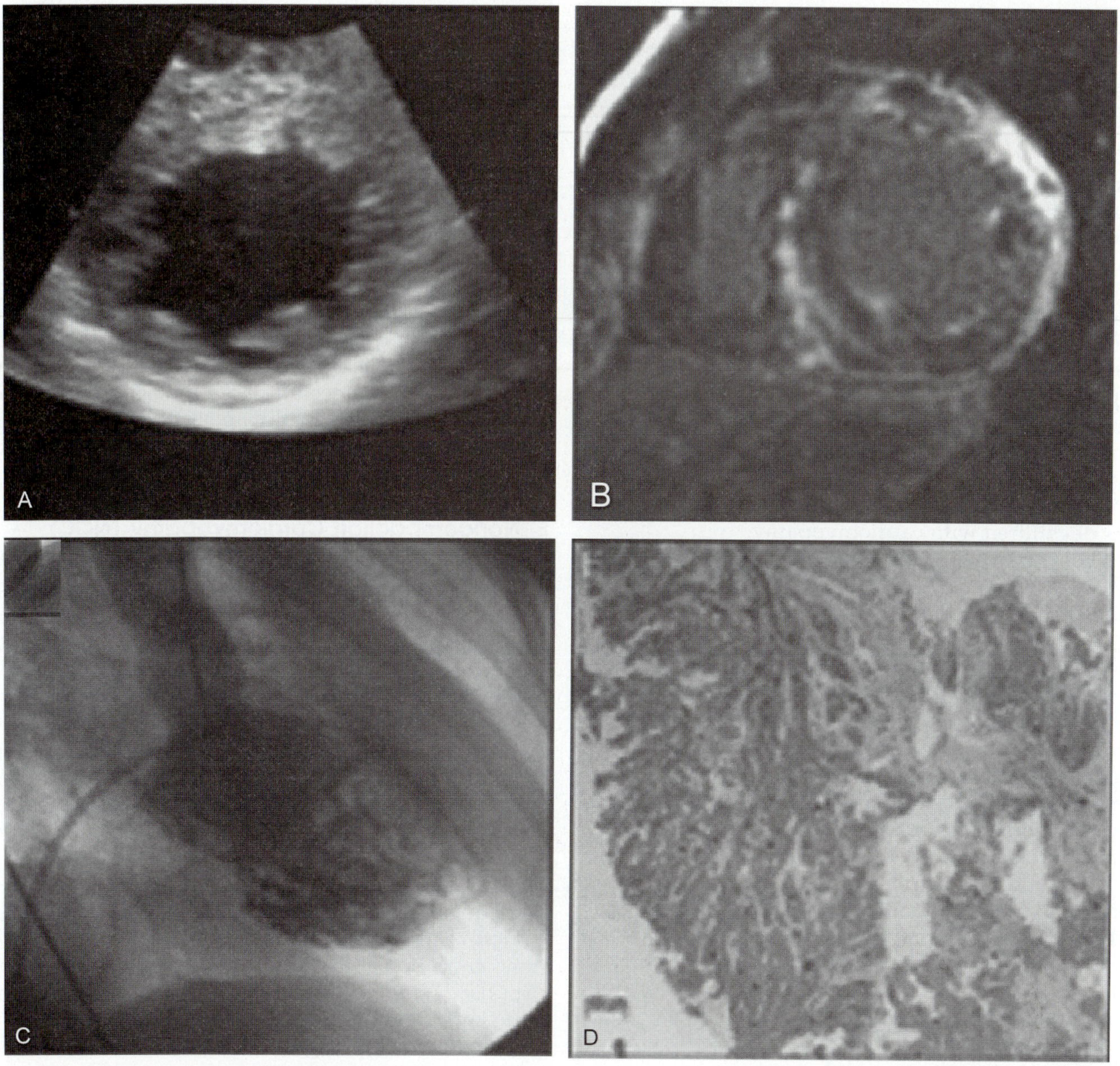

Fig. 28.59: *Noncompacted cardiomyopathy. (Panel A) Echocardiography at end-diastole of a mid-ventricular short-axis view showing deep intertrabecular recesses of LV myocardium. (Panel B) Delayed enhancement MRI acquired with diffuse myocardial hyper-enhancement occurring mainly in noncompacted areas. (Panel C) Left ventricular angiography, showing deep intertrabecular recesses. (Panel D) Histological specimen of a right ventricular biopsy which was taken from an area of hyperenhancement (haematoxylin and eosin stain); the disarray of myocardial architecture and infiltration of fibrotic tissue can be appreciated*

Attending School

The intellectual, psychological, and social benefits of attending school cannot be overestimated in the child with cardiomyopathy. Adjusting medication schedules so they do not interfere with school activities, discussing safe activity levels with school personnel, and providing tutoring to maintain academic performance are important interventions that can help a child to stay in school and keep up with their peers. Often close communication between the parents, medical care team, and the school nurse can help to keep a child up to date in school mixing with Friends.

Every effort should be made to allow a child with cardiomyopathy to spend time with friends. The child should also be allowed to participate in recreational activities whenever possible. However, an effort should be made to avoid contact with those who are acutely ill with fever, even though many children with cardiomyopathy are able to tolerate upper respiratory tract illnesses (common colds) well.

Adjusting to having a chronic illness is stressful for the child and the family. The child's reaction to having cardiomyopathy often depends on the stage of the child's development. Discussions about the disease should be tailored to the specific concerns of the child. Child-life professionals and pediatric psychiatrists are important resources to help children cope, and their services are often available through the treating center.

Acceptance of Child by Family Members

The impact of a diagnosis of cardiomyopathy is felt throughout the child's immediate and extended family. It is important for parents and other caregivers to realize that they are not alone in feeling the weight of responsibility that comes with taking care of a child with a chronic illness. Anticipating and/or preventing the stress imposed by an illness is an important part of caring for the child and family and personnel at the cardiomyopathy center can help identify issues that can lead to increased stress.

Practical solutions to problems giving medications, keeping track of appointments, and maintaining normal family life can often be found through discussions with nurse clinicians, the social worker, psychiatrist, and other parents of children with cardiomyopathy.

Dietic Management

All children with cardiomyopathy should follow a healthy diet. Certain types of cardiomyopathy are associated with an inability to digest certain types of food, and in these cases, a special diet is developed in consultation with metabolic specialists. In children with the dilated subtype of cardiomyopathy and heart failure, a low salt diet is recommended to avoid fluid retention.

Some children with heart failure may not grow well. In these cases, a diet that increases calories is recommended. Children who are taking some medications may have low levels of magnesium or potassium and a diet that has a higher amount of one or both of these two electrolytes may be recommended. Some children with severe heart failure can retain extra body fluid, and it may be necessary to limit the amount that a child can drink to prevent fluid from accumulating in the lungs.

Health Maintenance

Routine pediatric care is important for children with cardiomyopathy. Regular well child visits and standard childhood immunizations should be performed. The influenza vaccine should be administered on a yearly basis. Children under age 2 year should receive Synagis for protection against respiratory syncytial virus. A medical alert bracelet is an important safety measure for children with cardiomyopathy. In the event of an emergency, these bracelets allow medical personnel to know details about a child's illness, especially if a family member is not available.

What Does the Future Hold for "Rare" Cardiomyopathies?

Much progress has been made in our ability to diagnose rare cardiomyopathies in both the clinical and molecular arenas. However, much additional research is needed in this field. Areas of research to be highlighted over the next decade include:

1. Better understanding of these rare cardiomyopathy as a disease process and the characteristics of the disease as they relate to outcome, which will lead to better management strategies.
2. Increased clinical trials which will lead to new drug development and more effective therapies.
3. Molecular identification of novel genetic mutations as well as more precise diagnostic genetic testing/screening which will result in more accurate diagnosis. It is the expectation of the medical community that the data derived from exploring these avenues of scientific research will translate into a clinician's ability to tailor medical therapy based on a given child's precise diagnosis. Achieving this goal over the next couple of decades will represent a large milestone in the field of pediatric cardiomyopathy and will, hopefully, improve the ongoing care and prognosis of children afflicted with these heart muscle diseases.

E. Noncompaction Cardiomyopathy (NCC)

Noncompaction cardiomyopathy (NCC), also called spongiform cardiomyopathy, is a rare congenital cardiomyopathy that affects both children and adults. It results from the failure of myocardial development during embryogenesis.

During development, the majority of the heart muscle is a sponge-like meshwork of interwoven myocardial fibers. As normal development progresses, these trabeculated structures undergo significant compaction that transforms them from spongy to solid. This processis particularly apparent in the ventricles, and particularly so in the left ventricle. Noncompaction cardiomyopathy results when there is failure of this process of compaction. Because the consequence of noncompaction is particularly evident in the left ventricle, the condition is also called left ventricular noncompaction. Other hypotheses and models have been proposed, none of which is as widely accepted as the noncompaction model.

Symptoms can range, however, are often a result of a poor pumping performance by the heart. The disease can be associated with other problems with the heart and the body.

Diagnosis

Trabeculation of the ventricles is normal, as are prominent, discrete muscular bundles greater than 2 mm. In noncompaction, there is excessively prominent trabeculations. Chin et al described echocardiographic method to distinguish noncompaction for normal trabeculation. They described a ratio of the distance from the trough and peak, of the trabeculations, to the epicardial surface. Noncompaction is diagnosed when the trabeculations are more than twice the thickness of the underlying ventricular wall (Figs 28.52–28.59).

Genetics

The American Heart Association's 2006 classification of cardiomyopathies considers noncompaction cardiomyo-

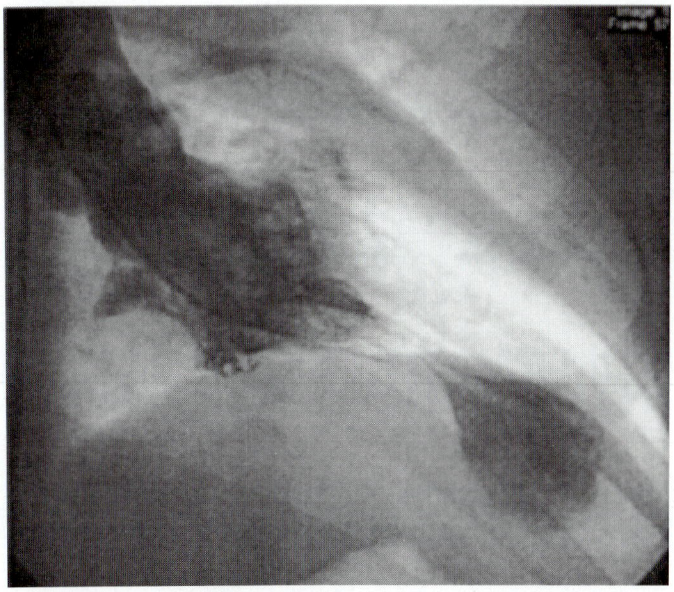

Fig. 28.60: *Left ventriculogram during systole displaying the characteristic apical ballooning with apical motionlessness in a patient with takotsubo cardiomyopathy*

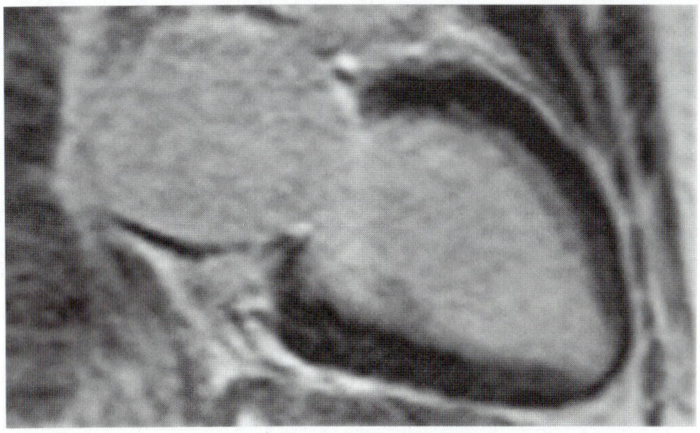

Fig. 28.61: *Takotsubo cardiomyopathy: no late enhancement. The modified Mayo Clinic criteria for diagnosis of takotsubo cardiomyopathy: transient hypokinesis, dyskinesis or akinesis of the left ventricular mid-segments with or without apical involvement. The regional wall motion abnormalities extend beyond a single epicardial vascular distribution. A stressful trigger is often present. Absence of obstructive coronary disease or angiographic evidence of acute plaque rupture. New electrocardiographic abnormalities either ST-segment elevation and/or T-wave inversion or modest elevation in cardiac troponin level. Absence of pheochromocytoma or myocarditis.*

pathy a genetic cardiomyopathy. Mutations in LDB3 (also known as "Cypher/ZASP") have been described in patients with the condition. There is recent information in which NCC has been seen in combination with 1q21.1 deletion syndrome.

Symptoms in NCC

Subjects symptoms from noncompaction cardiomyopathy range widely. It is possible to be diagnosed with the condition, yet not to suffer from any of the symptoms associated with heart disease. Likewise, it is possible to suffer from severe heart failure which even though the condition is present from birth, may only manifest itself later in life. Differences in symptoms between adults and children are also prevalent with adults more likely to suffer from heart failure and children from depression of systolic function.

Common symptoms associated with a reduced pumping performance of the heart include:

- Breathlessness
- Fatigue
- Swelling of the ankles
- Limited physical capacity and exercise intolerance.

Two conditions though that are more prevalent in noncompaction cardiomyopathy are: tachyarrhythmia which can lead to Sudden Cardiac Death and clotting of the blood in the heart.

Complications

The presence of NCC can also lead to other complications around the heart and elsewhere in the body. These are not necessarily common complications and no paper has yet commented on how frequently these complications occur with NCC as well.

- Cardiac
  - Abnormalities of the origin of the left coronary artery
  - Pulmonary atresia
  - Stenosis
  - Right or left ventricle obstruction
  - Hypoplastic left ventricle
  - Mitral regurgitation
- Neuromuscular (pertaining to both nerves and muscles)
  - Becker's muscular dystrophy
  - Mitochondrial myopathy
  - Polyneuropathy and metabolic myopathy
- Genetic related
  - Emery-Dreifuss muscular dystrophy
  - Myotubular cardiomyopathy
  - Barth syndrome

Prognosis in NCC

Due to noncompaction cardiomyopathy being a relatively new disease, its impact on human life expectancy is not very well understood. In a 2005 study which documented the long-term follow-up of 34 patients with NCC, 35% had died at the age of 42 +/– 40 months with a further 12% having to undergo a heart transplant due to heart failure. However, this study was based upon symptomatic patients referred to a tertiary care center, and so were suffering from more severe forms of NCC than might be found typically in the population. As NCC is a genetic disease, immediate family members are being tested as a precaution which is turning up more supposedly healthy people with NCC who are asymptomatic. The long-term prognosis for these people is currently unknown.

Management in NCC

These are similar to management programs for other types of cardiomyopathies which include the use of ACE

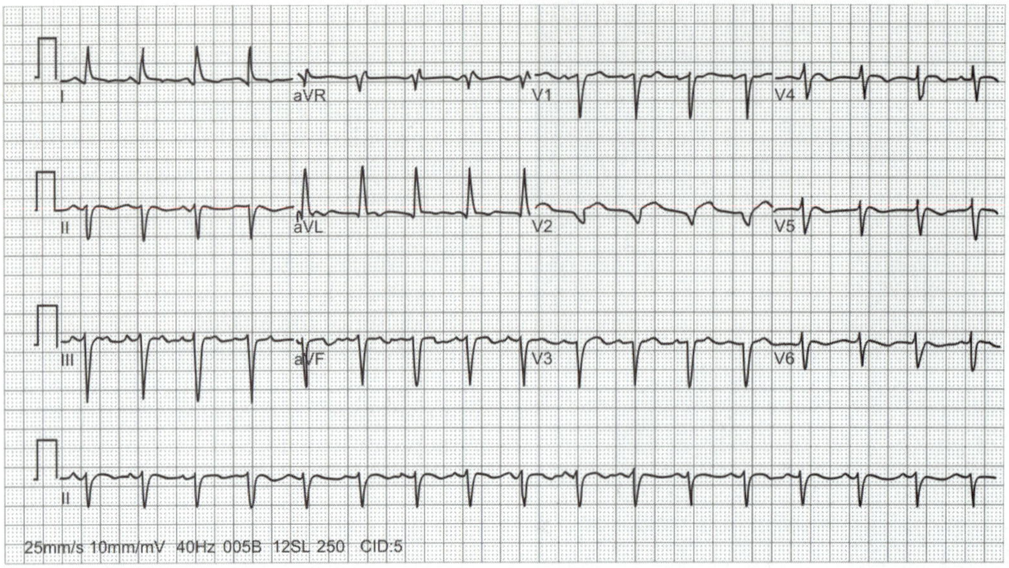

Fig. 28.62: *ECG showing sinus tachycardia and nonspecific ST and T wave changes from a patient with takotsubo cardiomyopathy*

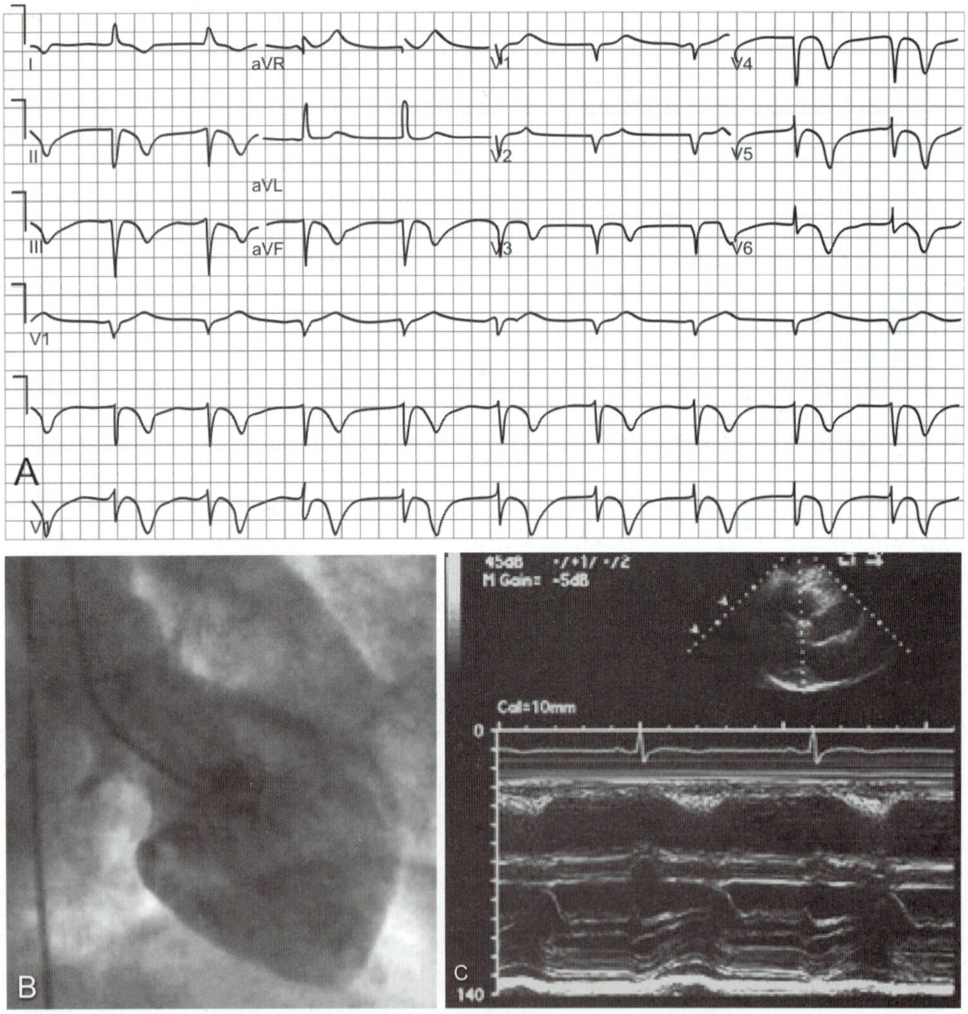

Fig. 28.63: *First episode of takotsubo cardiomyopathy. (A) ECG at time of admission consistent with ischemia. (B) Left ventriculography during first episode of takotsubo cardiomyopathy 6 years earlier at end-systolic phase showing similar features as the second presentation. (C) M-mode 2D echocardiography 4 years after the initial episode revealing normal function of the left ventricle and complete recovery*

inhibitors, beta-blockers and aspirin therapy to relieve the pressure on the heart, surgical options such as the installation of pacemaker is also an option for those thought to be at a high risk of arrhythmia problems.

In severe cases, where NCC has led to heart failure, with resulting surgical treatment including a heart valve operation, or a heart transplant.

F. Takotsubo Cardiomyopathy (Figs 28.60–28.63)

Takotsubo cardiomyopathy, also known as transient apical ballooning syndrome, apical ballooning cardiomyopathy, stress-induced cardiomyopathy, Gebrochenes-Herz-Syndrome, and simply stress cardiomyopathy, is a type of nonischemic cardiomyopathy in which there is a sudden temporary weakening of the myocardium (the muscle of the heart). Because this weakening can be triggered by emotional stress, such as the death of a loved one, a break-up, or constant anxiety, the condition is also known as broken heart syndrome. Stress cardiomyopathy is a well-recognized cause of acute heart failure, lethal ventricular arrhythmias, and ventricular rupture.

Clinical Presentation

The typical presentation of someone with takotsubo cardiomyopathy is a sudden onset of congestive heart failure associated with ECG changes suggestive of an anterior wall myocardial infarction. During the course of evaluation of the patient, a bulging out of the left ventricular apex with a hypercontractile base of the left ventricle is often noted. It is the hallmark bulging out of the apex of the heart with preserved function of the base that earned the syndrome its name "tako tsubo", or octopus trap in Japan, where it was first described. The cause appears to involve high circulating levels of catecholamines (mainly adrenaline/epinephrine). Evaluation of individuals with takotsubo cardiomyopathy typically includes a coronary angiogram, which will not reveal any significant blockages that would cause the left ventricular dysfunction. It provided that the individual survives their initial presentation, the left ventricular function improves within 2 months. Takotsubo cardiomyopathy is more commonly seen in post-menopausal women. Often there is a history of a recent severe emotional or physical stress.

Etiological Factors

The etiology of takotsubo cardiomyopathy is not fully understood, but several mechanisms have been proposed.

The exact etiology of takotsubo cardiomyopathy (TCM) is still unknown, but several theories have been proposed and are being investigated. These include multivessel coronary artery spasm, impaired cardiac microvascular function, impaired myocardial fatty acid metabolism, acute coronary syndrome with reperfusion injury, and endogenous catecholamine-induced myocardial stunning and microinfarction.

1. *Wrap around LAD:* The left anterior descending artery (LAD) supplies the anterior wall of the left ventricle in the majority of patients. If this artery also wraps around the apex of the heart, it may be responsible for blood supply to the apex and the inferior wall of the heart. Some researchers have noted a correlation between takotsubo and this type of LAD. Other researchers have shown that this anatomical variant is not common enough to explain takotsubo cardiomyopathy. This theory would also not explain documented variants where the midventricular walls or base of the heart does not contract (akinesis).
2. *Transient vasospasm:* Some of the original researchers of takotsubo suggested that multiple simultaneous spasms of coronary arteries could cause enough loss of blood flow to cause transient stunning of the myocardium. Other researchers have shown that vasospasm is much less common than initially thought. It has also been noted that when there are vasospasms, even in multiple arteries, that they do not correlate with the areas of myocardium that are not contracting.
3. *Microvascular dysfunction:* The theory gaining the most traction is that there is dysfunction of the coronary arteries at the level where they are no longer visible by coronary angiography. This could include microvascular vasospasm, however it may well also have some similarities to the diseases such as diabetes mellitus. In such disease conditions, the microvascular arteries fail to provide adequate oxygen to the myocardium.
4. *Mid-ventricular obstruction, apical stunning:* It has also been suggested that a mid-ventricular wall thickening with outflow obstruction is important in the pathophysiology.

It is likely that there are multiple factors at play which could include some amount of vasospasm, failure of the microvasculature, and an abnormal response to catecholamines (such as epinephrine and norepinephrine, released in response to stress).

Case series looking at large groups of patients report that some patients develop takotsubo cardiomyopathy after an emotional stress while others have a preceding clinical stressor (such as an asthma attack or sudden illness). Roughly one-third of patients have no preceding stressful event. A recent large case series from Europe found that takotsubo was slightly more frequent during the winter season. This may be related to two different possible/suspected pathophysiological causes: (1) coronary spasms of microvessels, which are more prevalent in cold weather, and (2) viral infections such as parvovirus B19 which occur more frequently during the winter season.

Diagnosis

Transient apical ballooning syndrome or takotsubo cardiomyopathy is found in 1.7–2.2% of patients presenting with acute coronary syndrome. While the original case reports reported on individuals in Japan, takotsubo cardiomyopathy has been noted more recently in the United States and Western Europe. It is likely that the syndrome went previously undiagnosed before it was described in detail in the Japanese literature.

The diagnosis of takotsubo cardiomyopathy may be difficult upon presentation. The ECG findings are often confused with those found during an acute anterior wall myocardial infarction. It classically mimics ST-segment elevation myocardial infarction, and is characterised by acute onset of transient ventricular apical wall motion abnormalities (ballooning) accompanied by chest pain, dyspnea, ST-segment elevation, T-wave inversion or QT-interval prolongation on ECG. Elevation of myocardial enzymes is moderate at worst and there is absence of significant coronary artery disease. The diagnosis is made by the pathognomonic wall motion abnormalities, in which the base of the left ventricle is contracting normally or is hyperkinetic while the remainder of the left ventricle is akinetic or dyskinetic. This is accompanied by the lack of significant coronary artery disease that would explain the wall motion abnormalities. Although, apical ballooning has been classically described as the angiographic manifestation of takotsubo, it has been shown that left ventricular dysfunction in this syndrome includes not only the classic apical ballooning, but also different angiographic morphologies such as mid-ventricular ballooning and rarely local ballooning of other segments (Figs 28.60 to 28.63).

The ballooning patterns were classified by Shimizu et al as takotsubo type for apical akinesia and basal hyper-kinesia, reverse takotsubo for basal akinesia and apical hyperkinesia, mid-ventricular type for mid-ventricular ballooning accompanied by basal and apical hyperkinesia and localised type for any other segmental left ventricular ballooning with clinical characteristics of takotsubo-like left ventricular dysfunction.

Prognosis

Despite the grave initial presentation in some of the patients, most of the patients survive the initial acute event, with a very low rate of in-hospital mortality or complications. The patients are expecting a favorable outcome once recovering from the acute stage of the syndrome, and the long-term prognosis is excellent. Even when ventricular systolic function is heavily compromised at presentation, it typically improves within the first few days and normalises within the first few months. Although infrequent, recurrence of the syndrome has been reported and seems to be associated with the nature of the trigger.

Treatment

The treatment of takotsubo cardiomyopathy is generally supportive in nature. Although patients with takotsubo heart disease may be hypotensive, treatment with inotropes will usually exacerbate the disease. Since the disease is due to a high catecholamine state, patients should not be given inotropes. Treatment recommendations include intra-aortic balloon pump, fluids, and negative inotropes such as beta-blockers or calcium channel blockers. In many individuals, left ventricular function normalizes within 2 months. Aspirin and other heart drugs also appear to help in the treatment of this disease, even in extreme cases.

BIBLIOGRAPHY

1. Hare JM. The dilated, restrictive, and infiltrative cardiomyopathies. In: Bonow RO, Mann DL, Zipes DP, Libby P, eds. Braunwald's Heart Disease: A Textbook of Cardiovascular Medicine. 9th ed. Philadelphia, Pa: Saunders Elsevier; 2011:chap 68.
2. Wexler RK, Elton T, Pleister A, Feldman D. Cardiomyopathy: An overview. Am Fam Physician. 2009;79:778-784. Bernstein D. Diseases of the myocardium. In: Kliegman RM, Behrman RE, Jenson HB, Stanton BF, eds. Nelson Textbook of Pediatrics. 18th ed. Philadelphia, Pa: Saunders Elsevier; 2007:chap 439.
3. Maron BJ. Hypertrophic cardiomyopathy. Zipes DP, Libby P, Bonow RO, Braunwald E, eds.Braunwald's Heart Disease: A Textbook of Cardiovascular Medicine. 8th ed. St. Louis, Mo: WB Saunders; 2007:chap 65.
4. Wexler RK, Elton T, Pleister A, Feldman D. Cardiomyopathy: An overview. Am Fam Physician. 2009;79:778-784.
5. Bernstein D. Diseases of the myocardium. In: Kliegman RM, Behrman RE, Jenson HB, Stanton BF, eds. Nelson Textbook of Pediatrics. 18th ed. Philadelphia, Pa: Saunders Elsevier;2007:chap 439.
6. Morrow DA, Boden WE. Stable ischemic heart disease. In: Bonow RO, Mann DL, Zipes DP, Libby P, eds. Braunwald's Heart Disease: A Textbook of Cardiovascular Medicine. 9th ed. Philadelphia, Pa; Saunders Elsevier;2011:chap 57.
7. Hare JM. The dilated, restrictive, and infiltrative cardiomyopathies. In: Libby P, Bonow RO, Mann DL, Zipes DP. Braunwald's Heart Disease: A Textbook of Cardiovascular Medicine. 8th ed. Philadelphia, Pa: Saunders Elsevier; 2007:chap 64.
8. Wexler RK, Elton T, Pleister A, Feldman D. Cardiomyopathy: An overview. Am Fam Physician. 2009;79:778-784.
9. Bernstein D. Diseases of the myocardium. In: Kliegman RM, Behrman RE, Jenson HB, Stanton BF, eds. Nelson Text
10. Behrman RE, Jenson HB, Stanton BF, eds. Nelson Textbook of Pediatrics. 18th ed. Philadelphia, Pa: Saunders Elsevier; 2007:chap 439.
11. Pignatelli RH, McMahon CJ, Dreyer WJ, et al. "Clinical characterization of left ventricular noncompaction in children: a relatively common form of cardiomyopathy". Circulation 2003; 108 (21): 2672–8.
12. Espinola-Zavaleta, Nilda.; Soto, Elena.; Castellanos, Luis Munoz; Játiva-Chávez, Silvio; Keirns, Candace. (2006). "Non-compacted Cardiomyopathy: Clinical-Echocardiographic Study". Cardiovasc Ultrasound 4 (1): 35. doi:10.1186/1476-7120-4-35.
13. Oechslin, Erwin; Jenni, Rolf (2005)). Non-compaction of the Left Ventricular Myocardium - From Clinical Observation to the Discovery of a New Disease. Archived from the original on 2007-09-29.
14. Engberding R, Bender F: Identification of a rare congenital anomaly of the myocardium by two-dimensional echocardiography: Persistence of isolated myocardial sinusoids. Am J Cardiol 1984 Jun 1;53(11):1733–4.
15. Chin TK, Perloff JK, Williams RG, et al: Isolated noncompaction of left ventricular myocardium. A study of eight cases. Circulation 1990 Aug;82(2):507–13.
16. Maron, Barry.; Towbin, Jeffrey.; Thiene, Gaetano; Antzelevitch, Charles; Corrado, Domenico.; Arnett, D; Moss,

AJ; Seidman, CE et al. "Contemporary Definitions and Classification of the Cardiomyopathies" (webpage). American Heart Association Journals (American Heart Association) 2006; 113 (14): 1807.

17. Vatta M, Mohapatra B, Jimenez S, et al. "Mutations in Cypher/ZASP in patients with dilated cardiomyopathy and left ventricular non-compaction". J. Am. Coll. Cardiol. 2003; 42 (11): 2014–27.
18. Weiford BC, Subbarao VD, Mulhern KM. "Noncompaction of the ventricular myocardium". Circulation 2004; 109 (24): 2965–71.
19. Lobo FV, Silver MD, Butany J, Heggtveit HA. Left ventricular involvement in right ventricular dysplasia/cardiomyopathy. Can J Cardiol. Nov 1999;15(11):1239–47.
20. Sen-Chowdhry S, Syrris P, Ward D, Asimaki A, Sevdalis E, McKenna WJ. Clinical and genetic characterization of families with arrhythmogenic right ventricular dysplasia/cardiomyopathy provides novel insights into patterns of disease expression. Circulation. Apr 3 2007;115(13):1710–20.
21. Burke AP, Farb A, Tashko G, Virmani R. Arrhythmogenic right ventricular cardiomyopathy and fatty replacement of the right ventricular myocardium: are they different diseases?. Circulation. Apr 28 1998;97(16):1571–80.
22. Basso C, Thiene G, Corrado D, Angelini A, Nava A, Valente M. Arrhythmogenic right ventricular cardiomyopathy. Dysplasia, dystrophy, or myocarditis?. Circulation. Sep 1 1996;94(5):983–91.
23. Bauce B, Basso C, Rampazzo A, et al. Clinical profile of four families with arrhythmogenic right ventricular cardiomyopathy caused by dominant desmoplakin mutations. Eur Heart J. Aug 2005;26(16):1666–75.
24. Dokuparti MV, Pamuru PR, Thakkar B, Tanjore RR, Nallari P. Etiopathogenesis of arrhythmogenic right ventricular cardiomyopathy. J Hum Genet. 2005;50(8):375–81.
25. Fidler LM, Wilson GJ, Liu F, Cui X, Scherer SW, Taylor GP, et al. Abnormal connexin43 in arrhythmogenic right ventricular cardiomyopathy caused by plakophilin-2 mutations. J Cell Mol Med. Oct 2009;13(10):4219–28.
26. Rampazzo A, Nava A, Malacrida S, et al. Mutation in human desmoplakin domain binding to plakoglobin causes a dominant form of arrhythmogenic right ventricular cardiomyopathy. Am J Hum Genet. Nov 2002;71(5):1200–6.
27. Syrris P, Ward D, Evans A, et al. Arrhythmogenic right ventricular dysplasia/cardiomyopathy associated with mutations in the desmosomal gene desmocollin-2. Am J Hum Genet. Nov 2006;79(5):978–84.
28. Francés RJ. Arrhythmogenic right ventricular dysplasia/cardiomyopathy. A review and update. Int J Cardiol. Jun 28 2006;110(3):279–87.
29. Thiene G, Corrado D, Basso C. Arrhythmogenic right ventricular cardiomyopathy/dysplasia. Orphanet J Rare Dis. Nov 14 2007;2:45.
30. Ferreira AC, Garcia SA, Pasquale MA, Canoniero MJ, Peter A. Arrhythmogenic right ventricular dysplasia in the elderly. Heart Dis. Nov-Dec 2003;5(6):393–6.
31. Richardson P, McKenna W, Bristow M, et al. Report of the 1995 World Health Organization/International Society and Federation of Cardiology Task Force on the Definition and Classification of cardiomyopathies. Circulation. Mar 1 1996;93(5):841–2.
32. Corrado D, Fontaine G, Marcus FI, et al. Arrhythmogenic right ventricular dysplasia/cardiomyopathy: need for an international registry. Study Group on Arrhythmogenic Right Ventricular Dysplasia/ Cardiomyopathy of the Working Groups on Myocardial and Pericardial Disease and Arrhythmias of the European Society of Cardiology and of the Scientific Council on Cardiomyopathies of the World Heart Federation. Circulation. Mar 21 2000;101(11):E101-6.
33. Hamid MS, Norman M, Quraishi A, et al. Prospective evaluation of relatives for familial arrhythmogenic right ventricular cardiomyopathy/dysplasia reveals a need to broaden diagnostic criteria. J Am Coll Cardiol. Oct 16 2002;40(8):1445–50.
34. Asimaki A, Tandri H, Huang H, et al. A new diagnostic test for arrhythmogenic right ventricular cardiomyopathy. N Engl J Med. Mar 12 2009;360(11):1075–84.
35. Burke AP, Robinson S, Radentz S, Smialek J, Virmani R. Sudden death in right ventricular dysplasia with minimal gross abnormalities. J Forensic Sci. Mar 1999;44(2):438–43.
36. Eshtehardi P, Koestner SC, Adorjan P, Windecker S, Meier B, Hess OM, Wahl A, Cook S. "Transient apical ballooning syndrome—clinical characteristics, ballooning pattern, and long-term follow-up in a Swiss population". Int. J. Cardiol. 2009; 135 (3): 370–5.
37. Bergman BR, Reynolds HR, Skolnick AH, Castillo D. "A case of apical ballooning cardiomyopathy associated with duloxetine". Ann Intern Med. 2008; 149 (3): 218–9.
38. Akashi YJ, Nef HM, Mollmann, H, Ueyama T. "Stress Cardiomyopathy". Annual Review of Medicine 2010; 61: 271–86.
39. Gianni, M, Dentali F et al. "Apical ballooning syndrome or takotsubo cardiomyopathy: a systematic review". European Heart Journal (Oxford University Press) 2006; 27 (13): 1523–1529.
40. Azzarelli S, Galassi AR, Amico F, Giacoppo M, Argentino V, Tomasello SD, Tamburino C, Fiscella A. "Clinical features of transient left ventricular apical ballooning". Am J Cardiol. 2006; 98 (9): 1273–6.
41. Ibáñez B, Navarro F, Farré J et al. "Tako-tsubo syndrome associated with a long course of the left anterior descending coronary artery along the apical diaphragmatic surface of the left ventricle." (in Spanish; Castilian) 2004.
42. Inoue, M, Shimizu M et al. "Differentiation between patients with takotsubo cardiomyopathy and those with anterior acute myocardial infarction". Circ J 2005;69 (1): 89–94.
43. Kurisu S, Sato H, Kawagoe T et al. "Tako-tsubo-like left ventricular dysfunction with ST-segment elevation: a novel cardiac syndrome mimicking acute myocardial infarction". American Heart Journal 2002; 143 (3): 448–55.
44. Tsuchihashi K; Ueshima K, Uchida T, Oh-mura N, Kimura K, Owa M, Yoshiyama M, Miyazaki S, Haze K, Ogawa H, Honda T, Hase M, Kai R, Morii I. Angina Pectoris-Myocardial Infarction Investigations in, Japan. "Transient left ventricular apical ballooning without coronary artery stenosis: a novel heart syndrome mimicking acute myocardial infarction. Angina Pectoris-Myocardial Infarction Investigations in Japan". J Am Coll Cardiol 2001; 38 (1): 11–8.12.
45. Desmet, WJ; Adriaenssens, BF, Dens, JA. "Apical ballooning of the left ventricle: first series in white patients". Heart (British Cardiac Society) 2003; 89 (9): 1027–31.

29 Peripheral Vascular Disease in Adolescents and Endovascular Therapy

Although peripheral vascular disease (PVD) generally manifests in adulthood, the process of atherosclerosis can begin in early childhood. For most children, atherosclerotic vascular changes are minor and can be minimized or even prevented with adherence to a healthy lifestyle. However, in some children, the process is accelerated because of the presence of identifiable risk factors (e.g. obesity and hypertension) and/or specific diseases that are associated with premature CVD (e.g. diabetes and Kawasaki disease).

Risk factors: Certain factors increase a child's risk of developing early atherosclerosis, including the following:

Overweight: Children and teenagers who are overweight or obese have a higher risk of developing high blood pressure, diabetes, and high cholesterol and lipids. In adults, these factors increase the risk for early atherosclerotic disease. Children who are overweight/obese are more likely to be overweight/obese as adults. In addition, there is increasing evidence that childhood obesity makes it more likely to have other risk factors that are associated with heart disease in early adulthood, such as high blood pressure or diabetes mellitus. The definitions of obesity and overweight for children and teenagers are described below.

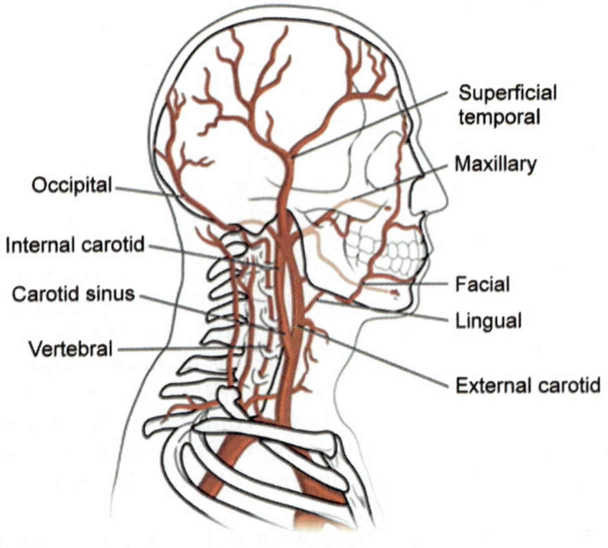

Fig. 29.1: *Illustration shows arteries of head and neck regions*

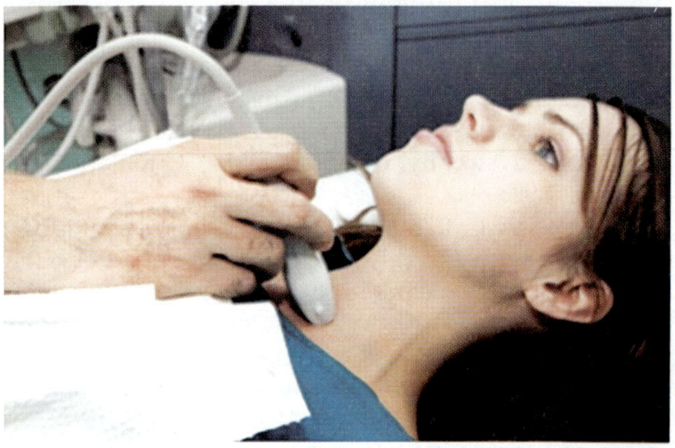

Fig. 29.2: *Ultrasound transducer kept over the carotid artery for obtaining record*

High blood pressure: Children and adolescents with high blood pressure are more likely to have high blood pressure as adults. High blood pressure in adulthood increases the risk of cardiovascular disease.

Family history of cardiovascular disease: Children whose parents or grandparents had a heart attack or stroke at an early age have twice the risk of developing cardiovascular disease. A family history of early-age cardiovascular disease is defined as a parent or grandparent who had a heart attack, a stroke, or peripheral vascular disease (blockages in the large blood vessels of the arms or legs) before the age of 56 years for men or 66 years for women.

Exposure to cigarette smoke: Smoking and exposure to smoking increases the risk of developing early cardiovascular disease. Children/teenagers who smoke

Table 29.1: *Risk factors for the development of peripheral arterial disease (PAD)*

Risk factor	*Feature of the risk factor*
Modifiable factor	
Smoking	Cigarette smoking is the most powerful risk factor for the development of PAD. It is dose-dependent and the risk declines within 6 months of quitting. A nonsmoker is 10 times less likely develop PAD than a smoker.
Blood lipid disorders	Plasma cholesterol levels of >5.2 mmol/L Increased plasma concentrations of low-density lipoprotein (LDL) cholesterol, low plasma concentrations of high-density lipoproteins (HDLs), and higher concentrations of plasma triglycerides all correlate with increased incidence of PAD. Familiar hypercholesteroplaemia (affecting 1:500 in UK) Familial combined hyperlipidaemia (affecting 1:250 in UK)
Diabetes mellitus (DM)	Type 2 DM increases risk of PAD by 1.5–4.0, due to the associated hypertension, hyperlipidaemia and altered vascular reactivity
Hypertension	Raised systolic blood pressure (BP) increases the risk of PAD and antherosclerosis by 4 due to endothelial injury caused by increased intra-arterial shear stresses at the blood-endothelium interface (raised systolic pressure are more predictive than raised diastolic pressures)
Obesity	Central obesity is an independent risk for PAD, but also predisposes to other risk factor for PAD, such as type 2 DM, hypertension
Homocysteine	Homocysteine is an amino acid that in high levels in associated with thromboembolism
Haemostatic variables	Increased levels of dotting factor VII, VIIIC and fibrinogen are associated with increased risk of atherosclerosis
Sedentary	Low levels of regular activity are associated with increased risk of PAD (higher levels of acitivtiy are associated with higher levels of plasma HDL-cholesterol and reduced blood pressures and facilitate the development of the collateral circulation)
Dietary	Low levels of antioxidant vitamins (vitamins C and E) and polyunsaturated fatty acids facilitate the formation of oxidized LDLs and thus predispose to the risk of
Type A behaviours (TABs)	People who tends to aggression, ambitiousness, restlessness, time urgency and high anxiety tend to an increased incidence of PAD, possibly due to increased levels of circulating catecholamines
Nonmodifiable or fixed factors	
Age and sex	Atherosclerosis is more common in males, and in postmenopausal women
Family history	Atherosclerosis shows familial patterns of incidence, possibly due to genetic factors and/or lifestyle choices and patterns
Early environment	Fetal origins hypothesis: adverse conditions in utero or infancy predispose to the risk of cardiovascular disease in later life (e.g. statistically, small-birth-weight babies have a higher incidence in adult life of hypertension, type 2 DM, altered plasma lipids, altered bone densities, altered stress responses, less elastic arteries, thicker-walled ventricles and "age" quicker)

themselves are likely to continue smoking into adulthood, thus increasing their risk of early cardiovascular disease.

Underlying medical problems: Certain underlying medical problems increase the risk of early cardiovascular disease. These include diabetes, chronic kidney disease, heart transplantation, Kawasaki disease with coronary aneurysms, and treatment for cancer during childhood. Children with these problems are treated especially vigorously with lifestyle changes and sometimes medications to lower their risk.

Peripheral arterial disease (PAD) involving the lower extremities is presumably a disease of the elderly. The awareness of PAD in the general population, and in younger adults in particular, is low. Atherosclerosis is the major cause of lower limb ischemia in the young. Young adults with clinical manifestations of premature lower extremity atherosclerosis (PLEA) typically have multiple cardiovascular risk factors and the majority are smokers, with strong family history of cardiovascular disease, and typically have chronic symptoms of claudication at diagnosis. Frequently these symptoms are either not reported in a timely manner by the patients or are attributed to other, presumably more common causes of leg pain in the young. More than 70% of patients with PLEA have angiographic evidence of severe aortoiliac disease. The results of surgical revascularizations in young adults are inferior to those reported in older patients. Younger adults typically require multiple revascularizations with relatively high amputation rate. We conclude that PAD should be considered in adults with multiple risk factors regardless of their age if appropriate symptoms are present. There is

Table 29.2: *Fontaine classification of peripheral arterial disease (PAD)*

Stage	*Characteristic symptoms*
1.	Clinically symptom-free vascular occlusion
2.	Exercise-induced ischaemia causing intermittent claudication. No pain at rest
3.	Ischaemia at rest, causing rest pain
4.	Ulceration and ischaemic gangrene

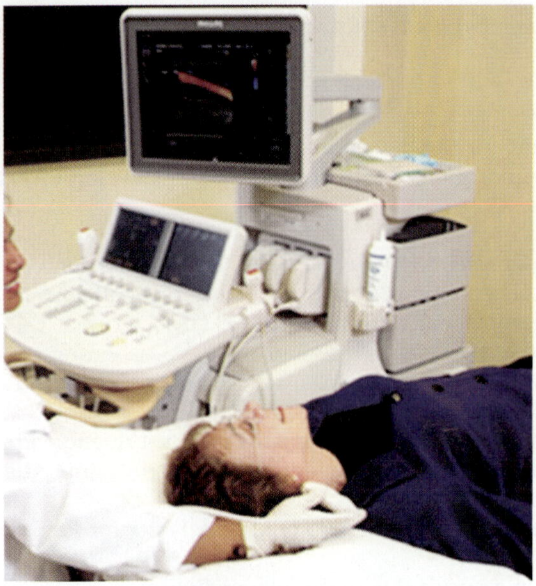

Fig. 29.3: *Carotid sonography is being conducted by a doctor on young patient with recurrent syncopal attacks*

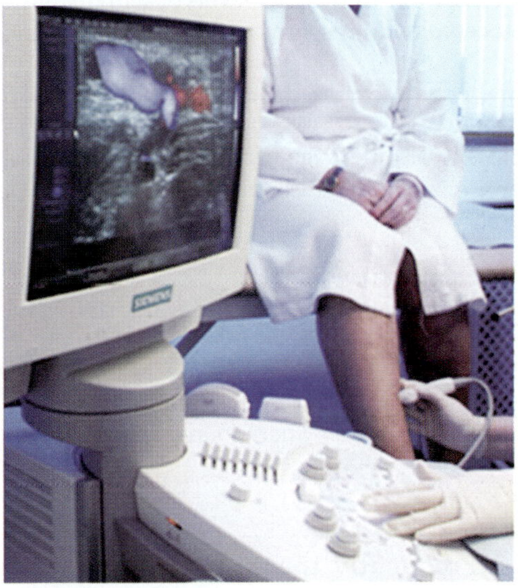

Fig. 29.4: *Doctor is examining peripheral venous system with Doppler technique*

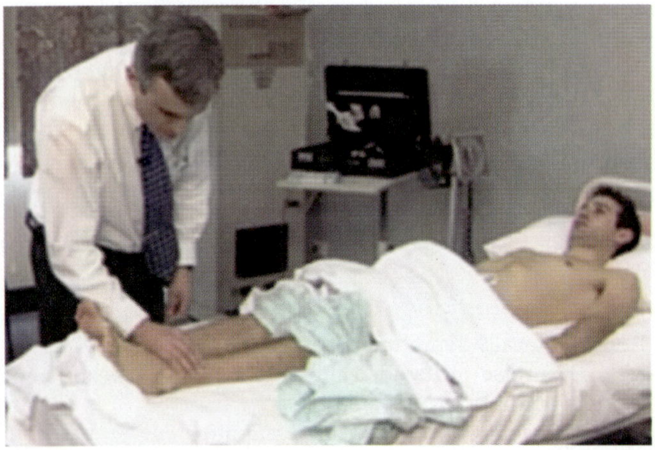

Fig. 29.5: *Physical examination of lower limb arteries by a doctor*

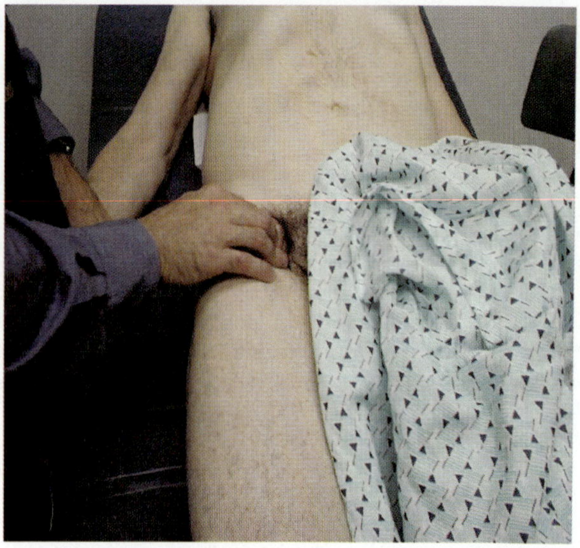

Fig. 29.6: *Palpation of right femoral artery in inguinal region*

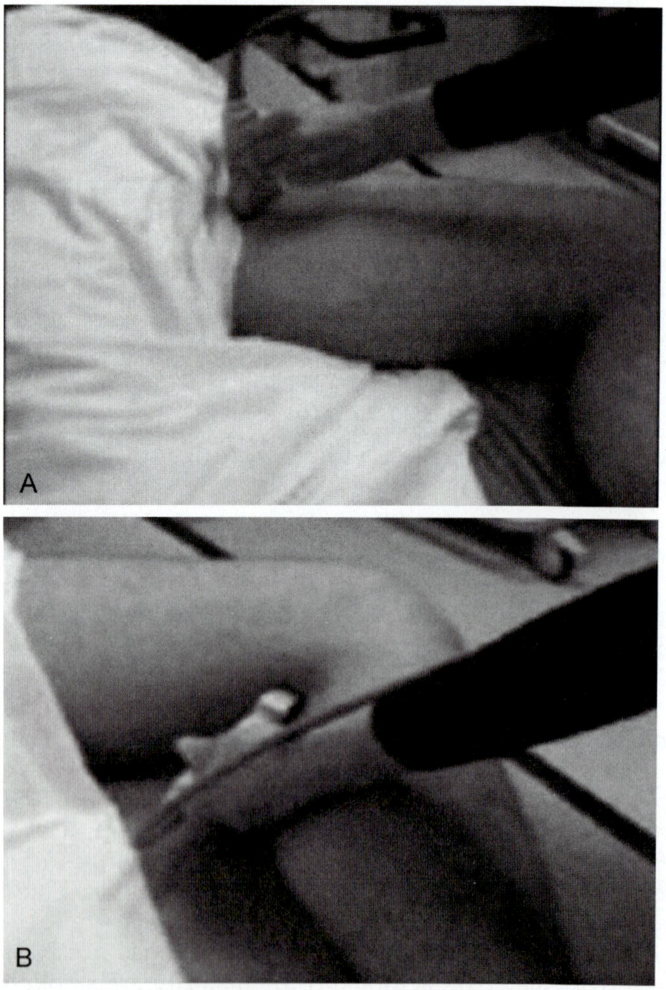

Fig. 29.7: *Patients position in obtaining US image of femoral vessel (A) and popliteal artery (B)*

Table 29.3: *Ankle-brachial index (ABI) results*

ABI number	*Diagnosis*	*What it means*
1.00–1.29	Normal	Your ABI is in the normal range and you are not likely to have PAD
0.91–0.99	Borderline	Your ABI is slightly lower than normal, but not low enough to diagnose PAD. Your doctor may want to measure your ABI again soon to make sure it is not getting worst, or measure your ABI after exercise.
0.41–0.90	Mild-to-moderate PAD	You have PAD. Working with your doctor to get your risk factors under control can prevent the disease from getting worse, and treatments are available to help to relieve your PAD symptoms.
0.40–less	Severe PAD	The blood flow in your legs is severely obstructed, and you may need immediate treatment to relieve your symptoms and prevent serious complications.

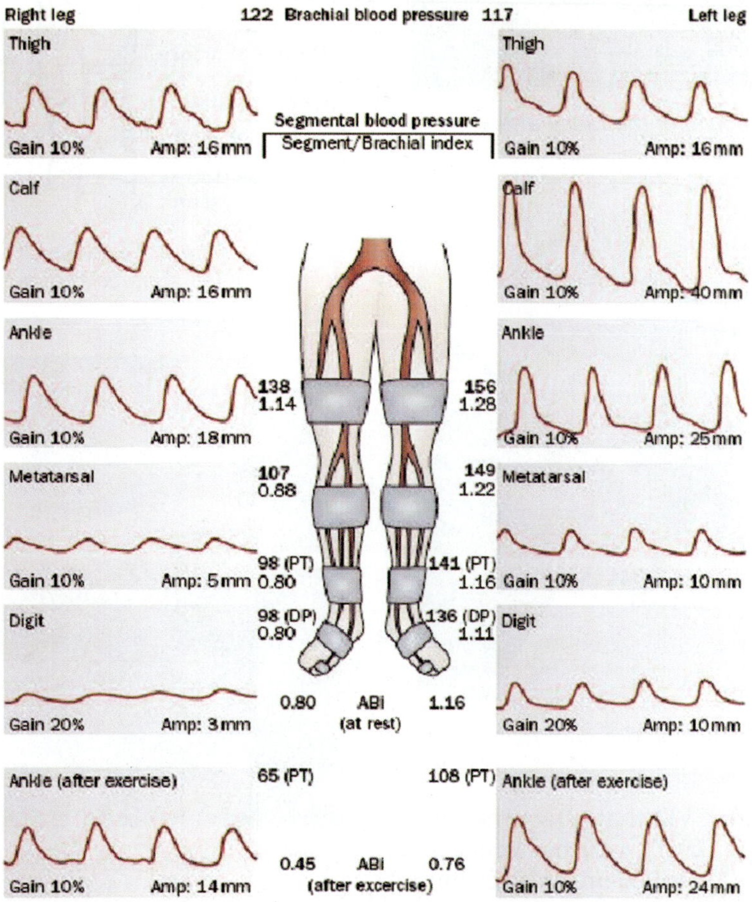

Fig. 29.8: *Segmental blood pressure, ABI, and PVRs at rest and after exercise. The tracings display PVRs taken at the thigh, calf, ankle, metatarsal and toe. The lowest diagram depicts an ankle PVR after exercise. The ABIs at rest are 0.80 on the right and 1.16 on the left. The patient walked on a treadmill for 3 min 20 sec. The exercise was ended because of right calf pain. The ABIs after exercise are 0.45 on the right and 0.76 on the left. The right ankle pressure is 98 mmHg at rest and decreases to 65 mmHg with exercise. The left ankle pressure is 141 mmHg at rest and decreases to 108 mmHg with exercise. The brachial artery systolic pressure is 122 mmHg at rest and augments to 143 mmHg with exercise. Note the pressure drop between the right thigh and the right calf, and the lack of augmentation of the right calf pulse volume waveform, which are consistent with right superficial femoral artery or popliteal artery disease. The left side was normal at rest but the decrease in ankle pressure after exercise indicates that there is peripheral artery disease in the left leg as well. The location of disease cannot be determined on the left. Abbreviations: ABI, ankle-brachial index; DP, dorsalis pedis; PT, posterior tibial; PVRs, pulse volume recordings*

a need for increased public health awareness for premature lower extremity atherosclerosis. Peripheral vascular disease (PVD) is a slow and progressive circulation disorder. It may involve disease in any of the blood vessels outside of the heart and diseases of the lymph vessels—the arteries, veins, or lymphatic vessels. Organs supplied by these vessels such as the brain, heart, and legs, may not receive adequate blood flow for ordinary function. However, the legs and feet are most commonly affected, thus the name peripheral vascular disease.

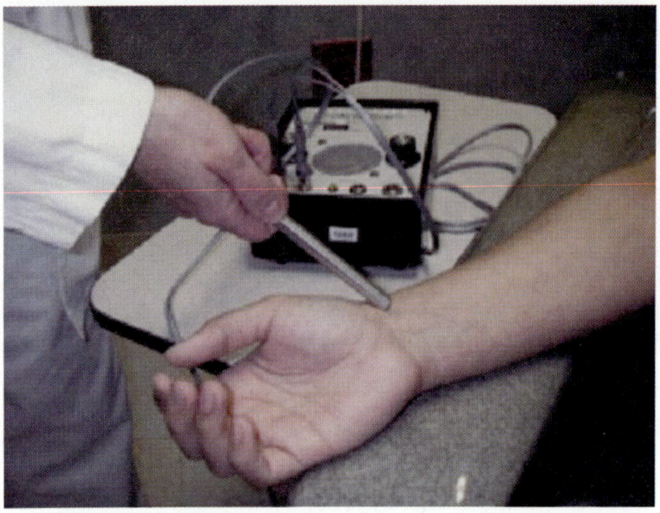

Fig. 29.9: *Doppler ultrasound of the radial artery*

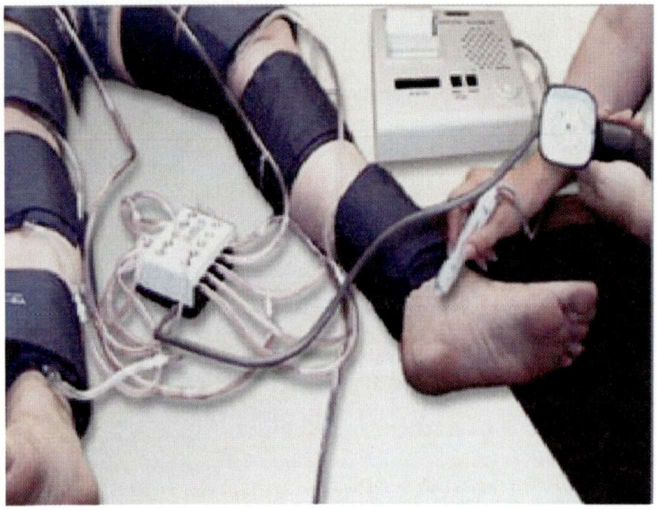

Fig. 29.10: *Measuring segmental blood pressure masurement*

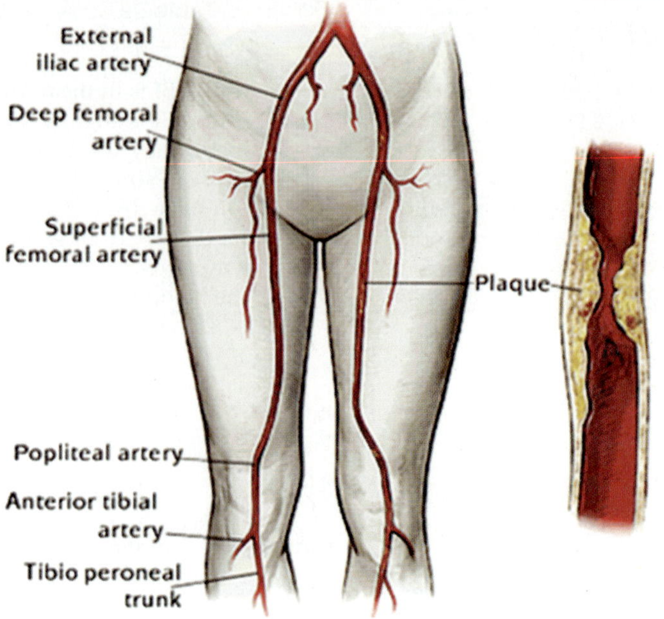

Fig. 29.11: *Different arteries of lower limbs with atherosclerotic occlusion of left superficial femoral artery*

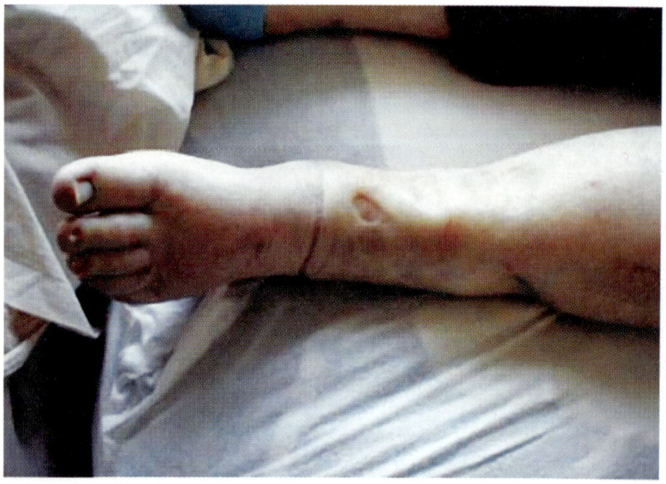

Fig. 29.12: *Massive edema. Note: Remaining imprint of fingers*

Conditions associated with PVD that affect the veins include deep vein thrombosis (DVT), varicose veins, and chronic venous insufficiency. Lymphedema is an example of PVD that affects the lymphatic vessels.

When PVD occurs in the arteries outside the heart, it may be referred to as peripheral arterial disease (PAD). However, the terms "peripheral vascular disease" and "peripheral arterial disease" are often used interchangeably. It's frequently found in people with coronary artery disease, because atherosclerosis, which causes coronary artery disease, is a widespread disease of the arteries.

Conditions associated with PAD may be occlusive (occurs because the artery becomes blocked in some manner) or functional (the artery either constricts due to a spasm or expands). Examples of occlusive PAD include peripheral arterial occlusion and Buerger's disease (thromboangiitis obliterans). Examples of functional PAD include Raynaud's disease, Raynaud's phenomenon, and acrocyanosis.

Pathophysiology and Risk Factors

PAD results from any disease causing stenosis or occlusion of the lower limb arteries with atherosclerosis disease being the most common etiology (Table 29.3).

Atherosclerosis is a complex process that involves endothelial dysfunction, lipid disturbances, platelet activation, thrombosis, oxidative stress, vascular smooth muscle activation, altered matrix metabolism, remodeling and genetic factors. Also, the role of inflammation in all stages of atherosclerosis development has been widely recognized. It usually affects arterial bifurcations due to the effect of flow disturbance leading to impaired endogenous atheroprotective mechanisms. Whilst this has allowed the identification of multiple potential circulating biomarkers, the complex and interwoven pathophysiology

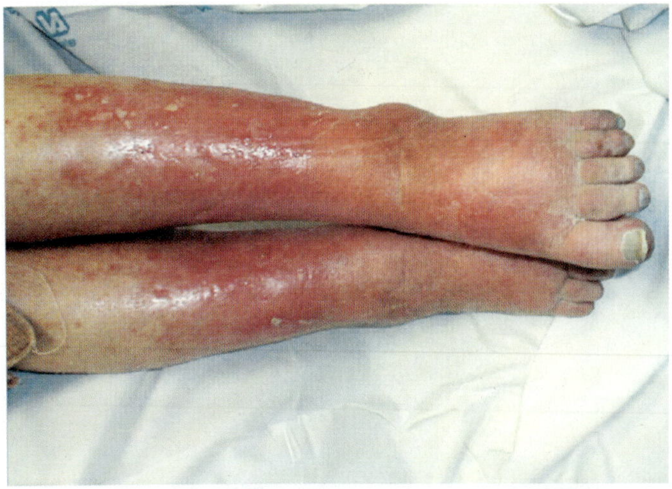

Fig. 29.13: *Swelling of both legs in patient with cellulitis*

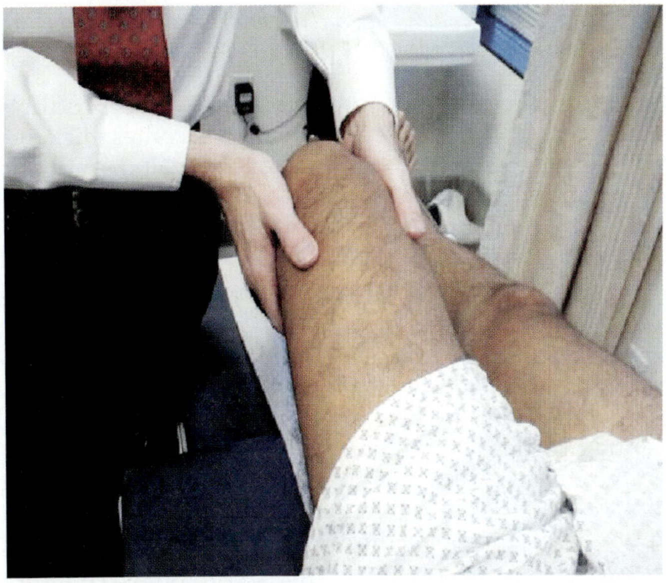

Fig. 29.14: *Palpation of left popliteal artery in popliteal fossa with slightly extended leg*

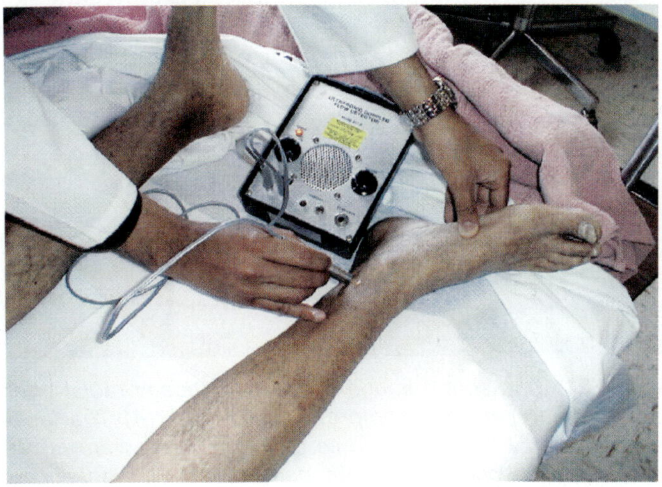

Fig. 29.15: *Swelling and discoloration of left leg in patient with venous stasis ulcer*

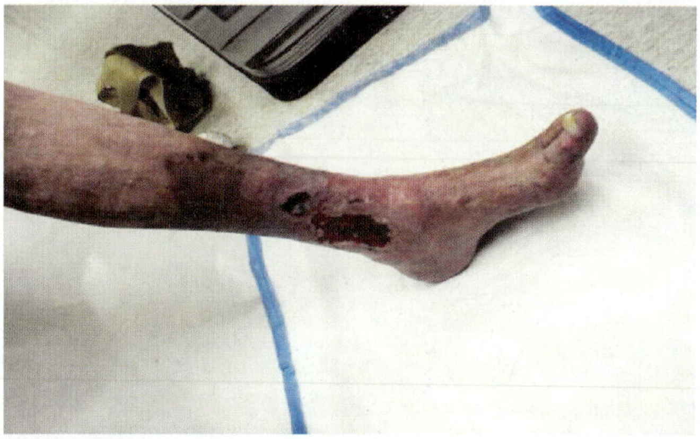

Fig. 29.16: *Swelling and discoloration of left leg in patient with venous stasis ulcer*

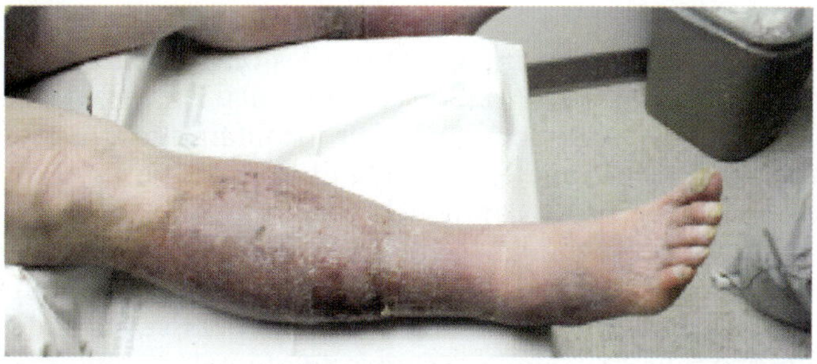

Fig. 29.17: *Swelling and discoloration of right leg in patient with venous insufficiency*

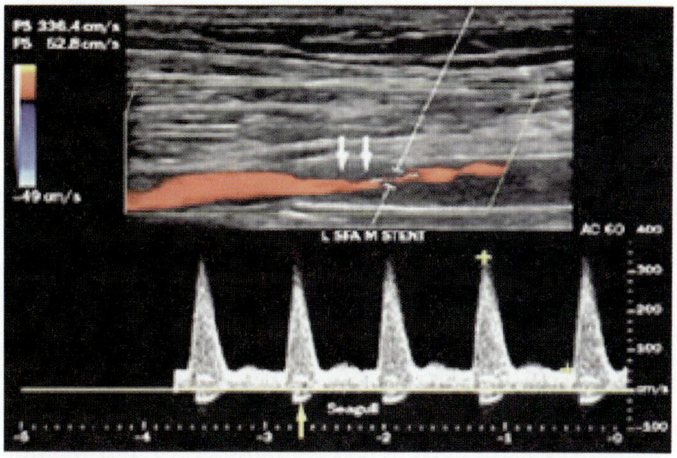

Fig. 29.18: *Duplex Ultrasonography of a left superficial femoral artery after stent implantation. Note that the flow velocity in the stent (peak systolic velocity 325 cm/s) is markedly increased and the color flow through the stent (in red) is reduced, indicating a severe stenosis. The spectral waveform also demonstrates the presence of a seagull bruit (yellow arrow), which also signifies that the stenosis is quite severe. The in-stent restenosis is caused by substantial intimal hyperplasia (white arrows)*

of plaque formation has limited the success of pharmacomodulating agents.

Atherosclerosis development commences in the teenage years as a result of endothelial dysfunction with the formation

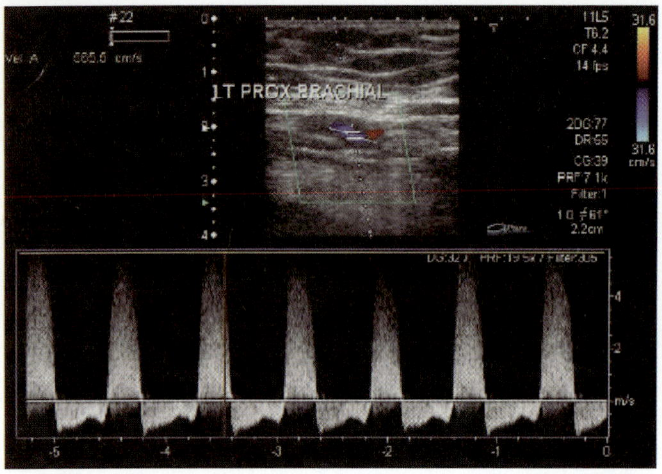

Fig. 29.19: *Doppler flow of brachial artery showing enhanced velocity in stenosis of this vessel*

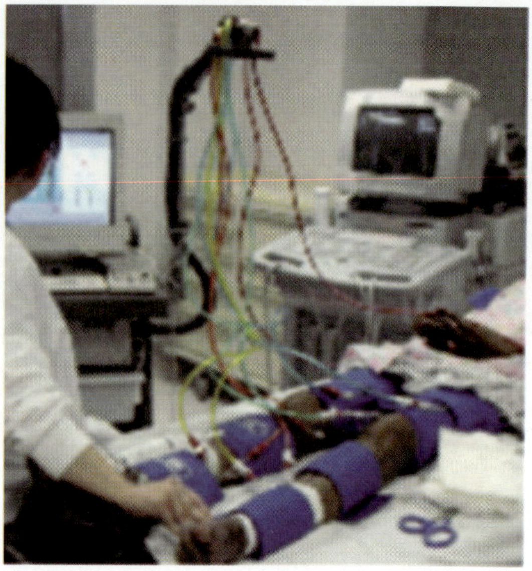

Fig. 29.20: *Pulse volume recording and segmental pressures measurements in patient with PVD*

of a fatty streak, an inflammatory lesion that affects the intima, causing the formation of foam cells. This progresses with time to development of a fibroproliferative atheroma and finally advanced lesion, containing a necrotic lipid core covered by a fibrous cap which may thin and rupture.

Risk factors for atherosclerosis include race; male gender; increasing age; smoking; diabetes mellitus; hypertension; dyslipidaemia; hypercoagulable and hyperviscous states; hyperhomocysteinaemia; systemic inflammatory conditions and chronic renal insufficiency.

Overall, PAD increases with smoking, African-American ethnicity, renal insufficiency, diabetes mellitus and hypercholesterolaemia, while it has been documented that developing critical limb ischaemia (CLI) is more likely with ankle-brachial index (ABI) <0.7, age over 65 years, smoking, and hypercholesterolaemia.

Etiological Factors in Peripheral Vascular Disease

PVD is often characterized by a narrowing of the vessels that carry blood to the leg and arm muscles. The most common cause is atherosclerosis (the buildup of plaque inside the artery wall). Plaque reduces the amount of blood flow to the limbs and decreases the oxygen and nutrients available to the tissue. Clots may form on the artery walls, further decreasing the inner size of the vessel and potentially blocking off major arteries.

Other causes of peripheral vascular disease may include trauma to the arms or legs, irregular anatomy of muscles or ligaments, or infection. People with coronary artery (arteries that supply blood to the heart muscle) disease are frequently found to also have peripheral vascular disease.

Conditions are Associated with Peripheral Vascular Disease

The term "peripheral vascular disease" encompasses several different conditions. Some of these conditions include, but are not limited to:

Atherosclerosis: Atherosclerosis is the build up of plaque inside the artery wall. Plaque is made up of deposits of fatty substances, cholesterol, cellular waste products, calcium and fibrin. The artery wall then becomes thickened and loses its elasticity. Symptoms may develop gradually, and may be few, as the plaque builds up in the artery. However, when a major artery is blocked, a heart attack, stroke, aneurysm, or blood clot may occur, depending on where the blockage occurs.

Buerger's disease (thromboangiitis obliterans): This is a chronic inflammatory disease in the peripheral arteries of the extremities leading to the development of clots in the small- and medium-sized arteries of the arms or legs and eventual blockage of the arteries. Buerger's disease most commonly occurs in men between ages 20 and 40 who smoke cigarettes. Symptoms include pain in the legs or feet, clammy cool skin, and a diminished sense of heat and cold.

Chronic venous insufficiency: This is a prolonged condition in which one or more veins don't adequately return blood from the lower extremities back to the heart due to damaged venous valves. Symptoms include discoloration of the skin and ankles, swelling of the legs, and feelings of dull, aching pain, heaviness, or cramping in the extremities.

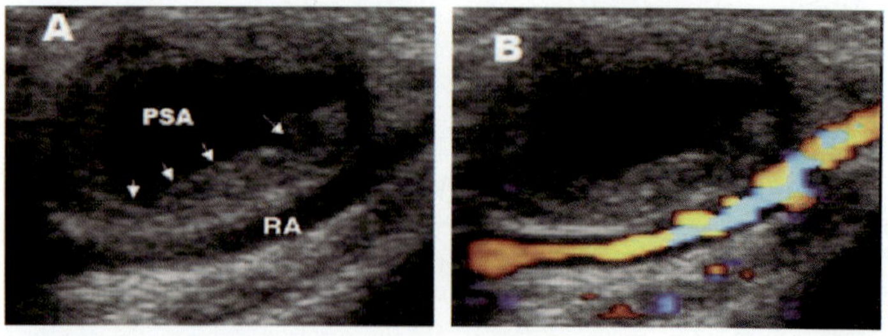

Fig. 29.21: *Ultrasound image of the thrombosed radial artery pseudoaneurysm after compression therapy. (A) The lesion presents partial thrombosis in its peripheral zone (arrows). (B) Color Doppler echocardiography demonstrates the absence of flow in the residual lesion, which does not communicate with the underlying radial artery*

Table 29.4: *Clinical tests used in the diagnosis of peripheral arterial disease (PAD)*

Test modality	*Diagnostic indicators*
Medical history	• Evidence of atherosclerosis, such as ischaemic heart disease, cerebrovascular disease • Risk of atherosclerosis, such as cigarette smoking, diabetes mellitus
Pulses in the lower limb	Popliteal, posterior tibial, dorsalis pedis and peroneal pulses • Pulse quality (bounding, full, normal, weak, absent) • Rate (beats/minute) • Regularity (regular, irregular, regularly irregular, irregularly irregular)
Presenting symptoms	• Cold, numb feet • Intermittent claudication • Rest pain • Painful ulceration
Ankle-brachial index (ABI)	• 0.9–1.1 = normal • 0.7–0.9 = PAD, some compromise of tissue viability • 0.5-0.7 = severe PAD, compromised tissue viability • <0.5 = threat of ischaemic gangrene/very poor tissue viability • >1.2 = calcification of tunica media of leg/foot artery, compromised tissue viability
Segmental systolic pressure	Serial measurement of systolic blood pressure along length of limb: • A sudden decrease indicates the location of the vascular obstruction
Venous filling time *Note:* This test is not valid if the patient has venous incompetence	The time it takes for veins to refill in a limb that has been drained of venous blood (with the patient supine, the leg is elevated to 45° for 1 minute, then the leg placed in a dependent position and the time taken for the dorsal foot veins to refill) • <15 seconds = normal • 20–30 seconds = moderate ischaemia • >40 seconds = severe ischaemia
Buerger's test	The observation of the change in skin colour in response to limb elevation and dependency (with the patient supine, the leg is elevated to 45° for 1 minute, then the leg is placed in a dependent position and the time taken for normal skin colour to return is noted) • <10 seconds = normal response • Patchy persistent rubor indicates limb ischaemia • Persistent pallor (>10 seconds) indicates limb ischaemia • Persistent cyanosis indicates limb ischaemia
Buerger's angle	The colour response of the sole of the foot to limb elevation (with the patient supine, the leg is elevated and the angle of limb elevation is noted when the skin of medial longitudinal arch shows pallor) • 60–70° = normal arterial supply to foot • < 45° = compromised arterial supply to foot • < 30° = severe compromised arterial supply to foot
Capillary refill time *Note:* This test is not valid if the patient has signs of current Raynaud's disease	The time taken for normal skin tone of a horizontal limb to return after the nail bed or digital pulp has been compressed by thumb pressure • <5 seconds = normal response • >5 seconds = some ischaemia • >15 seconds = marked ischaemia
Doppler sounds	• Triphasic = normal • Biphasic = normal/some loss of arterial elasticity • Monophasic = loss of arterial elasticity/arterial stenosis • Loud = high rate of blood flow • Quiet = slow rate of blood flow • No sound = no blood flow (proximal arterial occlusion)
Skin temperature *Note:* This test is not valid if the patient has signs of current Raynaud's disease	• ~ 31°C = normal foot skin temperature • <29°C = possible poor skin perfusion

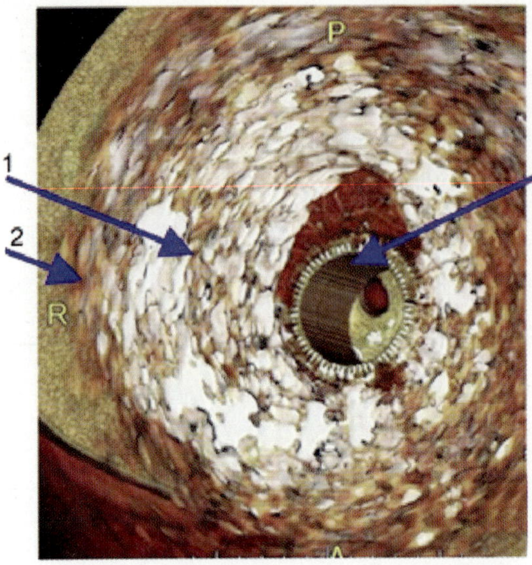

Fig. 29.22: *Sectional anatomical structures in superficial femoral artery. 1 = stent, 2 = artery and 3 = IUVS catheter*

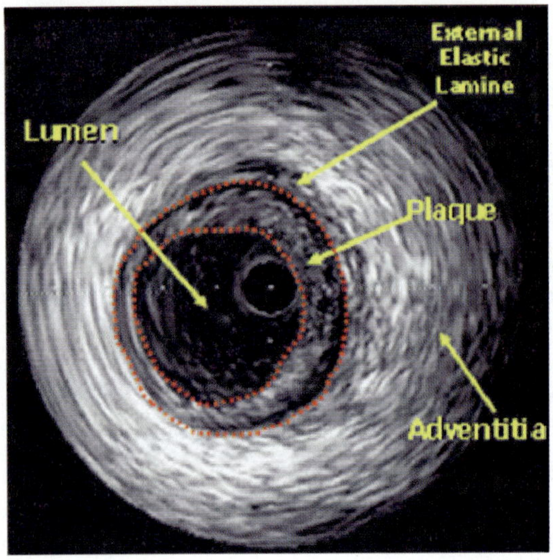

Fig. 29.23: *IUVS scan of an artery showing all the three layers and plaque inside two circles*

Deep vein thrombosis (DVT): DVT is a clot that occurs in a deep vein, and has the potential to dislodge, travel to the lungs, occlude a lung artery (pulmonary embolism), and cause a potentially life-threatening event. It is found most commonly in those who have undergone extended periods of inactivity, such as from sitting while traveling or prolonged bed rest after surgery. Symptoms may be absent or subtle, but include swelling and tenderness in the affected extremity, pain at rest and with compression, and raised vein pattern.

Raynaud's phenomenon: This is a condition in which the smallest arteries that bring blood to the fingers or toes constrict (go into spasm) when exposed to cold or as the result of emotional upset. Raynaud's most commonly occurs in women between ages 18 and 30. Symptoms include coldness, pain, and pallor (paleness) of the fingertips or toes.

Thrombophlebitis: Thrombophlebitis is a blood clot in an inflamed vein, most commonly in the legs, but it can also occur in the arms. The clot can either be close to the skin (superficial thrombophlebitis) or deep within a muscle (deep vein thrombosis). It may result from pooling of blood, venous wall injury, and altered blood coagulation. Symptoms in the affected extremity include swelling, pain, tenderness, redness and warmth.

Varicose veins: Dilated, twisted veins are caused by incompetent valves (valves that allow backward flow of blood) allowing blood to pool. It is most commonly found in the legs or lower trunk. Symptoms include bruising and sensations of burning or aching. Pregnancy, obesity, and extended periods of standing intensify the symptoms.

Risk Factors for Peripheral Vascular Disease

A risk factor is anything that may increase a person's chance of developing a disease. It may be an activity, diet, family history, or many other things. Risk factors for peripheral vascular disease include factors which can be changed or treated and factors that cannot be changed.

Risk factors that cannot be changed include:
- Age (especially older than age 50 year) (Table 29.5)
- History of heart disease
- Male gender
- Diabetes mellitus
- Postmenopausal women
- Family history of dyslipidemia (elevated lipids in the blood, such as cholesterol), hypertension, or peripheral vascular disease.

Risk factors that may be changed or treated include:
- Coronary artery disease
- Impaired glucose tolerance
- Dyslipidemia
- Hypertension (high blood pressure)
- Obesity
- Physical inactivity
- Smoking or use of tobacco products
- Those who smoke or have diabetes mellitus have the highest risk of complications from peripheral vascular disease because these risk factors also cause impaired blood flow.

Symptoms and Signs of Peripheral Vascular Disease?

Approximately half the people diagnosed with peripheral vascular disease are symptom free. For those experiencing symptoms, the most common first symptom is intermittent claudication in the calf (leg discomfort described as painful cramping that occurs with exercise and is relieved by rest). During rest, the muscles need less blood flow, so the pain disappears. It may occur in one or both legs depending on the location of the clogged or narrowed artery.

Other symptoms of peripheral vascular disease may include:
- Changes in the skin including decreased skin temperature, or thin, brittle shiny skin on the legs and feet

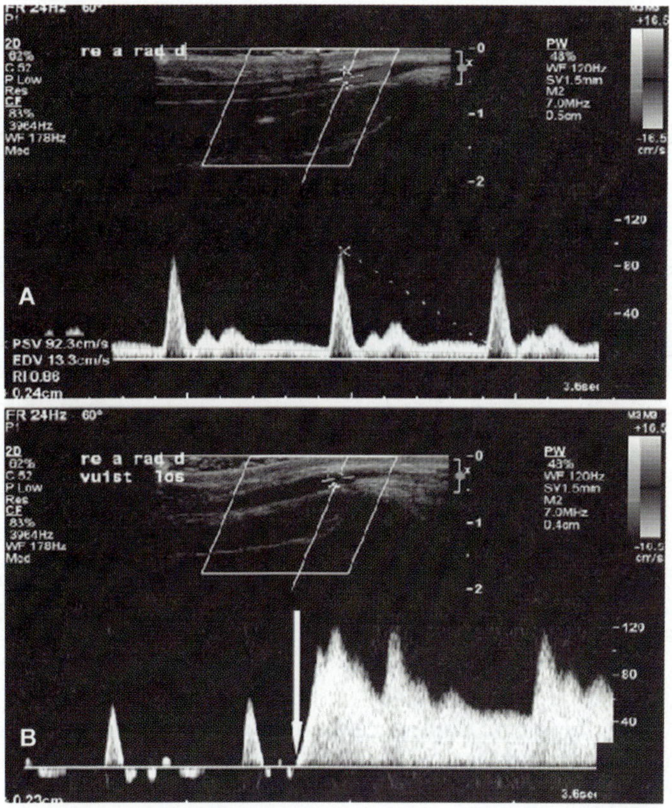

Fig. 29.24: *Duplex ultrasound assessment of radial artery flows at rest (A), during fist clenching (B) and during hyperemia after the fist clench has been released in a healthy volunteer. The arrow indicates the moment of fist clench release. Absence or diminished change in radial artery flow is associated with a higher risk of vascular access early failure and nonmaturation*

- Diminished pulses in the legs and the feet
- Gangrene (dead tissue due to lack of blood flow)
- Hair loss on the legs
- Impotence
- Nonhealing wounds over pressure points, such as heels or ankles
- Numbness, weakness, or heaviness in muscles
- Pain (described as burning or aching) at rest, commonly in the toes and at night while lying flat
- Pallor (paleness) when the legs are elevated
- Reddish-blue discoloration of the extremities
- Restricted mobility
- Severe pain
- Thickened, opaque toenails
- The symptoms of peripheral vascular disease may resemble other conditions. Consult your physician for a diagnosis.

Diagnosis of Peripheral Vascular Disease (Table 29.4)

In addition to a complete medical history and physical examination, diagnostic procedures for peripheral vascular disease may include any, or a combination, of the following:

Angiogram: This is an X-ray of the arteries and veins to detect blockage or narrowing of the vessels. This procedure involves inserting a thin, flexible tube into an artery in the leg and injecting a contrast dye. The contrast dye makes the arteries and veins visible on the X-ray (Figs 29.23, 29.29, 29.30, 29.33, 29.34 and 29.35).

Ankle-brachial index (ABI): An ABI is a comparison of the blood pressure in the ankle with the blood pressure in the arm using a regular blood pressure cuff and a Doppler ultrasound device. To determine the ABI, the systolic blood pressure (the top number of the blood pressure measurement) of the ankle is divided by the systolic blood pressure of the arm (Fig. 29.9 and Table 29.2).

Blood lipid profile: This blood test measures the levels of each type of fat in your blood: total cholesterol, LDL cholesterol, HDL cholesterol, triglycerides, and others.

Doppler ultrasound flow studies: This uses high-frequency sound waves and a computer to create images of blood

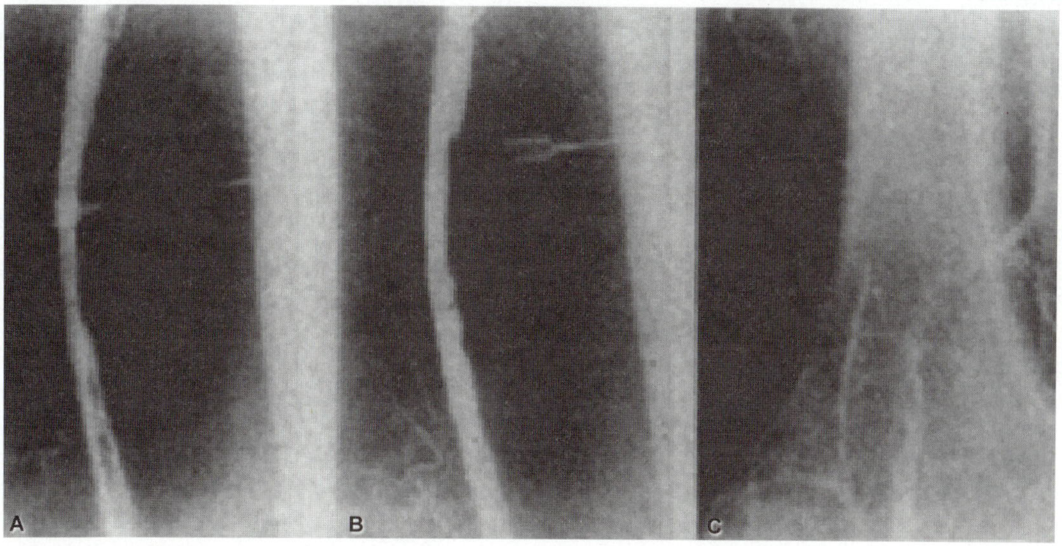

Fig. 29.25: *(A) Filling defect probably representing thrombus that partly occludes the superficial femoral artery; (B) disappearance of the filling defect after balloon angioplasty; (C) laser evidence of distal thrombus migration, resulting in occlusion of the trifurcation vessels*

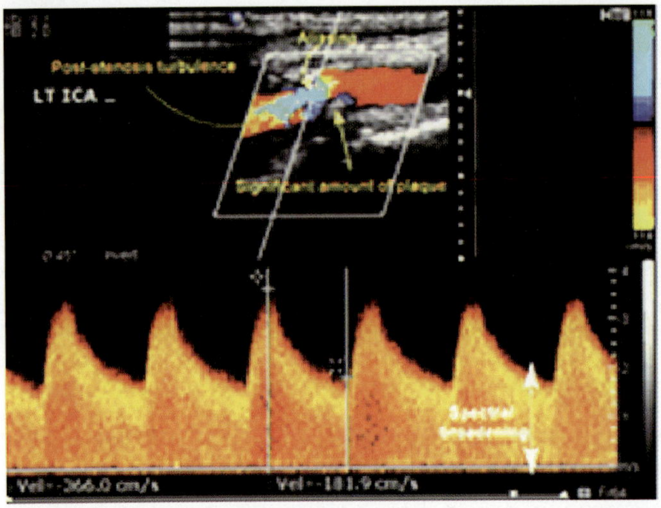

Fig. 29.26: *Severe stenosis (70% to near occlusion) of the ICA. Duplex US image of the left ICA shows a high PSV (366 cm/sec), a significant amount of visible plaque, the presence of aliasing despite a high color scale setting (114 cm/sec), color flow turbulence immediately distal to the stenotic segment, broadening of the PW Doppler spectrum, and a high end-diastolic velocity (182 cm/sec)*

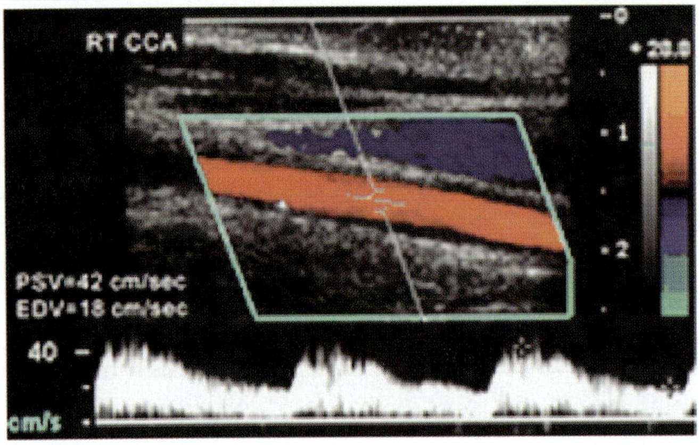

Fig. 29.27: *Severe stenosis of the innominate artery. PW Doppler spectral image of the right CCA shows a tardus-parvus waveform, which is suggestive of a severe stenosis proximal to the point of sampling*

vessels, tissues and organs. Doppler technique is used to measure and assess the flow of blood. Faintness or absence of sound may indicate an obstruction in the blood flow (Figs 29.1–29.5, 29.15–29.22).

Magnetic resonance angiography (MRA): This noninvasive diagnostic procedure uses a combination of a large magnet, radiofrequencies, and a computer to produce detailed images of organs and structures within the body. An MRA is often used to examine the heart and other soft tissues and to assess blood flow.

Treadmill exercise test: This test is given while a patient walks on a treadmill to monitor the heart during exercise.

Photoplethysmography (PPG): This examination is comparable to the ankle-brachial index except that it uses

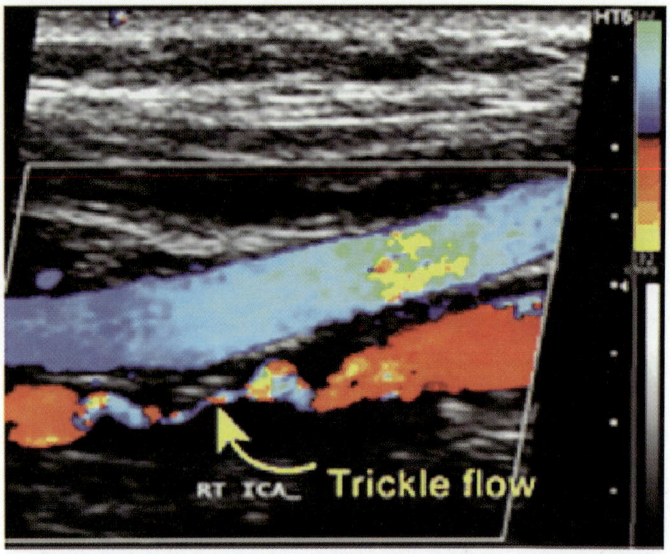

Fig. 29.28: *Trickle flow in the ICA. Color Doppler image shows a narrow patent channel (the string sign) in the right ICA. This finding is suggestive of near occlusion of the ICA*

a very tiny blood pressure cuff around the toe and a PPG sensor (infrared light to evaluate blood flow near the surface of the skin) to record waveforms and blood pressure measurements. These measurements are then compared to the systolic blood pressure in the arm.

Pulse volume recording (PVR) waveform analysis: This technique is used to calculate blood volume changes in the legs using a recording device that displays the results as a waveform.

Reactive hyperemia test: This test is similar to an ABI or a treadmill test but used for people who are unable to walk on a treadmill. While a person is lying on his or her back, comparative blood pressure measurements are taken on the thighs and ankles to determine any decrease between the two sites.

Segmental blood pressure measurements: This is a means of comparing blood pressure measurements using a Doppler device in the upper thigh, above and below the knee, at the ankle, and on the arm to determine any constriction in blood flow (Fig. 29.9).

Treatment for Peripheral Vascular Disease

There are two main goals for treatment of peripheral artery/vascular disease: control the symptoms and halt the progression of the disease to lower the risk for heart attack, stroke, and other complications.

Specific treatment will be determined by your physician based on:

- Age, overall health, and medical history
- Extent of the disease
- Signs and symptoms
- Tolerance for specific medications, procedures, or therapies
- Expectations for the course of the disease

Table 29.5: *Nonatherosclerotic causes of PAD*

Peripheral embolic
Aneurysm thrombosis or thromboembolism (aortic, popliteal)
Arteritis
Takayasu's disease
Thromboangiitis obliterans (Buerger's disease)
Giant cell arteritis
Polyarteritis nodosa
Fibromuscular dysplasia
Prior trauma or irradiation injury
Aortic coarctation
Endofibrosis of the external iliac artery (iliac artery syndrome in cryclists)
Primary vascular tumours
Pseudoxanthoma elasticus
Young patients
Adventitial cyst of the popliteal artery
Popliteal entrapment
Persistent sciatic artery

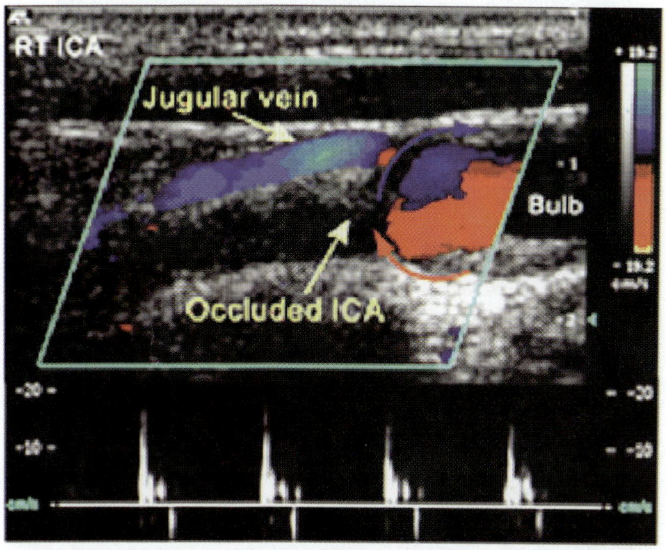

Fig. 29.29: *Thud flow. Color Doppler image of the right ICA and carotid bulb shows no flow in the ICA lumen and reversed flow in the bulb at the point of occlusion*

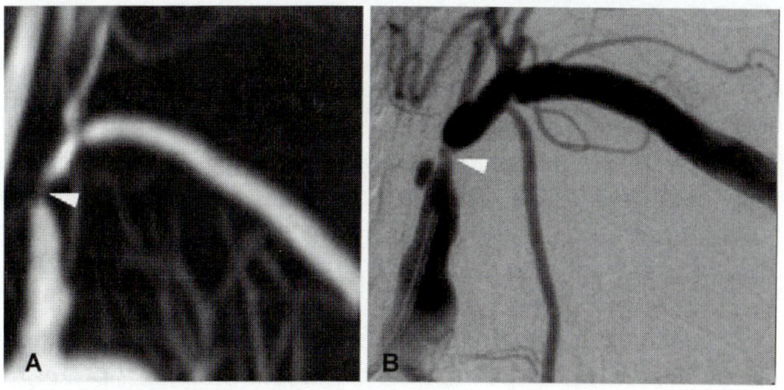

Fig. 29.30: *Typical example of a subclavian artery stenosis, initially detected by CE-MRA (A) and confirmed by DSA (B).The arrow indicates the location of the stenosis*

Treatment may include:

Lifestyle modifications to control risk factors including regular exercise, proper nutrition, and smoking cessation.

Aggressive treatment of existing conditions that may aggravate PVD, such as diabetes, hypertension and hyperlipidemia (elevated blood cholesterol).

Medications for improving blood flow, such as antiplatelet agents (blood thinners) and medications that relax the blood vessel walls.

Angioplasty: A catheter (long hollow tube) is used to create a larger opening in an artery to increase blood flow. Angioplasty may be performed in many of the arteries in the body. There are several types of angioplasty procedures, including:

Balloon angioplasty (a small balloon is inflated inside the blocked artery to open the blocked area) (Figs 29.34, 29.35, 29.37).

Atherectomy (the blocked area inside the artery is "shaved" away by a tiny device on the end of a catheter) (Fig. 29.30).

Laser angioplasty (a laser is used to "vaporize" the blockage in the artery) (Fig. 29.36).

Stent (a tiny coil is expanded inside the blocked artery to open the blocked area and is left in place to keep the artery open) (Figs 29.31, 29.34, 29.35, 29.27).

Vascular surgery: A bypass graft using a blood vessel from another part of the body or a tube made of synthetic material is placed in the area of the blocked or narrowed artery to reroute the blood flow (Fig. 29.38).

With both angioplasty and vascular surgery, an angiogram is often performed prior to the procedure.

Complications of Peripheral Vascular Disease

Complications of peripheral vascular disease most often occur because of decreased or absent blood flow. Such complications may include:

- Amputation (loss of a limb)
- Heart attack
- Poor wound healing
- Restricted mobility due to pain or discomfort with exertion
- Severe pain in the affected extremity
- Stroke (three times more likely in people with PVD).

By following an aggressive treatment plan for peripheral vascular disease, complications such as these may be prevented.

Prevention of Peripheral Vascular Disease

Steps to prevent PVD are primarily aimed at management of the risk factors for PVD. A prevention program for PVD may include:

- Smoking cessation including avoidance of second hand smoke and use of tobacco products.
- Dietary modifications including reduced fat, cholesterol, and simple carbohydrates (such as sweets), and increased amounts of fruits and vegetables.

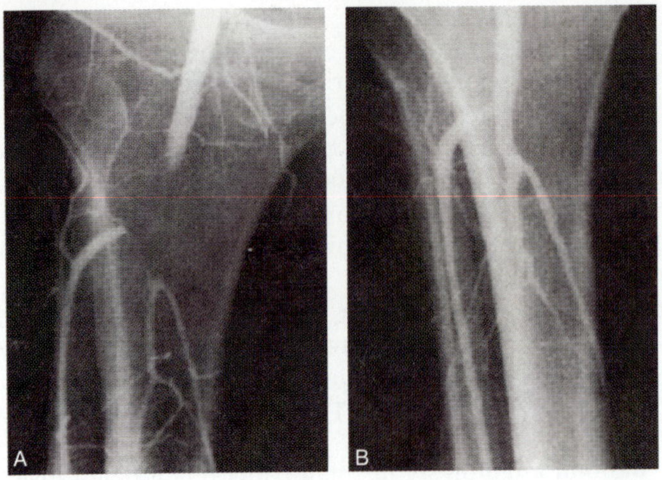

Fig. 29.31: (A) A newly formed thrombolic occlusion of the poplitial and trifurcation vessels. (B) treated successfully with urokinase infusion

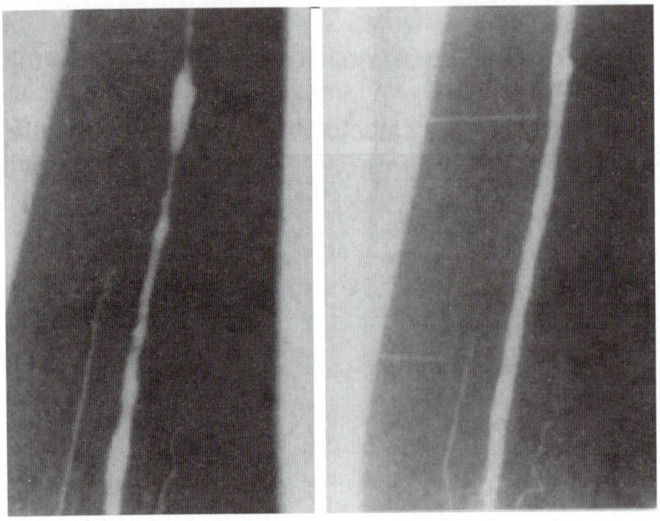

Fig. 29.32: Angiographic picture showing diffusely diseased segment of the superficial femoral artery (A) treated successfully with the atherectomy catheter (B)

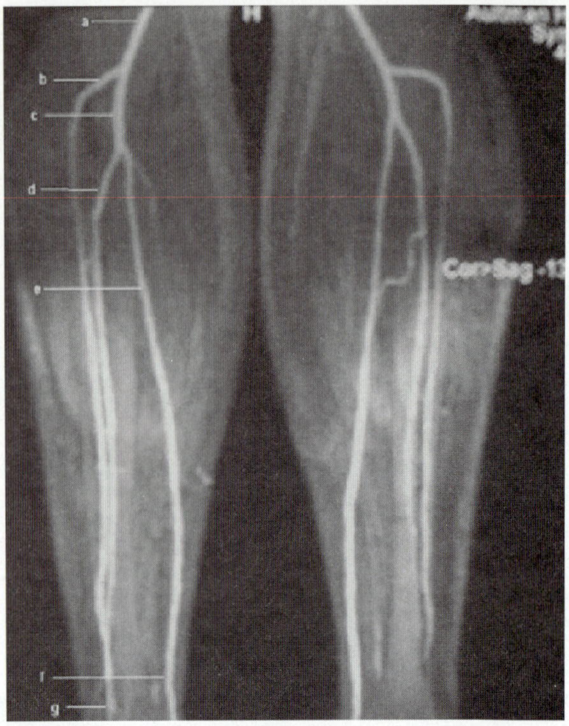

Fig. 29.33: Magnetic resonance angiogram (MRA) obtained by using the bolus-chase technique shows the normal anatomy of the lower extremity arterial vasculature

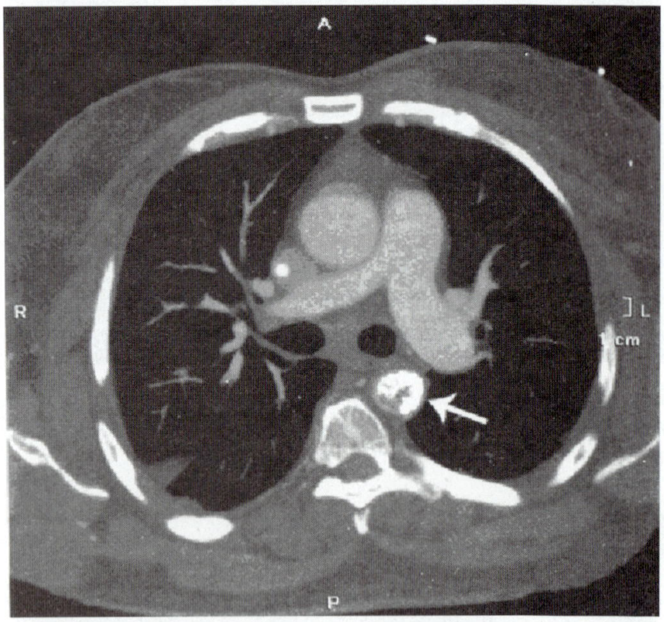

Fig. 29.34: 64 slice sagittal section at the level of calcific plaque revealed nondilated descending thoracic aorta, densely calcific and lumen filled with superadded thrombus (arrow)

- Treatment of dyslipidemia (high blood cholesterol levels) with medications as determined by your physician.
- Weight reduction
- Moderation in alcohol intake
- Medications as determined by your physician to reduce your risk for blood clot formation
- Exercise plan of a minimum of 30 minutes daily
- Control of diabetes mellitus
- Control of hypertension (high blood pressure)
- A prevention plan for PVD may also be used to prevent or lessen the progress of PVD once it has been diagnosed. Consult your physician for diagnosis and treatment.

Management of Children with Increased Risk of Atherosclerosis

The management of children with an increased risk of cardiovascular disease includes the following:

Lifestyle changes, including increased exercise, changes in diet, avoiding exposure to cigarette smoke, or weight loss.

If necessary, one or more medications to treat high cholesterol and/or high blood pressure.

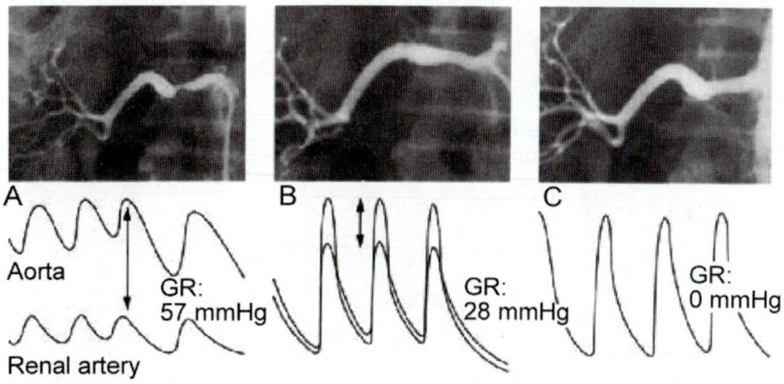

Fig. 29.35: *Treatment of renal artery stenosis with balloon angioplasty and stenting. (A) Angiogram showing substantial narrowing of the renal artery and a systolic pressure gradient of 57 mmHg. (B) After balloon angioplasty, the angiographic stenosis is improved with a residual translesional gradient of 28 mmHg. (C) Following stent placement, minor angiographic improvement is evident, but the hemodynamic gradient has completely resolved*

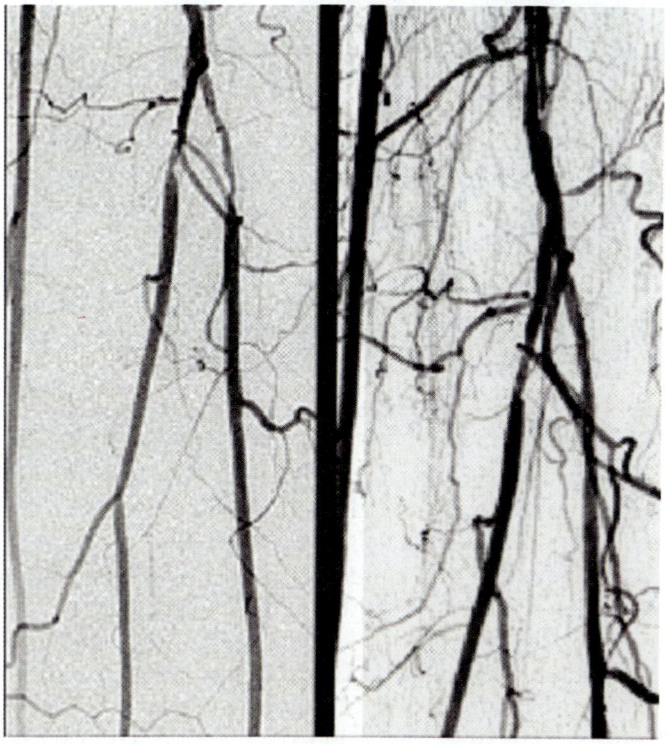

Fig. 29.36: *Angiography (Left) showing occluded femoral artery and fully revascularized after laser angioplasty (Right)*

Is treatment necessary? Treatment of atherosclerosis risk factors may prevent or delay the development of cardiovascular disease later in life. The decision about when to start treatment depends upon:

- The severity of risk for future heart disease
- The risk of side effects of the treatment
- The effectiveness of the treatment
- Making healthy lifestyle changes (diet, exercise, weight control, avoiding smoking) is effective and has few risks. The use of a medication(s) requires more careful consideration. For each child or teenager, the clinical provider will work to individualize a treatment plan that has the greatest potential benefits and fewest risks.

High Cholesterol and Lipids

Cholesterol and lipids are measured by testing the blood level of several components including total cholesterol, LDL (bad cholesterol), HDL (good cholesterol) and triglycerides. The most accurate time to measure these levels is before the first meal or drink of the day, 8–12 hours after the last meal (called fasting). The following levels are considered abnormal and may indicate a need for treatment:

- Total cholesterol is >200 mg/dL (5.18 mmol/L)
- Low-density lipoprotein (LDL) cholesterol is >130 mg/dL (3.36 mmol/L)
- High-density lipoprotein (HDL) cholesterol is <40 mg/dL, triglycerides (TG) is >130 mg/dL.

Initial treatment: The initial treatment for high cholesterol includes a combination of changes in diet and increased activity. These treatments are usually recommended for at least 6–12 months before considering the use of medication.

Diet: Parents of children with elevated low-density lipoprotein levels should offer their child a low-saturated fat, low-cholesterol diet. Increasing fruits and vegetables, whole grains, low-fat or nonfat dairy products, beans, fish, and lean proteins can help to meet this goal.

Children with high triglycerides should eat a diet without excessive carbohydrates, particularly "refined" carbohydrates (white rice, pasta, bread, desserts), which raise blood sugar and are low in fiber.

Meeting with a dietitian or nutritionist can help families to set realistic, individual goals and make long-lasting changes. In most cases, the entire family should change their diet together to maximize the child's chances of success. More than one visit with a nutritionist is often necessary.

Extent of daily activity: Increasing daily activity can help to decrease the risk of cardiovascular disease and improve cholesterol levels. Most expert groups recommend that children get 30–60 minutes of exercise 4–6 days per week.

For children who are not already active, the increase in activity should be gradual. For example, the initial goal may be to ride a bicycle outside for 10 minutes 3 times per week. Other options include joining a gym or YMCA, riding an exercise bike, or running on a treadmill; activity should be tailored to the child's age and interests.

Dietary supplements: Dietary supplements, such as fiber and omega-3 fatty acids, are sometimes recommended to decrease LDL cholesterol and triglyceride levels. However, the best source of fiber is from dietary sources, such as fruits, vegetables, and whole grains. The best source of omega-3 fatty acids is fish.

Medications

If changes in diet and activity do not decrease cholesterol levels enough after 6–12 months, or if a child's cholesterol or triglyceride levels are very high, one or more medications may be recommended. Medications do not permanently cure the problem but work to lower the child's risk factors.

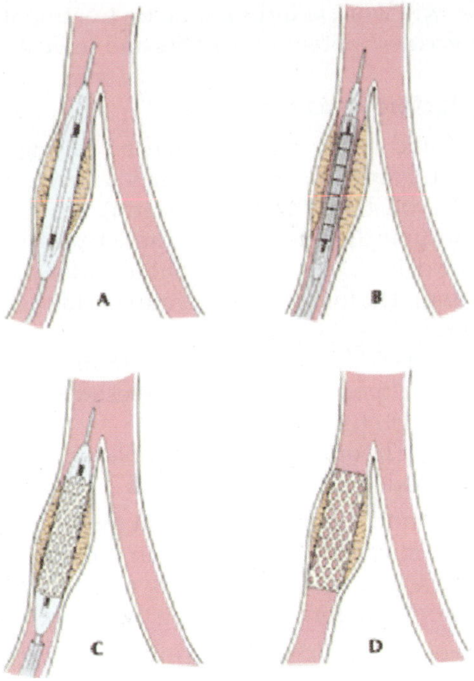

Fig. 29.37: *Schematic diagram of a peripheral artery being treated with angioplasty and stenting. (A) Balloon angioplasty of the blockage. (B) Positioning of a balloon-expandable stent. (C) Deployment of the stent. (D) Final result with the stent in place*

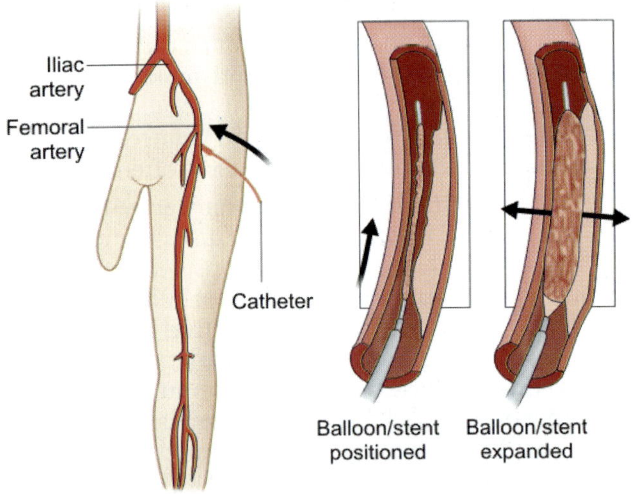

Fig. 29.38: *Management of illiac artery by stentoplasty*

Statins: The most commonly used medication to treat high cholesterol belongs to a class of drugs called statins. Several statins are approved for use in children. These medications are usually taken in pill form, once per day. More detailed information about use of statins in children is available separately.

High Blood Pressure

In children, the normal range for blood pressure (BP) is determined by the child's gender, age, and height. The

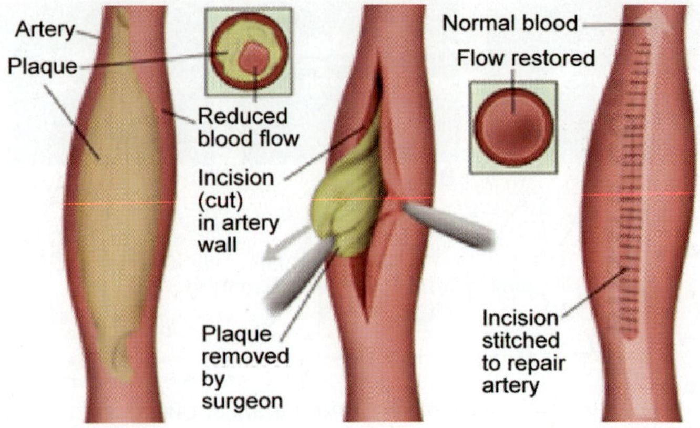

Fig. 29.39: *End-arterectomy. This surgical procedure involves the manual removal of plaque from the affected artery. It is generally used in case of arteries that are easily accessible, and is more commonly used in the treatment of carotid artery blockages*

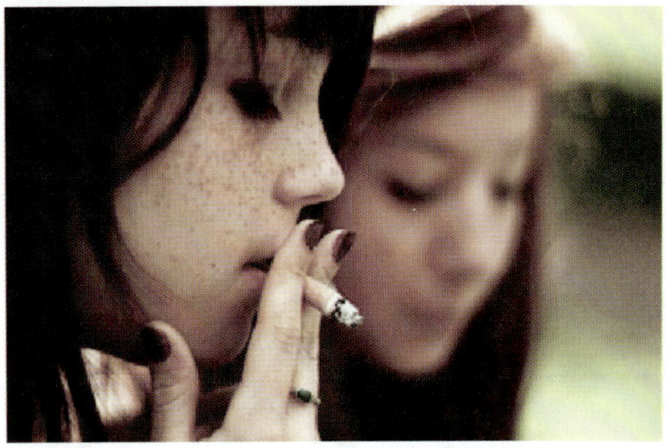

Fig. 29.40: *Stopping cigarette smoking not only prevents PAD but it can significantly regress the process of atherosclerosis*

normal range is expressed as a percentile, similar to charts used to track children's height and weight.

As an example, if a child's BP is at the 90th percentile, this means that 90% of children who are that age, gender, and height have a lower BP.

A child's blood pressure percentile can be calculated here for boys (calculator 1) or here for girls (calculator 2). Hypertension is defined as BP >95th percentile. Prehypertension is defined as BP >90–95th percentile or if BP exceeds 120/80 mmHg.

Blood pressure may change in response to an individual's emotions and environment. Hypertension (sustained high blood pressure) is not usually diagnosed until blood pressure is measured as high on three separate occasions when the child is calm and in a quiet environment.

When is treatment needed? Lifestyle changes (diet and increased activity) are initially recommended for most children with hypertension or prehypertension. One or more medications may be recommended if lifestyle changes are not effective if the blood pressure is very elevated or if the child has an underlying medical problem that causes high blood pressure.

Treatment of high blood pressure in children is discussed in detail in a separate topic.

Obesity

Body mass index (BMI) is a measure of weight in relation to height, and is currently the best way to determine whether a child (>2 years of age) is overweight or obese.

Because children grow in height as well as weight, a "normal" BMI depends upon the child's age and sex. A tool that calculates BMI for boys (calculator 3) and girls (calculator 4) is available here.

Children whose BMI is >85th percentile are considered to be overweight while children whose BMI is >95th percentile are considered to be obese.

Treatment is generally recommended for children whose BMI is >95th percentile for age and gender. Treatment usually includes making changes in diet, behavior, and increasing physical activity.

Cigarette Smoking

All patients and family members who smoke are counseled to quit smoking. Smoking, as well as exposure to second-hand smoke, has many health risks. Approaches to quitting smoking are described separately (Fig. 29.39).

Other Medical Conditions that Increase Risks

A number of medical conditions, such as diabetes, chronic kidney disease, and Kawasaki disease, increase a child's risk of developing cardiovascular disease. Careful management and monitoring of these conditions can reduce the child's risk. More information about these conditions is available separately.

BIBLIOGRAPHY

1. Diagnosis and management of peripheral arterial disease, Scottish Intercollegiate guidelines network-SIGN (2006)
2. Diagnosis and treatment of peripheral artery diseases, European society of cardiology (2011).
3. Peach G, Griffin M, Jones KG, et al. Diagnosis and management of peripheral arterial disease. BMJ. 2012 Aug 14;345:e5208.
4. Robless P, Mikhailidis DP, Stansby GP. Cilostazol for peripheral arterial disease. Cochrane Database Syst Rev. 2008 Jan 23;(1):CD003748.
5. The Edinburgh Claudication questionnaire.
6. Lower limb peripheral arterial disease, NICE Clinical Guideline (August 2012)
7. Mazari FA, Gulati S, Rahman MN, et al. Early outcomes from a randomized, controlled trial of supervised exercise, Ann Vasc Surg. 2010 Jan;24(1):69–79.
8. Watson L, Ellis B, Leng GC. Exercise for intermittent claudication. Cochrane Database Syst Rev. 2008 Oct 8;(4): CD000990.
9. No authors listed. MRC/BHF Heart Protection Study of cholesterol lowering with simvastatin in 20,536 high-risk individuals: a randomised placebo-controlled trial.; Lancet. 2002 Jul 6;360(9326):7–22.
10. Yusuf S, Sleight P, Pogue J, et al. Effects of an angiotensin-converting-enzyme inhibitor, ramipril, on cardiovascular events in high-risk patients. The heart outcomes prevention evaluation study Investigators. N Engl J Med. 2000 Jan 20;342(3):145–53.
11. Weiss N, Hilge R, Hoffmann U. Mild hyperhomocysteinemia: risk factor or just risk predictor for cardiovascular diseases? Vasa. 2004 Nov;33(4):191–203.
12. Vascular disease - clopidogrel and dipyridamole, NICE Technology Appraisal Guideline (December 2010).
13. Peripheral arterial disease - cilostazol, naftidrofyryl oxalate, pentoxifylline and inositol nicotinate; NICE Technology Appraisal Guideline (May 2011).
14. Mangiafico RA, Fiore CE. Current management of intermittent claudication: the role of pharmacological and Curr Vasc pharmacol. 2009 Jul;7(3):394–413.
15. Percutaneous atherectomy of femoropopliteal arterial lesions with plaque excision devices, NICE interventional procedure guideline (February 2011).
16. Ruffolo AJ, Romano M, Ciapponi A. Prostanoids for critical limb ischaemia. Cochrane Database Syst Rev. 2010 Jan 20;(1):CD006544.
17. Aronow WS. Office management of peripheral arterial disease. Am J Med. 2010 Sep;123(9):790–2.
18. Burns P, Gough S, Bradbury AW; Management of peripheral arterial disease in primary care. BMJ. 2003 Mar 15;326 (7389):584–8.
19. Santilli JD, Rodnick JE, Santilli SM. Claudication: diagnosis and treatment. Am Fam Physician. 1996;53:1245–53.
20. Dormandy J, Verstraete M, Andreani D, et al. Second European consensus document on chronic critical leg ischemia. Circulation. 1991;84(suppl 4):1–26.
21. Gordon T, Kannel WB. Predisposition to atherosclerosis in the head, heart, and legs. The Framingham study. JAMA. 1972;221:661–6.
22. Brown AL, Juergens JL. Arteriosclerosis and atherosclerosis. In: Allen EV, et al. Peripheral vascular disease. Philadelphia: Saunders, 1972;57–66.
23. DeBakey ME, Crawford ES, Garrett E, et al. Occlusive disease of the lower extremities in patients 16 to 37 years of age. Ann Surg. 1964;159:873–90.
24. Haid SP, Conn J Jr, Bergan JJ. Cystic adventitial disease of the popliteal artery. Arch Surg. 1970;101:765–70.
25. Haimovici H. Patterns of arteriosclerotic lesions of the lower extremity. Arch Surg. 1967;95:918–33.
26. Mavor GE. The pattern of occlusion in atheroma of the lower limb arteries. The correlation of clinical and arteriographic findings. Br J Surg. 1956;43:352–64.
27. Cutajar CL, Marston A, Newcombe JF. Value of cuff occlusion pressures in assessment of peripheral vascular disease. Br Med J. 1973;2(863):392–5.
28. Ouriel K, McDonnell AE, Metz CE, Zarins CK. Critical evaluation of stress testing in the diagnosis of peripheral vascular disease. Surgery. 1982;91:686–93.
29. Golledge J. lower-limb arterial disease. Lancet. 1997;350: 1459–65.
30. Welch HJ. chronic lower extremity ischemia. Compr Ther. 1997;23:534–8.
31. Cheshire NJ, Wolfe JH, Noone MA, Davies L, Drummond M. The economics of femorocrural reconstruction for critical

leg ischemia with and without autologous vein. J Vasc Surg. 1992;15: 167–74.

32. Albers M, Fratezi AC, De Luccia N. Assessment of quality of life of patients with severe ischemia as a result of infrainguinal arterial occlusive disease. J Vasc Surg. 1992; 16:54–9.
36. Eklund AE, Eriksson G, Olsson AG. A controlled study showing significant short-term effect of prostaglandin E1 in healing of ischaemic ulcers of the lower limb in man. Prostaglandins Leukot Med. 1982;8:265–71.
37. Schuler JJ, Flanigan DP, Holcroft JW, Ursprung JJ, Mohrland JS, Pyke J. Efficacy of prostaglandin E1 in the treatment of lower extremity ischemic ulcers secondary to peripheral vascular occlusive disease: results of a prospective randomized, double-blind, multicenter clinical trial. J Vasc Surg. 1984;1:160–70.
38. Taylor LM Jr, Porter JM. Current status of the reversed saphenous vein graft. In: Bergan JJ, Yao J, eds. Arterial surgery. New York: Grune and Stratton, 1987:494–501.
39. Taylor LM Jr, Edwards JM, Porter JM. Present status of reversed vein bypass grafting: five-year results of a modern series. J Vasc Surg. 1990;11:193–205.
40. Donaldson MC, Mannick JA, Whittemore AD. Femoral-distal bypass with in situ greater saphenous vein. Long-term results using the Mills valvulotome. Ann Surg. 1991;213:457–64.
41. Bergamini TM, Towne JB, Bandyk DF, Seabrook GR, Schmitt DD. Experience with in situ saphenous vein bypasses during 1981 to 1989: determinant factors of long-term patency. J Vasc Surg. 1991;13:137–47.
42. Quinones-Baldrich WJ, Prego AA, Ucelay-Gomez R, Freischlag JA, Ahn SS, Baker JD. Long-term results of infrainguinal revascularization with polytetrafluoroethylene: a ten-year experience. J Vasc Surg. 1992;16:209–17.

30 Deep Venous Thrombosis and Pulmonary Embolism

Symptomatic venous thrombosis and embolism (VTE) incidence is reported at a rate of 0.07 in every 10,000 children, which is significantly lower than the rate in adults. Pulmonary emboli in adolescents are rarely fatal, unlike in adults. VTE recurrence is also much lower in children. Young age has been shown to be protective of VTE, whereas central venous catheters are very important in pediatric venous thrombosis. The incidence of postthrombotic syndrome varies from 20% to 65%, with mild symptoms in most children. Cerebral and visceral vein thrombosis may lead to severe morbidity and death. Some factors of thrombophilia have a significant effect in the pediatric population; however, its overall significance is controversial. Most data on VTE treatment are extrapolated from studies in adults. Children with acute VTE should be treated with anticoagulation therapy. Treatment duration depends on the nature of the thrombosis and previous VTE events in venous insufficiency states, venous blood escapes from its normal antegrade path of flow and refluxes backward down the veins into an already congested leg. Venous insufficiency syndromes are most commonly caused by valvular incompetence in the low-pressure superficial venous system but may also be caused by valvular incompetence in the high-pressure deep venous system (or, rarely, both). In addition, they may result from the congenital absence of venous valves.

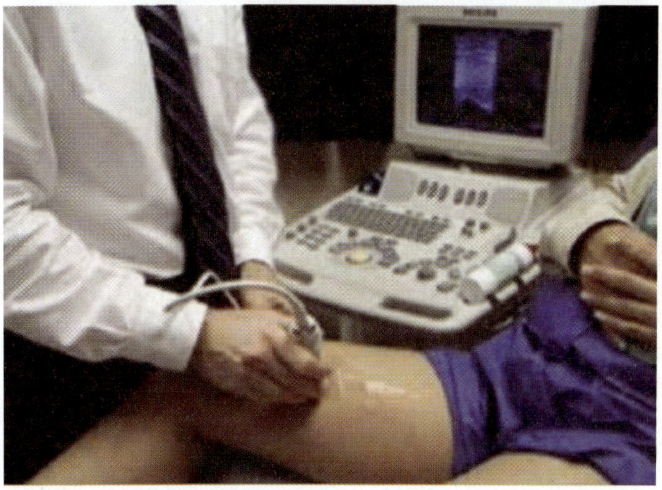

Fig. 30.1: Operator performing dual venous ultrasound examination for deep venous thrombosis and venous insufficiency in a young boy

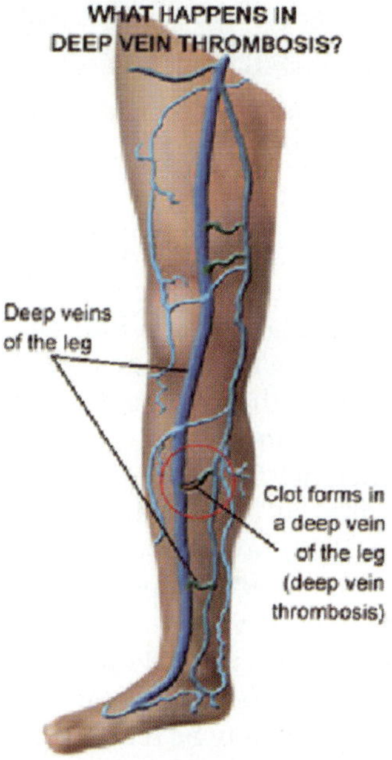

Fig. 30.2: *Anatomy of vein thrombosis*

Untreated venous insufficiency in the deep or superficial system causes a progressive syndrome [(chronic venous insufficiency (CVI)]. Historically, CVI was known as postphlebitic syndrome and postthrombotic syndrome, terms referring to the conditions that cause most cases. However, these terms have been largely abandoned because they do not include another common cause of the disease, the congenital absence of venous valves.

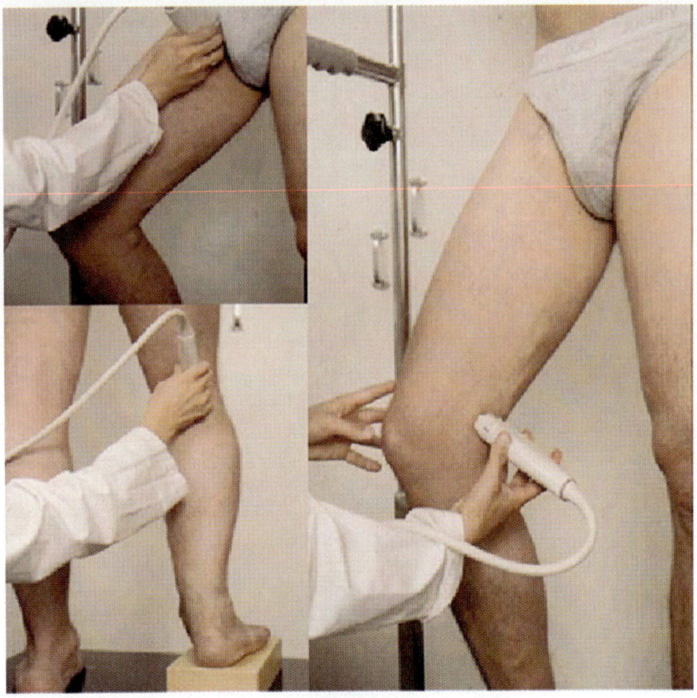

Fig. 30.3: *Duplex ultrasound investigation of the veins in chronic venous disease of the lower limbs*

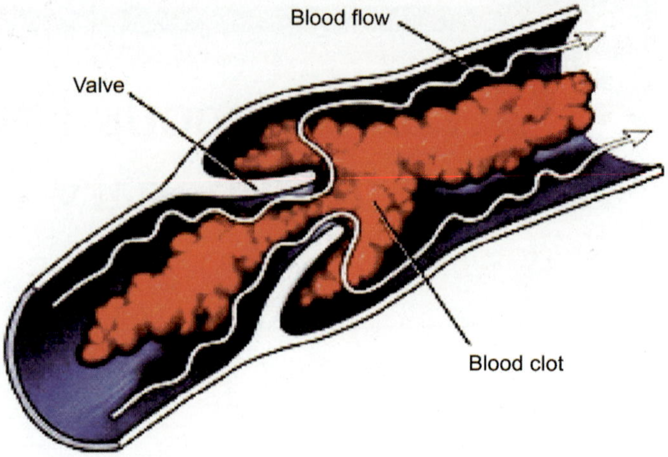

Fig. 30.4: *Obstructed blood flow due to blood clot and also depicts venus valve*

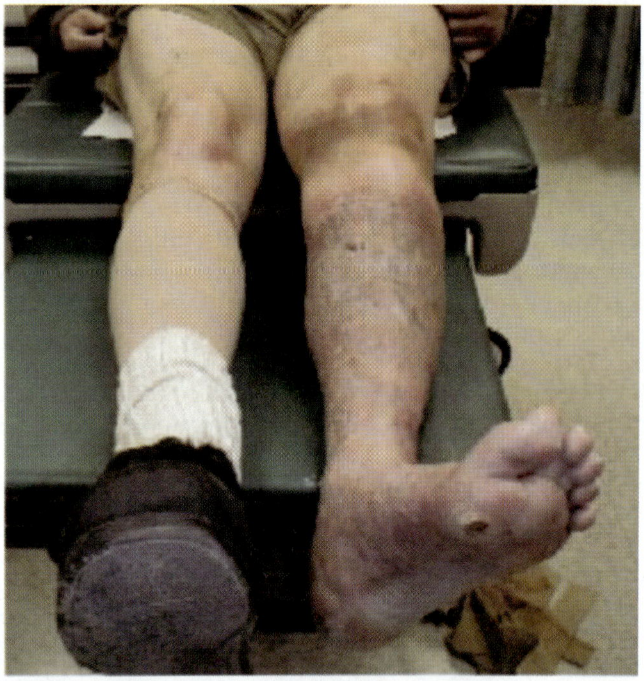

Fig. 30.5: *Deep vein thrombosis in teenager with history of smoking, alcoholism and drug addiction*

In addition to poor cosmesis, CVI can lead to chronic life-threatening infections of the lower extremities. Pain, especially after ambulation, is a hallmark of the disease. CVI causes characteristic changes, called lipodermatosclerosis, to the skin of the lower extremities, which lead to eventual skin ulceration.

Venous insufficiency is neither uncommon nor benign. Treatment is aimed at ameliorating the symptoms and, whenever possible, at correcting the underlying abnormality. Graduated compression is the cornerstone of modern therapy. Deep system disease is often refractory to treatment, but superficial system disease can usually be treated by ablating the refluxing vessels. Refluxing superficial vessels can safely be removed or ablated without sequelae.

Anatomy (Figs 30.2, 30.4, 30.6–30.8)

The venous network in the lower extremities commonly affected by CVI is divided into the following three systems (see the images below):

1. Superficial veins [including the great saphenous vein (GSV), the small saphenous vein (SSV), and their tributaries]
2. Deep veins (including the anterior tibial, posterior tibial, peroneal, popliteal, deep femoral, superficial femoral, and iliac veins)
3. Perforating or communicating veins, lower-leg venous anatomy, perforating veins of lower leg.

When the venous network is functioning correctly, every movement of the leg causes blood to be pumped inward and upward past a series of valves (see the image below). During ambulation, the normal pressure in the venous system of the lower leg is nearly zero. Immediately after ambulation, the early standing pressure in the normal leg remains low. Arterial inflow fills the leg veins slowly, and the only source of venous pressure is the hydrostatic pressure of a column of blood as high as the nearest competent valve.

In venous insufficiency, after prolonged standing, the veins are completely filled, and all the venous valves float open. At this time, high hydrostatic venous pressure results from the unbroken column of fluid that extends from the head to the foot. Failed valves cause the column of standing blood in the vein to remain high even during ambulation.

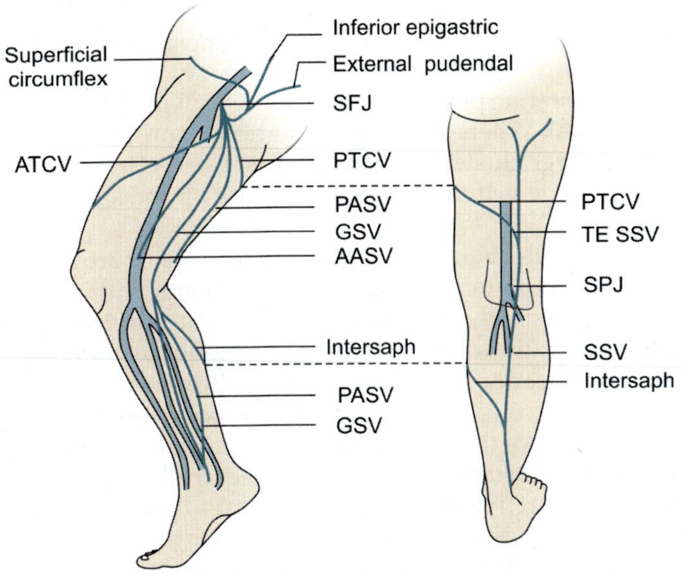

Fig. 30.6: *Superficial veins of the leg. Saphenofemoral junction (SFJ), great saphenous vein (GSV), anterior accessory saphenous vein (AASV), posterior accessory saphenous vein (PASV), anterior thigh circumflex vein (ATCV), posterior thigh circumflex vein (PTCV) saphenopopliteal junction (SPJ), small saphenous vein (SSV), thigh extension of the small saphenous vein (TE SSV), intersaphenous vein (Intersaph. V)*

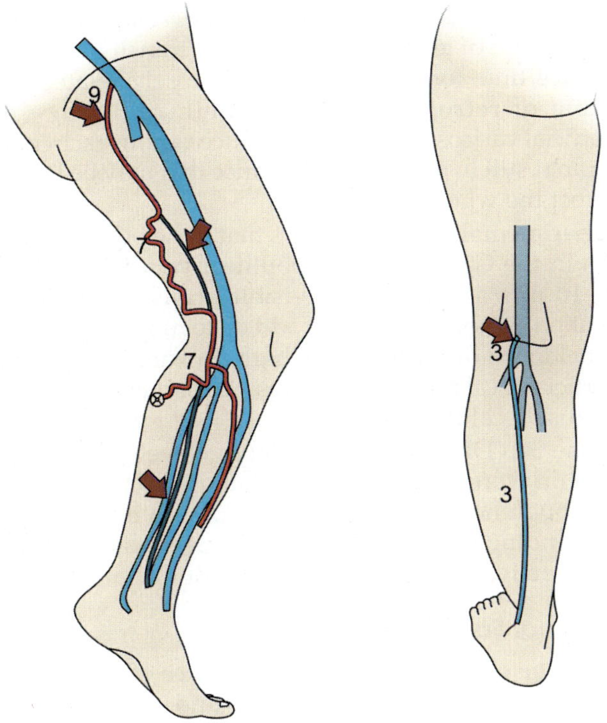

Fig. 30.7: *Duplex sampling sites. Assessment for reflux can be easily targeted so that relatively few locations along the superficial venous tree require color or spectral Doppler sampling. The patient below demonstrates primary varicose veins in the GSV territory with several tributaries. Arrows indicate the few locations which need to be tested*

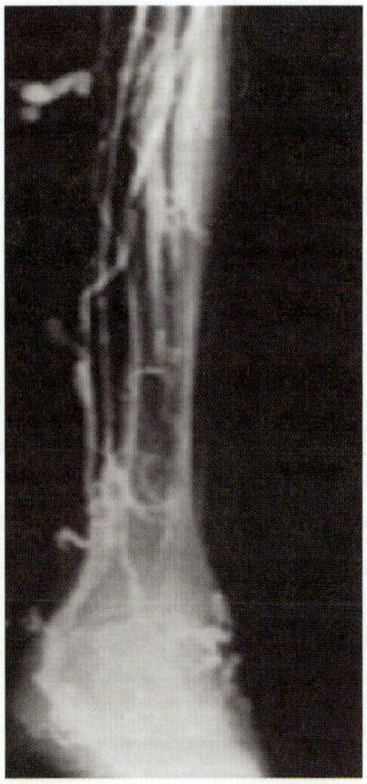

Fig. 30.8: *Venogram demonstrating incompetent perforating veins*

The hydrostatic pressure increases during and immediately after ambulation, which cause venous congestion.

Pathophysiology

Various mechanisms are associated with failure of superficial venous valves. Most commonly, congenitally weak vein walls dilate under normal pressures to cause secondary valve failure. Direct injury or superficial phlebitis may cause primary valve failure. Congenitally abnormal valves can also be incompetent at normal superficial venous pressures. Normal veins and normal valves may become excessively distensible under the influence of hormones (as in pregnancy) (Table 30.1).

High venous pressure is directly responsible for many aspects of venous insufficiency syndrome. Under normal conditions, two major mechanisms in the body operate to prevent venous hypertension. First, bicuspid valves in the veins prevent backflow and venous pooling. Deep venous thrombosis (DVT) commonly occurs at these valves, causing irreversible damage to the valve.

Second, during normal ambulation, calf muscles decrease venous pressures by approximately 70% in the lower extremities (*see* the image below). With rest, pressures return to normal in approximately 30 seconds. In diseased veins, ambulation decreases venous pressures by only 20%. When ambulation is stopped, pressure in the vein lumen increases slowly, returning to normal over a period of minutes.

- Increased venous pressure transcends the venules to the capillaries, impeding flow
- Low-flow states within the capillaries cause leukocyte trapping
- Trapped leukocytes release proteolytic enzymes and oxygen free radicals, which damage capillary basement membranes

Table 30.1: *Wells clinical score for DVT*

Clinical parameter score	*Score*
Active cancer (treatment ongoing, or within 6 mo or palliative	+1
Paralysis or recent plaster immobilization of the lower extremities	+1
Recently bedridden for >3 d or major surgery <4 wk	+1
Localized tenderness along the distribution of the deep venous system	+1
Entier leg sweelling	+1
Calf swelling >3 cm compared with the asymptomatic leg	+1
Pitting edema (greater in the symptomatic leg)	+1
Previous DVT documented	+1
Collateral superficial veins (nonvaricose)	+1
Alternative diagnosis (as likely or greater than that of DVT)	–2
Total of above	*Score*
High probability	≥3
Moderate probability	1 or 2
Low probability	? 0

Source: Adapted from JAMA. 1998 Apr 8:279(14):1094–9

- Plasma proteins (e.g. fibrinogen) leak into the surrounding tissues, forming a fibrin cuff.
- Interstitial fibrin and resultant edema decrease oxygen delivery to the tissues, resulting in local hypoxia.
- Inflammation and tissue loss result.

Most cases of superficial vein valve failure occur after primary points of high-pressure leakage develop between the deep system and the superficial system. High pressure leads to secondary valve failure when otherwise normal superficial veins become so widely dilated that the thin flaps of the venous valves can no longer make contact in the lumen of the vessel. Over time, these incompetent superficial veins become visibly dilated and tortuous, at which point they are recognized as varicose veins.

High pressure can enter the superficial veins as a result of the failure of key valves at any point of communication between the deep system and the superficial system. High-pressure leakage from the deep veins to the superficial system has two major sources, as follows:

- Junctional valve failure
- Perforator valve failure.

Junctional high-pressure disease most often results from failure of the primary valve at the junction between the GSV and the common femoral vein at the groin (saphenofemoral junction). Vein incompetence then proceeds distally from the groin, and patients perceive that a large vein is growing down their leg. A less common form of junctional reflux results from failure of the primary valve at the junction between the SSV and the popliteal vein at the knee (saphenopopliteal junction).

Perforator high-pressure disease results from failure of the valves of any perforating vein. The most common sites of primary perforator valve failure are in the midproximal thigh (Hunterian perforator) and in the proximal calf (Boyd perforators). When the primary high-pressure entry point is distal, large clusters of veins are first noticed in the lower leg with large veins eventually growing up the leg toward the groin.

Not all of the sequelae of venous insufficiency are related to venous hypertension, and not all patients with venous hypertension develop ulceration. Some patients with venous ulceration do not have marked venous hypertension.

Poor clearance of lactate, carbon dioxide, and other products of cellular respiration also contributes to the development of the syndrome. A defect in the clearance of extraneous substances can be quantified: if albumin labeled with a radioactive tracer is injected into the foot tissues, the clearance rate is markedly slowed by deep venous obstruction or by deep or superficial venous incompetence. Although this effect is referred to as venous stasis, the reduced clearance of cellular metabolites is not always due to true venous stasis. In many cases, the venous blood is moving at a normal speed, but a local recirculation of this venous blood upward through normal veins and downward through varicosities prolongs the average time required for the blood to pass from the heart and lungs through the legs and back to the central circulation.

The time required for an aliquot of radiolabeled blood to pass from the femoral artery through the leg and back to the central circulation is highly correlated with the development of leg ulcers. The aliquot transit time and the clearance time for an extremity are closely related to the volume of retrograde flow through refluxing veins. Superficial varicosities always produce venous recirculation and can result in prolonged clearance that may be localized or affect the whole leg.

Experimental evidence shows that if the peak retrograde flows in the GSV, SSV, and popliteal vein add up to less than 10 mL/s, progressive visible stasis dermatitis and ulceration do not occur. If they add up to more than 15 mL/s, the incidence of ulceration is high. In some cases, purely superficial local reflux with a pressure of more than 7 mL/s can cause local ulceration.

In the San Diego population study, levels of circulating P-selectin were found to be correlated with the severity of CVI though not with the incidence of CVI in general. The study findings suggest that the pathogenesis of CVI may include activation of platelets and endothelial cells.

Etiological Factors

CVI can be caused by congenital absence of or damage to venous valves in the superficial and communicating systems. It can also be caused by venous incompetence due to thrombus formation as favored by the Virchow triad (venous stasis, hypercoagulability, and endothelial trauma). Varicose veins rarely are associated with the development of CVI. Most cases of venous insufficiency are related to reflux through the superficial veins.

Chronic nonhealing wounds of the lower extremity have many different potential causes, but most chronic lower-extremity ulcers are of venous etiology. The majority of venous ulcers are caused by venous reflux that is purely or largely confined to the superficial venous system; only a minority are caused by chronic DVT or by valvular insufficiency in the deep veins.

Superficial Venous Insufficiency

In superficial venous insufficiency, the deep veins are normal, but venous blood escapes from a normal deep system and flows backwards through dilated superficial veins in which the valves have failed. More than 80% of varicose veins seen on the leg are caused by venous insufficiency or a leaky valve in the GSV which terminates near the inguinal ligament as it joins the common femoral vein.

The initial valve failure may occur at any level between the groin and the ankle, but the saphenofemoral junction is the high point of reflux in most patients with severe superficial venous insufficiency. Valve failure can be spontaneous in patients with congenitally weak valves. Congenitally normal valves can fail as a consequence of direct trauma, thrombosis, hormonal changes, or chronic environmental insult (e.g. prolonged standing).

Deep Venous Insufficiency

Deep venous insufficiency can be due to congenital valve or vessel abnormalities, but it most commonly occurs when the valves of the deep veins are damaged as a result of DVT. With no valves to prevent deep system reflux, the hydrostatic venous pressure in the lower extremity increases dramatically (Figs 30.5 and 30.9).

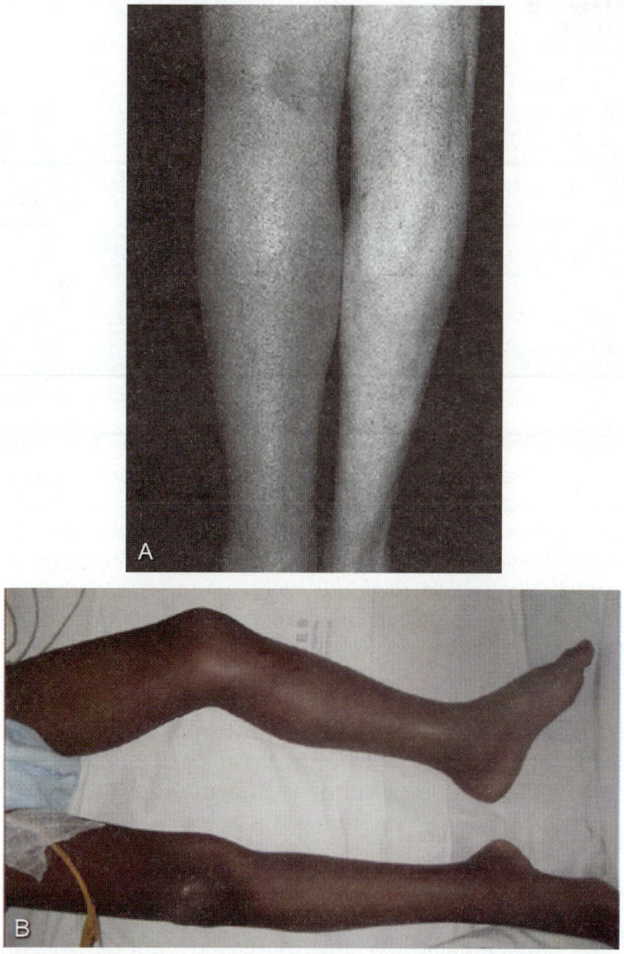

Fig. 30.9: *(Upper and lower) deep vein thrombosis in the left leg of two patients*

Klippel-Trénaunay-Weber Syndrome

A less common cause of venous insufficiency is Klippel-Trénaunay-Weber (KTW) syndrome, which involves port-wine stains, varicose veins, and bony or soft-tissue hypertrophy. Patients with pure Klippel-Trénaunay syndrome have only venous involvement whereas those with the Parkes Weber variant also have arteriovenous malformations.

The capillary hemangiomas (port-wine stains) of KTW syndrome, like those of other forms of venous insufficiency, can lead to local skin breakdown and ulceration, bleeding, and secondary infection. This can occur in any organ system of the body.

The sciatic vein is a large superficial vessel that is present during fetal development but usually does not persist. In patients with KTW syndrome, this vein may be noticed at birth, or it may become apparent later in life. The vein extends along the posterolateral aspect of the leg from the foot to the gluteal region. When present, it is invariably a reflux pathway rather than a pathway for antegrade flow. Patients with KTW syndrome may have atresia of the deep veins, as well as many abnormal venous pathways involving the deep and superficial venous systems. KTW syndrome can produce such severe venous insufficiency that the otherwise normal lymphatic system becomes overwhelmed by the amount of lymph production, which leads to secondary lymphedema.

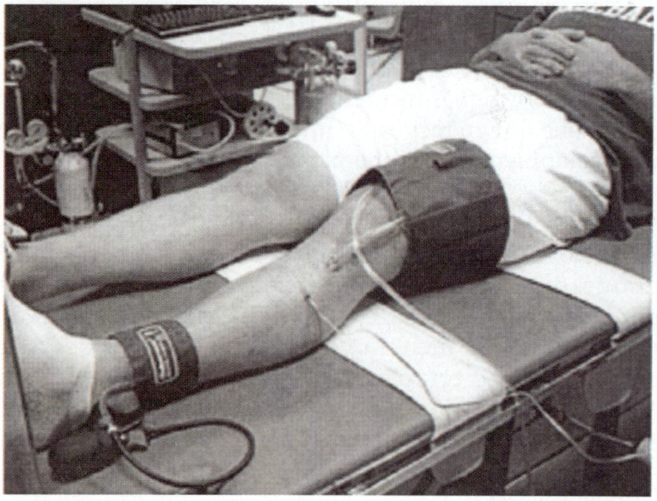

Fig. 30.10: *Laboratory setup showing the thigh and ankle cuffs of the plethysmograph with the mercury-in-rubber strain gauge secured to the midcalf region*

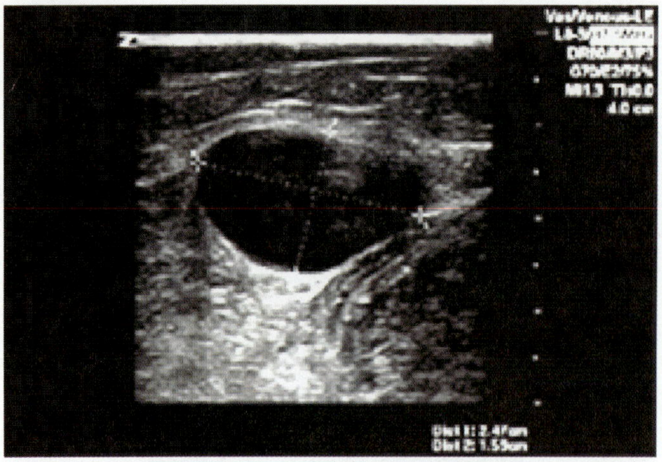

Fig. 30.11: *Paient is a 19 years adolescent that presented with swelling and aching of both lower extremities. He had bilateral varicose veins especially on the right with discoloration and stasis changes however no ulceration or previous ulceration was reported. He denied previous deep venous thrombosis or phlebitis.The patient was finally diagnosed as venous aneurysm of inferior vena cava*

Surgical attempts to treat the abnormal refluxing veins in KTW syndrome are fraught with peril because post-operative worsening of venous abnormalities is common.

Risk Factors

The incidence of CVI rises substantially with age. A history of DVT, which renders venous valves incompetent and thereby causes backflow and increased venous pressure, is a risk factor (Tables 30.2 and 30.3).

A sedentary lifestyle minimizes the pump action of calf muscles on venous return, causing higher venous pressure. CVI occurs more frequently in women who are obese. Vocations that involve standing for long periods predispose individuals to increased venous pressure in dependent lower extremities. A higher incidence of CVI is observed in men who smoke. Pregnancy is an important causative factor in the development of peripheral venous insufficiency.

Sex-related Demographics

The incidence and prevalence of deep and superficial venous disease depend on the age and sex of the population, but at any age, such disease is more common in women than in men. In younger men, the incidence is lower than 10%, compared with 30% in similarly aged women. In men older than 50 years, the incidence is 20%, compared with 50% in similarly aged women.

Clinical History

Patients with venous insufficiency often report subjective symptoms that are typically bothersome early in the disease, become less severe in the middle phases, and then worsen again with advancing age.

Even small telangiectasias are often symptomatic. More than one half of patients who present with telangiectasias smaller than 1 mm in diameter report symptoms that abate after treatment. Common symptoms include the following:
- Burning
- Swelling
- Throbbing
- Cramping
- Aching
- Heaviness
- Restless legs
- Leg fatigue.

Subjective complaints are also common in patients with truncal varices: 18% of patients with varicosities report frequent or continuous symptoms, whereas almost 50% complain of episodic symptoms.

In addition to poor cosmesis, varicose veins serve as indicators of venous hypertension, the most common reason for patient complaints regarding chronic venous insufficiency (CVI). Venous hypertension in muscles and fascial compartments of the lower leg from exercise and prolonged standing results in the characteristic ache of CVI. The discomfort is described as pain, pressure, burning, itching, dull ache, or heaviness in affected calves or legs.

Episodic pain and other symptoms associated with superficial venous disease may be temporally related to hormonal changes, both physiologic and pharmacologic. One half of all pregnant women with varicose veins complain of pain, and 17% are unable to remain upright for more than 1–2 hours at a time because of the severity of the pain.

Patients with deep system insufficiency are nearly always symptomatic. Leg aching, heaviness, and soreness are the most common subjective symptoms.

Pain caused by venous insufficiency often is improved by walking or by elevating the legs. Warmth tends to aggravate the symptoms of venous insufficiency, and cold tends to relieve them. Compression stockings usually ameliorate or prevent the pain of venous insufficiency.

In many ways, the behavior of the pain caused by venous insufficiency is the opposite of that of the pain caused by venous insufficiency. The pain of arterial insufficiency

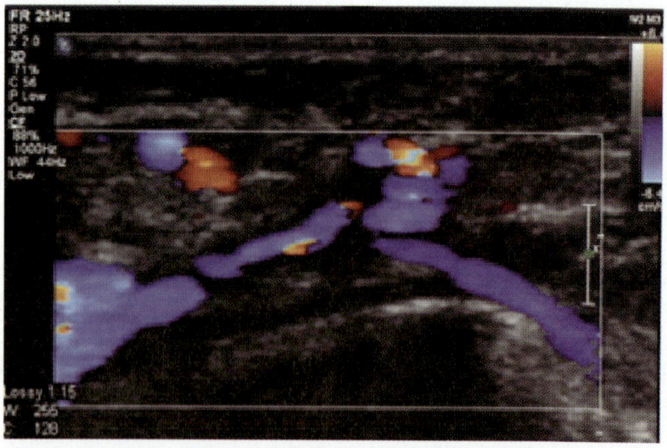

Fig. 30.12: *Chronic thrombosis of the common femoral vein is seen a year after it was diagnosed in a 4-month-old girl. Echogenic material is seen in the lumen of the partially recanalized vein. Irregular flow channels are seen through the old thrombus in the common femoral vein*

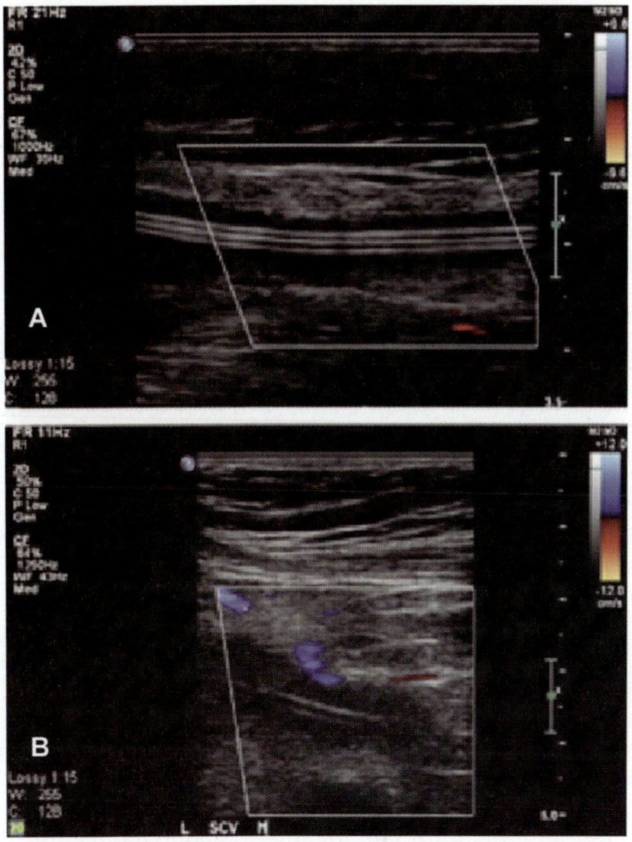

Fig. 30.13: *Ultrasound imaging shows catheter-induced thrombosis in the left arm of a 13-year-old girl. (A) Acute thrombosis of the basilic vein is seen around the catheter. No flow is seen in the dilated lumen, with the catheter being very bright in the center and the thrombus being echolucent around it. (B) Acute thrombosis of the subclavian vein is seen in the same patient. The catheter is seen in the lumen with absence of flow in the vein*

usually is worse with walking and worse when the legs are elevated. Cold tends to aggravate the symptoms of arterial insufficiency, whereas warmth tends to relieve them. Compression stockings usually aggravate the pain of arterial insufficiency.

The pain of venous obstruction is worse with walking or warmth but better with elevation of the legs. Compression stockings usually improve the pain of venous obstruction. Nonhealing ulcers are often noted around the medial malleolus, where venous pressure is maximal because of the presence of large perforating veins. Leg edema, resulting from damage done to capillary basement membranes by white blood cells (WBCs), may be reported. The characteristic skin changes of lipodermatosclerosis in the lower extremities include capillary proliferation, fat necrosis, and fibrosis of skin and subcutaneous tissues. Skin becomes reddish or brown because of the deposition of hemosiderin from red blood cells.

Physical examination: The most common physical signs of venous insufficiency are those attributed to the progressive syndromes of chronic venous stasis and chronic venous hypertension. These signs include the following:

- Edema
- Hyperpigmentation
- Venous dermatitis
- Chronic cellulitis
- Cutaneous infarction (atrophie blanche)
- Ulceration.

Swelling may result from acute venous obstruction [as in deep venous thrombosis (DVT)] or deep or superficial venous reflux. Alternatively, swelling may be completely unrelated to the venous system. Lower-extremity pitting edema is common in patients with venous insufficiency. Hepatic insufficiency, renal failure, cardiac decompensation, infection, trauma, and environmental effects can also cause lower-extremity pitting edema that may be indistinguishable from edema due to venous obstruction or venous insufficiency.

Lymphatic edema may be a sign of primary lymphatic outflow obstruction, or it may be secondary to the overproduction of lymph as a result of severe venous hypertension (a so-called venolymphatic syndrome).

Darkened, discolored, and stained skin may be a sign of venous stasis, arterial insufficiency, chronic infection, prior injury, or various other conditions (*see* the image below). Such discoloration is particularly likely to be a sign of chronic venous stasis if it is localized along the medial part of the ankle or the medial aspect of the lower leg; these areas are especially prone to venous hypertension because their drainage largely depends on the competence and patency of the entire great saphenous vein (GSV) and all the attached perforating veins. Normal veins are visibly distended at the foot and ankle and, occasionally, in the popliteal fossa; they usually are not visibly distended in the rest of the leg. Translucent skin may cause the normal veins to become visible in a bluish subdermal reticular

Table 30.2

Clinical features/risk factors	*Score*
Active cancer within 6 months (ongoing treatment or palliative)	1
Immobilization by paralysis or plaster dressings	1
Recent surgery (within 4 weeks) or bed rest longer than 3 days	1
Localized tenderness along distribution of the deep venous system	1
Calf swelling (>3-cm increase in calf circumference compared to asymptomatic leg) measured 10 cm below tibial tuberosity	1
Thigh and calf swelling (entire swollen leg)	1
Pitting edema confined to symptomatic leg	1
Collateral superficial veins (nonvaricosed)	1
Alternative diagnosis as likely or greater than that of DVT	–2

Pretest probability calculated as the total score: low ≤0; moderate 1 or 2; high ≥3. In the newer scoring system proposed by Wells et al, the probability of having a DVT is likely if a score of two or higher is obtained; a score of less than two indicates that the probability of acute DVT is unlikely. The more symptomatic leg is used if patients have symptoms in both legs pattern. A dilated vein above the ankle is usually evidence of venous pathology.

Nonhealing ulcerations may be due to deep or superficial venous insufficiency; other causes include arterial insufficiency, rheumatologic disorders, local trophic effects, unrecognized cancer, and various more exotic conditions. Nonhealing ulcers on the medial part of the ankle are most likely due to underlying venous stasis. Skin changes or ulcerations that are localized to the lateral aspect of the ankle are more likely to be related to prior trauma or arterial insufficiency than to pure venous insufficiency.

A long-standing venous ulcer rarely converts to a basal cell carcinoma or squamous cell carcinoma. The venous ulcer may develop collision lesions (e.g. basal cell carcinoma and stasis ulceration) at the same site.

The visual appearance of the lower extremities is a useful but not always reliable guide to the peripheral venous condition. Clinical findings in venous disease are also common to many other entities that affect the lower extremities. Physical examination alone is not a reliable means of assessing the venous system. Diagnostic testing nearly always is necessary to rule out deep venous obstruction, to assess the paths of reflux, and to guide treatment planning.

Trendelenburg Test

The trendelenburg test is a traditional part of the physical examination that may help in distinguishing distal venous congestion caused by superficial venous reflux from that caused by incompetence of the valves in the deep venous system.

To perform this test, elevate the patient's leg until all of the congested superficial veins collapse. Apply direct pressure to occlude the superficial veins below the point of suspected reflux from the deep system into the superficial varicosity. Most often, the GSV is manually occluded just below the saphenofemoral junction at the groin.

With the occlusion still in place, have the patient stand. If the distal varicosity remains empty or fills slowly, quickly remove the occluding hand or tourniquet. If the slow filling observed with occlusion is followed by rapid filling after the occlusion is removed, the principal high-pressure entry point into the superficial system is correctly identified.

Immediate refilling of the varicosity despite manual occlusion indicates that the principal entry point has not yet been identified or that more than 1 reflux pathway is involved. Extremely rapid refilling despite occlusion of the superficial reflux pathways suggests that the valves in the deep veins may be incompetent between the groin and the level at which the reflux escapes the deep system. The result is rapid filling of the superficial system.

If deep venous insufficiency is confirmed with results from further evaluations, the treatment options for the patient may be severely limited.

Complications

The local tissue sequelae of venous insufficiency are due to a combination of high venous pressures and reduced clearance of cellular metabolites from the lower extremity. Complications of untreated venous insufficiency include the following:

- Recruitment of veins: High venous pressures may cause the recruitment of adjacent normal veins into refluxing circuits
- DVT
- Pulmonary embolism (PE)
- Venous ulceration
- Secondary lymphedema.

Chronic pain, swelling, recurrent cellulitis, and chronic nonhealing leg ulcers (ulcer cruris) are the most common sequelae of venous insufficiency, but they are not the most severe.

Diagnostic Tests

Misdiagnosing venous disease often is lethal when venous thrombosis is involved, but it is rarely disastrous when the disease is caused by other conditions, because nonthrombotic venous disease is slowly progressive. Although morbidity results in a decreased quality of life and an inability to work, death is rare.

In addition to the conditions listed in the differential diagnosis, other problems to be considered include hepatic insufficiency and lymphedema.

- **Laboratory studies**
- Many patients with venous insufficiency have clinically unrecognized chronic recurrent varicose thrombosis due to stasis in areas with abnormal veins. Such patients may have elevated levels of D-dimer. This finding reduces the usefulness of that test for the evaluation of patients with suspected acute venous thromboembolic disease.
- Laboratory tests may be helpful in patients with venous insufficiency due to Klippel-Trénaunay-Weber (KTW) syndrome because such patients can develop consumptive thrombocytopenia.
- **Ultrasonography** (Figs 30.1, 30.2, 30.11–30.14, 30.20–30.22)
- Duplex ultrasonography is the study of choice for the evaluation of venous insufficiency syndromes. Color-flow duplex imaging uses the Doppler information to color code the two-dimensional sonogram. On the image, red indicates flow in one direction (relative to the transducer), and blue indicates flow in the other direction. On newer machines, the shade of the color may reflect the flow velocity (in the Doppler mode) or the flow volume (in the power Doppler mode).
- When used to evaluate patterns of venous reflux, ultrasonography is both sensitive and specific. Ultrasonographic reflux mapping is essential for the evaluation of peripheral venous insufficiency syndromes.
- A study from the United Kingdom compared 27 consecutive patients seen at a varicose vein clinic with 23 normal ambulatory volunteers and found evidence to suggest that the presence of pulsatile flow in the GSV might be a marker of severe chronic insufficiency of the superficial veins.
- In the diagnosis of deep venous thrombosis (DVT), ultrasonography has been shown to be superior to

contrast venography, and it has now replaced venography in this setting. Duplex ultrasonography is the initial diagnostic imaging modality of choice in patients with suspected DVT.

- **Venography** (Figs 30.15–30.19)
- Magnetic resonance venography (MRV) is the most sensitive and specific test for the assessment of deep and superficial venous disease in the lower legs and pelvis, areas not accessible by means of other modalities. MRV is particularly useful because it can help to detect previously unsuspected nonvascular causes of leg pain and edema when the clinical presentation erroneously suggests venous insufficiency or venous obstruction.
- Direct contrast venography is a labor-intensive and invasive imaging technique. In most centers, it has been replaced by duplex sonography for the routine evaluation of venous disease. However, the technique remains useful in difficult or confusing cases.
- An intravenous (IV) catheter is placed in a dorsal vein of the foot, and radiographic contrast material is infused into the vein. A superficial tourniquet is placed around the leg to occlude the superficial veins and force the contrast material into the deep veins.
- The assessment of reflux by means of direct contrast venography requires the passage of a catheter from the ankle to the groin with the selective introduction of contrast material into each segment of the vein.
- In nearly 15% of patients undergoing venography for detection of DVT, a new thrombosis is detected shortly after a contrast venogram shows negative results. The incidence of contrast-induced DVT in patients who undergo venography for the assessment of venous insufficiency is not known.
- **Venous plethysmography** (Fig. 30.10)
- Photoplethysmography uses infrared light to assess capillary filling during exercise. Increased capillary filling is indicative of venous reflux and, consequently, of incompetent veins.
- Outflow plethysmography involves placing and subsequently releasing a tourniquet on the lower extremity; the veins should quickly return to baseline pressures. Failure to do so indicates reflux.
- Physiologic venous function tests
- Physiologic tests of venous function are important in assessing the cause and severity of venous insufficiency. The physiologic parameters most often measured are the venous refilling time (VRT), the maximum venous outflow (MVO), and the calf muscle pump ejection fraction (MPEF).
- Venous refilling time
- The VRT is the time necessary for the lower leg to become suffused with blood after the calf muscle pump has emptied the lower leg as thoroughly as possible. When patients with healthy veins are in a sitting position, venous refilling of the lower leg occurs only by means of arterial inflow and requires at least 2 minutes.
- In patients with mild and asymptomatic venous insufficiency, some venous refilling occurs by means of reflux across leaky valves. These asymptomatic patients have a VRT of 40–120 seconds.
- In patients with significant venous insufficiency, venous refilling occurs through high-volume reflux and is fairly rapid. An abnormally fast VRT of 20–40 seconds is recorded, reflecting retrograde venous flow through failed valves in superficial or perforating veins. This degree of reflux may be associated with the typical symptoms of venous insufficiency. Patients often complain of nocturnal leg cramps, restless legs, leg soreness, burning leg pain, and premature leg fatigue.
- A VRT shorter than 20 seconds is markedly abnormal and is attributable to high volumes of retrograde venous flow. High-volume reflux may occur via the superficial veins, the large perforators, or the deep veins. Patients with this degree of reflux are nearly always symptomatic. When the VRT is shorter than 10 seconds, venous ulcerations are so common as to be considered virtually inevitable.

Table 30.3: *The following risk factors for DVT have been identified in many different epidemiologic studies*

General
- Age
- Immobilization longer than 3 days
- Pregnancy and the postpartum period
- Major surgery in previous 4 weeks
- Long plane or car trips (>4 h) in previous 4 weeks

Medical
- Cancer
- Previous DVT
- Stroke
- Acute myocardial infarction (AMI)
- Congestive heart failure (CHF)
- Sepsis
- Nephrotic syndrome
- Ulcerative colitis

Trauma
- Multiple trauma
- CNS/spinal cord injury
- Burns
- Lower extremity fractures

Vasculitis
- Systemic lupus erythematosus (SLE) and the lupus anticoagulant
- Behçet syndrome
- Homocystinuria

Hematologic
- Polycythemia rubra vera
- Thrombocytosis
- Inherited disorders of coagulation/fibrinolysis
- Antithrombin III deficiency
- Protein C deficiency
- Protein S deficiency
- Prothrombin 20210A mutation
- Factor V Leiden
- Dysfibrinogenemias and disorders of plasminogen activation

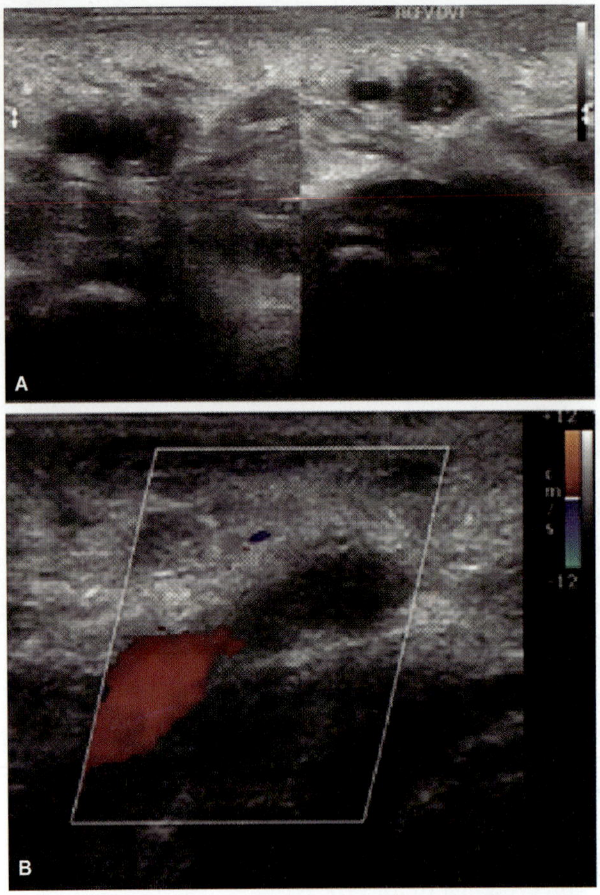

Fig. 30.14: *Acute thrombosis of the common femoral vein in 2-year-old boy is demonstrated by cross-sectional imaging of the femoral vessels. (A) The left panel shows a dilated common femoral vein with echolucent luminal material. The right panel shows that the common femoral vein is not compressible, despite the use pressure that reduced the common femoral artery diameter by half. (B) The common femoral vein from the same patient is viewed with color imaging. The vein is dilated, contains echolucent material, and has absence of flow in contrast to normal flow in the adjacent common femoral artery*

- Maximum venous outflow
- MVO testing is performed to detect an obstruction to venous outflow from the lower leg no matter what the cause. Its results are a measure of the speed with which blood can flow out of a maximally congested lower leg when an occluding thigh tourniquet is suddenly removed.
- A major advantage of MVO testing is that as a functional rather than anatomic test, it is sensitive to significant intrinsic or extrinsic venous obstruction due to any cause at almost any level. It can be used to detect obstructing thrombus in the calf veins, the iliac veins, and the vena cava, areas where ultrasonography and venography are insensitive. It can also be used to detect venous obstruction due to extravascular hematomas, tumors, and other extrinsic disease processes.
- The main disadvantage of MVO testing is that it is sensitive only for significant venous obstruction and not for partial obstruction. It is not useful for the detection of

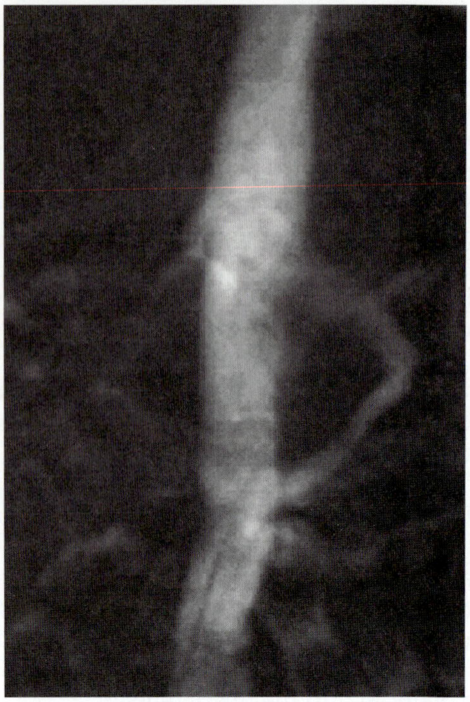

Fig. 30.15: *Anteroposterior image from an inferior vena cavographic examination demonstrates an inferior vena cava of normal diameter without thrombus. In addition, the inflow from the renal veins can be seen at the level of the L1 vertebral body*

reflux-induced venous insufficiency. A normal MVO result does not absolutely rule out DVT.
- Muscle pump ejection fraction
- The MPEF test is used to detect failure of the calf muscle pump to expel blood from the lower leg. Its results are highly repeatable, but a skilled operator is required to obtain clean, meaningful tracings.
- The patient is asked to stand on his or her tiptoes 10–20 times or to dorsiflex his or her ankle. The change in a physical parameter that reflects the blood volume in the calf is recorded as the calf muscle is pumped.

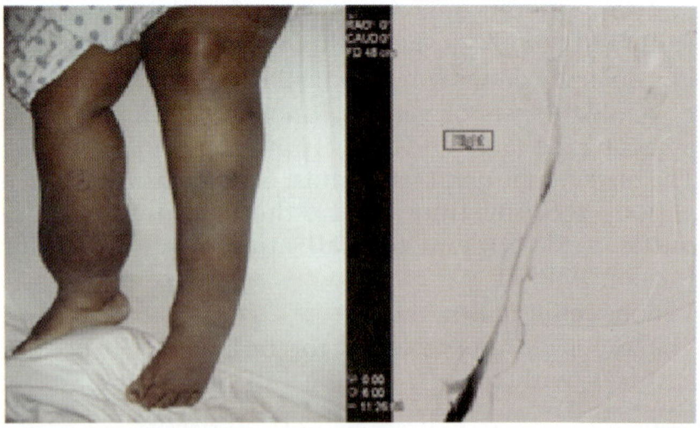

Fig. 30.16: *This patient had onset of leg swelling from early adolescence. Lymphatic delay was noted on the right side but was normal on the left. Venogram showed bilateral iliac vein stenoses. Right limb venogram is shown with severe diffuse iliac vein stenosis. Note the normal caliber of the femoral vein*

- In patients with normal veins and a normal calf muscle pump, 10–20 tiptoe motions or ankle dorsiflexions empties the venous capacitance circuit of the calf. In patients with muscle pump failure, severe proximal obstruction, or severe deep venous insufficiency, tiptoe motions or ankle dorsiflexions have little or no effect on the amount of blood remaining in the calf. Venous insufficiency due to this cause is difficult to treat.

Medical Treatment

Venous insufficiency is neither uncommon nor benign. Treatment is aimed at ameliorating the symptoms and, whenever possible, at correcting the underlying abnormality.

No oral medication has yet been proven useful for the treatment of venous disease. Graduated compression is the cornerstone of the modern treatment of venous insufficiency. Surgical or endovenous therapy is commonly reserved for those with discomfort or ulcers refractory to medical management. The primary goal of such therapy is to improve the venous circulation by correcting venous insufficiency by removing the major reflux pathways.

As yet, no treatment for deep venous insufficiency has been proved to be both safe and effective. Valvuloplasty is occasionally successful, but the incidence of postoperative deep venous thrombosis (DVT) is high. Venous bypass is successful in select patients. External vein valve banding devices and thermally induced collagen shrinkage procedures are being investigated in clinical trials. Restoration of valvular function to incompetent deep veins remains an important focus of research for vascular physicians.

Although deep system disease is often refractory to treatment, superficial system disease can usually be treated by ablating the refluxing vessels. Refluxing superficial vessels can safely be removed or ablated without sequelae; an incompetent vessel has already proved itself unnecessary because it is carrying venous blood in a retrograde direction. Antibiotics rarely are useful in patients with venous ulcerations.

Consultation with a phlebologist (a physician or vascular surgeon specializing in venous diseases) often yields new options for patients with chronic and seemingly refractory disease. Venous insufficiency syndromes can be diagnosed and treated by means of a variety of specialized techniques with which a generalist may not be familiar.

Graduated Compression and Other Physical Modalities

The standard approach has been to use gradient compression stockings that provide 30–40 or 40–50 mmHg of compression at the ankle, with gradually decreasing compression at more proximal levels of the leg. This amount of graduated compression is sufficient to restore normal venous flow patterns in many or most patients with superficial venous reflux and to improve venous flow, even in patients with severe deep venous incompetence.

The compression gradient is extremely important because nongradient stockings or high-stretch elastic bandages (e.g. ACE wraps) may cause a tourniquet effect that can exacerbate the venous insufficiency. The so-called antiembolic stockings that are commonly available in American hospitals do not provide sufficient compression to improve the venous return from the legs, and they are not particularly effective in preventing venous thromboembolism.

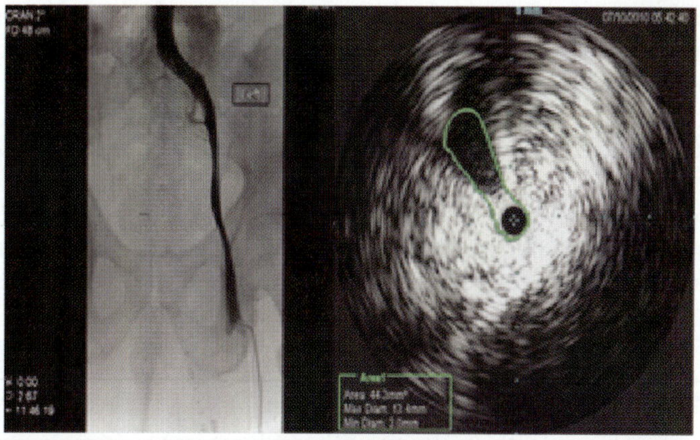

Fig. 30.17: *Venography is poorly sensitive to iliac vein obstruction. (Left) A venogram appears unremarkable. (Right) A tight stenosis is present, as shown by the IVUS image. Measured lumen area by IVUS planimetry was 44.3 mm². Normal value in adults is > 175 mm². A 75% stenosis can therefore be calculated to be present*

No patient with symptoms due to venous insufficiency should be without gradient compression hose, which can be prescribed by any physician. The prescription should specify 1 pair of calf-high (or thigh-high with waist attachment or panty-hose style) compression hose providing a pressure gradient of 30–40 mmHg with refills as needed.

A different approach to graduated compression was assessed in a 2012 study of 401 ambulatory patients with CVI, in which standard "degressive" compression stockings were compared with "progressive" compression stockings that applied maximal pressure over the calf. The investigators concluded that the progressive compressive stockings were superior with respect to improvement of pain and lower leg symptoms in patients with CVI as well as being easier to apply.

Additional physical measures may also be helpful. Leg elevation causes venous flow to be augmented by gravity, lowering venous pressures and ameliorating edema. In a sitting position, the patient's legs should be above the thighs; supine, they should be above the level of the heart. The Unna boot, first described in 1854, is now a mainstay of treatment for people with venous ulcers. Unna boots are rolled bandages that contain a combination of calamine lotion, glycerin, zinc oxide and gelatin.

Venous insufficiency is an especially common problem among postmenopausal women. In a randomized, controlled trial involving 65 postmenopausal women with venous insufficiency, the use of myofascial release therapy in combination with kinesiotherapy over a 10-week treatment period was found to yield significant improvements in basal metabolism, intracellular water, diastolic blood pressure, venous blood flow velocity, pain, and emotional role.

Venoablation

Venoablation is reserved for those with discomfort or ulcers refractory to medical management. The primary goal of surgical and endovenous approaches is to correct venous insufficiency by removing the major reflux pathways.

Techniques for venoablation include the following:

- Ligation with stripping
- Simple ligation and division
- Sclerotherapy (with or without ligation)
- Stab evulsion (with or without ligation)
- Radiofrequency ablation (RFA)
- Endovenous laser therapy (EVLT).

All methods of venoablation are effective (although there is some disagreement between the medical and the surgical literature as to the prevalence and timing of varicose recurrences). Once the overall volume of venous reflux is reduced below a critical threshold by any mechanism, venous ulcerations heal, and patient symptoms are resolved.

In general, vein ligation is reserved for cases of chronic venous insufficiency (CVI) involving reflux in the saphenous system that causes severe symptoms. Thus, a diagnosis of reflux must be established preoperatively, usually with photoplethysmography or duplex imaging.

Contraindications: In patients with symptomatic varicosities of the great saphenous vein (GSV), deep occlusion must be ruled out; it is an absolute contra-indication to vein ligation. Venography of the deep venous system before superficial vein ligation is imperative.

Sclerotherapy is performed by injecting or infusing a sclerosing substance into the refluxing vessel to produce endothelial destruction and fibrosis of the treated vessel. Injection of a sclerosing agent directly into veins usually is reserved for telangiectatic lesions rather than CVI. Phlebotonics have not been proven to be beneficial for CVI.

EVLT is performed by passing a laser fiber from the knee to the groin and then delivering laser energy along the entire course of the vein. Destruction of the vascular wall is followed by fibrosis of the treated vessel. It has been shown to yield excellent long-term (>5 years) results and a low rate of complications, which vary with the laser wavelength used.

RFA is performed by passing a special radiofrequency (RF) catheter from the knee to the groin and then carrying out controlled and preset heating of the targeted vessel until thermal injury causes shrinkage. The process is repeated every 7 cm along the course of the vein. Initial thermal injury is followed by fibrosis of the treated vessel. RFA has been shown to be effective, with a low rate of complications. It has produced excellent results that have been confirmed with up to 10 years of follow-up.

Subfascial endoscopic perforator surgery (SEPS) has also been employed to treat CVI. Endoscopic techniques are used to find and ligate perforating veins. Preliminary reports showed that after SEPS, the average healing time for ulcers was 42 days, with a recurrence rate of 3%, and that ulcers treated with SEPS healed 4 times faster than ulcers treated conventionally. In addition, the morbidity of SEPS was significantly lower than that of traditional operations.

Overall, approximately 8% of patients require surgical intervention for CVI. Different options are suitable for different conditions (see below). Careful monitoring of a patient's cardiac status and vital signs is extremely important. In addition, periodic monitoring of hemoglobin and hematocrit levels yields essential intraoperative data.

Varicose bleeding: Patients with varicose bleeding usually present to an emergency department (ED), where the traditional management is to oversew the involved vessel. Patients who have had significant blood loss may be admitted to the hospital, particularly if the bleeding varicosity is large and if the overlying tissue is friable. Oversewing a vessel almost always results in short-term control, but it can also cause short-term recurrence of hemorrhage because the procedure does nothing to ablate the dilated, superficial, thin-walled vessel that has ruptured.

Variceal hemorrhage is best managed by means of primary sclerotherapy with sodium tetradecyl sulfate. Tretbar reported a series of cases that were successfully treated by means of primary compression sclerotherapy over a 3-year period.

Superficial Venous Insufficiency

For superficial vein treatment, primary surgery offers a lower rate of early recurrence, whereas sclerotherapy produces fewer complications and offers higher rates of patient satisfaction both early and at follow-up. The lower likelihood of early recurrence after surgical treatment offsets the greater risk of complications.

Vein stripping with ligation of the saphenofemoral junction has long been the most commonly adopted surgical approach in cases of superficial venous insufficiency. At present, it is increasingly being replaced by endovenous ablation techniques such as RFA and EVLT.

The original approach to vein ligation for superficial vein disorders involved removal of the entire GSV system; this approach has largely been supplanted by the stab evulsion technique. In stab evulsion, several 2–3 mm incisions are made overlying the GSV at various levels. The vein is dissected from the underlying tissues, and any perforators are ligated. A small hook or blunt needle is used to extract as much of the vein as possible.

Typically, stab evulsion is limited to areas above the knee in the GSV system to avoid damage to the saphenous nerve or sural nerve. This technique is reserved for CVI in which reflux in the saphenous system occurs and causes severe symptoms. For this reason, it is mandatory to establish a diagnosis of reflux preoperatively.

Simple ligation and division of the incompetent vessels is not an effective way of treating failed perforating vessels, because this procedure is associated with a high incidence of early recurrence of reflux when it is applied to the GSV.

Skin grafts do not survive for very long unless the venous insufficiency has been treated, and after the venous insufficiency is ablated, the ulcer usually heals quickly, even without grafting.

Deep Venous Insufficiency

The decision to operate on a patient with venous obstruction in the deep veins should be made only after a careful assessment of symptom severity and direct measurement of both arm and foot venous pressures. Venography alone is not sufficient, because many patients with occlusive disease have extensive collateral circulation, which renders them less symptomatic. Clot lysis [e.g. with tissue plasminogen activator (TPA) or urokinase] and thrombectomy have been tried but have largely been abandoned because of extremely high recurrence rates.

For iliofemoral disease, the operation of choice is a saphenous vein crossover graft. In this procedure, the contralateral saphenous vein is mobilized and divided at its distal end, then tunneled suprapubically and anastomosed to the femoral vein on the diseased side (see the image below). The result is diversion of venous blood through the graft and into the intact contralateral venous system. Because of a relatively high failure rate (20%), ringed polytetrafluoroethylene (PTFE) grafts are used. Long-term patency has not been determined.

Venous insufficiency iliofemoral obstruction (Palma operation). Saphenous vein from contralateral leg tunneled subcutaneously to femoral vein of affected limb; cumulative patency of 75% at 5 years. Procedure relieves venous claudication but may not heal ulcers or relieve swelling.

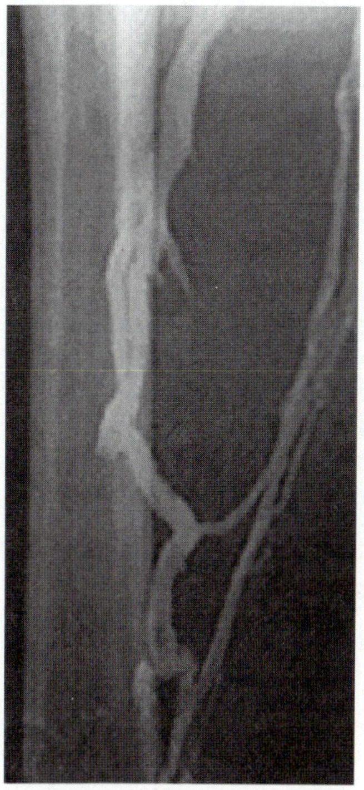

Fig. 30.18: Lower extremity venogram shows a nonocclusive chronic thrombus. The superficial femoral vein (lateral vein) has the appearance of 2 parallel veins, when in fact, it is 1 lumen containing a chronic linear thrombus. Although the chronic clot is not obstructive after it recanalizes, it effectively causes the venous valves to adhere in an open position, predisposing the patient to reflux in the involved segment

For occlusion of the superficial femoral vein, the Husni bypass, described by Warren in 1954 and Husni in 1983, may be considered. In this procedure, the ipsilateral GSV is harvested and used as an in-situ popliteal-femoral vein bypass. Because of its high failure rate (approximately 40%), the Husni bypass is performed infrequently. A minimally invasive technique using stents has been described.

Valvuloplasty is reserved for patients with a congenital absence of functional valves. A phlebotomy is performed, and the valve cusps are plicated. To ensure an adequate result, plicating 20–25% of each cusp is recommended. Addition of a PTFE sleeve around the operating site to maintain valve integrity is routine. When combined with ligation of perforating veins, valvuloplasty yields a superior outcome in 80% of cases after 5 years.

With vein segment transposition, a normally functioning vein that is in close proximity to the diseased vessel is identified. The incompetent vein is then dissected, mobilized, and transposed onto the normal vein distal to a functional valve.

With vein valve transplantation, a valve-containing segment of a competent axillary or brachial vein is mobilized and inserted into either the popliteal or the femoral system. The incompetent segment of the leg vein is excised and replaced with the transplant segment. Allograft or cadaveric vein transplants are being evaluated, with long-term results pending.

Complications of Surgical Ablation

Potential complications of surgical ablation of refluxing veins include the following:
- Infection
- Nerve injury (e.g. to sural or saphenous nerves)

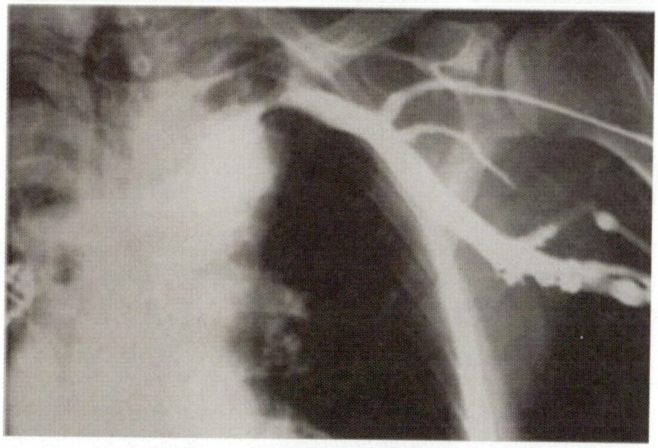

Fig. 30.19: Phlebogram of a patient in whom leads had been implanted on both sides due to repeated system infections. On the right, reoperation revealed complete occlusion of the brachiocephalic vein. Phlebography prior to left-side implantation showed subtotal stenosis of the subclavian vein

- Arterial injury
- Undesirable cosmetic outcomes

Potential complications of sclerotherapy include the following:

- Allergic reactions to sclerosants
- Cutaneous necrosis due to extravasation
- Inadvertent arterial injection (may cause loss of a limb)

Potential complications of RFA and EVLT include the following:

- Skin burns
- Thermal injury to adjacent tissues
- Inadvertent injury to deep veins.

Postprocedural Care

Anticoagulation with heparin (or low-molecular-weight heparin) in the immediate postoperative period and long-term prophylaxis with warfarin are recommended.

Observe patients frequently for wound infection after discharge, beginning 1 week postoperatively. Sutures or staples typically stay in 2–4 weeks, depending on the health of the skin at the operative site.

Increased pain or swelling is an indication for repeat duplex ultrasonography to rule out DVT.

Activity

Regular activity is an important ameliorating factor in patients with early or mild venous insufficiency syndrome. Prolonged standing or sitting can aggravate the symptoms of venous insufficiency. Patients with advanced disease do not tolerate activity well.

Walking or running, bicycling, and swimming are excellent activities for patients with an intact and

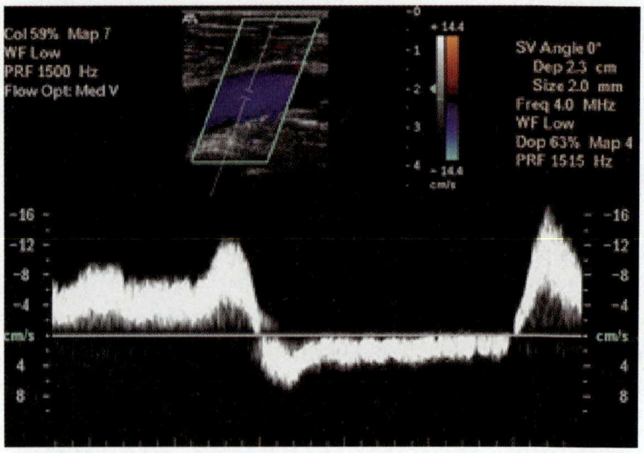

Fig. 30.21: *Refluxing deep vein. Reflux in the femoral vein elicited with a sustained Valsalva or simulated valsalva manoeuvre lasting three seconds*

functioning calf muscle pump. Patients with obstructed venous outflow usually experience increased pain and swelling with activity. Patients with muscle pump failure usually have a markedly reduced exercise tolerance because of early leg fatigue.

Prevention

In general, patients with venous insufficiency should avoid prolonged standing or sitting. Correction of the underlying problem prevents progression of the disease.

In patients with early venous insufficiency, progression to overt signs of disease (e.g. stasis dermatitis, skin breakdown, and ulceration) can virtually always be prevented with the use of compression hose that provide a pressure gradient of 30–40 mmHg between foot and knee.

Medication

No oral medication has yet been proven useful for the treatment of venous disease. Findings of prospective studies have not supported some manufacturers' claims about the effectiveness of their herbal products and nutritional supplements.

Sclerosing agents that are used to ablate refluxing veins and other anatomic structures can be grouped into several categories including fatty alcohols (detergents), osmotic agents, and caustic agents. The safest and most widely used sclerosing agents are detergents.

Sclerosing Agents

Sclerosing agents are used for the primary sclerosis of reflux pathways and for the ablation of friable thin-walled veins judged to be at high risk for rupture and hemorrhage.

Sodium Tetradecyl Sulfate (Sotradecol)

Primary sclerotherapy is the treatment of choice for ablation of refluxing superficial venous circuits in the absence of saphenofemoral junctional reflux. It is also the treatment of choice for ablation of venous bleeding sites and friable thin-walled varices. In general, a 1% concentration is most useful; in larger varicosities, a 3% concentration may be used as a liquid. Foam may be made by agitating a 1:4

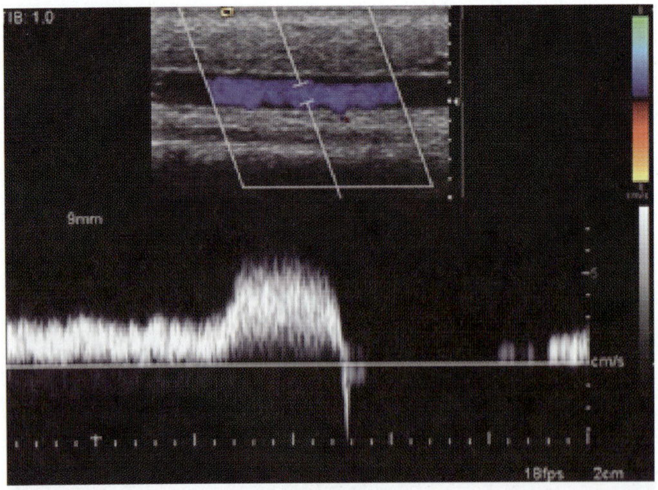

Fig. 30.20: *Competent superficial vein. Well optimised duplex image of flow in a competent superficial vein. Wide color box was used in order for a long segment of the vein to be visualised. Spectral waveform is large and clear. Spontaneous venous flow is seen in the left side of the spectral trace, followed by manual augmentation. There is a sharp "click" or "snap" of venous valve closure followed by a period of absent flow. Once arterial inflow refills the peripheral vascular bed, normal antegrade flow resumes again on the right side of the spectral Doppler trace*

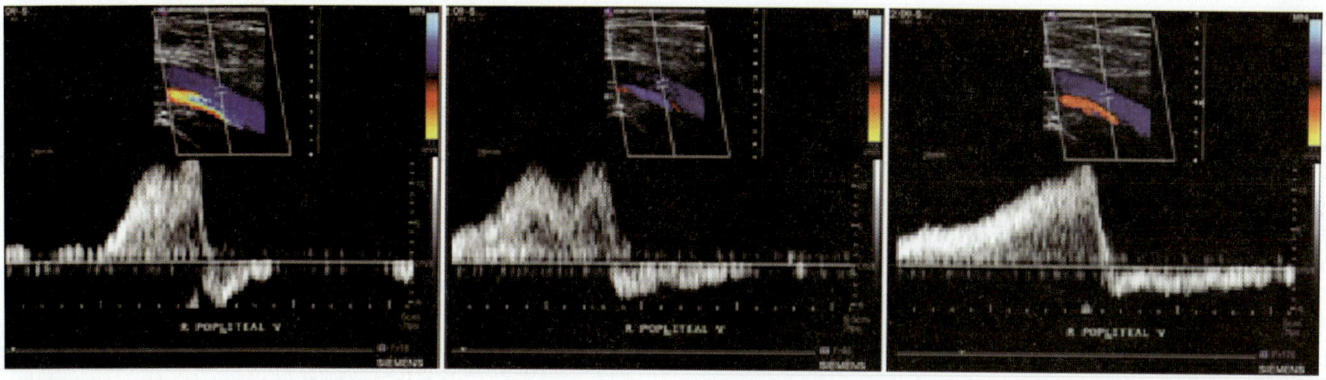

Fig. 30.22: *Variability of reflux response. The effect of the length of augmentation on the tendency of lower extremity veins to reflux. All images are obtained from the same sample site in the popliteal vein of the same patient. Left image: short augmentation resulting in reflux time of only 0.7 seconds. Middle image: longer augmentation resulting in reflux time of 1.5 seconds. Right image: prolonged augmentation resulting in continuous reflux for many seconds*

mixture of solution and air. When a foamed solution is used, a concentration of 0.25–0.5% is sufficient.

Prognosis

The syndromes of venous hypertension and reduced venous clearance are important causes of morbidity and disability in patients with varicose venous disease (see also Complications).

Without correction of the underlying cause, venous insufficiency is inexorably progressive. Subjective symptoms usually worsen over time.

In many patients, the skin eventually breaks down and nonhealing ulcers develop. A study by Abbade et al determined that long-standing and large ulcers and recurrences are the primary complications encountered by patients who have venous ulcers. Risk factors for these complications include severe lipodermatosclerosis, a previous history of ulcers, and time since first ulcer episode of 2 years or longer.

Chronic nonhealing leg ulceration can be debilitating. Approximately, 1 million Americans have an ulceration due to superficial venous disease, and approximately 100,000 are disabled because of their condition. Reflux need not be entirely eliminated for the ulceration to resolve. Ulcers will heal if the net volume and pressure of reflux are reduced below a threshold level. Tissue atrophy and staining are usually not reversible.

Patients have an increased lifetime risk of DVT and pulmonary embolism. Tsai et al examining the National Inpatient Sample from 1988–2000, found that DVT affected 1.3% of patients and that amputation was necessary in 1.2%, with an overall mortality of 1.6%.

As many as 50% of patients with untreated varicose veins develop superficial thrombophlebitis at some time. This is of grave concern because unrecognized DVT is present in as many as 45% of patients with what appears to be purely superficial phlebitis. The risk of DVT is 3 times higher in patients with superficial varicosities than in the general population.

Bed rest and intercurrent illness place patients with venous insufficiency at higher risk for DVT. Phlebitis develops in 60% of hospitalized patients with clinically evident superficial venous insufficiency, and in nearly one half of cases, the condition progresses to DVT. Approximately one half of patients with DVT have detectable pulmonary embolism, and the death rate in this group exceeds 1 in 3.

Venous insufficiency syndromes can also lead to death from hemorrhage. Bleeding from lower-extremity varicosities can be fatal; 23 such fatalities were reported in England and Wales in 1973, and although there is no central registry to tabulate the frequency with which it occurs, such cases are not unusual in the United States. Bleeding is not a rare problem, but it is often managed incorrectly.

Outcomes for different therapies have varied. Clot lysis (e.g. with tissue plasminogen activator or urokinase) and thrombectomy have been tried but have largely been abandoned because of the extremely high recurrence rates.

Saphenous vein crossover grafting for iliofemoral disease has a relatively high failure rate (20%), and thus, ringed polytetrafluoroethylene (PTFE) grafts are now being used. Long-term patency rates have not been determined. The Husni bypass for superficial femoral vein occlusion has an even higher failure rate (approximately 40%) and thus is now performed infrequently.

Surgery for CVI resulting from deep vein incompetence includes valvuloplasty and allograft or cadaveric vein transplant. Valvuloplasty for patients with congenital absence of functional valves, when combined with ligation of perforating veins, yields a superior outcome in 80% of cases after 5 years. Allograft or cadaveric vein transplants are undergoing further evaluation, with long-term results pending.

DIAGNOSIS OF DEEP VENOUS THROMBOSIS AND PULMONARY EMBOLISM

Venous thromboembolism manifests as deep venous thrombosis (DVT) or pulmonary embolism, and has a mortality rate of 6–12%. Well-validated clinical prediction rules are available to determine the pretest probability of DVT and pulmonary embolism. When the likelihood of

DVT is low, a negative D-dimer assay result excludes DVT. Likewise, a low pretest probability with a negative D-dimer assay result excludes the diagnosis of pulmonary embolism. If the likelihood of DVT is intermediate to high, compression ultrasonography should be performed. Impedance plethysmography, contrast venography, and magnetic resonance venography are available to assess for DVT, but are not widely used. Pulmonary embolism is usually a consequence of DVT and is associated with greater mortality. Multidetector computed tomography angiography is the diagnostic test of choice when the technology is available and appropriate for the patient. It is warranted in patients who may have a pulmonary embolism and a positive D-dimer assay result, or in patients who have a high pretest probability of pulmonary embolism, regardless of D-dimer assay result. Ventilation-perfusion scanning is an acceptable alternative to computed tomography angiography in select settings. Pulmonary angiography is needed only when the clinical suspicion for pulmonary embolism remains high, even when less invasive study results are negative. In unstable emergent cases highly suspicious for pulmonary embolism, echocardiography may be used to evaluate for right ventricular dysfunction, which is indicative of but not diagnostic for pulmonary embolism (Figs 30.27, 30.28).

Medical History

The challenge in dealing with pulmonary embolism is that patients rarely display the classic presentation of this problem, that is, the abrupt onset of pleuritic chest pain, shortness of breath, and hypoxia. Studies of patients who died unexpectedly from pulmonary embolism have revealed that often these individuals complained of nagging symptoms for weeks before death. Forty percent of these patients had been seen by a physician in the weeks prior to their death.

The following risk factors can be indications for the presence of pulmonary embolism:

- Venous stasis
- Hypercoagulable states
- Immobilization
- Surgery and trauma
- Pregnancy
- Oral contraceptives and estrogen replacement
- Malignancy
- Hereditary factors resulting in a hypercoagulable state
- Acute medical illness
- Drug abuse [intravenous (IV) drugs]
- Drug-induced lupus anticoagulant
- Hemolytic anemias
- Heparin-associated thrombocytopenia
- Homocystinemia
- Homocystinuria
- Hyperlipidemias
- Phenothiazines
- Thrombocytosis
- Varicose veins
- Venography
- Venous pacemakers
- Venous stasis
- Warfarin (first few days of therapy)
- Inflammatory bowel disease.

The PIOPED II study listed the following indicators for pulmonary embolism:

- Travel of 4 hours or more in the past month
- Surgery within the last 3 months
- Malignancy, especially lung cancer
- Current or past history of thrombophlebitis
- Trauma to the lower extremities and pelvis during the past 3 months.

Smoking

- Central venous instrumentation within the past 3 months
- Stroke, paresis, or paralysis
- Prior pulmonary embolism
- Heart failure
- Chronic obstructive pulmonary disease.

Physical Examination

Physical examination findings are quite variable in pulmonary embolism and, for convenience, may be grouped into four categories as follows:

- Massive pulmonary embolism
- Acute pulmonary infarction
- Acute embolism without infarction
- Multiple pulmonary emboli or thrombi.

The presentation of pulmonary embolism may vary from sudden catastrophic hemodynamic collapse to gradually progressive dyspnea. (Prior poor cardiopulmonary status of the patient is an important factor leading to hemodynamic collapse.) Most patients with pulmonary embolism have no obvious symptoms at presentation. In contrast, patients with symptomatic DVT commonly have pulmonary embolism confirmed on diagnostic studies in the absence of pulmonary symptoms. Sickle cell disease often creates a diagnostic difficulty with regard to pulmonary embolism. A chest infection is often the presenting symptom.

Patients with pulmonary embolism may present with atypical symptoms. In such cases, strong suspicion of pulmonary embolism based on the presence of risk factors can lead to consideration of pulmonary embolism in the differential diagnosis. These symptoms include the following:

- Seizures
- Syncope
- Abdominal pain
- Fever
- Productive cough
- Wheezing
- Decreasing level of consciousness
- New onset of atrial fibrillation
- Flank pain
- Delirium (in elderly patients)

The diagnosis of pulmonary embolism should be sought actively in patients with respiratory symptoms unexplained by an alternative diagnosis. The symptoms of pulmonary embolism are nonspecific; therefore, a high index of suspicion is required, particularly when a patient has risk factors for the condition.

Acute respiratory consequences of pulmonary embolism include the following:
- Increased alveolar dead space
- Hypoxemia
- Hyperventilation
- In patients with recognized pulmonary embolism, the incidence of physical signs has been reported as follows:
- Tachypnea (respiratory rate >16/min) (96%)
- Rales (58%)
- Accentuated second heart sound (53%)
- Tachycardia (heart rate >100/min) (44%)
- Fever (temperature >37.8°C) (43%)
- Diaphoresis (36%)
- S3 or S4 gallop (34%)
- Clinical signs and symptoms suggesting thrombophlebitis (32%)
- Lower extremity edema (24%)
- Cardiac murmur (23%)
- Cyanosis (19%)
- The PIOPED study reported the following incidence of common symptoms of pulmonary embolism:
- Dyspnea (73%)
- Pleuritic chest pain (66%)
- Cough (37%)
- Hemoptysis (13%).

Fever of less than 39°C may be present in 14% of patients; however, temperature higher than 39.5°C is not from pulmonary embolism. Chest wall tenderness upon palpation without a history of trauma, may be the sole physical finding in rare cases.

Pleuritic chest pain without other symptoms or risk factors may be a presentation of pulmonary embolism. Pleuritic or respirophasic chest pain is a particularly worrisome symptom. Pleuritic chest pain is reported to occur in as many as 84% of patients with pulmonary emboli. Its presence suggests that the embolus is located more peripherally and thus may be smaller.

Pulmonary embolism has been diagnosed in 21% of young, active patients who come to emergency departments (EDs) complaining only of pleuritic chest pain. These patients usually lack any other classical signs, symptoms, or known risk factors for pulmonary thromboembolism. Such patients often are dismissed inappropriately with an inadequate workup and a nonspecific diagnosis, such as musculoskeletal chest pain or pleurisy.

MASSIVE PULMONARY EMBOLISM

Patients with massive pulmonary embolism are in shock. They have systemic hypotension, poor perfusion of the extremities, tachycardia and tachypnea. In addition, patients appear weak, pale, sweaty, and oliguric and develop impaired mentation.

Signs of pulmonary hypertension, such as palpable impulse over the second left intercostal space, loud P2, right ventricular S3 gallop, and a systolic murmur louder on inspiration at left sternal border (tricuspid regurgitation), may be present.

Massive pulmonary embolism has been defined by hemodynamic parameters and evidence of myocardial injury rather than anatomic findings because the former is associated with adverse outcomes. Although previous studies of CT scans in the diagnosis of pulmonary embolus suggested that central obstruction was not associated with adverse outcomes, a new multicenter study clarifies this observation. Vedovati et al found no association between central obstruction and death or clinical deterioration in 579 patients with pulmonary embolus. However, when a subset of 516 patients who were hemodynamically stable was assessed, central localization of emboli was found to be an independent mortality risk factor while distal localization was inversely associated with adverse events. Thus, anatomic findings by CT scan may be important in assessing risk in hemodynamically stable patients with pulmonary embolus.

Acute Pulmonary Infarction

Approximately, 10% of patients have peripheral occlusion of a pulmonary artery, causing parenchymal infarction.

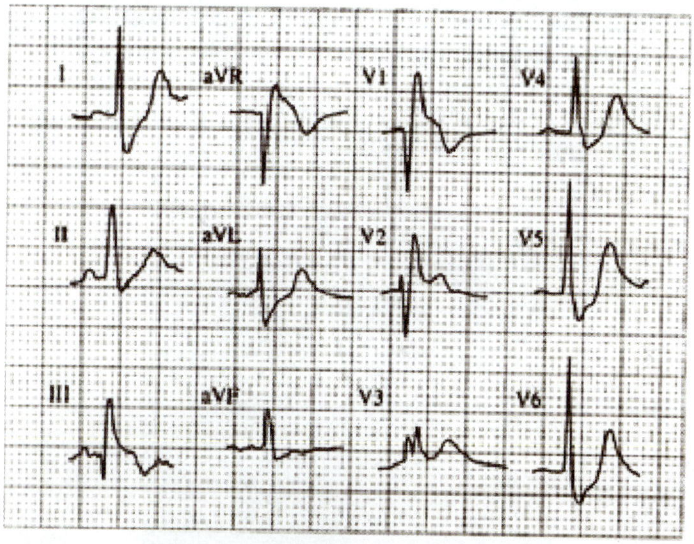

Fig. 30.23: *SI, Q3, T3 pattern. Right bundle-branch block (incomplete or complete). T wave inversion in the right precordial leads P pulmonale. Right-axis deviation in patient with acute pulmonary embolism*

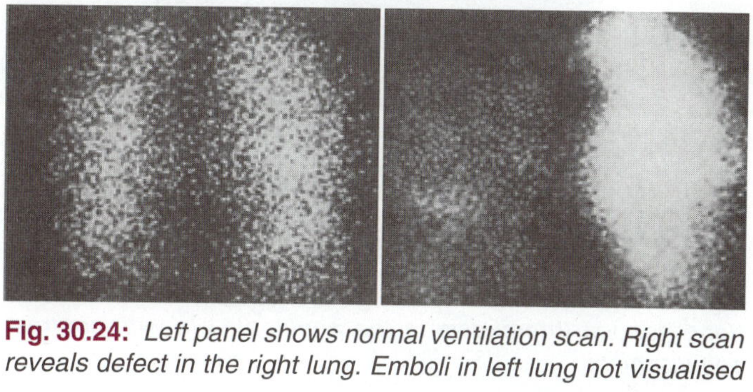

Fig. 30.24: *Left panel shows normal ventilation scan. Right scan reveals defect in the right lung. Emboli in left lung not visualised*

These patients present with acute onset of pleuritic chest pain, breathlessness and hemoptysis. Although the chest pain may be clinically indistinguishable from ischemic myocardial pain, normal ECG findings and no response to nitroglycerin rules out myocardial pain. Patients with acute pulmonary infarction have decreased excursion of the involved hemithorax, palpable or audible pleural friction rub, and even localized tenderness. Signs of pleural effusion, such as dullness to percussion and diminished breath sounds, may be present.

Acute Embolism without Infarction

Patients with acute embolism without infarction have nonspecific physical signs that may easily be secondary to another disease process. Tachypnea and tachycardia frequently are detected, pleuritic pain sometimes may be present, crackles may be heard in the area of embolization, and local wheeze may be heard rarely.

Multiple Pulmonary Emboli or Thrombi

Patients with pulmonary emboli and thrombi have physical signs of pulmonary hypertension and cor pulmonale. Patients may have elevated jugular venous pressure, right ventricular heave, palpable impulse in the left second intercostal space, right ventricular S3 gallop, systolic murmur over the left sternal border that is louder during inspiration, hepatomegaly, ascites, and dependent pitting edema. These findings are not specific for pulmonary embolism and require a high index of suspicion for pursuing appropriate diagnostic studies.

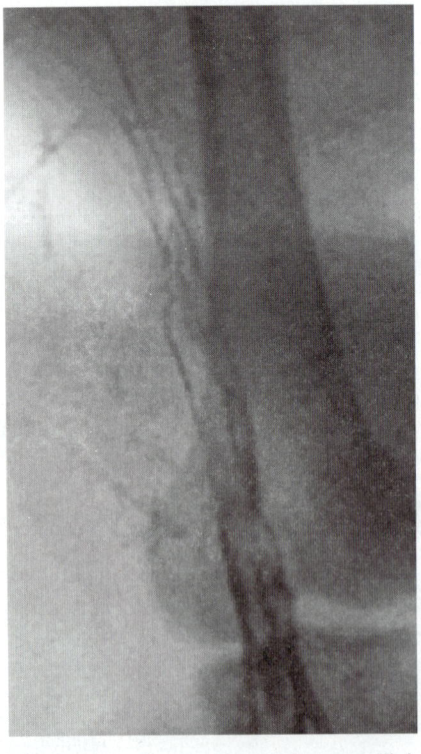

Fig. 30.25: *Lower extremity venogram shows outlining of an acute deep venous thrombosis in the popliteal vein with contrast enhancement*

Pulmonary Emboli in Children

Many physical findings are typically less marked in children than they are in adults, presumably because children have greater hemodynamic reserve and, thus, are better able to tolerate the significant hemodynamic and pulmonary changes.

Because of the rarity of pulmonary emboli in children, these patients are probably under diagnosed. For the same reason, much of the information pertaining to diagnosis and management of pulmonary embolism has been derived from adult practice.

Cough is present in approximately 50% of children with pulmonary emboli; tachypnea occurs with the same frequency. Hemoptysis is a feature in a minority of children with pulmonary emboli, occurring in about 30% of cases. Crackles are heard in a minority of cases.

Cyanosis and hypoxemia are not prominent features of pulmonary embolism. If present, cyanosis suggests a massive embolism leading to a marked ventilation-perfusion (V/Q) mismatch and systemic hypoxemia. Some case reports have described massive pediatric pulmonary embolism with normal saturation.

A pleural rub is often associated with pleuritic chest pain and indicates an embolism in a peripheral location in the pulmonary vasculature. Signs that indicate pulmonary hypertension and right ventricular failure include a loud pulmonary component of the second heart sound, right ventricular lift, distended neck veins, and hypotension. An increase in pulmonary artery pressure is reportedly not evident until at least 60% of the vascular bed has been occluded.

A gallop rhythm signifies ventricular failure while peripheral edema is a sign of congestive heart failure. Various heart murmurs may be audible including a tricuspid regurgitant murmur signifying pulmonary hypertension.

Fever is an unusual sign that is nonspecific, and diaphoresis is a manifestation of sympathetic arousal. Signs of other organ involvement in patients with sickle cell disease would be elicited, such as sequestration crisis, priapism, anemia and stroke.

Approach Considerations

Clinical signs and symptoms for pulmonary embolism are nonspecific; therefore, patients suspected of having pulmonary embolism—because of unexplained dyspnea, tachypnea, or chest pain or the presence of risk factors for pulmonary embolism—must undergo diagnostic tests until the diagnosis is ascertained or eliminated or an alternative diagnosis is confirmed. Further, routine laboratory findings are nonspecific and are not helpful in pulmonary embolism, although they may suggest another diagnosis.

A hypercoagulation workup should be performed if no obvious cause for embolic disease is apparent. This may include screening for conditions such as the following:

- Antithrombin III deficiency
- Protein C or protein S deficiency
- Lupus anticoagulant

- Homocystinuria
- Occult neoplasm
- Connective tissue disorders.

No particular strategy appears to be superior to another at present for the diagnosis of pulmonary embolism. More clinical studies are needed to evaluate the utility of new approaches to the condition's diagnosis. The availability of diagnostic tests, as well as cost-effectiveness analysis, local traditions, and the expertise of radiologists involved in the diagnosis, appears to be the considerations in the workup of a patient suspected of having pulmonary embolism.

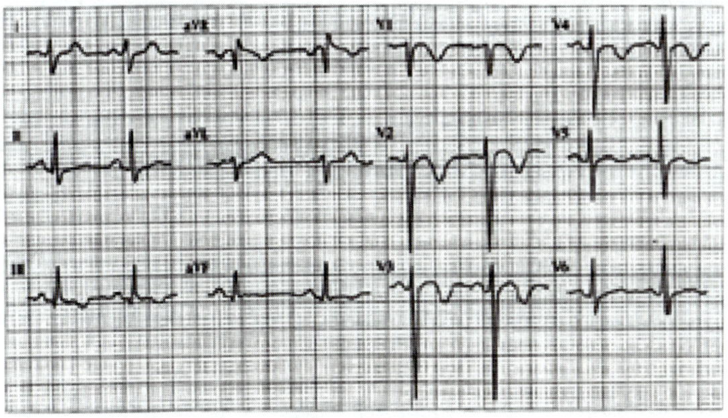

Fig. 30.26: *Acute pulmonary embolism: 10 days postoperatively the patient developed acute dyspnoea and hypotension (note the T wave inversion in the right precordial leads and lead III)*

Clinical Scoring Systems

Evidence-based literature supports the practice of determining the clinical probability of pulmonary embolism before proceeding with testing. A clinical practice guideline from the American academy of family physicians (AAFP) and the American College of Physicians (ACP) recommends that validated clinical prediction rules be used to estimate pretest probability of pulmonary embolism and to interpret test results. The guideline, current diagnosis of venous thromboembolism in primary care, advocates use of the Wells prediction rule for this purpose but notes that the Wells rule performs better in younger patients without comorbidities or a history of venous thromboembolism than in other patients.

One study assessed the performance of four clinical decision rules in addition to D-dimer testing to exclude acute PE. All 4 rules, Wells rule, simplified Wells rule, revised Geneva score, and simplified revised Geneva score, showed similar performance for excluding acute PE when combined with a normal D-dimer result.

D-Dimer Follow-Up on Low-to-Moderate Pretest Probability

When clinical prediction rule results indicate that the patient has a low or moderate pretest probability of pulmonary embolism, D-dimer testing is the usual next step.

D-dimer, a degradation product produced by plasmin-mediated proteases of cross-linked fibrin, is measured by a variety of assay types including quantitative, semiquan-

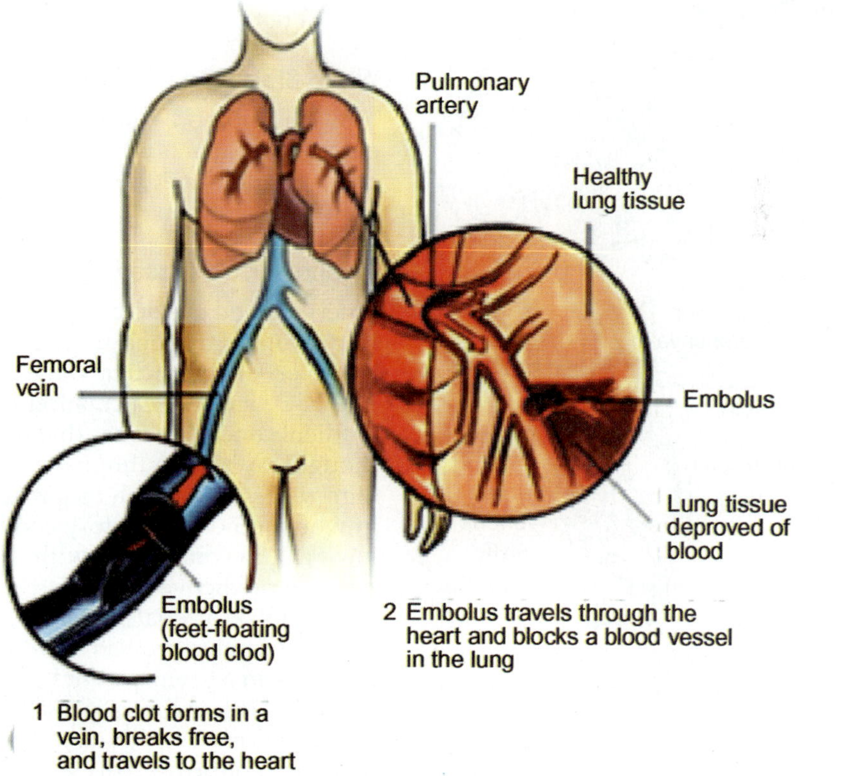

Fig. 30.27: *Immobilization (wearing a cast) coupled with a long flight can cause a blood clot to form in the large leg veins, a condition called deep vein thrombosis (DVT). It is the clot from a DVT that travels to the lung and causes the PE*

titative, and qualitative rapid enzyme-linked immunosorbent assays (ELISAs); quantitative and semiquantitative latex; and whole-blood assays. A systematic review of prospective studies of high methodologic quality concluded that the ELISAs—especially the quantitative rapid ELISA—dominate the comparative ranking among the D-dimer assays for sensitivity and negative likelihood ratio. The quantitative rapid ELISA has a sensitivity of 0.95 and negative likelihood ratio of 0.13; the latter is similar to that for a normal to near-normal lung scan in patients with suspected pulmonary embolism.

Negative results on a high-sensitivity D-dimer test in a patient with a low pretest probability of pulmonary embolism indicate a low likelihood of venous thromboembolism and reliably exclude pulmonary embolism. A large, prospective, randomized trial found that in patients with a low probability of pulmonary embolism who had negative D-dimer results, forgoing additional diagnostic testing was not associated with an increased frequency of symptomatic venous thromboembolism during the subsequent 6 months.

D-dimer testing is most reliable for excluding pulmonary embolism in younger patients who have no associated comorbidity or history of venous thromboembolism and whose symptoms are of short duration. However, it is of questionable value in patients who are older than 80 years, who are hospitalized, who have cancer, or who are pregnant, because nonspecific elevation of D-dimer concentrations is common in such patients.

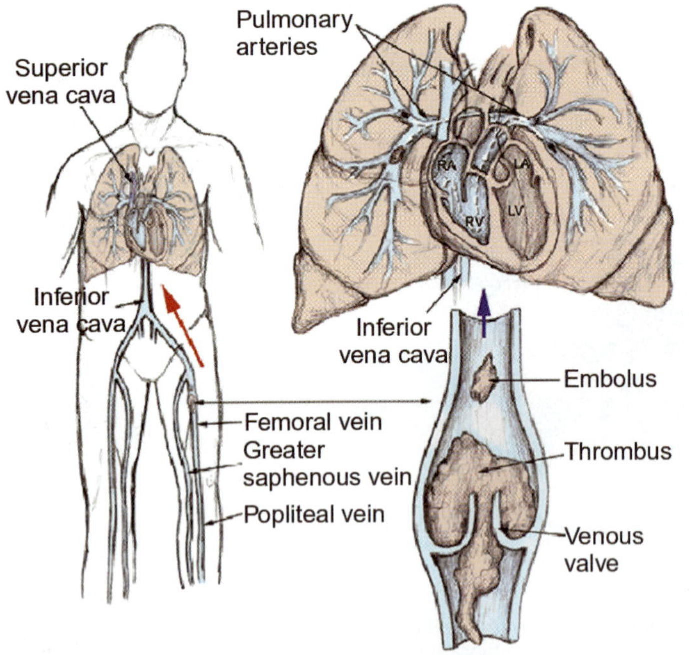

Fig. 30.28: *The pathophysiology of pulmonary embolism. Although pulmonary embolism can arise from anywhere in the body, most commonly it arises from the calf veins. The venous thrombi predominately originate in venous valve pockets (inset) and at other sites of presumed venous stasis. To reach the lungs, thromboemboli travel through the right side of the heart. RA, right atrium; RV, right ventricle; LA, left atrium; LV, left ventricle*

D-dimer testing should not be used when the clinical probability of pulmonary embolism is high, because the test has low negative predictive value in such cases.

Combining D-dimer results with measurement of the exhaled end-tidal ratio of carbon dioxide to oxygen ($etCO_2/O_2$) can be useful for diagnosis of pulmonary embolism. Kline et al found that, in moderate-risk patients with a positive D-dimer (>499 ng/mL), an $etCO_2/O_2 < 0.28$ significantly increased the probability of finding segmental or larger pulmonary embolism on computed tomography multidetector-row pulmonary angiography while an et CO_2/O_2); >0.45 predicted the absence of segmental or larger pulmonary embolism.

Because of the poor specificity, positive D-dimer measurements are generally not helpful in diagnosis. In addition, the use of D-dimers in children is not well studied. A small pediatric series reported that D-dimers findings are negative in 40% of patients. A retrospective series reported an elevated D-dimer in 86% of patients at presentation.

Ischemia-Modified Albumin Levels

A potential alternative to D-dimer testing is assessment of the ischemia-modified albumin (IMA) level, which data suggest is 93% sensitive and 75% specific for pulmonary embolism. Notably, in a study comparing the prognostic value of IMA to D-dimer testing, IMA assessment in combination with Wells and Geneva probability scores appeared to positively impact overall sensitivity and negative predictive value. The positive predictive value of IMA, in particular, is better than D-dimer. However, it should not be used alone.

White Blood Cell Count

The white blood cell (WBC) count may be normal or elevated in patients with pulmonary embolism, with a WBC count as high as 20,000 being not uncommon in patients with this condition.

Arterial Blood Gases

Arterial blood gas determinations characteristically reveal hypoxemia, hypocapnia, and respiratory alkalosis; however, the predictive value of hypoxemia is quite low. The PaO_2 and the calculation of alveolar-arterial oxygen gradient contribute to the diagnosis in a general population thought to have pulmonary embolism. Nonetheless, in high-risk settings such as patients in postoperative states in whom other respiratory conditions can be ruled out, a low PaO_2 in conjunction with dyspnea may have a strong positive predictive value.

The PO_2 on arterial blood gases analysis (ABG) has a zero or even negative-predictive value in a typical population of patients in whom pulmonary embolism is suspected clinically. This is contrary to what has been taught in many textbooks, and even though it seems counterintuitive, it is demonstrably true. This is because other etiologies that masquerade as pulmonary embolism are more likely to lower the PO_2 than pulmonary embolism. In fact, because other diseases that may masquerade as pulmonary embolism [e.g. chronic obstructive pulmonary disease (COPD), pneumonia, CHF] affect oxygen exchange more than does pulmonary embolism, the blood oxygen level often has an inverse predictive value for pulmonary embolism.

In most settings, fewer than half of all patients with symptoms suggestive of pulmonary embolism actually turn out to have pulmonary embolism as their diagnosis. In such a population, if any reasonable level of PaO_2 is chosen as a dividing line, the incidence of pulmonary embolism will be higher in the group with a PaO_2 above the dividing line than in the group whose PaO_2 is below the divider. This is a specific example of a general truth that may be demonstrated mathematically for any test finding with a Gaussian distribution and a population incidence of less than 50%.

Conversely, in a patient population with a very high incidence of pulmonary embolism and a lower incidence of other respiratory ailments (e.g. postoperative orthopedic patients with sudden onset of shortness of breath), a low PO_2 has a strongly positive-predictive value for pulmonary embolism.

The discussion above holds true not only for arterial PO_2 but also for the alveolar-arterial oxygen gradient and for the oxygen saturation level as measured by pulse oximetry. In particular, pulse oximetry is extremely insensitive, is normal in the majority of patients with pulmonary embolism, and should not be used to direct a diagnostic workup.

Troponin Levels

Serum troponin levels can be elevated in up to 50% of patients with a moderate to large pulmonary embolism, presumptively due to acute right ventricular myocardial stretch.

Although troponin assessment is not currently recommended as part of the diagnostic workup, studies have shown that elevated troponin levels in the setting of pulmonary embolism correlate with increased mortality. However, further studies need to be performed to identify subsets of patients with pulmonary embolism who might benefit from this testing.

A meta-analysis by Jimenez et al suggested that in acute symptomatic pulmonary embolism, elevated troponin levels do not distinguish between patients who are at high risk for death and those who are at low risk. Pooled results from studies including 1,366 normotensive patients with acute symptomatic pulmonary embolism showed that elevated troponin levels were associated with a 4.26-fold increased odds of overall mortality [95% confidence interval (CI), 2.13–8.50; heterogeneity chi2 = 12.64; degrees of freedom = 8; P = .125]. Summary receiver operating characteristic curve analysis showed a relationship between the sensitivity and the specificity of troponin levels to predict overall mortality (Spearman rank correlation coefficient = 0.68; P = .046). Pooled likelihood ratios (LRs) were not extreme [negative LR, 0.59 (95% CI, 0.39–0.88); positive LR, 2.26 (95% CI,1.66–3.07)].

Serum troponin, although seemingly marginal for purposes of diagnosis of pulmonary embolism, may contribute significantly to the ability to stratify patients by risk for short-term death or adverse outcome events when they reach the ED. In patients with pulmonary embolism and normal blood pressure specifically, elevated serum troponin level has been associated with right ventricular overload.

Leptin is another cardiovascular risk factor that may be associated with outcome in acute pulmonary embolism. Dellas et al conducted a prospective analysis of 264 patients with acute pulmonary embolus and found that serum leptin levels were inversely associated with the risk of adverse outcomes. Further study will be needed to confirm these findings and determine the clinical utility of leptin measurement.

Brain Natriuretic Peptide

Although brain natriuretic peptide (BNP) tests are neither sensitive nor specific, patients with pulmonary embolism tend to have higher BNP levels. BNP testing had a sensitivity and specificity of only 60% and 62%, respectively, in a case-control study of 2,213 hemodynamically stable patients with suspected acute pulmonary embolism.

Elevated levels of BNP or of its precursor, N-terminal pro-brain natriuretic peptide (NT-proBNP), do correlate with an increased risk of subsequent complications and mortality in patients with acute pulmonary embolism. One meta-analysis revealed that patients with a BNP level greater than 100 pg/mL or an NT-proBNP level greater than 600 ng/L had an all-cause in-hospital mortality rate 6- and 16-fold higher than those below these cutoffs, respectively. In a second smaller observational study, serum BNP levels greater than 90 pg/mL were associated with a higher rate of complications, such as the need for cardiopulmonary resuscitation, need for mechanical ventilation, need for vasopressor therapy, and death.

BNP testing is not currently recommended as part of the standard evaluation of acute pulmonary embolism, and future studies may aid in defining its role in this setting.

Elevated levels of brain-type natriuretic peptides (BNP) may also provide prognostic information. A meta-analysis demonstrated a significant association between elevated N-terminal–pro-BNP (NT-pro-BNP) and right ventricular function in patients with pulmonary embolism ($P < .001$), leading to an increased risk for complicated in-hospital course [odds ratio (OR) 6.8; 95% confidence interval (CI), 9.0–13] and 30-day mortality (OR 7.6; 95% CI, 3.4–17). Importantly, increased NT-pro-BNP alone does not justify more invasive treatment.

A recent study by Scherz et al analyzed a large sample of patients hospitalized with acute pulmonary embolism. Hyponatremia at presentation was common and was associated with a higher risk of 30-day mortality and readmission.

Venography

Venography is the criterion standard for diagnosing DVT. With the advent of noninvasive imaging, it has become less common in pediatric and adult practice.

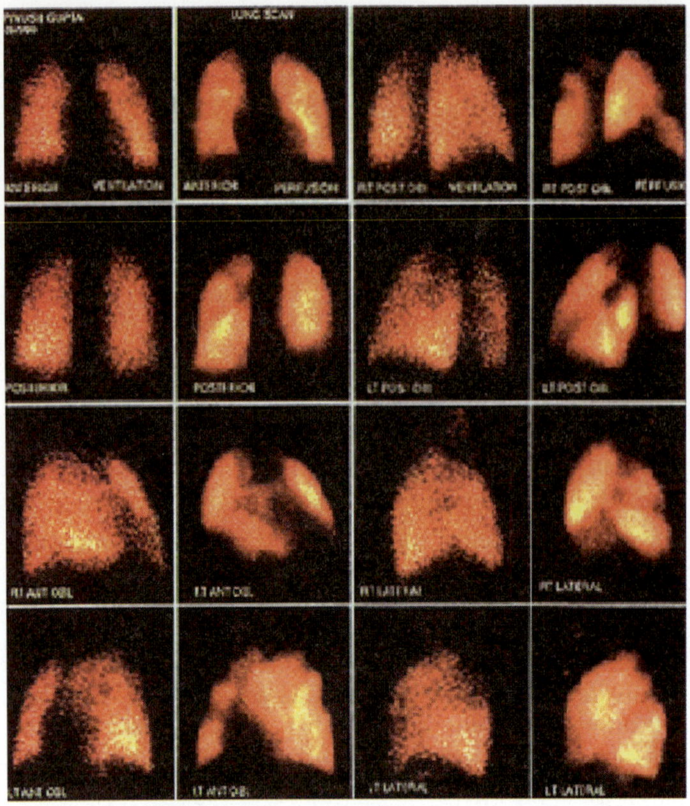

Fig. 30.29: *Ventilation perfusion scan of the patient showing reduced perfusion in right inferior and left upper lobes*

Angiography (Fig. 30.31)

Pulmonary angiography remains the criterion standard for the diagnosis of pulmonary embolism. Following injection of iodinated contrast, anteroposterior, lateral, and oblique studies are performed on each lung. Positive results consist of a filling defect or sharp cutoff of the affected artery (as shown in the image). Nonocclusive emboli are described as having a tram-track appearance. Abnormal findings on V/Q scans performed prior to angiography guide the operator to focus on abnormal areas. Angiography generally is a safe procedure. The mortality rate for patients undergoing this procedure is less than 0.5%, and the morbidity rate is less than 5%. Patients who have long-standing pulmonary arterial hypertension and right ventricular failure are considered high-risk patients. Negative pulmonary angiogram findings, even if false negative, exclude clinically relevant pulmonary embolism. A pulmonary angiogram shows the abrupt termination of the ascending branch of the right upper-lobe artery, confirming the diagnosis of pulmonary embolism. If multidetector-row computed tomography angiography (MDCTA) is unavailable, conduct pulmonary angiography. Long the criterion standard for pulmonary embolism diagnosis, pulmonary angiography is nevertheless more invasive and harder to perform than MDCTA, and for these reasons, it is rapidly being replaced. However, pulmonary angiography remains a useful diagnostic modality when MDCTA cannot be performed.

When pulmonary angiography has been performed carefully and completely, a positive result provides virtually a 100% certainty that an obstruction to pulmonary arterial blood flow exists. A negative pulmonary angiogram provides a greater than 90% certainty for the exclusion of pulmonary embolism.

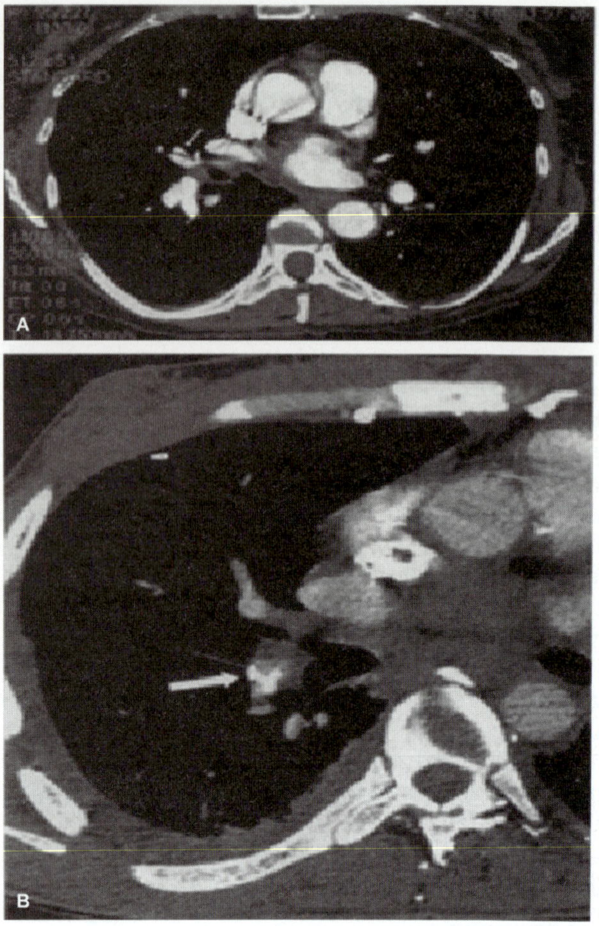

Fig. 30.30: *(A) CT scan showing septic emboli in both lungs. (B) Pulmonary embolism is also observed in left upper lobe (arrow)*

A positive angiogram is an acceptable end-point no matter how abbreviated the study. However, a complete negative study requires the visualization of the entire pulmonary tree bilaterally. This is accomplished via selective cannulation of each branch of the pulmonary artery and injection of contrast material into each branch, with multiple views of each area. Even then, emboli in vessels smaller than third order or lobular arteries are not seen.

Small emboli cannot be seen angiographically, yet embolic obstruction of these smaller pulmonary vessels is very common when postmortem examination follows a negative angiogram. These small emboli can produce pleuritic chest pain and a small sterile effusion even though the patient has a normal V/Q scan and a normal pulmonary angiogram.

In most patients, however, pulmonary embolism is a disease of multiple recurrences, with large and small emboli already present by the time the diagnosis is suspected. Under these circumstances, the V/Q scan and the angiogram are likely to detect at least some of the emboli.

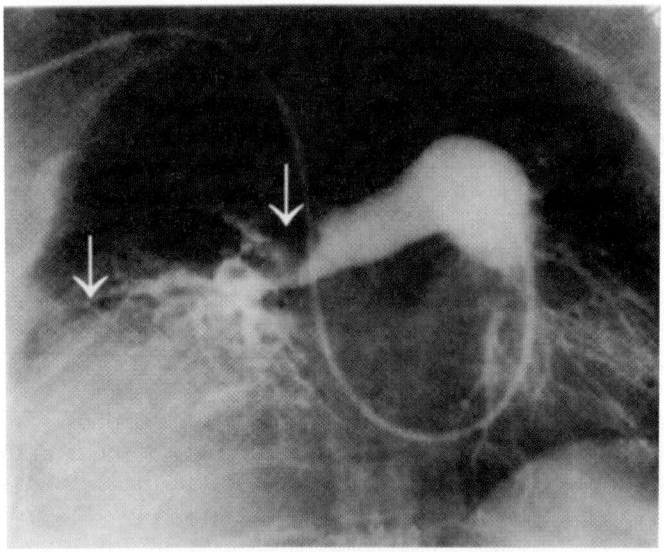

Fig. 30.31: *Pulmonary angiography showing massive thrombus in the right pulmonary artery with almost complete obstruction to the blood flow (arrow). Note also the elevation of right hemi-diaphragm (arrow)*

Pulmonary angiography demonstrates subsegmental vessels in more detail than does CT scanning, although the superimposition of the small vessels remains a limiting factor. As a result, the interobserver agreement rate for isolated subsegmental pulmonary embolism is only 45%.

Computed Tomography Scanning (Fig. 30.30)

Technical advances in CT scanning including the development of multidetector-array scanners, have led to the emergence of CT scanning as an important diagnostic technique in suspected pulmonary embolism. Contrast-enhanced CT scanning is increasingly used as the initial radiologic study in the diagnosis of pulmonary embolism, especially in patients with abnormal chest radiographs in whom scintigraphic results are more likely to be non-diagnostic.

Computed tomography angiography (CTA) is the initial imaging modality of choice for stable patients with suspected pulmonary embolism. The American College of Radiology (ACR) considers chest CTA to be the current standard of care for the detection of pulmonary embolism. A study by Ward et al determined that a selective strategy in which CTA is used after compression ultrasonography is cost-effective for patients with a high pretest probability of pulmonary embolism. This strategy may reduce the need for CTA and help to eliminate adverse effects associated with CTA.

Toward a goal of reducing unnecessary CTA and associated radiation exposure, Drescher et al studied the effect of implementing a computerized decision support system for pulmonary embolism evaluation in the ED. Before implementation, the rate of positive pulmonary embolism diagnosis for CTAs performed was 8.3%; after, the positivity rate rose to 12.7%. The positive yield would have been higher (16.7%) had emergency physicians adhered in all cases to the outcome of the decision support system; in 27% of cases they did not.

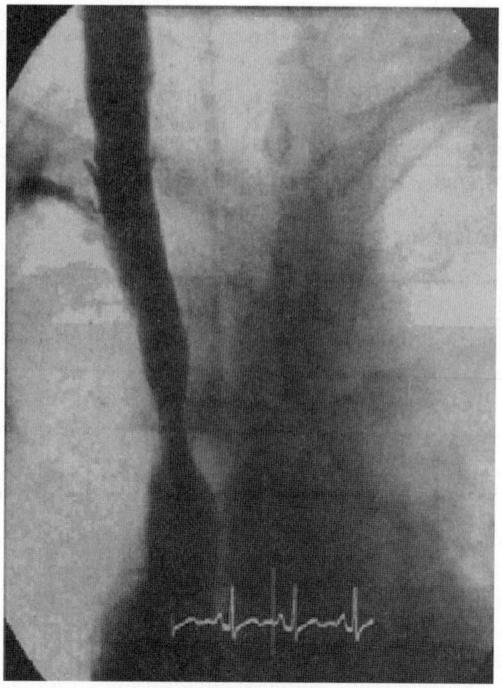

Fig. 30.32: *Superior venogram before stent deployment shows narrowing of the SVC*

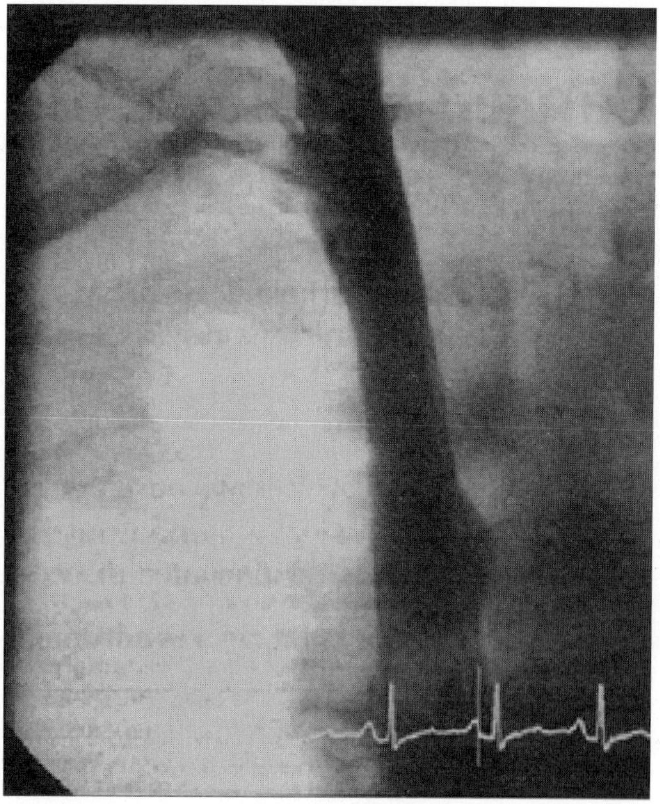

Fig. 30.33: *Check angiogram showing no residual stenosis and good antegrade flow in the SVC (see Fig. 30.32)*

Like pulmonary angiography, CT scanning shows emboli directly, but it is noninvasive, cheaper than pulmonary

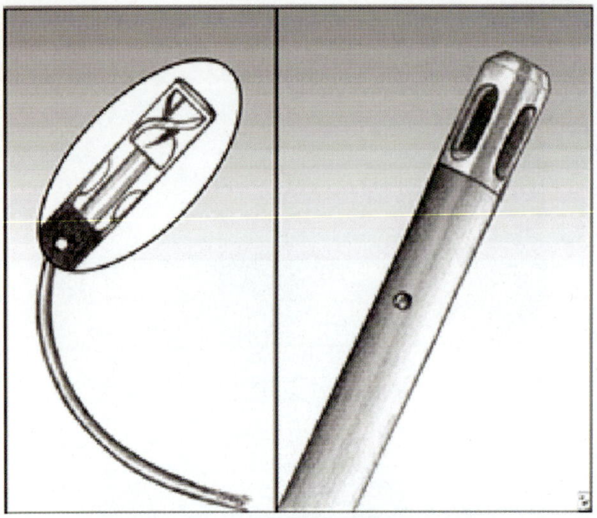

Fig. 30.34: *Two views of a commercially available thrombectomy device. The Helix Clot Buster (Microvena Corp, Plymouth, MN) works by creating a vortex with a spinning self-contained propeller that macerates the clot. No thrombolytic agent (i.e. tissue plasminogen activator) is necessary when this device is used, but adjunct thrombolytic medications can be useful. Competing devices are available from Boston Scientific, Cordis Endovascular, Possis Medical, and other manufacturers*

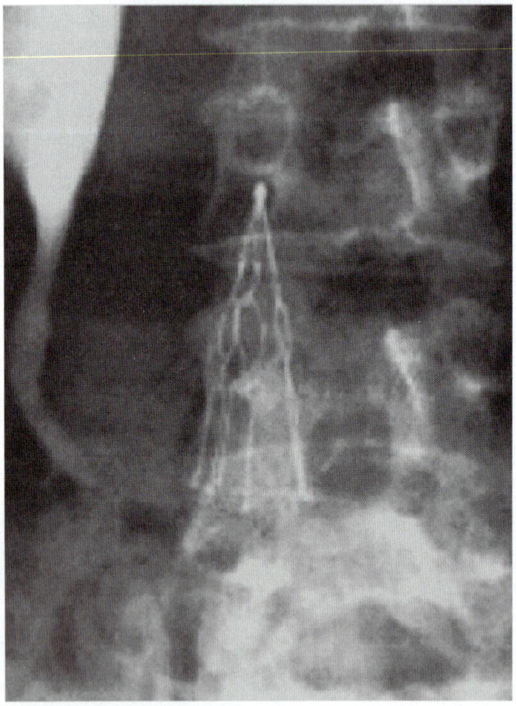

Fig. 30.35: *Showing Greenfield filter for the prevention of thromboembolism out of DVT from the lower limb veins*

angiography, and widely available. CT scanning is the only test that can provide significant additional information related to alternate diagnoses; spiral (helical) CT scanning results may suggest an alternative diagnosis in up to 57% of patients. This is a clear advantage of CT scanning over pulmonary angiography or scintigraphy.

A study of multidetector computed tomography (MDCTA) for detection of right ventricular dysfunction in 457 patients with acute pulmonary embolism found reasonable correlation with echocardiography, the reference standard. The criterion selected, a right-to-left ventricular dimensional ratio of 0.9 or more at MDCTA, had 92% sensitivity for right ventricular dysfunction. The combination of quantatative assessment of ventricular dimensions by CT and measurement of biomarkers may provide additional diagnostic accuracy for the presence of right ventricular dysfunction.

Chest Radiography

Chest radiographs are abnormal in most cases of pulmonary embolism, but the findings are nonspecific. Common radiographic abnormalities include atelectasis, pleural effusion, parenchymal opacities, and elevation of a hemidiaphragm. The classic radiographic findings of pulmonary infarction include a wedge-shaped, pleura-based triangular opacity with an apex pointing toward the hilus **(Hampton hump)** or decreased vascularity (Westermark sign). These findings are suggestive of pulmonary embolism but are infrequently observed.

A prominent central pulmonary artery **(knuckle sign)**, cardiomegaly (especially on the right side of the heart), and pulmonary edema are other findings. In the appropriate clinical setting, these findings could be consistent with acute cor pulmonale. A normal-appearing chest radiograph in a patient with severe dyspnea and hypoxemia, but without evidence of bronchospasm or a cardiac shunt, is strongly suggestive of pulmonary embolism.

The ACR recommends chest radiography as the most appropriate study for ruling out other causes of chest pain in patients with suspected pulmonary embolism. Initially, the chest radiographic findings are normal in most cases of pulmonary embolism. However, in later stages, radiographic signs may include a Westermark sign (dilatation of pulmonary vessels and a sharp cutoff), atelectasis, a small pleural effusion, and an elevated diaphragm. Generally, chest radiographs cannot be used to conclusively prove or exclude pulmonary embolism; however, radiography and electrocardiography may be useful for establishing alternative diagnoses.

Ventilation-Perfusion Scanning

V/Q scanning of the lungs is an important modality for establishing the diagnosis of pulmonary embolism. However, V/Q scanning should be used only when CT scanning is not available or if the patient has a contraindication to CT scanning or intravenous contrast material. Children generally have a more homogenous perfusion scan; thus, deficits in perfusion are more likely to represent real or significant pulmonary embolism than they are in adults (Figs 30.24 and 30.29).

The high probability criteria are as follows:

Two large (>75% of a segment) segmental perfusion defects without corresponding ventilation or chest radiographic abnormalities.

One large segmental perfusion defect and 2 moderate (25–75% of a segment) segmental perfusion defects without corresponding ventilation or radiographic abnormalities.

Four moderate segmental perfusion defects without corresponding ventilation or chest radiographic abnormalities.

The intermediate-probability criteria are as follows:

- One moderate to fewer than two large segmental perfusion defects without corresponding ventilation or chest radiographic abnormalities.
- Corresponding V/Q defects and radiographic parenchymal opacity in lower lung zone.
- Single moderate matched V/Q defects with normal chest radiographic findings.
- Corresponding V/Q and chest radiography small pleural effusion.
- Difficult to categorize as normal, low, or high probability.

Low probability criteria are as follows:

- Multiple matched V/Q defects, regardless of size, with normal chest radiographic findings
- Corresponding V/Q defects and radiographic parenchymal opacity in upper or middle lung zone
- Corresponding V/Q defects and large pleural effusion
- Any perfusion defects with substantially larger radiographic abnormality
- Defects surrounded by normally perfused lung (stripe sign)
- More than 3 small (< 25% of a segment) segmental perfusion defects with normal chest radiographic findings
- Nonsegmental perfusion defects (cardiomegaly, aortic impression, enlarged hila)
- The normal finding is the presence of no perfusion defects and perfusion outlines the shape of the lung seen on a chest radiograph.
- The very low-probability criterion is the presence of 3 small (< 25% of a segment) segmental perfusion defects with normal chest radiographic findings.

Electrocardiography (Figs 30.24 and 30.26)

The most common ECG abnormalities in the setting of pulmonary embolism are tachycardia and nonspecific ST-T wave abnormalities. The finding of S1 Q3 T3 is nonspecific and insensitive in the absence of clinical suspicion for pulmonary embolism. The classic findings of right heart strain and acute cor pulmonale are tall, peaked P waves in lead II (P pulmonale); right axis deviation; right bundle-branch block; an S1 Q3 T3 pattern; or atrial fibrillation. Unfortunately, only 20% of patients with proven pulmonary embolism have any of these classic electrocardiographic abnormalities. If electrocardiographic abnormalities are present, they may be suggestive of pulmonary embolism, but the absence of such abnormalities has no significant predictive value.

Magnetic Resonance Imaging

With magnetic resonance imaging (MRI), evidence of pulmonary emboli may be detected by using standard or gated spin-echo techniques. Pulmonary emboli demonstrate increased signal intensity within the pulmonary artery. By obtaining a sequence of images, this signal that is originating from slow blood flow may be distinguished from pulmonary embolism. However, this remains a problem in pulmonary hypertension.

Magnetic resonance angiography is performed following intravenous administration of gadolinium. Gadolinium-based contrast agents [gadopentetate dimeglumine (Magnevist), gadobenate dimeglumine (MultiHance), gadodiamide (Omniscan), gadoversetamide (OptiMARK), gadoteridol (ProHance)] have been linked to the development of nephrogenic systemic fibrosis (NSF) or nephrogenic fibrosing dermopathy (NFD). The disease has occurred in patients with moderate to end-stage renal disease after being given a gadolinium-based contrast agent to enhance MRI or magnetic resonance angiography scans. NSF/NFD is a debilitating and sometimes fatal disease. Characteristics include red or dark patches on the skin; burning, itching, swelling, hardening, and tightening of the skin; yellow spots on the whites of the eyes; joint stiffness with trouble moving or straightening the arms, hands, legs, or feet; pain deep in the hip bones or ribs; and muscle weakness.

MRI has a sensitivity of 85% and specificity of 96% for central, lobar, and segmental emboli; MRI is inadequate for the diagnosis of subsegmental emboli.

Few data are available regarding the use of MRI in children suspected of having a pulmonary embolism. Its use in these patients should be considered investigational at this time.

Few investigators have reported the feasibility of MRI in the evaluation of pulmonary embolism. However, the role of MRI is mostly limited to the evaluation of patients who have impaired renal function or other contraindications for the use of iodinated contrast material. Newer blood-pool contrast agents and respiratory navigators may enhance the role of MRI in the diagnosis of pulmonary embolism.

Echocardiography

This modality generally has limited accuracy in the diagnosis of pulmonary embolism. Transesophageal echocardiography may identify central pulmonary embolism, and the sensitivity for central pulmonary embolism is reported to be 82%. Overall sensitivity and specificity for central and peripheral pulmonary embolism is 59% and 77%.

Echocardiography (ECHO) provides useful information. It may allow diagnosis of other conditions that may be confused with pulmonary embolism, such as pericardial effusion. ECHO allows visualization of the right ventricle and assessment of the pulmonary artery pressure. ECHO serves a prognostic function; the mortality rate is almost 10% in the presence of right ventricular dysfunction and 0% in the absence of right ventricular dysfunction. (Vanni et al reported that a right ventricular strain pattern is associated with a worse short-term outcome.) ECHO may be used to identify the presence of right-chamber emboli.

The subcostal view is preferred at initial screening for mechanical activity and pericardial fluid and for gross assessment of global and regional abnormalities. To obtain a subcostal view, place the transducer on the left subcostal margin with the beam aimed at the left shoulder. The parasternal view allows visualization of the aortic valve, proximal ascending aorta, and posterior pericardium and permits determination of left ventricular size. It is particularly helpful when the subcostal view is difficult to obtain. To obtain a parasternal view, place the transducer in the left parasternal area between the second and fourth intercostal spaces. The plane of the beam is parallel to a line drawn from the right shoulder to the left hip.

Several echocardiographic findings have been proposed for noninvasive diagnosis of right ventricular dysfunction at the bedside, including right ventricular enlargement and/or hypokinesis of the free wall, leftward septal shift, and evidence of pulmonary hypertension. If right ventricular dysfunction is seen on cardiac ultrasonography, the diagnosis of acute submassive or massive pulmonary embolism is supported. While the presence of right ventricular dysfunction can be used to support the clinical suspicion of pulmonary embolism, prognostic information can be obtained by assessing the severity of right ventricular dysfunction.

Duplex Ultrasonography

The diagnosis of pulmonary embolism can be proven by demonstrating the presence of a DVT at any site. This may sometimes be accomplished noninvasively by using duplex ultrasonography. To look for DVT using ultrasonography, the ultrasonographic transducer is placed against the skin and pressed inward firmly enough to compress the vein being examined. In an area of normal veins, the veins are easily compressed completely closed while the muscular arteries are extremely resistant to compression. Where DVT is present, the veins do not collapse completely when pressure is applied using the ultrasonographic probe.

A negative ultrasonographic scan does not rule out DVT, because many DVTs occur in areas that are inaccessible to ultrasonographic examination. Before an ultrasonographic scan can be considered negative, the entire deep venous system must be interrogated using centimeter-by-centimeter compression testing of every vessel. In two thirds of patients with pulmonary embolism, the site of DVT cannot be visualized with ultrasonography, so a negative duplex ultrasonographic scan does not markedly reduce the likelihood of pulmonary embolism.

Approach Considerations

Immediate therapeutic anticoagulation is initiated for patients with suspected DVT or pulmonary embolism. Anticoagulation therapy with heparin reduces mortality rates from 30% to less than 10%.

The current eighth edition of the American College of Chest Physicians (ACCP) guidelines for antithrombotic and thrombolytic therapy are summarized as follows:

All patients with pulmonary embolism require rapid risk stratification (grade 1C).

Thrombolytic therapy should be used in patients with evidence of hemodynamic compromise, except in the face of major contraindications due to bleeding risks (grade 1B). Do not delay thrombolysis in this population, owing to the potential for the development of irreversible cardiogenic shock.

Thrombolytic therapy is suggested in select high-risk patients who do not have hypotension and are at low risk for bleeding (grade 2B).

Assessment of pulmonary embolism severity, prognosis, and risk of bleeding dictate whether thrombolytic therapy should be started. Thrombolytic therapy is not recommended for most patients (grade 1B).

Immediate full anticoagulation is mandatory for all patients suspected of having have DVT or pulmonary embolism. Diagnostic investigations should not delay empirical anticoagulant therapy. Current guidelines recommend starting unfractionated heparin (UFH), low-molecular weight heparin (LMWH), or fondaparinux (all grade 1A) in addition to an oral anticoagulant (warfarin) at the time of diagnosis, and to discontinue UFH, LMWH, or fondaparinux only after the international normalized ratio (INR) is 2.0 for at least 24 hours, but no sooner than 5 days after warfarin therapy has been started (grade 1C recommendation). The recommended duration of UFH, LMWH, and fondaparinux is based on evidence suggesting that the relatively long half-life of factor II, along with the short half-lives of protein C and protein S, may provoke a paradoxical hypercoagulable state if these agents are discontinued prematurely.

Even in patients who are fully anticoagulated, however, DVT and pulmonary embolism can and often do recur. New pulmonary embolism in the hospital can occur in the following patients despite therapeutic anticoagulation:

- Patients who have nonfloating DVT without pulmonary embolism at presentation (3%).
- Patients who present with a floating thrombus but have no pulmonary embolism (13%).
- Patients who present with pulmonary embolism but have no floating thrombus (11%).
- Patients who present with pulmonary embolism who have a floating thrombus visible at venography (39%).

Deciding how to treat a venous thrombosis that may lead to a pulmonary embolism is difficult. A survey of Canadian pediatric intensivists reported 4 patient factors commonly used to determine if a venous thrombosis is clinically important.

Clinical Suspicion of a Pulmonary Embolism

Symptoms

Detection of thrombosis on clinical examination.

Presence of an acute or chronic cardiopulmonary comorbidity that affects the patient's ability to tolerate a pulmonary embolism.

Anticoagulants are the treatment of choice in most children with pulmonary emboli. Thrombolytics are rarely used. To date, little data are available regarding the use of LMWH in children with thromboembolic disease.

Thrombolysis

The ACCP guidelines recommend that all patients with pulmonary embolism require rapid risk stratification (grade 1C). Thrombolytic therapy should be used in patients with evidence of hemodynamic compromise, except in the face of major contraindications due to bleeding risks (grade 1B). Do not delay thrombolysis in this population, owing to the potential for the development of irreversible cardiogenic shock. Thrombolytic therapy is suggested in select high-risk patients who do not have hypotension and are at low risk for bleeding (grade 2B). Assessment of pulmonary embolism severity, prognosis, and risk of bleeding dictate whether thrombolytic therapy should be started. Thrombolytic therapy is not recommended for most patients (grade 1B).

Although most studies demonstrate the superiority of thrombolytic therapy with respect to the resolution of radiographic and hemodynamic abnormalities within the first 24 hours, this advantage disappears 7 days after treatment. Controlled clinical trials have not demonstrated benefits in terms of reduced mortality rates or earlier resolution of symptoms when currently compared with heparin. A large, retrospective review suggests that the use of thrombolytic therapy in unstable patients with pulmonary embolism may lead to reduced mortality when compared to anticoagulation therapy alone. Concurrent use of thrombolytic therapy and vena cava filters in such patients may reduce mortality even further.

Until randomized clinical trials demonstrate a clear morbidity or mortality benefit, the role of thrombolytic therapy in the management of acute pulmonary embolism will remain controversial. The currently accepted indications for thrombolytic therapy include hemodynamic instability or right ventricular dysfunction demonstrated on ECHO.

Anticoagulation

Unfractionated Heparin Therapy

In patients with massive pulmonary embolism, if concerns regarding subcutaneous absorption arise, severe renal failure exists, or if thrombolytic therapy is being considered, IV UFH is the recommended form of initial anticoagulation (grade 2C).

The efficacy of heparin therapy depends on achieving a critical therapeutic level of heparin within the first 24 hours of treatment. The critical therapeutic level of heparin is 1.5 times the baseline control value or the upper limit of normal range of the activated partial thromboplastin time (aPTT). This level of anticoagulation is expected to correspond to a heparin blood level of 0.2–0.4 U/mL by the protamine sulfate titration assay and 0.3–0.6 by the antifactor X assay. Each laboratory should establish the minimal therapeutic level for heparin, as measured by the aPTT, to coincide with a heparin blood level of at least 0.2 U/mL for each batch of thromboplastin reagent being used.

If IV UFH is chosen, an initial bolus of 80 U/kg or 5,000 U followed by an infusion of 18 U/kg/h or 1,300 U/h should be given, with the goal of rapidly achieving and maintaining the aPTT at levels that correspond to therapeutic heparin levels. Fixed-dose and monitored regimens of subcutaneous UFH are available and are acceptable alternatives.

Low-Molecular-Weight Heparin Therapy

Current guidelines for patients with acute nonmassive pulmonary embolism recommend LMWH over UFH (grade 1A).

LMWHs have many advantages over UFH. These agents have a greater bioavailability, can be administered by subcutaneous injections, and have a longer duration of anticoagulant effect. A fixed dose of LMWH can be used, and laboratory monitoring of aPTT is not necessary.

Trials comparing LMWH with UFH have shown that LMWH is at least as effective and as safe as UFH. The studies have not pointed to any significant differences in recurrent thromboembolic events, major bleeding, or mortality between the two types of heparin.

LMWH can be administered safely in an outpatient setting. This has lead to the development of programs in which clinically stable patients with pulmonary embolism are treated at home, at substantial cost savings.

An international, open-label, randomized trial compared outpatient and inpatient treatment (both using the LMWH enoxaparin as initial therapy) of low-risk patients with acute pulmonary embolism and concluded that outpatient treatment was noninferior to inpatient treatment.

Factor Xa Inhibitors

Rivaroxaban (Xarelto) is an oral factor Xa inhibitor approved by the FDA in November 2012 for the treatment of DVT or PE, and to reduce risk of recurrent DVT and PE following initial treatment.

Approval for this indication was based on studies totaling 9,478 patients with DVT or PE. Participants were randomly assigned to receive rivaroxaban, a combination of enoxaparin and a vitamin K antagonist (VKA) (e.g. warfarin), or a placebo. Study endpoints were designed to measure the number of patients who experienced recurrent symptoms of DVT, PE, or death after receiving treatment. Additionally, results from extended treatment demonstrated a reduced risk of recurrent DVT and PE. Approximately, 1.3% in the rivaroxaban group experienced recurrent DVT or PE compared with 7.1% in the placebo group.

The results of the Einstein-PE study provide an important advance in the treatment of symptomatic pulmonary embolism. In a prospective, open-label study, 4,832 patients were randomized to receive either rivaroxaban or enoxaparin followed by an adjusted-dose vitamin K antagonist for 3, 6, or 12 months. Treatment with a fixed-dose regimen of rivaroxaban was noninferior to standard therapy and had a satisfactory safety profile.

Data from a pooled analysis of the EINSTEIN-PE and EINSTEIN-DVT studies in the treatment of DVT or pulmonary embolism suggest that rivaroxaban is as effective in preventing VTE recurrence as administration of enoxaparin followed by a vitamin-K antagonist. Rivaroxaban may also be associated with less bleeding, particularly in elderly patients and those with moderate renal impairment.

This advance thus offers the prospect of a safe and effective regimen of anticoagulation for patients with the advantages of simplicity and cost-effectiveness in comparison to current management strategies.

Fondaparinux

Fondaparinux is a synthetic polysaccharide derived from the antithrombin binding region of heparin. Fondaparinux catalyzes factor Xa inactivation by antithrombin without inhibiting thrombin.

Fondaparinux has not been directly compared with subcutaneous UFH or LMWH. However, once-daily fondaparinux was found to have similar rates of recurrent pulmonary embolism, bleeding, and death as IV UFH, according to one randomized open-label study of 2,213 patients with symptomatic pulmonary embolism.

With the exception of patients presenting with massive pulmonary embolism (defined by hemodynamic compromise), LMWH or fondaparinux is recommended over IV UFH. This is because of a more predictable bioavailability, more rapid onset of full anticoagulant effect, and the benefit of not typically needing to monitor anticoagulant effect. However, if uncertainty arises regarding the accuracy of dosing, factor Xa levels can be monitored to determine efficacy.

In cases in which an anticoagulant with a shorter half-life is more desirable (i.e. patients at particularly high risk of bleeding) or in patients with impaired renal function, IV UFH may be preferred (grade 2C).

Warfarin Therapy

The anticoagulant effect of warfarin is mediated by the inhibition of vitamin K–dependent factors, which are II, VII, IX and X. The peak effect does not occur until 36–72 hours after drug administration, and the dosage is difficult to titrate.

A prothrombin time ratio is expressed as an INR and is monitored to assess the adequacy of warfarin therapy. The recommended therapeutic range for venous thromboembolism is an INR of 2–3. This level of anticoagulation markedly reduces the risk of bleeding without the loss of effectiveness. Initially, INR measurements are performed on a daily basis; once the patient is stabilized on a specific dose of warfarin, the INR determinations may be performed every 1–2 weeks or at longer intervals.

Duration of Anticoagulation Therapy

A patient with a first thromboembolic event occurring in the setting of reversible risk factors, such as immobilization, surgery, or trauma, should receive warfarin therapy for at least 3 months. No difference in the rate of recurrence was observed in either of two studies comparing 3 versus 6 months of anticoagulant therapy in patients with idiopathic (or unprovoked) first events. The current recommendation is anticoagulation for at least 3 months in these patients; the need for extending the duration of anticoagulation should be reevaluated at that time.

The current ACCP guidelines recommend that all patients with unprovoked pulmonary embolism should undergo a risk-to-benefit evaluation to determine if long-term therapy is needed (grade 1C). Long-term treatment is recommended for these patients who do not have risk factors for bleeding and in whom accurate anticoagulant monitoring is possible (grade 1A).

Patients who have pulmonary embolism and preexisting irreversible risk factors, such as deficiency of antithrombin III, protein S and C, factor V Leiden mutation, or the presence of antiphospholipid antibodies, should be placed on long-term anticoagulation.

Heparin-induced Thrombocytopenia

Heparin-induced thrombocytopenia (HIT) is a transient prothrombotic disorder initiated by heparin. The main features of HIT are (1) thrombocytopenia resulting from immunoglobulin G-mediated platelet activation and (2) in vivo thrombin generation and increased risk of venous and arterial thrombosis.

The highest frequency of HIT, 5%, has been reported in postorthopedic surgery patients receiving up to 2 weeks of unfractionated heparin. HIT occurred in approximately 0.5% of postorthopedic surgery patients receiving LMWH for up to 2 weeks.

HIT may manifest clinically as extension of the thrombus or formation of new arterial thrombosis. HIT should be suspected whenever the patient's platelet count falls to less than 100,000/µL or less than 50% of the baseline value, generally after 5–15 days of heparin therapy. The definitive diagnosis is made by performing a platelet activation factor assay.

The treatment of patients who develop HIT is to stop all heparin products including catheter flushes and heparin-coated catheters, and to initiate an alternative, nonheparin anticoagulant, even when thrombosis is not clinically apparent. Preferred agents include direct thrombin inhibitors, such as lepirudin or argatroban. Start warfarin while the patient receives an alternative, nonheparin anticoagulant and only when the platelet count has recovered to at least 100,000/µL (preferably to 150,000/µL).

Resistance to Heparin

Few patients with venous thromboembolism require large doses of heparin for achieving an optimal activated partial thromboplastin time (aPTT). Those patients who do require them have increased plasma concentrations of factor VIII and heparin-binding proteins. Increased factor VIII concentration causes dissociation between aPTT and plasma heparin values. The aPTT is suboptimal, but patients have adequate heparin levels upon protamine titration. This commonly occurs in patients with a concomitant inflammatory disease.

Monitoring the antifactor Xa assay results in this situation is safe and effective and results in less escalation of the heparin dose when compared with monitoring with aPTT. Whenever a therapeutic level of aPTT cannot be achieved with large doses of UFH, either determination of plasma heparin concentration or therapy with LMWH should be instituted.

Embolectomy

Guidelines from the American Heart Association (AHA) advise that either catheter embolectomy and fragmentation or surgical embolectomy is reasonable for patients with massive pulmonary embolism who have contraindications to fibrinolysis or who remain unstable after receiving fibrinolysis. If these procedures are not available locally, it is reasonable to consider transferring the patient to an institution with experience in one of these procedures, providing the transfer can be accomplished safely.

In patients with submassive acute pulmonary embolism, either catheter embolectomy or surgical embolectomy may be considered if they have clinical evidence of an adverse prognosis (i.e. new hemodynamic instability, worsening respiratory failure, severe right ventricular dysfunction, or major myocardial necrosis). These interventions are not recommended for patients with low-risk or submassive acute pulmonary embolism who have minor right ventricular dysfunction, minor myocardial necrosis, and no clinical worsening.

Vena Cava Filters (Figs 30.34 and 30.35)

The current grade 1A recommendation is that patients with acute pulmonary embolism should not routinely receive vena cava filters in addition to anticoagulants. An ideal IVC filter should be easily and safely placed using a percutaneous technique, biocompatible and mechanically stable, and able to trap emboli without causing occlusion of the vena cava.

IVC interruption by the insertion of an IVC filter (Greenfield filter) is only indicated in the following settings:

Patients with acute venous thromboembolism who have an absolute contraindication to anticoagulant therapy (e.g. recent surgery, hemorrhagic stroke, significant active or recent bleeding).

Patients with massive pulmonary embolism who survived but in whom recurrent embolism invariably will be fatal.

Patients who have objectively documented recurrent venous thromboembolism, adequate anticoagulant therapy not withstanding.

In patients with a time-limited indication for IVC filter placement (e.g. a short-term contraindication to anticoagulation), it is reasonable to select a retrievable IVC filter and evaluate the patient periodically for filter retrieval. After placement of an IVC filter, AHA guidelines recommend that anticoagulation be resumed once contraindications to anticoagulation or active bleeding complications have resolved.

Supportive Care

Compression Stockings

For patients who have had a proximal DVT, the use of elastic compression stockings provides a safe and effective adjunctive treatment that can limit or prevent extension of the thrombus. Stockings with a pressure of 30–40 mmHg at the ankle, worn for 2 years following diagnosis, are recommended (grade 1A) to reduce the risk of postphlebitic syndrome.

True gradient compression stockings are highly elastic, providing a gradient of compression that is highest at the toes and gradually decreases to the level of the thigh. This reduces capacitive venous volume by approximately 70% and increases the measured velocity of blood flow in the deep veins by a factor of 5 or more. Compression stockings of this type have been proven effective in the prophylaxis of thromboembolism and are also effective in preventing progression of thrombus in patients who already have DVT and pulmonary embolism.

A 1994 meta-analysis calculated a DVT risk odds ratio of 0.28 for gradient compression stockings (as compared to no prophylaxis) in patients undergoing abdominal surgery, gynecologic surgery or neurosurgery.

Other studies found that gradient compression stockings and LMWH were the most effective modalities in reducing the incidence of DVT after hip surgery; they were more effective than subcutaneous UFH, oral warfarin, dextran, or aspirin.

The ubiquitous white stockings known as antiembolic stockings or "Ted hose" produce a maximum compression of 18 mmHg. Ted hose rarely are fitted in such a way as to provide even that inadequate gradient compression. Because they provide such limited compression, they have no efficacy in the treatment of DVT and pulmonary embolism, nor have they been proven effective as prophylaxis against a recurrence.

True 30–40 mmHg gradient compression pantyhose are available in sizes for pregnant women. They are recommended by many specialists for all pregnant women because they not only prevent DVT, but they also reduce or prevent the development of varicose veins during pregnancy.

Additional Support Therapies

Activity is recommended as tolerated. Early ambulation is recommended over bed rest when feasible (grade 1A recommendation).

Pharmacologic support of the cardiovascular system may be necessary. Dopamine and dobutamine are the usual inotropic agents. Mechanical ventilation may be necessary to provide respiratory support and as adjunctive therapy for a failing circulatory system.

Children with sickle cell disease who present with pulmonary symptoms require treatment with a macrolide and cephalosporin antibiotic. Their clinical status should be closely monitored in order to anticipate those children who may develop acute chest syndrome. Transfusion with packed red blood cells (either simple or exchange) improves oxygenation immediately, helping to break the vicious cycle outlined above.

IV fluids may help or may hurt the patient who is hypotensive from pulmonary embolism, depending on which point on the starling curve describes the patient's condition. A cautious trial of a small fluid bolus may be attempted, with careful surveillance of the systolic and diastolic blood pressures and immediate cessation if the situation worsens after the fluid bolus. Improvement or normalization of blood pressure after fluid loading does not mean the patient has become hemodynamically stable.

Individuals with acute, submassive pulmonary embolisms have low levels of endogenous activated protein C. A study by Dempfle et al determined that administering drotrecogin alfa (activated) along with therapeutic doses of enoxaparin enhanced the inhibition of fibrin formation in these patients. Drotrecogin alfa was withdrawn from the worldwide market October 25, 2011 after analysis of the Recombinant Human Activated Protein C Worldwide Evaluation in Severe Sepsis (PROWESS)-SHOCK clinical trial. Drotrecogin alfa failed to demonstrate a statistically significant reduction in 28-day all-cause mortality in patients with severe sepsis and septic shock. Trial results observed a 28-day all-cause mortality rate of 26.4% in patients treated with activated drotrecogin alfa compared with 24.2% in the placebo group of the study.

Complications of Pulmonary Embolism

Complications of pulmonary embolism include the following:

- Sudden cardiac death
- Obstructive shock
- Pulseless electrical activity
- Atrial or ventricular arrhythmias
- Secondary pulmonary arterial hypertension
- Cor pulmonale
- Severe hypoxemia
- Right-to-left intracardiac shunt
- Lung infarction
- Pleural effusion
- Paradoxical embolism
- Heparin-induced thrombocytopenia
- Thrombophlebitis.

Prevention of Pulmonary Embolism

Preventing idiopathic outpatient pulmonary embolism is difficult if not impossible. That said, the majority of pulmonary embolisms occur in hospitalized patients. The incidence in these cases can be reduced through appropriate prophylaxis, achieved mechanically or via the administration of heparin, LMWH or warfarin.

The incidence of venous thrombosis, pulmonary embolism, and death can be significantly reduced by embracing a prophylactic strategy in high-risk patients. Prevention of DVT in the lower extremities inevitably reduces the frequency of pulmonary embolism; therefore, populations at risk must be identified, and safe and efficacious prophylactic modalities should be used.

The QThrombosis algorithm is intended to identify currently asymptomatic adults at greatest future risk of venous thrombosis based on established risk factors. According to the study in which it was developed and validated, QThrombosis estimates the absolute risk of venous thrombosis at 1 year and 5 years into the future, information that can be used to guide prophylaxis and medication decisions.

Future Research

Advances over the past several decades have significantly improved physicians' ability to diagnosis pulmonary embolism and have refined the treatment of this disorder. However, several areas need further research and properly conducted therapeutic trials. The role of LMWH and the optimal duration of anticoagulant therapy in different subgroups of patients with venous thromboembolism require further study.

Because warfarin therapy results in bleeding, future studies should determine whether less intense warfarin therapy is effective in preventing recurrences of pulmonary embolism.

Whether drugs that inhibit the action of thrombin (e.g. hirudin) are useful in treating patients with venous thromboembolic disease also needs to be determined by future trials.

Long-term Monitoring

PT should be measured on a regular basis; the goal is an INR of 2–3.

The length of treatment depends on the presence of risk factors. If no underlying risk factors are present, therapy can be stopped within 1–2 months. If risk factors are present, especially anticardiolipin antibodies, therapy should continue for at least 4–6 months.

Long-term anticoagulation is essential for patients who survive an initial DVT or pulmonary embolism. The optimum total duration of anticoagulation is controversial, but general consensus holds that at least 6 months of anticoagulation is associated with significant reduction in recurrences and a net positive benefit.

Patients may have treatment initiated using concomitant warfarin and unfractionated heparin for 5 days in the hospital, with discharge on warfarin alone when the international normalized ratio (INR) is 2. Alternatively, patients may be discharged on concomitant therapy with a LMWH and warfarin for at least 5 days. The LMWH is then discontinued in the outpatient setting when the INR reaches 2.

Medication

Immediate therapeutic anticoagulation is initiated for patients with suspected deep venous thrombosis (DVT) or pulmonary embolism (PE). Anticoagulation therapy with heparin reduces mortality rates from 30% to less than 10%. Anticoagulation is essential, but anticoagulation alone does not guarantee a successful outcome. DVT and PE may recur or extend despite full and effective heparin anticoagulation. Chronic anticoagulation is critical to prevent relapse of DVT or PE following initial heparinization. Heparin works by activating antithrombin III to slow or prevent the progression of DVT and to reduce the size and frequency of PE. Heparin does not dissolve existing clot.

The current eighth edition of the American College of Chest Physicians (ACCP) guidelines for antithrombotic and thrombolytic therapy are summarized as follows:

All patients with pulmonary embolism require rapid risk stratification (grade 1C).

Thrombolytic therapy should be used in patients with evidence of hemodynamic compromise, except in the face of major contraindications due to bleeding risks (grade 1B). Do not delay thrombolysis in this population, owing to the potential for the development of irreversible cardiogenic shock.

Thrombolytic therapy is suggested in select high-risk patients who do not have hypotension and are at low risk for bleeding (grade 2B).

Assessment of pulmonary embolism severity, prognosis, and risk of bleeding dictate whether thrombolytic therapy should be started. Thrombolytic therapy is not recommended for most patients (grade 1B).

The current ACCP guidelines recommend that all patients with unprovoked pulmonary embolism should undergo a risk-to-benefit evaluation to determine if long-term therapy is needed (grade 1C). Long-term treatment is recommended for these patients who do not have risk factors for bleeding and in whom accurate anticoagulant monitoring is possible (grade 1A).

Anticoagulants

Heparin augments the activity of antithrombin III and prevents the conversion of fibrinogen to fibrin. Full-dose LMWH or full-dose unfractionated IV heparin should be initiated at the first suspicion of DVT or PE.

With proper dosing, several LMWH products have been found safer and more effective than unfractionated heparin both for prophylaxis and for treatment of DVT and PE. Monitoring the aPTT is neither necessary nor useful when giving LMWH, because the drug is most active in a tissue phase and does not exert most of its effects on coagulation factor IIa.

Many different LMWH products are available around the world. Because of pharmacokinetic differences, dosing is highly product specific. Several LMWH products are approved for use in the United States: enoxaparin (Lovenox), dalteparin (Fragmin), and tinzaparin (Innohep). Enoxaparin and tinzaparin are currently approved by the FDA for treatment of DVT. Dalteparin is FDA approved for prophylaxis and has approval for cancer patients. Each of the other agents has been approved by the FDA at a lower dose for prophylaxis, but all appear to be safe and effective at some therapeutic dose in patients with active DVT or PE.

Fractionated LMWH administered subcutaneously is now the preferred choice for initial anticoagulation therapy. Unfractionated IV heparin can be nearly as effective but is more difficult to titrate for therapeutic effect. Warfarin maintenance therapy may be initiated after 1–3 days of effective heparinization.

The weight-adjusted heparin dosing regimens that are appropriate for prophylaxis and treatment of coronary artery thrombosis are too low to be used unmodified in the treatment of active DVT and PE. Coronary artery thrombosis does not result from hypercoagulability but rather from platelet adhesion to ruptured plaque. In contrast, patients with DVT and PE are in the midst of a hypercoagulable crisis, and aggressive countermeasures are essential to reduce mortality and morbidity rates.

Enoxaparin (Lovenox)

Exonaparin was the first low-molecular-weight heparin (LMWH) released in the United States. It was approved by the FDA for both treatment and prophylaxis of DVT and PE. Enoxaparin enhances the inhibition of factor Xa and thrombin by increasing antithrombin III activity. In addition, it preferentially increases the inhibition of factor Xa. LMWH has been used widely in pregnancy, although clinical trials are not yet available to demonstrate that it is as safe as unfractionated heparin. Except in overdoses, checking PT or aPTT has no utility, as aPTT does not correlate with anticoagulant effect of fractionated LMWH. Factor Xa levels can be monitored if concern arises about whether the dose is adequate.

Dalteparin (Fragmin)

Dalteparin is an LMWH with many similarities to enoxaparin but with a different dosing schedule. It is approved for DVT prophylaxis in patients undergoing abdominal surgery. Except in overdoses, checking PT or aPTT has no utility, as aPTT does not correlate with anticoagulant effect of fractionated LMWH. LMWH. Factor Xa levels can be monitored if concern arises about whether the dose is adequate.

Tinzaparin (Innohep)

Tinzaparin is approved for treatment of DVT in hospitalized patients. Enhances inhibition of factor Xa and thrombin by increasing antithrombin III activity. In addition, preferentially increases inhibition of factor Xa.

Heparin (Hep-Lock U/P, Hep-Lock, Hep-Flush-10)

Heparin augments the activity of antithrombin III and prevents conversion of fibrinogen to fibrin. It does not actively lyse but is able to inhibit further thrombogenesis. Heparin prevents the reaccumulation of a clot after spontaneous fibrinolysis. When UFH is used, the aPTT should not be checked until 6 hours after the initial heparin bolus because an extremely high or low value during this time should not provoke any action.

Warfarin (Coumadin, Jantoven)

Warfarin (Coumadin) interferes with the hepatic synthesis of vitamin K–dependent coagulation factors. It is used for the prophylaxis and treatment of venous thrombosis, pulmonary embolism, and thromboembolic disorders.

Never administer warfarin to patients with thrombosis until after they have been fully anticoagulated with heparin (the first few days of warfarin therapy produce a hypercoagulable state). Failing to anticoagulate with heparin before starting warfarin causes clot extension and recurrent thromboembolism in approximately 40% of patients, compared with 8% of those who receive full-dose heparin before starting warfarin. Heparin should be continued for the first 5–7 days of oral warfarin therapy, regardless of the PT time, to allow time for depletion of procoagulant vitamin K–dependent proteins.

Tailor the warfarin dose to maintain an INR in the range of 2.5–3.5. The risk of serious bleeding (including hemorrhagic stroke) is approximately constant when the INR is 2.5–4.5 but rises dramatically when the INR is over 5. In the United Kingdom, a higher INR target of 3–4 often is recommended.

Evidence suggests that 6 months of anticoagulation reduces the rate of recurrence to half of the recurrence rate observed when only 6 weeks of anticoagulation is given. Long-term anticoagulation is indicated for patients with an irreversible underlying risk factor and recurrent DVT or recurrent pulmonary embolism.

Procoagulant vitamin K-dependent proteins are responsible for a transient hypercoagulable state when warfarin is first started and stopped. This is the phenomenon that occasionally causes warfarin-induced necrosis of large areas of skin or of distal appendages. Heparin is always used to protect against this hypercoagulability when warfarin is started; when warfarin is stopped, however, the problem resurfaces, causing an abrupt, temporary rise in the rate of recurrent venous thromboembolism.

At least 186 different foods and drugs reportedly interact with warfarin. Clinically significant interactions have been verified for a total of 26 common drugs and foods including 6 antibiotics and 5 cardiac drugs. Every effort should be made to keep the patient adequately anticoagulated at all times because procoagulant factors recover first when warfarin therapy is inadequate.

Patients who have difficulty maintaining adequate anticoagulation while taking warfarin may be asked to limit their intake of foods that contain vitamin K.

Foods that have moderate to high amounts of vitamin K include Brussels sprouts, kale, green tea, asparagus, avocado, broccoli, cabbage, cauliflower, collard greens, liver, soybean oil, soybeans, certain beans, mustard greens, peas (black-eyed peas, split peas, chick peas), turnip greens, parsley, green onions, spinach and lettuce.

Fondaparinux Sodium (Arixtra)

Fondaparinux sodium is a synthetic anticoagulant that works by inhibiting factor Xa, a key component involved in blood clotting. It provides a highly predictable response and has a bioavailability of 100%. The drug has a rapid onset of action and a half-life of 14–16 hours, allowing for sustained antithrombotic activity over a 24-hour period. Fondaparinux sodium does not affect prothrombin time or activated partial thromboplastin time, nor does it affect platelet function or aggregation.

Thrombolytics

Class Summary

Thrombolysis is indicated for hemodynamically unstable patients with pulmonary embolism. Thrombolysis dramatically improves acute cor pulmonale. Thrombolytic therapy has replaced surgical embolectomy as the treatment for hemodynamically unstable patients with massive pulmonary embolism.

Fibrinolytic regimens currently in common use for pulmonary embolism include two forms of recombinant tPA, alteplase and reteplase, along with urokinase and streptokinase. Alteplase usually is given as a front-loaded infusion over 90 or 120 minutes. Urokinase and streptokinase usually are given as infusions over 24 hours or more. Reteplase is a new-generation thrombolytic with a longer half-life; it is given as a single bolus or as two boluses administered 30 minutes apart.

Of the four drugs, the faster-acting agents reteplase and alteplase are preferred for patients with pulmonary embolism because the condition of patients with pulmonary embolism can deteriorate extremely rapidly.

Many comparative clinical studies have shown that administration of a 2-hour infusion of alteplase is more effective (and more rapidly effective) than urokinase or streptokinase over a 12-hour period. One prospective, randomized study comparing reteplase and alteplase found that total pulmonary resistance (along with pulmonary artery pressure and cardiac index) improved significantly after just one half hour in the reteplase group as compared with 2 hours in the alteplase group. Fibrinolytic agents do not seem to differ significantly with respect to safety or overall efficacy.

Streptokinase is least desirable of all the fibrinolytic agents because antigenic problems and other adverse reactions force the cessation of therapy in a large number of cases.

Empiric thrombolysis may be indicated in selected hemodynamically unstable patients, particularly when the clinical likelihood of pulmonary embolism is overwhelming and the patient's condition is deteriorating. The overall risk of severe complications from thrombolysis is low and the potential benefit in a deteriorating patient with pulmonary embolism is high. Empiric therapy especially is indicated when a patient is compromised so severely that he or she will not survive long enough to obtain a confirmatory study. Empiric thrombolysis should be reserved, however, for cases that truly meet these definitions, as many other clinical entities (including aortic dissection) may masquerade as pulmonary embolism, yet may not benefit from thrombolysis in any way.

Newborns may be relatively resistant to thrombolytics because of their lack of fibrinogen activity.

Reteplase (Retavase)

Reteplase is a second-generation recombinant tissue plasminogen activator (recombinant tPA) that forms plasmin after facilitating cleavage of endogenous plasminogen. In clinical trials, reteplase has been shown to be comparable to the recombinant tPA alteplase in achieving TIMI, 2 or 3 patency, at 90 minutes. Reteplase is given as a single bolus or as two boluses administered 30 minutes apart.

As a fibrinolytic agent, reteplase seems to work faster than its forerunner, alteplase, and may be more effective in patients with larger clot burdens. It has also been reported to be more effective than other agents in lysis of older clots. Two major differences help to explain these improvements. Because reteplase does not bind fibrin as tightly as does alteplase, this allows reteplase drug to diffuse more freely through the clot. Another advantage seems to be that reteplase does not compete with plasminogen for fibrin-binding sites, allowing plasminogen at the site of the clot to be transformed into clot-dissolving plasmin.

The FDA has not approved reteplase for administration to patients with pulmonary embolism. Studies of the drug's use for pulmonary embolism have employed the same dose approved by the FDA for coronary artery fibrinolysis.

Alteplase (Activase, Cathflo Activase)

Alteplase, a recombinant tPA, is used in the management of acute myocardial infarction (AMI), acute ischemic stroke, and pulmonary embolism. Alteplase is most often used to treat patients with pulmonary embolism in the ED. It is usually given as a front-loaded infusion over 90–120 minutes. It is FDA approved for this indication. Most ED personnel are familiar with alteplase's use because it is widely employed in the treatment of patients with AMI. An accelerated 90-minute regimen is widely used, and most believe it is safer and more effective than the approved 2-hour infusion. An accelerated-regimen dose is based on patient weight.

Heparin therapy should be instituted or reinstituted near the end of or immediately following infusion when the aPTT or thrombin time returns to twice normal or less.

Urokinase (Abbokinase, Kinlytic)

Urokinase is a direct plasminogen activator produced by human fetal kidney cells grown in culture. It acts on the endogenous fibrinolytic system and converts plasminogen to the enzyme plasmin, which, in turn, degrades fibrin clots, fibrinogen, and other plasma proteins. An advantage of urokinase is that it is nonantigenic; however, it is more expensive than streptokinase, which limits its use. When urokinase is used for localized fibrinolysis, it is given as a local, catheter-directed, continuous infusion directly into area of the thrombus with no loading dose. When it is used for pulmonary embolism, a loading dose is necessary.

Streptokinase (Streptase)

Streptokinase acts with plasminogen to convert plasminogen to plasmin. Plasmin degrades fibrin clots, fibrinogen, and other plasma proteins. An increase in fibrinolytic activity that degrades fibrinogen levels for 24–36 hours takes place with IV infusion of streptokinase. The agent is highly antigenic, and it is highly likely that treatment will be interrupted due to allergic drug reactions. Chills, fever, nausea, and skin rashes are frequent (up to 20%). Blood pressure and heart rate drop in approximately 10% of cases during or shortly after treatment.

Late complications may include purpura, respiratory distress syndrome, serum sickness, Guillain-Barré syndrome, vasculitis, and renal or hepatic dysfunction.

BIBLIOGRAPHY

1. Lilienfeld DE. Decreasing mortality from pulmonary embolism in the United States, 1979–1996. Int J Epidemiol. 2000;29:465–9.
2. Ramzi DW, Leeper KV. DVT and pulmonary embolism: part I. Diagnosis. Am Fam Physician. 2004;69:2829–36.
3. Bauer KA. The thrombophilias: well-defined risk factors with uncertain therapeutic implications. Ann Intern Med. 2001;135:367–73.
4. Hyers TM, Agnelli G, Hull RD, Morris TA, Samama M, Tapson V, et al. Antithrombotic therapy for venous thromboembolic disease. Chest. 2001;119(1 suppl):176S–93S.
5. Brandjes DP, Buller HR, Heijboer H, Huisman MV, de Rijk M, Jagt H, et al. Randomised trial of effect of compression stockings in patients with symptomatic proximal-vein thrombosis. Lancet. 1997;349:759–62.
6. Raschke RA, Reilly BM, Guidry JR, Fontana JR, Srinivas S. The weight-based heparin dosing nomogram compared with a "standard care" nomogram. A randomized controlled trial. Ann Intern Med. 1993;119:874–81.
7. Juergens CP, Semsarian C, Keech AC, Beller EM, Harris PJ. Hemorrhagic complications of intravenous heparin use. Am J Cardiol. 1997;80:150–4.
8. Hull RD, Raskob GE, Rosenbloom D, Panju AA, Brill-Edwards P, Ginsberg JS, et al. Heparin for 5 days as compared with 10 days in the initial treatment of proximal venous thrombosis. N Engl J Med. 1990;322:1260–4.
9. Hull RD, Raskob GE, Brant RF, Pineo GF, Elliott G, Stein PD, et al. Low-molecular-weight heparin vs heparin in the treatment of patients with pulmonary embolism. American-Canadian Thrombosis Study Group. Arch Intern Med. 2000;160:229–36.
10. Levine M, Gent M, Hirsh J, Leclerc J, Anderson D, Weitz J, et al. A comparison of low-molecular-weight heparin administered primarily at home with unfractionated heparin administered in the hospital for proximal deep-vein thrombosis. N Engl J Med. 1996;334:677–81.
11. Savage KJ, Wells PS, Schulz V, Goudie D, Morrow B, Cruickshank M, et al. Out-patient use of low molecular weight heparin (dalteparin) for the treatment of deep vein thrombosis of the upper extremity. Thromb Haemost. 1999;82:1008–10.
12. Kovacs MJ, Anderson D, Morrow B, Gray L, Touchie D, Wells PS. Outpatient treatment of pulmonary embolism with dalteparin. Thromb Haemost. 2000;83:209–11.
13. Crowther MA, Harrison L, Hirsh J. Reply. Warfarin: less may be better. Ann Intern Med. 1997:127:333.
14. Ridker PM, Goldhaber SZ, Danielson E, Rosenberg Y, Eby CS, Deitcher SR, et al. Long-term, low-intensity warfarin therapy for the prevention of recurrent venous thromboembolism. N Engl J Med. 2003;348:1425–34.
15. Kearon C, Ginsberg JS, Kovacs MJ, Anderson DR, Wells P, Julian JA, et al. Comparison of low-intensity warfarin therapy

with conventional-intensity warfarin therapy for long-term prevention of recurrent venous thromboembolism. N Engl J Med. 2003;349:631–9.

16. Kovacs MJ, Rodger M, Anderson DR, Morrow B, Kells G, Kovacs J, et al. Comparison of 10-mg and 5-mg warfarin initiation nomograms together with low-molecular-weight heparin for outpatient treatment of acute venous thromboembolism. A randomized, double-blind, controlled trial. Ann Intern Med. 2003;138:714–9.
17. Pinede L, Ninet J, Duhaut P, Chabaud S, Demolombe-Rague S, Durieu I, et al. Comparison of 3 and 6 months of oral anticoagulant therapy after a first episode of proximal deep vein thrombosis or pulmonary embolism and comparison of 6 and 12 weeks of therapy after isolated calf deep vein thrombosis. Circulation. 2001;103:2453–60.
18. Lee AY, Levine MN, Baker RI, Bowden C, Kakkar AK, Prins M, et al. Low-molecular-weight heparin versus a coumarin for the prevention of recurrent venous thromboembolism in patients with cancer. N Engl J Med. 2003;349:146–53.
19. Konstantinides S, Geibel A, Heusel G, Heinrich F, Kasper W. Heparin plus alteplase compared with heparin alone in patients with submassive pulmonary embolism. N Engl J Med. 2002;347:1143–50.
20. Decousus H, Leizorovicz A, Parent F, Page Y, Tardy B, Girard P, et al. A clinical trial of vena caval filters in the prevention of pulmonary embolism in patients with proximal deep-vein thrombosis. N Engl J Med. 1998;338:409–15.
21. Aklog L, Williams CS, Byrne JG, Goldhaber SZ. Acute pulmonary embolectomy: a contemporary approach. Circulation. 2002;105:1416–9.
22. Geerts WH, Heit JA, Clagett GP, Pineo GF, Colwell CW, Anderson FA Jr, et al. Prevention of venous thromboembolism. Chest. 2001;119(1 suppl):132S–75S.
23. Pineo GF. Prevention of venous thromboembolic disease. Accessed online February 3, 2004.

31 Cardiovascular Emergencies in Children and Adolescents

Compared with adults, cardiac emergencies are infrequent in children and clinical presentation is often quite variable. In adults, cardiac emergencies are most commonly related to complications of coronary artery disease; however, in pediatric cases, the coronaries are only rarely the underlying problem. Pediatric cardiac emergencies comprise a range of pathology including but not limited to undiagnosed congenital heart disease in the infant; complications of palliated congenital heart disease in children; arrhythmias related to underlying cardiac pathology in the

Table 31.1: *Common cardiovascular emergencies in children and adolescents*

1. Congenital heart diseases
   A. Acyonotic
      Left-sided obstructive disorders HLHS
      Dissection of aorta, Marfan syndrome
   B. Cyanotic heart diseases:
      Tetrology of fallot, D-TGV, TAPVC, abstein anomaly
2. Acquired heart disease, rheumatic heart disease hypertensive heart disease, myocarditis infective endocarditis, Kawasaki's disease, pulmonary embolism
3. Coronary artery anomalies, i.e. ALCAPA
4. Heart failure
5. Cardiac arrhythmia
6. Cardiac tamponade
7. Postoperative cardiac emergencies
8. Cardiomyopathies
9. Toxicological emergencies
10. Electrolyte imbalance

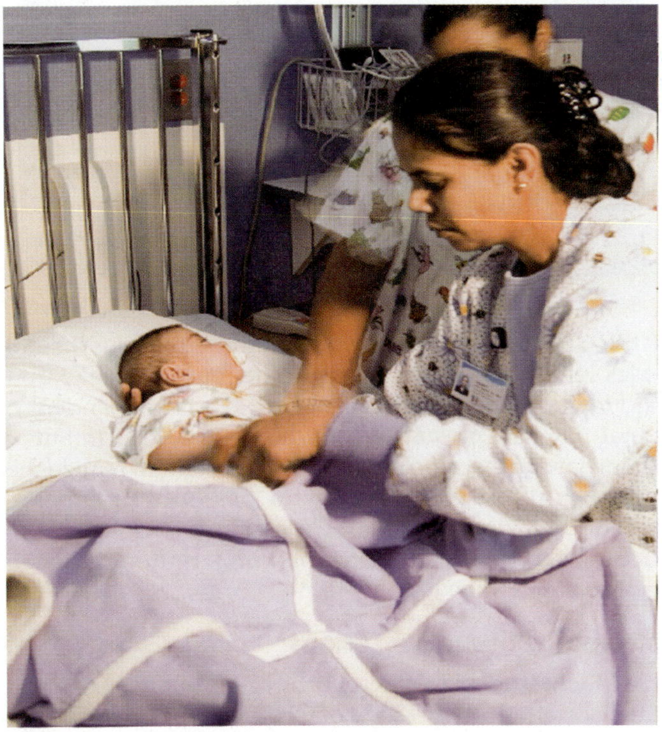

Fig. 31.1: *Cardiologist and attending nurse are connecting life supports to a child admitted in emergency department with intractable heart failure*

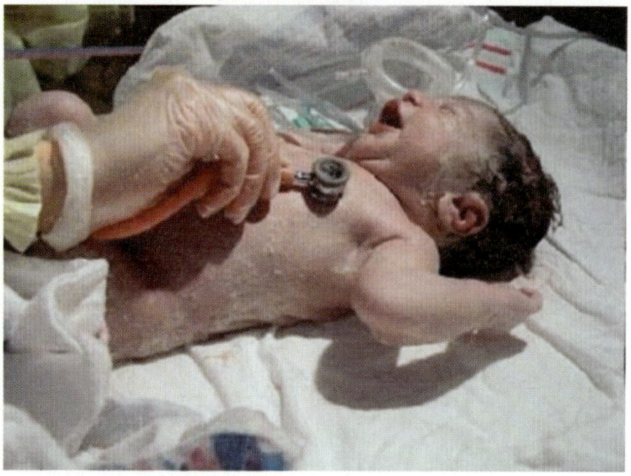

Fig. 31.2: *Emergency physician is attending a child admitted in emergency department*

teenager and acquired heart disease. The emergency room physician and pediatric intensivist will usually be the first and second lines of care for pediatric cardiac emergencies and thus it is imperative that they have knowledge of the diverse presentations of cardiac disease in order to increase the likelihood of delivering early appropriate therapy and referral. The objective of this review is to outline cardiac emergencies in the pediatric population and contrast the presentation with adults.

In adults, cardiac disease is not uncommon and the majority of causes of sudden cardiac death are due to atherosclerotic coronary artery disease. However, cardiac death in children is a rare occurrence and the cause differs based on the age of the child. For infants less than 1 year of age, ductal dependent congenital heart disease is the most common cause, and after the first year and into early adulthood acquired heart conditions, such as myocarditis, cardiomyopathy and aortic dissection in patients with Marfan's syndrome. The objective of this review is to outline cardiac emergencies in the pediatric population and contrast the presentation with adults. The emergency room physician and pediatric intensivist will usually be the first and second lines of care for pediatric cardiac emergencies and thus it is imperative that they have knowledge of the diverse presentations of cardiac disease in order to increase the likelihood of delivering early appropriate therapy and referral (Table 31.1).

Ductal Dependent Lesions

Congenital heart diseases (CHD) are rare conditions, and the mortality is highest among infants and children and among the severe cardiac defects, such as hypoplastic left heart syndrome (HLHS). In the majority of the cases, mortality can be attributed to the underlying heart defect. Infants with severe CHD can initially be asymptomatic, with a relatively benign physical examination prior to discharge from the newborn nursery, due to the patency

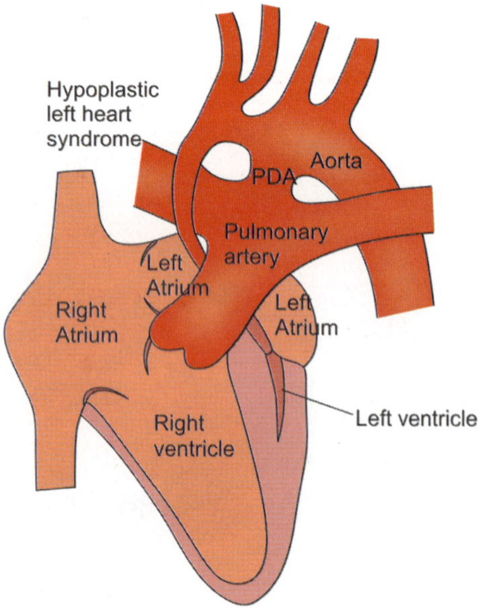

Fig. 31.3 *Anatomical features of hypoplastic left heart syndrome (HLHS)*

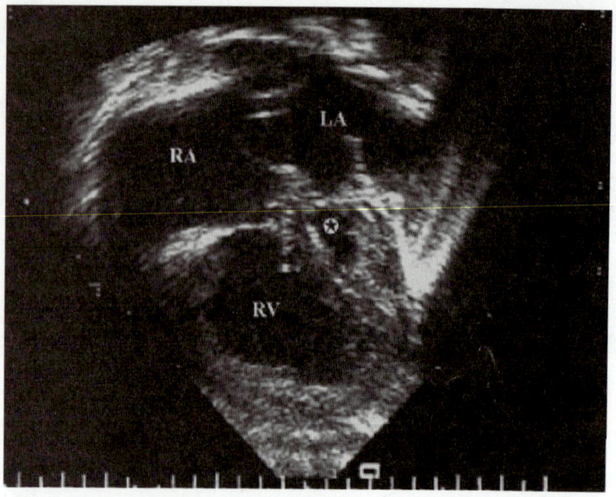

Fig. 31.4: *This echocardiographic still frame shows a four-chamber view of the heart in a patient with hypoplastic left heart syndrome (HLHS). A large right ventricle (RV) and hypoplastic left ventricle (star) are seen. RA, right atrium; LA, Left atrium*

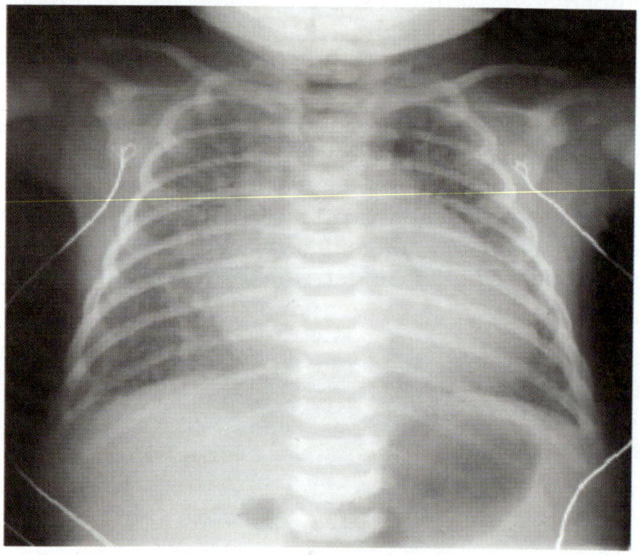

Fig. 31.5: *CXR - HLHS. The radiograph shows pulmonary venous congestion in an infant with hypoplastic left heart syndrome (HLHS)*

of the ductus arteriosus. The ductus arteriosus usually closes within the first 2 weeks of life, but some take up to six. However, in infants with heart disease dependent on ductal patency, closure of the ductus can lead infants to become abruptly critically ill. It is important to realize then that any infant ≥ 6 weeks who presents in shock or profoundly cyanotic might be secondary to closure of the ductus arteriosus in conjunction with a right or left-sided obstructive cardiac lesion.

Left-sided Obstructive Lesions

These include *HLHS*, critical aortic stenosis, and coarctation of the aorta represent 12.4% of CHD. In HLHS for example as the PDA closes, pulmonary overcirculation develops and systemic hypoperfusion, circulatory collapse and shock ensue. The patient will present with respiratory distress,

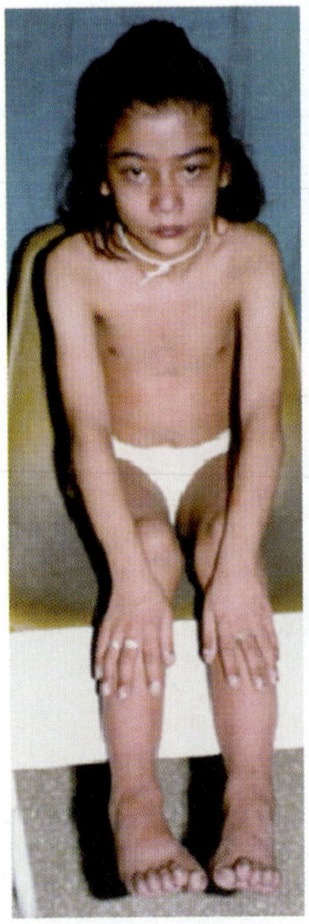

Fig. 31.6: *Showing central cyanosis and digital clubbing in a child with R-L shunt*

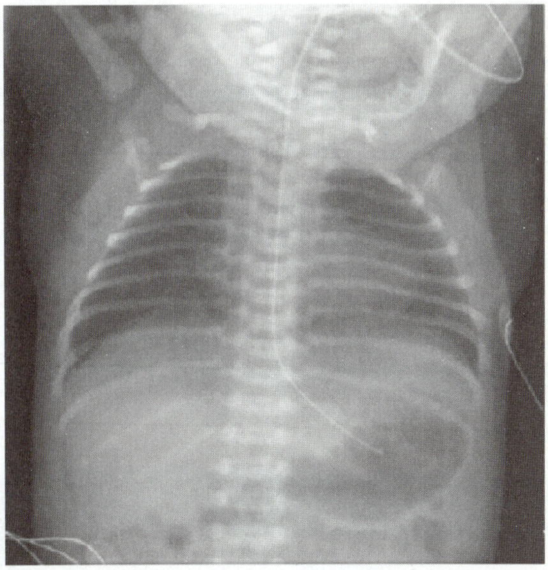

Fig. 31.7: *In TOF radiologically, the heart size is usually normal. There is elevation of the cardiac apex, secondary to right ventricular hypertrophy. The cardiac silhouette is often described as "boot-shaped". The lung fields are usually clear and in cases of severe outflow tract obstruction may appear oligaemic. There may be a concavity of the left border of the heart usually occupied by the pulmonary artery. The radiological appearances can vary depending on other associated cardiac lesions. For example, if collateral vessels are present between the aorta and the pulmonary circulations, there may be pulmonary plethora*

hepatomegaly, tachycardia, and signs of poor perfusion. Additionally, in critical coarctation of the aorta femoral pulses are weak or absent and there is a blood pressure differential between the upper and the lower extremities reflecting the gradient across the stenotic aortic segment. Prostaglandin infusion is necessary to reopen the PDA and basic resuscitative measures (ABC's) should be initiated. Oxygen therapy can either help or hurt the patient and should be used judiciously, directed by the underlying anatomy and anticipated oxygen saturation for the heart defect. For example, to achieve a pulmonary circulation to systemic circulation flow ratio of 1:1, an oxygen saturation of 75–80% may be desired (such as in HLHS). In this lesion, administration of oxygen to obtain a "normal" saturation of 100% would be detrimental, as the oxygen effect of reduced pulmonary vascular resistance compromises systemic perfusion. Of note, in patients with critical coarctation, blood supply to the lower extremities will be extremely compromised such that an IO in the tibia may not be adequate and a right upper extremity or scalp IV may provide better access until a surgical cut down can be obtained.

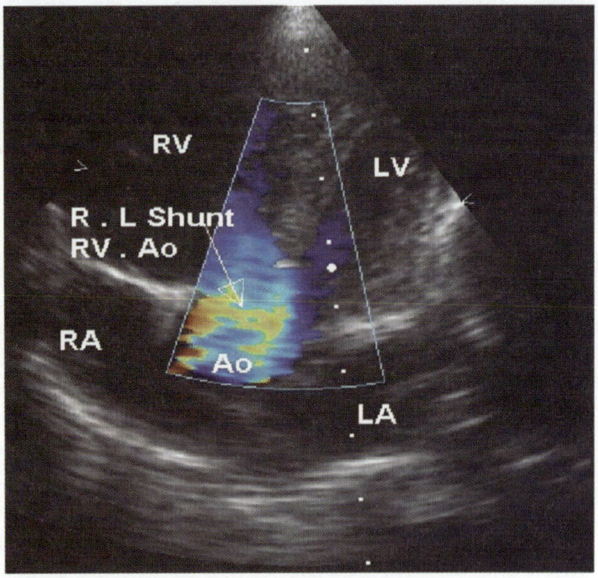

Fig. 31.8: *Apical five chamber view in tetralogy of fallot in systole with right to left shunt*

I. APPROACH TO THE PEDIATRIC PATIENT WITH CYANOSIS

The presentation of a child who is cyanotic can be dramatic. Appropriate management requires a logical approach to reach a general division of the various diagnoses that can be associated with cyanosis. Differentiation must be made to determine if the etiology of the hypoxemia is secondary to respiratory or cardiac disease. Pneumothorax, airway obstruction, and severe bronchospasm are examples of the most common respiratory causes for cyanosis.

General Approach to the Cyanotic Child with Suspected Cardiac Disease (Figs 31.6–31.27)

Understanding some general concepts of cardiac physiology in each of the cyanotic heart lesions will guide the emergency physician to the appropriate management plan. Children with a cyanotic heart defect are hypoxic

Table 31.2: *Pulmonary blood flow in cyanotic congenital heart defects*

Decreased pulmonary blood flow
- Tetralogy of Fallot
- Tetralogy of Fallot with pulmonary atresia
- Pulmonary atresia with intact ventricular septum
- Critical pulmonary stenosis
- Ebstein's malformation of the tricuspid valve Tricuspid atresia with pulmonary stenosis

Normal to slightly increased pulmonary blood flow
- Transposition of the great arteries

Increased pulmonary blood flow
- Total anomalous pulmonary venous connection
- Truncus arteriosus

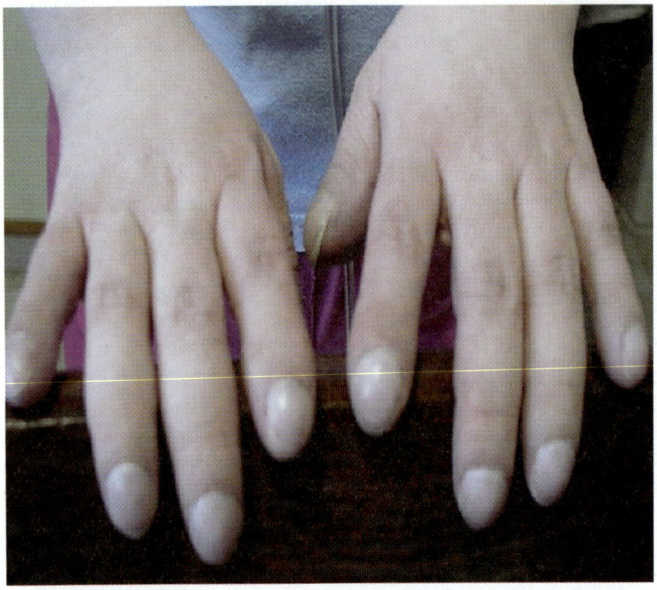

Fig. 31.9: *Clubbing in the fingers of a 18-year-old female with Eisenmenger syndrome (VSD, R-L shunt)*

because systemic venous blood bypasses the alveolar capillary bed and enters the systemic circulation. The degree of cyanosis is partly determined by the amount of pulmonary venous blood that mixes with the desaturated systemic return. This mixing can occur at various levels, in the atrium, in the ventricles, or across the ductus arteriosus. For most of the lesions with decreased pulmonary blood flow, the major determinant to the degree of desaturation is the severity of obstruction of flow to the pulmonary circulation. For the other lesions, the amount of mixing of saturated and desaturated blood will dictate the degree of cyanosis.

A. Patient Presentation

As with acyanotic and obstructive lesions, the age of the child at the time of presentation with previously unrecognized cyanosis is helpful in narrowing the list of differential diagnoses. Children with cyanotic congenital heart disease usually present within the first few months after birth. Infants with complete transposition of the great arteries, tricuspid atresia, or pulmonary atresia with intact

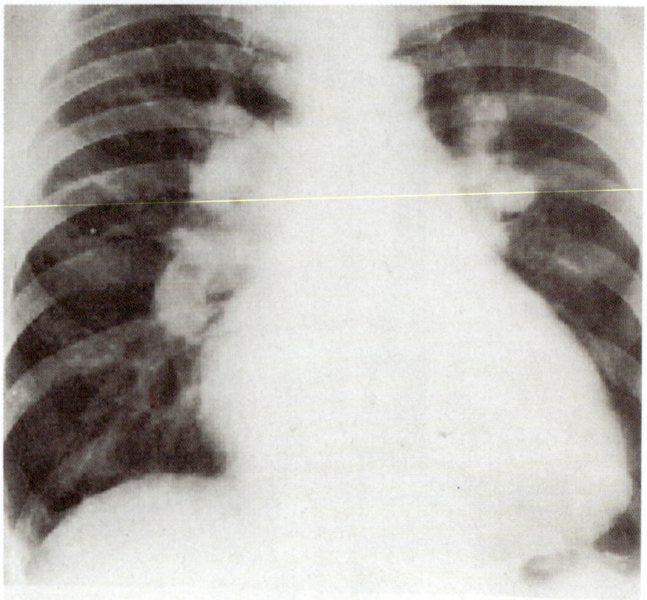

Fig. 31.10: *In atrial septal defect (ASD[2]) with elevated pulmonary vascular resistance, there is a marked disparity between the size of the hilar arteries and the peripheral pulmonary vessels, indicating increase in pulmonary vascular resistance. The right ventricular pressure was almost at systemic levels*

Table 31.3: *Treatment of hypercyanotic spells in tetralogy of Fallot*

- Knee to chest position
- Supplemental oxygen
- Morphine sulfate (0.1 mg/kg 1 m or SC)

If not responding to above:
- Obtain IV access
- Repeat morphine sulfate if agitaged
- IV fluid bolus 00 mL/kg)
- Phenylephrine infusion (0.5–5.0 (~kg/min titrate to effect)
- $NaHCO_3$ (1 mEq/kg IV)
- Propranolol (0.5–0.10) mg/kg IV(maximum dose 1 mg)

If remains criticat:
- Consider general anethesia and paralytic agent.
- Urgent consultation with cardiothoracic surgery is needed for

ventricular septum will usually present in the first week after birth if not shortly after delivery. Associated lesions such as large ventricular septal defects may lessen the degree of cyanosis and thus delay presentation. The timing of presentation for some lesions is determined by the development of obstruction to pulmonary blood flow. In tetralogy of fallot, the initial degree of pulmonary stenosis may be quite mild and the patient may experience signs and symptoms related to a large left-to-right shunt. The infundibular stenosis, however, can be progressive leading to decrease in pulmonary blood flow and greater right-to-left shunting. In an older previously healthy child, new onset cyanosis is extremely unlikely to be the result of undiagnosed cyanotic heart lesion.

1. **Patient history:** In the newborn, there may not be much history apart from the cyanosis. Obviously, any

respiratory symptoms should suggest a pulmonary process; however, this does not exclude cardiac disease. In the child who has known congenital heart disease

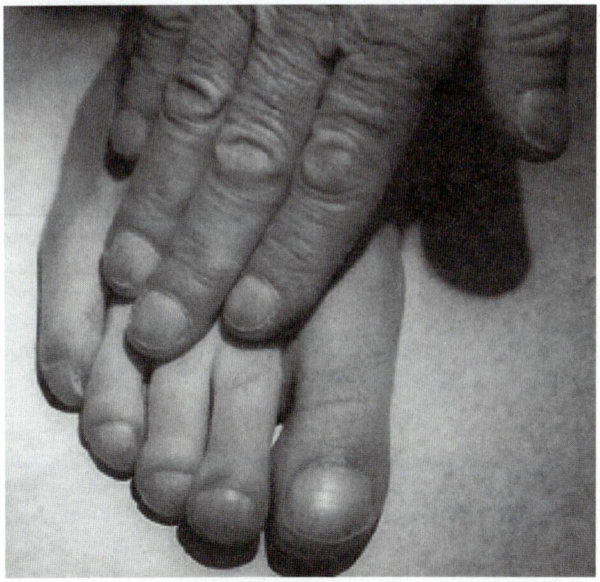

Fig. 31.11: *17-year-old adolescent with unrepaired large PDA, Eisenmenger's syndrome, and right-to-left shunting at the ductal level producing differential cyanosis. The transcutaneous oxygen saturation in the fingers was 92% and in the toes 84%. The central hematocrit was 65%. Clubbing is more apparent in the toes than in the fingers*

information regarding the underlying cardiac defect, current medications, and most importantly previous surgeries altering the physiology can be crucial in guiding the emergency physician to the appropriate treatment. If the child is chronically cyanotic, most families will know the "baseline" oxygen saturation for their child. Comparing this information with the current measured saturation will help to determine if there is any acute disease process or interval change. Specific problems seen in children who have undergone corrective or palliative surgery will be discussed separately.

2. **Physical examination:** The examination should always include an accurate documentation of the patient's vital signs. Shock can present with cyanosis because of poor perfusion and venous stasis. Examination of the oral mucosa will usually determine the presence or absence of central cyanosis. It should be noted that central cyanosis can be masked by the presence of significant anemia. Auscultation of the lung fields will determine if there is evidence of pulmonary disease. Children with cyanotic heart defects most often have clear lung fields, with the possible exception of total anomalous pulmonary venous connection when rales may be present. Many infants with significant cyanosis will also have an increased respiratory rate without signs of distress-so-called happy tachypnea-caused by the CNS response to hypoxemia.

The absence of a heart murmur does not exclude the presence of congenital heart disease. The presence of a

Table 31.4: *Aetiological factors in heart failure in infants and children*

1. Common causes of heart failure in the structurally normal heart		
Prenatal	***Neonates and infants***	***Childhood***
Anemia Arrhythmia Arteriovenous fistula Cardiomyopathy Twin-twin transfusion	Anemia Arrhythmia Arteriovenous fistula Dilated cardiomyopathy Endocrionpathies Hypoglycemia Hypothyroidism Hypoxic ischemic injury Hypertension Infection/sepsis Kawasaki syndrome	Acquired valve disorders Anemia Arrhythmia Dilated cardiomyopathy Hypertension Renal failure Restrictive cardiomyopathy
2. Common causes of heart failure in patients with congenital heart disease		
Prenatal	***Neonates and infants***	***Children***
Atrioventricular valve regurgitation Mitral stenosis with intact atrial septum	Systemic outflow obstruction Aortic valve stenosis Coarctation of the aorta Subaortic stenosis Systemic inflow obstruction Pulmonary venous stenosis Systemic ventricular volume overload Aortic or mitral regurgitation Atrial/ventricular septal defect Mitral stenosis Patent ductus arteriosus	Aortic regurgitation Mitral regurgitation Mitral stenosis Pulmonary vein stenosis

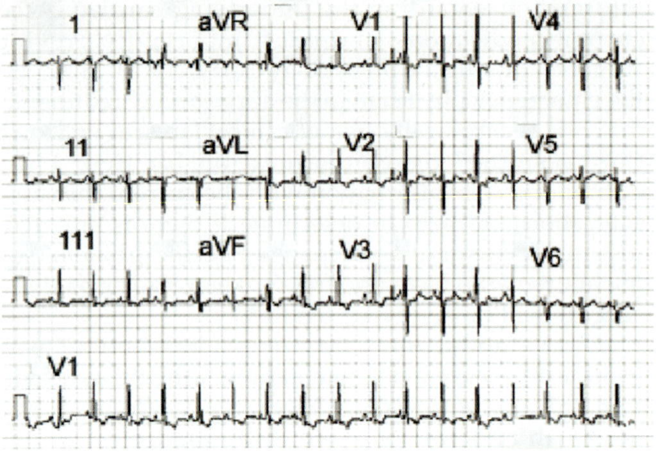

Fig. 31.12: 20-year-old patient with large conoventricular ventricular septal defect and Eisenmenger's syndrome. The aortic oxygen saturation was 72% and hematocrit 74%. The tracing shows right-axis deviation, right atrial enlargement, right ventricular hypertrophy, and right ventricular strain (inverted T waves in the anterior leads)

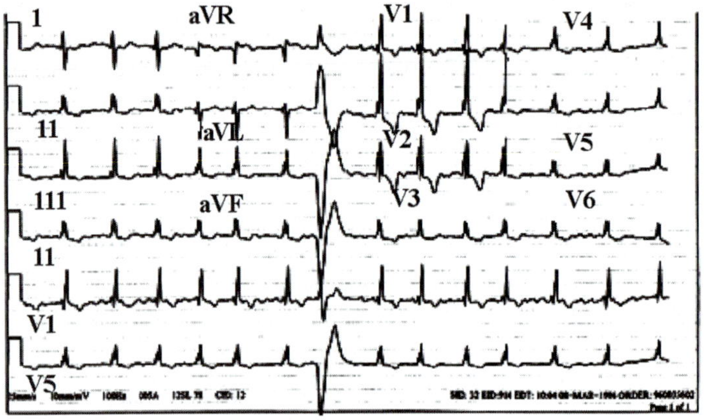

Fig. 31.13: Electrocardiogram of a 12-year-old girl with Eisenmenger complex, demonstrating atrial fibrillation with right axis deviation, right ventricular hypertrophy, right bundle-branch block, and premature ventricular beat

specific type or location of a murmur simply may indicate an associated defect and not the primary anomaly. In the majority of cyanotic defects, the second heart sound is single and loud; total anomalous pulmonary venous connection and Ebstein's malformation of the tricuspid valve are the exceptions, where the second heart sound is usually widely split.

B. Patient Assessment

1. **Pulse-oximetry and arterial blood gas measurement:** Transcutaneous pulse-oximetry is usually readily available and accurate to determine the level of hypoxia. In some situations, a transcutaneous saturation cannot be obtained or the accuracy of the measurement is doubtful, such as in a poorly perfused child. In these situations, an arterial blood gas analysis is essential to determine the oxygenation, ventilation, and acid-base status of the patient.

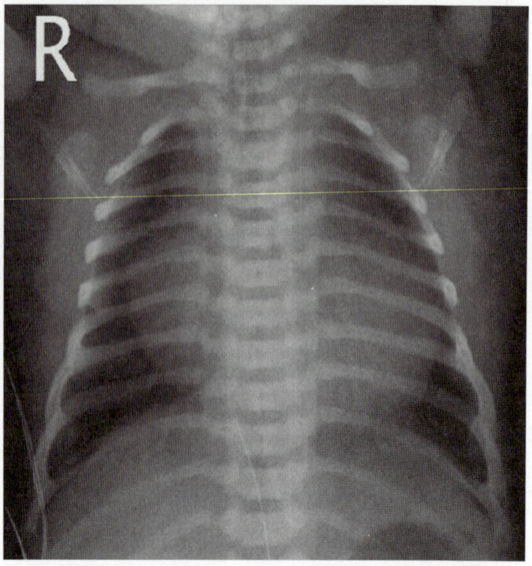

Fig. 31.14: X-ray chest PA view pulmonary atresia. The cardiac silhouette may be normal size, or enlarged (in this case shown to the left, this was from right atrial enlargement due to poor communication between right and left atria via a restricted foramen ovale). Fistulae from the right ventricle to the coronary circulation may be present, particularly if the right ventricle and tricuspid valve are small

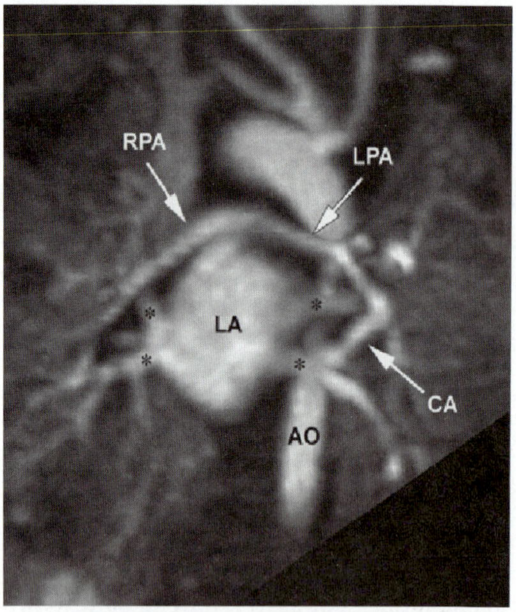

Fig. 31.15: Pulmonary atresia with intact ventricular septum in a 1-day-old girl. MR angiographic images demonstrate that the pulmonary arteries (LPA, RPA) are hypoplastic, confluent, and supplied by a single collateral artery (CA) from the descending aorta (AO). LA, left atrium; PV, pulmonary veins. A right ventricle-pulmonary artery conduit was planned, but the patient died before surgery could be performed

2. **Radiographic findings:** A CXR is important to differentiate the varied cyanotic congenital heart defects as well as to exclude the presence of pulmonary disease. It should be obtained on all patients with the initial presentation of cyanosis. The importance of comparing

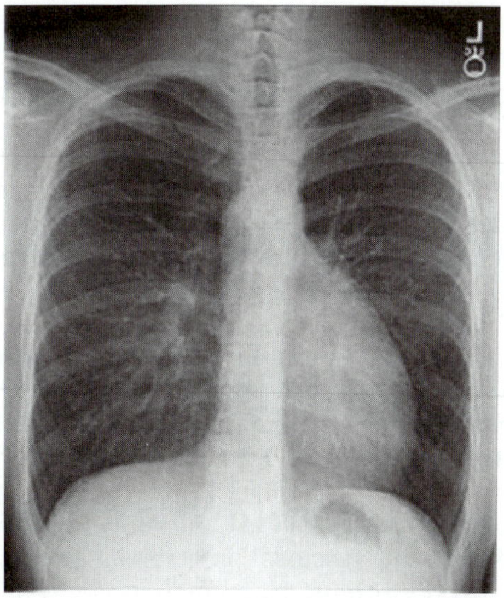

Fig. 31.16: *X-ray showing characteristic finding in case of transposition of the great vessels which is called egg on side sign*

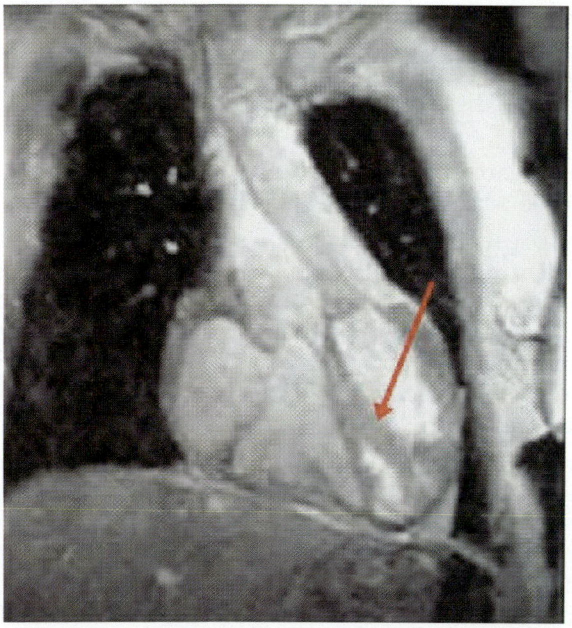

Fig. 31.17: *This gradient echo cine image in the coronal plane shows the great vessels arising in a parallel fashion, a finding that represents transposition of the great arteries (TGA). Notice that the ventricle on the patients left is markedly trabeculated and a moderator band (arrow) is present; this therefore represents the morphologic right ventricle. In L-TGA , the morphological right ventricle is located in the usual location of the left ventricle and gives rise to the aorta. This configuration is also known a congenitally corrected transposition*

the present study to any previous CXRs, if available, cannot be more strongly emphasized. Chronic pulmonary changes may mimic an infiltrate, and progressive changes in cardiac size and pulmonary vascularity in the patient with known heart disease may be diagnostic of the underlying pathology.

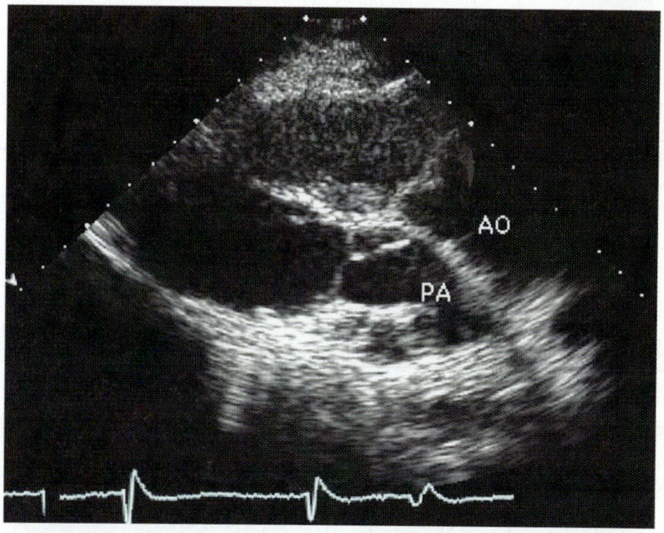

Fig. 31.18: *TGV-D echo shows parallel position of aorta and pulmonary artery. Aorta is placed anteriorly*

Table 31.5: *Signs and symptoms of heart failure in infants and children*

History		
	Infants	
		Take longer to feed with frequent breaks
		Fall asleep shortly after beginning to feed
		Sweat excessively with feeds, cry
		Breathe harder and faster than normal
		Not gaining weight well
	Older children	
		Anorexia
		Decreased exercise tolerance
		Orthopnea
		Chronic nonproductive cough
Physical findings		
	Infants	
		Tachypnea
		Retrations, grunting, nasal flaring
		Wheezing
		Tachycardia
		Gallop rhythm
		Hepatomegaly
		Cool extremities
		Decreased capillary refill
		Diminished peripheral pulses
		Mottled skin
		Peripheral cyanosis
		Central cyanosis (if congestive heart failure is severe)
	Older children and adolescents	
		Rales
		Peripheral edema
		Ascites
		Systemic venous distention

The presence of the stomach on the opposite side of the cardiac silhouette, as in left-sided stomach bubble with dextrocardia, suggests a high probability of a complex heart defect.

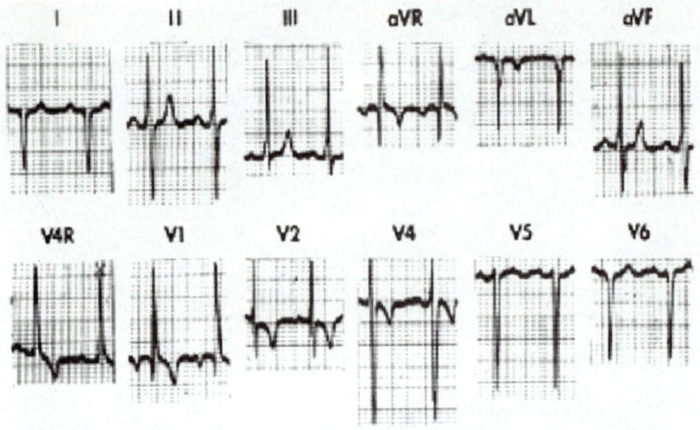

Fig. 31.19: *ECG showing right-axis deviation, right ventricular hypertrophy, almost QS pattern in leads 1, aVL V5 and V6 in a patient with D-transposition of great arteries*

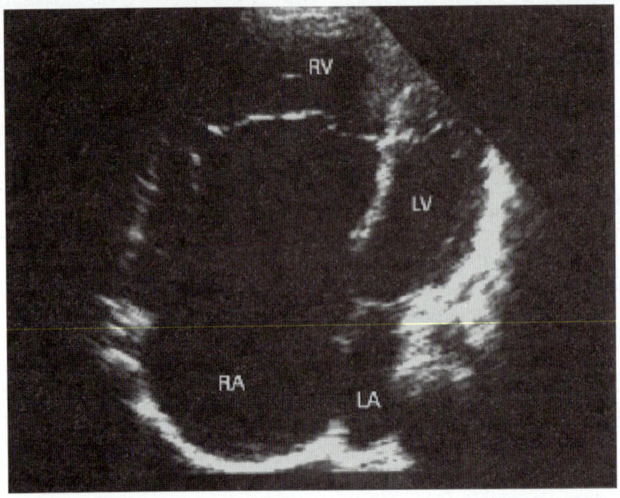

Fig. 31.20: *Four chamber view in a patient with Ebstein's anomaly of the tricuspid valve showing it to be apically displaced. The left ventricle (LV) and atrium (LA) are small and the right atrium (RA) large consisting of the true atrium and the "atrialised" right ventricle (RV)*

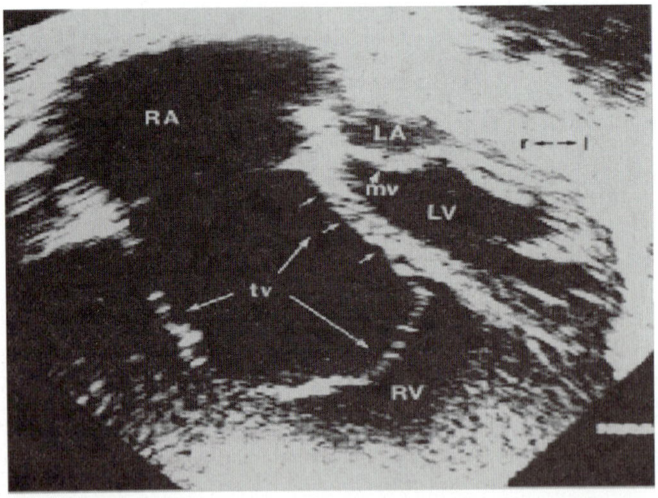

Fig. 31.21: *Inverted apical four chamber echocardiographic view of RA, RV, LA and LV depicting anatomical placement of mitral and tricuspid valves with significant displacement of tricuspid valve, almost atrilization of RV, reduced cavity of RV, comparatively small-sized LV and LA in patient with Ebstein anomaly*

The shape of the cardiac silhouette may guide the physician to the correct cardiac diagnosis. Patients with tetralogy of fallot classically have a "boot-shaped" heart because of absence of the pulmonary artery knob and upturned apex. In transposition of the great arteries, the silhouette has been described as an "egg on a string," a shape caused by the narrow mediastinum resulting from the abnormal orientation of the aorta and pulmonary artery. The cardiac shape on the CXR should be used only to collaborate the physical findings and history of the patient. Unlike the anomalies presenting with CHF, the pulmonary vascularity in cyanotic lesions can be normal, increased or decreased. The appearance of the **right-sided obstructive lesions** such as severe tetralogy of fallot and pulmonary atresia with intact ventricular septum depend on ductal patency to provide blood flow to the pulmonary artery. As the ductus closes, infants develop progressive and rapid cyanosis not improved with oxygen administration and respiratory distress. Prostaglandins should be started immediately to reopen the ductus arteriosus in order to provide pulmonary blood flow through left to right shunting (aorta across the PDA to pulmonary artery), as opposed to the right to left shunt on left-sided obstructive lesions. In these lesions, 100% oxygen is useful to improve pulmonary blood flow and increase dissolved O_2 content. Pulmonary vascular markings will reflect the physiology of the patient.

3. **Electrocardiogram:** As in the patient with acyanotic heart disease with CHF, the ECG is usually not diagnostic.

   The presence or absence of sinus rhythm should be determined. Any ventricular hypertrophy, atrial enlargement, and axis deviation should be noted. It should be emphasized that the age of the patient will determine the normal criteria in interpreting any ECG from a child. Tachyarrhythmias do not typically present with cyanosis.

4. **Oxygen challenge test:** The patient who presents to the emergency department with cyanosis should be treated with oxygen supplementation. However, a few caveats should be noted. **First,** children with pulmonary pathology usually have a greater response to oxygen supplementation than children with cyanotic heart disease. **Second, in older patients with pulmonary hypertension.** Eisenmenger's physiology), oxygen may blunt their respiratory drive. Such patients should be closely monitored. Finally, as noted in the previous section, oxygen supplementation in the patient with cyanosis and evidence of CHF should be used cautiously. In a young infant, if cyanotic heart disease is suspected, an oxygen challenge test should be performed. The oxygen challenge test starts with documentation of the patient's arterial oxygen level in room air. Oxygen at a concentration at or near 100% is then delivered. Mter approximately 10–20 min, a repeat PO_2 is measured. If the PO_2 increases to greater than 100 mmHg, the most likely cause of the cyanosis is pulmonary disease. The lack of a significant rise in oxygen tension strongly suggests an underlying cyanotic heart lesion.

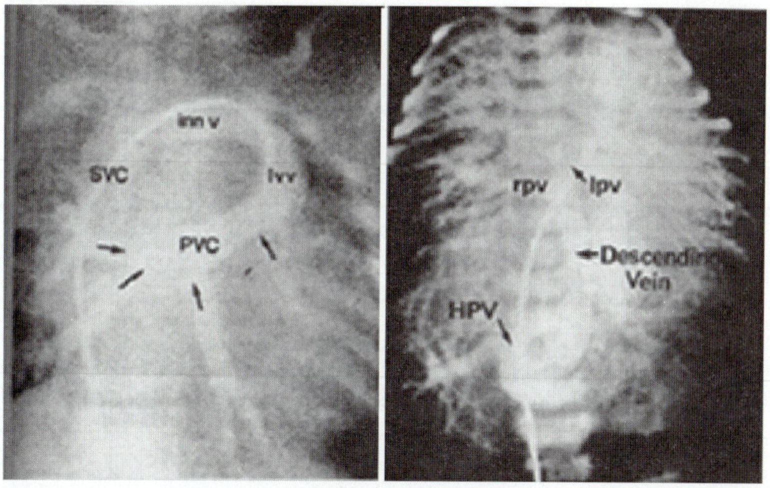

Fig. 31.22: *Contrast angiography showing contrast material entering into pulmonary artery (PA) showing return of pulmonary venous blood. (B) Left-sided vertical vein with subsequent opacification of the right SVC (RSVC) in patient with total anomalous pulmonary venous connection*

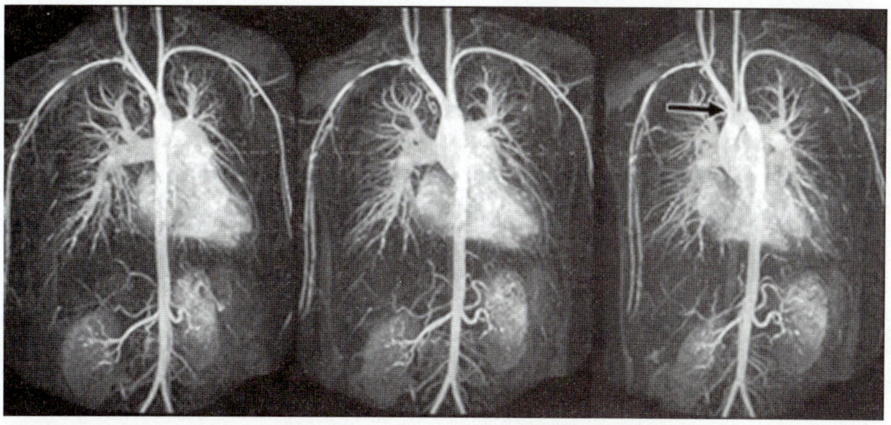

Fig. 31.23: *Images in patient with cyanosis secondary to total anomalous pulmonary venous return (type II, drainage into coronary sinus) and large ASD. Coronal MPs from high-spatial-resolution MR angiography, flip angle, 30°) in anterioposterior projection and with ± 15° rotation. Branching of right and left carotid arteries from brachiocephalic artery (arrow), which can merely be suspected with the time-resolved image series, is clearly visualized. (c) Diastolic (left) and systolic (right) image frames from double-oblique four chamber cine SSFP MR imaging sequence (2.4/1.2; flip angle, 65°) show the large ASD (white arrows). An enlarged right ventricle (*) with right ventricular myocardial hypertrophy (black arrows) can also be appreciated*

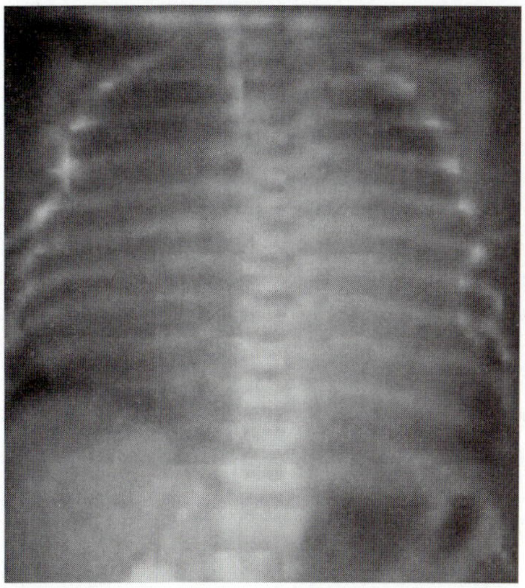

Fig. 31.24: *The radiograph demonstrate marked cardiac enlargement (a "carpet" heart) in patient with TAPVC*

5. **Laboratory studies:** Measurement of the hemoglobin and hematocrit is important, for several reasons. As mentioned earlier, the presence of anemia can mask the presence of significant cyanosis. The finding of polycythemia strongly supports the presence of long-standing hypoxemia, whether secondary to cardiac or pulmonary disease.

C. *Patient Management* (Table 31.3)

The specific management of the cyanotic infant or child depends considerably on the underlying pathology. For example, in tetralogy of fallot, the degree of obstruction is extremely variable and is the key determinant of the degree of cyanosis. Furthermore, any surgical intervention may markedly change the expected physiology of the individual lesion. The general approach to these defects will be based on the underlying pathophysiology.

1. **Cyanotic lesions with decreased pulmonary blood flow:** The general pathophysiologic aberration in this group is a decrease in blood flow to the lungs for oxygenation.

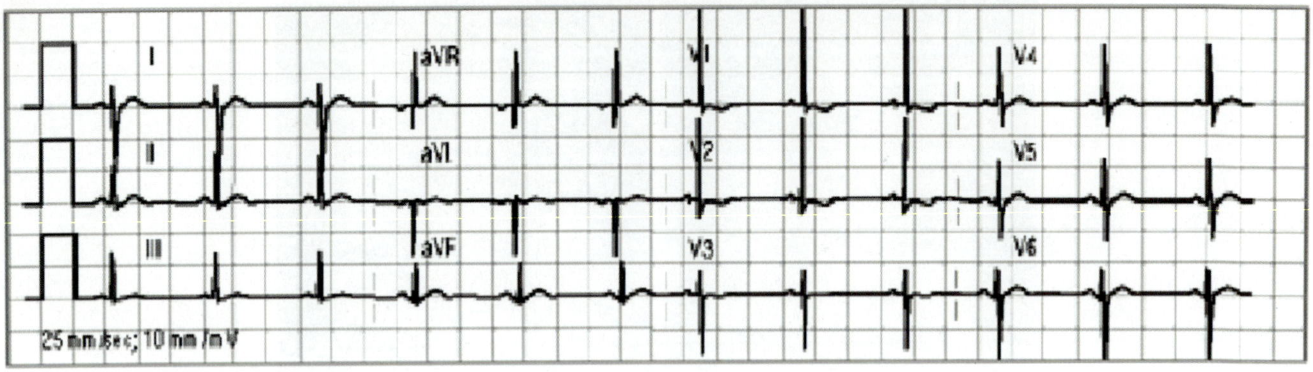

Fig. 31.25: *ECG. There is typically right ventricular hypertrophy with right-axis deviation in a younger patient with TOF*

Table 31.6: *Medical management strategies of congestive heart failure in pediatric patients*

1. Remove any precipitating or aggravating factors:
   - Transfuse for severe anemia
   - Treat arrhythmias
   - Restrict fluid and salt.
2. Reduce metabolic demands:
   - Reduce fever
   - Bed rest
   - Sedate agitated patient!
   - Endotracheal intubation and ventilation.
3. Relieve pulmonary congestion:
   - Diuresis (furosemide 1 mg/kg IVIPO)
   - Mechanical ventilation with positive end expiratory pressure
   - Morphine sulfate (0.05–0.10 mg/kg IVIIM).
4. Improve myocardial performance and oxygen delivery:
   - Inotropes (debutamine, dopamine)
   - Afterload reduction (nitroprusside)
   - Preload reduction (nitroprusside, nitroglycerin)
   - Oxygen (use cautiously in suspected left-to-right shunt lesions)
   - Prostaglandin El (0.1 (~g/kg/min) for left heart obstructive lesions. Correct metabolic acidosis with NaHCOa (1–2 mEq/kg).

This results in a relatively smaller amount of oxygenated pulmonary venous return mixing with the desaturated systemic venous blood. The ratio of the two will determine the oxygen level in the systemic circulation. The most common lesions in this category include tetralogy of fallot, tricuspid atresia with pulmonary stenosis, pulmonary atresia with intact ventricular septum, and critical pulmonary stenosis.

Therapy for this group of patients should enhance the pulmonary blood flow either by decreasing the degree of obstruction or by augmenting the pulmonary blood flow. The former effect is usually difficult to achieve on an acute medical basis and requires an interventional catheter or surgical procedure. Augmentation of pulmonary blood flow may also be quite difficult medically in the older infant and child, with the possible exception of tetralogy of fallot, which will be discussed separately.

Newborn infants presenting with severe cyanosis and decreased pulmonary blood flow often can benefit greatly from opening or dilation of the ductus arteriosus with prostaglandin E (PGE). The patent ductus can supply an alternative source offlow to the pulmonary circulation, bypassing any existing central obstruction. As in the critical left-sided obstructive lesions discussed earlier, PGE is administered by continuous intravenous infusion at a rate of 0.1 mcg/kg/min. The major side effects of PGE1

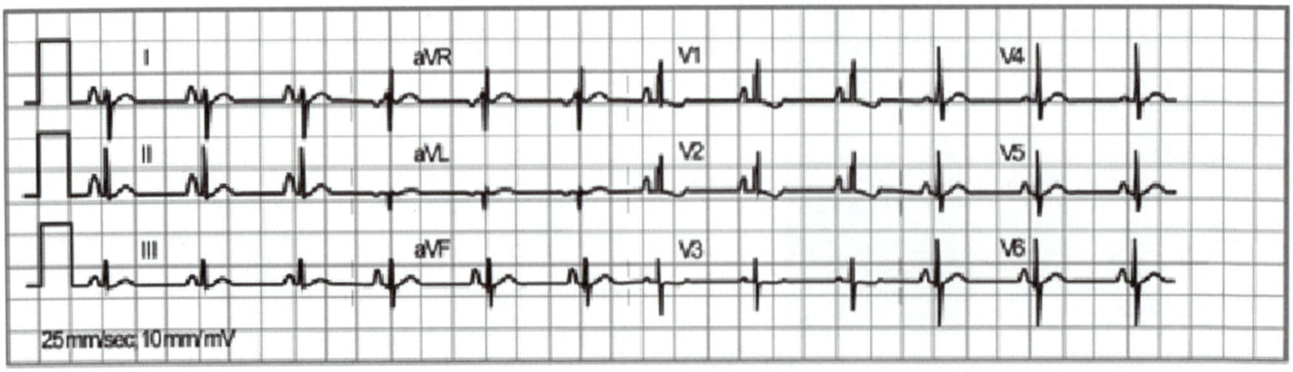

Fig. 31.26: *ECG showing right-axis deviation and right ventricular hypertrophy in TAPVC*

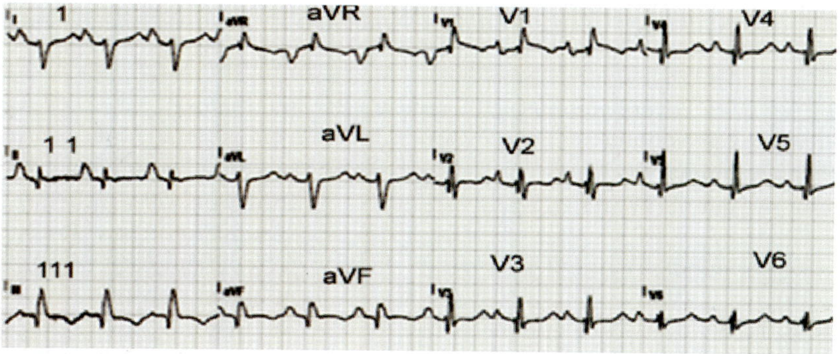

Fig. 31.27: *The electrocardiogram showed sinus rhythm, signs of right atrial hypertrophy, and a right bundle-branch block in Ebstein anomaly*

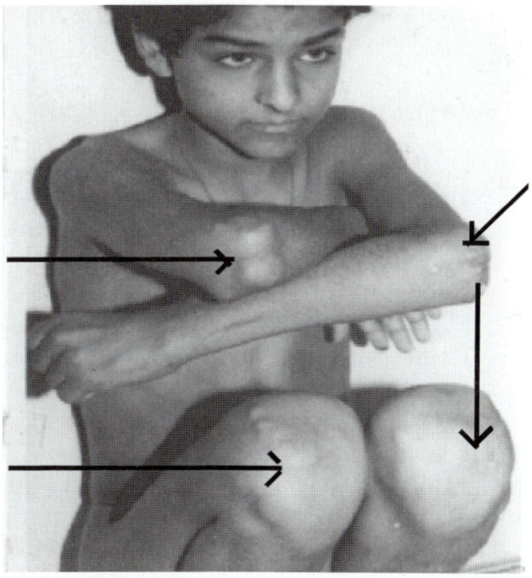

Fig. 31.28: *Subcutaneous nodules (arrows) in a young child with acute rheumatic fever*

administration are hypotension secondary to vasodilation, apnea, and irritability. All patients receiving PGE, should be carefully monitored for these adverse effects. The medical staff should be prepared to intervene in anticipation of potential apnea or hypotension.

Again, any patient who will require transfer to another hospital should be electively intubated and ventilated prior to transport.

a. **Tetralogy of Fallot:** Patients with unrepaired tetralogy of Fallot can be at risk for a hypercyanotic or "tet" spell. Hypercyanotic episodes usually occur in the early waking hours. With agitation, the infant may become tachycardic and cyanotic. As a result of the hypoxemia, the infant may become more agitated and thus more cyanotic. Accompanying respiratory distress is usually present. Some clinicians hypothesize that there is constriction of the right ventricular outflow tract (RVOT), which causes further compromise in pulmonary blood flow. Regardless of the mechanism, the relative amount of blood that exits the heart consists of a progressively smaller proportion of oxygenated blood. With continued agitation, this cycle

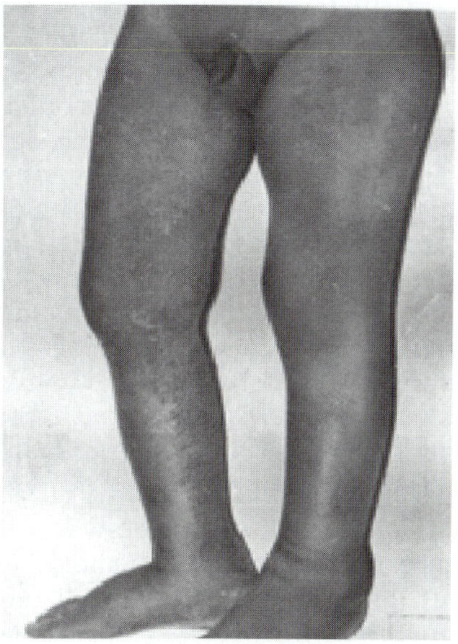

Fig. 31.29: *Edema of ankles and lower legs in patient with congestive cardiac failure*

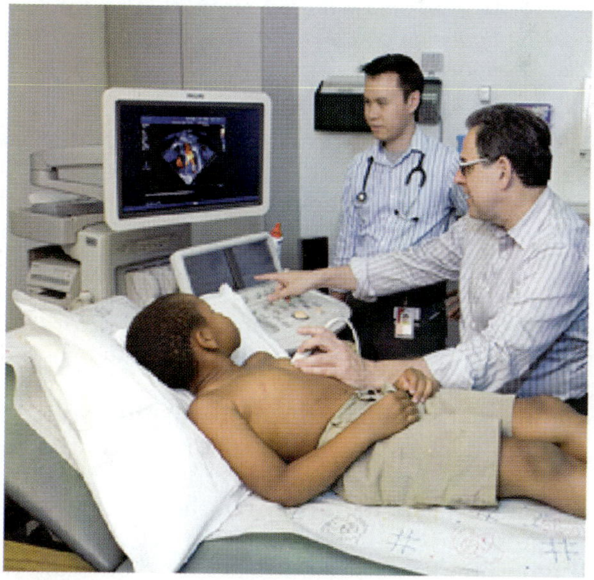

Fig. 31.30: *Echocardiographic evaluation of heart disease in a young child who was admitted into emergency department with cyanosis and heart failure*

Table 31.7: *Medications to maintain cardiac output and for postresuscitation stabilization*

Medication	*Dose range*	*Comment*
Amrinone	0.75–1 mg/kg IV/IO over 5 minutes; may repeat × 2; then; 2–20 μg/kg per minute	Inodilator
Dobutamine	2–20 μg/kg per minute IV/IO	Inotrope; vasodilator
Dopamine	2–20 μg/kg per minute IV/IO	Inotrope; chronotrope; renal and splanchnic vasodilator in low doses; pressor in high doses
Epinephrine	0.1–1 μg/kg per minute IV/IO	Intrope; chronotrope; vasodilator in low doses; pressor in higher doses
Milrinone	50–75 μg/kg IV/IO over 10–60 min then 0.5–0.75 μg/kg per minute	Inodilator
Norepinephrine	0.1–2 μg/kg per minute	Inotrope; vasopressor
Sodium nitroprusside	1–8 μg/kg per minute	Vasodilator; prepare only in D5W

IV indicates intravenous; and IO, intraosseous.
Alternative formula for calculating an infusion:
Infusion rate (mL/h) = [weight (kg) × dose (μg/kg/min) × 60 (min/h)]/concentration μg/mL).

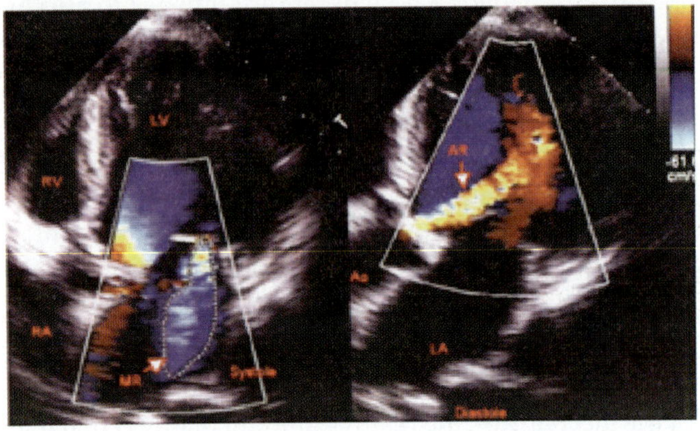

Fig. 31.31: *Colour Doppler echocardiogram showing aortic regurgitation (AR) and mitral regurgitation (MR). MR jet is seen in the left atrium (LA) in the systolic frame on the left side of the image, while AR jet is seen in the left ventricle (LV) in the diastolic frame on the right side of the image. RA, right atrium; RV, right ventricle; Ao, aorta*

can perpetuate and may lead to death. The presence of a hypercyanotic episode is truly a medical emergency. The approach to the management of the patient with a hypercyanotic spell is given in after an initial episode, the child is at marked risk for having recurrent episodes. Therefore, the occurrence of a hypercyanotic spell is an indication for surgical intevention, and appropriate arrangement for admission to a tertiary center should be made.

b. **Ebstein's malformation of the tricuspid valve:** Most patients are diagnosed with this condition in the newborn period because of cyanosis and the presence of a murmur. The cyanosis tends to improve in the first few days of life as pulmonary vascular resistance decreases. The CXR will typically demonstrate marked cardiomegaly even in a newborn infant because of severe insufficiency of the abnormal tricuspid valve and right atrial dilation. Cyanosis, particularly associated with exercise, can return when the child is older. Treatment is limited and most often involves anticongestive therapy with diuretics and digoxin if CHF exists. There is a 5–20% incidence of an accessory bypass tract resulting in Wolff-Parkinson-White (WPW) syndrome in patients with Ebstein's anomaly. These patients can present with peripheral cyanosis if tachyarrhythmias are present. As in all patients with WPW, the presence of atrial flutter/fibrillation secondary to the stretched atrium is especially concerning. Rapid antegrade conduction via the bypass tract can result in ventricular fibrillation. A patient with Ebstein's anomaly and hemodynamic instability should have an ECG to evaluate for any evidence of WPW and tachyarrhythmias.

2. **Cyanotic lesions with normal to slightly increased pulmonary vascularity:** Complete transposition of the great arteries (TGA) is the primary congenital heart defect in this category. The primary reason for the cyanosis in the newborn is the presence of parallel circulatory pathways instead of the pulmonary and systemic circulations functioning in series. The systemic venous blood flows through the right atrium and through the right ventricle, and then is ejected back into the systemic circulation. Parallel to this, the pulmonary venous blood circulates through the left atrium, the left ventricle, and then the pulmonary artery. The degree of mixing between the circulations across the foramen ovale, ductus arteriosus, and/or ventricular septal defect, if present, will determine the level of cyanosis. Almost all patients with simple TGA will present as newborns with intense cyanosis. Children with complicated forms of TGA can present at a later age from a lesser degree of cyanosis.

The lack of mixing of blood between the parallel circulation can lead to death. The immediate therapy should be oriented at improving the mixing of blood. Again, prostaglandin El (PGE) infusion represents the major therapeutic advance that can be life-saving. In this situation, the patent ductus is not necessary to augment diminished

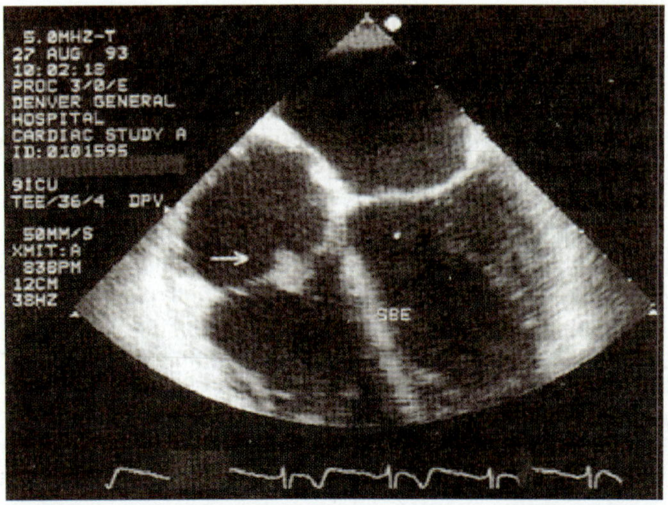

Fig. 31.32: *TEE four chamber view showing large mobile vegetation on tricuspid valve (arrow)*

pulmonary or systemic blood flow, but serves as a site to allow oxygenated blood to reach the systemic circulation and vice versa. The dosage and side effects are similar to those previously outlined. Rarely, the administration of PGE1 does not result in a rise in oxygen levels. In these patients, immediate transfer to a center with expertise in pediatric cardiology for balloon atrial septostomy is needed. Administration of fluid boluses and aggressive correction of metabolic acidosis are intermediate palliative resuscitative maneuvers.

3. Cyanotic lesions with increased pulmonary vascularity: In this group of defects, the cyanosis is often variable and could be quite mild, depending on the amount of pulmonary blood flow. CHF often develops in those patients with unrestricted pulmonary blood flow. This category includes persistent truncus arteriosus, tricuspid atresia without pulmonary stenosis, and total anomalous pulmonary venous return. In patients presenting with mild cyanosis, CHF, and increased pulmonary vascularity on CXR, treating with high-concentration oxygen may result in a rapid decompensation caused by worsening of the CHF. This is similar to the infant or child with a large left-to-right shunt lesion without cyanosis. The hypoxemia is usually mild in this situation and not lifethreatening. Immediate management should be directed toward improving the CHF, primarily with diuretics.

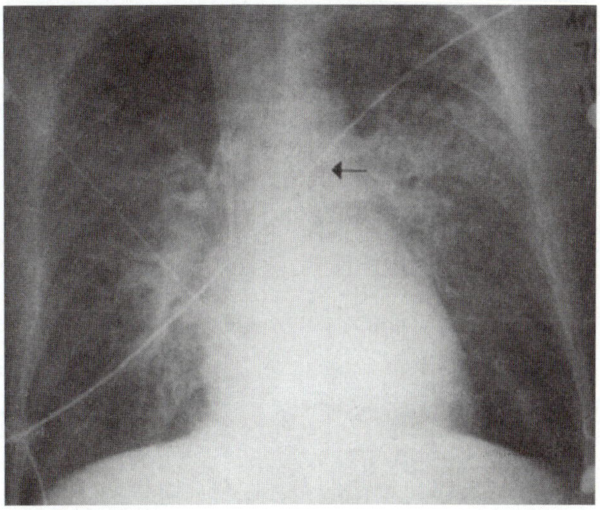

Fig. 31.33: *Cardiogenic alveolar oedema. Symmetrical air space opacity with perihilar predominance is one characteristic pattern produced by cardiogenic oedema*

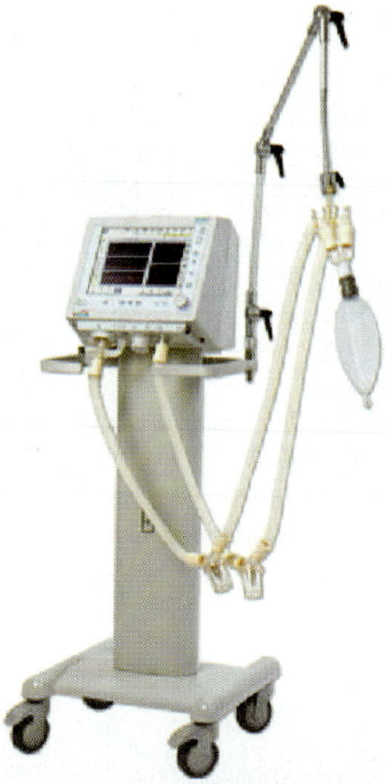

Fig. 31.34: *Invasive and noninvasive ventilation for adult, pediatric and neonate (including premature) patients. Designed and developed for the intensive respiratory care of neonatal and pediatric patient*

II. APPROACH TO THE PEDIATRIC PATIENT WITH CONGESTIVE HEART FAILURE (CHF)

Heart failure is a pathophysiologic condition that results when the pump function of the myocardium is unable to meet the metabolic demands of the body. In infancy and childhood, this condition usually occurs from abnormal work imposed on a normal myocardium from excessive volume or pressure loads. However intrinsic alterations in myocardial contractile performance can also exist. Both physiologic states can exist as a result of congenital or acquired diseases (Figs 31.35–31.41).

A. Patient Presentation

The age at presentation can provide important information regarding the specific etiology ofthe CHF. The timing of key events in the transition from fetal to postpartum circulation has a significant influence on the onset of heart failure when certain underlying structural defects exist. Closure of the ductus arteriosus typically occurs in the first few days of life; however, it may remain patent for several weeks. In left-sided obstructive lesions such as coarctation

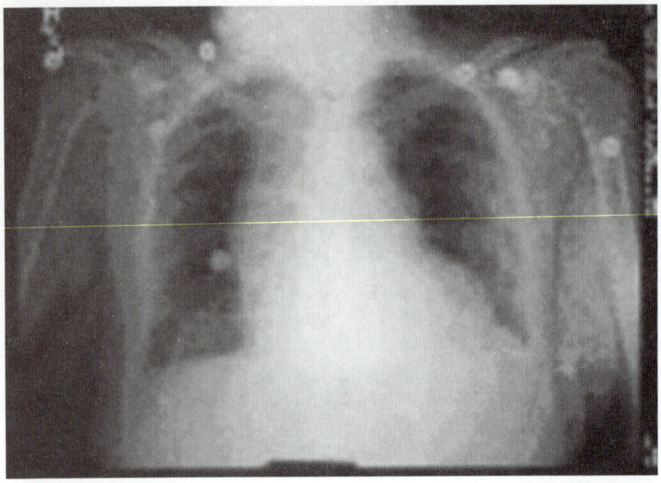

Fig. 31.35: *Chest radiograph shows signs of congestive heart failure (CHF)*

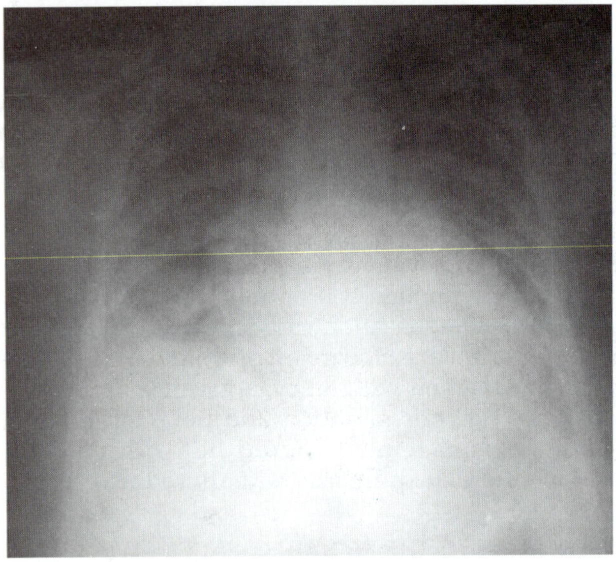

Fig. 31.36: *X-ray chest frontal view showing pulmonary edema in a patient with cardiogenic shock as a result of acute myocarditis in a 12-years-old child*

of the aorta and hypoplastic left heart syndrome, as in the fetus, the ductus arteriosus permits perfusion of the systemic circulation by output from the right ventricle. Constriction of the ductus results in decreased systemic perfusion to all or portions of the body with resultant CHF. In isolated coarctation, the left ventricle may experience a severe, acute rise in afterload as the result of an increase in the degree of obstruction caused by closure of ductal tissue in the juxtaductal aorta. Development of signs and symptoms of heart failure follow closely. Another major alteration in transitional circulation is the progressive decrease in pulmonary vascular resistance that occurs over the first few weeks to months of life. In cardiac anomalies characterized by left-to-right shunts, the degree of shunting is directly related to the relaxation of the pulmonary vascular bed. It is unusual for heart failure to develop in patients even with large defects before the third week of life. The presence of associated lesions, atrioventricular valve regurgitation, and anemia may hasten the development of symptoms. Another congenital anomaly that may present with the fall in pulmonary vascular resistance is anomalous left coronary artery from the pulmonary artery.

Older infants and children rarely present with CHF secondary to undiagnosed congenital heart disease. Diagnoses such as new-onset cardiomyopathy, myocarditis, or pericarditis are more likely.

The clinical manifestations of heart failure in infants and children may be quite different from those of adolescents and adults. A detailed discussion of the compensatory mechanisms, such as myocardial hypertrophy, ventricular dilatation, and increased adrenergic activity, are beyond the scope of this chapter. The specific signs and symptoms that result from failure of these adaptive mechanisms vary with the underlying pathologic process.

1. **History:** A careful, detailed history can often be the most useful information in helping the clinician determine the presence of CHF. Many of the physical findings, particularly in infants, can mimic those of more common pediatric ailments such as bronchiolitis. Specific areas of investigation should be the patient's feeding habits and intake, the presence of significant sweating, the breathing pattern and growth.

   Feeding represents the most significant form of exercise and energy expenditure for an infant. The earliest sign of CHF is increased respiratory effort during feeding that may or may not exist during rest. The increased respiratory demands often result in the need for frequent breaks between sucking and thus prolong the time required for feeding. The act of feeding may also be accompanied by significant diaphoresis caused by the increased energy expenditure and increased adrenergic state. Older children and adolescents in CHF often complain of anorexia.

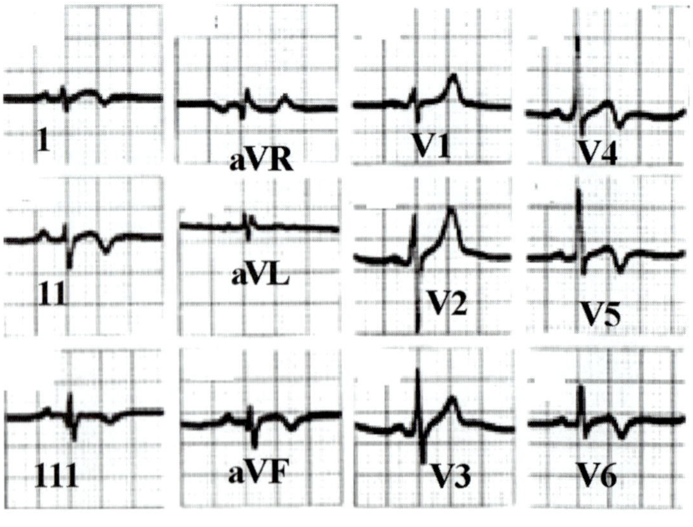

Fig. 31.37: *The T waves are deeply and symmetrically inverted in I, II, III, and V4-6, suggesting a diffuse myocardial inflammatory process in a young patient with acute viral myocarditis*

Table 31.8: *Medications for pediatric resuscitation and arrhythmias*

Medication	*Dose*	*Remarks*
Adenosine	0.1 mg/kg (maximum 6 mg) Repeat: 0.2 mg/kg (maximum 12 mg)	Monitor ECG Rapid IV/IO bolus
Amiodarone	5 mg/kg IV/IO; repeat upto 15 mg/kg Maximum: 300 mg	Monitor ECG and blood pressure Adjust administration rate to urgency (give more slowly when perfusing rhythm present) Use caution when administering with other drugs that prolong QT (consider expert consultation)
Atropine	0.02 mg/kg IV/IO 0.03 mg/kg ET* Repeat once if needed Minimum dose: 0.1 mg Maximum single dose: • Child 0.5 mg • Adolescent 1 mg	Higher doses may be used with organophosphate poisoning
Calcium chloride (10%)	20 mg/kg IV/IO (0.2 mL/kg)	Slowly Adult dose: 5–10 mL
Epinephrine	0.01 mg/kg (0.1 mL/kg 1:10,000) IV/IO 0.1 mg/kg (0.1 mL/kg 1:1,000) ET* Maximum dose: 1 mg IV/IO; 10 mg ET	May repeat: q 3–5 min
Glucose	0.5–1 g/kg IV/IO	D10W: 5–10 mL/kg D25W: 2–4 mL/kg D50W: 1–2 mL/kg
Lidocaine	Bolus: 1 mg/kg IV/IO Maximum dose: 100 mg Infusion: 20–50½ g/kg per minute ET*: 2–3 mg	
Magnesium sulfate	25–50 mg/kg IV/IO over 10–20 min; faster in torsades Maximum dose: 2 g	
Naloxone	<5 years or 20 kg: 0.1 mg/kg IV/IO/ET* 5 years or >20 kg: 2 mg IV/IO/ET*	Use lower doses to reverse respiratory depression associated with therapeutic opioid use (1–15½ g/kg)
Procainaminde	15 mg/kg IV/IO over 30–60 min Adult dose: 20 mg/min IV infusion upto	Monitor ECG and blood pressure Use caution when administering with other drugs that prolong QT (consider expert consulation)
Sodium bicarbonate	1 mEq/kg per dose IV/IO slowly	After adequate ventilation

IV indicates intravenous; IO, intraosseous; and ET, via endotracheal tube
* Flush with 5 mL of normal saline and follow with 5 ventilations

Somatic growth, particularly weight, is often affected. Infants with chronic CHF typically are underweight and undernourished. There are several underlying causes of this phenomenon. The alterations in feeding usually result in decreased caloric intake while the increased work of the heart and respiratory muscles creates a state of increased metabolic demand. Congestion of the gastrointestinal tract results in malabsorption of nutrients. Finally, the redistribution of regional blood flow seen in severe heart failure results in decreased flow and perfusion to organs such as the skin and skeletal muscle. In older children and adolescents, there may be weight loss due to anorexia or weight gain secondary to fluid retention.

2. **Physical examination:** Tachypnea is one of the most consistent physical findings in infants with CHF regardless of the underlying etiology. AB the degree of CHF increases, alveolar and bronchiolar edema result in more labored respiratory effort, accompanied by the development of retractions, nasal flaring, and grunting. It is extremely important to note that wheezing can be a sign of heart failure in infants and should not be simply excuse'd as bronchiolitis or virals, syndrome in this age group. The presence ofrales is rare in infants and becomes more common with advancing age. Chronic cough may also be present at any age. Central cyanosis can be seen as the result of impaired gas exchange. This is typically an indicator of moderately severe CHF. Peripheral

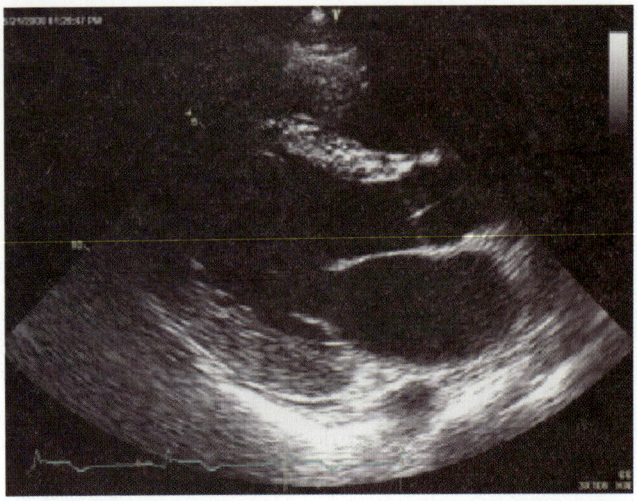

Fig. 31.38: *Two dimensional parasternal long-axis view depicting disproportionate thickening, increased echogenicity, and dyskinesis of the inferolateral wall relative to the septum; findings are consistent with tissue oedema*

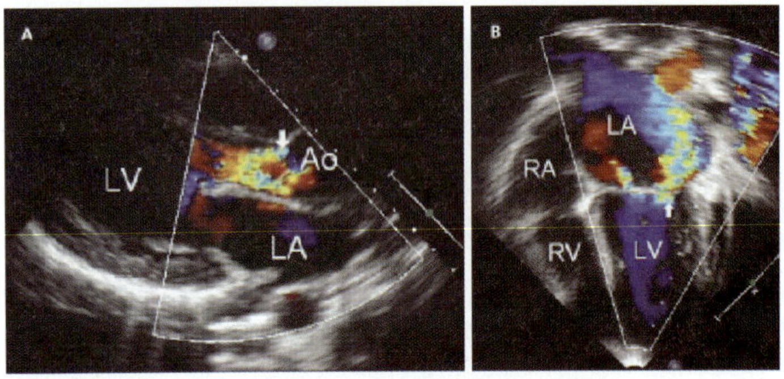

Fig. 31.39: *Two dimensional color and spectral Doppler echocardiographic studies of patients with acute myocarditis show moderate to severe aortic valve insufficiency wihout stenosis (A, arrow) and bowing of the anterior mitral leaflet with severe insufficiency wihout stenosis (B, arrow)*

Table 31.9: *Aetiological classification of cardiomyopathy*

Dilated cardiomyopathy
- Idiopathic cardiomyopathy
- Noncompacted myacardium
- Postpartum cardiomyopathy
- Hemachromatosis
- Infectious
- Postviral myocarditis
- Human immunodeficiency
- Legionella infection
- Sepsis (gram negative)
- Toxic cardiomyopathy
- Adriamycin
- Alcohol
- Carbon monoxide poisoning
- Other chemotherapy

High-output cardiomyopathy
- Tachycardia-mediated cardiomyopathy
- Thyrotoxicosis
- Nutritional (beriberi, thiamine deficiency)
- Peripheral left to right shunt lesions
- Anemia

Hypertrophic cardiomyopathy
- Asymmetric septal hypertrophy
- Idiopathic hypertrophic cardiomyopathy)
- Atypical hypertrophic cardiomyopathy

Restrictive cardiomyopathy
- Idiopathic
- Infiltrative
- Amyloidosis
- Glycogen storage diseases
- Hemachromatosis
- Postradiation therapy
- Endocardial fibroelastosis

Other
- Friederich ataxia
- Muscular dystrophies

cyanosis can also be seen secondary to poor peripheral perfusion.

Sinus tachycardia represents a compensatory mechanism resulting from increased adrenergic tone. In pathologic conditions where there is diminished stroke volume (i.e. dilated cardiomyopathy) or congenital defects with large left-to-right shunts, systemic cardiac output is maintained by increased heart rate. Caution should be taken not to confuse a compensatory sinus tachycardia with a supraventricular tachyarrhythmia presenting with heart failure. In general, infants with sustained heart rates of more than 230 bpm should be strongly suspected of having a tachyarrhythmia.

Cardiac murmurs can be highly variable depending on the underlying lesion and are typically nondiagnostic. The absence of these findings in no way excludes heart disease, because infants and children with significant dilated cardiomyopathy may have few to no auscultatory abnormalities.

Palpation of the chest may demonstrate a hyperactive precardium with displacement of the left ventricular (LV) impulse or the presence of a right ventricular (RV) heave or tap. These findings are also nonspecific and can be found in numerous cardiac etiologies.

Peripheral pulses may be diminished to some degree in all infants and children with CHF. In infants less than 1 month of age, the finding of markedly diminished, absent, or differential pulses between upper and lower extremities should strongly suggest obstructive lesions of left ventricular outflow. In lesions such as patent ductus arteriosus (PDA) and arteriovenous malformations, peripheral pulses may be bounding. There is a wide pulse pressure because of the large diastolic runoff into the low-resistance pulmonary or venous circulations. Other findings of low systemic perfusion include cool extremities, mottled skin, and delayed capillary refill.

Peripheral edema, venous distention, and ascites in older children, as in adults, are signs of systemic venous congestion associated with significant right heart failure.

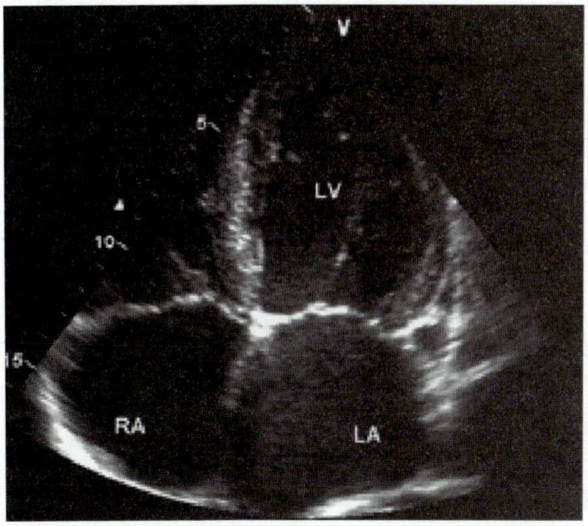

Fig. 31.40: *Dilated cardiomyopathy in a 20-year-adolescent with AIDS. Apical four chamber echocardiographic view shows marked enlargement of all four chambers as well as spontaneous echo contrast ("smoke") in the left-sided chambers because of a very low ejection fraction and sluggish flow. LA, left atrium; LV, left ventricle; RA, right atrium; RV, right ventricle*

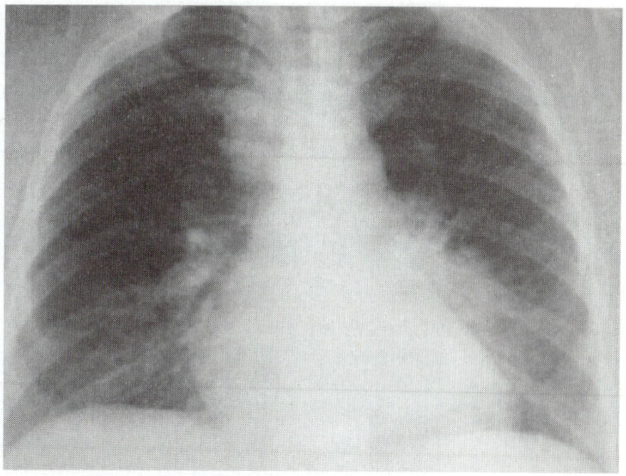

Fig. 31.41: *Chest radiograph in a patient presenting with heart failure, which was subsequently found to be the result of dilated cardiomyopathy. Although cardiac size is at the upper limit of normal, left ventricular function is poor, causing severe pulmonary edema with bilateral alveolar edema and marked dilatation of the superior vena cava*

These findings are extremely unusual in infants. Enlargement ofthe liver due to passive congestion is the most common finding in infancy and can be seen in both right and left heart failure. Hepatomegaly should be distinguished from liver displacement secondary to lung hyperinflation and flattening of the diaphragm seen with bronchiolitis. In addition to an increased span, the liver may be pulsatile in the presence of significant right atrioventricular valve regurgitation. In newborns with severe CHF, jaundice may be secondary to liver congestion and impaired bilirubin metabolism.

B. Patient Assessment

1. **Radiologic studies:** Any patient suspected of having CHF should have a routine chest X-ray (CXR) performed including any infant presenting with wheezing for the first time. With the exception of obstructed total anomalous pulmonary venous return, cardiomegaly should be present. There should and a variable degree of pulmonary vascular congestion depending on the severity of the heart failure and the underlying pathology. Significant cardiomegaly in the absence of pulmonary vascular congestion should raise the possibility of a large pericardial effusion. Other findings may include hyperinflated lung fields and pleural effusions (Fig. 31.41).
2. **Electrocardiogram:** There are no specific ECG findings that are diagnostic of CHF. Ventricular hypertrophy, atrial enlargement, axis deviation, and T wave changes are relatively nonspecific indicators of the underlying etiology. An exception would be the presence of significant left-axis deviation with a mean frontal-plane QRS axis between –60° and –150°, which strongly suggests the presence of an atrioventricular septal defect, either as an isolated defect or as part of a more complex condition. The ECG can be extremely helpful in determining the presence of an underlying arrhythmia or myocardial ischemia, which can be seen in anomalous left coronary artery from the pulmonary artery or Kawasaki disease (Figs 31.31, 31.37).
3. **Laboratory studies:** In patients with evidence of significant respiratory or cardiovascular compromise, an arterial blood gas (ABG) analysis can detect the presence and degree of metabolic or respiratory acidosis, hypoxemia, and the presence of impending respiratory failure. Serum electrolytes may reveal underlying life-threatening dearangements, especially hypokalemia in patients already receiving chronic therapies such as furosemide and digoxin. Hyponatremia may be present secondary to excessive water retention.

A complete blood count with differential analysis can demonstrate evidence of severe anemia or infection as an underlying cause. It should be noted that patients in CHF can have a leukocytosis with a slight left shift.

Echocardiography: It would be very helpful in the diagnosis of anatomical placement of chambers and their relationship with great vessels, cardiac hypertrophy, origin of coronary arteries and inflammation of myocardium and aneurysms of coronary arteries as seen in Kawasaki disease (Figs 31.31, 31.38–31.40).

C. Patient Management

Because of the large number of potential underlying etiologies, CHF cannot be treated uniformly in all pediatric patients. After the diagnosis of heart failure has been established, therapeutic interventions should be aimed at removing any precipitating or aggravating causes, decreasing metabolic demands, relieving pulmonary congestion, and improving systemic perfusion and oxygen delivery require identification of the specific diagnosis and often surgical intervention, both of which may not be readily available in the emergency setting.

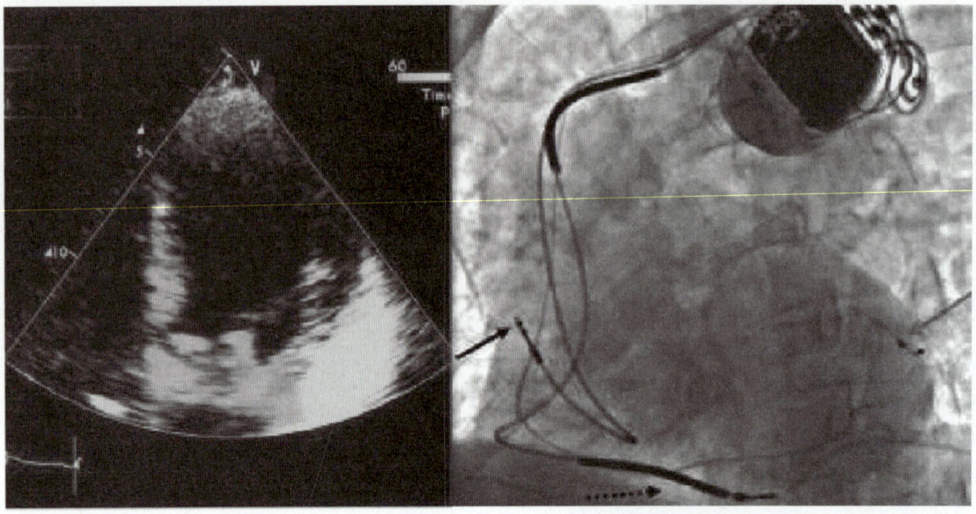

Fig. 31.42: *(Left) echo cardiography showing diastolic wall motion defect in cardiac failure. (Right) CRT in dilated cardiomyopathy*

1. **Remove precipitating or aggravating causes:** Treat any underlying arrhythmias when present. Tachyarrhythmias should be converted to normal sinus rhythm by medical therapy, electrical cardioversion or defibrillation. The specitic treatment for various arrhythmias is discussed later in the chapter. Life-threatening bradyarrhythmias should be treated with an external pacemaker, isoproterenol infusion, or with temporary transvenous pacing when available. Significant anemia should be corrected.
2. **Decrease metabolic demands:** Endotracheal intubation with mechanical ventilation is crucial. Patients who are not in need intubation should be oxygenated by whatever means possible, guided by blood gases or pulse-oximetry. In cases of severe pulmonary edema, endotracheal intubation with the use of positive end-expiratory pressure (PEEP) may help control the pulmonary edema and improve gas exchange.
   Reduce fever if present using antipyretics. Agitated patients should be sedated. Morphine sulfate administered in doses of 0.05–0. 10 mg/kg IV or 1M can be used for patients who, are particularly restless. Apnea can develop with narcotics administration especially in infants.
3. **Relieve pulmonary congestion:** Diuresis should be initiated by pharmacologic therapy. Loop diuretics, such as furosemide, are usually effective. Doses starting at 1 mg/kg given IV or 1M should be used in cases of severe CHF with pulmonary edema. In less severe failure, oral dosing at 1–2 mg/kg two to four times daily should be adequate. Other diuretics, such as thiazide diuretics and aldosterone antagonists, should be reserved for chronic therapy. Aggressive treatment with loop diuretics will increase potassium loss and may result in significant hypokalemia. Electrolytes should be monitored closely. Morphine therapy can be used to improve pulmonary hemodynamics. In addition to the previously mentioned sedative effects, morphine both reduces systemic arterial resistance and increases systemic venous capacitance. This will decrease both the afterload and the preload imposed on the myocardium and may improve pulmonary edema.
4. **Improve systemic perfusion and oxygen delivery:** Systemic perfusion or cardiac output is determined by the physiologic principles of preload, afterload, contractility and heart rate. Therapy aimed at improving cardiac output should address these determinants.
   a. **Inotropic agents:** In the acute setting, parenteral agents are most efficacious in augmenting myocardial performance. Betal-adrenergic receptor agonists are the inotropic agents of choice. Dobutamine infused at rates of 10–20 mcg/kg/min produces a positive inotropic effect with minimal chronotropic changes. Stimulation of beta-adrenergic receptors produces peripheral vascular dilatation, reducing left ventricular afterload and further augmenting cardiac output. Other agents,

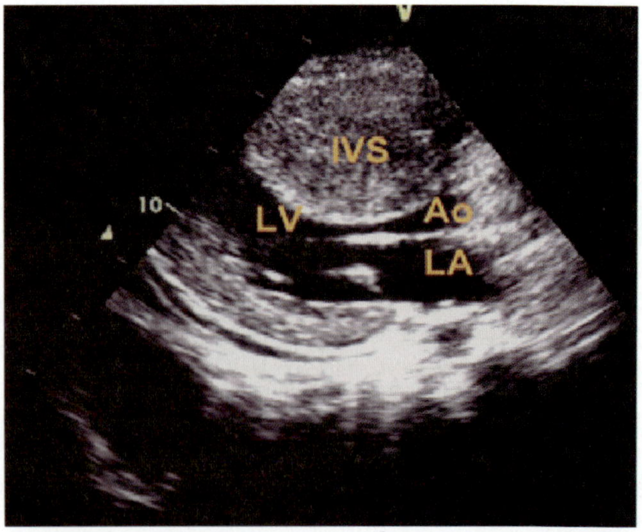

Fig. 31.43: *Transthoracic echocardiogram showing diffuse hypertrophy variant of hypertrophic cardiomyopathy (HCM). This pattern of hypertrophy is classically seen in younger patients. Ao, aorta; IVS, interventricular septum; LA, left atrium; LV, left ventricle*

such as isoproterenol, have similar effects, but their potent chronotropic effects often limit their use. Low-dose dopamine (3–6 mcg/kg/min) also produces vasodilation through stimulation of dopaminergic receptors with selectivity for the renal, mesenteric, cerebral, and coronary vascular beds. Higher-dose dopamine should be avoided because of the potential negative effects on intracardiac shunting and increased afterload placed on the ventricular myocardium. Digoxin should be reserved for more stable patients and long-term therapy.

b. **Vasodilator therapy**: Vasodilators can influence after-load and/or preload, depending on their site of action. AB with inotropic agents, N vasodilators that are titratable and short-acting are preferable. Sodium nitroprusside affects both the arterial and venous vascular beds. Nitroglycerin has primarily venodilatory properties. The major adverse reaction to initiation of any vasodilator is hypotension. Hypotension can be avoided by initiating low-dose therapy and titrating as tolerated. An initial infusion of nitroprusside at 0.25–0.5 mcg/kg/min can be used safely in most patients. If hypotension occurs, treating with volume expansion and concurrently decreasing or discontinuing therapy is usually adequate. In rare situations, vasoconstrictors may be necessary.

c. **Oxygen therapy:** As CHF worsens, gas exchange at the alveoli becomes progressively impaired. Administration of humidified oxygen may improve oxygen delivery to the peripheral tissues. It should be emphasized strongly that oxygen therapy in patients with large left-to-right shunt lesions such as ventricular septal defect, PDA or atrioventricular septal defect may actually result in acute worsening of their condition. This occurs as a result of oxygen's ability to lower pulmonary vascular resistance and raise systemic vascular resistance, both serving to increase the amount of left-to-right shunting.

d. **Prostaglandin therapy**: When there is evidence from the history and clinical findings to suggest a ductal-dependent circulation such as in coarctation, interrupted aortic arch, critical aortic stenosis, or hypoplastic left heart syndrome in a newborn infant, prostaglandin E1 (PGE1) is often life-saving. Ductal dilation permits improved systemic perfusion via the right ventricle while decreasing pulmonary congestion. PGE1 should be administered by continuous N infusion at a rate of 0.1 mcg/kg/min. The major side effects of PGE1 administration are hypotension secondary to vasodilation, respiratory depression with apnea, and irritability, with the latter two symptoms related to CNS effects. If the patient is not already intubated prior to initiation of therapy, the patient should be placed on cardiorespiratory monitors and equipment and personnel should be readily available in anticipation of potential apnea. Any patient who will require transfer to another hospital should be electively intubated and ventilated before transport.

5. **Correct metabolic derangements:** Many infants with left-sided obstructive lesions present with metabolic acidosis due to poor tissue perfusion and lactic acid production. Often, reestablishing distal perfusion with prostaglandin will have a major influence on correcting this problem. In the setting of severe acidosis, however, myocardial performance is greatly diminished and correction of the acidosis with sodium bicarbonate in 1–2 mEq/kg aliquots is necessary.

D. Patient Disposition:

The prognosis for an infant or child presenting with CHF is highly variable and depends a great deal on the underlying pathology. The long-term outlook, therefore, relies upon a specific and accurate diagnosis. This may not always be available in the emergency setting because of the need for specialized diagnostic testing such as two dimensional echocardiography and cardiac catheterization, and the need for trained physicians including pediatric cardiologists and cardiothoracic surgeons, to interpret and implement more diagnosis-specific interventions. Unfortunately, these personnel and technologies are typically available only at regional tertiary care pediatric *centers. Regardless of the etiology, the morbidity and mortality of CHF can be significantly altered by appropriate recognition and initial management in the emergency department.*

Whereas ductal dependent lesions typically present early after ductal closure within the first 2 weeks of life, other CHD usually present in 4–6 weeks after birth when the pulmonary vascular resistance has fallen, such as a large ventricular septal defect. Congestive heart failure (CHF) ensues from the significant left to right shunt and pulmonary congestion. Infants typically present with poor feeding, failure to thrive, tachypnea and diaphoresis. Symptoms of older children are more typical adult symptoms of decreased exercise tolerance and dyspnea. Of note, dependent edema in children is very difficult to assess and more often a very late finding. Increased jugular venous pressure is difficult to assess in infants secondary to their short necks and liver size is used as a surrogate marker. CHF is usually related to one of the following conditions: anomalous left coronary artery arising from the pulmonary artery (ALCAPA), congenital cardiomyopathy, myocarditis, lesions resulting from a large intracardiac shunt (e.g. ventricular sepal defect) or extracardiac shunt (vein of Galen malformation), or arrhythmias.

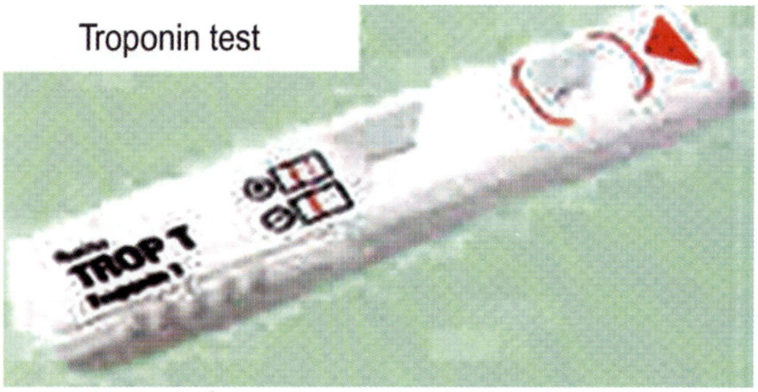

Fig. 31.44: *Apparatus for performing Trop T test for acute myocardial injury in emergency department*

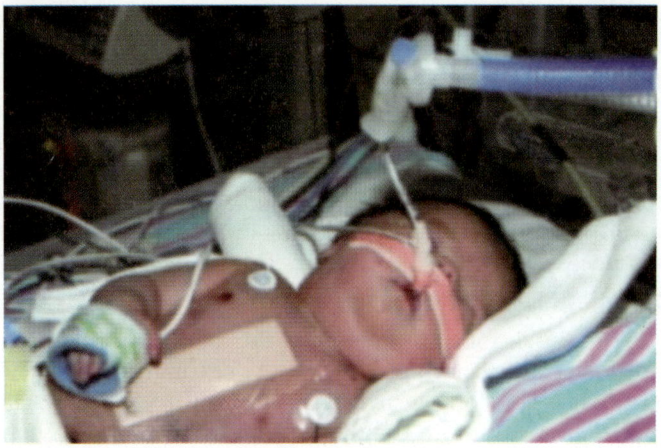

Fig. 31.45: *An amazing Tennessee baby has become one of the smallest babies in the world to have heart bypass surgery. Tiny 4 pound Cole Latch underwent surgery at Le Bonheur Children's Medical Center in Memphis, Tenn., to repair a congenital heart defect. The 1-month-old was born prematurely and had a cardiopulmonary bypass less than a week later. "He was born at 35 weeks with a knot in his umbilical cord"*

ALCAPA is a type of CHD that typically presents at 2–3 months of age when pulmonary artery (PA) pressure decreases. ALCAPA is one of the most common causes of myocardial ischemia and infarction in children, specifically anterolateral infarct pattern and is associated with high mortality, where 90% of untreated patients die within the first year of life. Infants typically present with episodes of irritability (angina pain) and diaphoresis particularly during feeding (when myocardial oxygen consumption increases), signs of CHF, and a murmur of mitral regurgitation. Although mortality is high without treatment, prompt diagnosis and surgical treatment have excellent results with improvement in myocardial function overtime.

Some patients with ALCAPA may survive undetected through adolescence and adulthood due to the development of significant collateral circulation from the right coronary artery to the LCA. However, these collaterals may not be sufficient to perfuse the left ventricle, and these patients are at risk of chronic mitral regurgitation, ischemic cardiomyopathy, and sudden cardiac death from malignant ventricular arrhythmias in 80–90% of cases. Surgical intervention is recommended, even in asymptomatic adult patients with ALCAPA and preserved left ventricular function discovered incidentally, due to the potential for progressive LV dysfunction and sudden death.

MYOCARDITIS

Myocarditis is an often insidious, inflammatory disease of the myocardium preceded by a nonspecific flu-like illness. Myocarditis may have a fulminant presentation characterized by acute severe hemodynamic compromise with severe congestive heart failure or cardiogenic shock. It is the most common cause of dilated cardiomyopathy in children. The symptoms can range from being asymptomatic to cardiovascular collapse and death. It is a potentially fatal disease, accounting for 22% of unexpected deaths in persons less than 20 years, with more staggering statistics for infants and children as high as 75 and 25%, respectively. Recognition and diagnosis is imperative, but may prove challenging since the clinical presentation is varied and can be similar to other common conditions, such as gastroenteritis, asthma and pneumonia. In one series, the initial evaluating physician diagnosed asthma or pneumonia in more than 50% of patients who actually had myocarditis. In contrast, cardiac symptoms of chest pain are more common in adults. In the European study of epidemiology and treatment of cardiac inflammatory diseases, 526 adults diagnosed with acute or chronic myocarditis of the 3,055 patients screened by endomyocardial biopsy, 32% presented with chest pain, 72% with dyspnea, and 18% had an arrhythmia. In adults, myocarditis should be considered as a possible diagnosis among many cardiac syndromes, whereas in children the clinician needs to consider myocarditis among cardiac and noncardiac

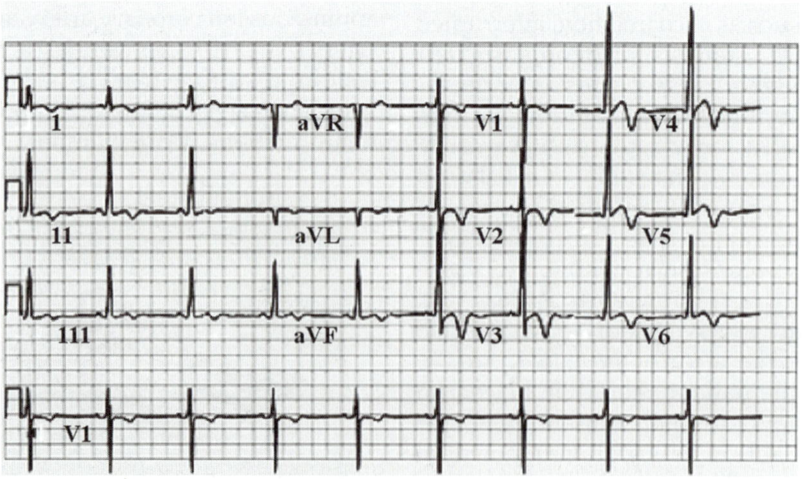

Fig. 31.46: *ECG from a 20-year-old adolescent with apical hypertrophic cardiomyopathy. Note elevated QRS voltages associated with left ventricular hypertrophy and inverted T waves in all precordial leads*

Table 31.10: *World Health Organization/International Society and Federation Cardiology classification of nonischemic cardiomyopathies*

Cardiomyopathy	*Characteristics*
Dilated	Dilatation and impared constraction of the left ventricle or both ventriles, nonspecification histology. Arrhythmias thromboembolism, and sudden deadth are common.
Hypertrophic	Left and/or right ventricular hypertrophy, which is usually asymmetric and involves the interventricular septum with left ventricular volume is normal or reduced includes myocyte hypertrophy and disarry surrounding areas of increased loose connective tissue. Arrhythmias and premature sudden death are common.
Restrictive	Restrictive filling and reduced diastolic volume of either or both ventricles with normal or near normal systolic function and wall thickness, increased interstitial fibrosis may be present, it may be idiopathic or assocaited with other disease (e.g. amyloidosis)
ARVC	Progressive fibrofatty replacement of right ventricular myocardium, initially with typical regional and later global right and some left ventricular involvement, with relative sparing of the septum. Presentation with arrhythmias and sudden death is common, particularly in the young.
Unclassified	Unclassified cardiomyopathies includes a few cases that do not fit readily into any group. Some disease may present with fearures of more than one type of cardiomyopathy.
Specific	The term specific cardiomyopathies is not used to described heart muscle disease that are associated with specific cardiac or systemic disorders (e.g. hypertensive, cardiomyopathy)

presentations. ALCAPA, for example, should be on the differential in a 2–3 month old infant with presentations such as colic or respiratory distress, although EKG findings should help to differentiate them. The long-term prognosis is favorable if recognized quickly and managed aggressively with a heart failure regimen and possibly mechanical circulatory support as a bridge to transplantation or recovery (Fig. 31.37).

CARDIOMYOPATHIES (Tables 31.9 and 31.10)

Cardiomyopathies are a heterogeneous group of myocardial diseases that causes significant disability and death. They are characterized by inappropriate ventricular hypertrophy or dilatation and are associated with electrical dysfunction or systolic and/or diastolic ventricular dysfunction.

Dilated Cardiomyopathy (Fig. 31.40)

Dilated cardiomyopathy (DCM) is a heart muscle disease characterized by dilation of the left ventricle and systolic dysfunction. Progressive heart failure ensues with resultant sudden and heart failure related death. DCM is the most common reason for heart transplantation in children and adults. In children, myocarditis is the most frequently identified cause followed by neuromuscular diseases, whereas in adults the most common causes are idiopathic DCM, idiopathic myocarditis and coronary artery disease. The long-term prognosis regardless of the cause may be progressive with approximately 54% of affected individuals within 5 years of diagnosis die or require a heart transplant. The worst outcomes were found among older children, children who had CHF symptoms, and LV dysfunction at the time of presentation. Almost two-thirds of children present with congestive heart failure. Infants may present with failure to thrive, colic, or a conglomeration of symptoms of low cardiac output, such as poor perfusion, decreased distal pulses, pallor, and tachypnea, and on examination a diffuse or displaced cardiac apex, soft heart sounds, a gallop rhythm, hepatomegaly, and a mitral regurgitant murmur may be present. Adolescents may experience syncopal events, fatigue, exercise intolerance, dyspnea, pallor and tachycardia. GI symptoms of nausea, vomiting and abdominal pain are also frequently noted.

Hypertrophic Cardiomyopathy (Fig. 31.43)

Unfortunately cardiac arrest and sudden death may be the first presentation of hypertrophic cardiomyopathy (HCM) It is the most common cause of sudden cardiac death in the young and can lead to progressive heart failure across all ages. The clinical presentation is varied. Young people, typically athletes aged 10–35 years old are the most common group to experience a cardiac arrest or sudden cardiac death. Evidence has shown that sudden death is primarily due to complex ventricular tachyarrhythmias, bradyarrhythmias, and supraventricular arrhythmias that lead to ventricular fibrillation or hypotension, and these events are exacerbated when there is left ventricular outflow tract obstruction or ischemia. Additionally, patients can present with symptoms related to poor diastolic function with preserved systolic function that include exertional chest pain and dyspnea, palpitations, presyncope, or syncope. The disease can then progress to end stage congestive heart failure heralded by systolic dysfunction, or patients can have atrial fibrillation associated complications, particularly embolic stroke.

Cardiac Arrhythmias (Figs 31.47–31.63, 31.76, 31.77, 31.85–86, 31.89 and Tables 31.8, 31.11)

Arrhythmias are far more common among adults than children, but are equally as important for the clinician be able to recognize the abnormal rhythm, respond immediately and treat appropriately. Of adults presenting to the emergency room with an acute myocardial infarction, 90% have a rhythm abnormality and 25% have a conduction disturbance. Most pediatric arrhythmias occur among children with congenital and acquired heart disease, and symptoms of congestive heart failure or cyanosis precede the dysrhythmia. In children whose initial presentation is an arrhythmia, the underlying problem is a primary conduction disorder in a structurally normal heart. Children admitted to the cardiac intensive care unit for the medical management of heart disease, and particularly after cardiac surgery, certain catheterization procedures, and pre- and posttransplantation are at high risk for arrhythmias due to the underlying pathophysiology and medical and surgical interventions involved.

The tachyarrhythmias can be characterized as supraventricular or ventricular. The most common symptomatic pediatric arrhythmia is supraventricular tachycardia (SVT) with an incidence of 1 in every 250–1,000 children. In infants, half are due to idiopathic causes, a quarter caused by congenital heart disease such as Ebstein's anomaly, and 10–20% due to Wolff-Parkinson-White (WPW) syndrome, a type of AV reentrant tachycardia characterized on EKG by a delta wave, wide QRS, and short PR interval. It should be suspected if there is a regular and rapid heart rate usually greater than 180 bpm in older children and greater than 220 bpm in infants. On the electrocardiogram, the QRS is considered narrow complex with indiscernible p waves or retrograde p waves due to an accessory AV pathway. Patients with bundle-branch block may be confused with VT. Most infants are hemodynamically stable in SVT, although within 48 hours congestive heart failure may develop with rapid deterioration occurring in 50%. The infant may appear lethargic, tachypneic, fussy, and mottled with signs of poor perfusion including cool extremities and hypotension. Older children rarely present in CHF and are usually able to articulate their symptoms of racing heart beat, chest pain, dizziness and lightheadedness. A 12 lead EKG and rhythm strip should be obtained and an immediate clinical assessment should be made to determine if the patient is cardiovascularly stable or unstable. For hemodynamically unstable SVT with poor perfusion and severe heart failure, adenosine (0.1 mg/kg/dose max. 6 mg increased to 0.2 mg/kg/dose, max. 12 mg), pushed and flushed quickly, can be given and/or immediate synchronized cardioversion (0.5 J/kg then increased up to 1 J/kg) if IV access is not immediately available. For stable SVT, vagal maneuvers such as valsalva or ice to the face may be attempted first. Adenosine can then be used if those maneuvers are unsuccessful.

Ventricular fibrillation (VF) and pulseless ventricular tachycardia (VT) are the common causes of cardiac arrest

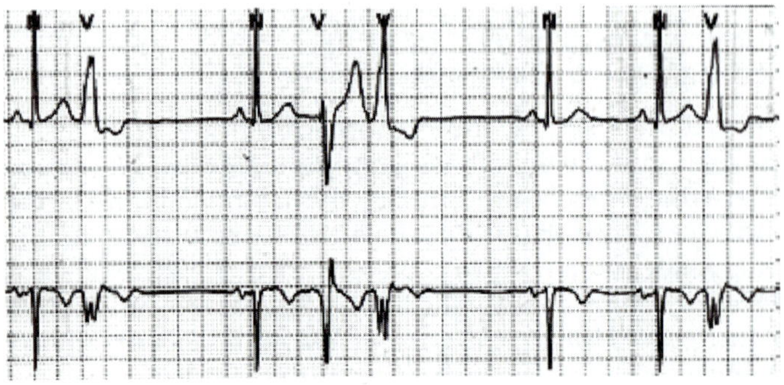

Fig. 31.47: *Polymorphic VPC on Holter after mustard operation*

in adults and often due to coronary artery disease. Fourteen percent of children compared to 23% of adults had VF or pulseless VT as the first documented rhythm during in-hospital cardiac arrest. However, this is still much higher than many clinicians would have thought as the cause of cardiac arrest in children and demonstrates that those caring for children need to be capable of administering rapid defibrillation. The incidence of VF/VT as the first recorded rhythm in out of hospital arrest in children varies by age, from 4 to 5% in infants and children to 15% in adolescents. In children, there is a cardiac origin in 21–71% of cases, such as in palliated congenital heart disease and cardiomyopathies. The incidence of VT after congenital heart surgery is low but can lead to a fatal outcome in an already hemodynamically unstable period. Intractable VT in the postoperative period, particularly after surgery involving manipulation of the coronary arteries, (i.e. arterial switch operation for d-transposition of the great arteries) should raise suspicion for myocardial ischemia and the possible need for surgical revision. In conduction disorders, such as in long QT syndrome, torsades de pointes (a polymorphic VT) is characteristic and can degenerate into VF and sudden death. WPW also can rarely lead to sudden death in high-risk patients after preexcited atrial fibrillation with a rapid ventricular response that leads to VF.

On EKG, VT is a wide QRS complex tachycardia that can be monomorphic or polymorphic, and VF has a fine or coarse chaotic rhythm with no discernible QRS complexes. Defibrillation is the treatment for VT/VF along with prompt and effective CPR. There is clear evidence in adult cardiac arrest caused by ventricular arrhythmia that the rates of survival decreases with increasing time to defibrillation, and mortality increases by 7–10% every minute defibrillation is delayed.

Kawasaki Disease (Fig. 31.64)

Kawasaki disease does not usually present as a critical emergency; however, timely recognition and treatment can prevent the leading cause of acquired heart disease in children in the United States and fatal cardiac events in adults. Kawasaki disease is an acute vasculitis of unknown cause that predominantly affects children under 5 years of age. In 15 to 25% of untreated children, coronary artery aneurysms and progressive stenosis develop which can lead to significant morbidity and mortality from ischemic heart disease, myocardial infarction or sudden death. The disease is diagnosed based on clinical criteria of at least 5 days of fever and at least four of the main clinical features including: polymorphous rash; limbic sparing nonexudative conjunctivitis; mucocutaneous changes (e.g. strawberry tongue, dry cracked lips); cervical lymphadenopathy; and extremity changes with acute edema of the hands and feet or palmar erythema and after 2–3 weeks of illness periungual desquamation of the fingers and toes. There are also other supplemental laboratory and other clinical findings that are characteristic of the disease. Children with a protracted febrile illness greater than 5 days with two to three of the clinical features of Kawasaki, incomplete

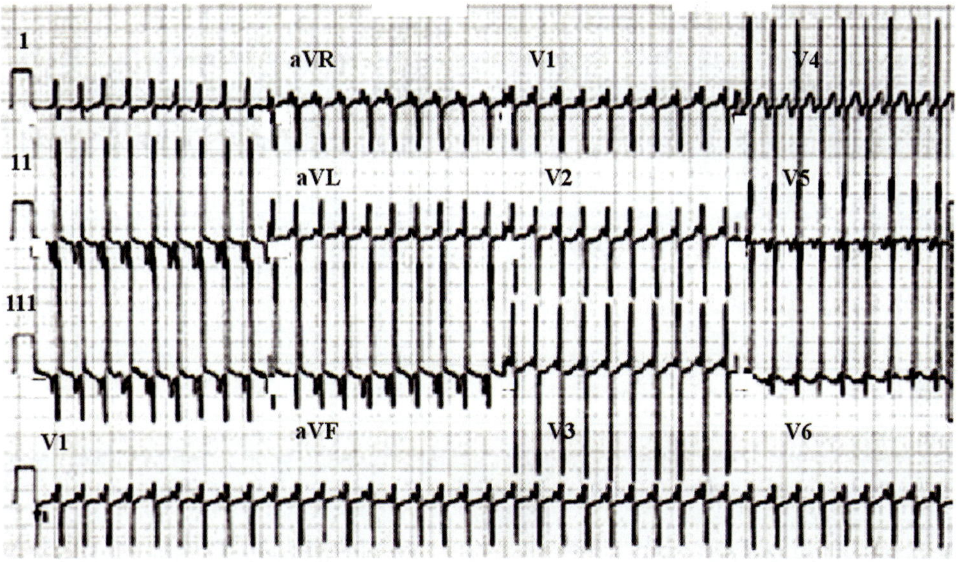

Fig. 31.48: *Permanent junctional reciprocating tachycardia. An incessant arrhythmia with a characteristic appearance. Note the very long RP interval and the deeply inverted P waves in leads II, III and aVF. This is a type of orthodromic atrioventricular (AV) reentry over a relatively slowly conducting concealed right posteroseptal pathway*

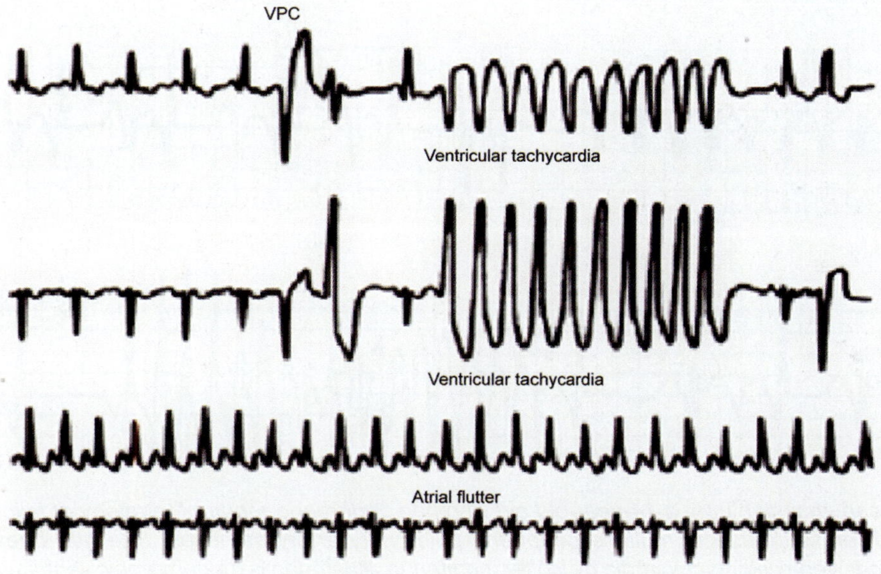

Fig. 31.49: *Holter recording from a 15-year-old adolescent with dilated cardiomyopathy. The upper tracing shows nonsustained ventricular tachycardia; the lower shows sustained atrial flutter. The patient remained asymptomatic throughout*

Kawasaki should be considered. Moreover, the AHA recommends that an infant less than 6 months with fever greater than 7 days and laboratory signs of systemic inflammation even without clinical features should have an echocardiogram. Mortality is principally due to the cardiac sequelae. During the acute phase of the disease, in addition to coronary arteritis, pericarditis, myocarditis, and valvar heart disease can develop. Myocarditis can lead to myocardial dysfunction and children can present hypotensive and in cardiogenic shock. Arrhythmias can be associated as well as PR prolongation and nonspecific ST and T wave changes noted on electrocardiogram. There are specific guidelines associated with the acute and long-term management of Kawasaki disease. Treatment consist of IVIG 2 g/kg over 12 hours and high dose aspirin 80–100 mg/kg/day in 4 doses for 48–72 hours after fever defervescence, then low dose 3–5 mg/kg/day. Patients with persistent fever (36 hours after initial IVIG) or recurrent fever should be retreated with IVIG. The long-term management should be tailored based on the degree of coronary artery involvement and the risk for ischemic events.

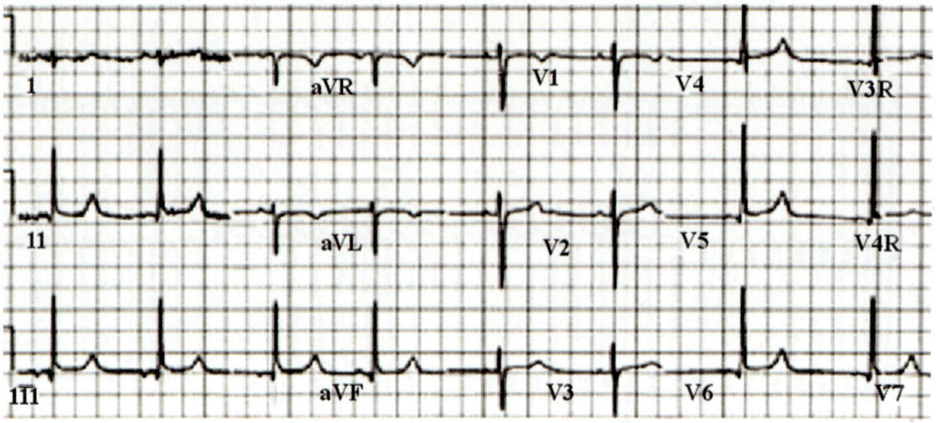

Fig. 31.50: *Exercise in a young athlete. The QTc prolonged with exercise stress testing in the recovery period to 520 milliseconds, confirming the impression of long QT syndrome (LQTS)*

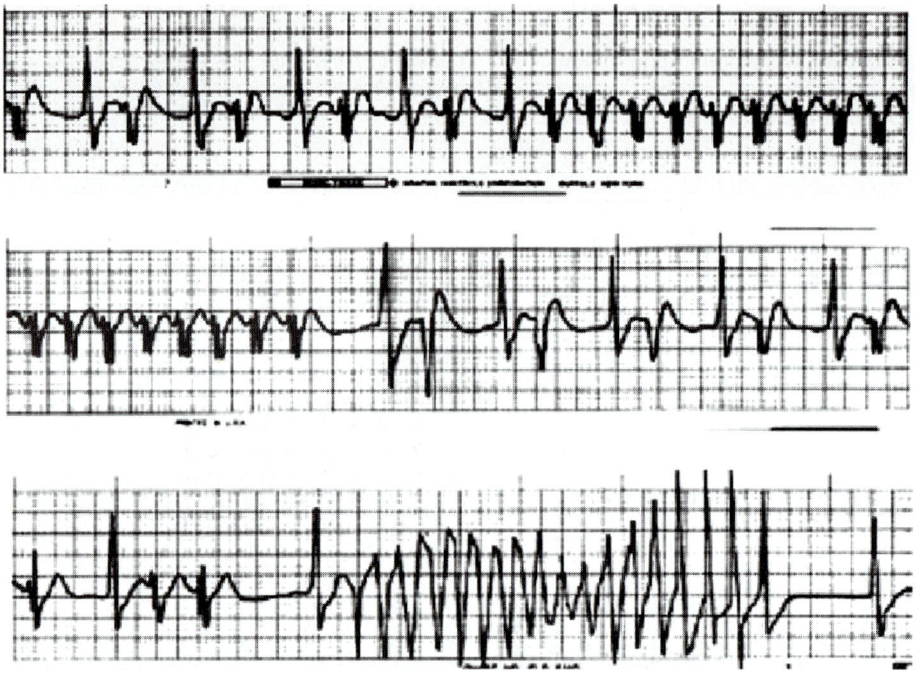

Fig. 31.51: *A continuous rhythm strip from a 14-year-old girl who had undergone repair of tetralogy of fallot but who had persistently elevated right ventricular pressure due to multiple peripheral pulmonary artery stenoses. She had been placed on quinidine for asymptomatic nonsustained ventricular tachycardia by Holter monitoring. Illustrated is monomorphic ventricular bigeminy, nonsustained monomorphic ventricular tachycardia, and a 4 second episode of polymorphic ventricular tachycardia (torsade de pointes). The latter was a proarrhythmic response to the quinidine*

Aortic Disease and Dissection

Aortic dissection is rare in infants and children, and is associated with inherited disorders such as Marfan syndrome and other connective tissue disorders, and after balloon dilation of coarctation and recoarctation, complication of cardiopulmonary bypass at the aortic cannulation site, and in young adults with a bicuspid aortic valve and ascending aortic dilation. In contrast, atherosclerosis is the main cause of aortic aneurysms and dissection in adults, with hypertension being the main risk factor (Figs 31.65 and 31.66).

The clinical presentation in aortic dissection will vary based on the origin and extension of the dissection. Typically, there is abrupt onset of sharp pain that may change in location, followed by congestive cardiac failure due to severe aortic regurgitation. Patients may present with syncope, cardiac tamponade, stroke, limb ischemia with pulse deficits, paraplegia, and if renal or mesenteric arteries are involved may result in oliguria/anuria or have persistent abdominal pain. A diastolic murmur of aortic regurgitation and the typical wide pulse pressure is present in half of patients with proximal dissection. Aortic rupture into the pericardium with cardiac tamponade (i.e. friction

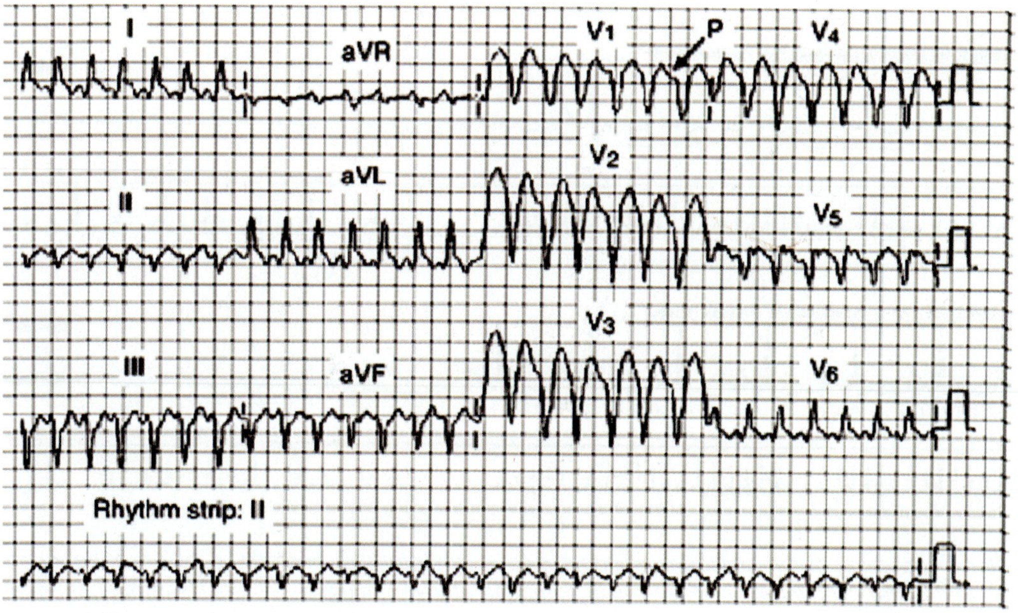

Fig. 31.52: *ECG showing broad QRS ventricular tachycardia. The QRS duration is 160 msec. An independent P wave can be seen in V1 (arrow). There is a leftward mean frontal axis shift*

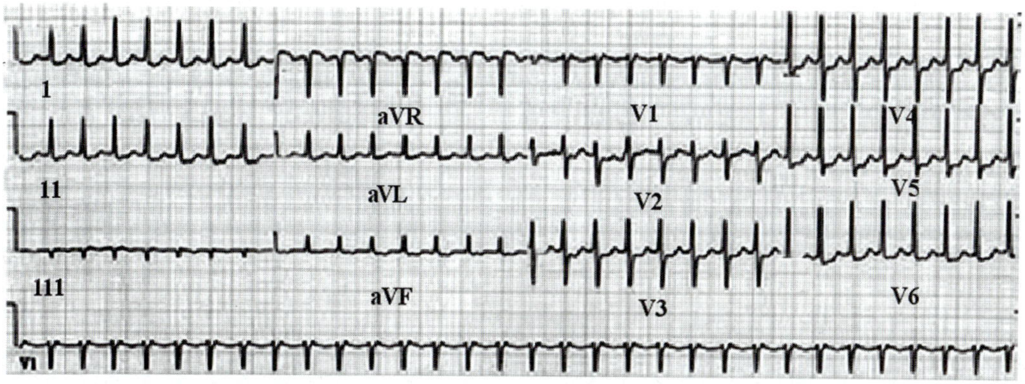

Fig. 31.53: *ECG showing hemodynamically stable supraventricular tachycardia*

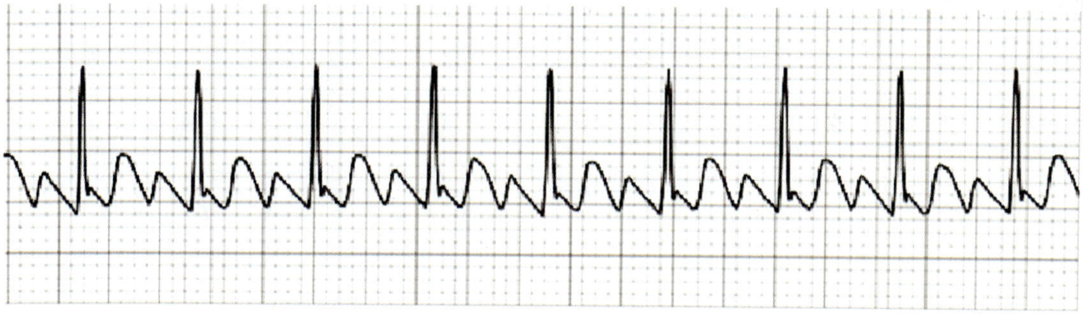

Fig. 31.54: *Atrial flutter: narrow QRS complexes are associated with regular flutter waves*

rub, muffled heart sounds, hypotension, jugular venous distention, pulsus paradoxus) or the pleural space are indications for surgical emergencies.

A detailed history and physical examination should be performed; a patient with stigmata of Marfan syndrome or other connective tissue disease would raise the index of suspicion for dissection compared to other possible diagnoses (such as acute coronary syndrome, pericarditis, pulmonary embolism and cholecystitis). An EKG is important to differentiate acute myocardial infarction to prevent the administration of thrombolytic therapy that would be detrimental in aortic dissection. Although, 20% of patients with dissection involving the ascending aorta have evidence of ischemia or infarction

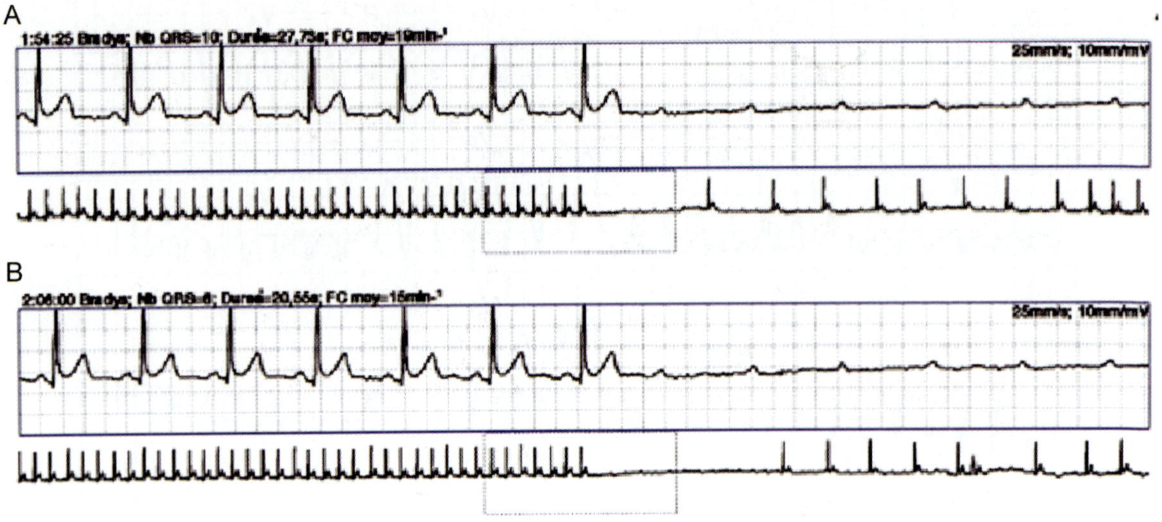

Fig. 31.55: *(A, B) Holter recording of two episodes of spontaneous syncope that occurred a few minutes apart. The two episodes were very similar and were characterized by sudden-onset complete atrioventricular (AV) block without changes in P-P cycle length, which constantly remained 720 ms and long ventricular asystole of 7 and 11 s (top and bottom, compressed traces, respectively)*

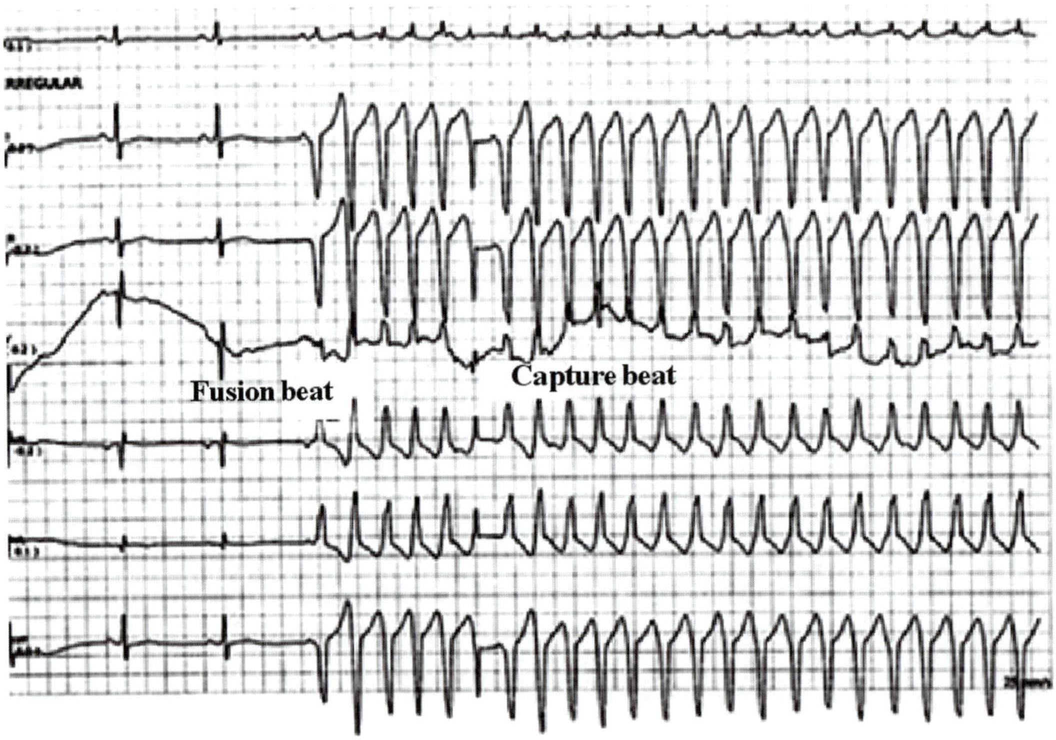

Fig. 31.56: *ECG showing morphology of ventricular tachycardia (VT)*

as the dissection extends into the coronary ostium, and in this situation, additional imaging studies should be preformed to confirm the dissection if the index of suspicion is high. Diverse imaging modalities can be used to detect aortic dissection. Transthoracic and transesophageal echocardiography can be useful in the emergency room and operating room for emergent decision making. CT scans are the most often used technique in patients with suspected aortic dissection and have a high sensitivity and specificity. Branch vessel involvement can be accurately identified with contrast angiography, and should be used in patients with neurological symptoms, acute renal failure, and limb and mesenteric ischemia.

Patients should be in an intensive care unit with blood pressure and heart rate monitoring. Fluid repletion, pain relief (e.g. morphine) and blood pressure lowering drugs, starting with a beta-blocker and adding intravenous sodium nitroprusside for severe hypertension are important initial therapies. Surgical management in

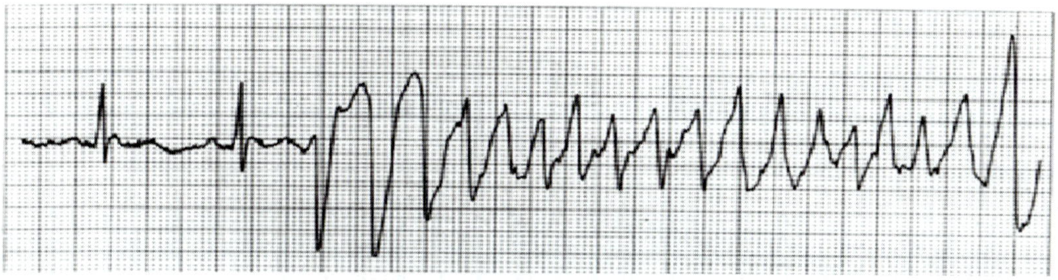

Fig. 31.57: *ECG showing torsades de pointes*

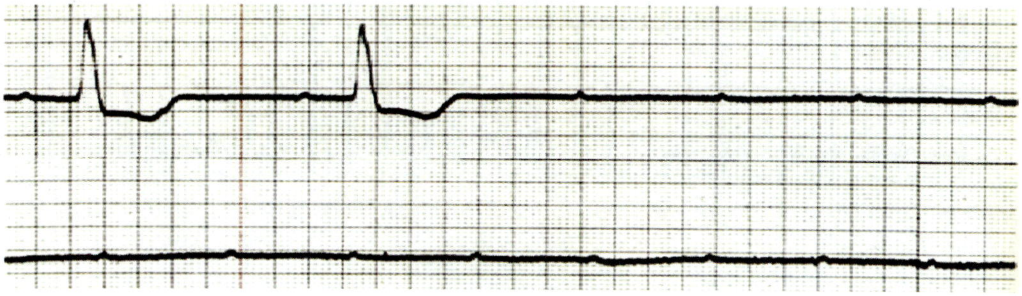

Fig. 31.58: *ECG showing complete A-V dissociation in patient with Stokes-Adam attack*

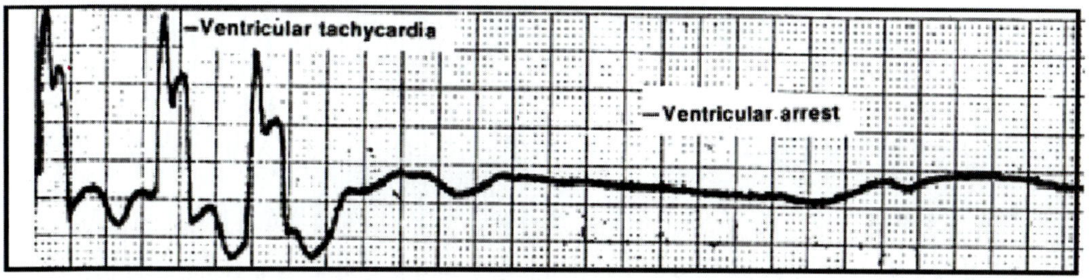

Fig. 31.59: *Graph showing the features of ventricular tachycardia ending in a long asystole (cardiac arrest)*

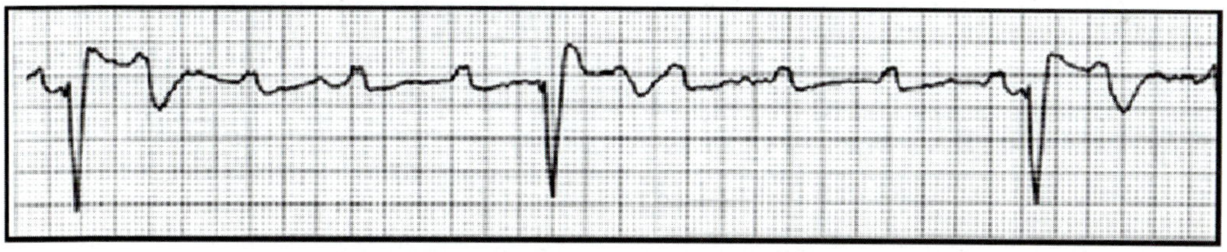

Fig. 31.60: *ECG trace showing acute myocardial infarction with complete heart block*

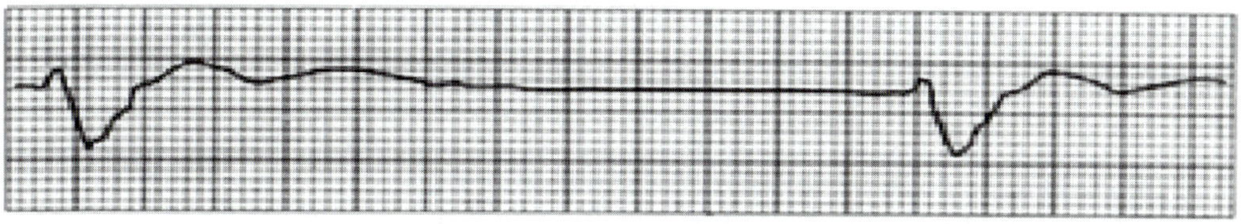

Fig. 31.61: *ECG showing broad and slow rhythm in association with pulseless electrical activity*

children is guided by similar principles as adults, with the emphasis on prophylactic intervention in patients with underlying dilation to prevent dissection.

Pulmonary Embolism

Pulmonary embolism (PE) is an uncommon cardiovascular emergency in children although relatively common in

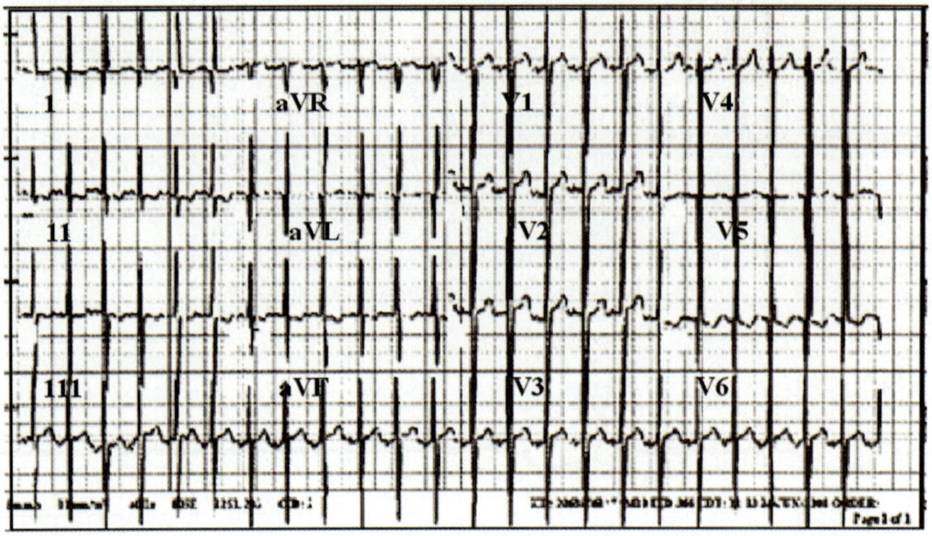

Fig. 31.62: *EKG of an 8-month-old who initially presented to the ER with respiratory distress and wheezing, and echocardiogram confirmed ALCAPA. EKG shows deep (3 mm) and wide (30 ms) Q waves in I, aVL, V6, absent Q waves in II, III, aVF, and ST segment changes*

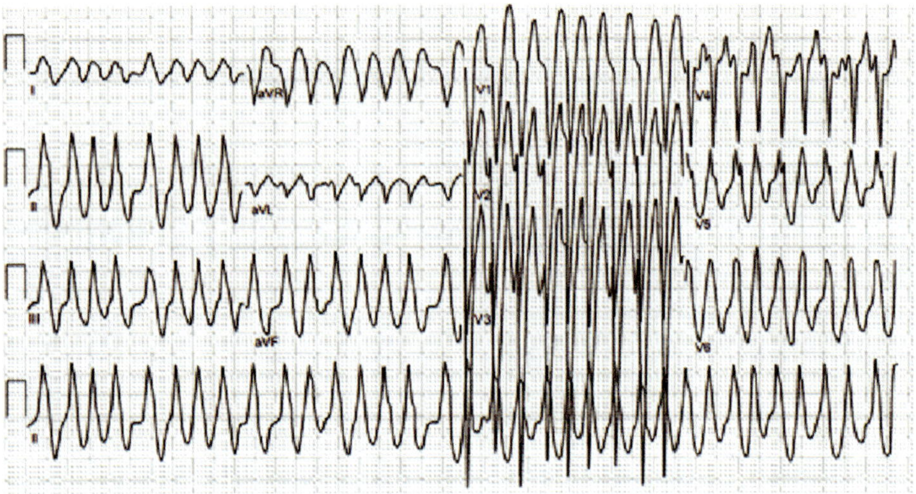

Fig. 31.63: *ECG morphology showing preexcited atrial fibrillation*

adults. However, adolescent females with collagen vascular diseases or on birth control increase the risk as well as the increasing population of obese teenagers. Acute but often reversible right ventricular failure can result from pulmonary arterial occlusion by thromboemboli. The hemodynamic consequences of PE results when large and/ or multiple emboli (occluding >30–50% of pulmonary arterial bed) acutely increase pulmonary vascular resistance, and the afterload that the right ventricular has to pump against is too high leading to RV failure. This can lead to sudden death or syncope with systemic hypotension that might progress to shock and death from acute RV collapse. The mortality rate is higher in children and they are more likely to be diagnosed at autopsy, where approximately 60% presented with sudden death. The most common predisposing factors were central venous catheters, malignancy, cardiac or other major surgery, and infection/sepsis. Furthermore, thrombosis in children is more likely to originate in the upper extremity veins. Children typically present with dyspnea and hypoxemia, findings which are nonspecific and often difficult to differentiate from symptoms attributable to the underlying disease. Adolescents have similar presenting complaints to adults including pleuritic chest pain, dyspnea, cough and hemoptysis although there is often a delay in the diagnosis in adolescents (Figs 31.67–31.69, 31.73).

The goal of diagnosis and appropriate treatment is to decrease mortality by preventing potentially lethal recurrent large thrombi. Clinical signs, symptoms and laboratory studies are not sensitive or specific to confirm or exclude PE, but should increase the index of suspicion to proceed with additional imaging. Such as, an

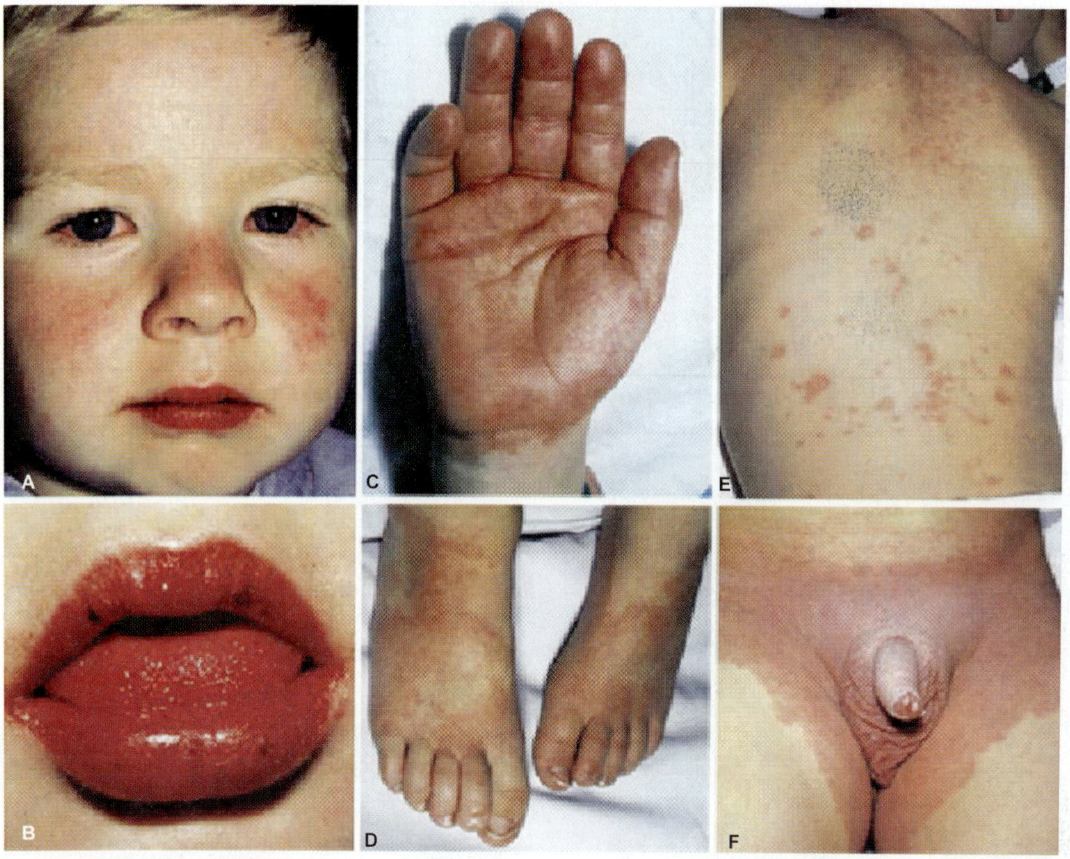

Fig. 31.64: *Photographs of a 4-year-old boy show the typical features of Kawasaki's disease. These features include bilateral nonexudative conjunctivitis (Panel A); dry, fissured, erythematous lips and a "strawberry" tongue (Panel A and B); erythematous and edematous hands and feet (Panel C and D); an erythematous truncal rash (Panel E); and a desquamating perineal rash (Panel F). the patient also had anterior cervical lymphadenopathy and sterile pyluria but none of the other complications of the disease. The child recovered uneventfully after receiving treatment with intravenous immune globulin and aspirin*

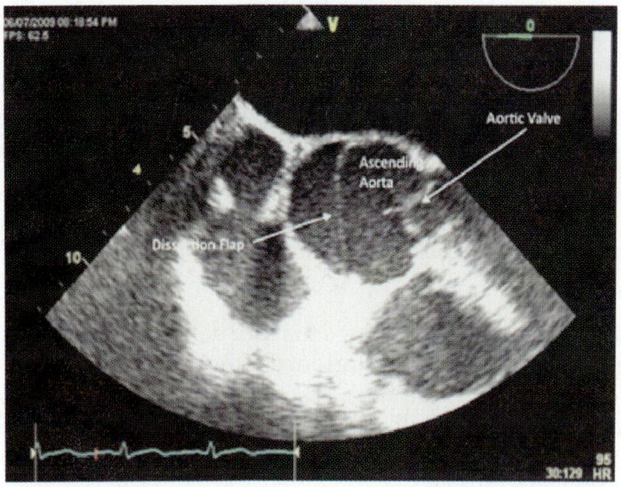

Fig. 31.65: *Transesophegeal echocardiogram (TEE) was performed. The TEE confirmed a 5.5 cm aortic aneurysm with a dissection flap in the sinuses of Valsalva extending distally to the sinotubular junction. The dissection did not involve the coronary arteries, but did extend in to the aortic arch and further into the thoracic aorta. There was minimal aortic insufficiency but a left pleural effusion (assumed to be a hemothorax) was present. It was also noted that the aortic arch and descending aorta were dilated and aneurismal*

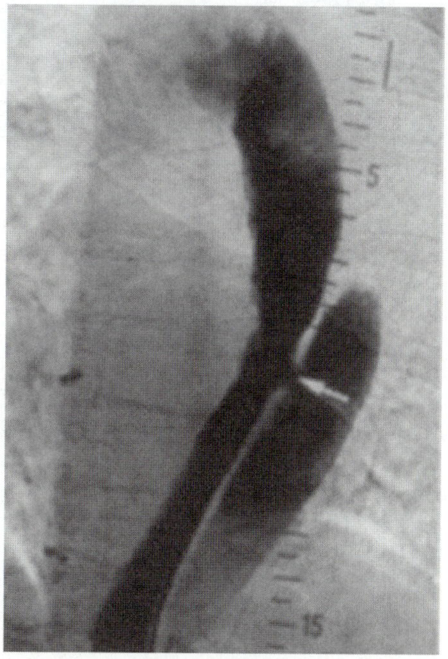

Fig. 31.66: *Left anterior oblique DSA image obtained at 45° shows the intimal tear (arrow) located in the proximal descending thoracic aorta 10 cm distal to the origin of the left subclavian artery*

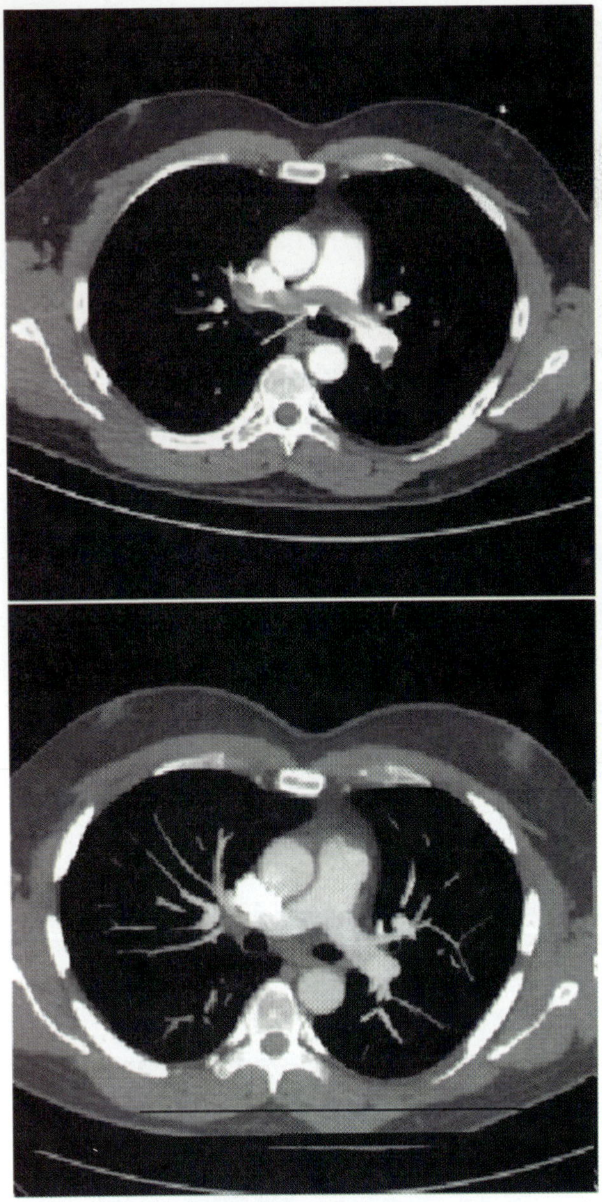

Fig. 31.67: *(Upper) CT pulmonary angiogram (axial slice) revealing thrombus (arrowed) in the main pulmonary artery at the saddle extending across the origin of both right and left pulmonary arteries. (Lower) repeat CTPA at 3 months confirming complete resolution of the thrombus*

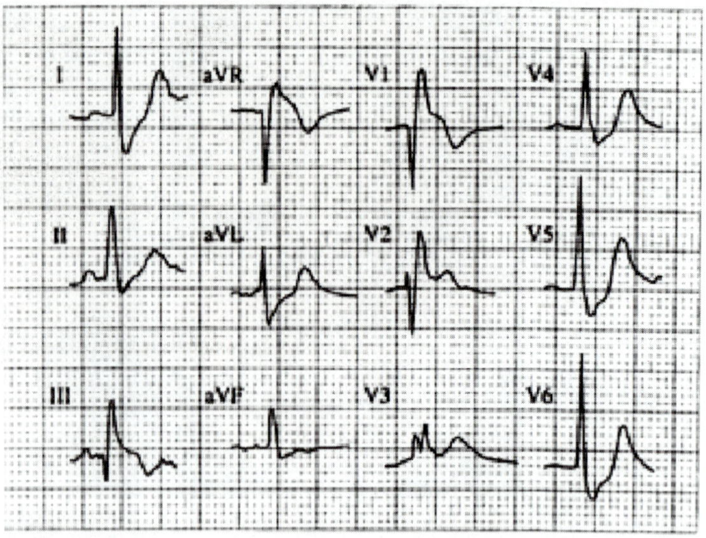

Fig. 31.68: *ECG shows SI, Q3, T3 pattern right-bundle branch block (incomplete or complete). T wave inversion in the right precordial leads P pulmonale right-axis deviation in patient with acute pulmonary embolism*

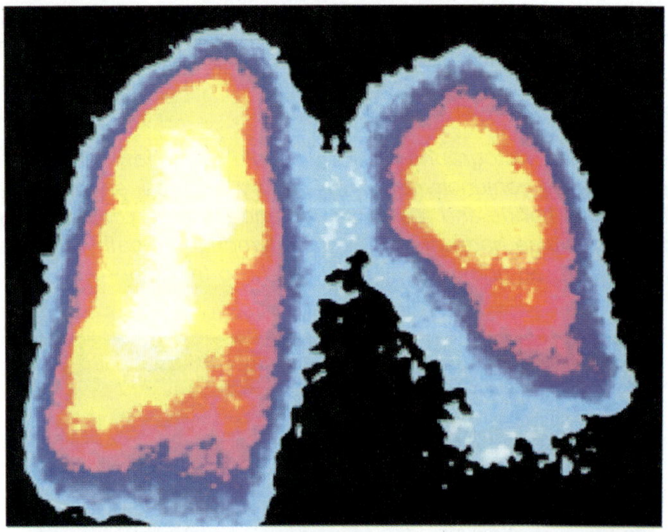

Fig. 31.69: *Pulmonary embolism. Coloured frontal chest scintigram (gamma scan) of a pulmonary embolism in the right lower lung*

electrocardiogram may show RV strain (classic S1, Q3, T3, new onset incomplete or complete RBBB), but this finding is not specific to PE and may be present in other causes of RV strain.

Diagnostic imaging include venous ultrasonography to detect DVT; echocardiography to detect right heart thrombi, a right to left shunt through a patent foramen ovale (an indication of elevated right-sided pressures), and right ventricular dysfunction (RV dilation, hypokinesis, increased velocity of the tricuspid regurgitation jet) findings which were associated with greater than twofold increased risk of PE-related mortality; V/Q lung scan is useful when the scan is normal or indicates high probability, but most patients do not have findings that are definitive; pulmonary angiography is the gold standard although it is an invasive specialized technique with associated risks that should be reserved for the small subgroup of patients in whom the diagnosis of PE cannot be made by other noninvasive imaging modalities.

Heparin followed by oral anticoagulation therapy is the standard treatment for PE. In children, the use of thrombolytic therapy, such as tissue plasminogen activator (tPA), and surgical or transvenous catheter embolectomy may be considered in hemodynamically unstable patients at high risk of death due to RV failure. This can quickly reduce the RV afterload by recanalization of the occluded pulmonary arterial bed.

Table 31.11: *Conditions that cause pulseless electrical activity*

Condition	*Clues*	*Management*
Hypovolemia	History, flat nedc veins	Volume infuston
Hypoxia	Cyanosis, bood gases, airway problems	Ventilation
Cardiac tamponade	History (trauma, renal failure, thoracic malignancy), no pulse with CPR. Vein distention; impending tamponade-fachycardia, hypotension low pulse pressure-changing to sudden bradycardia as terminal event	Pericardiocentesis
Tension pneumothorax	History (asthma, ventilator, chronic obstructive pulmonary disease, trauma) no pulse with CPR, neck vein distention, tracheal deviation	Needle decompression
Hypothermia	History of exposure to cold, central body temperature	Wraming
Massive pulmonary embolism	History, no pulse felt with CPR	Pulmonary arteriogram, surgical embolectomy thrombolytics
Drug overdose (tricyclics. diagoxin, b-blockers calcium	Bradycardia, history of ingestion, empty bottles at the scene, pupils, neurologic examination	Drug screens, intubation, lavage, activated charcoal, lactulose per local protocols
Hyperkalemia	History of renal failure diabetes, recent dialysis dialysis fistulas, medications	Calcium chloride (immediate): then combination of insulin glucose sodium bicarbonate; then sodium polystyrene sulfonate and sorbitol; dialysis (long term)
Preexisting acidosis	History of bicarbonate responsive pr-eexisting acidosis renal failure	Sodium bicarbonate, hypervenflation
Acure massive MI	History, ECG, enzymes	Treat for cardiogenic shock

CPR, cardiopulmonary resuscitation; ECG, electrocardiography; MI, myocardial infarction. From Wnard CA 1997.

Hypertensive Emergencies in Children

Hypertensive emergencies though uncommon in children, are potentially life-threatening. While targeting blood pressure reduction to below the 90th percentile for age, gender and height, mean arterial blood pressure should be gradually lowered by one-fourth of the planned reduction over 8–12 h, a further fourth over the next 8–12 h, and the final 50% over the 24 h after that. Frequent invasive or non-invasive blood pressure monitoring is essential, as is monitoring for sensorial alteration and loss of papillary reflexes. Few antihypertensive agents have been examined in children. Continuous intravenous infusions of short-acting drugs such as nitroprusside, labetalol and nicardipine are preferred to intravenous boluses of hydralazine or diazoxide. If severe symptoms are absent, oral agents such as nifedipine, clonidine, minoxidil, hydralazine, labetalol, captopril and prazosin may be used. Nicardipine and labetalol are particularly suited in emergencies with intracranial bleeding or ischemic stroke while furosemide,

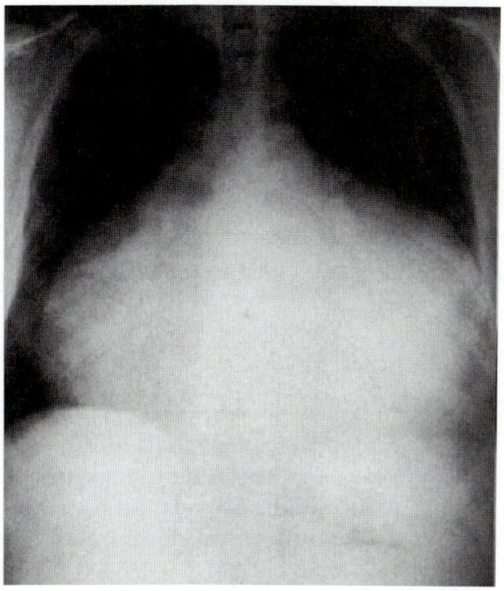

Fig. 31.70: *This anteroposterior-view chest radiograph shows a massive, bottle-shaped heart and conspicuous absence of pulmonary vascular congestion in patient with pericardial effusion large*

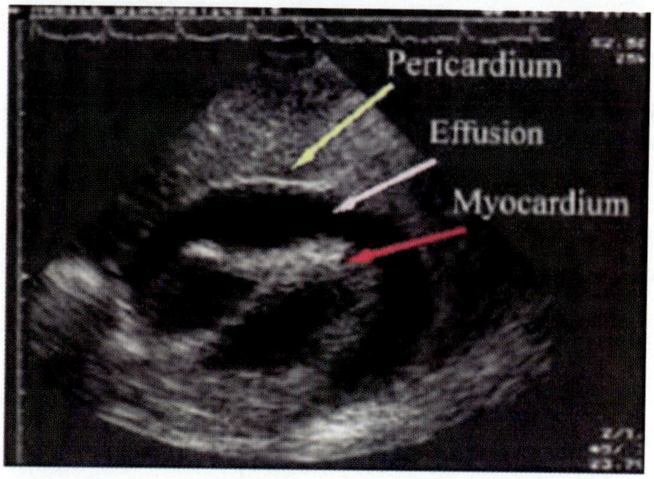

Fig. 31.71: *Echo scan showing pericardial sac filled with fluid leading to cardiac tamponade*

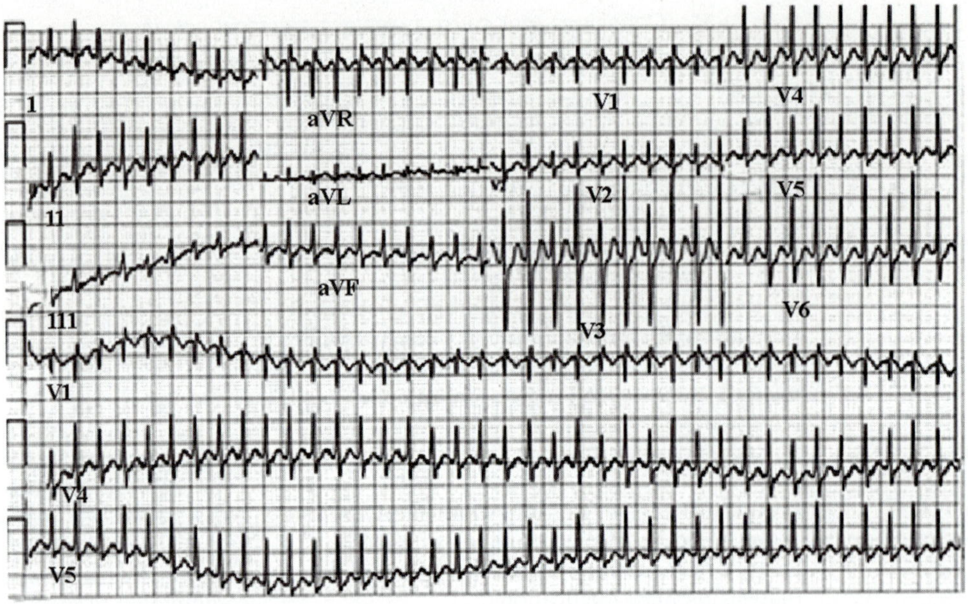

Fig. 31.72: *Electrical alternans during sinus rhythm implies cardiac tamponade. However, electrical alternans is well known to accompany some cases of SVT, atrial flutter, or ventricular tachycardia, in the absence of any pericardial problems*

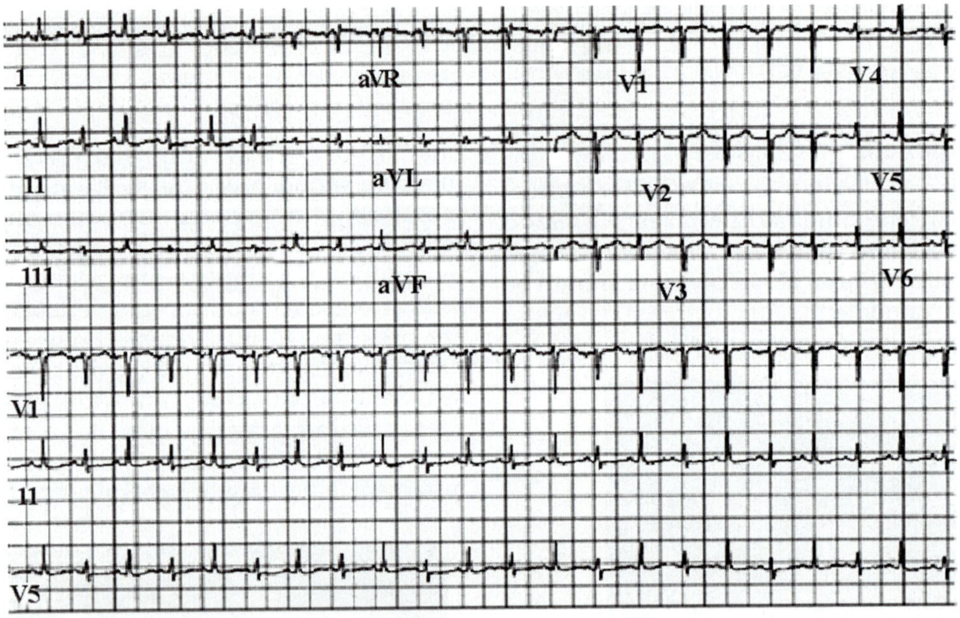

Fig. 31.73: *A 15-year-adolescent on warfarin for postoperative pulmonary embolism presented with chest pain and was found to be in cardiac tamponade due to an atraumatic haemopericardium*

sodium nitroprusside and nitroglycerine are useful in congestive cardiac failure. Therapy with oral antihypertensive drugs should be instituted within 6–12 h of parenteral therapy and the latter gradually withdrawn over the next 12–48 h. Oral agents have limited application as primary therapy, except when administration of intravenous infusion is likely to be delayed. This article provides a summary of the clinical approach to evaluation and management of severe symptomatic hypertension in children.

Cardiac Tamponade (Figs 31.70–31.72)

Cardiac tamponade occurs when fluid builds up between the heart muscle and the surrounding tissue (called the pericardium). This fluid compresses the heart. Because of this, enough blood cannot be pumped in and out of the heart.

This condition can be life-threatening. With proper treatment, prognosis is good. Cardiac tamponade can recur after treatment though the widespread use of central venous catheters in the treatment of pediatric patients has

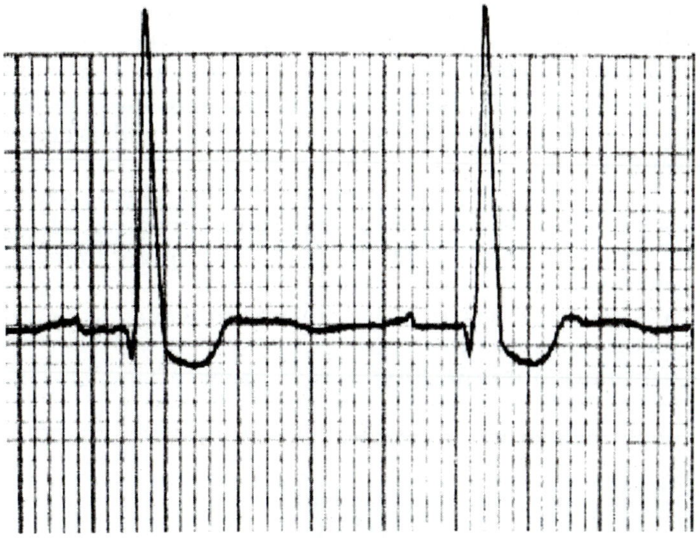

Fig. 31.74: *ECG shows a downsloaping ST segment depression in multiple leads that are shaped like the "reverse check mark sign" or a "scooped out" appearance.*

caused an increased incidence of complications. A rare, but potentially fatal complication occurs when the heart is perforated by the catheter tip causing a cardiac tamponade. This perforation of the heart generally is associated with the insertion procedure, but may also occur after some time because of displacement of the catheter tip. Proper positioning of the catheter tip in the superior vena cava and a high index of suspicion are essential in preventing this serious complication. Contrast-enhanced chest X-ray after insertion of the catheter must be performed to ascertain a correct position of the tip.

Causes

Cardiac tamponade can be caused by a variety of factors and conditions including:

- Pericarditis (an inflammation of the sac that surrounds the heart) caused by bacterial or viral infections
- Bleeding into the pericardium, caused by injury
- Ruptured heart muscle
- Cancer in or near the heart.

Risk Factors

These factors increase your chance of developing this condition. Tell your doctor if you have any of these risk factors:

- Heart surgery
- Tumors in the heart
- Heart attack
- Injury to the heart
- End-stage lung cancer
- Kidney failure
- Radiation therapy to the chest
- Hypothyroidism
- Systemic lupus erythematosus.

Symptoms

Symptoms vary from mild to severe. They typically include one or more of the following:

- Fatigue or drowsiness
- Shortness of breath, rapid breathing, or difficulty breathing
- Dizziness or light-headedness
- Chest pai
  - That extends to the neck, shoulders, or abdomen
  - Sharp or stabbing pain
  - Pain that is worsened by coughing or deep breathing
- Discomfort that can be relieved by sitting upright or leaning forward
- Swelling of the abdomen, veins in the arms or legs, or other areas
- Pale skin, or skin that is blue- or gray-tinted

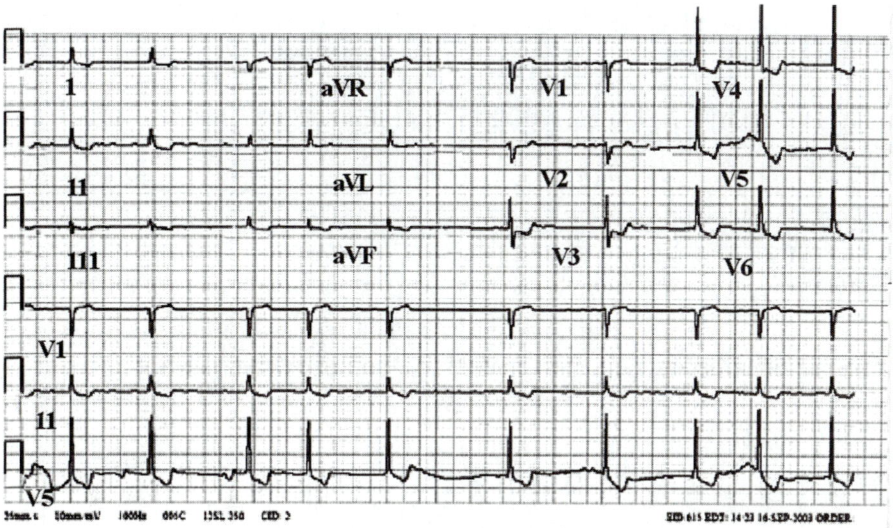

Fig. 31.75: *ECG showing (1) atrial fibrillation with bradycardia (2) ST segment depression consistent with digoxin effect it shows a downsloaping ST segment depression in multiple leads that are shaped like the "reverse check mark sign" or a "scooped out" appearance. This pattern is typical of digoxin. This may occur at normal digoxin levels in some patients, but becomes more common as the digoxin level increases*

- Rapid heartbeat
- Anxiety or restlessness
- Low blood pressure
- Fainting
- Feeling of weakness
- General malaise.

Diagnosis

Your doctor will ask about your symptoms and medical history. You will also be examined. If you have a significant change in blood pressure between breaths, this is one way your doctor will diagnose this condition.

The following tests are also used for diagnosis:

- **Echocardiogram:** A test that uses high-frequency sound waves (ultrasound) to examine the size, shape, and motion of the heart. This is the primary test used to diagnose and manage cardiac tamponade (Fig. 31.71).
- **Cardiac catheterization:** A tube-like instrument inserted into the heart through a vein or artery (usually in the arm or leg) to detect problems with the heart and its blood supply.
- **Chest X-ray:** A test that uses radiation to take a picture of structures inside the body, especially bones (Fig. 31.70)
- **CT scan:** A type of X-ray that uses a computer to make pictures of structures inside the chest
- **MRI scan:** A test that uses magnetic waves to make pictures of structures inside the chest
- **Coronary angiography:** X-rays taken after a dye is injected into the arteries; allows the doctor to look for abnormalities in the arteries

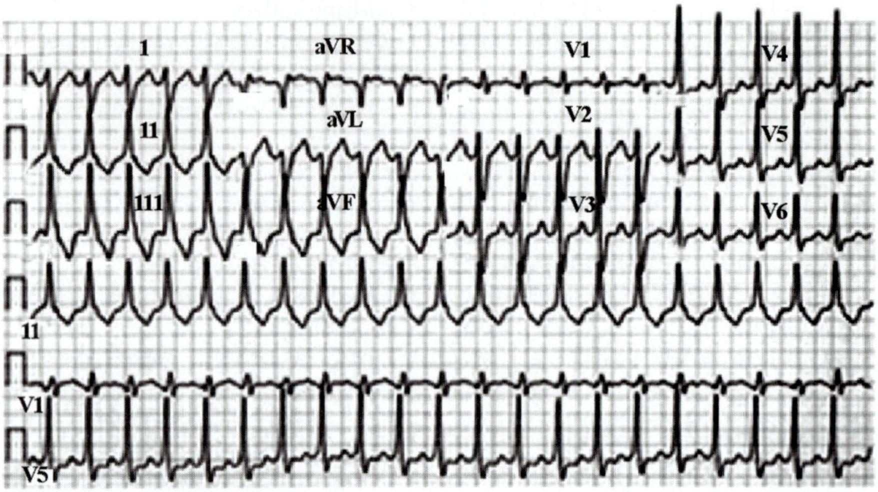

Fig. 31.76: *Electrocardiogram illustrating left ventricular outflow tract ventricular tachycardia (LVOT VT). The S wave in LI and R-wave transition in V1 suggest LVOT VT. In addition, an R:S amplitude ratio of 30% and an R:QRS duration ratio of 50% are seen. Presence of an S wave in leads V5 and V6 suggests an infravalvular origin of the tachycardia*

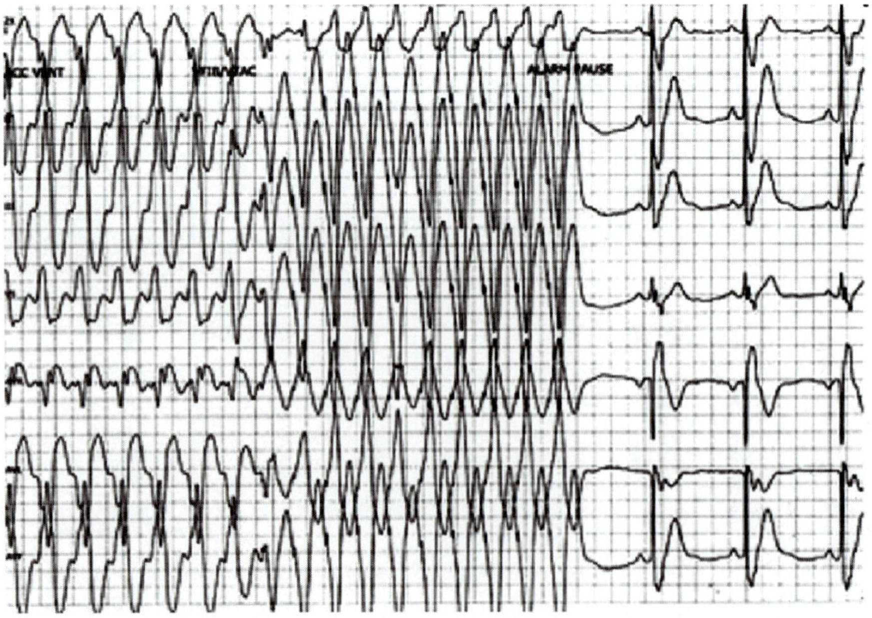

Fig. 31.77: *ECG showing ventricular tachycardia which has been terminated with ventricular burst pacing from the ICD*

- **Electrocardiogram (ECG):** A test that records the heart's activity by measuring electrical currents through the heart muscle (Fig. 31.72).

Treatment

This is a serious condition. It can be life-threatening and requires immediate hospitalization and treatment.

Treatments are administered to:
- Save the patient's life
- Improve heart function
- Relieve symptoms

Treatments that are administered for cardiac tamponade include:
- Pericardiocentesis: A procedure to drain the fluid around the heart
- Fluids to maintain normal blood pressure
- Antibiotics
- Medications to help increase blood pressure to normal levels
- Oxygen to reduce workload on the heart
- Surgery to remove or cut part of the pericardium.

Toxicological Emergencies in Children

Digoxin Toxicity

It is a disorder that is characterized by poisoning due to consumption of excessive amounts of digoxin, a chemical found in plants of the genus *Digitalis.* Poisoning may also occur due to intake of small amounts of digoxin over an extended period of time.

Digoxin Toxicity Diagnosis

Patients suspected of having this condition should undergo an ECG examination. A measurement of serum digoxin concentrations should be carried out. Measurement is, however, only truly reflective after completion of distribution (4–6 hours after last dosage). It usually requires two levels to make sure of the distributed levels.

Signs and Symptoms of Digoxin Toxicity

The symptoms of digoxin toxicity range from obvious to nonspecific. Obvious signs of digoxin poisoning may include vomiting, nausea, hypotension, or hypothyroidism. It can be difficult to recognize digoxin toxicity in patients, however, since the symptoms may be attributed to the underlying condition for which digoxin is prescribed.

Signs and symptoms of life-threatening or potentially life-threatening digoxin toxicity include but are not limited to
- Severe ventricular arrhythmias
- Including sinus ventricular tachycardia or fibrillation
- Progressive bradycardia
- Second- or third-degree heart block not responsive to atropine
- Serum potassium levels exceeding 5.5 mEq/L in adults or 6 mEq/L in children with rapidly progressive signs and symptoms of digoxin toxicity
- Neurologic symptoms (e.g. visual disturbances, disorientation, and confusion)

Diagnosing digoxin toxicity can also be difficult because about 30% of patients with digoxin toxicity have no symptoms. It may be helpful to know who's at risk for digoxin toxicity and the side effects of digitalis treatment to facilitate proper diagnosis.

Diagnosing Digoxin Toxicity

Which patients may be at higher risk for digoxin toxicity? Recognizing digoxin toxicity may be difficult, but it may help to know what to look for. Patients at risk of digoxin toxicity are typically older and have comorbidities.

Risk factors for digoxin toxicity include:
- Advanced age (>80 years)
- Decrease in renal clearance or loss of renal function due to chronic disease
- Hypokalemia
- Hypomagnesemia
- Hypothyroidism
- Multiple concomitant prescription drugs
- Macrolide antibiotics
- Drugs that impair renal function
- Drugs that cause hypokalemia.

When diagnosing digoxin toxicity, pay attention to these risk factors. Patients undergoing digoxin therapy who exhibit these risk factors should be closely monitored so that any signs of digoxin poisoning are identified early to ensure timely treatment.

ECG Changes in Digoxin Toxicity (Figs 31.74 and 31.75)

In case of digitalis use and digitalis toxicity, some characteristic electrocardiographic (ECG) changes can be seen. At therapeutic levels, digoxin gives rise to characteristic changes in ECG readings such as scooping of the ST segments or prolongation of the PR segment. On the other hand, digitalis toxicity may give rise to myriad changes in ECG readings.

Digoxin Toxicity Management

It can be difficult to conduct treatment of digitalis toxicity. This is due to the fact that the condition of the heart of a

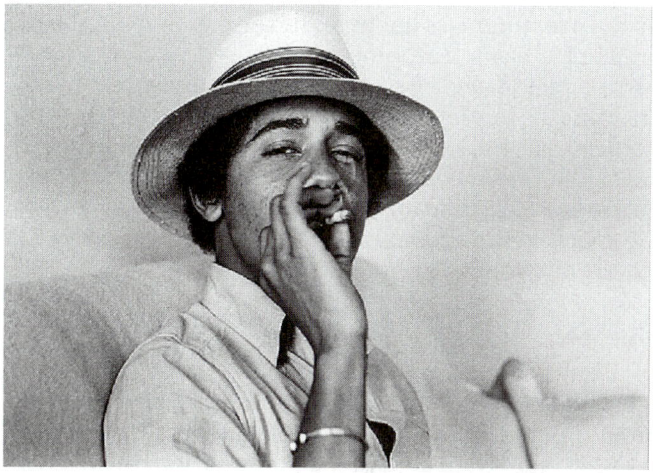

Fig. 31.78: *Adolescent is busy in cocaine cigarette smoking*

diseased individual is highly fragile due to toxic effects of digoxin. Cure may include nonserious treatment such as,

- Monitoring cardiac condition
- Use of intravenous fluids
- Use of potassium supplements.

Medications may also be used to bind digoxin in the intestine. This will help to prevent absorption of the chemical into the bloodstream. Digibind is a popular drug of this type. It is used as an antidote for digoxin toxicity.

It is not advisable to induce vomiting in DT sufferers as it can put further stress on hearts with reduced cardiac rate. It is also unwise to stimulate vomiting in patients suffering from other damaging conditions.

In emergency cases, afflicted individual should necessarily be assisted in breathing to keep them alive for long enough to receive treatment. Cure, in such cases, can involve removing the contents of the stomach with the aid of tubes. In cases where toxic effects have developed occurred over an extended time period, drugs may be required to reverse the harmful effects.

Effective management of this condition depends on early recognition of its association with dysrhythmia and/or any noncardiac manifestation. Generally, management involves:

- Assessment of the severity of the problem
- Assessment of the cause of toxicity, such as reduced renal clearance, the prescribed dosage, concurrent medications
- Assessing whether over-dosage is intentional or accidental
- Considering factors that influence treatment, such as age, chronicity of digoxin intoxication, medical history, existing renal insufficiency and/or heart disease
- Taking ECG changes into account
- Constant hemodynamic assessment involving cardiac monitoring and 12-lead ECG
- Immediate electrolyte level measurement.

Treatment of digitalis toxicity should include the withdrawal of the cardiac glycoside and the elimination of all factors enhancing the toxic effects of digitalis. When the arrhythmia is causing haemodynamic instability or when there is ventricular irritability, treatment with anti-arrhythmic agents is indicated. Potassium chloride, lidocaine and diphenylhydantoin are the drugs of choice in the treatment of tachyarrhythmias and ventricular premature beats. Atropine can be used to counteract the vagal effect of digitalis in bradycardia and heart block. If atropine is ineffective, the placement of a temporary artificial pacemaker may be necessary. When congestive heart failure is a complication, the use of a vasodilator to decrease ventricular preload and afterload will improve the mechanical efficiency of the heart, increase cardiac output and relieve pulmonary congestion.

DigiFab

DigiFab® Digoxin immune fab (ovine) is a sterile, purified, lyophilized preparation of digoxin-immune ovine Fab (monovalent) immunoglobulin fragments.

Each vial of DigiFab® digoxin immune fab (ovine), which will bind approximately 0.5 mg digoxin, contains 40 mg of

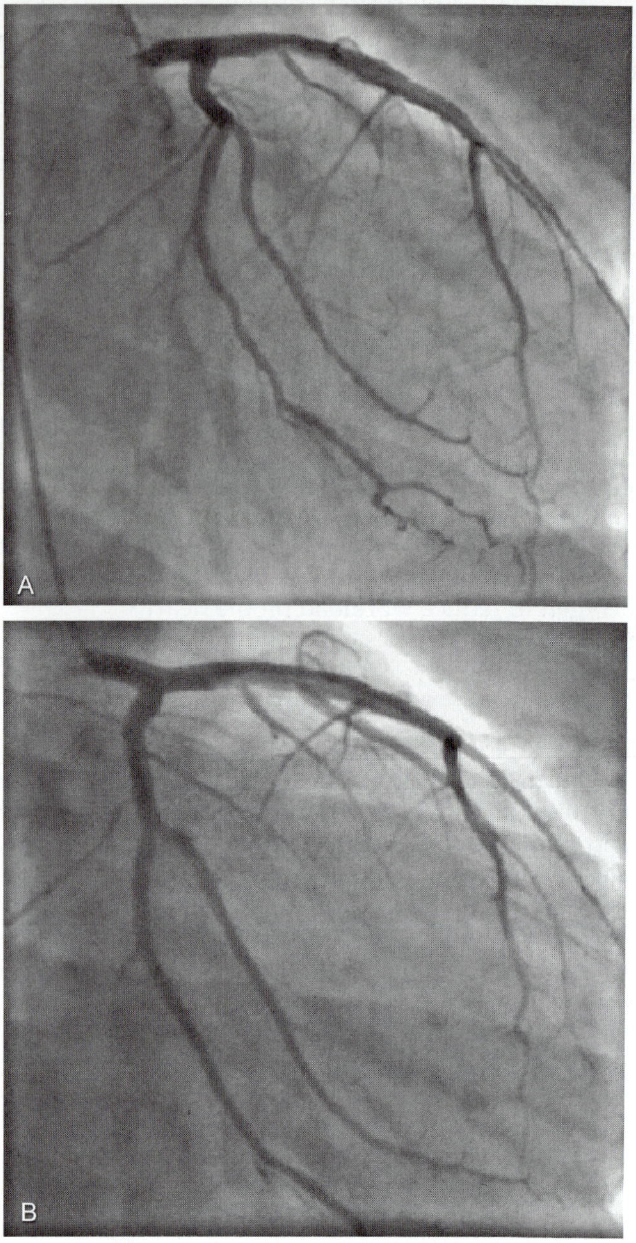

Fig. 31.79: *Coronary artery dissection secondary to cocaine abuse coronary angiography, on the second day, revealed a dissection extending from the proximal to mid-segment of left anterior descending (LAD) coronary artery with normal left circumflex and right coronary arteries (A and B). Left ventriculogram showed moderate left ventricular systolic dysfunction primary percutaneous intervention was not considered due to late presentation and ECG evidence of completed infarct, as well as insignificant symptoms. In view of possible cocaine-induced vasospasm related anterolateral STEMI, it was decided to manage the patient conservatively with nitrate infusion, diltiazem, dual antiplatelet and low molecular weight heparin (LMWH) after consultation with a specialist. Subsequently, he had two more admissions with chest pain and a small rise in troponin levels. His case was, therefore, re-discussed, where a decision to perform a repeat diagnostic coronary angiogram was suggested before any further intervention. Fortunately, his repeat coronary angiogram revealed spontaneously healed dissection*

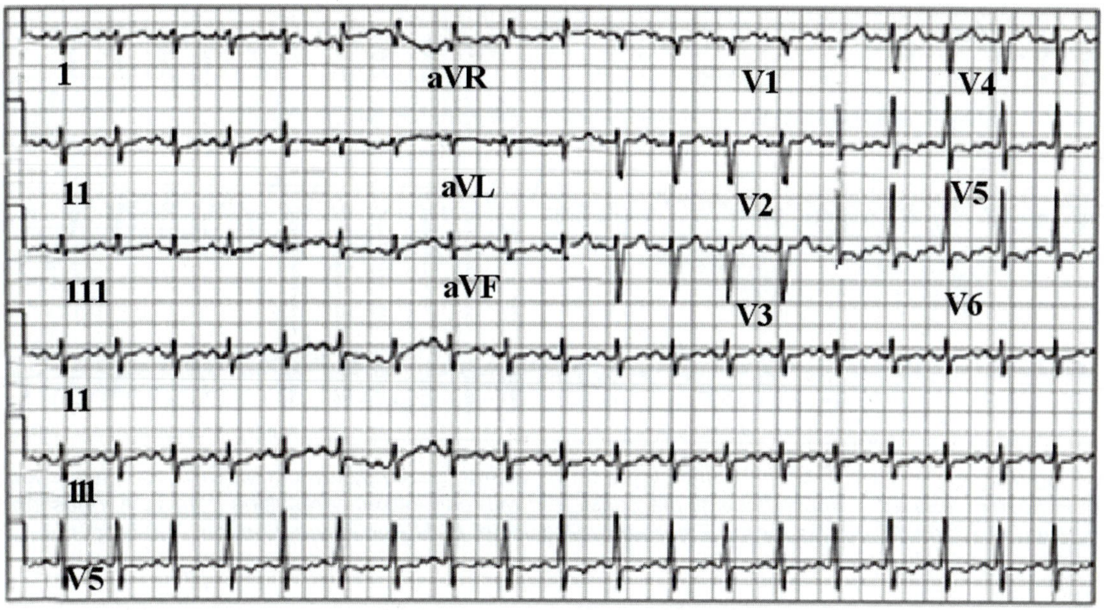

Fig. 31.80: *An 18-year-old girl has abused cocaine and alcohol for 4 years. She has been followed for 2 years for a dilated cardiomyopathy, presumably precipitated by substance abuse, but she frequently fails to keep her appointments. She has no structural abnormalities of the heart. The ECG shows sinus tachycardia, right atrial enlargement, and right-axis deviation.*

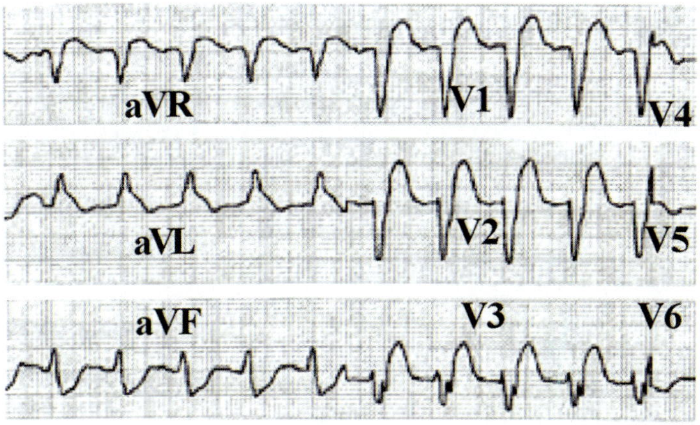

Fig. 31.81: *ECG myocardial infarction in cocaine user. ST elevation in aVL V1–V4 in AMI*

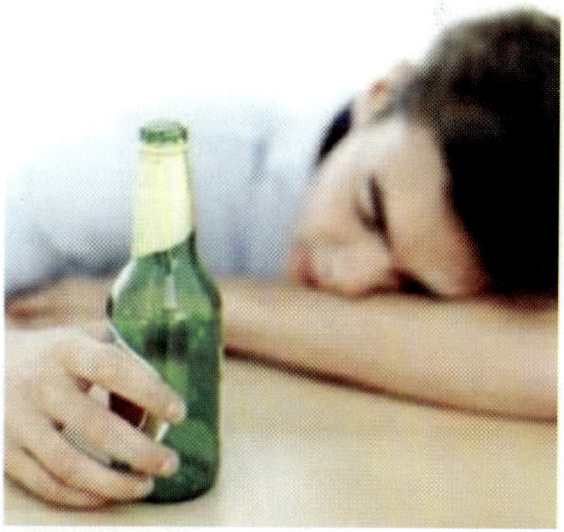

Fig. 31.82: *An adolescent had cansumed over dose of alcohol with drowsiness*

digoxin immune Fab, 75 mg (approx) of mannitol USP, and 2 mg (approx) sodium acetate USP as a buffering agent.

The product contains no preservatives and is intended for intravenous administration after reconstitution with 4 mL of sterile water for injection USP.

DigiFab® Digoxin Immune Fab (Ovine) 1:

- Rapidly binds to and neutralizes digoxin with measurable results
- Rapidly reduces levels of free digoxin to undetectable:
  - More than 40% of digoxin excreted by 24 hours
  - 93% of patients resolved their digoxin poisoning by 20 hours.

Cocaine Abuse Among Adolescents

Cocaine is a naturally occurring alkaloid that increases dopamine concentrations in the reward centers of the brain. There has been a marked increase in cocaine abuse over the last two decades. A neuropsychological stimulant, cocaine also reduces somnolence, increases alertness and improves concentration. However, cocaine abuse has many pathophysiological consequences. These fall broadly into four groups: (1) pathology associated with a drug abusing lifestyle, (2) pathology that occurs whilst intoxicated with (but not directly due to) the drug, (3) pathology associated

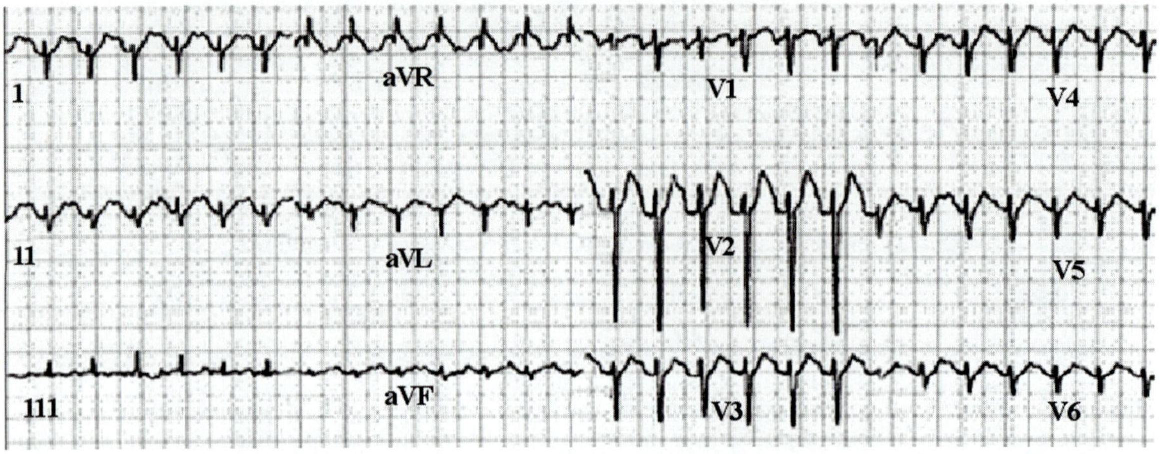

Fig. 31.83: *(TCA ingestion)—12-lead ECG with a sinus tachycardia characterized by a widened QRS complex, deep S wave in lead I, and prominent R wave in lead aVR. These findings are consistent with cardiotoxicity resulting from TCA ingestion. Reprinted with permission from Mattu A, Brady WJ: ECGs for the Emergency Physician. BMJ Publishing, London, 2004, pg 110.*

with drug administration and (4) pathology resulting from pharmacological action of the drug. This review provides a detailed description of the physiological, pharmacological, and pathological effects of cocaine, and highlights the forensic and medicolegal implications of cocaine abuse.

Effect of Cocaine on Cardiovascular System (Figs 31.79–31.81)

Cardiac complications are the commonest cause of death amongst cocaine users, 16 and can occur after acute or chronic abuse. Chest pain, myocardial ischaemia and infarction, cardiac dysrhythmias and sudden death have been reported. Myocarditis and aortic rupture may also occur, but rarely.

Ischaemia and infarction usually occur in chronic abusers, but infarction can occur after initial use of cocaine. Cocaine (usually) has a positive inochronotropic action on the heart, through peripheral and central stimulation of the

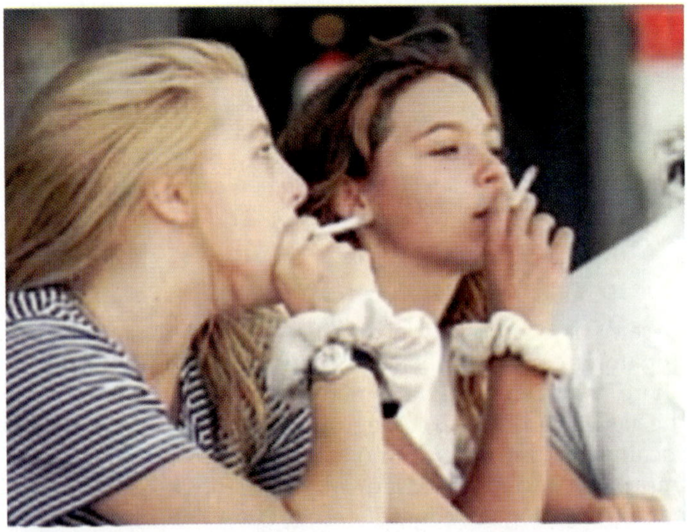

Fig. 31.84: *By raising the age restriction on tobacco purchases, we can deter many young people from ever starting this bad habit and save them years of health complications*

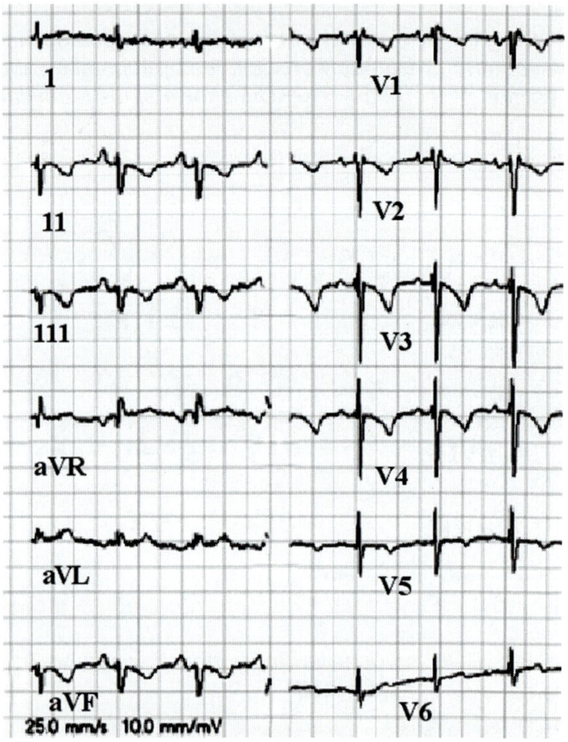

Fig. 31.85: *12-lead ECG from a patient with severe CO poisoning (CO hemoglobin of 39.1%) showing signs of myocardial ischemia as suggested by T-wave inversion in the precordial and inferior limb leads. An elevated troponin level (troponin I level of 11.8 ng/L) confirmed the presence of myocardial injury*

sympathetic nervous system, and increased adrenal medullary epinephrine production. Heart rate, blood pressure, systemic vascular resistance, and left ventricular rate-pressure product are acutely increased, and myocardial oxygen demand is increased in parallel. However, myocardial oxygen delivery is reduced due to raised left ventricular end diastolic pressure, myocardial arteriolar vasoconstriction, reduced coronary diastolic filling time during tachycardia and cocaine-induced

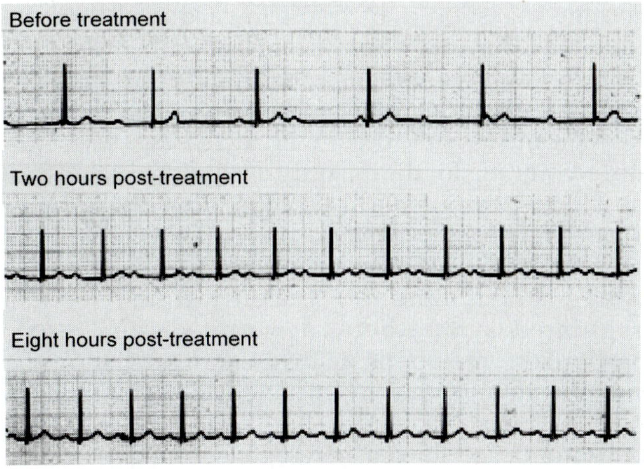

Fig. 31.86: *Yellow oleander poisoning: electrocardiogram showing resolution of cardiac arrhythmia after treatment*

coronary artery vasospasm Myocardial ischaemia results from the imbalance between oxygen supply and demand. Q or non-Q wave infarcts may ensue. Coronary artery dissection has been reported. Spasm may be worsened by the coadministration of cigarette smoke (which elevate carboxyhaemoglobin levels and increase blood viscosity, which further reduces myocardial oxygen supply).

Infarction is made more likely by the prothrombotic effects of cocaine. Platelet aggregation and activation are enhanced, and fibrinolysis is decreased (by an increase in levels of endogenous tissue plasminogen activator inhibitor).

Underlying heart disease is not a prerequisite for the development of cocaine-related ischaemia and infarction, but its presence significantly increases the likelihood of infarction and worsens the prognosis after infarction. Coronary atherosclerosis reduces the arterial endothelial release of coronary vasodilators (nitric oxide and prostacycline), enhancing coronary vasospasm at the site of atherosclerotic plaque. In addition, endothelial damage may occur after coronary vasospasm, promoting further atherosclerotic change and thrombosis. Moreover, platelet activation releases smooth muscle growth factors, which promote vascular hyperplasia and coronary luminal occlusion. Indeed, cocaine appears to be an independent accelerant of coronary atherosclerosis.

Cocaine-related chest pain annually accounts for 37,000 admissions to hospital in the United States. The pain is commonly described as sharp, stabbing or pleuritic, and may represent ischaemia secondary to coronary vasospasm. Chest pain is invariably present prior to cocaine-related infarction. 6% with chest pain proceed to infarction. 4% die after infarction, 4–12% develop life-threatening arrhythmias, and congestive cardiac failure occurs in 5–7%. Electrocardiography is only sensitive for infarction in a third of cases of cocaine-related chest pain (compared to 61% of noncocaine-related chest pain though abnormalities

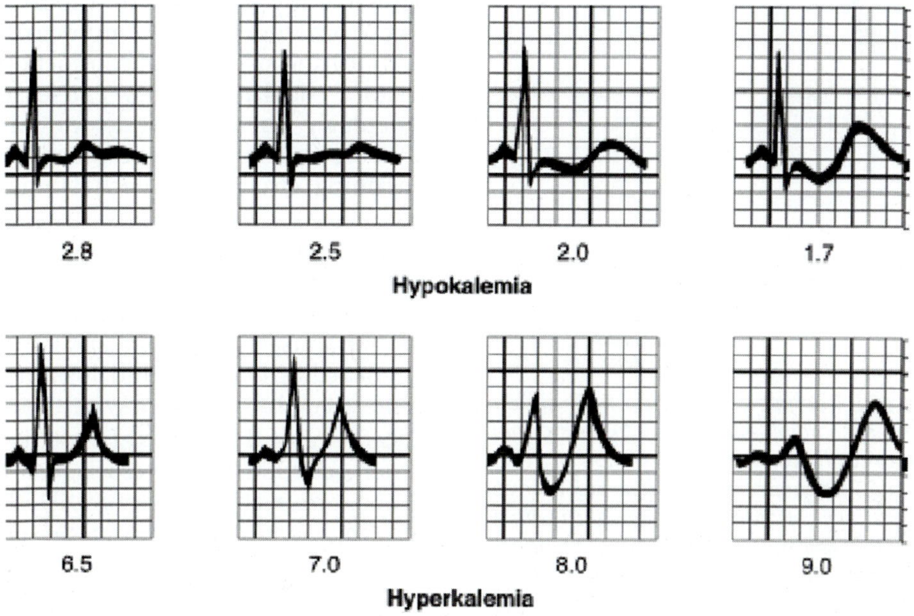

Fig. 31.87: *(Upper) in patients with hypokalemia. Cardiac effects of hypokalemia are usually minimal until serum K concentrations are < 3 mEq/L. Hypokalemia causes sagging of the ST segment, depression of the T wave, and elevation of the U wave. With marked hypokalemia, the T wave becomes progressively smaller and the U wave becomes increasingly larger. Sometimes, a flat or positive T wave merges with a positive U wave, which may be confused with QT prolongation (Bottom) in patient with hyperkaelemia showing of conduction characterized by an increased PR interval and shortening of the QT interval as well as tall, symmetric, peaked T waves are visible initially. K > 6.5 mEq/L causes further slowing of conduction with widening of the QRS interval, disappearance of the P wave, and nodal and escape ventricular arrhythmias. Finally, the QRS complex degenerates into a sine wave pattern, and ventricular fibrillation or asystole ensues*

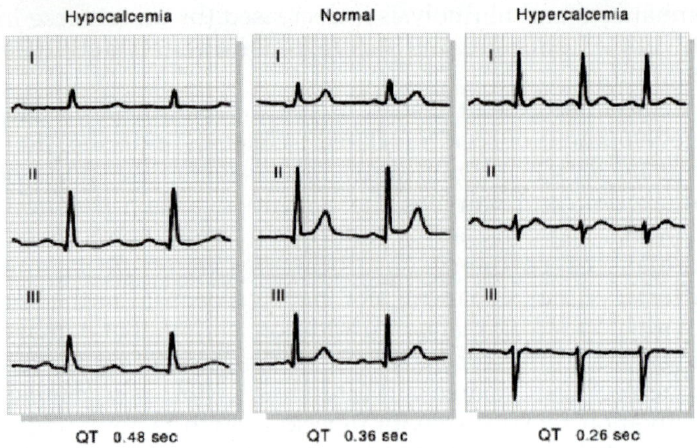

Fig. 31.88: *Prolongation of the QT interval is typical of hypocalcemia. Hypercalcemia may cause shortening of the QT interval, (From Goldberger AL: Clinical Electrocardiography. A simplified approach 6th ed. St. Louis, CB Mosby, 1999)*

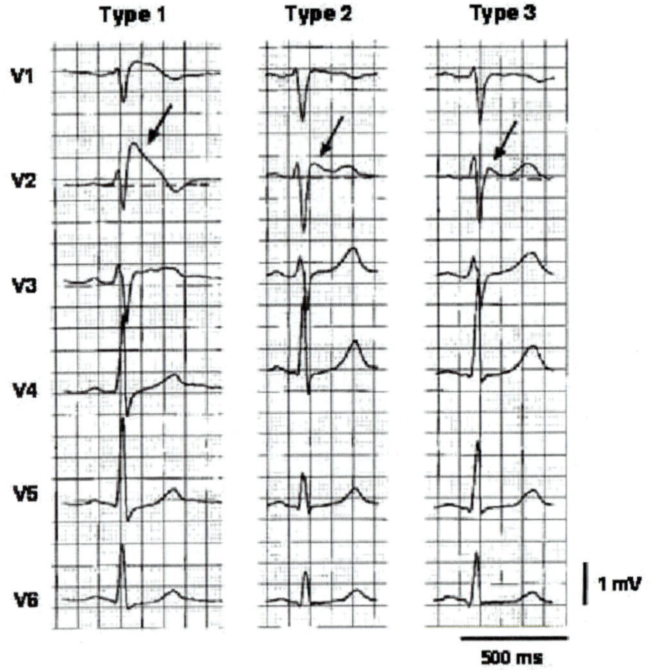

Fig. 31.89: *Three types of ST-segment elevation in Brugada syndrome, as shown in the precordial leads on ECG. Left panel shows a type 1 ECG pattern with pronounced elevation of the J point (arrow), a coved-type ST segment, and an inverted T wave in V1 and V2. The middle panel illustrates a type 2 pattern with a saddleback ST-segment elevated by >1 mm. The right panel shows a type 3 pattern in which the ST segment is elevated < 1 mm. According to a consensus report (Antzelevitch, 2005), the type 1 ECG pattern is diagnostic of Brugada syndrome. (Modified from Wilde, 2002)*

are seen in two-thirds. CK and CK-MB levels may be raised in cocaine users who have not had an infarct (due to increased motor activity, seizures, hyperthermia, and rhabdomyolysis). Troponin I levels may be more beneficial in diagnosing cocaine-related myocardial infarction.

Cocaine ingestion may result in cardiac dysrhythmia. Initial ingestion may be associated with bradycardia, although tachycardia is most common multifocal ventricular ectopics, ventricular tachycardia, ventricular fibrillation and asystole occur with increasing dose. Sudden death, accounting for the majority of cocaine-related deaths, is most likely attributable to a combination of dysrhythmia and cardiomyopathy. Several mechanisms contribute to cocaine induced dysrhythmia: myocardial ischaemia, raised plasma catecholamine concentrations, centrally upregulated sympathetic nervous system outflow, hyperpyrexia, metabolic acidosis and cardiac myocyte membrane stabilization by cocaine (by interference with transmembranal Na^+ and Ca^{2+} flux). Intracardiac nerve impulses undergo slowed, heterogeneous depolarizations, with prolonged repolarisations. More recently, cocaine and cocaethylene have been shown to effectively block HERG-related (Human ether-a-go-go-related gene) potassium channels, thereby suppressing the delayed-rectifier potassium current [I(K)] resulting in prolongation of cardiac repolarisation. Reentrant dysrhythmias occur, and may be promoted by the formation of myocardial contraction bands which are noncontracting, disorganised, amorphous masses of cardiac myofibrils that are associated with prolonged, high intake of cocaine (amongst other causes). Massive doses of cocaine can result in ventricular standstill.

Left ventricular hypertrophy occurs in 54% of cocaine abusers and regional wall motion abnormalities in 21%. Contractile dysfunction may occur with prolonged, high dose abuse, secondary to the effects of catecholamines, progressive myocytolysis, and focal fibrosis (in response to recurrent episodes of myocardial ischaemia and infarction) and myocardial contraction band formation. In addition, cocaine directly causes myocyte apoptosis (particularly during episodes of oxidative stress). Poor contractile function may be reversible by reducing (and maintaining) circulating catecholamine levels to the normal range.

Cocaine-related myocarditis may occur in a to toxic, dose-dependent manner, secondary to a hypersensitivity (dose-independent) reaction. Toxic myocarditis was found in 20% of cocaine abusers at autopsy, and is manifest by small areas of myocardial necrosis and loss of cardiac myofibrils. Cocaine-related chest pain may be a symptom of myocarditis.

Cocaine-related episodes of hypertension, in the presence of atherosclerotic blood vessels, can result in potentially fatal aortic dissection or rupture. This usually involves the ascending aorta. Aortic root dissection may impinge coronary artery blood flow, leading to further myocardial infarction.

Alcohol Abuse by Adolescents (Figs 31.80–31.82)

Alcohol induces a number of pathologic changes to the heart. The classic manifestation is heart failure from dilated cardiomyopathy. Dilated cardiomyopathy is an irreversible process in which the ventricular wall thickness is normal but the ventricular chambers are enlarged, giving the appearance of thinned walls (shown). Patients have sub-

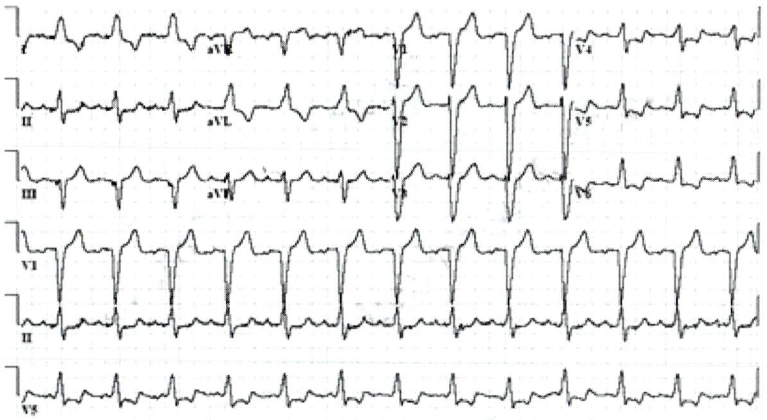

Fig. 31.90: *The ECG findings of hypercalcemia include: (1) A shortened QT interval (2) A shortened ST segment*

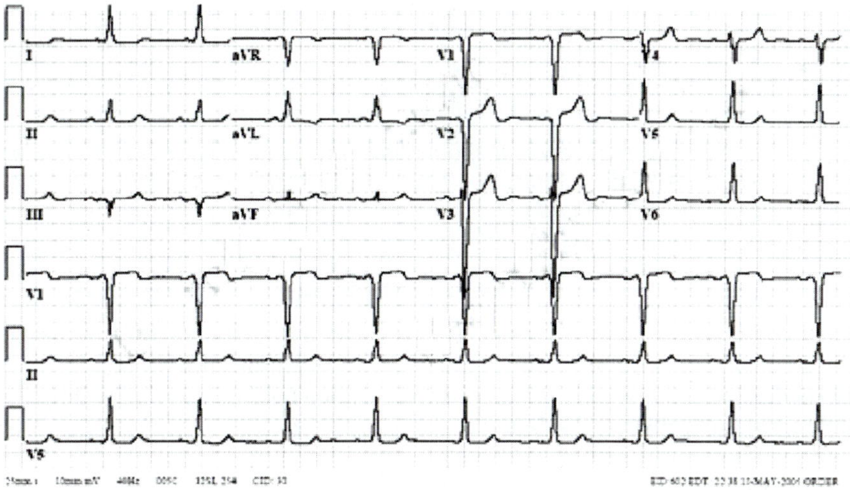

Fig. 31.91: *The ECG findings of hypocalcemia include: (1) A prolonged QT interval, (2) A lengthened ST segment*

sequent systolic dysfunction and are at risk for arrhythmias, thromboembolism, and sudden death. Holiday heart syndrome refers to the development of rhythm disturbances after alcohol use in patients without structural heart disease. Atrial fibrillation is the most common disturbance, and most cases are self-limiting.

Smoking tobacco by adolescents: Smoking harms nearly every organ of the body. Smoking causes many diseases and reduces the health of smokers in general.

Smoking Causes Death (Fig. 31.84)

- The adverse health effects from cigarette smoking account for an estimated 443,000 deaths, or nearly one of every five deaths, each year in the United States.
- More deaths are caused each year by tobacco use than by all deaths from human immunodeficiency virus (HIV), illegal drug use, alcohol use, motor vehicle injuries, suicides, and murders combined.
- Smoking causes an estimated 90% of all lung cancer deaths in men and 80% of all lung cancer deaths in women.
- An estimated 90% of all deaths from chronic obstructive lung disease are caused by smoking.

Smoking and Increased Health Risks

Compared with nonsmokers, smoking is estimated to increase the risk of

- Coronary heart disease by 2 to 4 times
- Stroke by 2 to 4 times
- Men developing lung cancer by 23 times
- Women developing lung cancer by 13 times
- Dying from chronic obstructive lung diseases (such as chronic bronchitis and emphysema) by 12 to 13 times.

Smoking and Cardiovascular Disease

- Smoking causes coronary heart disease, the leading cause of death in the United States.
- Cigarette smoking causes reduced circulation by narrowing the blood vessels (arteries) and puts smokers at risk of developing peripheral vascular disease (i.e. obstruction of the large arteries in the arms and legs that can cause a range of problems from pain to tissue loss or gangrene).
- Smoking causes abdominal aortic aneurysm (i.e. a swelling or weakening of the main artery of the body the aorta—where it runs through the abdomen).

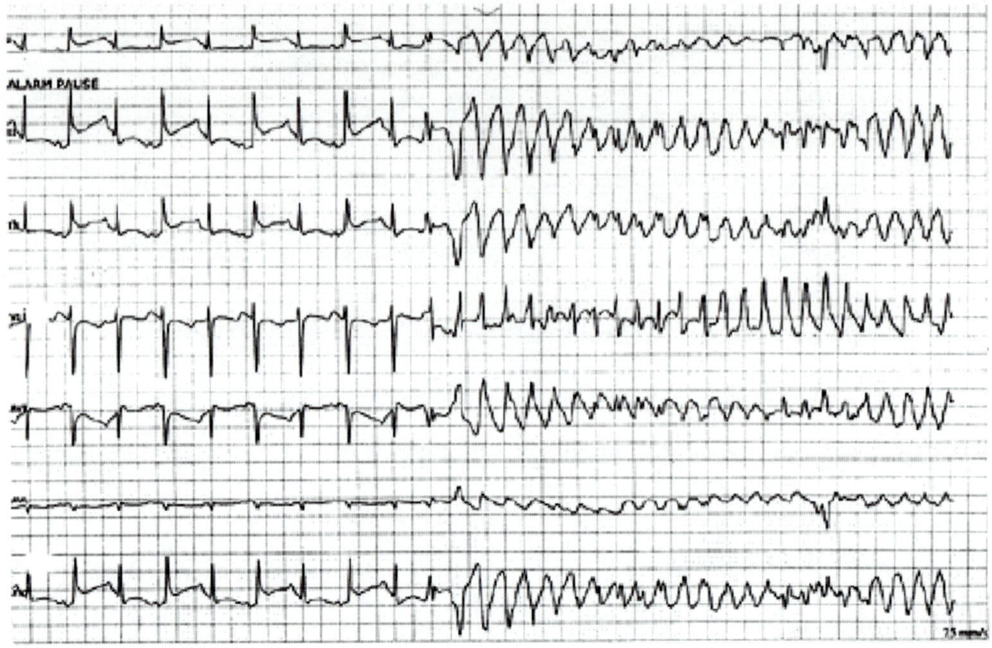

Fig. 31.92: *Patients with hypokalemia or hypomagnesemia should have the condition corrected as these disorders can exaggerate the degree of QTc prolongation and increase the potential for TdP. Special attention should be given to electrolyte and acid-base balance in patients experiencing severe or prolonged diarrhea or in patients receiving concomitant diuretics*

Tricyclic Antidepressant Overdose

The first report of the adverse effects of tricyclic overdose was in 1959 and came within 2 years of their clinical usefulness having been recognized. Now tricyclics are identified as one of the most frequently ingested substances in self-poisoning along with paracetamol, benzodiazepines and alcohol. They are second only to analgesics as the commonest drug taken in fatal drug overdose. There is also evidence that the number of deaths relative to the number of prescriptions issued is significantly higher for tricyclics in comparison to other antidepressants.

Cardiovascular Effects (Fig. 31.83)

The commonest cardiovascular effect is a sinus tachycardia, which is attributable to the inhibition of norepinephrine reuptake and the anticholinergic action. However, the most important toxic effect of tricyclics is the slowing of depolarization of the cardiac action potential by inhibition of the sodium current and this delays propagation of depolarization through both myocardium and conducting tissue. This results in prolongation of the QRS complex and the PR/QT intervals with a predisposition to cardiac arrhythmias. This inhibition of sodium flux into myocardial cells can occur to such an extent that depressed contractility can result and this, coupled with the reduction in peripheral resistance, contributes to hypotension. The overall incidence of serious cardiovascular arrhythmias is low. In one series four patients from 153 admitted to an intensive care unit had either a nodal or ventricular arrhythmia and only 3 of 225 patients admitted to another intensive care unit developed arrhythmias. Hypotension is more common with an incidence of 14– 51% having been reported.

Management Plan for Treatment of Tricyclic Overdose

1. Assess and treat ABCs as appropriate.
2. Examine for clinical features
   - Check urea and electrolytes—look for low potassium
   - Check arterial blood gases—look for acidosis
   - Perform electrocardiograph—look for QRS>0.16 seconds.
3. Consider gastric lavage only if within 1 hour of a potentially fatal overdose.
4. Give 50 grams of charcoal if within 1 hour of ingestion.
5. Give sodium bicarbonate (50 ml of 8.4%) if:
   i. pH <7.1
   ii. RS >0.16 seconds
   iii. Arrhythmias
   iv. Hypotension.
6. **Arrhythmias:** Avoid antiarrhythmics
   - Correct hypoxia, hypotension, acidosis, hypokalaemia
   - Give sodium bicarbonate.
7. **Hypotension:** Give intravenous fluids
   - Consider inotropes
8. **Cardiac arrest:** Prolonged resuscitation may be successful
9. **Monitoring:** Patients who display signs of toxicity should be monitored for a minimum of 12 hours.

Effect of Electrolyte Imbalance on Cardiovascular System

Electrolytes, or ions, are the charged particles in body fluids that help transmit electrical impulses for proper nerve, heart, and muscle function. The number of positive ions, called cations, and negative ions, called anions, is supposed to be equal. Anything that upsets this balance can have life-threatening consequences (Figs 31.87, 31.88, 31.90–31.92).

There's a long list of conditions that lead to electrolyte imbalances including dehydration, diabetic ketoacidosis, cancer, and even head injury. But, renal disease is at the top of the list. It's the kidneys' job to control fluid, electrolyte, and acid-base balance. Because too much or too little of any one of the electrolytes quickly becomes a major problem of its own, doing everything possible to maintain the proper balance is a vital component of patient care. Therefore, monitoring electrolytes and checking for signs of an imbalance should be an integral part of your nursing assessment. Here, then, is a review of the role each electrolyte plays, the causes of imbalances, and the corrective measures required.

Understanding Sodium's Effect on Water Balance

Sodium (Na), the most abundant cation in extracellular fluid, plays a key role in transmitting nerve impulses. It also helps to maintain serum concentration, or osmolality.

Water follows salt in the body, so a gain or loss in sodium results in a gain or loss in water. For instance, when you eat too much salt, the rise in serum osmolality triggers thirst and the release of antidiuretic hormone (ADH) from the pituitary gland. Thirst leads you to drink, while ADH signals the kidneys to hang onto water. The opposite is also true: low serum osmolality from too little salt stops thirst and inhibits ADH release, allowing more water to be excreted by the kidneys.

Hypernatremia occurs when either too much water is lost or too much salt is taken in. You'll find a list of normal values and causes of electrolyte imbalances. The elderly are particularly at risk for hypernatremia following surgery or a fever because of volume depletion, and because of a diminished thirst mechanism. All patients on fluid restrictions and those receiving diuretic therapy, hypertonic IV solutions, or tube feedings are at risk, as well. So, too, are patients with diabetes, because of dehydration related to their hyperglycemia.

Regardless of the cause, patients with hypernatremia may appear thirsty, tachycardic and lethargic. As their cells become more dehydrated, patients may develop disorientation, weakness, irritability and muscle twitching. Urine output is generally low as the body tries to compensate by hanging onto water. The exception is untreated diabetes insipidus, where a lack of ADH results in a high urine output—possibly as much as 20 liters in 24 hours. Regardless, though, of whether urine output is high or low, seizures, coma, or death may result if hypernatremia is left untreated. Correcting the situation requires that you focus on the underlying cause. That may be as simple as replacing volume orally or by the IV administration of isotonic solutions such as normal saline. Or it may be as complex as putting the patient on dialysis. Part of your routine nursing care for the hypernatremic patient will involve monitoring serum sodium and osmolality and administering fluids based on the results. You'll also carefully monitor intake and output, and avoid overhydration. The flip side of the sodium equation is hyponatremia, which usually occurs when the body loses more sodium than water or when excess water dilutes the normal sodium concentration. Dilutional hyponatremia can be caused by excess fluid intake, and conditions such as congestive heart failure or syndrome of inappropriate antidiuretic hormone secretion (SIADH). The neurological symptoms of hyponatremia are similar to those of hypernatremia—lethargy and confusion—with the possible addition of nausea and vomiting resulting from cerebral edema. Other signs and symptoms depend upon the cause. Patients who've lost sodium through diarrhea, certain diuretics, suctioning, or laxatives, for example, may show signs of dehydration, including tachycardia and hypotension. Those with dilutional hyponatremia may show signs of fluid overload, such as hypertension and difficulty breathing.

Treatment depends upon both the degree of sodium deficiency and the cause. In cases of mild hyponatremia, an increased intake of dietary sodium may be ordered, while patients who are both hyponatremic and hypovolemic may receive IV fluid replacement using solutions containing normal saline. Those with mild dilutional hyponatremia from over administration of free water may need nothing more than the restriction of fluid intake. This approach is also appropriate for patients with hyponatremia caused by SIADH. Severe hyponatremia, however, is a medical emergency: permanent neurological damage can occur when serum sodium falls below 110 mEq/L. Giving hypertonic saline (3% NaCl) solution is the treatment of choice, but must be done with caution: a rapid increase in serum sodium can cause fluid overload and cardiac failure, as well as cerebral osmotic demyelination syndrome—a condition caused by osmotic injury to myelinated nerve fibers that leads to paralysis and death.

Potassium (K), Magnesium (Mg), Calcium (Ca), and Phosphorus (PO_4) Imbalances

These can also alter the electrical equilibrium of the cells. The end result? Serious changes in cardiac conduction that can quickly turn lethal. Let's look at each of these electrolytes and the implications that an imbalance will have on your care (Fig. 31.92).

Potassium: This electrolyte is the major intracellular cation. The 2% that's found in extracellular fluid is crucial to neuromuscular and cardiac function. Normally, elevated serum potassium stimulates the release of aldosterone, a hormone produced by the adrenal gland. In the kidneys, aldosterone triggers the excretion of potassium and the retention of sodium until serum potassium levels return to normal. But when the kidneys aren't functioning properly, that correction doesn't take place. Not surprisingly, renal disease is the most common cause of hyperkalemia, but acidosis, aldosterone deficiency, sodium depletion, and excess oral intake of potassium supplements are among a number of other possible causes. Signs and symptoms of hyperkalemia include abdominal cramping, fatigue, lethargy, and muscle weakness or paralysis. Severe hyperkalemia will slow cardiac impulse conduction, producing classic changes on ***EKG Tall, peaked T waves are often seen first, followed by a prolonged PR interval***

and widened QRS complex, signifying delayed conduction, and a shortened QT interval. Left untreated, the excess potassium will continue to suppress conduction until cardiac arrest occurs. Severe hyperkalemia requires rapid action: stop any potassium administration, and give IV calcium chloride or calcium gluconate, as ordered, to stimulate conduction. The doctor may also order IV sodium bicarbonate, insulin and 50% dextrose, or albuterol to try to shift potassium out of the bloodstream and back into the cells. Depending upon their kidney function, patients with hyperkalemia that is not severe may be given IV diuretics to promote potassium excretion by the kidneys or a resin such as sodium polystyrene sulfonate (Kayexalate) that will bind potassium in the gut. But if these efforts fail, hemodialysis may be required in addition to treating the underlying cause. When it comes to hypokalemia, diuretic therapy with inadequate potassium replacement is the most common cause, but patients who lose large amounts of potassium through nasogastric suctioning and diarrhea, for instance, are also at risk. Interestingly, so, too, are patients who were recently hyperkalemic—especially when acidosis is the cause or they're given too much of a drug that brings the potassium down. In acidosis, as pH returns to normal, potassium returns to the cells, lowering serum potassium and increasing the risk of hypokalemia.

Symptoms of hypokalemia include muscle weakness or tenderness, leg cramps, drowsiness, confusion, loss of appetite, abdominal distention, and abnormal cardiac conduction.

Look for flattened or inverted T waves and a depressed ST segment on an EKG tracing. The lack of potassium makes cardiac muscle irritable, increasing the risk of premature atrial and/or ventricular contractions that can trigger ventricular tachycardia, which can progress to fibrillation and death. Initial treatment of hypokalemia, especially when it is accompanied by cardiac symptoms, focuses on replacing potassium. But, this requires great care: given too rapidly, IV potassium can cause cardiac arrest, so never administer it by IV push. Follow your institution's protocol, using a pump, if possible, to regulate the infusion so that it runs in over at least an hour when 15–20 mEqs are mixed in 100 mL of solution. Because potassium is very irritating to tissues, administration through a central line is recommended. For the same reason, you should give oral preparations with food to reduce gastric irritation and abdominal discomfort. Report continued complaints of abdominal pain or distention to the physician. This could be a sign of upper GI ulcers caused by potassium.

Magnesium: This cation is found primarily in the cells and is responsible for reactions that involve muscle function, energy production, and carbohydrate and protein metabolism. Renal failure is the major cause of hypermagnesemia. Other causes include excessive intake of magnesium-containing antacids and laxatives and conditions that produce acidosis such as diabetic ketoacidosis.

Signs of hypermagnesemia include lethargy, altered mental status that can progress to coma, respiratory depression, and muscle weakness. Impaired cardiac conduction and contractility produce bradycardia and hypotension and can progress to a full cardiac arrest.

EKG changes include a prolonged PR interval, widened QRS complex, and lengthened QT interval. If a patient's renal function is normal, treatment may include diuretics to promote magnesium loss. Calcium gluconate given intravenously can help counteract muscle weakness and improve cardiac function. Patients with severe hypermagnesemia and renal failure may need hemodialysis. The other side of the magnesium equation is hypomagnesemia. It's common in critically ill patients and is associated with high mortality rates. Diuretic therapy, chronic alcoholism, cirrhosis, pancreatitis, and preeclampsia can all cause excessive magnesium loss, as can losses from the GI tract through nasogastric suctioning, fistula drainage, and diarrhea. Signs and symptoms of hypomagnesemia include muscle weakness or tremors, anorexia, nausea, and dizziness, as well as neurologic changes including lethargy, confusion, and coma. Like hypokalemia, hypomagnesemia increases cardiac muscle irritability and the potential for ventricular dysrhythmias, especially in patients with a recent MI.

EKG changes associated with low serum magnesium are similar to those seen in hypokalemia: a flat or inverted T wave and ST segment depression. There is also a shortened QT interval treatment focuses on giving the patient magnesium—either in IV or oral form—as ordered to return levels to normal. This is especially important in patients recovering from an acute MI. Research has shown that maintaining adequate serum magnesium levels in these patients can significantly improve ventricular function and reduce mortality rates.

Calcium and phosphorus: These two electrolytes are inversely related in the blood: when calcium levels are high, phosphorus levels are low, and vice versa. Calcium is a cation with multiple functions, including transmitting nerve impulses, maintaining cell wall permeability, and activating the body's clotting mechanism. It's also involved in contracting cardiac and smooth muscle, generating cardiac impulses, mediating cardiac pacemaker function, and forming bones and teeth. Phosphorus, the major intracellular anion, also plays a major role in bone formation. It's necessary for energy production in the cells and for carbohydrate, protein, and fat metabolism, as well. Phosphorous also helps to maintain acid-base balance by buffering hydrogen ions. Parathyroid hormone (PTH) is responsible for regulating calcium and phosphorus. When calcium levels are low, PTH increases calcium reabsorption, and blocks phosphorus from being reabsorbed. Hypocalcemia can result from diarrhea, diuretics, or acute pancreatitis. It can also be caused by malignancies that steal calcium for abnormal bone formation, conditions that affect the parathyroid gland and thus interfere with PTH production, and disorders that interfere with the availability of calcitrol, such as vitamin D deficiency and malabsorption syndromes. The drop in calcium that occurs in the presence of these disorders triggers a concomitant rise in phosphorus. But, there are primary triggers for hyperphosphatemia to watch for, as well. Hyperphosphatemia can occur in patients with normal renal function if they abuse laxatives that are high in phosphorus or have too much of the mineral in their diet. Both hypocalcemia and hyperphosphatemia can cause lethargy, fatigue, bone or joint pain, and sudden seizures. Low calcium levels also produce neuromuscular symptoms including tremors, cramps, and numbness or tingling in the extremities and around the mouth. Patients may also complain of nausea, abdominal distention, vomiting, or constipation and develop cardiac symptoms including life-threatening ventricular dysrhythmias (Figs 31.88, 31.90, 31.91).

EKG tracings will show prolonged ST segments and QT intervals. Decreased cardiac output and vascular smooth muscle relaxation produce decreases in BP that can progress to circulatory collapse.

Treatment focuses on increasing calcium and lowering phosphorus. Give IV calcium gluconate or calcium chloride or oral preparations, as ordered. Aluminum hydroxide gels that bind to phosphorus are given to increase elimination through the bowel. Patients with normal renal function may also receive the diuretic acetazolamide (diamox) to promote renal excretion of phosphorus. When necessary, hemodialysis is used to quickly correct hyperphosphatemia. Now let's take a look at the clinical picture for hypercalemia and hypophosphatemia. Causes of hypercalcemia include excessive use of dietary supplements containing calcium and vitamin D, which increase calcium reabsorption, and hyperparathyroidism. A primary cause of low serum phosphorus is chronic alcoholism. Symptoms of hypercalcemia and hypophosphatemia include lethargy, fatigue, changes in mental status, anorexia, nausea, diminished bowel sounds, and constipation. Patients may also complain of bone pain; flank and thigh pain is associated with stones formed by excess calcium in the kidneys.

Cardiovascular effects include hypertension and conduction abnormalities, seen as AV blocks on EKG, that can progress to cardiac arrest. IV saline infusions and diuretics are given to lower serum calcium through increased renal excretion. Steroids may also be administered to decrease intestinal reabsorption of calcium and mithramycin (Mithracin) is given to stimulate calcium deposits in bones. Phosphorus replacements can be given orally or by IV infusion.

Acid-base Balance must be Maintained

Chloride (Cl) and bicarbonate (HCO_3) are the major extracellular anions. While both play an important role in maintaining acid-base balance, bicarbonate is by far the star of the show. Bicarbonate is the body's major buffer system. It helps keep the ratio between acids and bases in a tight range that's numerically expressed as the pH (normal pH is 7.35–7.45). A rise in pH above normal (alkalosis) or below normal (acidosis) causes cellular damage and can eventually lead to a patient's death. For its part, chloride exists in an inverse relationship with bicarbonate. When there's too little chloride, bicarbonate builds up, and metabolic alkalosis results. The flip side of this—too much chloride—is a bit more complicated. If chloride is high and sodium is normal, the patient may be acidotic. If chloride is high and the sodium is also high, the patient is likely to be dehydrated. One way to determine the cause of an acid-base imbalance is by calculating the anion gap. To calculate this gap, you need to take your patient's lab results and add the chloride and bicarbonate values. Then, subtract the sum of the two from the value for sodium. The normal anion gap range is 8–12.5. A high anion gap (>12) is indicative of conditions such as diabetic- or alcohol-induced ketoacidosis. A high anion gap may also be your first indication of lactic acidosis in patients with shock or sepsis. A normal anion gap with elevated chloride levels should also raise a flag for acidosis. That's because in cases of diarrhea and renal tubular acidosis, bicarbonate is lost, and chloride is retained to maintain electrical neutrality. Either way, interventions focus on treating the underlying cause of the acidosis. A low anion gap indicates alkalosis and hypochloremia from vomiting, nasogastric suctioning, or diuretic therapy. But, other causes of alkalosis include Cushing's syndrome, excessive aldosterone secretion, and hypokalemia. Massive blood transfusions, over-administration of IV fluids containing bicarbonate, and excessive intake of antacids containing sodium bicarbonate can also cause bicarbonate levels to rise. Again, treatment focuses on resolving the underlying cause. Patients with alkalosis may receive acetazolamide. The drug lowers bicarbonate levels by increasing its excretion in the urine and prevents the formation of new bicarbonate. Prolonged use can lead to acidosis, however, so watch bicarbonate levels closely. Your careful attention to bicarbonate, chloride, and the other electrolytes mentioned here, can have a tremendous impact on your patient's well-being. Understanding what the lab values mean in relation to changes in a patient's condition can be a challenge. But, getting a firm handle on things will ensure that you take the necessary steps to correct imbalances before the situation becomes dire.

BIBLIOGRAPHY

1. Drory Y, Turetz Y, Hiss Y, Lev B, Fisman EZ, Pines A, Kramer MR. Sudden unexpected death in persons <40 years of age. Am J Cardiol 1991;68:1388–92.
2. Litherthson RR. Sudden death from cardiac causes in children and young adults. N Engl J Med 1996;334:1039–44.
3. Boneva RS, Botto, LD, Moore CA, Yang Q, Correa A, Erickson JD. Mortality associated with congenital heart defects in the United States: trends and racial disparities, 1979–1997. Circulation 2001;103:2376–81.
4. Colletti JE, Homme JL, Woodridge DP. Unsuspected neonatal killers in emergency medicine. Emerg Med Clin North Am 2004;22:929–60.
5. Schamberger MS. Cardiac Emergencies in Children. Pediatr Ann 1996;25:339–44.
6. Massin MM, Malekzadeh-Milani SG, Van Aerschot I, Dessy H. Management of cardiac emergencies in children. Minerva Pediatr 2009;61:163–73.

7. Park MK. Pediatric Cardiology for Practitioners. 5 th ed. Missouri: Mosby; 2008. p. 62–4,314–5.
8. Moodie DS, Fyfe D, Gill CC, Cook SA, Lytle BW, Taylor PA, et al. Anomalous origin of the left coronary artery from the pulmonary artery (Bland-White-Garland syndrome) in adult patients: long-term follow-up after surgery. Am Heart J 1983; 106:381–8.
9. Alexi-Meskishvilla V, Berger F, Weng Y, Lange PE, Hetzer R. Anomalous origin of the left coronary artery from the pulmonary artery in adults. J Card Surg 1995;10:309–15.
10. Selzman CH, Zimmerman MA, Campbell DN. ALCAPA in an adult with preserved left ventricular function. J Card Surg 2003;18:25–8.
11. Towbin JA, Lowe AM, Colan SD, Sleeper, LA, Orav EJ, Clunie S, et al. Incidence, Causes, and Outcomes of Dilated Cardiomyopathy in Children. JAMA 2006;296:1867–76.
12. Chang Y, Chao, H, Hsia S, Yan D. Myocarditis presenting as gastritis in children. Pediatr Emerg Care 2006;22:439–40.
13. Freedman SB, Haladyn JK, Floh A, Kirsh JA, Taylor G. Thull-Freedman J. Pediatric myocarditis: emergency department clinical findings and diagnostic evaluation. Pediatrics 2007;120:1278–85.
14. Mahrholdt H, Wagner A, Deluigi CC, Kispert E, Hager S, Meinhardt G, et al. Presentation, patterns of myocardial damage, and clinical course of viral myocarditis. Circulation 2006;114:1581–90.
15. Hufnagel G, Pankuweit S, Richter A, Schonian U, Maisch B. The European Study of Epidemiology and Treatment of Cardiac Inflammatory Diseases (ESETCID): First Epidemiological Results. Herz 2000;25:279–85.
16. Johnsrude CL, Perry JC, Cecchin F, Smith EO, Fraley K, Friedman RA, et al. Differentiating anomalous left main coronary artery from the pulmonary artery in infants from myocarditis and dilated cardiomyopathy by electrogram. Am J Cardiol 1995;75:71–4.
17. Amabile N, Fraisse A, Bouvenot J, Chetaille P, Ovaert C. Outcome of acute fulminant myocarditis in children. Heart 2006;92:1269–73.
18. Chau EM, Chow W, Chiu CS, Wang E. Treatment and outcome of biopsy-proven fulminant myocarditis in adults. Int J Cardiol 2006;110:405–6.
19. Gupta S, Markman DW, Drazner MH, Mammen P. Fulminant myocarditis. Nat Clin Pract Cardiovasc Med 2008;5:693–706.
20. McCarthy RE, Boehmer JP, Hruban RH, Hutchins GM, Kasper EK, Hare JM, et al. Long-term Outcome of Fulminant Myocarditis as Compared with Acute (Nonfulminant) Myocarditis. N Engl J Med 2000;342:690–5.
21. Cooper LT. Myocarditis. N Engl J Med 2009;360:1526–38.
22. Towbin JA, Lowe AM, Colan SD. Incidence, causes, and outcomes of dilated cardiomyopathy in children. JAMA 2006;296:1867–76.
23. Kapser EK, Agema W, Hutchins GM, Deckers JW, Hare JM, Baughman KL. The causes of dilated cardiomyopathy: a clinicopathologic review of 673 consecutive patients. J Am Coll Cardiol 1994;23:586–90.
24. Codd MB, Sugrue DD, Gersh BJ, Melton LJ. Epidemiology of idiopathic dilated and hypertrophic cardiomyopathy: A population-based study in Olmsted County, Minnesota, 1975–1984. Circulation 1989;80:564–72.
25. Kantor PF, Mertens LL. Clinical practice: Heart failure in children. Part I: clinical evaluation, diagnostics testing, and initial medical management. Eur J Pediatr 2010;169:269–79.
26. Towbin JA, Bowles NE. The failing heart. Nature 2002; 415:227–33.
27. Monserrat L, Elliott PM, Gimeno JR, Sharma S, Penas-Lado M, McKenna WJ. Non-sustained ventricular tachycardia in hypertrophic cardiomyopathy: an in dependent marker of sudden death in young patients. J Am Coll Cardiol 2003;42:873–9.
28. Maron BJ, Fananapazir L. Sudden cardiac death in hypertrophic cardiomyopathy. Circulation 1992;85:I–57–I–63.
29. Maron BJ, McKenna WJ, Danielson GK, Kappenberger LJ, Kuhn HJ, Seidman CE, et al. American College of Cardiology/European Society of Cardiology Expert Consensus Document on Hypertrophic Cardiomyopathy: A Report of the American College of Cardiology Foundation Task Force on Clinical Expert Consensus Documents and the European Society of Cardiology Committee for Practice Guidelines. J Am Coll Cardiol 2003;42:1687–713.
30. Decker JA, Rossano JW, O'Brian Smith E, Cannon B, Clunie SK, Gates C, et al. Risk factors and mode of death in isolated hypertrophic cardiomyopathy in children. J Am Coll Cardiol 2009;54:250–4.
31. Caglar S, Leffler S. Prevalence of life-threatening arrhythmias in ED patients transported to the radiology suite while monitored by telementry. Am J Emerg Med 2006;24:655–7.
32. Hoffmam TM, Wernovsky G, Wieand TS, Cohen MI, Jennings AC, Vetter VL, et al. The Incidence of Arrhythmias in a Pediatric Cardiac Intensive Care Unit. Ped Cardiol 2002;23:598–604.
33. Samson RA, Atkins DL. Tachyarrhythmias and defibrillation. Pediatr Clin North Am 2008;55:887–907.
34. Doniger SJ, Sharieff GQ. Pediatric dysrrhythmias. Pediatr Clin North Am 2006;53:85–105.
35. Manole MD, Saladino RA. Emergency department management of the pediatric patient with supraventricular tachycardia. Pediatr Emerg Care 2007;23:176–85.
36. Nadkarni VM, Larkin GL, Peberdy MA, Carey SM, Kaye W, Mancini ME, et al. First documented rhythm and clinical outcome from in-hospital cardiac arrest among children and adults. JAMA 2006;295:50–7.
37. Atkins DL, Everson-Stewart S, Sears GK, Daya M, Osmond MH, Warden CR, et al. Epidemiology and outcomes from out-of-hospital cardiac arrest in children: the resuscitation outcomes consortium epistry cardiac arrest. Circulation 2009;119:1484–91.

32 Chest Pain in Children and Adolescents

Chest pain comes in many varieties, ranging from a sharp stab to a dull ache. Some types of chest pain can be described as crushing or burning. In certain cases, the pain travels up the neck, pierces through to the back or radiates down one or both arms.

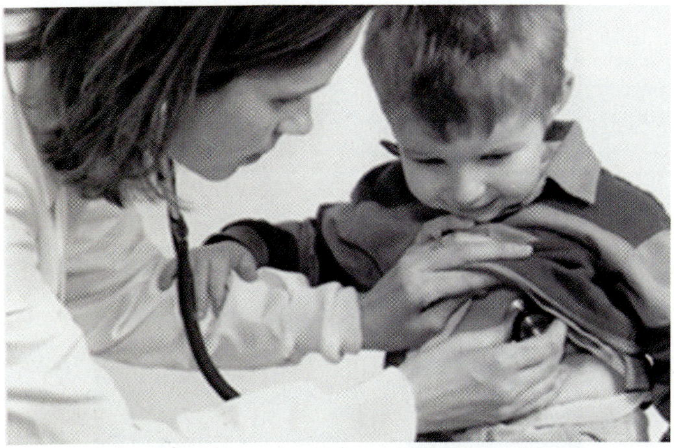

Fig. 32.1: *Doctor is examining a young child with chest pain*

Many different types of problems can cause chest pain. The most life-threatening ones involve the heart or lungs. Because it can be difficult to determine what exactly is causing chest pain, is best to seek immediate medical help.

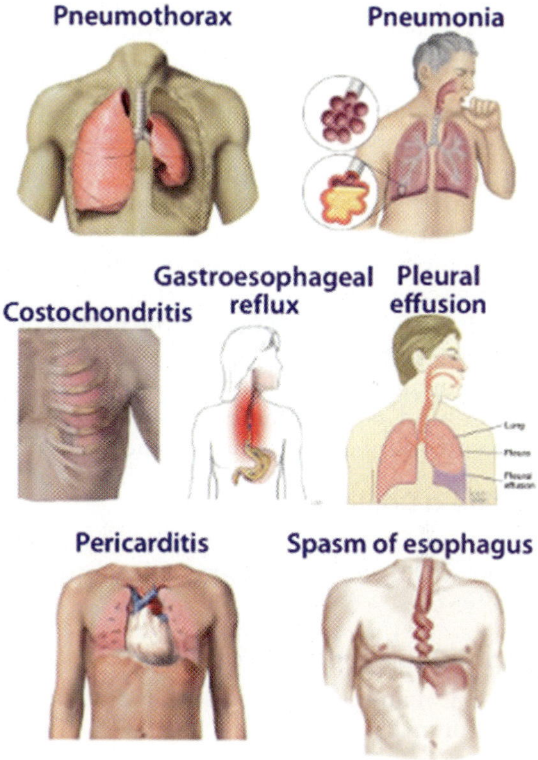

Fig. 32.2: *Various causes of chest pain*

Symptoms (Figs 32.1–32.5)

A wide range of health problems can cause chest pain. In many cases, the underlying cause has nothing to do with your heart—though there's no easy way to tell without seeing a doctor.

Heart-related Chest Pain (Figs 32.3 and 32.9)

Although chest pain is commonly attributed to heart disease, many heart patients experience a vague discomfort and they often specifically mention that pain does not seem to be an adequate description. In general, chest discomfort related to a heart attack or another heart problem may be associated with one or more of the following:

- Pressure, fullness or tightness in your chest
- Crushing or searing pain that radiates to your back, neck, jaw, shoulders and arms—particularly your left arm
- Pain that lasts more than a few minutes, goes away and comes back or varies in intensity
- Shortness of breath, sweating, dizziness or nausea

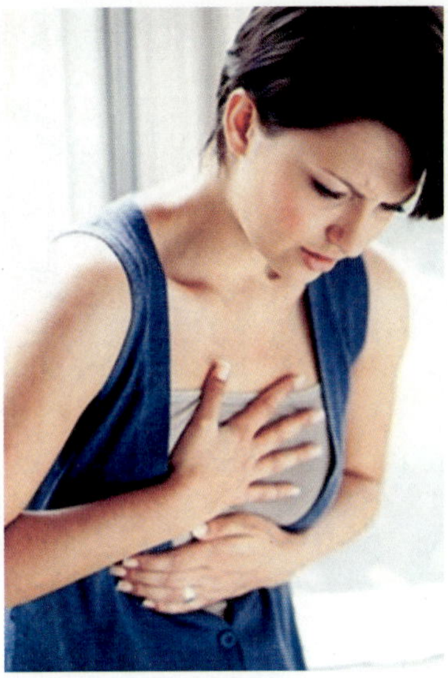

Fig. 32.3: *Chest pain in a teenage girl*

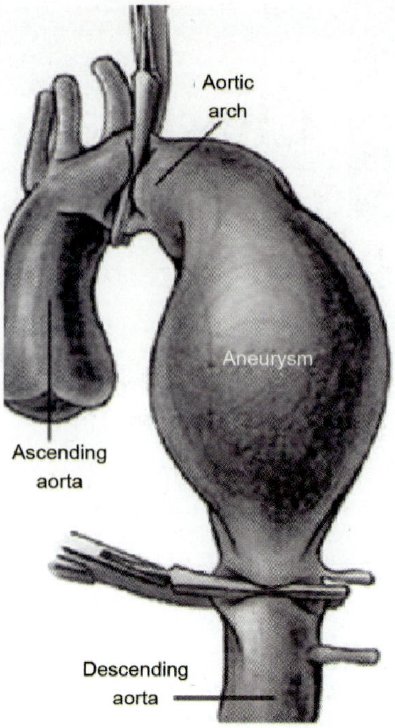

Fig. 32.4: *Aneurysm in Marfan syndrome*

Other types of Chest Pain

It can be difficult to distinguish chest pain due to a heart problem from other types of chest pain. However, chest pain that is less likely due to a heart problem is more often associated with:

- A sour taste or a sensation of food re-entering your mouth
- Trouble swallowing
- Pain that gets better or worse when you change your body position
- Pain that intensifies when you breathe deeply or cough
- Tenderness when you push on your chest.

The classic symptoms of heartburn—a painful, burning sensation behind your breastbone—can be caused by problems with your heart or your stomach.

When to See a Doctor

If you have new or unexplained chest pain or suspect you're having a heart attack, call for emergency medical help immediately.

Etiological Factors in Chest Pain

Chest pain has many possible causes, all of which deserve medical attention.

Heart-related Causes (Tables 32.1 and 32.2)

Examples of heart-related causes of chest pain include:

- **Heart attack:** A heart attack is a result of a blood clot that's blocking blood flow to your heart muscle.
- **Angina:** Thick plaques can gradually build up on the inner walls of the arteries that carry blood to your heart. These plaques narrow the arteries and restrict the heart's blood supply, particularly during exertion (Fig. 32.13).
- **Aortic dissection:** This life-threatening condition involves the main artery leading from your heart—your aorta. If the inner layers of this blood vessel separate, blood will be forced between the layers and can cause the aorta to rupture.

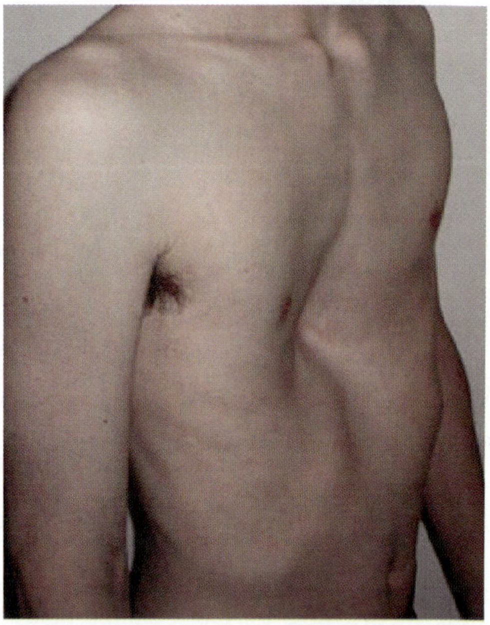

Fig. 32.5: *Chest pain in young boy with pectus excavatum*

- **Pericarditis:** This condition, an inflammation of the sac surrounding your heart, is short-lived and often related to a viral infection (Figs 32.6 and 32.10).

Digestive Causes

Chest pain can be caused by disorders of the digestive system, including:

- **Heartburn:** This painful, burning sensation behind your breastbone occurs when stomach acid washes up from your stomach into the esophagus–the tube that connects your throat to your stomach (Figs 32.9, 32.19 and 32.20).

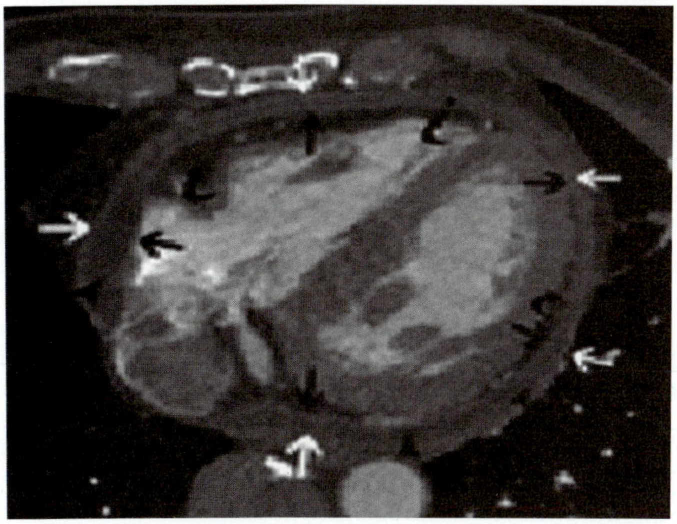

Fig. 32.6: *Acute pericarditis. Axial CT image of a 18-year-old adolescent shows thickening and enhancement of the visceral (black arrows) and parietal pericardial layers (white arrows) surrounding small amount of pericardial fluid (arrowheads). Epicardial fat is indicated by curved arrows. Small pleural effusions are present*

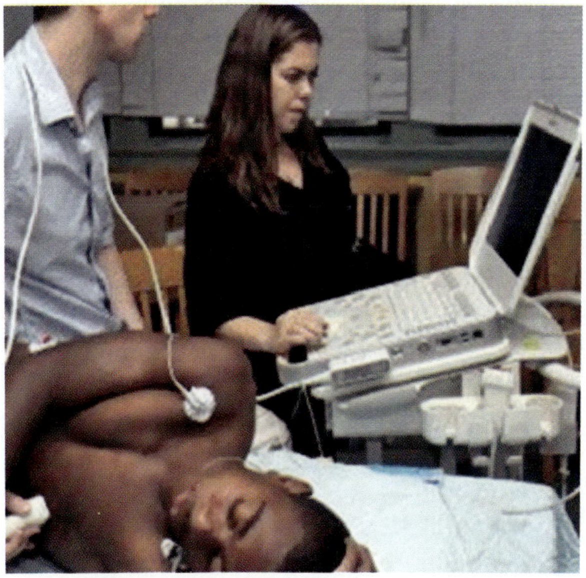

Fig. 32.7: *Child is being examined by the doctors with echocardiography for acute chest pain*

- **Swallowing disorders:** Disorders of the esophagus can make swallowing difficult and even painful.
- **Gallbladder or pancreas problems.** Gallstones or inflammation of your gallbladder or pancreas can cause abdominal pain that radiates to your chest.

Muscle and Bone Causes (Fig. 32.5)

Some types of chest pain are associated with injuries and other problems affecting the structures that make up the chest wall. Examples include:

- **Costochondritis:** In this condition, the cartilage of your rib cage, particularly the cartilage that joins your ribs to your breastbone, becomes inflamed and painful.
- **Sore muscles:** Chronic pain syndromes, such as fibromyalgia, can produce persistent muscle-related chest pain.
- **Injured ribs:** A bruised or broken rib can cause chest pain.

Lung-related Causes

Many lung disorders can cause chest pain, including:

- **Pulmonary embolism:** This cause of chest pain occurs when a blood clot becomes lodged in a lung (pulmonary) artery, blocking blood flow to lung tissue.

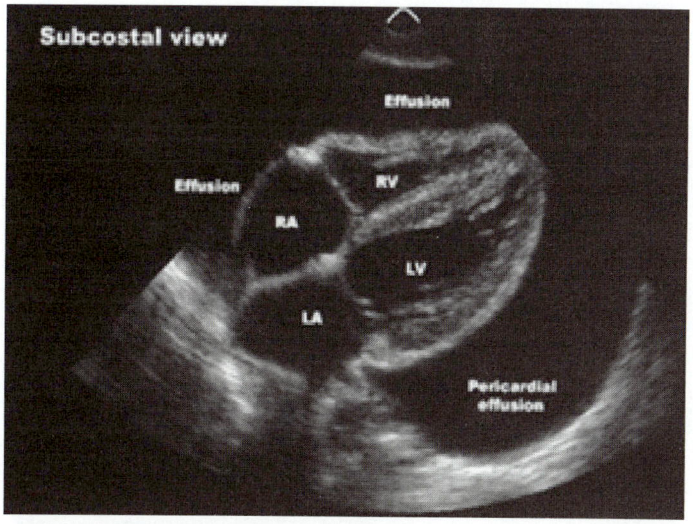

Fig. 32.8: *Subcostal view. Echocardiogram showing the presence of pericarditis with pericardial effusion*

Table 32.1: *Uncommon serious conditions in chest pain*

Condition	*Finding*
Myocardial ischaemia	Abnormal pulse or blood pressure, arrhythmia, ST segment elevation or depression, raised troponins
Pericarditis	Positional plain, pericardial rub, widespread saddle-shaped ST elevation
Pericardial effusion	Hypotension, distended neck veins, muffled heart sound, pulsus paradoxus, globular enlarged cardiac silhouette or CXR
Pulmonary embolus	Tachypnoea, tachycardia, hypoxia, haemoptysis, nonspecific ST and T wave changes in anterior chest leads most common ECG finding, classical S1Q3T3 pattern is uncommon. may seen mirror CXR abnormalities-usually normal
Aortic dissection	Differential limb BP's CXR findings include: widen-end mediastinum, left pleural cap and deviated trachea and main stem bronchi. Signs of myocardial is ischaemia or pericardial tamponade if complicated by these events

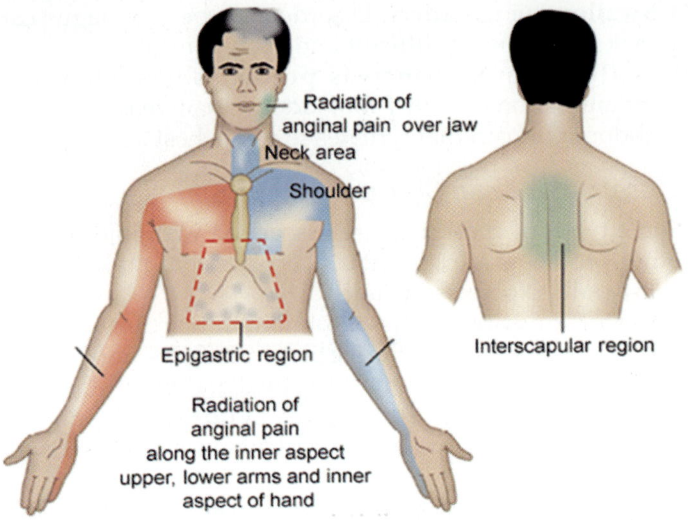

Fig. 32.9: *Diagrammatic representation of regional distribution of anginal pain*

- **Pleurisy:** If the membrane that covers your lungs becomes inflamed, it can cause chest pain that's made worse when you inhale or cough.
- **Collapsed lung:** The chest pain associated with a collapsed lung typically begins suddenly and can last for hours. A collapsed lung occurs when air leaks into the space between the lung and the ribs.
- **Pulmonary hypertension:** High blood pressure in the arteries carrying blood to the lungs (pulmonary hypertension) also can produce chest pain.

Other Cause

Chest pain can also be caused by:

- **Panic attack:** If you experience periods of intense fear accompanied by chest pain, rapid heartbeat, rapid breathing, profuse sweating and shortness of breath, you may be experiencing a panic attack.
- **Shingles:** Caused by a reactivation of the chickenpox virus, shingles can produce pain and a band of blisters from your back around to your chest wall.

Preparing for Your Appointment

Call for an ambulance or have someone drive you to an emergency room if you experience new or unexplained chest pain or pressure that lasts for more than a few moments. Don't waste any time for fear of embarrassment if it's not a heart attack. Even if there's another cause for your chest pain, you need to be seen right away.

What You can Do

On the way to the hospital, share the following information with the emergency caregivers:

- **Symptoms:** Describe your signs and symptoms in detail, noting when they started and whether anything makes the pain better or worse.
- **Medical history:** Have you ever had chest pain before? What caused it? Do you or any close family members have a history of heart disease or diabetes?
- **Medications:** Having a list of all the medications and supplements you regularly take will be helpful to the emergency workers. You might want to prepare such a list in advance to carry in your wallet or purse.

Once you're at the hospital, it's likely that your medical evaluation will move ahead rapidly. Based on results from an electrocardiogram (ECG) and blood tests, your doctor may be able to quickly determine if you are having a heart attack - or give you another explanation for your symptoms. You'll probably have a number of questions at this point. If you haven't received the following information, you may want to ask:

- What is likely causing my symptoms or condition?

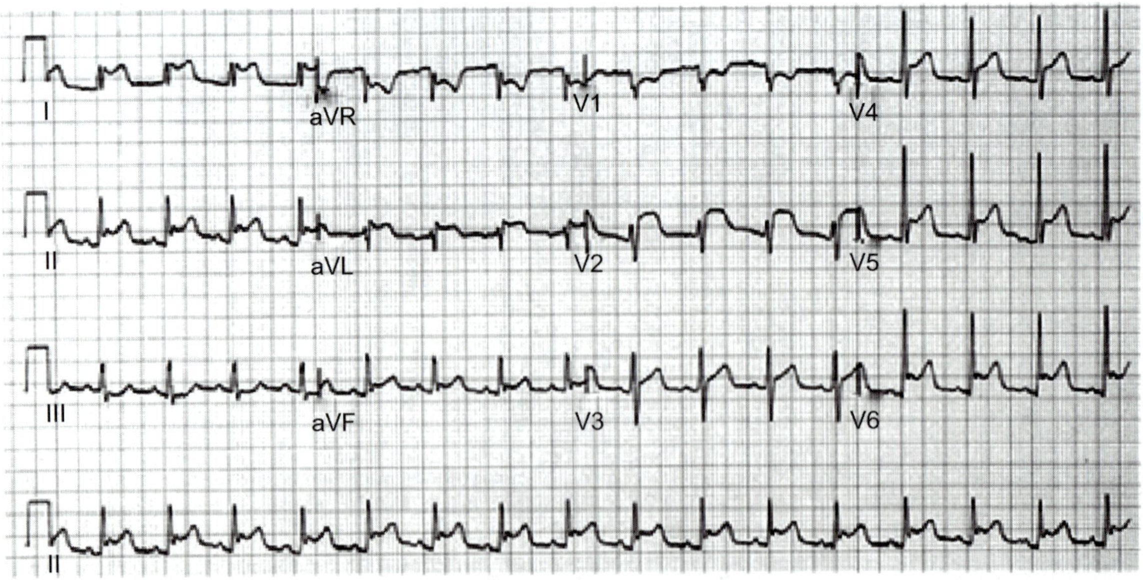

Fig. 32.10: *ECG features of acute pericarditis 1. Diffuse concave up ST segment elevation. 2. T waves are concordant with ST segment. 3. ST segment depression in aVR and V1. 4. PR segment depression. 5. Absence of reciprocal ST segment depression*

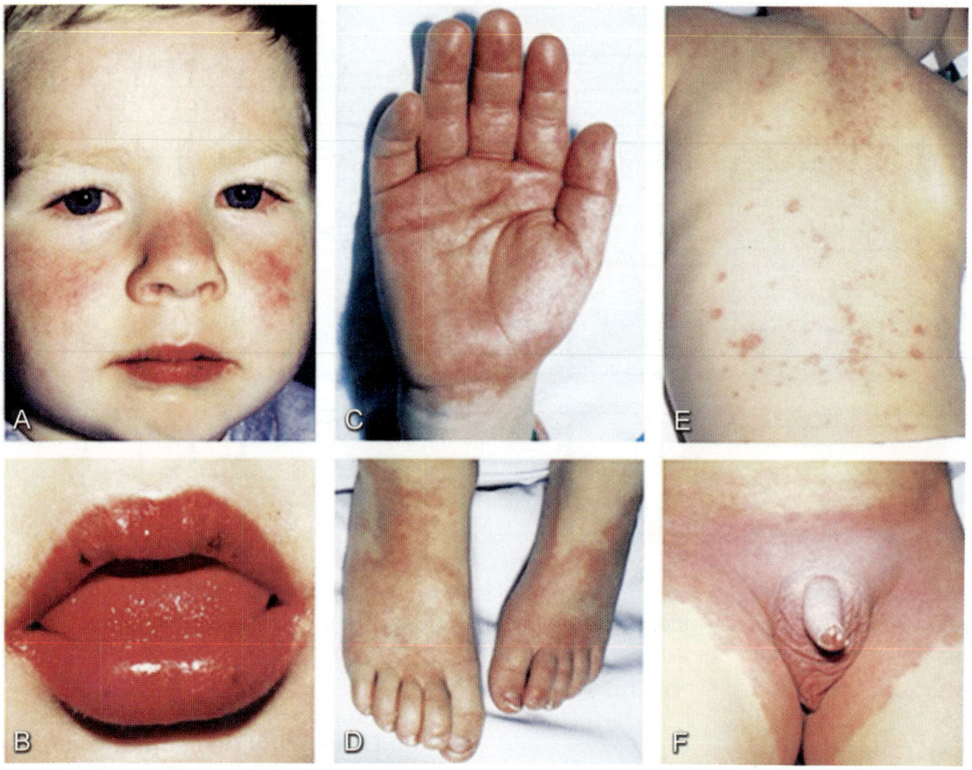

Figs 32.11A to F: *Photographs of a 4-year-old boy show the typical features of Kawasaki's disease. These features include bilateral nonexudative conjunctivitis (Panel A); dry, fissured, erythematous lips and a "strawberry" tongue (Panels A and B); erythematous and edematous hands and feet (Panels C and D); an erythematous truncal rash (Panel E); and a desquamating perineal rash (Panel F). the patient also had anterior cervical lymphadenopathy and sterile pyuria but none of the other complications of the disease. The child recovered uneventfully after receiving treatment with intravenous immune globulin and aspirin*

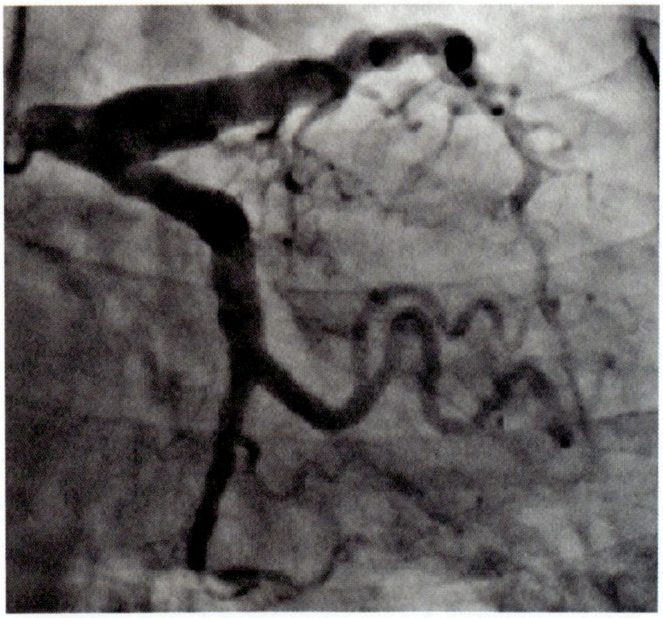

Fig. 32.12: *RAO caudal view showing aneurysmal left anterior descending and left circumflex coronary arteries in an adolescent with Kawasaki's disease*

- Are there other possible causes for my symptoms or condition?
- What kinds of tests do I need?
- Do I need to be hospitalized?
- What treatments do I need right now?
- Are there any risks associated with these treatments?
- What are the next steps in my diagnosis and treatment?
- Do I need to follow any restrictions after returning home?
- Should I see a specialist?

Don't hesitate to ask any additional questions that occur to you during your medical evaluation.

What to expect from the doctor

A doctor who sees you for chest pain may ask:
- When did your symptoms start? Have they gotten worse over time?
- Where does your pain seem to start?
- Does your pain radiate to any other parts of your body?
- What words would you use to describe your pain?
- Are you having any trouble breathing?
- Do your symptoms include dizziness or light headedness?
- Do your symptoms include vomiting?
- Do you have high blood pressure? If so, do you take medicine for it?
- Do you or did you smoke? How much?
- Do you use alcohol or caffeine? How much?
- Do you use illicit drugs, such as cocaine?

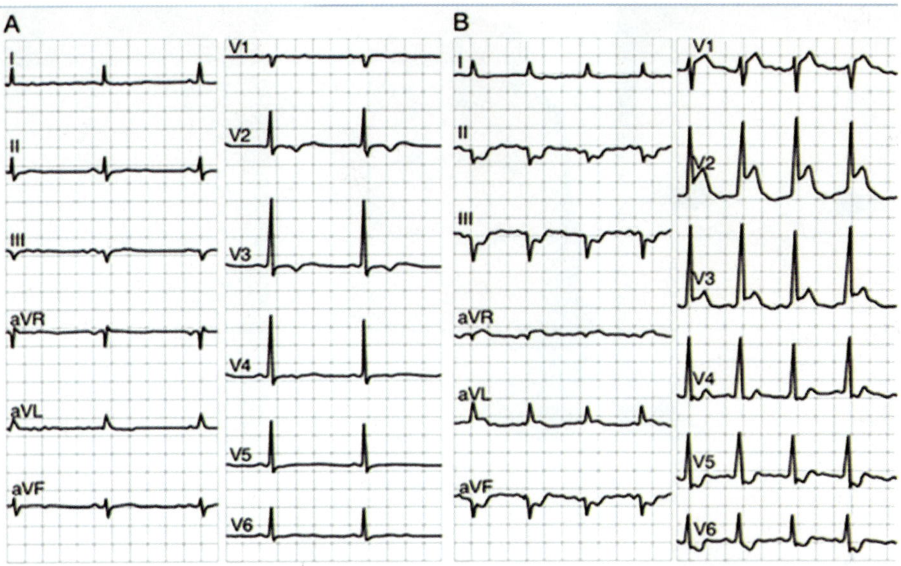

Fig. 32.13: *ECG on admission showing mild T wave inversion in the precordial leads (A). ECG tracing during exercise stress test at maximal workload demonstrating left-axis deviation and pronounced ST segment elevation in the precardial leads (5 mm in V2) (B). in an adolescent with chest pain syndrome*

Tests and Diagnosis

Chest pain doesn't always signal a heart attack. But, that's what emergency room doctors will test for first because it's potentially the most immediate threat to your life. They may also check for life-threatening lung conditions—such as a collapsed lung or a clot in your lung.

1. *Immediate Tests*

Some of the first tests you may undergo include:

- **Electrocardiogram (ECG):** This test records the electrical activity of your heart through electrodes attached to your skin. Because injured heart muscle doesn't conduct electrical impulses normally, the ECG may show that a heart attack has occurred or is in progress (Figs 32.10–32.13A ad B).
- **Blood tests:** Your doctor may order blood tests to check for increased levels of certain enzymes normally found in heart muscle. Damage to heart cells from a heart attack may allow these enzymes to leak, over a period of hours, into your blood.
- **Chest X-ray:** An X-ray of your chest allows doctors to check the condition of your lungs and the size and shape of your heart and major blood vessels. A chest X-ray can also reveal lung problems such as pneumonia or a collapsed lung.
- **Echocardiogram:** An echocardiogram uses sound waves to produce a video image of your heart in motion. In some cases, a small device may be passed down your throat to obtain better views of different parts of your heart (Figs 32.7 and 32.8).

Table 32.2: *Risk factors for serious or life-threatening conditions*

Risk factor	*Condition to consider*
Major chest trauma	Pneumothorax, haemothorax, cardiac or pulmonary contusion, mediastinal disruption.
Prior cardiac disease or surgery	Myocardial ischaemia, arrhythmia, pericarditis, pericardial effusion.
Hypercoaguable states (primary clotting disorders, neoplasms, pregnancy, contraceptive pill use prolonged immobility or post-surgery, cental venous catheters, connective tissue disease, past history or strong family history of thromboembolic disease)	Pulmonary embolus
Sickle cell disease	Acute chest syndrome
Chronic respiratory disease	Pneumothorax
Kawasaki disease	Coronary aneurysm and myocardial ischaemia
Familial hyperlipidaemia syndromes	Myocardial ischaemia
Cocaine or stimulant use	Myocardial ischaemia
Connective tissue disease	Pericarditis and pericardial effusion, aortic dissection

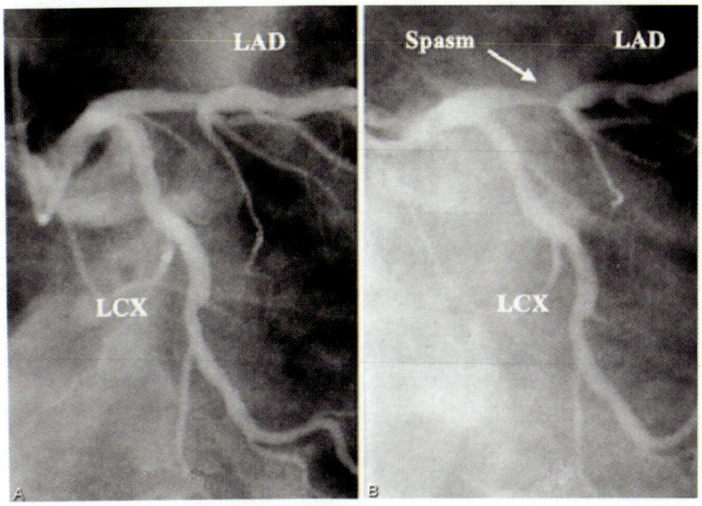

Figs 32.14A and B: *Angiographic images of the left coronary artery (right anterior oblique) demonstrating a nonsignificantly diseased proximal LAD (A) developing a spontaneous sustained spasm (B) in an adolescent with chest pain syndrome*

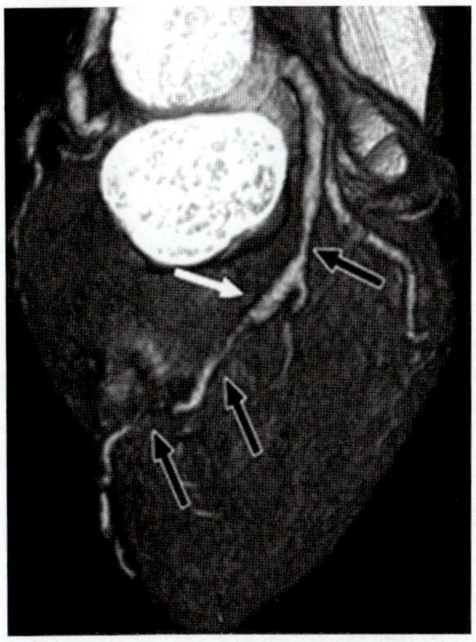

Fig. 32.15: *18-year-old man with Kawasaki disease. Volume-rendering MDCT image shows braid like appearance with multifocal aneurysmal change (white arrow) and stenosis (black arrows) at left anterior descending artery*

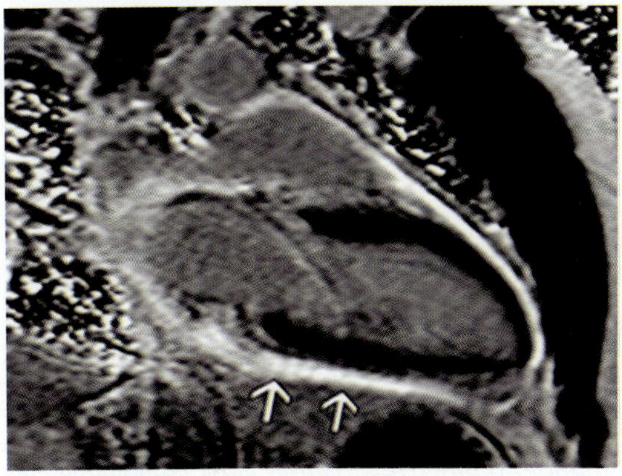

Fig. 32.16: *Pericarditis. Two chamber DE-MRI demonstrates diffuse, intense pericardial enhancement, more prominent inferiorly, consistent with acute pericarditis*

- **Computerized tomography (CT scan):** Different types of CT scans can be used to check your heart arteries for signs of calcium, which indicate areas where plaque blockages are accumulating. CT scans can also be done with dye to check your heart and lung arteries for blockages and other problems (Figs 32.6, 32.15 and 32.18).
- **Magnetic resonance imaging (MRI):** MRI is an imaging technique that uses magnetic fields and radio waves to create cross-sectional images of your body. MRI of the heart is sometimes done to look for evidence of damage to the heart or aorta (Fig. 32.16).
- **Stress tests:** These measure how your heart and blood vessels respond to exertion, which may indicate if your pain is related to your heart. There are many kinds of stress tests. You may be asked to walk on a treadmill or pedal a stationary bike while hooked up to an ECG. Or you may be given a drug intravenously to stimulate your heart in a way similar to exercise (Figs 32.13A and B).
- **Coronary catheterization (angiogram):** This test helps doctors identify individual arteries to your heart that may be narrowed or blocked. A liquid dye is injected into the arteries of your heart through a catheter—a long, thin tube that's fed through an artery, usually in your groin, to arteries in your heart. As the dye fills your arteries, they become visible on X-ray and video (Figs 32.14, 32.21A and B).

Management of Chest Pain

Treatment will vary depending on the underlying cause of your chest pain.

Medications

Drugs used to treat some of the most common causes of chest pain include:

- **Artery relaxers:** Nitroglycerin—usually taken as a tablet under the tongue—relaxes heart arteries, so blood can flow more easily through the narrowed spaces. Some blood pressure medicines also relax and widen blood vessels.
- **Clot-busting drugs:** If you are having a heart attack, you may receive drugs that work to dissolve the clot that is blocking blood from reaching your heart muscle.
- **Blood thinners:** If you have a clot in an artery feeding your heart or lungs, you'll be given drugs that inhibit blood clotting—to help prevent more clots from forming.
- **Antacids:** If your chest pain is caused by stomach acid splashing up your esophagus, the doctor may suggest medications that reduce the amount of acid in your stomach (Figs 32.19 and 32.20).
- **Antianxiety drugs:** If you are experiencing panic attacks, your doctor may prescribe antianxiety drugs to help control your symptoms.

Surgical and other Procedures

Procedures used to treat some of the most dangerous causes of chest pain include (Figs 32.21A and B):

- **Balloons and stents:** If your chest pain is caused by a blockage in an artery feeding your heart, doctors insert narrow tubing into a large blood vessel in your groin

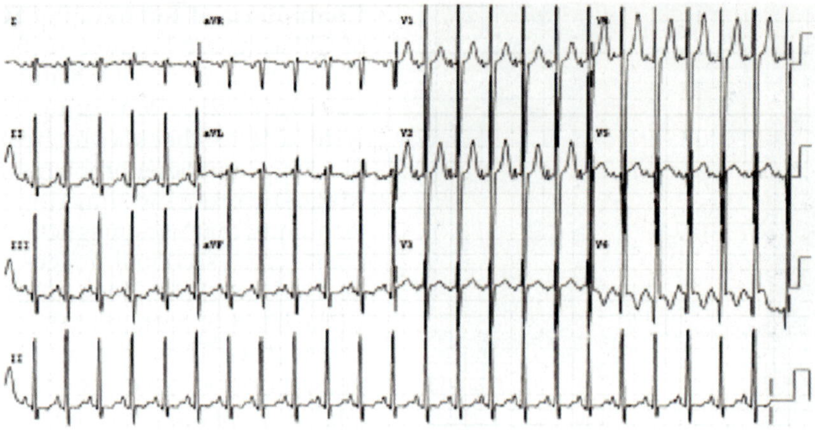

Fig. 32.17: *ECG from day 1 of presentation in patient with ALCAPA. Typical prominent Q waves are present in lead V6. Conversely, typical abrupt loss of R waves in midprecordial leads and prominent Q waves in leads I and aVL associated with ALCAPA are not present*

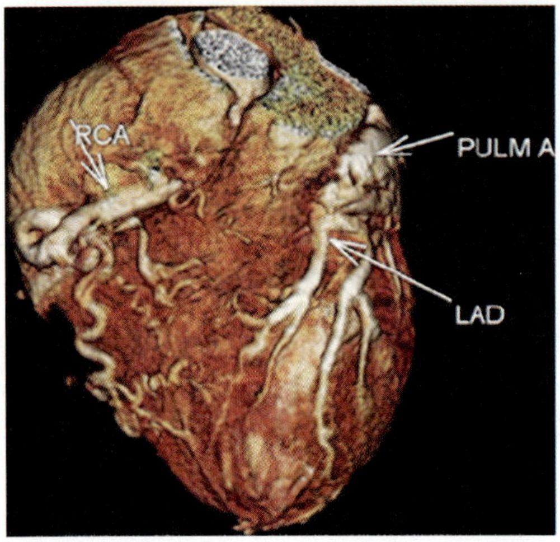

Fig. 32.18: *CT angiography volume rendered image. Right coronary artery is dilated and tortious with a large number of collaterals feeding the left coronary system. Left coronary artery is emerging from pulmonary artery trunk. The left anterior descending artery and their diagonal branches are also dilated and tortuous*

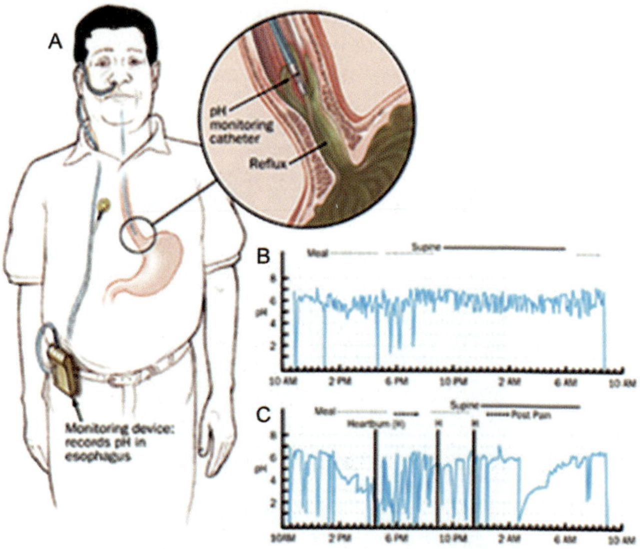

Figs 32.20A to C: *(A) pH monitor placement. Inset shows the catheter position in the esophagus; (B) normal pH monitor tracing; (C) abnormal continuous pH monitor tracing*

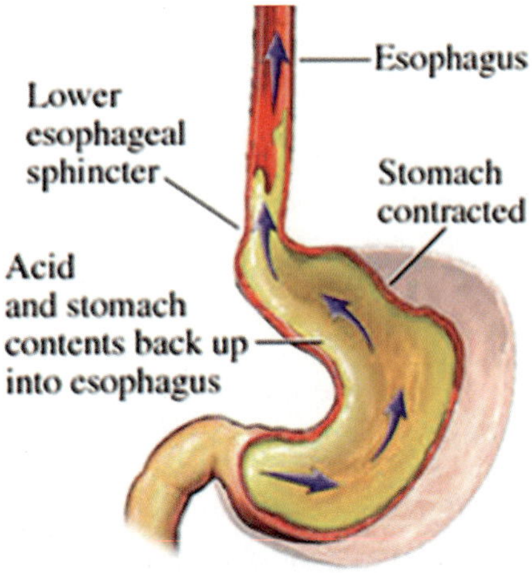

Fig. 32.19: *Illustration showing gastroesophageal reflux disease (GERD disorder that results from food and stomach acid backing up into the esophagus from the stomach as one of the causes of chest pain*

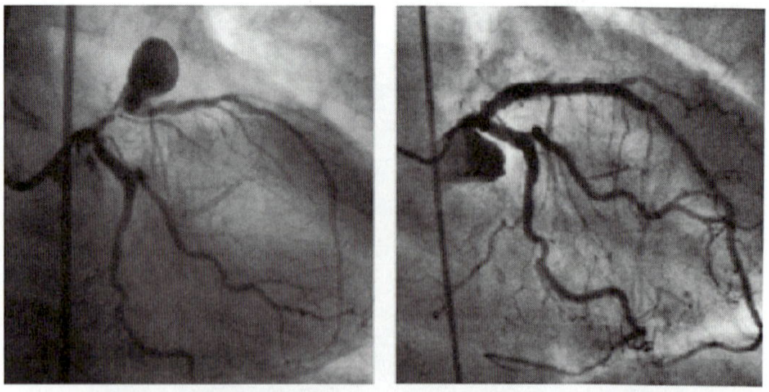

Figs 32.21A and B: *Coronary angiography revealed a large saccular aneurysm of the proximal left anterior descending coronary artery (Left). The covered stent completely closed the entrance of the aneurysm, and no contrast medium was seen entering the aneurysm in the final angiographic images (Right) in patient with Kawasaki's disease*

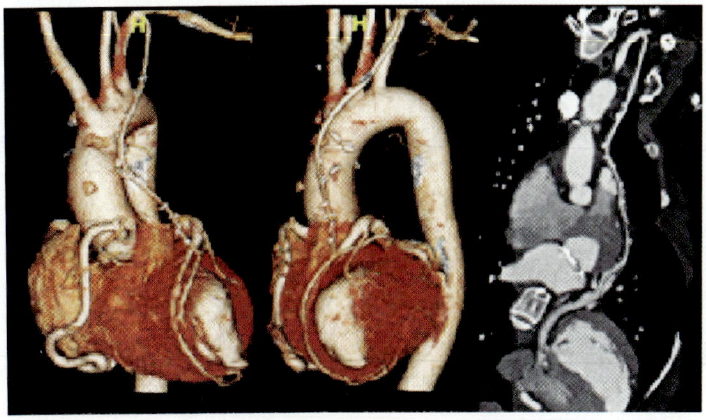

Fig. 32.22: *CT angio showing left main coronary artery to pulmonary artery closure with CABG (LIMA to LAD) in patient with ALCAPA*

and then thread it up to the blockage. They then deploy a balloon to reopen the artery. In many cases, a small wire mesh tube (stent) is inserted to keep the artery open.

- **Bypass surgery:** During this procedure, surgeons take a blood vessel from another part of your body and use it to create an alternative route for blood to go around the blocked artery (Fig. 32.22).
- **Dissection repair:** You may need emergency surgery to repair an aortic dissection-a life-threatening condition that can result in the rupture of the artery that carries blood from your heart to the rest of your body.
- **Lung reinflation:** If you have a collapsed lung, doctors may insert a tube in your chest, which allows the lung to reinflate.

BIBLIOGRAPHY

1. Selbst SM. Chest pain in children. Pediatrics 1985; 75:1068.
2. Selbst SM, Ruddy RM, Clark BJ, et al. Pediatric chest pain: a prospective study. Pediatrics 1988; 82:319.
3. Brown RT. Costochondritis in adolescents. J Adolesc Health Care 1981; 1:198.
4. Brunswick AF, Boyle JM, Tarica C. Who sees the doctor? A study of urban black adolescents. Soc Sci Med Med Psychol Med Sociol 1979; 13A:45.
5. Pantell RH, Goodman BW Jr. Adolescent chest pain: a prospective study. Pediatrics 1983; 71:881.
6. Fyfe DA, Moodie DS. Chest pain in pediatric patients presenting to a cardiac clinic. Clin Pediatr (Phila) 1984; 23:321.
7. Rowland TW, Richards MM. The natural history of idiopathic chest pain in children. A follow-up study. Clin Pediatr (Phila) 1986; 25:612.
8. Selbst SM, Ruddy R, Clark BJ. Chest pain in children. Follow-up of patients previously reported. Clin Pediatr (Phila) 1990; 29:374.
9. Driscoll DJ, Glicklich LB, Gallen WJ. Chest pain in children: a prospective study. Pediatrics 1976; 57:648.
10. Kocis KC. Chest pain in pediatrics. Pediatr Clin North Am 1999; 46:189.
11. Tunaoglu FS, Olguntürk R, Akcabay S, et al. Chest pain in children referred to a cardiology clinic. Pediatr Cardiol 1995; 16:69.
12. Anzai AK, Merkin TE. Adolescent chest pain. Am Fam Physician 1996; 53:1682.
13. Zavaras-Angelidou KA, Weinhouse E, Nelson DB. Review of 180 episodes of chest pain in 134 children. Pediatr Emerg Care 1992; 8:189.
14. Selbst SM. Evaluation of chest pain in children. Pediatr Rev 1986; 8:56.
15. Evangelista JA, Parsons M, Renneburg AK. Chest pain in children: diagnosis through history and physical examination. J Pediatr Health Care 2000; 14:3.
16. Saleeb SF, Li WY, Warren SZ, Lock JE. Effectiveness of screening for life-threatening chest pain in children. Pediatrics 2011; 128:e1062.
17. Epstein SE, Gerber LH, Borer JS. Chest wall syndrome. A common cause of unexplained cardiac pain. JAMA 1979; 241:2793.
18. Porter GE. Slipping rib syndrome: an infrequently recognized entity in children: a report of three cases and review of the literature. Pediatrics 1985; 76:810.
19. Mooney DP, Shorter NA. Slipping rib syndrome in childhood. J Pediatr Surg 1997; 32:1081.
20. Taubman B, Vetter VL. Slipping rib syndrome as a cause of chest pain in children. Clin Pediatr (Phila) 1996; 35:403.
21. Heinz GJ, Zavala DC. Slipping rib syndrome. JAMA 1977; 237:794.
22. Coleman WL. Recurrent chest pain in children. Pediatr Clin North Am 1984; 31:1007.
23. Pickering D. Precordial catch syndrome. Arch Dis Child 1981; 56:401.
24. Friedman SB. Conversion symptoms in adolescents. Pediatr Clin North Am 1973; 20:873.
25. Smith MS. Psychosomatic symptoms in adolescence. Med Clin North Am 1990; 74:1121.
26. Asnes RS, Santulli R, Bemporad JR. Psychogenic chest pain in children. Clin Pediatr (Phila) 1981; 20:788.
27. Kashani JH, Lababidi Z, Jones RS. Depression in children and adolescents with cardiovascular symptomatology: the significance of chest pain. J Am Acad Child Psychiatry 1982; 21:187.
28. Neill WA, Hattenhauer M. Impairment of myocardial O2 supply due to hyperventilation. Circulation 1975; 52:854.
29. Wiens L, Sabath R, Ewing L, et al. Chest pain in otherwise healthy children and adolescents is frequently caused by exercise-induced asthma. Pediatrics 1992; 90:350.
30. Damore DT, Dayan PS. Medical causes of pneumomediastinum in children. Clin Pediatr (Phila) 2001; 40:87.
31. Stack AM, Caputo GL. Pneumomediastinum in childhood asthma. Pediatr Emerg Care 1996; 12:98.
32. Chalumeau M, Le Clainche L, Sayeg N, et al. Spontaneous pneumomediastinum in children. Pediatr Pulmonol 2001; 31:67.
33. Orenstein DM, Winnie GB, Altman H. Cystic fibrosis: a 2002 update. J Pediatr 2002; 140:156.
34. Hall JR, Pyeritz RE, Dudgeon DL, Haller JA Jr. Pneumothorax in the Marfan syndrome: prevalence and therapy. Ann Thorac Surg 1984; 37:500.
35. Ravilly S, Robinson W, Suresh S, et al. Chronic pain in cystic fibrosis. Pediatrics 1996; 98:741.
36. Berezin S, Medow MS, Glassman MS, Newman LJ. Chest pain of gastrointestinal origin. Arch Dis Child 1988; 63:1457.
37. Glassman MS, Medow MS, Berezin S, Newman LJ. Spectrum of esophageal disorders in children with chest pain. Dig Dis Sci 1992; 37:663.

38. Long WB, Cohen S. The digestive tract as a cause of chest pain. Am Heart J 1980; 100:567.
39. Bernstein D, Coupey S, Schonberg SK. Pulmonary embolism in adolescents. Am J Dis Child 1986; 140:667.
40. Buck JR, Connors RH, Coon WW, et al. Pulmonary embolism in children. J Pediatr Surg 1981; 16:385.
41. Goldsby RE, Saulys AJ, Helton JG. Pediatric pulmonary artery thromboembolism: an illustrative case. Pediatr Emerg Care 1996; 12:105.
42. Evans DA, Wilmott RW. Pulmonary embolism in children. Pediatr Clin North Am 1994; 41:569.
43. Brenner JI, Ringel RE, Berman MA. Cardiologic perspectives of chest pain in childhood: a referral problem? To whom? Pediatr Clin North Am 1984; 31:1241.
44. Graneto JW, Turnbull TL, Marciniak SA. An unusual cause of chest pain in an adolescent presenting to the emergency department. Pediatr Emerg Care 1997; 13:33.45.
45. Vaughan CJ, Casey M, He J, et al. Identification of a chromosome 11q23.2–q24 locus for familial aortic aneurysm disease, a genetically heterogeneous disorder. Circulation 2001; 103:2469.
46. Ratnapalan S, Brown K, Benson L. Children presenting with acute pericarditis to the emergency department. Pediatr Emerg Care 2011; 27:581.
47. Karaaslan T, Gudinchet F, Payot M, Sekarski N. Congenital aneurysm of sinus of valsalva ruptured into right ventricle diagnosed by magnetic resonance imaging. Pediatr Cardiol 1999; 20:212.
48. Ivy D, Kaye J, Flitter D, Wiggins J. Variant angina in an adolescent. Pediatr Cardiol 1994; 15:45.
49. Wilkes D, Donner R, Black I, Carabello BA. Variant angina in an 11 year old boy. J Am Coll Cardiol 1985; 5:761.
50. Perry RF, Garlisi AP, Allison EJ, et al. Acute myocardial infarction in a 16–year-old boy with no predisposing risk factors. Pediatr Emerg Care 1997; 13:413.
51. Mahle WT, Campbell RM, Favaloro-Sabatier J. Myocardial infarction in adolescents. J Pediatr 2007; 151:150.
52. Bisset GS 3rd, Schwartz DC, Meyer RA, et al. Clinical spectrum and long-term follow-up of isolated mitral valve prolapse in 119 children. Circulation 1980; 62:423.
53. Freed LA, Levy D, Levine RA, et al. Prevalence and clinical outcome of mitral-valve prolapse. N Engl J Med 1999; 341:1.
54. Arfken CL, Lachman AS, McLaren MJ, et al. Mitral valve prolapse: associations with symptoms and anxiety. Pediatrics 1990; 85:311.
55. Hollander JE, Todd KH, Green G, et al. Chest pain associated with cocaine: an assessment of prevalence in suburban and urban emergency departments. Ann Emerg Med 1995; 26:671.
56. Woodward GA, Selbst SM. Chest pain secondary to cocaine use. Pediatr Emerg Care 1987; 3:153.
57. Isner JM, Estes NA 3rd, Thompson PD, et al. Acute cardiac events temporally related to cocaine abuse. N Engl J Med 1986; 315:1438.
58. Lantner, IL. Adolescent chest pain (letter). Pediatrics 1983; 72:916.
59. Friedman GD, Siegelaub AB, Dales LG. Cigarette smoking and chest pain. Ann Intern Med 1975; 83:1.

33 Myocardial Infarction in Children and Adolescents

Acute myocardial infarction is rare in childhood and adolescence. Although adults acquire coronary artery disease from lifelong deposition of atheroma and plaque, which causes coronary artery spasm and thrombosis, children usually have either an acute inflammatory condition of the coronary arteries or an anomalous origin of the left coronary artery. Intrauterine myocardial infarction also does occur, often in association with coronary artery stenosis (Fig. 33.1).

Pathophysiology

Whatever the etiology, the final common pathway of acute myocardial infarction includes myocardial ischemia (resulting in hypoxia), release of inflammatory cytokines, and cell death. The terminal event is often a cardiac arrhythmia, either ventricular tachycardia deteriorating to ventricular fibrillation or extreme bradycardic arrest. The onset of the terminal event is heralded by a loss of peripheral circulation and consciousness and by cardiovascular collapse and cardiac arrest (Figs 33.4 and 33.6A to E).

Incidence

According to the Centers for Disease Control and Prevention (CDC), annual mortality rates in the United States from all causes in the pediatric population range from 22 deaths per 100,000 population in children aged 5–14 years to 756 deaths per 100,000 population in infants younger than 1 year. (Compare this to 90 deaths per 100,000 in persons aged 15–24 y and 2,538 deaths 100,000 in individuals aged 65–74 y.

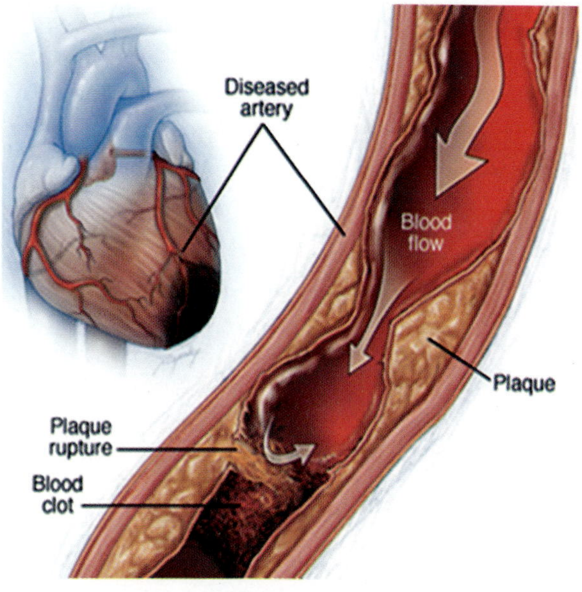

Fig. 33.1: *Involvement of different stages in the pathogenesis of acute myocardial infarction*

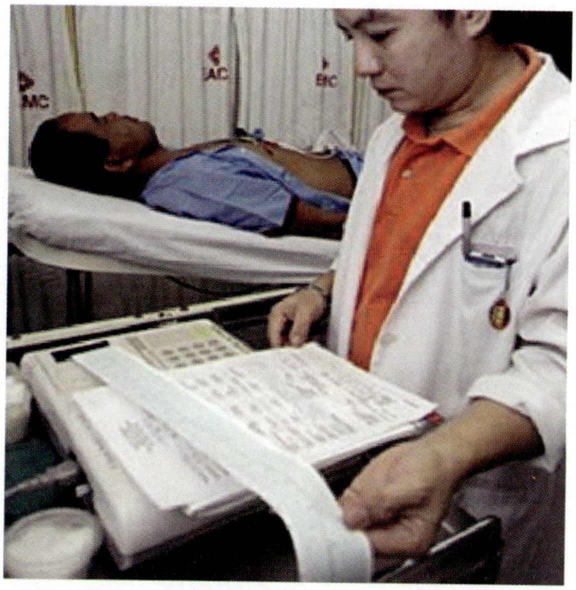

Fig. 33.2: *ECG is being taken in a young patient with cardiac chest pain*

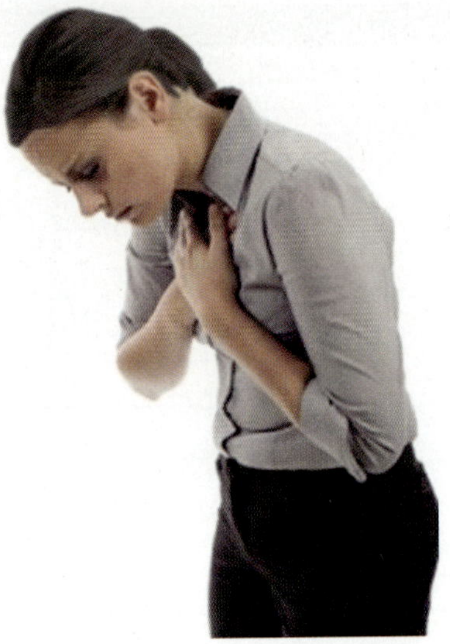

Fig. 33.3: *An adolescent is having acute chest pain prior to acute myocardial infarction*

The CDC also reports that the mortality rate from acute myocardial infarction is 0.2 deaths per 100,000 population in persons aged 15–24 years and fewer than 0.2 deaths per 100,000 in infants younger than 1 year. (Compare this to 1.4 deaths per 100,000 population in persons aged 25–34 y and 262 deaths per 100,000 population in individuals aged 65–74 y.

One study used data from the Nationwide Inpatient Sample (NIS) from 1998–2001 to determine the incidence and outcomes of adolescent acute myocardial infarction and revealed an incidence of 157 cases per year, or 6.6 events per 1 million patient-years. Within the subset of adolescents with acute myocardial infarction, the incidence was higher in individuals aged 16–18 years than in individuals aged 13–15 years.

Mortality/Morbidity

Acute myocardial infarction affects a small subset of children at risk for sudden cardiac death. Sudden cardiac death is defined as any natural death from cardiac causes that occurs from minutes to 24 hours after onset of symptoms.

- The early mortality rate can be high, depending on the cause, the speed of diagnosis, and the availability of therapeutic interventions.
- Unlike adult myocardial infarction secondary to ischemic and atherogenic disease, children with myocardial infarction who survive are less likely to have significant prolonged illness or disability.
- Some data suggest the hospital survival for acute myocardial infarction in adolescents is excellent (mortality rate is 0.8%).

Sex and Age

One study from the NIS suggests a significant male preponderance in adolescent acute myocardial infarction (80%).

The etiology of myocardial infarction determines the age of incidence.

- Anomalous origin of the left coronary artery from the pulmonary artery (ALCAPA) may occur as unexplained sudden death in a neonate.
- Coronary artery ostial stenosis may occur after repair of a dextro-transposition of the great arteries (D-TGA) in the neonatal period. In childhood, infarction may occur years after arterial switch due to kinking of the coronary arteries, possibly in association with aortic root dilation.
- Thrombotic coronary artery occlusion from Kawasaki disease may occur in early childhood.
- Sudden death from an aberrantly coursing left main coronary artery with its origin at the right sinus of Valsalva may occur in athletes who are exercising.

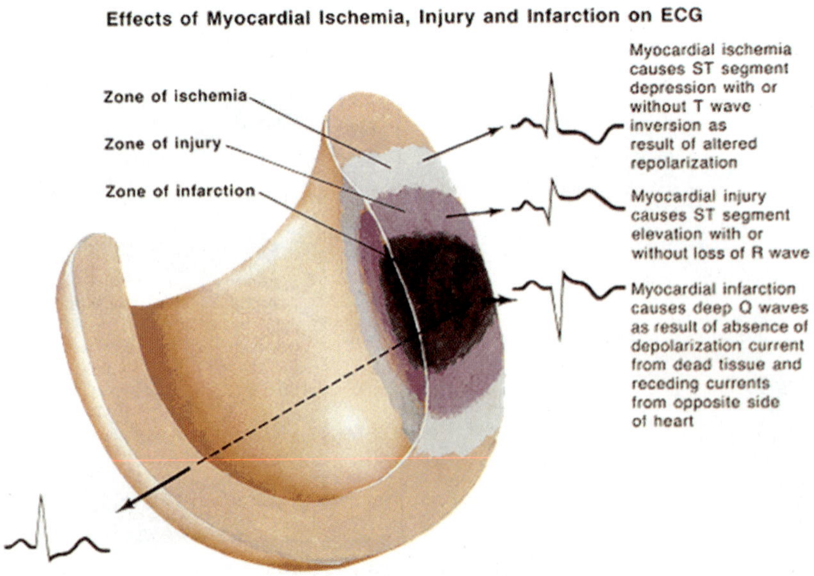

Fig. 33.4: *Zones of ischemia injury and infarction*

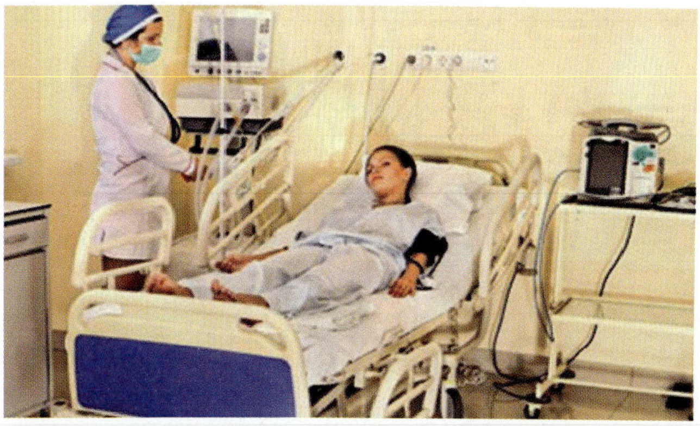

Fig. 33.5: *A young child is under treatment in CCU for acute myocardial infarction as a result of anomalous origin of left coronary artery from pulmonary artery (ALCAPA)*

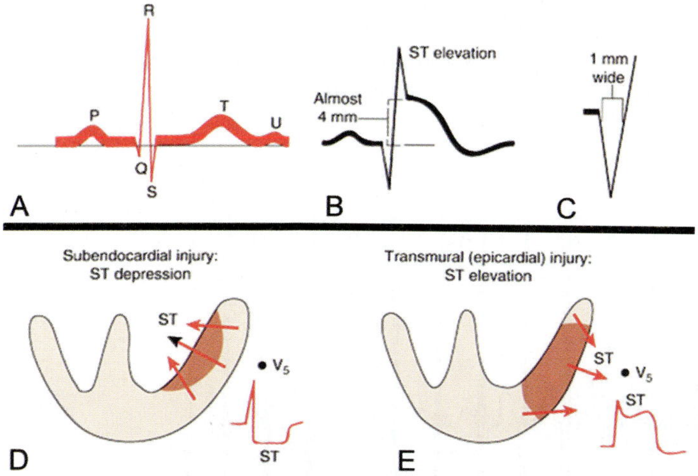

Figs 33.6A to E: *(Top) (A) ECG tracing showing normal P, Q,R,S and T waves. (B) ST elevation with acute ischemia. (C) Q wave with acute myocardial infarction. (Bottom) Current-of-injury patterns with acute ischemia. With predominant subendocardial ischemia (D), the resultant ST segment is directed toward the inner layer of the affected ventricle and the ventricular cavity. Overlying leads therefore record ST-segment depression. With ischemia involving the outer ventricular layer (E) (transmural or epicardial injury), the ST vector is directed outward. Overlying leads record ST-segment elevation [adapted from Braunwald E, Zipes DP, Libby P. (2002)]*

- Coronary insufficiency may develop in patients with Marfan syndrome, Takayasu arteritis, or cystic medial necrosis with aortic root dilatation, aneurysm formation, and dissection into the coronary artery.
- Although very rarely, traumatic myocardial infarction can occur in patients at any age but is more likely to occur in ambulatory patients.
- **Accelerated atherosclerosis** is known to occur in orthotopic cardiac transplant recipients on immunosuppressive therapy and can occur in early adolescence.
- **Coronary artery spasm** as a cause of acute typical chest pain with associated cardiac enzyme elevation has been increasingly recognized in adolescents with otherwise normal coronary arteries.
- The incidence of substance abuse and smoking are higher in adolescents with acute myocardial infarction than in adolescents admitted to the hospital for other conditions.

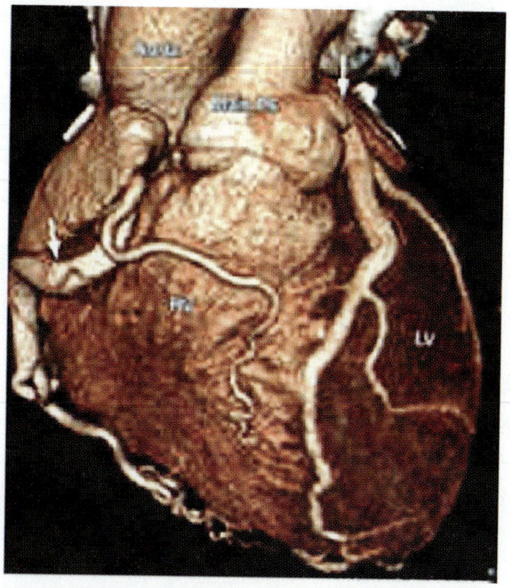

Fig. 33.7: *A three dimensional, volume-rendered coronary CTA image shows the anomalous origin of the left main coronary artery from the main pulmonary artery (PA) (white arrow). Note the ectatic left and right (white arrow) coronary arteries. LV, left ventricle; RV, right ventricle*

History

Patients who experience myocardial infarction in whom sudden death does not occur may present with a prodrome that can include any of the following features:

- Chest pain (angina) (Fig. 33.3)
- Palpitation
- Dyspnea
- Evidence of poor cardiac output
- Weakness
- Dizziness
- Mental confusion
- Irritability
- Orthostasis
- Presyncope
- Syncope.

Physical Examination

Examination findings vary, depending on the degree of disability and duration of ischemia.

- Altered level of consciousness
  - Lethargy
  - Unconsciousness
  - Irritability
- Pulse abnormalities
  - Tachycardia
  - Bradycardia
  - Dysrhythmia
- Respiratory embarrassment

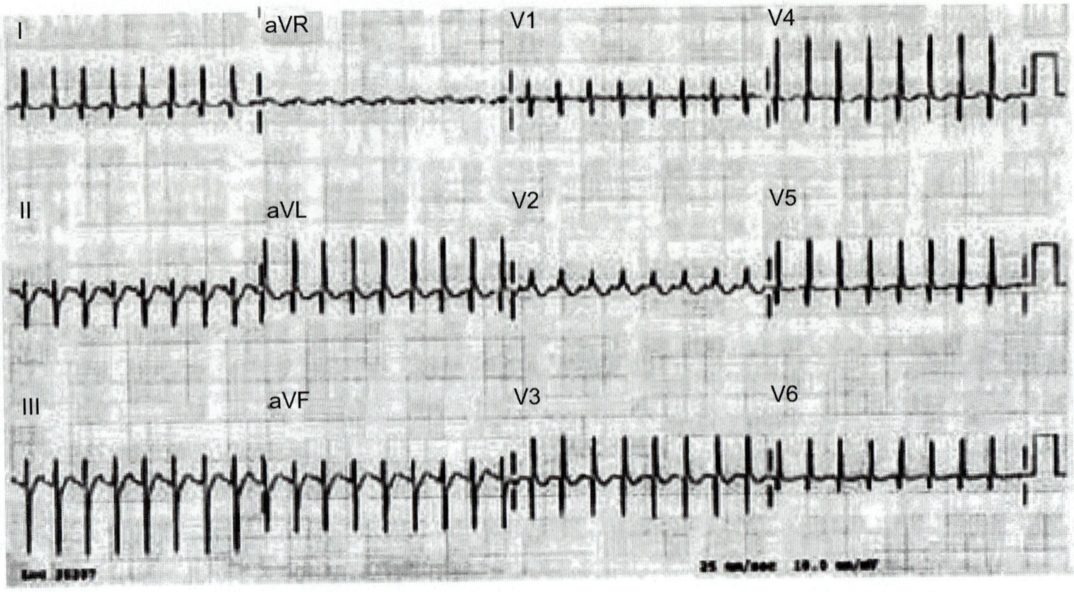

Fig. 33.8: *Electrocardiogram in an infant with anomalous origin of the left coronary artery from the pulmonary artery, demonstrating pathologic q waves in leads I and aVL and diffuse ST-T wave changes consistent with an anterolateral infarction*

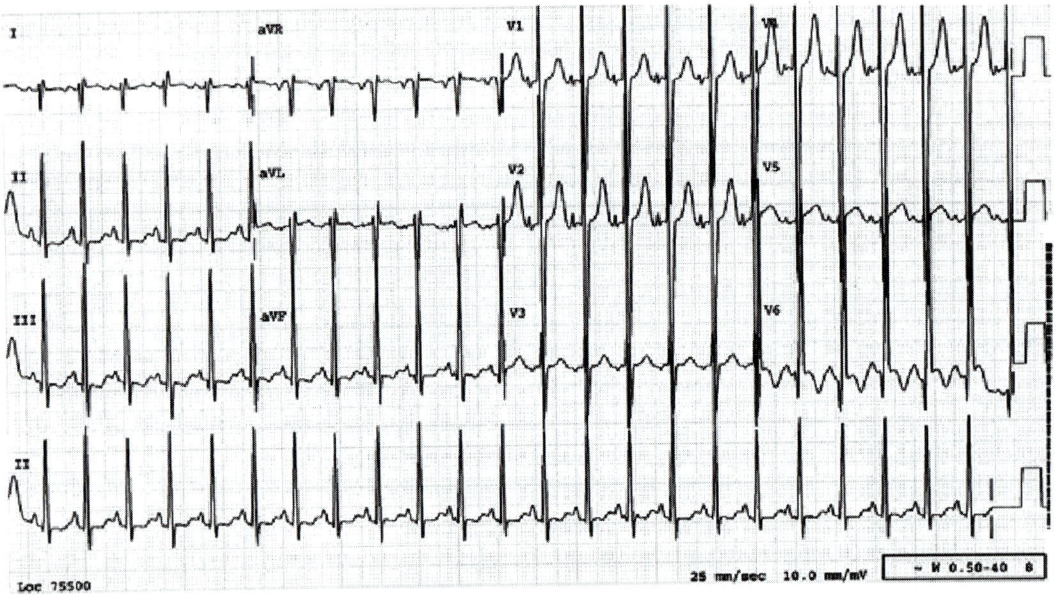

Fig. 33.9: *ST elevation in Leads 1,aVL ,V1-V3 and T inversion in leads 1,aVL ,V5-V6 in anomalous origin of the left coronary artery from the pulmonary artery (ALCAPA)*

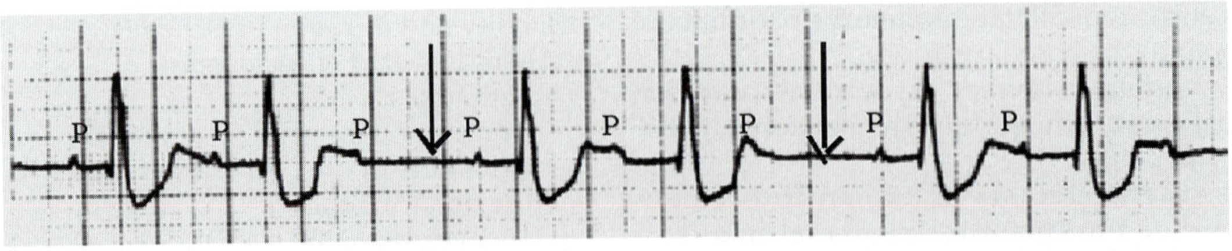

Fig. 33.10: *Mobitz type 1 (Wenckebach) second-degree heart block in an acute myocardial infarction. The patient had a recent inferior infarct. The Wenckebach cycles are indicated in each of which progressive prolongation of the P-R interval culminates in a dropped beat (arrow)*

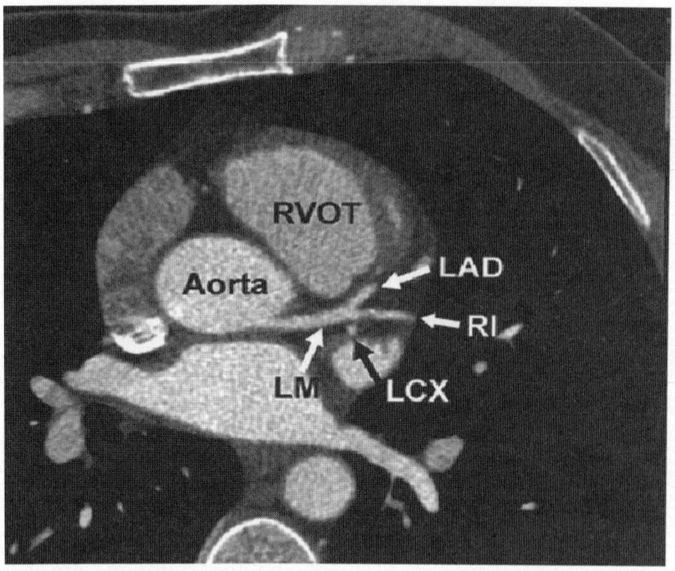

Fig. 33.11: *Axial CT image (0.75 mm section thickness) shows the left main (LM) coronary artery at the level of the ostium. The left main artery arises from the left valsalva sinus, courses posterior to the right ventricular outflow tract (RVOT), and bifurcates into the left anterior descending (LAD) and the left circumflex (LCX) branches. In about 15% of patients, a separate intermediate branch, or ramus intermedius (RI), also arises from the left main coronary artery*

  - Apnea
  - Bradypnea
  - Tachypnea
  - Hyperpnea
  - Nasal flaring
  - Grunting
  - Head bobbing
  - Retractions (supraclavicular, intercostal, subcostal)
  - Paradoxic respirations
  - Rales
  - Rubs
  - Rhonchi
  - Consolidation
- Cardiac examination abnormalities
  - Hyperdynamic precordium
  - Broad cardiac impulse
  - Displaced apical beat
  - S3
  - S4
  - Holosystolic murmur at the apex (mitral insufficiency)
  - Holosystolic murmur at the left lower sternal border (tricuspid insufficiency)
  - Loud pulmonic closure sound (P2, pulmonary hypertension)
  - Diastolic murmur of aortic/pulmonary insufficiency
  - Diastolic rumble of increased tricuspid/mitral flow
- Hypotension and signs of low cardiac output
  - Cool skin
  - Prolonged capillary refill time (CRFT)
  - Diaphoresis
  - Poor turgor
  - Peripheral cyanosis
- Signs of cor pulmonale (right heart failure)
  - Jugular vein distention
  - Hepatosplenomegaly
  - Hepatojugular reflux
  - Ascites
  - Peripheral edema

Etiological Factors

Two leading causes of acute myocardial infarction in children are anomalous left coronary artery from the pulmonary artery (ALCAPA) and Kawasaki disease.

- **ALCAPA**
  - Infants with ALCAPA develop irritability with dyspnea, tachycardia, diaphoresis, and vomiting while feeding. Irritability is secondary to anginal pain caused by a coronary artery steal phenomenon to the anomalous origin of the left coronary artery. The flow in this vessel, which has its distribution over the left ventricular myocardium, is retrograde to the main pulmonary artery.
  - The diagnosis of ALCAPA is suspected in irritable anxious infants presenting with pain while feeding (a modified stress test). Electrocardiography (ECG) demonstrates classic findings of deep Q waves, peaked T waves, and/or ST segment changes consistent with ischemia, injury, or infarction. Confirmation of the anomaly may be obtained using high-quality two dimensional and Doppler echocardiography or cardiac catheterization with angiography. A high degree of suspicion must predominate to make this diagnosis.
- **Kawasaki disease**
  - Kawasaki disease is an acquired disease of unknown etiology, and it can affect all cardiac tissues (pericardium, endocardium, myocardium, valvular, conductive). The pathogenetic mechanism is attributable to a high degree of immune activation. Since the introduction of intravenous gammaglobulin to standard therapy for Kawasaki disease, the incidence of acute myocardial infarction due to Kawasaki disease has decreased.
  - Coronary artery involvement occurs in 15–25% of children with Kawasaki disease within 1–3 weeks of onset. In patients with untreated Kawasaki disease, sudden death has resulted from acute myocardial infarction caused by ruptured coronary artery aneurysms or thromboses.
  - Detrimental changes in arterial wall hemodynamics are present and persist after acute Kawasaki disease which may predispose to long-term cardiovascular events.
- **Other conditions:** Other, often rarer, conditions that predispose children to acute myocardial infarction have been described, as follows:
  - *Coronary artery ostial stenosis or coronary artery kinking:* These may present after arterial switch repair of dextro-transposition of the great arteries (D-TGA) in the neonatal period or may develop years later, possibly, related to aortic root dilation. These may also occur status post Ross procedure for aortic valve disease.

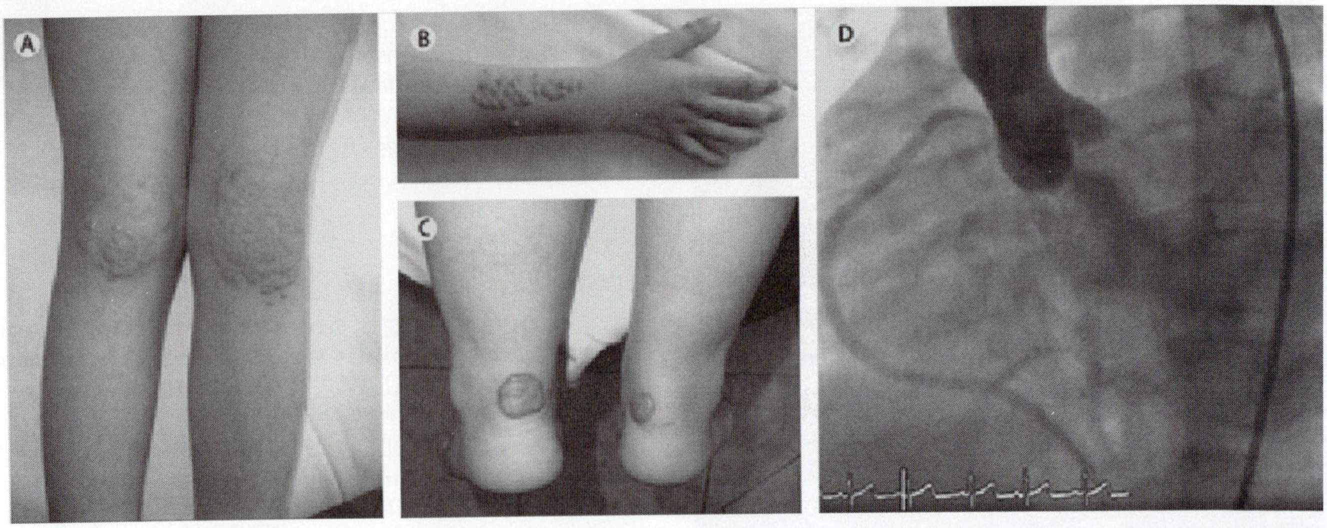

Figs 33.12A to D: *Homozygous familial hypercholesterolaemia. Tendon xanthomas at the knees (A), wrist (B), and achilles (C). Coronary angiography (D) showing occlusion of the left main coronary artery; the radiocontrast fills only the right coronary artery and its branches*

- ***Other abnormalities of coronary structure or course:*** Left main coronary artery atresia is a rare anomaly that can masquerade as dilated cardiomyopathy. Coronary ostial stenoses can be seen in patients with Williams syndrome, most commonly accompanying supravalvar aortic stenosis, but can rarely occur in isolation. Infarction can present in utero in these cases.
- *Sudden death:* Sudden death due to an aberrantly coursing left main coronary artery with its origin at the right sinus of valsalva may present in athletes who are exercising.
- *Coronary insufficiency:* This may develop in patients with Marfan syndrome, Takayasu arteritis, or cystic medial necrosis with aortic root dilatation, aneurysm formation, and dissection into the coronary artery.
- *Traumatic myocardial infarction:* Although very rare, traumatic myocardial infarction can occur in patients of any age but is more likely to occur in ambulatory and adolescent patients.
- *Atherosclerosis:* Accelerated coronary artery atherosclerosis is known to occur in orthotopic cardiac transplant recipients on immunosuppressive therapy.
- Familial homozygous hypercholesterolemia

Cocaine intoxication

- Accelerated coronary atherosclerosis due to juvenile diabetic dyslipidemia or nephrotic syndrome
- Accelerated coronary vascular disease associated with chronic kidney disease and renal failure
- Accelerated atherogenesis after treatment for childhood cancer
- Inflammatory conditions including viral and eosinophilic myocarditis and systemic lupus erythematosus (SLE): dyslipidemia frequently occurs in children with SLE and is often under recognized and under treated.

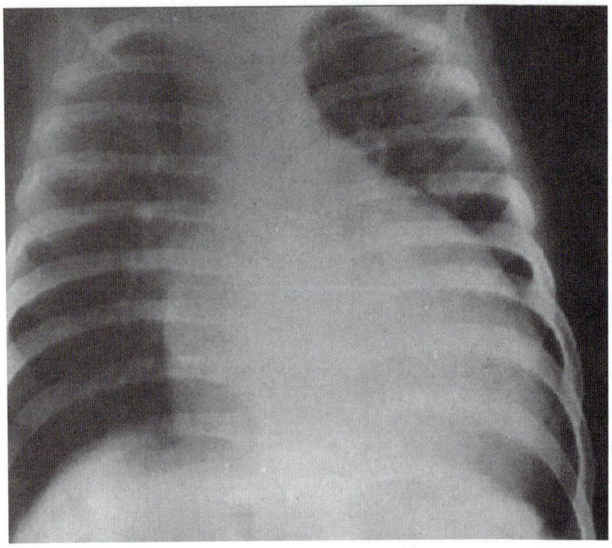

Fig. 33.13: *Radiographic finding of infant with ALCAPA shows cardiomegaly and pulmonary congestion*

- Sickle cell disease
- Prothrombotic defects (such as protein C deficiency and prothrombin gene mutations), especially in conjunction with other coronary anomalies
- Coronary artery spasm in adolescents
- Complications of dilated or ischemic cardiomyopathy
- D-TGA
    - For patients undergoing the Jatene arterial switch procedure, the presence of an intramural coronary artery course in patients with D-TGA may prohibit arterial repair.
    - Hypothetically, manipulation of the intramural coronary artery may cause damage and resultant inflammation, kinking, thrombosis, and myocardial ischemia or infarction (see Transposition of the Great Arteries).

– **Tetralogy of Fallot**
  - Surgical repair of pulmonary outflow obstruction often involves patching of the right ventricular outflow tract and resecting of the obstructing right ventricular muscle. An estimated 2–9% of patients with tetralogy of Fallot have coronary arterial anomalies, possibly affecting the timing of or approach to surgical repair.
  - The most common anomaly (4% of patients) is the origin of the left anterior descending (LAD) coronary artery from the right coronary artery (RCA), which then courses across the pulmonary outflow tract. Inadvertent transection of this vessel yields disastrous consequences. Frequently, the conus branch of the RCA is large and supplies a significant portion of right ventricular infundibular muscle.
  - Surgical techniques to avoid transection include limited incisions, varied tunneling techniques, and, perhaps, conduit placement. Cardiologists must predefine these abnormalities by noninvasive or invasive study (*see* Tetralogy of Fallot with Pulmonary Atresia).

– Pulmonary atresia with an intact ventricular septum
  - Primitive embryonic sinusoidal connections to coronary vasculature [most commonly affected is the RCA, then the LAD system, and, less frequently, the distal extent of the circumflex (Cx) coronary artery] may demonstrate severe intimal thickening, occlusion, or interruption.
  - In most patients, endocardial fibroelastosis, myocardial fibrosis, and acute myocardial infarction are observed (*see* Pulmonary Atresia with Intact Ventricular Septum).

Differential Diagnosis

- Acidosis, metabolic
- Acidosis, eespiratory
- Acute lymphoblastic leukemia
- Acute respiratory distress syndrome
- Afebrile pneumonia syndrome
- Anemia, acute
- Anomalous left coronary artery from the pulmonary artery
- Anomalous left coronary artery from the pulmonary artery: surgical perspective
- Aortic stenosis, valvar
- Aortic valve insufficiency
- Aortopulmonary septal defect
- Ascites
- Aspiration syndromes
- Atrioventricular block, third degree, acquired
- Atrioventricular septal defect, complete
- Atrioventricular septal defect, unbalanced
- Bacteremia
- Bundle-branch block, left
- Bundle-branch block, right
- Cardiomyopathy, dilated

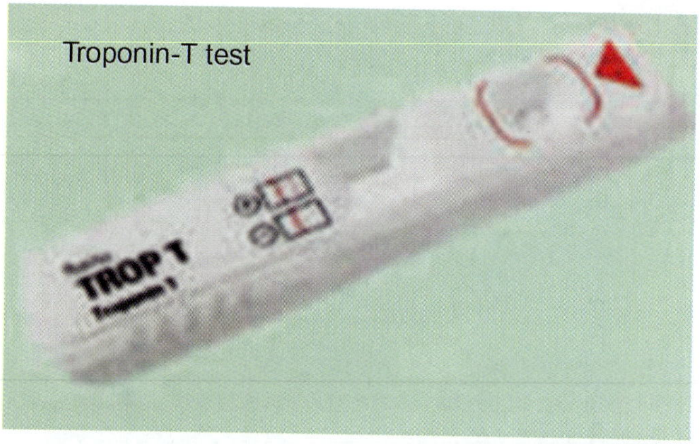

Fig. 33.14: *Trop T kit for diagnosis of myocardial infarction*

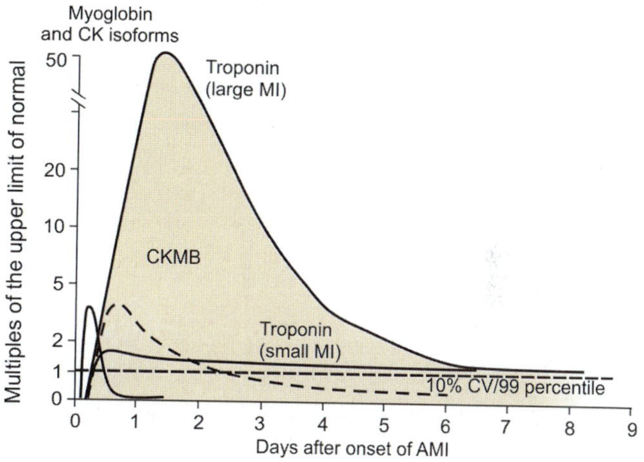

Fig. 33.15: *Progressive daily changes in CKMB and tropon levels after myocardial infarction*

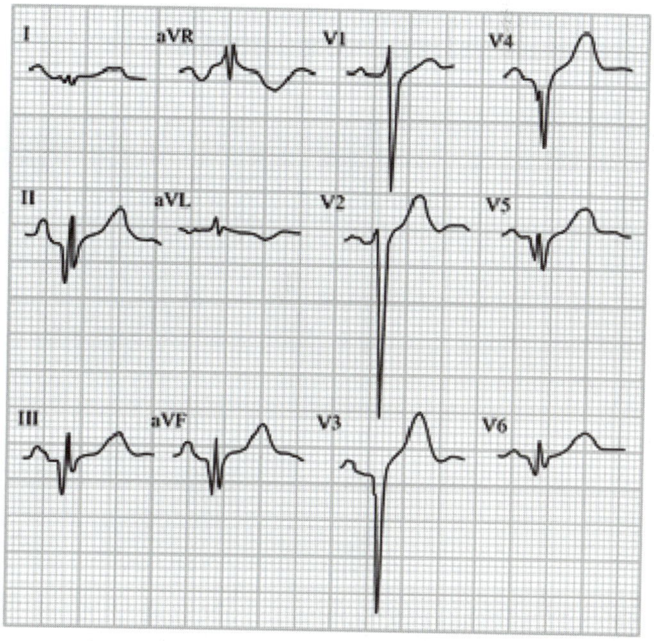

Fig. 33.16: *Pathological Q waves in inferior and anterior leads*

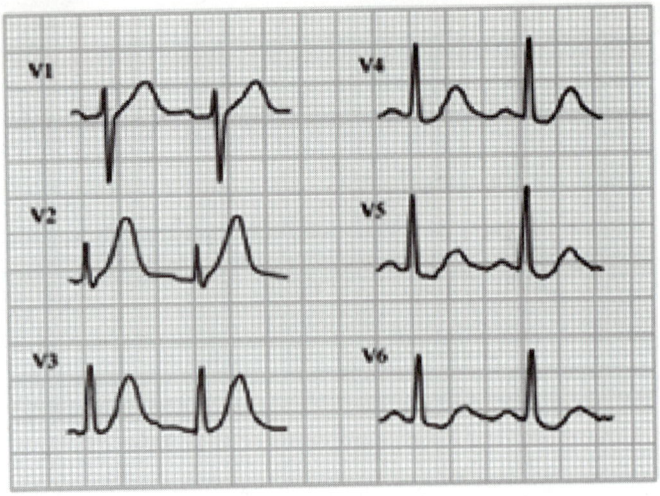

Fig. 33.17: *Hyperacute T waves in acute myocardial infarction*

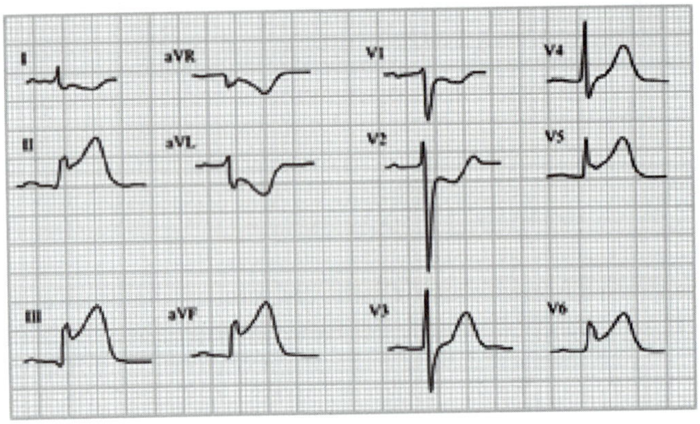

Fig. 33.18: *An inferolateral myocardial infarction with reciprocal changes in leads I, aVL, V1 and V2*

- Carnitine deficiency
- Child abuse and neglect: failure to thrive
- Child abuse and neglect: physical abuse
- Coarctation of the aorta
- Coarctation of the aorta and interrupted aortic arch
- Surgical perspective
- Colic
- Congenital coronary abnormalities: surgical perspective
- Coronary artery anomalies
- Coronary artery fistula
- Cyclic vomiting syndrome
- Dehydration
- Diabetic ketoacidosis
- Ebstein anomaly
- Endocardial fibroelastosis
- Endocarditis, bacterial
- Failure to thrive
- Fever in the toddler
- Fever in the young infant
- Fever without a focus
- Heart failure, congestive
- Hypoplastic left heart syndrome
- Infantile polyarteritis nodosa
- Interrupted aortic arch
- Intussusception
- Kawasaki disease
- Long QT syndrome
- Lyme disease
- Marfan syndrome
- Mitral stenosis, acquired
- Mitral stenosis, congenital
- Mitral valve insufficiency
- Myocarditis, nonviral
- Myocarditis, viral
- Pneumococcal bacteremia
- Pneumonia
- Pulmonary atresia with ventricular septal defect
- Respiratory distress syndrome
- Rheumatic heart disease
- Shock
- Shock and hypotension in the newborn
- Single ventricle
- Sinus of valsalva aneurysm

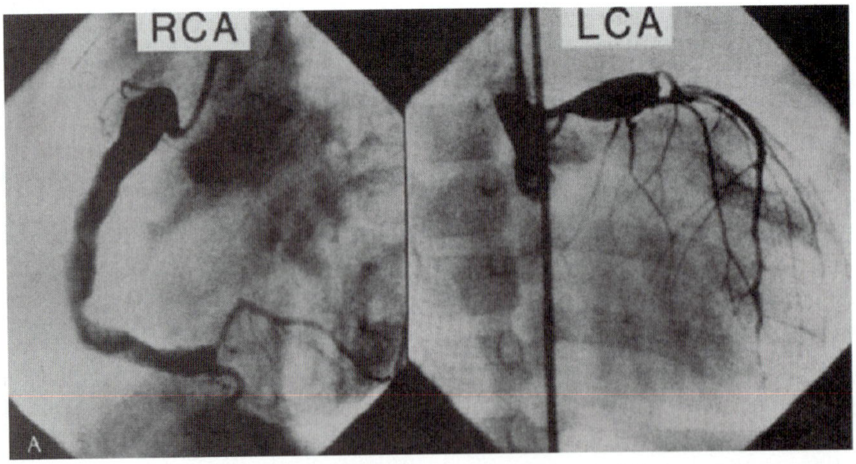

Fig. 33.19: *Coronary angiography showing longitudinal dilatation of the right coronary artery (RCA) and the saccular aneurysm at the proximal site of the left anterior descending coronary artery (LCA) in a young child with mucocutaneous lymph node syndrome (Kawasaki disease)*

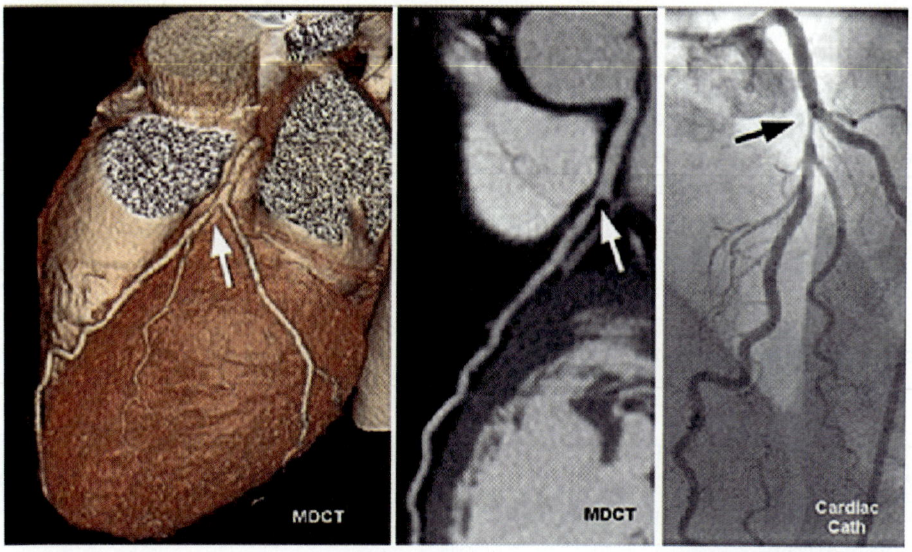

Fig. 33.20: *CT angiogram demonstrating proximal narrowing of the LAD*

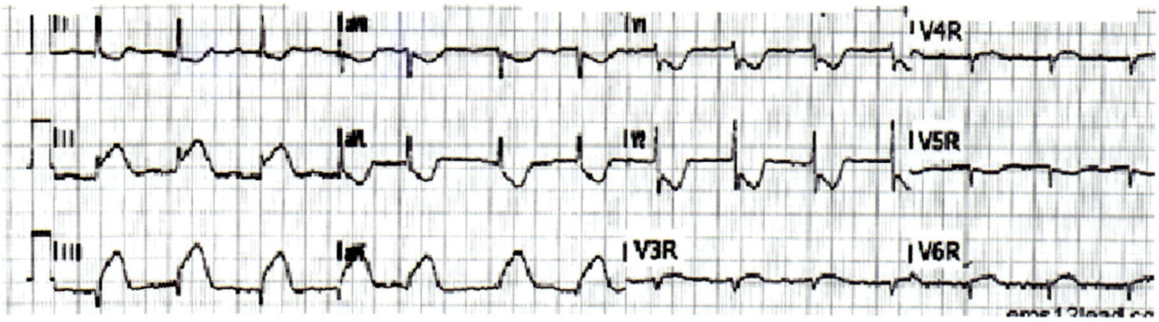

Fig. 33.21: *ECG Showing ST elevation in V3 and V4 ,11,111 and aVF In a patient with right ventricular infarction*

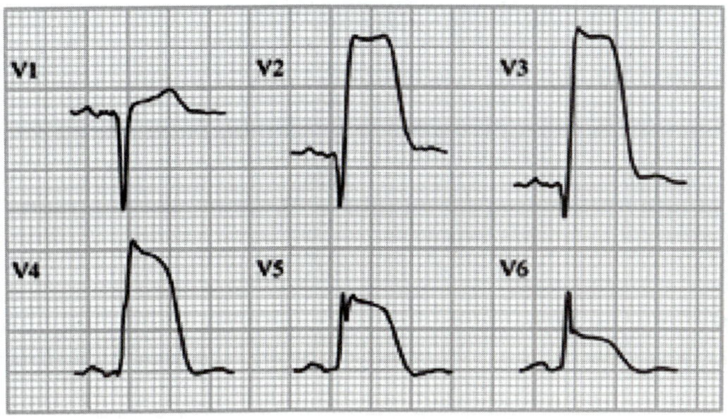

Fig. 33.22: *Anterior myocardial infarction with gross ST segment elevation (showing "tombstone" R waves)*

- Sudden infant death syndrome
- Supraventricular tachycardia, atrial ectopic tachycardia
- Supraventricular tachycardia, atrioventricular node re-entry
- Supraventricular tachycardia, junctional ectopic tachycardia
- Syncope
- Takayasu arteritis
- Tetralogy of fallot with absent pulmonary valve
- Tetralogy of fallot with pulmonary atresia
- Tetralogy of fallot: surgical perspective
- Tricuspid atresia
- Vascular ring and sling: surgical perspective
- Ventricular fibrillation
- Ventricular tachycardia.

Laboratory Studies

The following studies are indicated in pediatric patients with myocardial infarction:

- Testing of cardiac enzymes is the criterion standard for identification of myocardial cell death by measuring the following levels:
  - Serum glutamic-oxaloacetic transaminase (SGOT)
  - Lactate dehydrogenase (LDH) and isoenzymes
  - Creatine kinase (CK)
  - CK-MB isoforms
  - Troponin I and troponin T

  Levels of acute-phase reactants are elevated in the early stages of Kawasaki disease.
  - WBC
  - C-reactive protein

- Erythrocyte sedimentation rate (ESR)
- Thrombocytosis
- 1-antitrypsin (A1AT).

Evaluation for heritable forms of thrombophilia, such as prothrombin G20210 and C677T MTHFR gene mutations, and protein C deficiencies should be considered in young patients with myocardial ischemia.

Imaging Studies

- **Chest radiography:** This is indicated to reveal cardiomegaly with or without pulmonary venous congestion (Fig. 33.13).
- Echocardiography
  - Two dimensional echocardiography may be used to identify the following:
    - ♦ The abnormal origin of the left coronary artery from the main pulmonary artery
    - ♦ Chamber enlargement
    - ♦ Systolic and diastolic dysfunction
    - ♦ Coronary artery ectasia or aneurysm
    - ♦ A flail mitral valve leaflet and ruptured papillary muscle
    - ♦ Segmental wall motion abnormality
- **Mural or intraventricular thrombi**
  - In experienced hands, color-flow Doppler mapping can have the following uses:
    - ♦ Can be diagnostic for anomalous left coronary artery from the pulmonary artery (ALCAPA), demonstrating retrograde flow from the anomalous left coronary into the pulmonary trunk
    - ♦ Demonstrates direction of coronary artery flow
    - ♦ Quantifies mitral insufficiency
    - ♦ In conjunction with spectral Doppler, quantifies pulmonary hypertension
  - **Tissue Doppler imaging (TDI):** TDI is an echocardiographic technique that can noninvasively evaluate myocardial contraction and relaxation. Data suggest that TDI may have a role in early detection of graft failure due to coronary vasculopathy in orthotopic transplant recipients.
- **CT and MRI** (Figs 33.7, 33.11, 33.20, 33.29A and B, 33.37, 33.38)
  - **Multislice CT angiography** has been shown to be useful in identifying coronary ostial or arterial stenoses in pediatric patients following the arterial switch operation for dextrotransposition of the great arteries (D-TGA).
  - MRI can reveal coronary origins, anatomy and coronary artery abnormalities, and infarction in patients with Kawasaki disease.
  - Cardiac MRI has been used to determine myocardial viability and prognosis in a case of in uteromyocardial infarction.
- **Myocardial perfusion imaging:** This may be useful in evaluating myocardial ischemia and infarction in various disease states.
- **Electrocardiography (ECG):** As in adult patients, ECG in the younger group of population too gives valuable

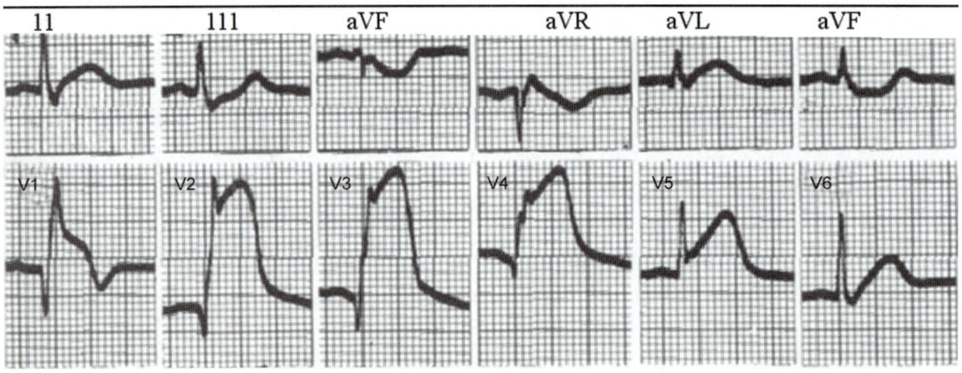

Fig. 33.23: *Acute anterior myocardial infarction; see ST elevation in V1–5 and loss of the normal upward concavity of the ST segment in 1,aVL and V6 with reciprocal changes in 2,3,and aVF. Q waves have developed in the right chest leads, and the pattern of RBBB has appeared, indicating extension upto septal wall*

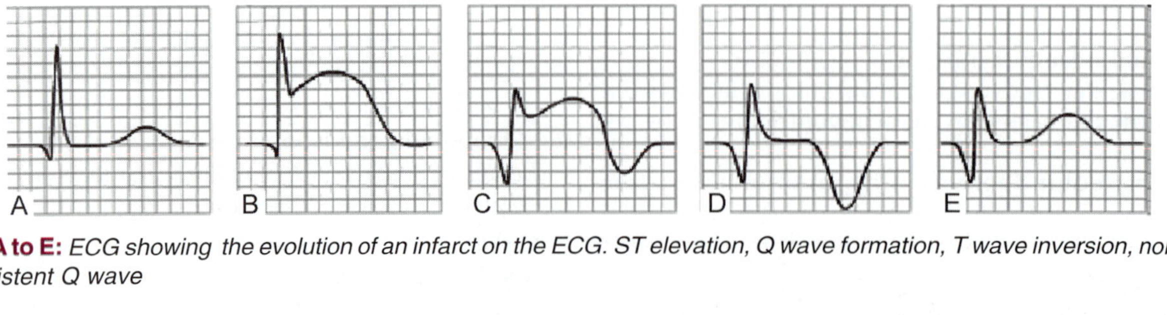

Figs 33.24A to E: *ECG showing the evolution of an infarct on the ECG. ST elevation, Q wave formation, T wave inversion, normalisation with a persistent Q wave*

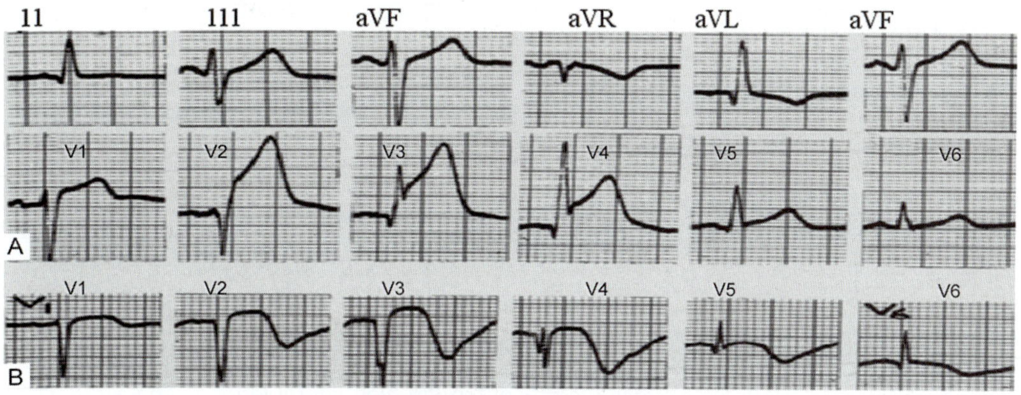

Figs 33.25A and B: *Acute extensive anterior myocardial infarction: see in (A) probable LAH in the limb leads with high ST take-off and tall T- waves in precordial leads (B) Two days later, coving of ST segment with deep inversion of T and U waves while simultaneously R waves have dwindled in V1–2, a QS complex has appeared in V3, and a Q waves have deepened in V4-6*

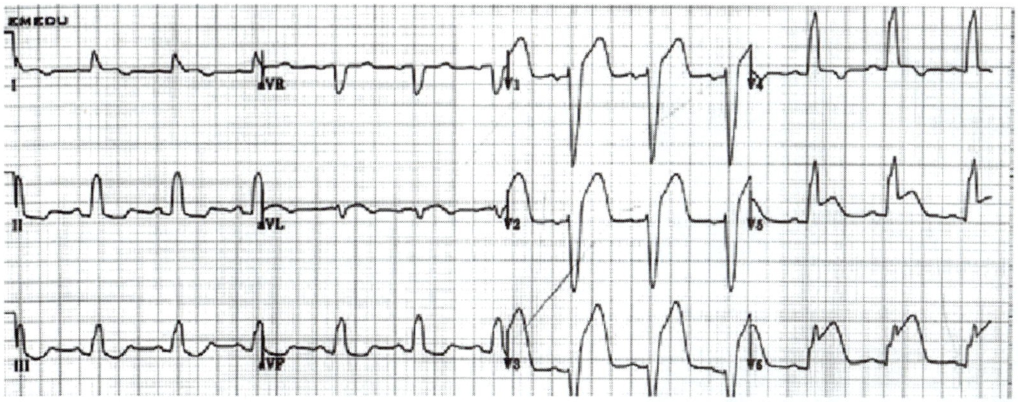

Fig. 33.26: *ECG showing acute anteroseptal myocardial infarction: see the tall T waves in V2–V4*

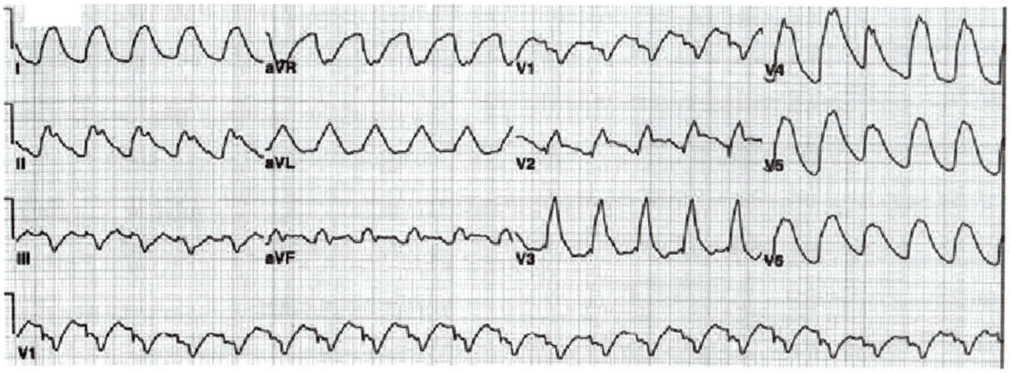

Fig. 33.27: *ECG showing in wide complex tachycardia in acute myocardial infarction*

information regarding myocardial ischemia and myocardial infarction

- **Exercise myocardial perfusion s**tress testing has been shown to be safe and useful in assessing myocardial perfusion and for risk stratification in children with Kawasaki disease.

Procedures (Figs 33.19, 33.20, 33.29, 33.36A to F, 33.37 and 33.38)

- **Angiographic evaluation of the coronary artery** system should be urgently performed but with caution because of the inherent instability of the diseased myocardium.
  - Definitive diagnosis of an anomalous left coronary artery from the pulmonary artery is made.
  - Aortography demonstrates an enlarged right coronary artery (RCA) system with collateralization to the left coronary artery and reflux of contrast into the pulmonary arterial system (ALCAPA).

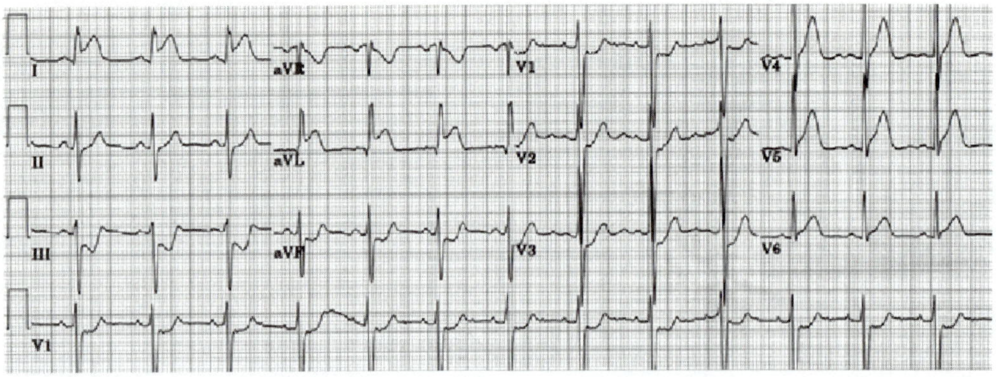

Fig. 33.28: *ECG shows high lateral STEMI: ST elevation is present in the high lateral leads (I and aVL). There is also subtle ST elevation with hyperacute T waves in V5–6. There is reciprocal ST depression in the inferior leads (III and aVF) with associated ST depression in V1–3 (which could represent anterior ischaemia or reciprocal change).This pattern is consistent with an acute infarction localised to the superior portion of the lateral wall of the left ventricle (high lateral STEMI). The culprit vessel in this case was an occluded first diagonal branch of the LAD*

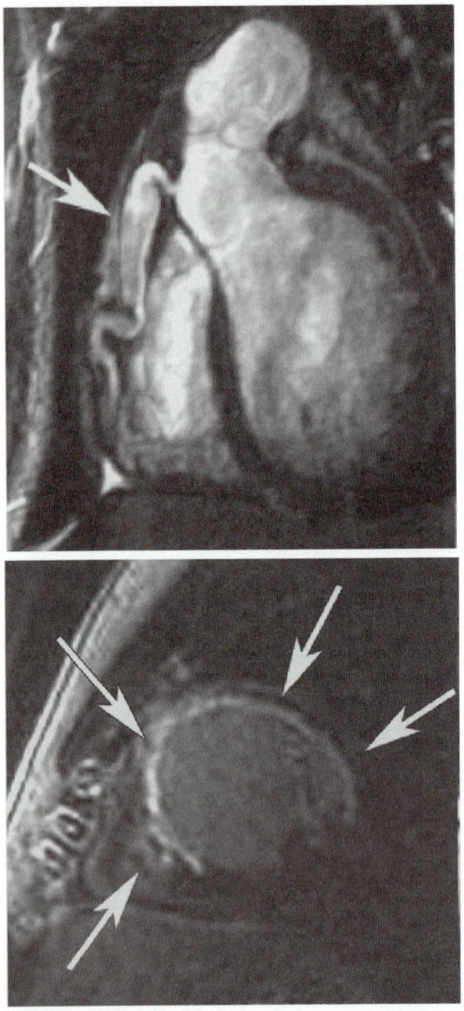

Fig. 33.29: *Kawasaki syndrome in an 18-year-old adolescent. (Top) Maximum intensity projection steady-state free precession image shows a 1.5 cm aneurysm (arrow) at the origin of the right coronary artery. There was also an aneurysm in the distribution of the left coronary artery with thrombosis; this aneurysm resulted in an extensive infarction of the left anterior descending artery (bottom) Short-axis delayed enhancement MR image shows wall thinning and delayed enhancement (arrows) due to infarction*

- Coronary aneurysm, ectasia, or both is frequently identified in patients with Kawasaki disease.
- Hemodynamic (oximetric) measurements may demonstrate the following:
  - ♦ Decreased systemic venous oxygen content is consistent with low cardiac output.
  - ♦ A small left-to-right shunt may be demonstrated by oximetry in the main pulmonary artery if ALCAPA is the diagnosis.
  - ♦ Elevated left atrial pressures are secondary to reduced left ventricular compliance, significant mitral valve insufficiency, or both.

- Successful percutaneous transluminal coronary angioplasty for proximal coronary stenoses following the arterial switch procedure has been reported in a small number of patients with apparent excellent results 3–5 years later.
- Postcatheterization effects that require precautions include hemorrhage, vascular disruption after balloon dilation, pain, nausea and vomiting, and arterial or venous obstruction from thrombosis or spasm.
- Possible complications include rupture of blood vessel, tachyarrhythmias, bradyarrhythmias, and vascular occlusion.
- The use of cardiac catheterization and percutaneous coronary interventions appears to be less in adolescents with acute myocardial infarction (29%) than in adults (40–50%) with acute myocardial infarction in review of the NIS. This may be due to a higher incidence of coronary vasospasm and subendocardial acute myocardial infarction in adolescents.

Medical Care (Fig. 33.5)

Medical care for a disease or condition that predisposes children to acute myocardial infarction can be found in anomalous left coronary artery from the pulmonary artery and Kawasaki disease. The primary treatment in patients with anomalous left coronary artery from the pulmonary artery (ALCAPA) is surgical. Surgical revascularization may also be necessary in patients with Kawasaki disease who develop significant coronary stenoses or occlusion.

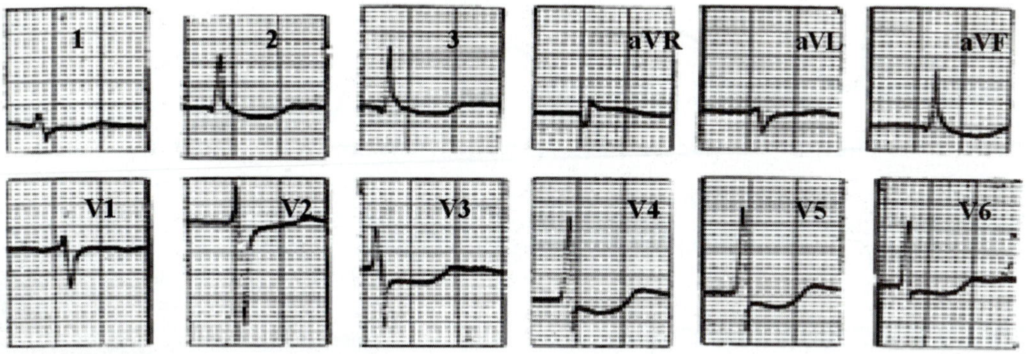

Fig. 33.30: *ECG showing classical subendocardial (non-Q-wave) infarction manifested by abnormal ST-segment depression in all leads except AVR, which showed ST-segment elevation*

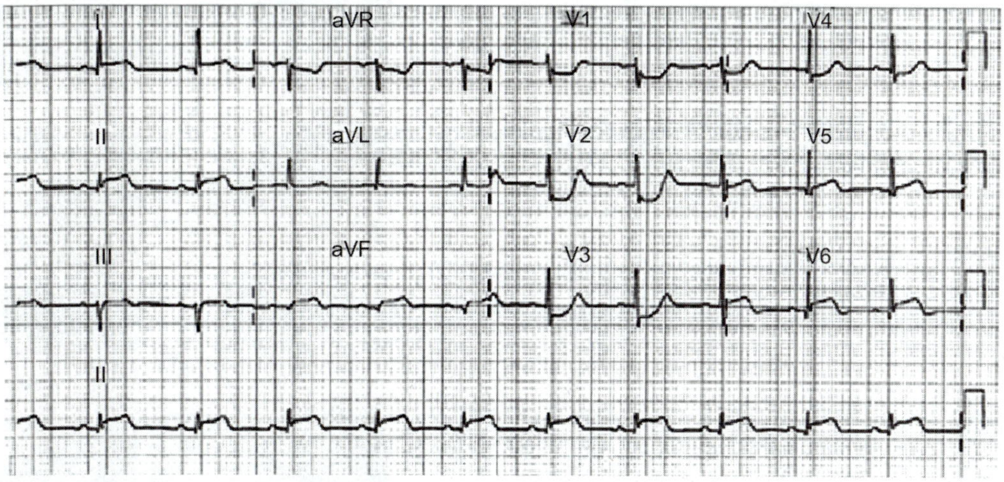

Fig. 33.31: *ECG showing inferoposterolateral STEMI: ST elevation is present in the inferior (II, III and aVF) and lateral leads (I, V5–6).ST depression in V1–3 with tall, broad R waves and upright T waves and a R/S ratio > 1 in V2 indicate concomitant posterior infarction (this patient also had ST elevation in the posterior leads V7–9).These changes are consistent with a massive infarction involving the inferior, lateral and posterior walls of the left ventricle.The culprit vessel is very likely to be an occluded proximal circumflex artery*

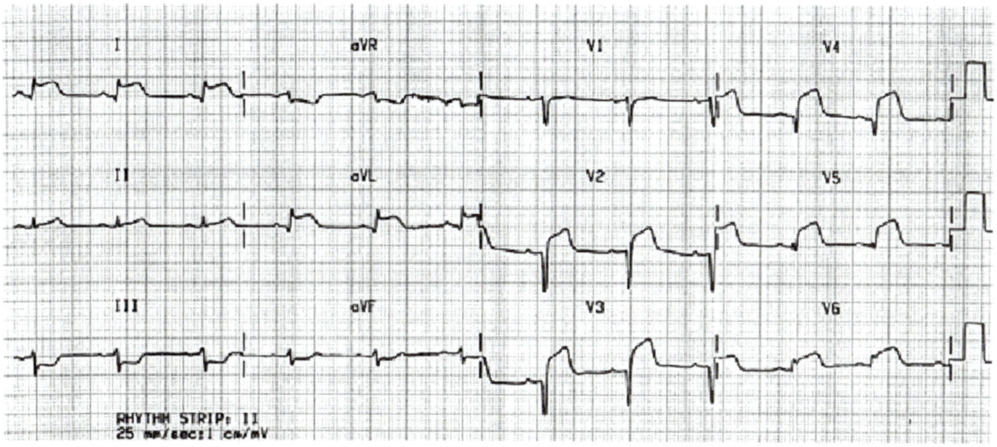

Fig. 33.32: *ECG showing anterolateral STEMI:ST elevation is present in the anterior (V2–4) and lateral leads (I, aVL, V5–6). Q waves are present in both the anterior and lateral leads, most prominently in V2–4. There is reciprocal ST depression in the inferior leads (III and aVF). This pattern indicates an extensive infarction involving the anterior and lateral walls of the left ventricle. ST elevation in the precordial leads plus the high lateral leads (I and aVL) is strongly suggestive of an acute proximal LAD occlusion (this combination predicts a proximal LAD lesion 87%)*

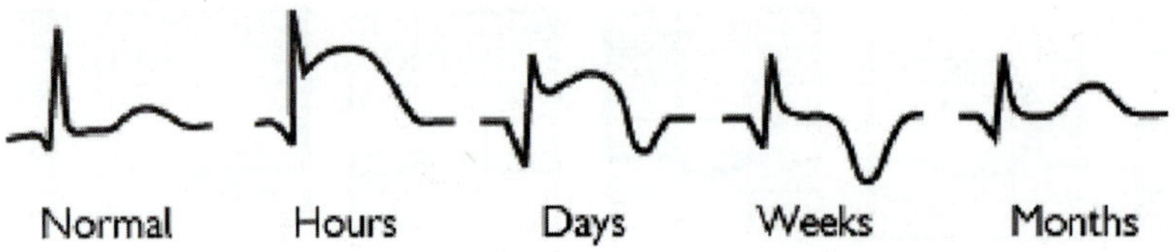

Fig. 33.33: *ECG changes following MI*

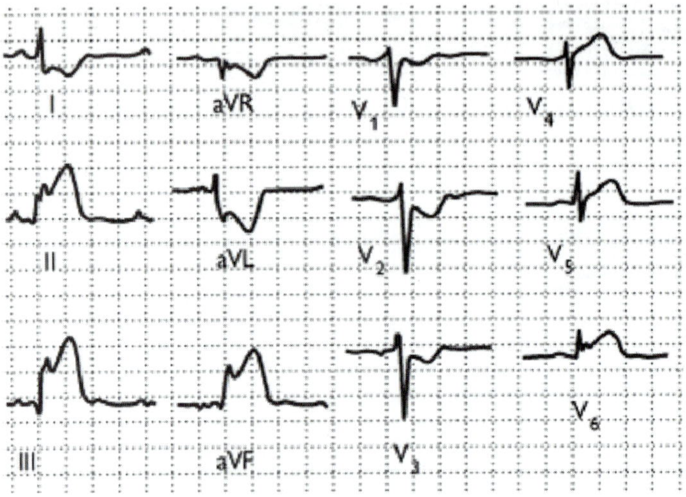

Fig. 33.34: *Acute inferolateral infarction with "reciprocal" ST changes in I, aVL, and V2–3*

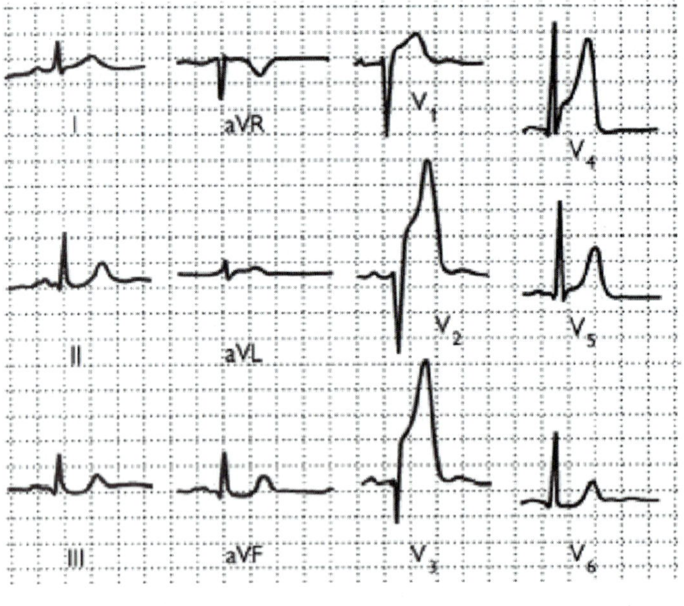

Fig. 33.35: *Acute anteroseptal infarction with minimal "reciprocal" ST changes in III and aVF*

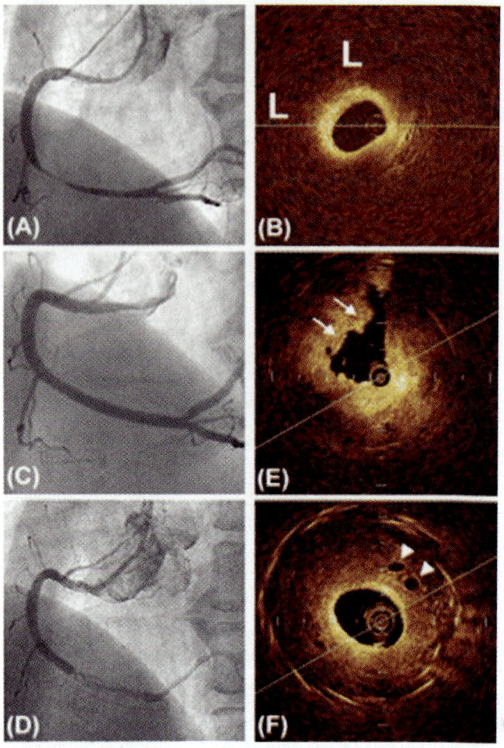

Figs 33.36A to F: *Coronary angiography showed a 90% stenosis in the mid-right coronary artery (Panel A) and optical coherence tomography (OCT: LightLabTM) was performed to assess plaque morphology. OCT revealed diffusely bordered signal poor region with overlying signal-rich band at the culprit site (L indicates lipid core in Panel B). Two sirolimus-eluting stents (CypherTM; 3.0 × 33 and 3.0 × 33 mm) were deployed in the culprit lesion and excellent angiographic results were obtained (Panel C). The final intravascular ultrasound also demonstrated the well-expanded and apposed stents with no plaque protrusion. The patient was prescribed aspirin 100 mg and ticlopidin 200 mg orally daily for 1 year. Twelve months follow-up coronary angiography showed a 99%; stenosis with contrast filling defect in the stents (Panel D). At this site, OCT revealed a low-backscattering projections irregular mass protruding into the lumen (white arrows in Panel E) with some microchannels (white arrow heads in Panel F). This finding may suggest that organized thrombus was the main component of restenotic tissue 12 months after sirolimus-eluting stent implantation*

- Intensive and acute care of the infant with symptoms of coronary artery ischemia or injury is initially directed at reducing myocardial oxygen demands while administering oxygen, fluids, or blood products and endotracheal intubation and correction of acid-base status and paralysis to reduce the work of breathing.
- Treatment of congestive heart failure (CHF) includes carefully administering diuretics, afterload reduction medications and inotropic drugs.
- Aggressive afterload reduction may be deleterious in patients with ALCAPA. Right coronary artery (RCA) perfusion may be reduced during aggressive afterload

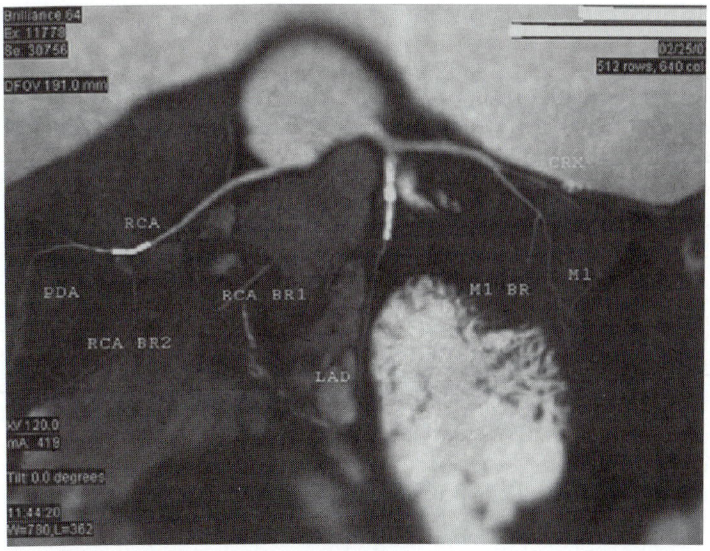

Fig. 33.37: *Computed tomographic angiogram showing patency of the stent in the right coronary artery and left anterior descending artery*

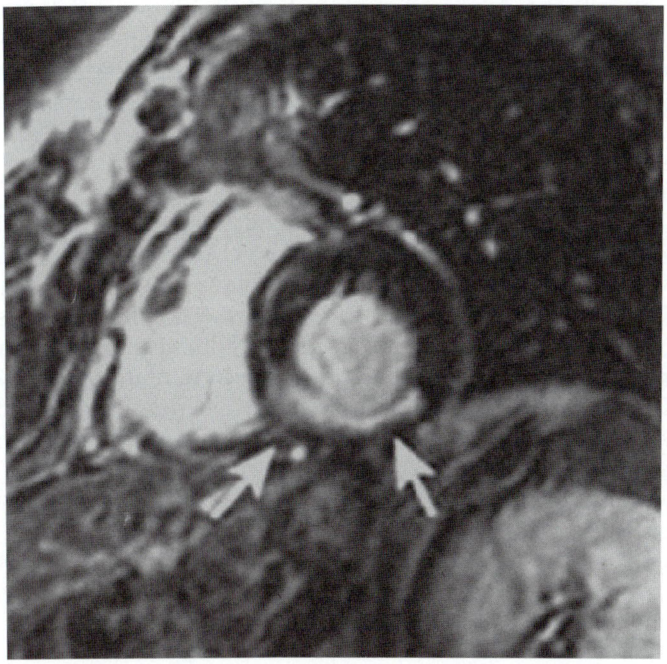

Fig. 33.38: *Transmural infarct area in right coronary artery territory. Breath-hold short-axis ECG gated inversion recovery gradient echo image obtained about 10 minutes after the injection of gadolinium contrast agent, clearly indicates infarct enhancement in the right coronary artery territory (arrows). This area is nonviable*

reduction, leading to decreased left coronary blood flow.
- Conversely, inotropic support may increase myocardial oxygen consumption significantly, which, in the presence of reduced myocardial blood flow, may worsen ischemia.
- Spontaneous resolution of CHF symptoms is rare. **Surgical revascularization** is usually necessary in the event of acute myocardial infarction (Fig. 33.39).
- Percutaneous transluminal coronary angioplasty for proximal coronary stenoses following the arterial switch procedure for dextrotransposition of the great arteries (D-TGA) has been reported.

Predischarge Exercise Testing

In patients with spontaneous postinfarction angina, congestive heart failure, hypotension, or malignant ventricular arrhythmia, exercise testing should generally be deferred and coronary angiography should be performed. However, in patients without these high-risk characteristics, exercise testing is generally recommended before discharge from the hospital to assess a patient's functional capacity and ability to return to activities of daily living and work. Most data indicating that predischarge exercise testing can identify patients at increased risk for cardiac events after discharge are from the prethrombolytic era, when the risk of adverse cardiac events was much higher. In the modern era, in which thrombolytic therapy or primary coronary angioplasty is frequently performed and in which aspirin, beta-blockers, ACE inhibitors, and lipid-lowering agents are routinely administered—all of which reduce the frequency of adverse events in the years after discharge it is difficult to identify patients at risk, because the adverse event rate is so low. Nonetheless, exercise testing is generally recommended to provide a measure of comfort to both the patient and the physician, to help determine the appropriateness of medical therapy, and to facilitate entry of the patient into a cardiac rehabilitation program.

Although predischarge exercise testing has been the standard of care in the United States for some time, only recently has a study examined whether therapy based on the results of a predischarge exercise test improves clinical outcome. The Danish Trial in acute myocardial infarction (DANAMI) was the first study to examine the usefulness of exercise testing in patients treated with thrombolytic agents (a low-risk group) and to provide support for what has been the standard of care in the United States. The results of this study revealed that clinical outcome was improved in patients who received angiography and coronary angioplasty, compared with those who received medical therapy alone. Use of the results of exercise testing to decide whether or not to employ revascularization in patients without spontaneous angina is less common outside of the United States. Patients with acute myocardial infarction who do not receive thrombolytic therapy or do not undergo primary angioplasty are at greater risk for adverse events after discharge from the hospital, and predischarge exercise testing is of even greater utility in such patients.

Prognostic variables indicating increased risk during exercise testing are exercise-induced angina or ST segment depression, particularly when it occurs during exercise at a low work load, and an abnormal drop in systolic blood pressure. However, electrocardiographic, symptomatic, and scintigraphic risk markers of ischemia (e.g. ST segment depression, angina, or a reversible perfusion defect) are less sensitive for identifying morbid and fatal outcomes than markers of left ventricular dysfunction or heart failure (e.g. exercise duration, impaired systolic blood pressure response, and peak left ventricular ejection fraction). The patients at greatest risk are those unable to exercise; such patients have the highest mortality after discharge. The type of exercise test that should be performed has been the subject of controversy. It is generally recommended that only simple treadmill testing be performed before discharge; in patients with abnormalities in the baseline ECG, stress testing with perfusion imaging or stress echocardiography may be helpful. In patients without widespread abnormalities on the ECG, perfusion imaging or stress echocardiography is generally deferred until at least 4 weeks after discharge, when a more vigorous exercise test can be performed. Whether the predischarge treadmill test should be a low-level test or a more vigorous symptom-limited test is unclear. It has been shown that a symptom-limited Bruce protocol exercise test detects ischemia more frequently than a submaximal test; however, it is not known which test has the greater positive and greater negative-predictive value for identifying patients at risk. Currently, a lower-level exercise test is preferred, although a more vigorous test may be appropriate in patients likely to resume a more active and vigorous lifestyle shortly after discharge and in whom a low-level test may not cause the patient to expend the amount of energy he or she will be using during activities of daily living. There has been concern that the use of beta blockers before the predischarge exercise test may mask the presence of significant coronary artery disease and prevent the identification of high-risk patients. This concern does not appear to be significant enough to outweigh the benefits of early beta-blocker therapy.

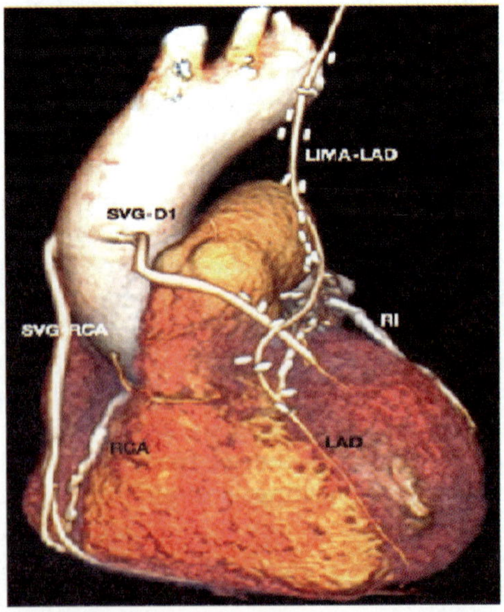

Fig. 33.39: *CABG: MD CT 64 slices of the LV and aorta showing CABG with intact grafts from ascending aorta to the proximal of of the obstructed right coronary artery and left anterior descending artery in the process of perfusion plan in the management of ischemic myocardium as a result of myocardial infarction*

Secondary Prevention

Lipid-Lowering Therapy

Recent studies have demonstrated that in patients with coronary artery disease, lipid-lowering therapy with HMG-CoA (3-hydroxy-3-methylglutaryl coenzyme A) reductase inhibitors reduces not only fatal and nonfatal infarction but also mortality from all causes. The Scandinavian Simvastatin survival study revealed a 42% reduction in cardiac mortality and a 30% reduction in all-cause mortality in 4,444 men and women with coronary artery disease over the 5.4 years of the study.

The reductions in mortality were similar in patients in the lowest and those in the highest quartiles of serum low-density lipoprotein (LDL) cholesterol. It has been demonstrated that postinfarction patients with an LDL cholesterol level at or above 130 mg/dL benefit from lipid-lowering therapy within as little as 2 years after the initiation of such therapy initial measurement of cholesterol should be made within 24 hours after myocardial infarction; measurement of lipids 24 hours or more after myocardial infarction can be misleading in that cholesterol levels may be reduced below baseline levels during this period and remain low for up to 1 month. Early initiation of statins may be more beneficial than later initiation. Exercise, weight reduction in overweight patients, avoidance of dietary saturated fat and cholesterol, and smoking cessation have all been reported to favorably influence blood lipid levels and should be recommended whether or not lipid-lowering medications are prescribed.

Several prospective, randomized trials revealed that warfarin therapy reduces mortality after discharge from the hospital in patients with acute myocardial infarction. However, in these studies, in which warfarin therapy was compared with placebo, aspirin was not administered in either arm of the study. The Coumadin aspirin reinfarction study (CARS) revealed that the risk of reinfarction in patients treated with aspirin alone was similar to that in patients treated with aspirin and either low-dose (1 mg) or higher-dose (3 mg) warfarin Warfarin is also ineffective at preventing coronary reocclusion in patients in whom thrombolytic therapy was successful. The routine administration of warfarin is not currently recommended to prevent reinfarction in patients who have survived myocardial infarction.

Antiarrhythmic Therapy

Although Holter monitoring before discharge can help to identify patients at increased risk for sudden cardiac death, antiarrhythmic therapy has not been shown to decrease the risk of death in such patients, and in fact, it increased mortality in the Cardiac Arrhythmia Suppression Trial (CAST). Since CAST, several prospective, randomized studies have been performed that have examined the role of amiodarone in patients at increased risk for sudden death. Taken together, the results of those studies do not indicate that amiodarone reduces mortality. Further studies are needed before the routine use of amiodarone can be recommended in high-risk patients, such as those included in these trials.

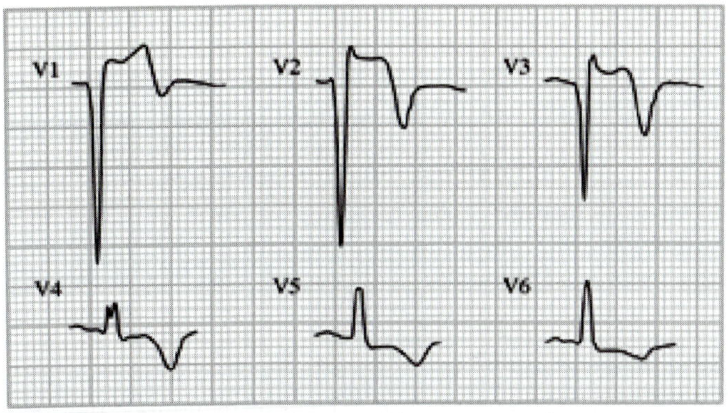

Fig. 33.40: *ECG showing long-standing ST segment elevation and T wave inversion associated with a previous anterior myocardial infarction (echocardiography showed a left ventricular aneurysm)*

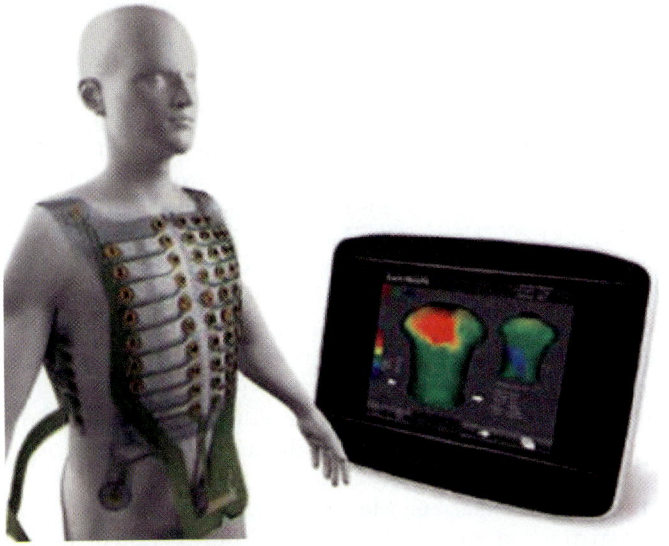

Fig. 33.41: *Heartscape 80-lead 3D ECG system. Heartscape 80-lead 3D ECG System. The concept is not entirely new, as it is the successor to the PRIME ECG system which has the same amount of leads, and has been available since 2003. The Heartscape 3D ECG System aims to give a 360° electrocardiographic view of the heart, to helping in identifying myocardial infarcts without ST-segment elevation on traditional 12-lead ECGs, and in patients with left bundle-branch block. Compared to traditional 12-lead ECG's, the system has shown to be more sensitive while retaining comparable specificity in detecting acute infarcts*

Automated, Implantable Cardioverter-Defibrillator

Automated implantable cardioverter-defibrillators are of proven benefit in patients with coronary artery disease, reduced left ventricular ejection fraction, nonsustained ventricular tachycardia, and inducible ventricular tachycardia. It has been proposed that patients with a prior myocardial infarction and advanced left ventricular dysfunction may benefit from prophylactic implantation of a defibrillator (in the absence of electrophysiologic testing to induce arrhythmias). Prophylactic implantation of a defibrillator is a recommended therapy in this patient population.

Risk-Factor Modification

An important and often neglected aspect of medical care after a myocardial infarction is the identification and modification of risk factors for atherosclerosis. Hypertension and hypercholesterolemia should be treated. Cessation of smoking has been shown to prolong life in patients who have survived a myocardial infarction; behavior modification and group therapy can increase the likelihood of kicking the habit. Cardiac rehabilitation and the establishment of a healthier lifestyle with an exercise program can further reduce the likelihood of a return to smoking. Hypercholesterolemia should be aggressively treated as described above.

Although there are few data that conclusively indicate that patients who participate in a cardiac rehabilitation program after discharge have increased survival, an exercise rehabilitation program appears to improve a patient's sense of well-being and hasten return to work and leisure activities. A cardiac rehabilitation program can also help to improve diet and aid weight reduction in overweight patients, help smokers refrain from smoking, and help to establish an exercise program that the patient can maintain long after the formal rehabilitation program has ended. Thus, participation in a cardiac rehabilitation program often leads to the establishment of a healthier lifestyle.

Long-Term Prognosis

Long-term prognosis after myocardial infarction is determined primarily by the severity of left ventricular dysfunction, the presence and degree of residual ischemia, and the potential for malignant ventricular arrhythmia. These adverse prognostic factors are related to each other but are also independently associated with death after discharge. Age is also an important determinant of outcome. Most deaths that occur in the first year after discharge occur in the first 3 months, a fact that stresses the importance of assessing risk and optimizing therapy before discharge from the hospital. However, there can be substantial improvement in ventricular function in the weeks and months after acute myocardial infarction, particularly in patients in whom early reperfusion was achieved. Therefore, measurement of ventricular function 2–3 months after myocardial infarction is a more accurate predictor of long-term prognosis than measurement of left ventricular function in the acute stages.

BIBLIOGRAPHY

1. Concheiro-Guisan A, Sousa-Rouco C, Fernandez-Santamarina I, Gonzalez-Carrero J. Intrauterine myocardial infarction: unsuspected diagnosis in the delivery room. Fetal Pediatr Pathol. Jul-Aug 2006;25(4):179–84.
2. CDC. National Vital Statistics Report: Acute myocardial infarction. 1998 Nov; 47(9). Available at: http://

www.disastercenter.com/cdc/aacutcar.html. Accessed September 30, 2008.
3. Mahle WT, Campbell RM, Favaloro-Sabatier J. Myocardial infarction in adolescents. J Pediatr. Aug 2007;151(2):150–4.
4. Oglesby P. The international cooperative study on epidemiology. Circulation. Jun 1970;41(6):895–7.
5. Lane JR, Ben-Shachar G. Myocardial infarction in healthy adolescents. Pediatrics. Oct 2007;120(4):e938–43.
6. Safi M, Taherkhani M, Badalabadi RM, Eslami V, Movahed MR. Coronary aneurysm and silent myocardial infarction in an adolescent secondary to undiagnosed childhood Kawasaki disease. Exp Clin Cardiol. Spring 2010;15(1):e18–9.
7. Hunley TE, Kon V, Jabs K. Myocardial infarction in chronic kidney disease. Pediatrics. Jul 2008;122(1):223–4.
8. Ardoin SP, Sandborg C, Schanberg LE. Management of dyslipidemia in children and adolescents with systemic lupus erythematosus. Lupus. 2007;16(8):618–26.
9. Koestenberger M, Nagel B, Gamillscheg A, Temmel W, Cvirn G, Beitzke A. Myocardial infarction in an adolescent: anomalous origin of the left main coronary artery from the right coronary sinus in association with combined prothrombotic defects. Pediatrics. Aug 2007;120(2):e424–7.
10. Fyfe DA, Ketchum D, Lewis R, et al. Tissue Doppler imaging detects severely abnormal myocardial velocities that identify children with pre-terminal cardiac graft failure after heart transplantation. J Heart Lung Transplant. May 2006;25(5): 510–7.
11. Tacke CE, Kuipers IM, Groenink M, Spijkerboer AM, Kuijpers TW. Cardiac magnetic resonance imaging for noninvasive assessment of cardiovascular disease during the follow-up of patients with kawasaki disease. Circ Cardiovasc Imaging. Nov 1 2011;4(6):712–20.
12. Whitham JK, Hasan BS, Schamberger MS, Johnson TR. Use of cardiac magnetic resonance imaging to determine myocardial viability in an infant with in utero septal myocardial infarction and ventricular noncompaction. Pediatr Cardiol. Sep 2008;29(5):950–3.
13. Gazit AZ, Avari JN, Balzer DT, Rhee EK. Electrocardiographic diagnosis of myocardial ischemia in children: is a diagnostic electrocardiogram always diagnostic?. Pediatrics. Aug 2007;120(2):440–4.
14. Towbin JA, Bricker JT, Garson A Jr. Electrocardiographic criteria for diagnosis of acute myocardial infarction in childhood. Am J Cardiol. Jun 15 1992;69(19):1545–8.
15. Lim CW, Ho KT, Quek SC. Exercise myocardial perfusion stress testing in children with Kawasaki disease. J Paediatr Child Health. Jul-Aug 2006;42(7–8):419–22.
16. Sugahara Y, Ishii M, Muta H, Iemura M, Matsuishi T, Kato H. Warfarin therapy for giant aneurysm prevents myocardial infarction in Kawasaki disease. Pediatr Cardiol. Mar 2008;29(2):398–401.
17. Ahn YK, Jeong MH, Bom HS, et al. Myocardial infarction with Moyamoya disease and pituitary gigantism in a young female patient. Jpn Circ J. Aug 1999;63(8):644–8.
18. Bagby GC Jr, Goldman RD, Newman HC, Means JF. Acute myocardial infarction due to childhood lymphoma. N Engl J Med. Aug 17 1972;287(7):338–40.
19. Berenson GS, Srinivasan SR, Hunter SM, et al. Risk factors in early life as predictors of adult heart disease: the Bogalusa Heart Study. Am J Med Sci. Sep 1989;298(3):141–51.
20. Berry CL. Myocardial ischaemia in infancy and childhood. J Clin Pathol. Jan 1967;20(1):38–41.
21. Bex JP, Laborde F, Baillot F, Martelli H, Hazan E. Myocardial infarction in an infant without coronary artery birth anomalies. Arch Mal Coeur Vaiss. May 1980;73(5):535–7.
22. Burns JC, Shike H, Gordon JB, et al. Sequelae of Kawasaki disease in adolescents and young adults. J Am Coll Cardiol. Jul 1996;28(1):253–7.
23. Celermajer DS, Sholler GF, Howman–Giles R, Celermajer JM. Myocardial infarction in childhood: clinical analysis of 17 cases and medium-term follow-up of survivors. Br Heart J. Jun 1991;65(6):332–6.
24. Coggon D, Margetts B, Barker DJ, et al. Childhood risk factors for ischaemic heart disease and stroke. Paediatr Perinat Epidemiol. Oct 1990;4(4):464–9.
25. Dhillon R, Clarkson P, Donald AE, et al. Endothelial dysfunction late after Kawasaki disease. Circulation. Nov 1 1996;94(9):2103–6.
26. Esterly JR, Oppenheimer EH. Some aspects of cardiac pathology in infancy and childhood. IV. Myocardial and coronary lesions in cardiac malformations. Pediatrics. Jun 1967;39(6):896–903.
27. Fukuda T, Ishibashi M, Shinohara T, et al. Follow-up assessment of the collateral circulation in patients with Kawasaki disease who underwent dipyridamole stress technetium-99m tetrofosmin scintigraphy. Pediatr Cardiol. Sep-Oct 2005;26(5):558–64.
28. Garcia RE, Moodie DS. Routine cholesterol surveillance in childhood. Pediatrics. Nov 1989;84(5):751–5.
29. Gattorno M, Falcini F, Ravelli A, et al. Outcome of primary antiphospholipid syndrome in childhood. Lupus. 2003;12(6):449–53.
30. Gunal N, Kara N, Cakar N, et al. Cardiac involvement in childhood polyarteritis nodosa. Int J Cardiol. Aug 8 1997;60(3):257–62.
31. Haitas B, Baker SG, Meyer TE, et al. Natural history and cardiac manifestations of homozygous familial hypercholesterolaemia. Q J Med. Jul 1990;76(279):731–40.
32. Hancock SL, Donaldson SS, Hoppe RT. Cardiac disease following treatment of Hodgkin's disease in children and adolescents. J Clin Oncol. Jul 1993;11(7):1208–15.
33. Hawkins MM, Kingston JE, Kinnier Wilson LM. Late deaths after treatment for childhood cancer. Arch Dis Child. Dec 1990;65(12):1356–63.
34. Isaka N, Nakano T. Myocardial infarction in childhood. Ryoikibetsu Shokogun Shirizu. 1996;(12):679–83.
35. Israels SJ, Michelson AD. Antiplatelet therapy in children. Thromb Res. 2006;118(1):75–83.
36. Kampmann C, Kuroczynski W, Trubel H, et al. Late results after PTCA for coronary stenosis after the arterial switch procedure for transposition of the great arteries. Ann Thorac Surg. Nov 2005;80(5):1641–6.
37. Kondo C. Myocardial perfusion imaging in pediatric cardiology. Ann Nucl Med. Oct 2004;18(7):551–61.
38. Kovacs CS, Sanfilippo AJ, Burggraf GW. Anterior wall myocardial infarction in a 15-year-old diabetic female associated with spontaneously resolving coronary thrombosis. Can J Cardiol. Sep 1992;8(7):733–6.
39. Kreutzer U, Krulls-Munch J, Angres M, Schiessler A. Successful resuscitation of a patient with ventricular

fibrillation in Bland-White-Garland syndrome in adulthood. A case report. Z Kardiol. Jul 1998;87(7):560–5.
40. L'Ecuyer TJ, Poulik JM, Vincent JA. Myocardial infarction due to coronary abnormalities in pulmonary atresia with intact ventricular septum. Pediatr Cardiol. Jan-Feb 2001;22(1):68–70.
41. Lindblade CL, Kirkpatrick EC, Ebenroth ES. Eosinophilic myocarditis presenting with pediatric myocardial infarction. Pediatr Cardiol. Jan-Feb 2006;27(1):162–5.
42. Long WA, Willis PW 4th, Henry GW. Childhood traumatic infarction causing left ventricular aneurysm: diagnosis by two dimensional echocardiography. J Am Coll Cardiol. Jun 1985;5(6):1478–83.
43. Mavrogeni S, Papadopoulos G, Douskou M, et al. Magnetic resonance angiography, function and viability evaluation in patients with Kawasaki disease. J Cardiovasc Magn Reson. 2006;8(3):493–8.
44. McMahon CJ, Nihill MR, Denfield S. Neoaortic root dilation associated with left coronary artery stenosis following arterial switch procedure. Pediatr Cardiol. Jan-Feb 2003;24(1): 43–6.

34 Percutaneous Coronary Interventions (Balloon Angioplasty and Stentoplasty)

Gruentzig's first successful coronary angioplasty treatment on a human was performed in 1977, in Zurich, Switzerland. He expanded a short, about 3 mm, nonbranching section of the left anterior descending (LAD) artery (the front branch of the left coronary artery) which supplies the front wall and tip of the heart (*see* Coronary Circulation) which had a high-grade stenosis, about 80%, of the lumen. Dr Grüntzig presented the results of his first four angioplasty cases at the 1977 American Heart Association (AHA) meeting, which led to widespread acknowledgment of his pioneering work (Figs 34.1 and 34.2).

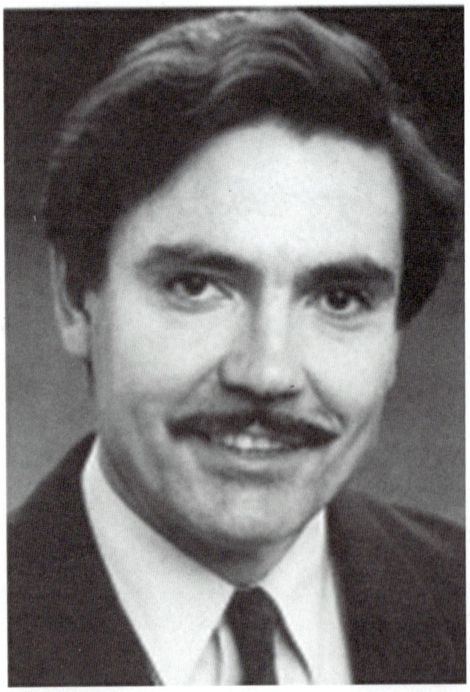

Fig. 34.1: *Andreas Roland Gruentzig (June 25, 1939 October 27, 1985) was a German cardiologist who first developed successful balloon angioplasty for expanding lumens of narrowed arteries*

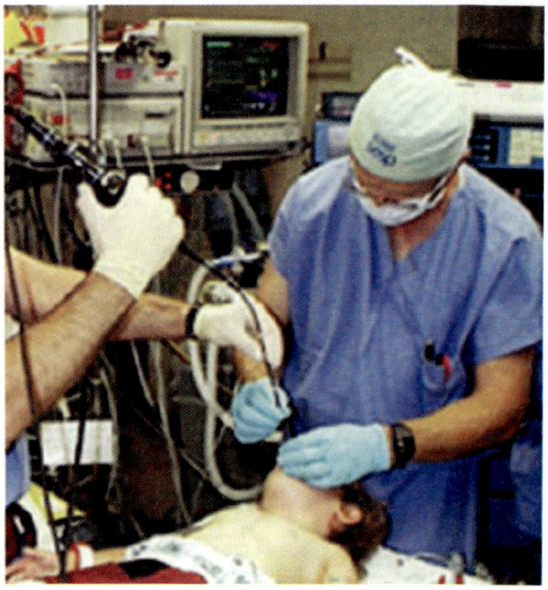

Fig. 34.2: *Showing doctors inducing anesthesia prior to interventional procedure on a child*

The immediate results of this treatment, despite using only a carefully *kitchen built* catheter (crude by current standards), was quite good. The patient became and remained angina free after this treatment. This initial patient's result was electively rechecked, by angiography at Emory University, on the 10 year anniversary of the initial treatment. The LAD narrowing, after this 10 year timespan, remained almost perfectly expanded. There was minimal residual narrowing, probably less than 10%, as seen in similar angle and multiple different views comparing with photographs of the original, 10 years earlier, before and after results. The excellent results of this initial and subsequent patients were critical to the rapid development and growing acceptance of the angioplasty treatment option. Dr Grüntzig recognized multiple important issues early: (a) the treatment would not be readily accepted by most physicians, especially bypass

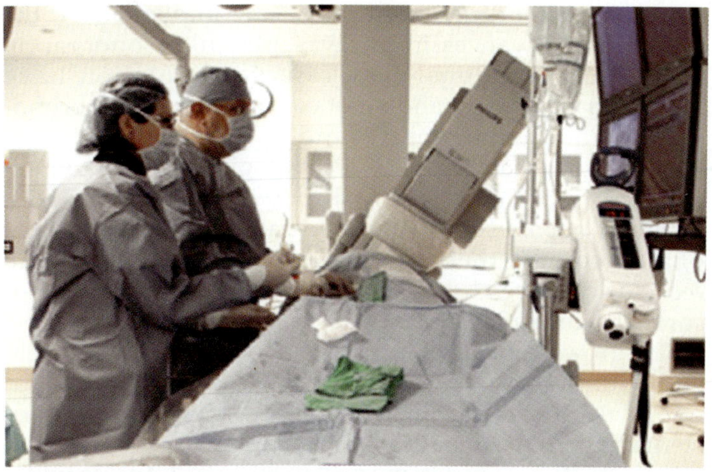

Fig. 34.3: *Interventional laboratory for conducting percutaneous coronary interventions*

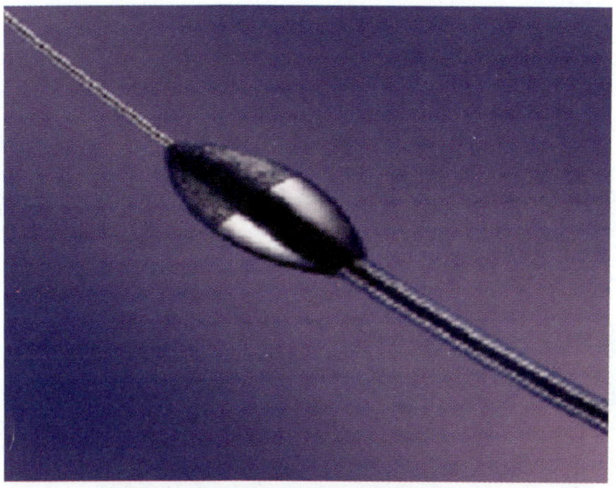

Fig. 34.4: *Percutaneous transluminal coronary angioplasty (PTCA). The rotational atherectomy catheter (Rotablator) is a device designed for the removal of plaque from coronary arteries. This device, which has a diamond-studded burr at its tip, rotates at about 160,000 rpm and is particularly well suited for ablation of calcific or fibrotic plaque material*

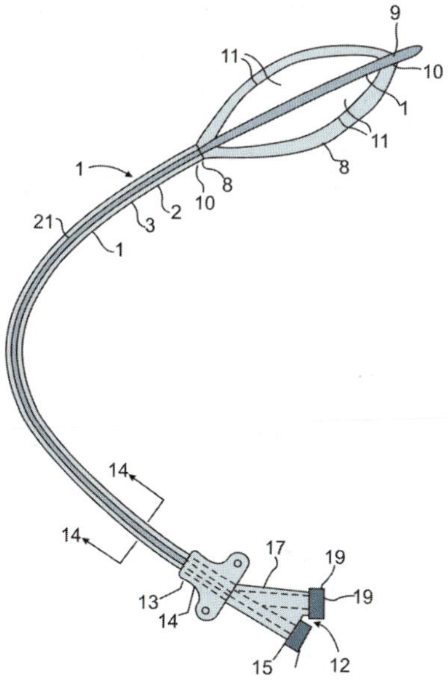

Fig. 34.5: *A balloon catheter is a type of "soft" catheter with an inflatable "balloon" at its tip which is used during a catheterization procedure to enlarge a narrow opening or passage within the body. The deflated balloon catheter is positioned, then inflated to perform the necessary procedure, and deflated again in order to be removed*

surgeons, (b) it could easily lead to bad outcomes without great care in selection of which patients/lesions to treat and of the treating physicians, and (c) it required careful teaching of the technique and its potential difficulties and pitfalls to other physicians, so as to proactively reduce the occurrence of poor results. Understanding these issues and tireless effort on his part are widely recognized in cardiology for being of fundamental importance to the ultimate success of the technique.

By about 1990, lumen stenosis of the coronary arteries was more commonly treated by the angioplasty technique than by coronary artery bypass surgery. This treatment approach is now referred to as plain old balloon angioplasty (POBA).

In the 1990s, further major improvements, both immediate and especially long-term became possible with better understanding of disease as a result of clinical research trials using IVUS and the development of stents to mechanically support POBA results.

Since the later 1990s, most angioplasties also involve a stent over the angioplasty balloon; the balloon is hydraulically (typically 6 up to 25 atmospheres of internal pressure) expanded, then deflated and removed while the stent remains behind to mechanically support the lumen remaining in the new, more open shape as created by the hydraulically expanded balloon.

Gruentzig's success remains a major breakthrough and great contribution to the field of medicine in demonstrating that doctors could work inside of the arteries safely without the need for open surgery. By utilizing the arterial circulation as a "therapeutic highway", many types of devices and drugs can now be delivered directly to the heart, kidneys, carotid arteries, brain, legs and aorta without the need for major surgery and general anesthesia.

Since the first human percutaneous transluminal coronary angioplasty (PTCA) procedure was performed in 1977, the use of percutaneous coronary intervention (PCI) has increased dramatically, becoming one of the most common medical interventions performed.

The technique, originally developed in Switzerland by Andreas Gruentzig, has transformed the practice of revascularization for coronary artery disease (CAD). Initially used in the treatment of patients with stable angina and discrete lesions in a single coronary artery, coronary angioplasty has multiple indications today including unstable angina, acute myocardial infarction (MI), and multivessel coronary artery disease. With the combination of sophisticated equipment, experienced operators, and modern drug therapy, PCI has evolved into an effective nonsurgical modality for treating patients with coronary artery disease.

Recent advances in guidewires, stents, and devices to cross chronically occluded arteries are evolving, so that more patients with chronic total occlusions (CTOs) are now being successfully treated percutaneously.

Improvements in catheter technique and the development of new devices, wires, stents, drug-eluting stents, and medications have occurred parallel to advances in the understanding of cardiovascular physiology, the pathogenesis of atherosclerosis, and the body's response to vascular injury. Intracoronary stents and atherectomy devices were developed to increase the success rate of, and decrease the complications associated with, conventional balloon dilation and to expand the indications for revascularization. These devices have enabled the intervention list to safely treat more complex coronary lesions and restenosis.

Stents have evolved to a level where the problems of restenosis seen with bare metal stents are a less frequent occurrence after drug-eluting stents are implanted. At the same time, advances in intravascular ultrasonography (IVUS) and fractional flow reserve evaluation have improved the understanding of coronary plaque morphology, plaque vulnerability, and coronary physiology. Furthermore, many of these technologies are able to help to identify patients who will benefit most from PCI, coronary bypass surgery, or medical therapy. Adjunctive pharmacologic therapies aimed at preventing acute reocclusion have also improved the safety and efficacy of coronary angioplasty.

The growth of PCIs has been remarkable and will likely be sustained, as new technologies have resulted in improved outcomes. Since 1994, the use of intracoronary stents has risen dramatically, and now with drug-eluting stents, stents are used in more than 80% of PCI cases in the United States. Innovations in PCIs over the past 2 decades have been paralleled by a dramatic reduction in 30 day death, myocardial infarction, and target-vessel revascularization rates.

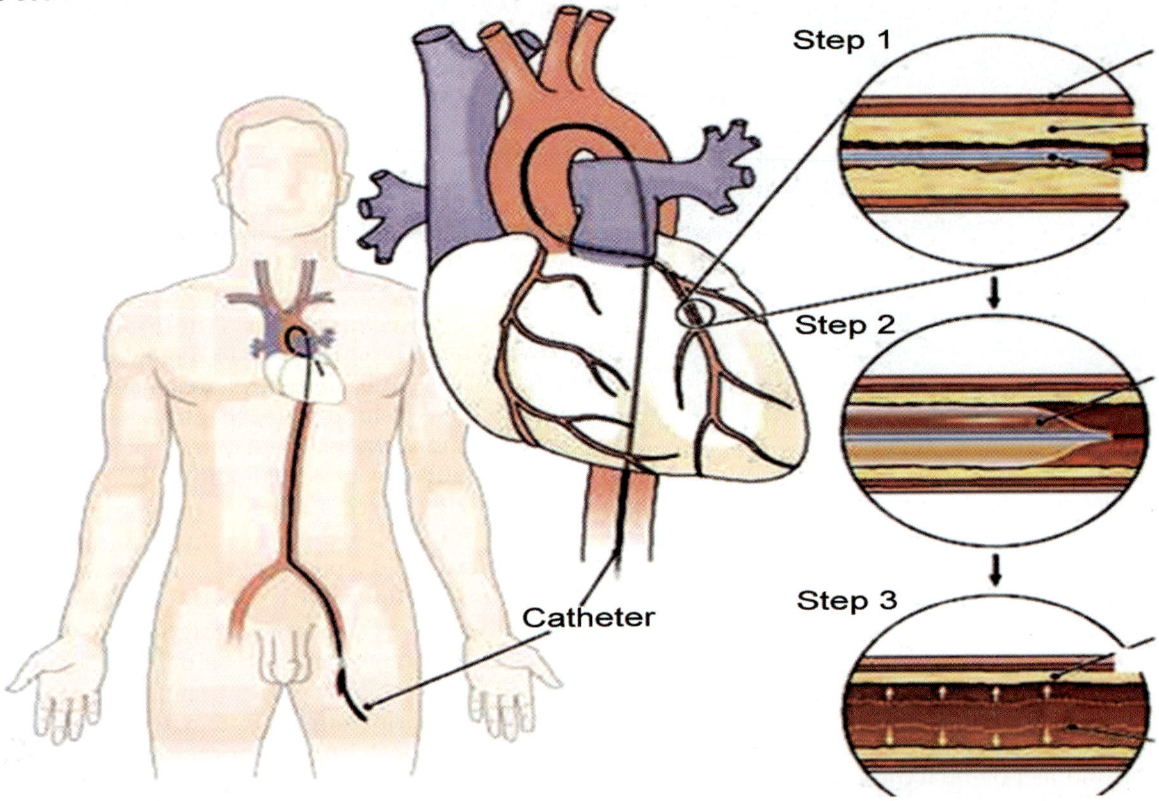

Fig. 34.6: ***Angioplasty procedure Step 1.*** *While the patient is awake and pain-free (local anesthesia), a catheter is inserted into an artery at the top of the leg (the femoral artery). The procedure begins with the doctor injecting some local anesthesia into the groin area and putting a needle into the femoral artery (the blood vessel that runs from the heart down the leg). Once the needle is inserted, a guide wire is placed through the needle, into the blood vessel. Following this step, the guidewire is left in the blood vessel and the needle is removed. A large needle called an introducer is then placed over the guidewire and the guidewire is removed.* ***Angioplasty procedure Step 2.*** *Next, a diagnostic catheter, which is a long narrow tube, is advanced through the introducer over a 0.035" guidewire, into the blood vessel. This catheter is then guided to the aorta and the guidewire is removed. Once the catheter is placed in the opening or ostium of one of the coronary arteries, the doctor injects dye and takes a series of X-rays films.* ***Angioplasty procedure Step 3.*** *After visualising the culprit vessel an appropriate sized balloon over the catheter is inserted and the vessel is then dilated with desired pressure to its fullest intraluminal size .This procedure can greatly improve the blood flow through the coronary arteries and to the heart tissue in about 90% of patients and may eliminate the need for coronary artery bypass surgery. The outcome is relief from chest pain symptoms and an improved exercise capacity. In 2 out of 3 cases, the procedure is considered successful with complete elimination of the narrowing or blockage*

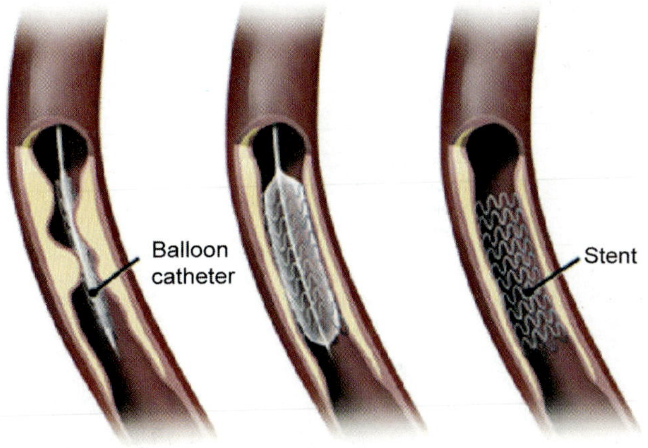

Fig. 34.7: *Illustration showing atheromated blocked coronary artery opened with stentoplasty*

Indications for PCI

Clinical Indications for PCI Include the following:

- Acute ST elevation myocardial infarction (STEMI)
- Non-ST elevation acute coronary syndrome
- Stable angina
- Anginal equivalent (e.g. dyspnea, arrhythmia, dizziness/ syncope)
- Asymptomatic or mildly symptomatic patients with objective evidence of a moderate to large area of viable myocardium or moderate to severe ischemia on noninvasive testing.
- Angiographic indications include hemodynamically significant lesions in vessels serving viable myocardium (vessel diameter >1.5 mm).

Contraindications to PCI

Clinical contraindications include significant comorbidities (relative contraindication).

Angiographic contraindications include the following:

- Left main stenosis in a patient who is a surgical candidate [coronary artery bypass graft (CABG) surgery is still the preferred treatment for left main stenosis; however, this area is rapidly evolving toward safe and feasible PCI options]
- Diffusely diseased small-caliber artery or vein graft
- Other coronary anatomy not amenable to percutaneous intervention.

Preparation in Percutaneous Coronary *Balloon Angioplasty* (Figs 34.3–34.6, 34.8, 34.10)

Equipment

The original description of angioplasty by Dotter and Judkins described enlargement of the vessel lumen through a mechanism of atheromatous plaque compression. This mechanism is also partially responsible for luminal enlargement with balloon angioplasty. In addition, however, improvement in luminal diameter following balloon angioplasty also results from stretching of the vessel wall by the balloon. Balloon inflation actually results in overstretching of the vessel wall and partial disruption of not only the intimal plaque but also the media and adventitia, resulting in enlargement of the lumen and the outer diameter of the vessel.

Axial redistribution of plaque material also contributes to improvements in lumen diameter. Atherectomy devices and, subsequently, intracoronary stents were developed, in part, to decrease the early and late loss in luminal diameter observed with conventional balloon angioplasty.

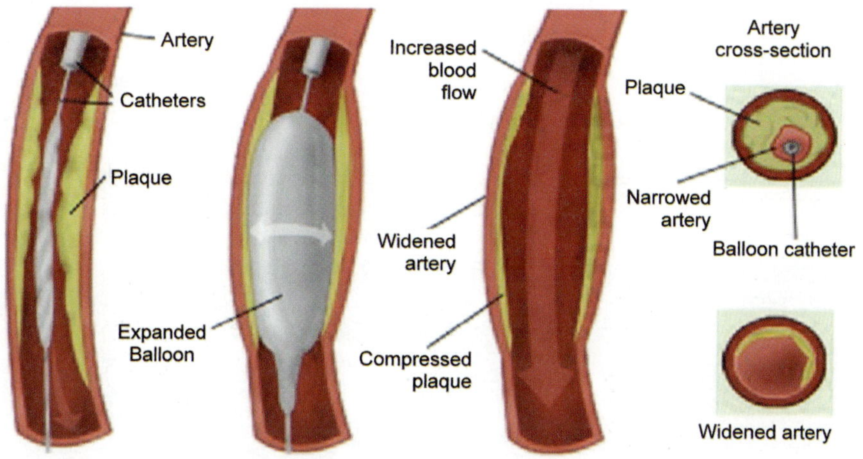

Fig. 34.8: *Balloon angioplasty. Angioplasty is a minimally invasive procedure used to open up clogged arteries in almost any part of the body. In balloon angioplasty, a small balloon is guided to the site of blockage, and inflated to compress the plaque and thus widen the artery. A small incision is made in the groin or wrist, following the administration of local anesthesia. A balloon-tipped catheter (balloon catheter) is then inserted into an artery of the leg or arms. The balloon catheter is threaded to the blockage site under X-ray guidance. Once at the site of blockage, a dye may be inserted at the site so as to determine the exact location of the blockage. The balloon catheter is then positioned at the precise location, and the balloon is inflated. As a result the surrounding plaque gets compressed, thus widening the arterial lumen. The balloon is then deflated and removed along with the catheter*

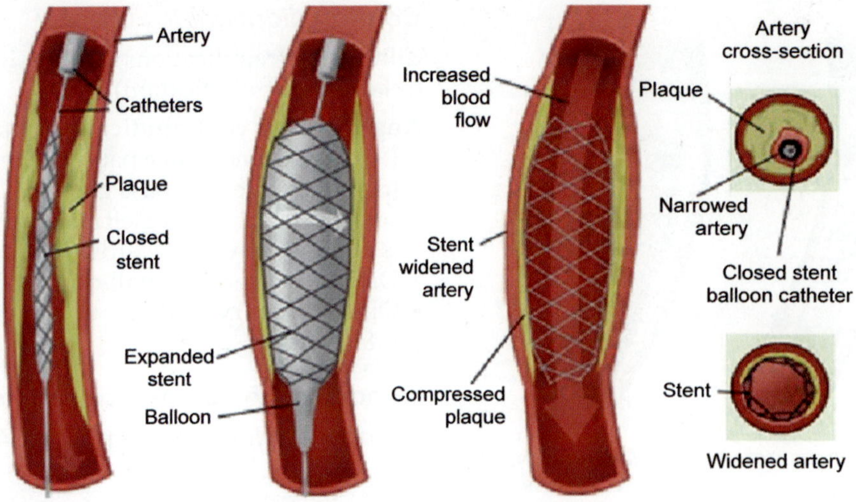

Fig. 34.9: *Stent angioplasty. This procedure is similar to balloon angioplasty, but involves the use of a small, expandable metallic mesh called stent, along with the balloon. The stent is placed around the balloon in a compressed form, and this assembly is placed at the tip of a catheter. It is then guided to the site of blockage as done during a balloon angioplasty. When the balloon is inflated, the stent expands and compresses the plaque. The balloon is then deflated and removed, leaving behind the stent which acts as a support and helps to keep the artery open*

Several different balloon catheter designs have existed (over-the-wire, monorail, fixed wire) with balloon materials that have different compliance characteristics allowing various degrees of expansion with increasing pressure. Irrespective of the balloon design, a steerable guidewire precedes the balloon into the artery and allows navigation through a considerable portion of the coronary tree. The development of balloon catheters that bend, allowing easy advancement through tortuous vascular segments (trackability), and that have increased shaft stiffness (pushability), allowing the catheter to be forced through stenotic lesions, has increased their versatility significantly. Another evolving feature of catheter design has been a reduction in the diameter of the deflated balloon, allowing easier passage through very stenotic lesions.

Improvements in catheter design have been partially responsible for the improved success rates of PCIs. The balloon catheter also serves as an adjunctive device for many other interventional therapies including atherectomy and coronary stents.

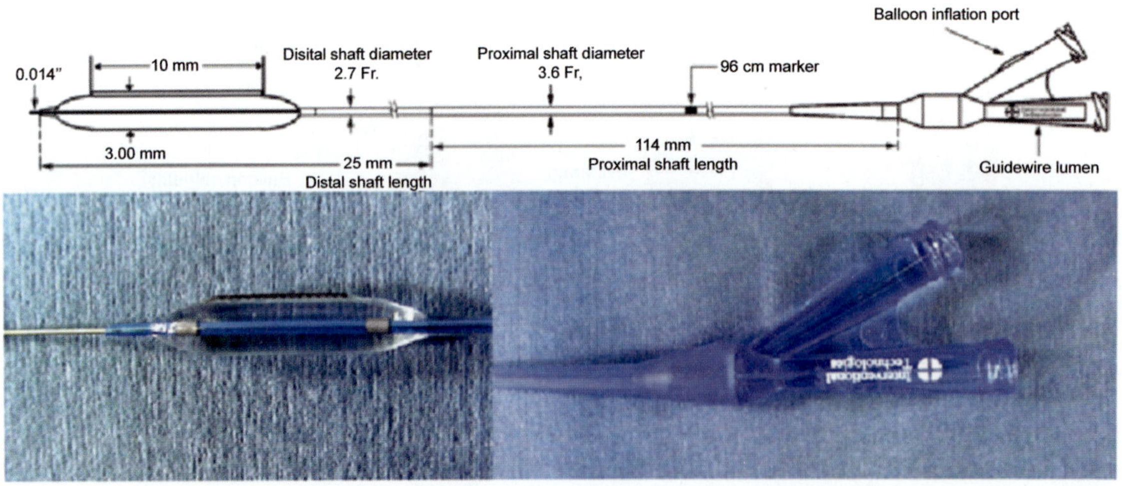

Fig. 34.10: *Athertomy device The SBC is an over-the-wire type catheter with a single blade attached to the surface of a noncompliant balloon. The blade is 10 mm in length and runs along the same side and axis as the balloon inflation port. The polysulfone balloon shaft is 3.6 Fr proximal and 2.7 Fr distal and is compatible with a 6 Fr guiding catheter. The working height and width of the blade are identical to those used for the current Cutting Balloon, namely 0.005–0.006 inches in height and 0.003 inches thick*

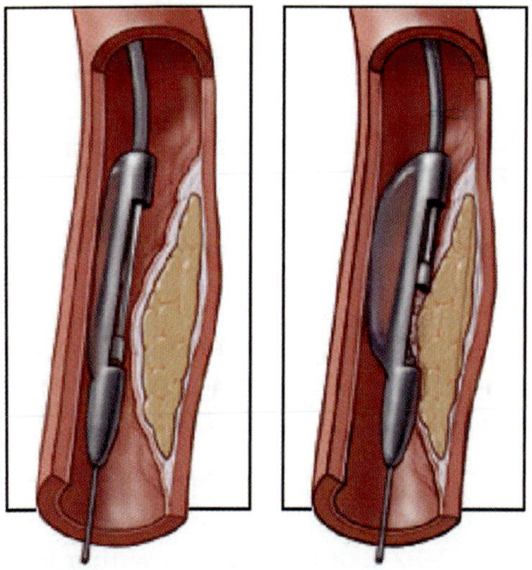

Fig. 34.11: *Diagram showing working of directional atherotomy device in removing the plaque from the occluded artery*

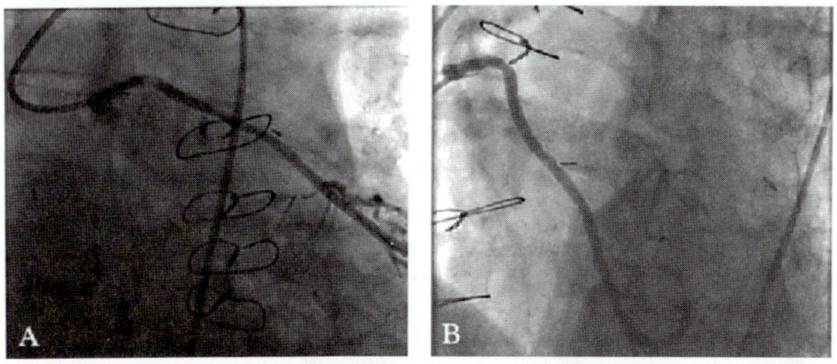

Figs 34.12A and B: *(A) Vein graft deply intubated to allow the rotablator burr to be advanced. (B) Final result after rotational atherectomy and stent placement*

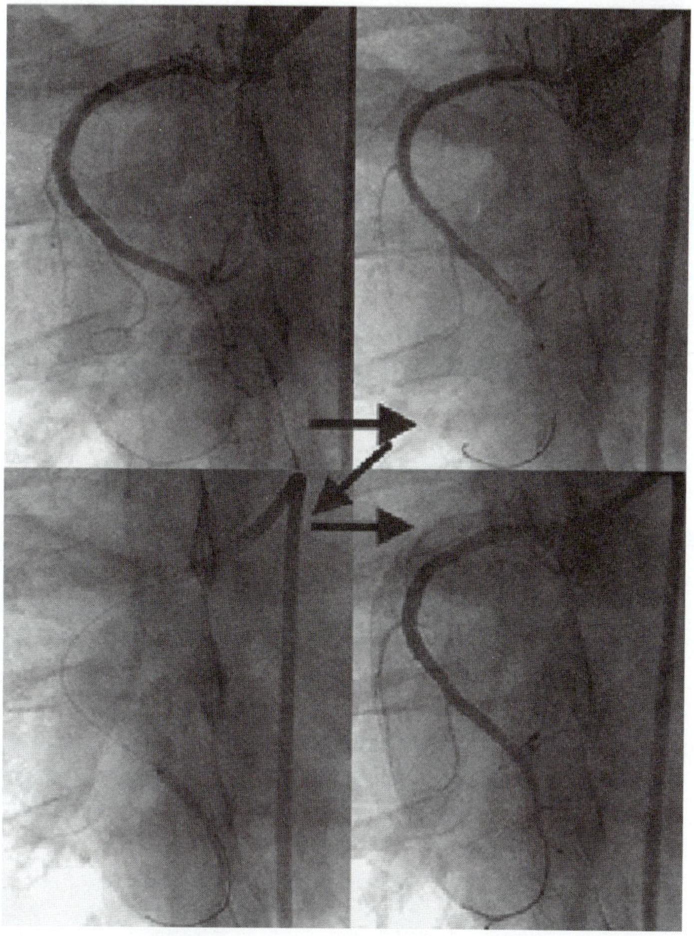

Fig. 34.13: *Angiogram with rotational set black arrow explaining as how occluded vessel has been shown to restore near normal lumen after atherotomy procedure*

Atherectomy Devices and Coronary Stents

As a result of technical challenges, suboptimal clinical outcomes, and the significant rates of restenosis following percutaneous coronary artery balloon angioplasty, two innovative types of devices were developed: (1) those used for atherectomy and (2) coronary stents (Figs 34.7, 34.9, 34.11–34.18A–C).

The idea behind atherectomy devices was to physically remove atheroma, calcium, and excess cellular material from the site of a coronary occlusion or stenosis. Both mechanical and laser-based approaches are used. An alternative approach developed at about the same time was intracoronary stent placement, based on the notion that permanent implantation of a scaffold to hold open the coronary artery at the site of an intervention would improve outcomes. Long-term outcomes from atherectomy alone have been disappointing and, in most cases, little better than balloon angioplasty. Stents, particularly stents coated with materials to reduce inflammatory and cell growth responses, have resulted in greatly improved outcomes.

Long-term outcomes from atherectomy alone have been disappointing and little better than balloon angioplasty in most cases. Stents, particularly stents coated with materials to reduce inflammatory and cell growth responses, have

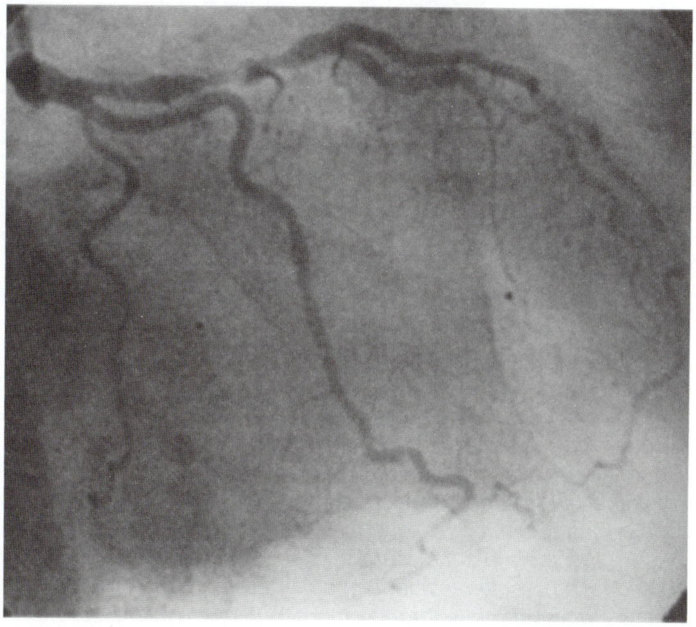

Fig. 34.14: *Coronary angiography revealed diffuse irregular 73% luminal narrowing of the proximal left anterior descending coronary artery*

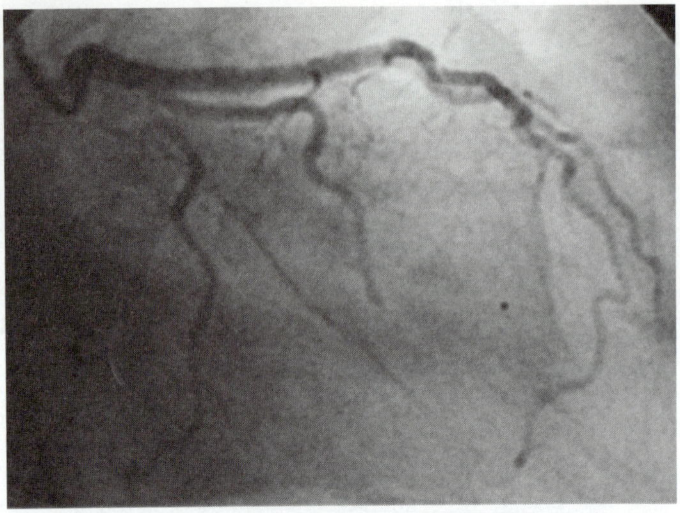

Fig. 34.15: *One day after percutaneous transluminal coronary angioplasty with stenting, a follow-up coronary angiography revealed the patent stents of the left main coronary artery and proximal left anterior descending coronary artery with remaining thrombotic occlusion of the distal intermediate branch*

resulted in greatly improved outcomes. Atherectomy is still used for specific, niche indications, but the most common intracoronary device used today is a stent.

The rotational atherectomy catheter (rotablator) is designed for the removal of plaque from coronary arteries. This device (*see* the image below), which has a diamond-studded burr at its tip, rotates at about 160,000 rpm and is particularly well suited for ablation of calcific or fibrotic plaque material.

Percutaneous transluminal coronary angioplasty (PTCA). The rotational atherectomy catheter (Rotablator) is a device designed for the removal of plaque from coronary arteries. This device, which has a diamond-studded burr at its tip, rotates at about 160,000 rpm and is particularly well suited for ablation of calcific or fibrotic plaque material.

Unlike other atherectomy devices that rely on tissue cutting, the rotational atherectomy device relies on plaque abrasion and pulverization. Rotational atherectomy is successful in 92–97% of these cases, with a low incidence of major complications. It causes dislodgement of particles into the microcirculation, which occasionally may lead to infarction and no reflow (impaired distal coronary flow). Currently, the use of rotational atherectomy is largely confined to fibrotic or heavily calcified lesions that can be wired but not crossed or dilated by a balloon catheter.

The excimer laser, rotational atherectomy, and balloon angioplasty comparison (ERBAC) study showed that

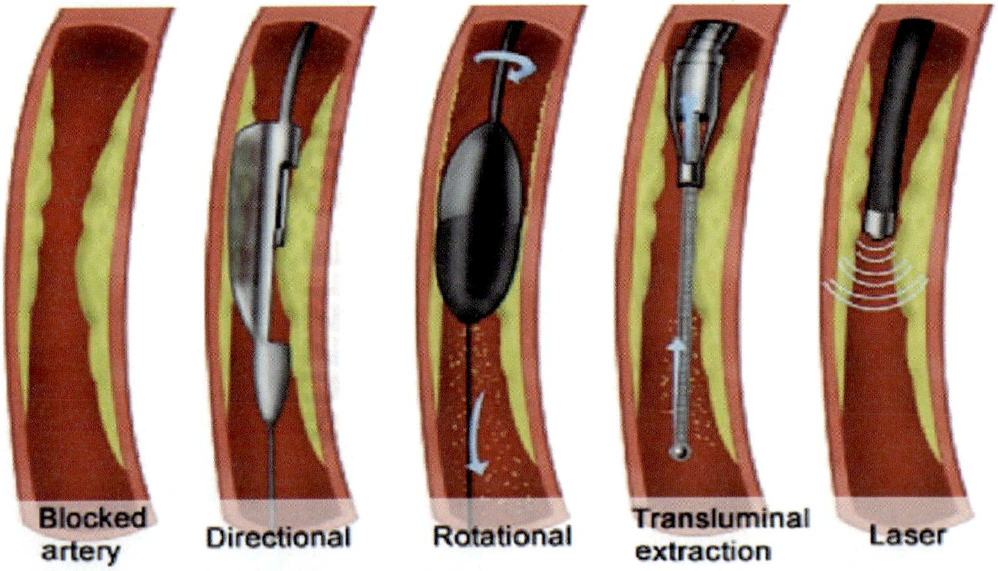

Fig. 34.16: *Atherectomy this is a minimally invasive procedure that involves the use of specialized catheters for mechanical removal of plaque from the arterial walls. The plaque is either scraped out or pulverized with the help of tiny blades. The design and working of these devices ensures that the arterial wall remains damage-free. The catheter is inserted into an artery in the leg or arm, through an incision in the groin or wrist. It is then routed to the blockage site, and the plaque is mechanically scraped out. Depending on the type of device or catheter used, atherectomy procedures employed are: "Directional: here, the catheter has a scraping blade attached to it along with a low pressure balloon on the opposite side. Once at the blockage site the balloon is inflated, as a result of which the blade is pushed towards the plaque. The plaque is then scraped out, and the catheter is rotated to ensure complete plaque removal. The plaque fragments are collected in a chamber present at the tip of the device. "Rotational: a rotational atherectomy catheter has small, diamond-tipped, rotating edges which disintegrate the plaque into microscopic fragments. These fragments flow through the circulatory system, and are removed from the body through normal waste-removal processes. "Transluminal extraction: the catheter used in this procedure has two stainless steel, rotating blades attached to a hollow tube. At the site of blockage, the rotating blades grind the plaque, and the resultant fragments are collected into the hollow tube by vacuum suction. "Laser: in this procedure, a laser-tipped catheter is used to vaporize the plaque. The resultant molecules are removed by the body via liver and kidneys*

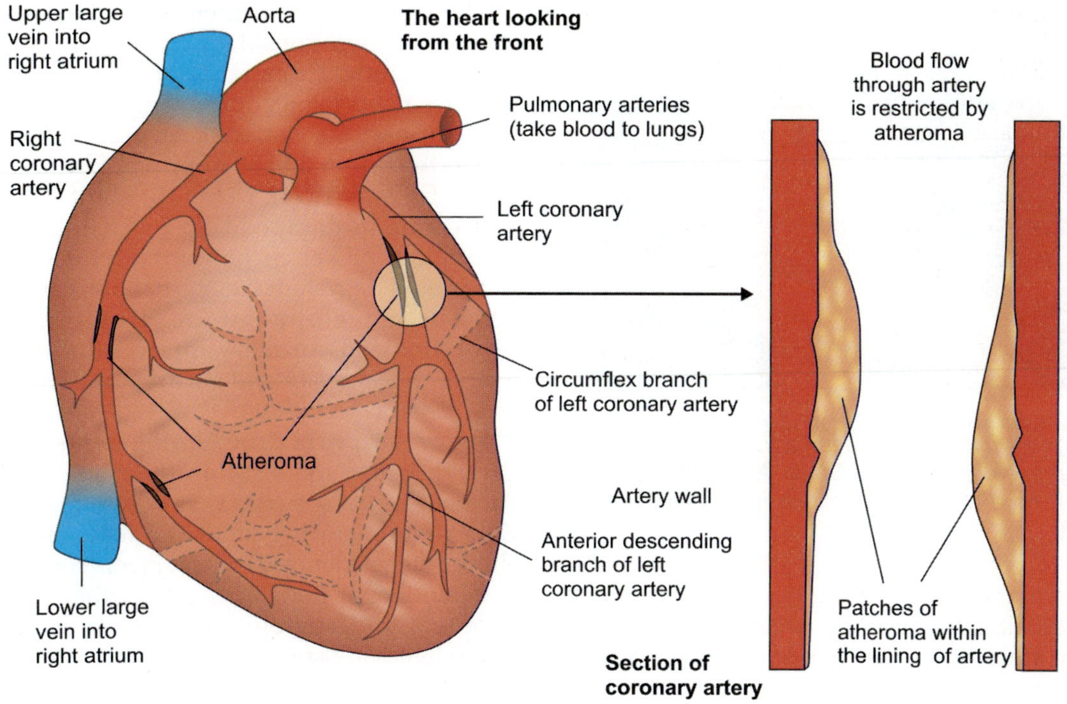

Fig. 34.17: *Diagram showing (Left) anatomical localisation of atherosclerosed coronary arteries and morphology of section of atheromatous coronary artery (Right)*

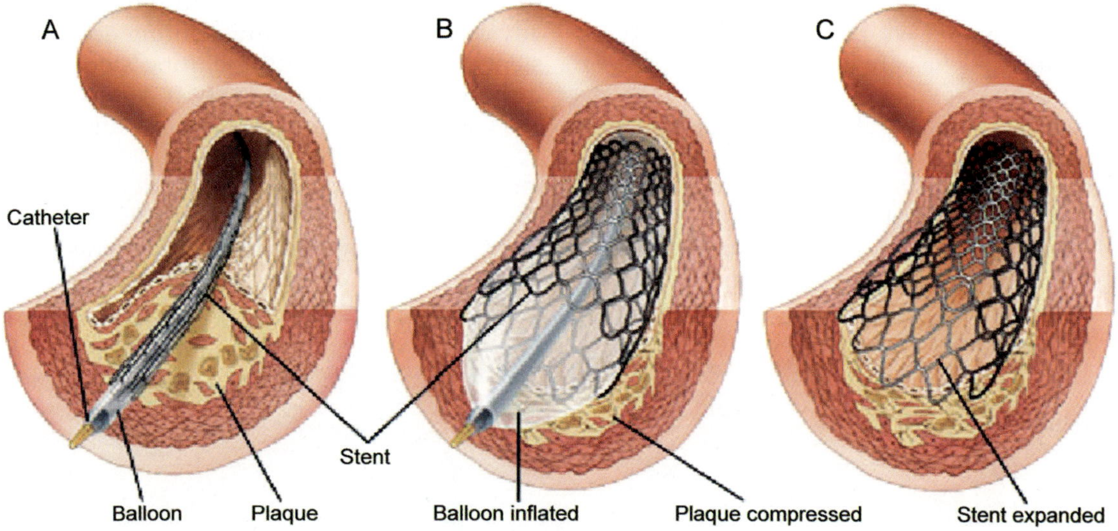

Figs 34.18A to C: *Stepwise opening of obstructed coronary artery after stent has been installed in the lumen of the artery*

rotational atherectomy was associated with a higher short-term success rate than balloon angioplasty (90% vs 80%), but major ischemic complications and repeat revascularization were higher 6 months after treatment (46% vs 37%).

A meta-analysis failed to show any significant difference in mortality, major adverse cardiovascular events (MACE), or revascularization rates in patients treated with rotational atherectomy, laser, or cutting balloon angioplasty when compared with balloon angioplasty alone. In some cases, rotational atherectomy was actually associated with an increase in periprocedural myocardial infarction. However, none of these trials compared stent-related outcomes. In fact, many of these devices may be used to facilitate stent delivery in complex lesions, especially when balloon angioplasty alone has failed.

Since 1987, directional coronary atherectomy (DCA) has been used to debulk coronary plaques. A steel fenestrated cage housing a cup-shaped blade is positioned against the coronary lesion by a low-pressure positioning balloon, allowing any protruding plaque to be removed.

Atherectomy is typically followed by balloon dilation and stenting. The acute gain, therefore, is a combination of the

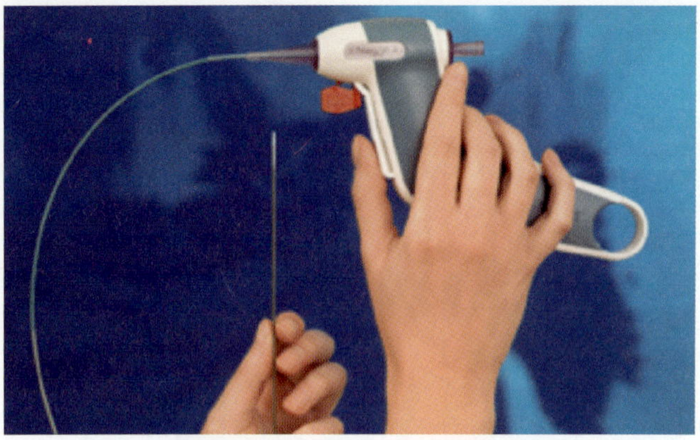

Fig. 34.19: *Self-expanding nitinol stent pulsar-18 fracture resistant by design asymmetrical s-shape articulations and peak-to-valley design prevent fish-scaling. Small design modifications allow for better fatigue resistance through improved axial and bending flexibility*

removal of atheromatous plaque and radial displacement of plaque from dilation. Major complication rates associated with directional atherectomy are low and similar to those associated with conventional balloon angioplasty. Other complications (e.g. distal embolization of plaque, transient side-branch occlusion, coronary vasospasm, the no-reflow phenomenon, non-Q-wave myocardial infarction) are greater with DCA than with balloon angioplasty. Because of the increased complication rates and the greater technical demands of DCA compared with balloon angioplasty or stenting, the use of DCAs has greatly decreased in recent years.

A 2006 meta-analysis demonstrated that DCA is superior to stenting alone with regard to acute angiographic results and target-lesion revascularization with a similar prevalence of late MACEs. There was, however, a higher prevalence of early MACEs with DCA before stenting, which probably related to distal embolization.

Although initial excitement about the development of laser atherectomy was considerable, it is not used widely because of the technical demands of this device and no clear improvements in outcome over therapy with other devices. Intracoronary stents have been used widely since the early 1990s (the original FDA approval for intracoronary stents in the US was 1994). Many different stents are available and differ in composition (e.g. stainless steel, cobalt chromium, nickel chromium), architectural design, and stent delivery system (i.e. the balloon catheter that delivers it). The development of drug-eluting stents has revolutionized coronary intervention to the extent that balloon angioplasty and bare metal stents did in the 1980s and 1990s.

Today, 4 types of drug-eluting stents are available in the United States, the sirolimuseluting stent (Cypher), the Paclitaxel-eluting stent (Taxus), and the newer-generation Zotarolimus-eluting stent (Endeavor) and Everolimus-eluting stent (Xience V). These stents comprise a metal stent with a polymer that elutes a drug that reduces neointimal hyperplasia. Drug-eluting stents have been extensively tested in a wide spectrum of coronary lesions, all of which have demonstrated significant reductions in restenosis and target-lesion revascularization rates when compared with bare metal stents (Figs 34.19–34.22).

The zotarolimus-eluting stent and everolimus-eluting stent have improved deliverability, thinner struts, and a thinner polymer layer, and they may have clinical advantages over sirolimus-eluting and paclitaxel-eluting stents. Studies with drug-eluting stents are ongoing and include efforts to define safety and outcomes in every range of PCI setting, such as stable and unstable lesions, small vessels, vein grafts, chronic total occlusions, primary PCI, and comparing drug-eluting stent technologies with a coronary artery bypass graft (CABG) in left main coronary artery disease and in diabetes patients with multivessel coronary artery disease.

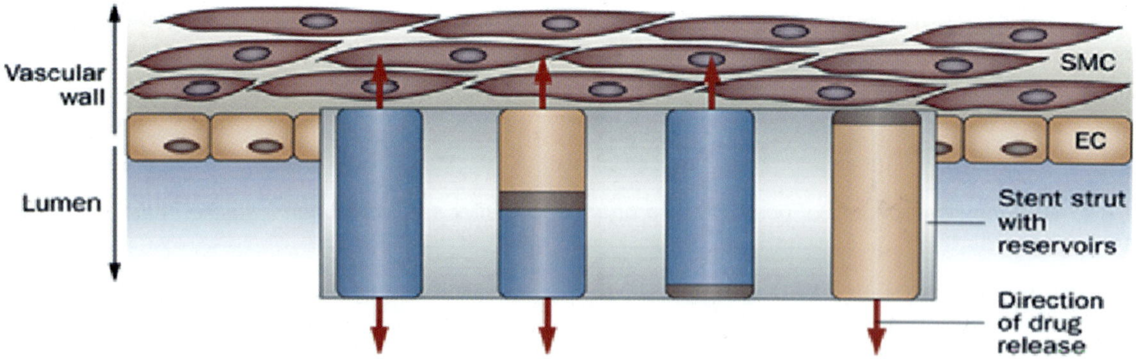

Fig. 34.20: *This technology allows a targeted therapeutic approach by, for example, delivery of an agent that inhibits SMC proliferation via the ablumenal route of the stent surface. Concomitantly, an agent that promotes endothelial recovery can be released via the lumenal route. Furthermore, downstream drug delivery to tissue seems to be feasible (preferably at the lumenal side). The lateral view of a stent strut in the blood vessel exemplifies the diversity of drug delivery options (from left to right): bidirectional delivery of one drug to both the ablumenal and lumenal side (blue), ablumenal delivery of one drug (orange) and lumenal delivery of a different drug (blue) where the drugs are separated in the reservoir to avoid mixing, or ablumenal delivery of one drug only (blue) and lumenal delivery of one drug only (orange). Reservoirs are sealed and drugs are separated by a layer of biodegradable polymer (brown disk). Abbreviations: EC, endothelial cell; SMC, smooth muscle cell*

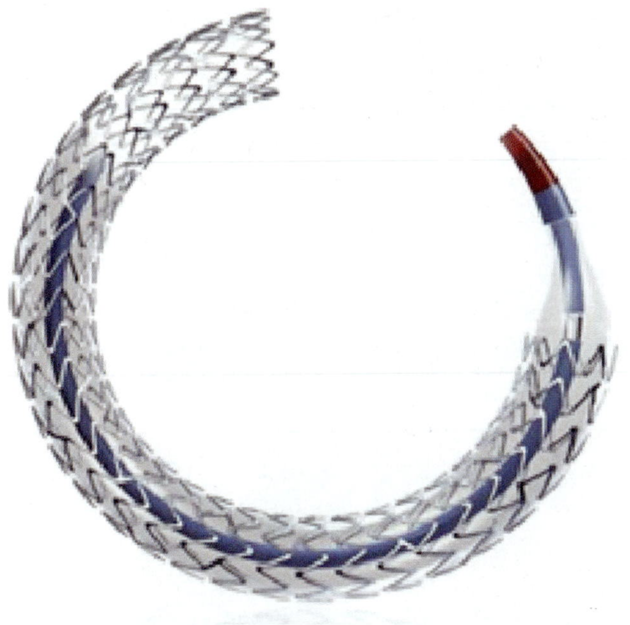

Fig. 34.21: *Promus premier stent system is designed to provide physicians improved drug-eluting stent performance in treating patients with coronary artery disease. It is the only platform to feature a customised platinum chromium stent architecture, the market-leading everolimus drug coating and fluorinated co-polymer, and an enhanced stent delivery system*

Although stents are conventionally placed after balloon predilation, a meta-analysis by Piscione et al suggests that, in selected coronary lesions, direct stenting may lead to better outcomes. Myocardial infarction rates were lower with direct stenting (3.16% vs 4.04% with conventional stenting) while rates of target vessel revascularization were similar.

Ancillary devices

In addition to balloons, stents, and atherectomy devices, other devices such as thrombus extraction catheters and distal embolic protection devices have found roles in PCI. In the TAPAS trial (Thrombus Aspiration during Percutaneous coronary intervention in acute myocardial infarction), which studied the use of thrombus aspiration during primary PCI for ST elevation myocardial infarction, thrombus aspiration with an Export catheter before stenting had a reduced all-cause mortality (4.7% vs 7.6%) and reduced cardiac death (3.6% vs 6.7%) at 1 year compared with conventional PCI.

In a pooled analysis of data from three prospective randomized trials, De Vita et al found that although increasing time to treatment was associated with a decreased rate of optimal reperfusion in patients receiving standard PCI, this trend was not seen in patients treated with thrombus aspiration. De Vita et al concluded that the use of thrombus aspiration limits the adverse effects that prolonged time to treatment has on myocardial reperfusion.

The use of distal embolic protection during saphenous vein graft intervention has become the standard of care. The SAFER trial (saphenous vein graft angioplasty free of emboli randomized) initially proved the benefit of embolic protection in reducing 30 days rates of major adverse cardiac events (MACE) (9.6% vs 16.5%, $P = 0.004$), myocardial infarction (8.6% vs 14.7%), and no reflow (3% vs 9%).

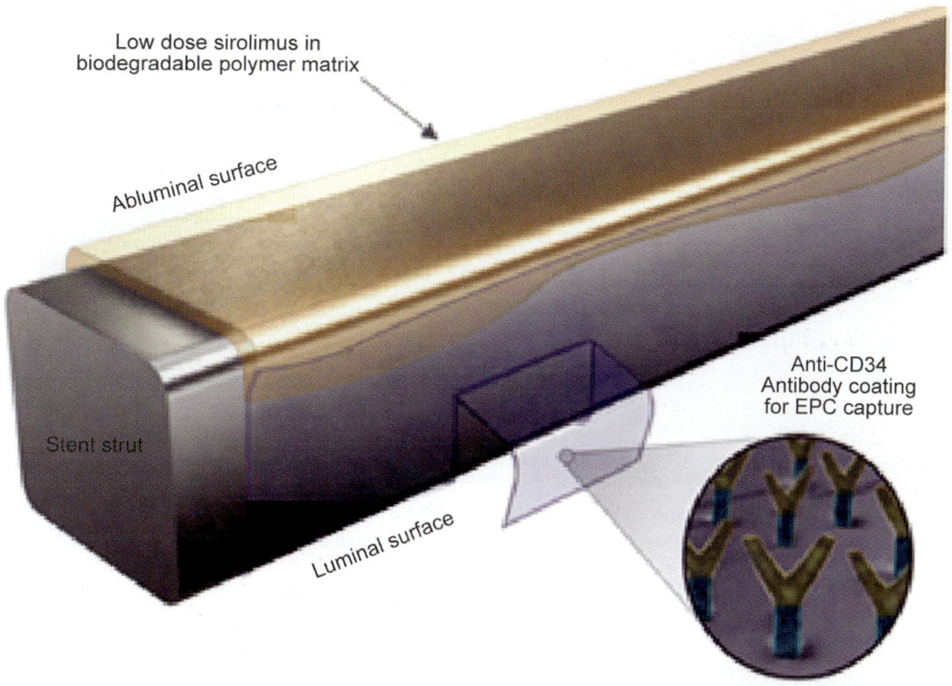

Fig. 34.22: *The combo dual therapy device is hailed by OrbusNeich (Hoevelaken, Netherlands) as the first example of a dual therapy stent. The product combines abluminal sirolimus drug elution for the control of neointimal proliferation with the company's proprietary genous pro-healing technology to promote endothelial coverage. On the luminal side of the stent are immobilized antibodies that capture circulating endothelial progenitor cells*

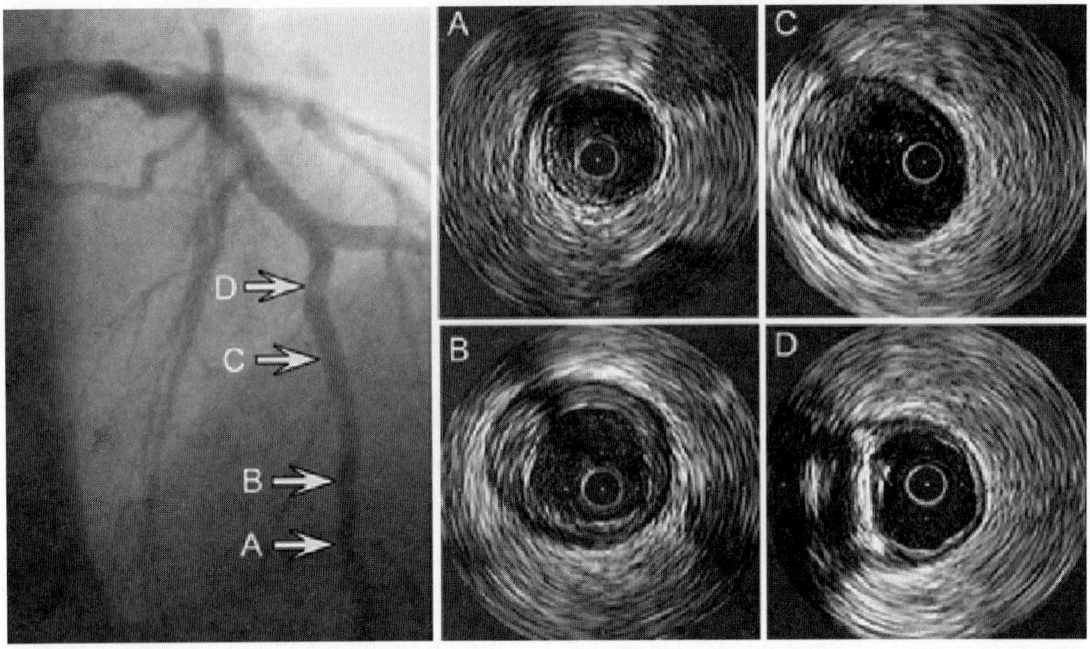

Fig. 34.23: *Intravascular ultrasound (IVUS) at multiple sites in an angiographically normal artery. The four images obtained from sites A through D exhibit various degrees of atherosclerotic involvement, despite a normal-appearing angiogram. The IVUS images were obtained via a motorized pullback*

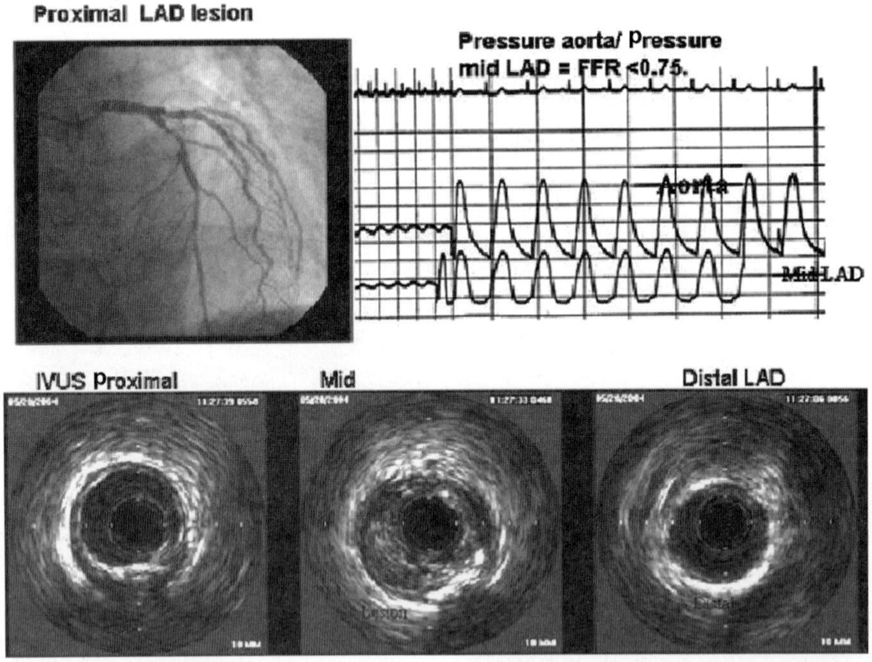

Fig. 34.24: *Fractional flow ratio (FFR). Pressure wire is advanced across left anterior descending (LAD) stenosis and intracoronary adenosine is given. FFR ratio is recorded at baseline and then after adenosine push is given. Here, LAD lesion and FFR postadenosine is shown*

Intravascular Ultrasonography (Figs 34.23, 34.24, 34.26A and B, 36.27A–F and 36.32A–D)

Coronary angiography provides a display of luminal narrowing in multiple planes and is useful in guiding coronary interventions. However, angiography cannot provide information about the vessel wall, which is where the atherosclerotic process resides. Intravascular ultrasonography (IVUS) (*see* the image below) was developed to provide information about the plaque, the vessel wall, and the degree of luminal narrowing. It provides a tomographic cross-section of the vessel, allowing operators to gather significant qualitative and quantitative

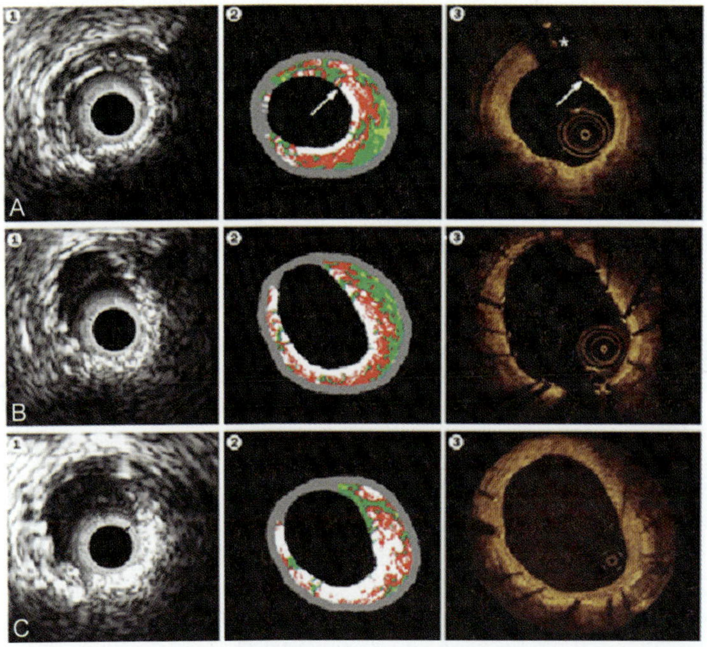

Fig. 34.25: *Matched grayscale IVUS (1), IVUS-VH (2) and OCT (3) images of the IVUS-derived, thin-capped fibroatheroma (A) before stenting with the vProtect® Luminal Shield, (B) immediately after treatment with the vProtect® Luminal Shield and (C) at the 6-month follow-up appointment. The arrow in panel a part 2 indicates the necrotic core in contact with the lumen. The arrow in panel a part 3 indicates the thin fibrous cap, and the asterisk indicates a guidewire artifact. In the IVUS-VH images (parts 2): red, necrotic core; dark green, fibrotic tissue; light green, fibrofatty tissue; and white, dense calcium. Abbreviations: IVUS, intravascular ultrasound; IVUS-VH, intravascular ultrasound virtual histology; OCT, optical coherence tomography*

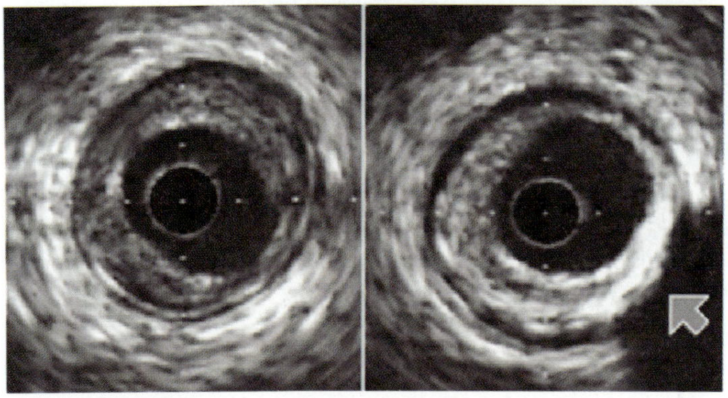

Fig. 32.26: *Differing plaque morphologies by intravascular ultrasound. (Left) A soft atheroma is characterized by a plaque less echogenic than the surrounding adventitia. (Right) A hard atheroma is characterized by dense fibrous tissue more echogenic than the surrounding adventitia. A portion of the fibrous atheroma is calcified (arrow)*

information that is potentially valuable in assessing stenosis severity and the true extent of atherosclerotic involvement. Identification of the lumen border and the media-adventitia interface form the key landmarks during interpretation. Plaque can be distinguished from the lumen by differences in echogenicity. In addition to providing information about the amount and distribution of plaque, IVUS can identify features of plaque composition, such as calcification and lipid collections, which may not be appreciated by angiography alone. Frequent uses of IVUS include the assessment of indeterminate lesions and the evaluation of adequate stent deployment. The latter has become increasingly important, since proper deployment of drug-eluting stents is critical to reduction in rates of thrombosis. Recent developments in ultrasonography (e.g. virtual histology) and other technologies (e.g. optical coherence tomography, plaque thermography) have led to ways of characterizing and identifying vulnerable segments of plaque that may pose a risk for future cardiac events (Figs 34.25A to C).

Coronary Physiologic Assessment

Intracoronary Doppler pressure wires are able to characterize coronary lesion physiology and to estimate lesion severity. Comparison of pressure distal to a lesion with aortic pressure enables determination of fractional flow reserve (FFR) (*see* the image below). A measurement below 0.75–0.80 during maximal hyperemia (induced via administration of adenosine) is consistent with a hemodynamically significant lesion. This determination is useful in deciding whether to perform PCI in an angiographic intermediate lesion. Clinical data, namely the DEFER study, support using this approach, with a low event rate seen in medically managed patients with angina and an FFR measurement greater than 0.75.

Fractional flow ratio (FFR): Pressure wire is advanced across left anterior descending (LAD) stenosis and intracoronary adenosine is given. FFR ratio is recorded at baseline and then after adenosine push is given. Here, LAD lesion and FFR postadenosine is shown (Fig. 34.24).

The fractional flow reserve versus angiography for guiding PCI in patients with multivessel coronary artery disease (FAME) trial showed that routine measurement of FFR during angioplasty reduced the risk of death, myocardial infarction, or repeat revascularization by 30% and death or myocardial infarction by 35%, compared with the current practice of using angiography to guide stenting decisions. In this study, a cut-off of FFR greater than 0.80 was used to define a nonischemic lesion. Two-year follow-up of the FAME trial showed continuing significant reductions in the combined end-point of death and myocardial infarction with the use of FFR compared with standard angiography-guided PCI.

This form of physiologic lesion assessment is also useful for defining optimal stenting, assessing the angiographic severity of jailed side branch lesions, helping guide the decision for multivessel percutaneous coronary intervention (PCI) or coronary artery bypass graft (CABG) in multiple intermediate lesions, and assessing the severity of instant restenosis. FFR measurements have excellent correlation with IVUS analysis, especially when determining lesion severity, such as in ambiguous left main coronary artery anatomy.

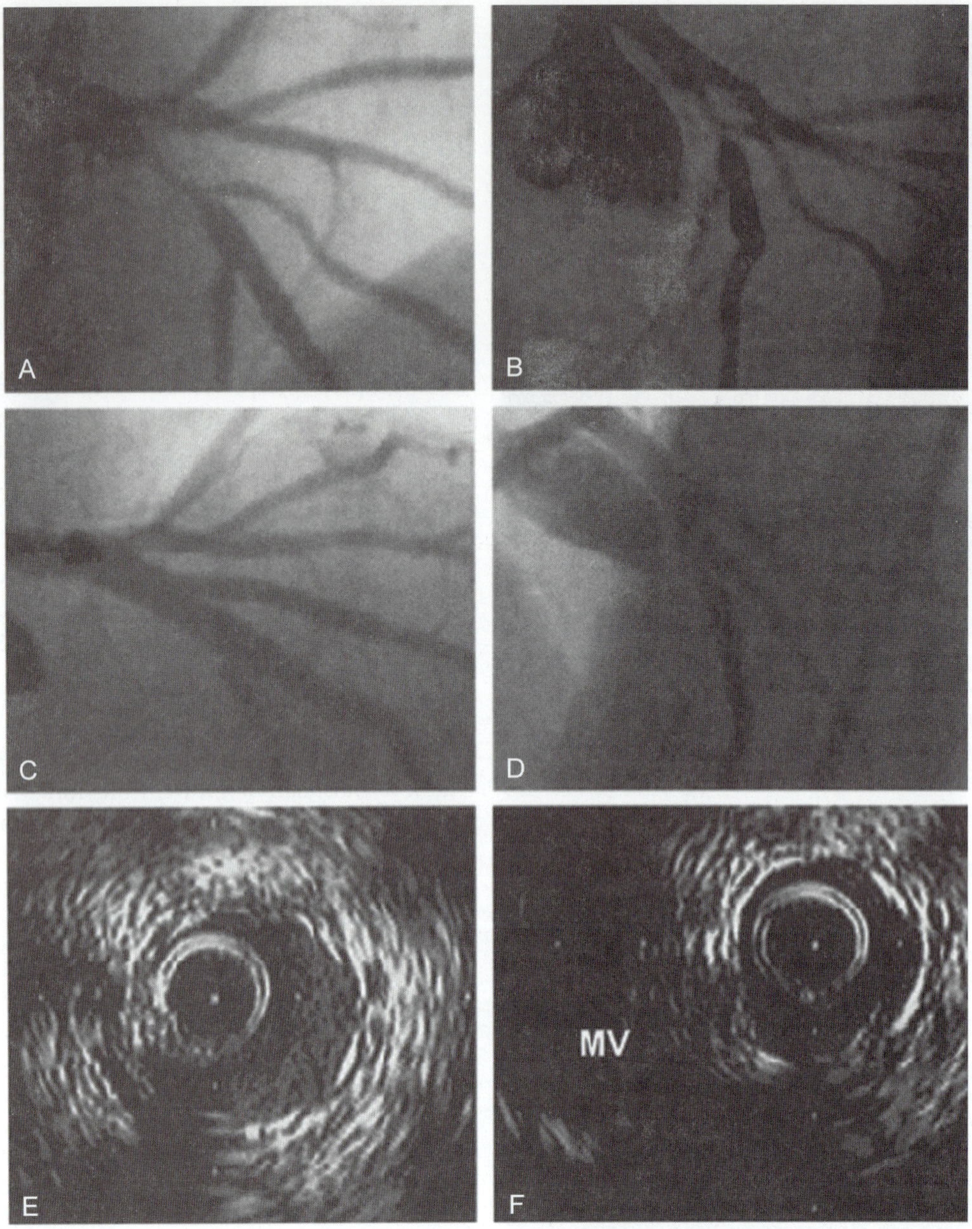

Figs 34.27A to F: *(A, B) Preprocedure angiograms showing a "true bifurcation" lesion (type D) in the proximal left anterior descending coronary artery/first diagonal branch in the cranial and left anterior oblique (LAO) views, respectively. (C, D) Final angiograms showing optimal angiographic result after crush-stenting at the bifurcation lesion (cranial and LAO views, respectively). (E) Intravascular ultrasound image showing the distal portion of the side branch (SB) (first diagonal) stent. (F) Intravascular ultrasound of the SB ostium showing stent underexpansion. MV, main vessel*

Adjunctive therapies in the catheterization laboratory: Aspirin and heparin have been the traditional adjunctive medical therapies for patients undergoing coronary angioplasty and have been shown to decrease complications following the procedure. Since 1994, several new antithrombotic drugs have been developed that have advantages over standard heparin therapy. Although it is an effective anticoagulant, heparin has several limitations including variable pharmacokinetics requiring careful monitoring, inhibition by substances released from activated platelets, and an inability to inhibit fibrin-bound thrombin.

To address these limitations, several direct thrombin inhibitors have been developed. Hirudin and bivalirudin (angiomax) were evaluated in 2 multicenter trials, and both agents were found to be slightly better than heparin in preventing ischemic complications during balloon angioplasty, but they had no effect on restenosis rates.

Low-molecular-weight heparins are also being substituted for standard heparin in some centers in patients with acute coronary syndromes and during coronary interventions. Newer factor IX and factor Xa inhibitors are being evaluated as potential alternative anticoagulants. However, trials have failed to show a significant difference in efficacy of factor Xa inhibition compared with unfractionated heparin (UFH).

With an improved understanding of how stents should be deployed, warfarin is no longer necessary. Patients receiving stents are now treated with a combination of aspirin and clopidogrel, and with this therapy, the incidence of subacute thrombosis is approximately 1%. Today, this combination is given to all stent patients for a minimum of 4 weeks after a bare metal stent and a minimum of 12 months when a drug-eluting stent is used. Issues remain as to whether the duration of aspirin and clopidogrel should be longer in drug-eluting stent patients. The authors advocate that a baby aspirin should be maintained for life and clopidogrel should be considered for life in drug-eluting stent patients, unless bleeding contraindications restrict its use. Other considerations with antiplatelet therapy during PCI include the cost of clopidogrel, the proper loading dose, and timing of the initial dose relative to cardiac catheterization.

In elective situations, clopidogrel is most effective when given prior to PCI. In acute situations, this may not be practical, and clopidogrel is therefore often given after PCI. Concerns still exist regarding the risk of bleeding and platelet transfusion requirements in patients taking clopidogrel who require an urgent coronary artery bypass graft (CABG). However, as emergent CABG is rare, there

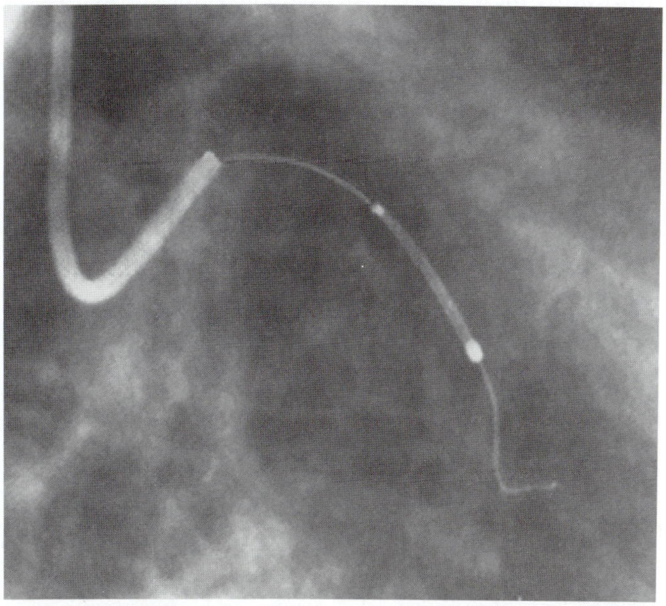

Fig. 34.28: *Coronary angioplasty. X-ray angiogram of a balloon catheter and stent (white tipped tube, centre right) being placed within a coronary artery of a heart. They will be used to treat stenosis (narrowing) of the artery. The flexible catheter used to place them there is seen snaking down from top left. The inflation of the balloon catheter will expand the artery and restore normal blood flow. The stent is a hollow tube mesh, expanded by the balloon catheter, that stays in the artery and supports it after the balloon catheter has been withdrawn. Arterial stenosis may arise from arterial disease. X-ray angiography injects a radio-opaque contrast medium to highlight blood vessels on X-rays*

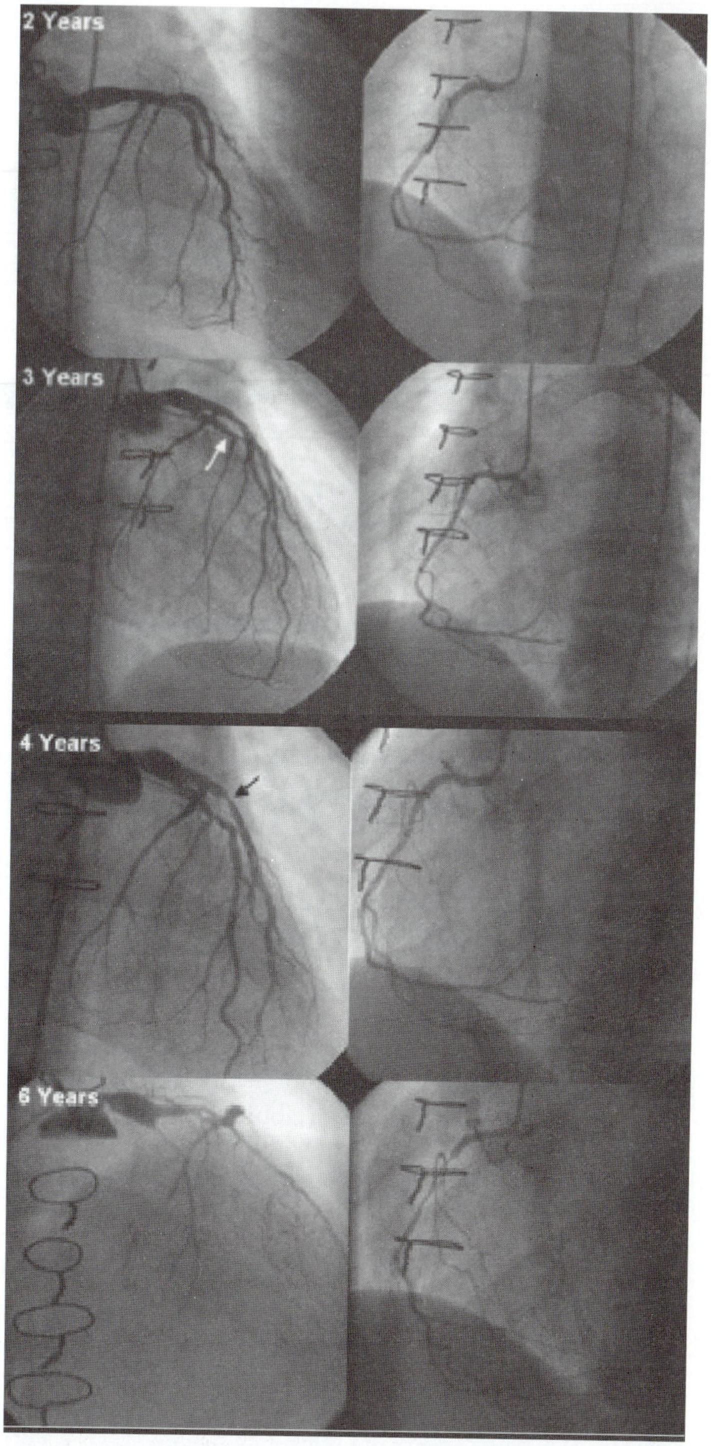

Fig. 34.29: *The progressive nature of allograft vasculopathy. At 2 years after heart transplantation, there is ectasia of the left main coronary artery but no evidence of allograft vasculopathy. At 3 years, the left anterior descending coronary artery developed mild disease at the bifurcation of the septal artery (white arrow). At 4 years, the first obtuse marginal branch of the circumflex has an additional lesion (black arrow). At 6 years, the left anterior descending coronary artery is occluded totally and the circumflex is diseased severely. The right coronary is also diseased diffusely including the smaller secondary branches, with abrupt cut-off in some of them. Unfortunately, this patient had a fatal myocardial infarction a few weeks after the last angiogram*

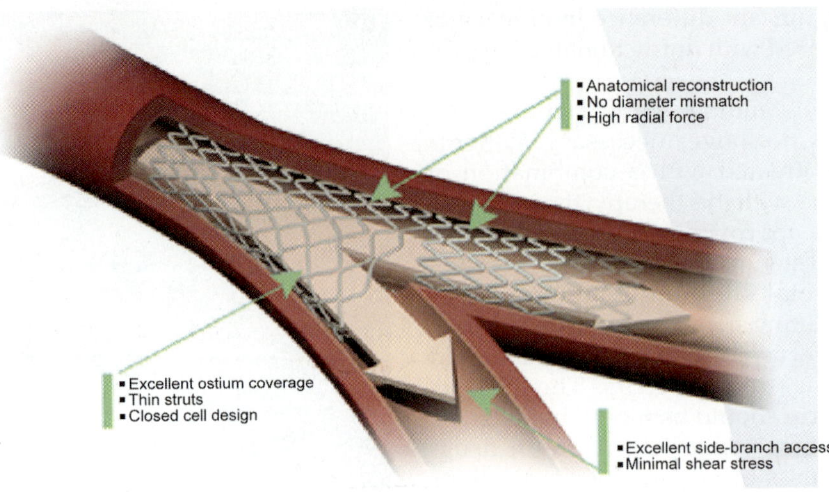

Fig. 34.30: *Features of a bifurcated self-expanding coronary stents*

may be time to risk-stratify patients and to give clopidogrel before cardiac catheterization. If CABG is required, the effect of clopidogrel usually diminishes within 5 days.

Another important consideration is the dose of clopidogrel. If given 2 hours prior to PCI, 600 mg is recommended; if given more than 2 hours prior to PCI, then 300 mg is recommended. Some centers have even given 900 mg instead of 600 mg. At present, the ACC/AHA guidelines recommend giving 300 mg up to 6 hours prior to PCI. Development of newer intravenous antiplatelet therapies with shorter half-lives may help overcome these issues. Aspirin, 325 mg, should be given prior to all PCIs and then maintained at 81 mg daily.

Clopidogrel is a prodrug that is metabolized to the active form of the drug by the cytochrome (CYP) 450 enzyme system in the liver. Recent research has demonstrated that genetic variation at the CYP450 2C19 locus results in decreased metabolic activation of clopidogrel and increased risk of adverse cardiovascular events. This led to a recent update to the package insert for clopidogrel (plavix) that includes a "black box" warning for use in patients who are "poor metabolizers" (individuals who have two abnormal alleles at the CYP 2C19 locus; approximately 2–4% of white patients). Individuals with one abnormal allele have intermediate metabolism of clopidogrel to the active metabolite.

In a meta-analysis of 9 studies and almost 10,000 patients, Mega et al found that carriage of even one reduced-function CYP2C19 allele in patients treated with clopidogrel after percutaneous coronary intervention was associated with a significantly increased risk of major adverse cardiovascular events, particularly stent thrombosis.

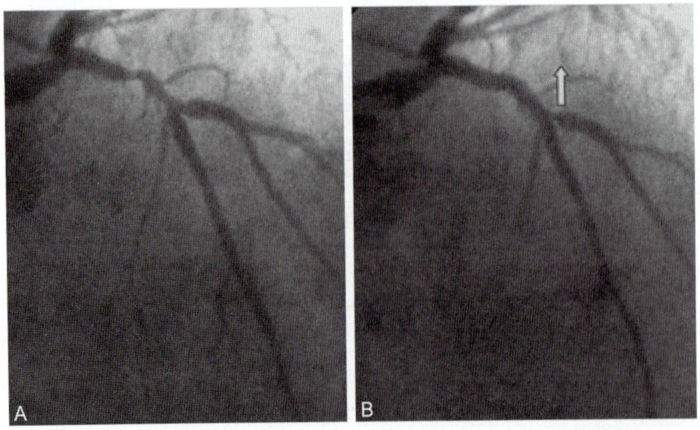

Fig. 34.31: *(A) Type 3 LAD/ diagonal bifurcation lesion. (B) After stenting the LAD across the diagonal branch with a jailed wire in the diagonal artery; the diagonal artery ostium is pulled up by the stent and the jailed wire*

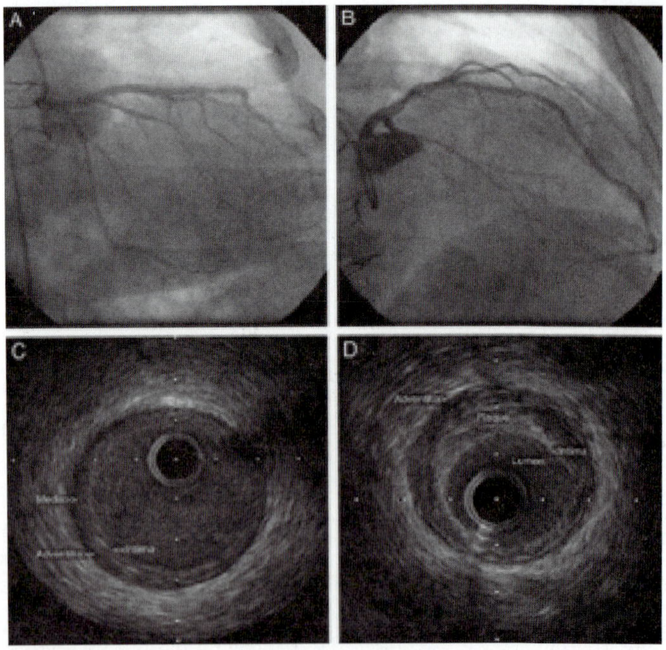

Fig. 34.32: *Intravascular ultrasound images of the anterior descending artery in a patient transplanted 5 years previously, showing both the concentric intimal thickening typical of cardiac allograft vasculopathy (C) and an eccentric plaque typical of atherosclerotic coronary disease (D). Coronary angiography did not suggest disease in this artery (A and B)*

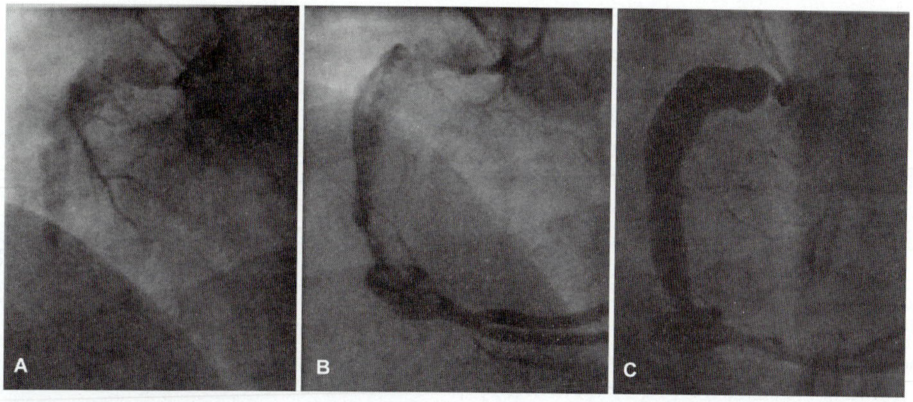

Fig. 34.33: *Occlusion of the RCA. Angiogram of occluded right coronary artery (RCA) aneurysm in a 20 yrs-old adolescent who experienced a Kawasaki disease-compatible illness at age 6 years (diagnosed as nonspecific viral illness) and was asymptomatic until his myocardial infarction. (A) Injection of the occluded RCA, (B) RCA after percutaneous transluminal coronary angioplasty with re-established distal flow. Note smooth appearance of distal branches of the RCA. (C) Patent RCA aneurysm 1 month after percutaneous transluminal coronary angioplasty, aspirin, and warfarin therapy maintaining an international normalized ratio of 2 to 2.5*

The best treatment strategy for platelet inhibition in patients who are poor or intermediate metabolizers has not been established, but alternative antiplatelet strategies should be considered.

A consensus statement issued by the American College of Cardiology, American College of Gastroenterology, and American Heart Association in November 2010 addresses the issue of concomitant use of proton pump inhibitors (PPIs), which are CYP2C19 inhibitors, and thienopyridine antiplatelet drugs, such as clopidogrel.

Clopidogrel findings and recommendations are listed below:

- Clopidogrel reduces major CV events compared with placebo or aspirin
- Dual antiplatelet therapy with clopidogrel and aspirin, compared with aspirin alone, reduces major CV events in patients with established ischemic heart disease, and it reduces coronary stent thrombosis but is not routinely recommended for patients with prior ischemic stroke because of the risk of bleeding.
- Clopidogrel alone, aspirin alone, and their combination are all associated with increased risk of GI bleeding
- Patients with prior GI bleeding are at highest risk for recurrent bleeding on antiplatelet therapy; other risk factors include advanced age, concurrent use of anticoagulants, steroids, or NSAIDs (including aspirin), and *Helicobacter pylori* infection; risk increases as the number of risk factors increases.
- Use of proton pump inhibitors (PPIs) or histamine (H2) receptor antagonists (H2RAs) reduces the risk of upper GI bleeding compared with no therapy; PPIs reduce upper GI bleeding to a greater degree than do H2RAs.
- PPIs are recommended to reduce GI bleeding in patients with a history of upper GI bleeding; PPIs are appropriate in patients with multiple risk factors for GI bleeding who require antiplatelet therapy.
- Routine use of either a PPI or an H2RA is not recommended for patients at lower risk of upper GI bleeding, who have much less potential to benefit from prophylactic therapy.

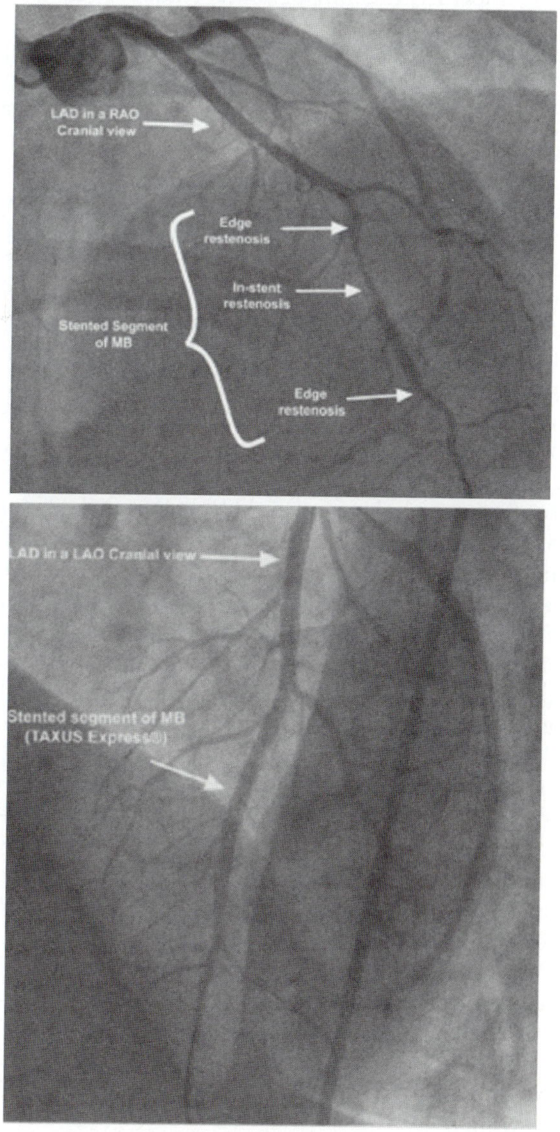

Fig. 34.34: *Stent restenosis of LAD artery in myocardial bridging (bottom) shows successful stenting of segment in myocardial bridging (MB). Top showing stenosed segment of MB*

- Clinical decisions regarding concomitant use of PPIs and thienopyridines must balance overall risks and benefits, considering both CV and GI complications.
- Pharmacokinetic and pharmacodynamic studies, using platelet assays as surrogate end-points, suggest that concomitant use of clopidogrel and a PPI reduces the antiplatelet effects of clopidogrel; the strongest evidence for an interaction is between omeprazole and clopidogrel; it is not established that changes in these surrogate end-points translate into clinically meaningful differences.
- Observational studies and a single randomized clinical trial have shown inconsistent effects on CV outcomes of concomitant use of thienopyridines and PPIs; a clinically important interaction cannot be excluded, particularly in certain subgroups, such as poor metabolizers of clopidogrel.
- The role of either pharmacogenomic testing or platelet function testing in managing therapy with thienopyridines and PPIs has not yet been established.

Prasugrel is a thienopyridine adenosine diphosphate (ADP) receptor inhibitor that inhibits platelet aggregation. It has been shown to reduce new and recurrent myocardial infarctions. The loading dose is 60 mg PO once, and maintenance is 10 mg PO qd (given with aspirin 75–325 mg/d). Prasugrel is indicated to reduce thrombotic cardiovascular events (including stent thrombosis) with acute coronary syndrome that is managed with PCI. It is used specifically for unstable angina or non-ST-segment elevation myocardial infarction (NSTEMI) or with acute ST-segment elevation myocardial infarction (STEMI) when managed with primary or delayed PCI.

Additional information from the TRITON TIMI 38 trial analyzed whether the type, size and timing of myocardial infarction affected prasugrel's ability to reduce new or recurrent myocardial infarction. TRITON TIMI 38 included 13,608 patients with acute coronary syndrome randomized to either prasugrel or clopidogrel. Prasugrel significantly reduced the overall risk of myocardial infarction compared with clopidogrel for any type of myocardial infarction (e.g. procedure-related, nonprocedural, and consistently across myocardial infarction size). Significant, sometimes fatal, bleeding occurred more frequently with prasugrel than with clopidogrel.

All types of percutaneous coronary interventions result in disruption of the coronary endothelium, which leads to platelet activation. Activated platelets bind to the vessel wall (adhesion) and to each other (aggregation) and release numerous vasoactive compounds. Aspirin blocks the cyclooxygenase pathway and reduces thrombotic complications after balloon angioplasty. However, despite heparin and aspirin therapy, thrombotic complications are not eliminated. Further studies identified the importance of the GP IIb/IIIa receptor, which binds fibrinogen and mediates the cross-linking of platelets and platelet aggregation.

The introduction of GP IIb/IIIa receptor inhibitors has had a major influence on current treatment strategies in the catheterization laboratory, such as the following:

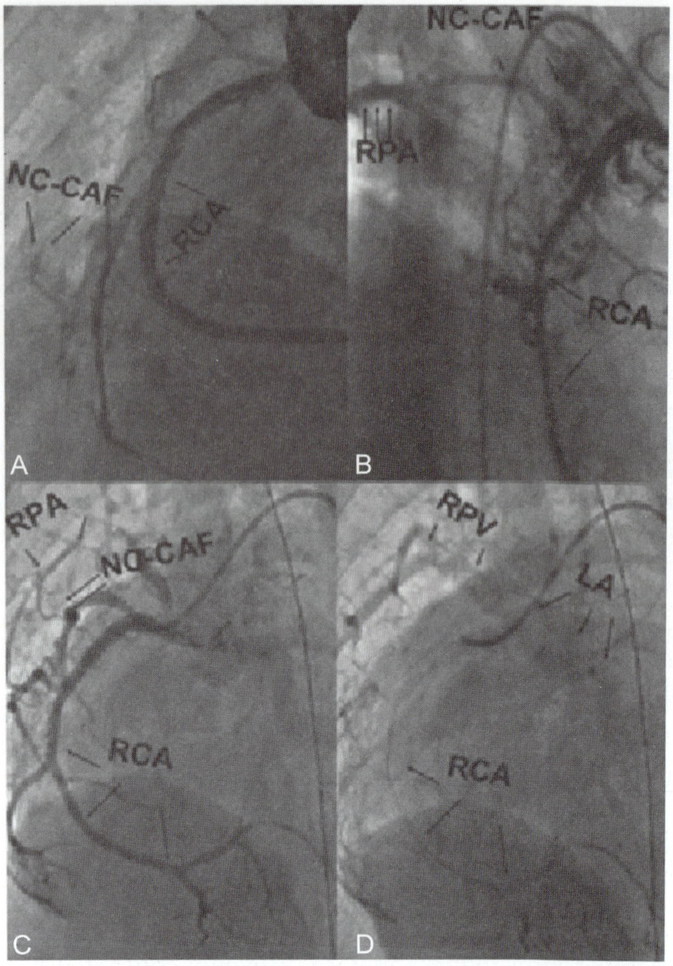

Fig. 34.35: *Examples of noncameral coronary artery fistulae (NC-CAFs) are shown in three patients: (A) a small NC-CAF from the right coronary artery (RCA) with flow into the right lung field, but no clear identification of a pulmonary vessel; (B) a moderate NC-CAF with a diffuse connection originating from the RCA and filling an identifiable right pulmonary artery (RPA) branch; and (C-D) a large NC-CAF from the RCA (C) filling a RPA branch, (d) and then on levophase of the same angiogram, filling of left atrium (LA) is clearly identified*

- Abciximab, tirofiban, and eptifibatide have all been shown to reduce ischemic complications in patients undergoing balloon angioplasty and coronary stenting.
- In primary PCI, GP IIb/IIIa receptor inhibitors have also been shown to improve flow and perfusion and to reduce adverse events.
- Abciximab may improve outcomes in patients when given prior to their arrival in the catheterization laboratory for primary PCI.
- A meta-analysis of GP IIb/IIIa inhibitor trials showed a significant reduction in early mortality rates when these agents are used during coronary intervention; the combined end point of death or myocardial infarction was also reduced significantly at 30 days.
- The EVA-AMI trial (Eptifibatide vs Abciximab in primary PCI for acute ST elevation myocardial infarction) compared the efficacy of 2 glycoprotein (GP) IIb/IIIa

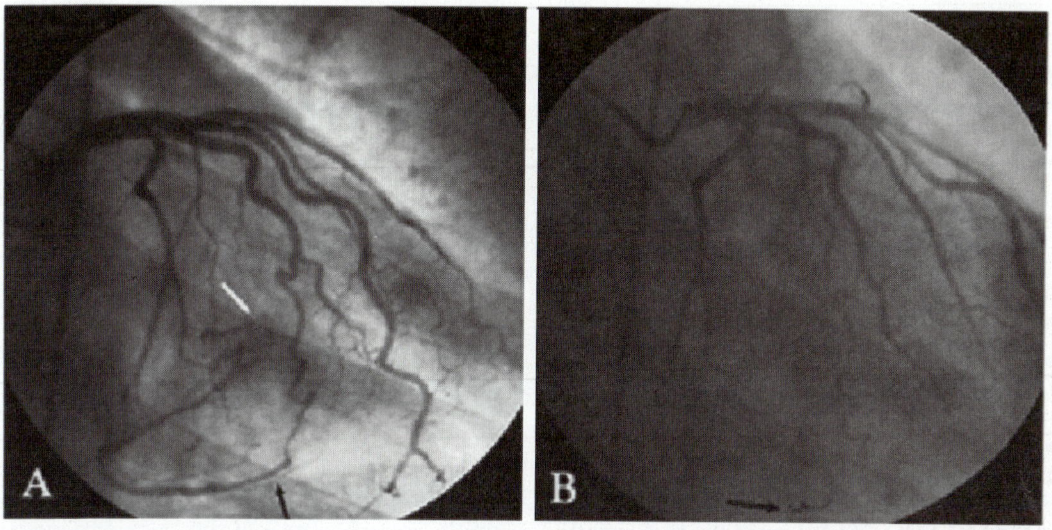

Fig. 34.36: *(A) Shows a coronary angiography of the left coronary system in a right anterior oblique angiographic view. After contrast injection, flow from a coronary artery fistula originating from the distal ramus intermedius coronary artery (black arrow) and draining into the left ventricular chamber (white arrow) is visualized. No obstructive coronary artery disease is noted. (B) microcoil embolization of the distal ramus intermedius coronary artery fistual (arrow) is shown after a single coil delivery through a microcatheter positioned in the proximal segment of the fistula. After contrast injection into the left coronary artery, no contrast filling is visualized via the fistula into the left ventricular chamber, indicating the successful coronary artery fistula closure*

inhibitors as adjunct to PCI in 427 patients with STEMI; results showed double-bolus eptifibatide followed by a 24 hour infusion was as effective as single-bolus abciximab followed by a 12 hour infusion for ST-segment resolution.

- These agents are effective at reducing ischemic complications of PCIs; however, they have not been shown to improve outcome in saphenous vein graft PCI.
- One meta-analysis of 22 studies including 10,123 patients evaluated the use of GP IIb/IIIa inhibitors during elective PCI in patients pretreated with clopidogrel. The analysis found that use of GPIIb/IIIa inhibitors had no effect on mortality or major bleeding but were associated with a decrease in the incidence of nonfatal myocardial infarction and an increase in the rate of minor bleeding.

Post-Procedure Outcome of PCI

A major 2009 task force report viewed favorably, in general, the use of coronary revascularization for patients with acute coronary syndromes and combinations of significant symptoms and/or ischemia. However, revascularization of asymptomatic patients or patients with low-risk findings on noninvasive testing and minimal medical therapy were viewed less favorably (Figs 34.27A and B, 34.38A–B, 34.39A and B).

Acute Myocardial Infarction (AMI)

The recognition that intracoronary thrombosis is the primary mechanism of vessel occlusion in acute myocardial infarction and that prompt restoration of vessel patency provides significant clinical benefit has led to the development of aggressive new treatments for this disorder.

Thrombolytic therapies, such as front-loaded tissue plasminogen activator (tPA), reteplase (r-PA), and tenecteplase (TNK), open approximately 80% of infarct-related vessels within 90 minutes, but only 50% will have normal (TIMI grade 3) flow. In addition, 10% of vessels opened by thrombolysis either reocclude or are the source for recurrent symptoms of angina. Because of these limitations to thrombolytic therapy, several randomized trials have evaluated mechanical revascularization, so-called primary angioplasty, in the setting of acute myocardial infarction.

An analysis of 23 trials confirms the superiority of primary angioplasty over fibrinolytic therapy in terms of adverse events and mortality reduction in both the short-term and long-term. Overall, primary PCI was associated with significant reductions in death, recurrent myocardial infarction, reinfarction, and the combined endpoint of death, myocardial infarction and stroke.

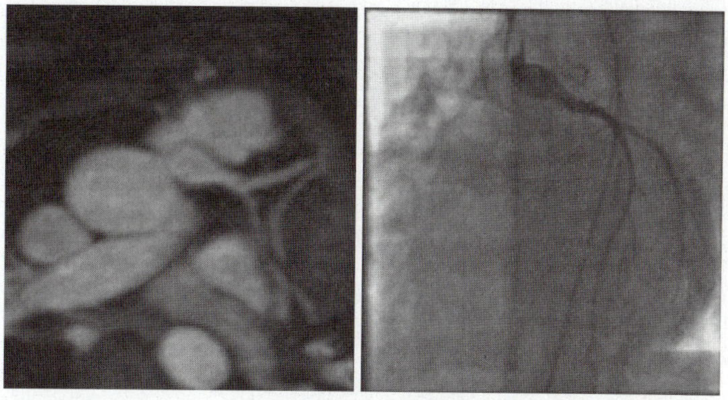

Fig. 34.37: *3D b-SSFP whole heart images, magnetic resonance coronary angiography MRCA (left) shows large patent, reconstructed, re-implanted left coronary artery into the left coronary sinus. Findings confirmed on X-ray coronary angiography (right)*

In the situation where patients are transferred from outside hospitals, primary angioplasty is often preferred to onsite fibrinolytic therapy for patients with the following: expected door-to-balloon time less than 90 minutes and symptom duration less than 3 hours, symptom duration more than 3 hours, cardiogenic shock, contraindications to fibrinolytic therapy, and age older than 75 years. The use of thrombolytic therapy and then referral for intentional PCI (facilitated PCI) has not been shown to be superior to primary PCI and may actually worsen outcomes with increased risk of stroke and bleeding (ASSENT 4).

Recent data suggest that early use of GP IIb/IIIa inhibitors may help to achieve earlier infarct vessel patency and better outcomes during PCI. Whether this is so for all of these agents is being assessed in several studies. One meta-analysis has shown that abciximab is associated with a 46% reduction in death and reinfarction in primary PCI patients and the AHA/ACC STEMI guidelines currently recommend early use of abciximab in these patients. When fibrinolytic therapy is given but fails to produce ST resolution, then immediate PCI (rescue PCI) is recommended.

Some of the most important considerations in providing effective primary PCI relate to the logistical issues and barriers that are known to exist. The PCI system or network, ambiguity of leadership and organization, protocols/care, pathways/interfacility transfer, and reimbursement issues are the main areas of contention. Studies of the US primary PCI sites that are considered the best (those sites that deliver door-to-balloon times consistently within 90 minutes, which is currently about 5% of the US myocardial infarction population) have identified the key determinants of shorter door-to-balloon times as the following: ECG being performed within 10 minutes, the emergency department independently making the decision to engage the catheterization laboratory team, and interdisciplinary teamwork.

The key factor for effective primary PCI is timely reperfusion therapy. Studies from the National Registry of Myocardial Infarction (NRMI) data have shown that shortening door-to-balloon time to less than 90 minutes is associated with a reduction in mortality. In certain situations, timely reperfusion may be best achieved with fibrinolytic therapy if delays are likely in accessing primary PCI.

From a procedural perspective, because primary PCI involves a thrombotic plaque, the potential risk of more complications exists, especially no reflow and distal embolization. These patients should achieve final TIMI 3 flow. Stenting plus GP IIb/IIIa inhibition has been shown to improve outcomes, reducing target vessel revasculari-

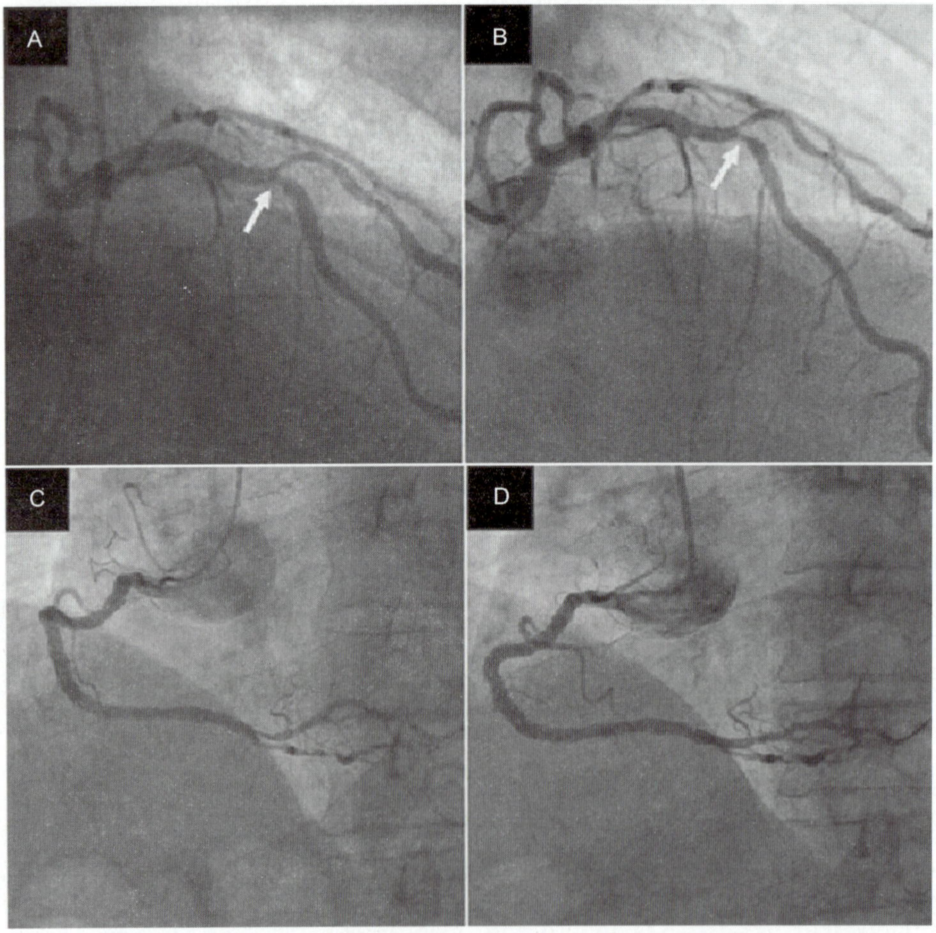

Fig. 34.38: *(Upper) Follow-up coronary angiogram showed stent fracture with abundant movement and displacement of fractured fragment over 1 mm during cardiac cycle (type 4). Severe stenosis at the fracture site (B) was shown compared to previous coronary angiogram (A) 3 years ago. (lower) After 2 years, his symptoms returned due to RCA obstruction (C) He was then stented successfully (D)*

zation and myocardial infarction rates in comparison with balloon angioplasty. The use of adjunctive antithrombotic approaches including early GP IIb/IIIa inhibition use and mechanical thrombectomy, has shown benefit. Important issues remain as to which type of stent to use (drug-eluting or bare metal), and timing of antiplatelet therapy (both IV and oral) might provide better outcomes for certain patients.

Stone and colleagues studied the safety and efficacy of drug-eluting stents and bare-metal stents in patients with STEMI undergoing primary PCI. Patients (n = 3006) were assigned in a 3:1 ratio to receive paclitaxel-eluting stents or otherwise identical bare-metal stents. Paclitaxel-eluting stents significantly reduced angiographic evidence of restenosis and recurrent ischemia necessitating repeat revascularization, compared with bare-metal stents, at 12-month follow-up. Rates of death and stent thrombosis were similar for the 2 groups.

Complications Associated with PCI (Figs 34.39A and B)

Early registries of balloon angioplasty results showed complication rates that were much higher than those typically observed today. With advancements in technique, devices, and adjuvant medical therapy, percutaneous transluminal coronary intervention is now associated with mortality and emergency bypass rates of less than 1%. The rate of nonfatal myocardial infarction following coronary angioplasty ranges from 5–15%, whereas the rate following stent placement is 2–5%. Restenosis after balloon angioplasty requiring a second revascularization procedure is a major limitation occurring in about 15–30% of patients, depending on the definition of restenosis applied. However, with drug-eluting stents, restenosis rates are now less than 10%.

Reduction in the complications of balloon angioplasty has been complemented by improvements in the acute success rate. Registries, such as the National Heart, Lung, and Blood Institute (NHLBI) coronary angioplasty registry from the early 1980s, reported primary success rates of 61%. Today, success rates are 95–99% with the use of stents and adjunctive pharmacotherapy.

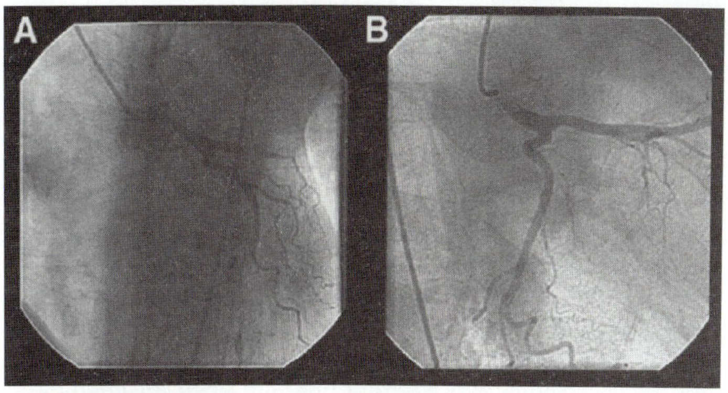

Figs 34.39A and B: *(A) Coronary angiogram confirming a severe ostial stenosis of the LMCA, with extensive right-to-left collaterals to the left anterior descending (LAD) and left anterior circumflex (LCX) vessels. (B) Coronary angiogram showing the final result of the percutaneous coronary intervention*

The mechanism by which balloon angioplasty or stenting improves luminal diameter is associated with significant local trauma to the vessel wall, which can, in turn, lead to occlusive complications in a minority of patients. Coronary artery dissection typically results from the vessel injury secondary to balloon expansion. Animal and postmortem studies have shown that localized dissection at the site of balloon expansion is a common occurrence, detected angiographically in as many as 50% of patients immediately following the procedure. Such small dissections probably are necessary to obtain adequate lumen expansion, rarely interfere with antegrade blood flow, or are important. Angiographic follow-up typically shows no residual evidence of a dissection as early as 6 weeks after angioplasty in most of the cases studied. However, larger dissections can lead to complications.

Abrupt Vessel Closure

It may occur in as many as 5% of balloon angioplasty cases and typically develops when there is compression of the true lumen by a large dissection flap, thrombus formation, superimposed coronary vasospasm, or a combination of these processes. The presence of large coronary dissections immediately after balloon angioplasty is associated with a fivefold increase in the risk of abrupt closure. This underscores the importance of a good postprocedure angiographic result on clinical outcomes.

Since the introduction and use of intracoronary stents and newer antiplatelet drugs, the incidence of abrupt closure has significantly decreased (to < 1%). Microembolization of plaque debris or adherent thrombus may also cause acute complications during angioplasty and may contribute to postprocedure cardiac enzyme elevation and chest pain in some patients.

In less than 1% of patients undergoing angioplasty, microembolization of the platelet-rich thrombus may cause diffuse distal arteriolar vasospasm secondary to the release of vasoactive agents, resulting in the phenomenon of no-reflow. This complication is difficult to treat but may respond to intracoronary calcium channel antagonists, adenosine, or nitroprusside. Patients undergoing balloon angioplasty of saphenous vein graft lesions and primary angioplasty in the setting of acute myocardial infarction with a large amount of adherent thrombus are at greatest risk of distal embolization.

Coronary perforation or rupture following balloon angioplasty.

It is very rare (< 1%) and is typically associated with the use of ablative devices or oversized balloons.

Restenosis

Following balloon angioplasty or stent implantation, the vessel wall undergoes a number of changes. Platelets and fibrin adhere to the site within minutes of vessel injury. Within hours to days, inflammatory cells infiltrate the site and vascular smooth muscle cells begin to migrate toward the lumen.

The vascular smooth muscle cells then hypertrophy and excrete an extensive extracellular matrix. During this period of vascular smooth muscle cell proliferation, endothelial cells colonize the surface of the lumen and regain their normal function. Over the course of several weeks to months, multiple forces interact to cause remodeling of the vessel wall with either a decrease in lumen diameter (negative remodeling) or an increase in lumen diameter (positive remodeling). The amount of late loss in lumen diameter is dependent on the amount of neointimal proliferation and the degree of remodeling following intervention. After 6 months, the repair process stabilizes and the risk of restenosis decreases significantly.

Mechanism of Restenosis Following Percutaneous Transluminal Coronary Angioplasty (PTCA)

Several studies have shown that the lumen diameter or area after treatment is one of the major predictors of restenosis. The use of coronary artery stents has decreased the rate of restenosis by improving the acute gain achieved and by minimizing negative remodeling. Depending on the definition used, angiographic restenosis has been reported in as many as 50% of patients within 6 months after balloon angioplasty, necessitating repeat target vessel revascularization (TVR) in approximately 20–30% of patients. Drug-eluting stents have reduced restenosis rates to less than 10%. Poststent lumen diameter and lesion complexity are still the major predictors of restenosis with these newer stents.

Stent Thrombosis

While drug-eluting stents have significantly reduced restenosis events, concerns of stent thrombosis with these newer stents still exist. In fact, the rate of thrombosis with a drug-eluting stent is virtually identical to that for a bare metal stent at 1 year (0.5–0.7%). However, late stent thrombosis (>1 y) continues to occur with a drug-eluting stent, while it is exceedingly rare for a bare metal stent.

The biggest factor contributing to stent thrombosis is interruption of antiplatelet therapy. Current guidelines recommend a minimum of 1 year of dual antiplatelet therapy for drug-eluting stents and a month for bare metal stents. Drug-eluting stents take longer to endothelialize on the coronary vessel wall than bare metal stents, and discontinuing dual antiplatelet therapy may expose patients to an increased risk for stent thrombosis over time. In some clinical situations (such as before urgent noncardiac surgery where antiplatelet therapy may have to be discontinued and in patients with known or potential medicine compliance issues), implanting a bare metal stent may be preferred during PCI rather than using a drug-eluting stent. Another important factor is final stent diameter and area.

Underdeployment or incomplete apposition of the drug-eluting stent may also increase the risk for stent thrombosis. This is not to say that drug-eluting stents are unsafe. In fact, there is no difference in long-term rates of death and myocardial infarction between drug-eluting and bare metal stents; however, there is a striking reduction in restenosis. Stone and colleagues found that although stent thrombosis is infrequent, it results in higher rates of myocardial infarction and death. The more frequent target lesion revascularization results in a lower rate of myocardial infarction and death. Although late stent thrombosis is a risk with drug-eluting stents, the noticeable reduction in restenosis may offset the risk.

Optical Coherence Tomography

The technique is based on optical technology and commercially available fiber-optic components adapted for ophthalmic use. OCT is a noninvasive technique that does not utilize ionizing radiation to provide in vivo images. OCT has numerous potential clinical applications and, in effect, creates "optical biopsies" of tissues. It has also been used in the detection, characterization and management of skin tumors and other dermatological diseases, cardiology and intravascular disease. OCT may be able to contribute to early diagnosis of vulnerable atherosclerotic lesions (Figs 34.40 to 34.44A–F).

Non-invasive imaging modalities such as magnetic resonance and computerized tomography are currently under intense investigation. Catheter-based diagnostic techniques, however, can provide structural information with higher resolution than noninvasive methods. Intravascular magnetic resonance is being actively investigated for plaque detection and characterization. Intravascular ultrasound magnetic resonance is being actively investigated for plaque detection and characterization. Intravascular ultrasound (IVUS) is widely used in interventional cardiology. A recent publication suggests a correlation between the presence of echolucent zones in coronary plaques on IVUS images and acute coronary events. Preliminary angioscopic studies have suggested that the presence of yellow plaques with a glistening surface correlates with acute events. More quantitative approaches which measure molecular absorption overtones of lipid or the Raman shift of cholesterol, may provide unique signals

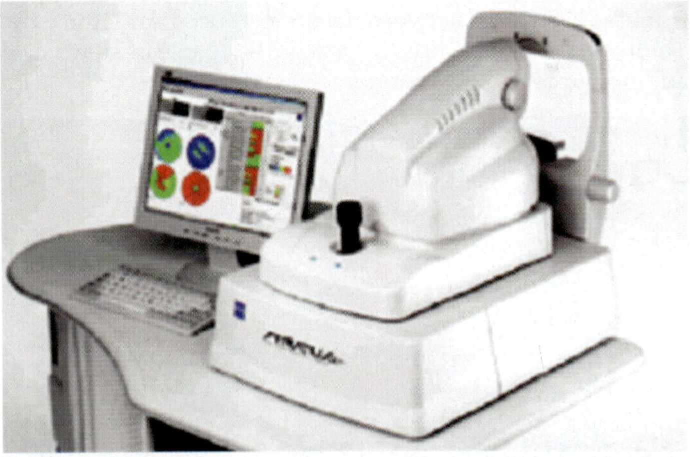

Fig. 34.40: *Photograph showing machine used for analysis of optical coherence tomography in vascular diseases of the body. Optical coherence tomography is a new imaging modality capable of obtaining cross sectional images of coronary vessels with a high resolution of about 10 mm which is estimated about 10-fold greater than that of IVUS*

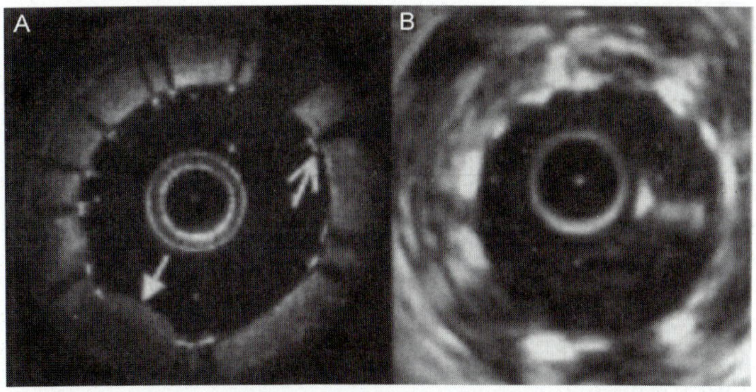

Fig. 34.41: *(A) Optical coherence tomographic image showing tissues prolapse (arrows) (B) Neither of these small features is readily apparent in the corresponding intravascular ultrasound image*

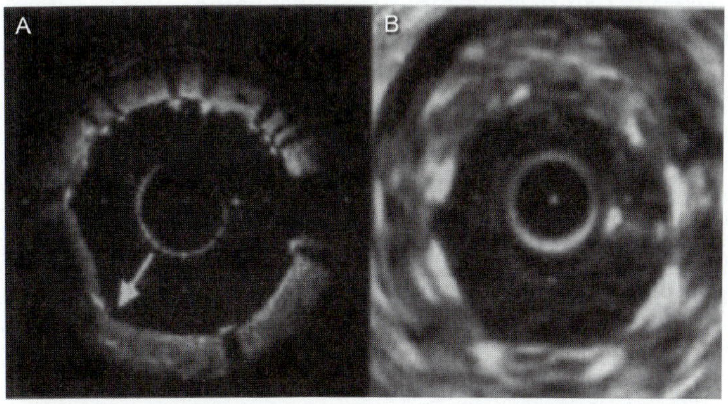

Fig. 34.42: *(A) Optical coherence tomography (OCT) and (B) IVUS of a patient with in-stent restenosis*

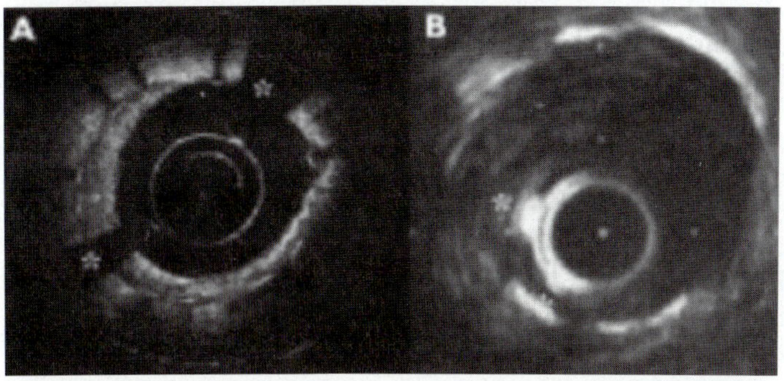

Figs 34.43A and B: *(A) Stent showing irregular spacing between adjacent struts acquired with optical coherence tomography and with intravascular ultrasound, (B) At locations of greater strut separation the pronounced angulation observed in the vessel wall (arrow in A) may corresspond to increased focal stress*

from vessel walls to identify large lipid pools. Based on the hypothesis that local inflammation within vulnerable plaques may lead to local elevations in temperature, a temperature-sensing catheter has been used to study temperature heterogeneity and temperature differences between atherosclerotic plaque and healthy vessel walls Intravascular optical coherence tomography (OCT) has recently been proposed as a high-resolution imaging method for plaque characterization. Optical coherence tomography is an optical analog of ultrasound imaging because it measures the amplitude of backscattered light (optical echoes) returning from a sample as a function of delay. In vitro studies have shown that the resolution of OCT (10–20 µm) can resolve the thin fibrous caps thought to be responsible for plaque vulnerability. Additionally, the intrinsic optical properties of typical plaque constituents have provided sufficient contrast in these studies for OCT to differentiate between lipid, calcium and fibrous tissue. Recent experiments performed in vivo have demonstrated intravascular OCT imaging of normal rabbit aortas (13) and swine coronary arteries (14). Here, we present the first application, to our knowledge, of intracoronary OCT in living patients. The goals of this study were: (1) to demonstrate the feasibility and safety of OCT imaging in patients and (2) to assess OCT images of human coronary pathology acquired in vivo by comparison with IVUS images obtained from corresponding locations. A catheter-based imaging technology called optical coherence tomography (OCT) can successfully identify the characteristics of coronary plaques in patients with various cardiac symptoms. The report from researchers at Massachusetts General Hospital (MGH) will appear in the journal Circulation. "More than 1.2 million people die from coronary artery disease every year, a quarter of them before or soon after arriving at the hospital", says Ik-Kyung Jang, MD, PhD, director of cardiovascular clinical research in the MGH cardiology division and lead author of the current study. "The ability to identify dangerous plaques before they rupture and produce a heart attack or sudden cardiac death will be crucial to innovative preventive therapies". Plaques are deposits of fats, cholesterol and other materials that collect in major arteries, restricting or sometimes blocking blood flow. While some plaques are relatively stable, others are vulnerable to rupture and release their contents into the bloodstream, causing a blood clot to form. Heart attacks and other acute coronary events usually result from the rupture of high-risk, vulnerable plaques in coronary arteries, and the characteristics of those plaques have been determined primarily by autopsy studies. **OCT** uses infrared light delivered via fiberoptic catheter to produce high-resolution, cross-sectional images of blood vessels. Study co-authors Guillermo Tearney, MD, PhD, of the MGH pathology department and the Wellman Center for Photomedicine at MGH, and Brett Bouma, PhD, also of the Wellman Center, developed the use of OCT to visualize coronary arteries including vulnerable plaques. The technology developed in their laboratory was used for this first study to examine the structure of plaques in patients with cardiac disease. The study enrolled patients scheduled to undergo cardiac catheterization for whom angiograms or other imaging techniques had identified the arterial lesion responsible for their symptoms. Participants either had experienced a recent heart attack or had acute coronary syndrome (ACS), a set of symptoms associated with reduced blood supply to the heart muscle. A third group had stable angina, chest pain that occurs with physical or mental stress, which is not usually related to plaque

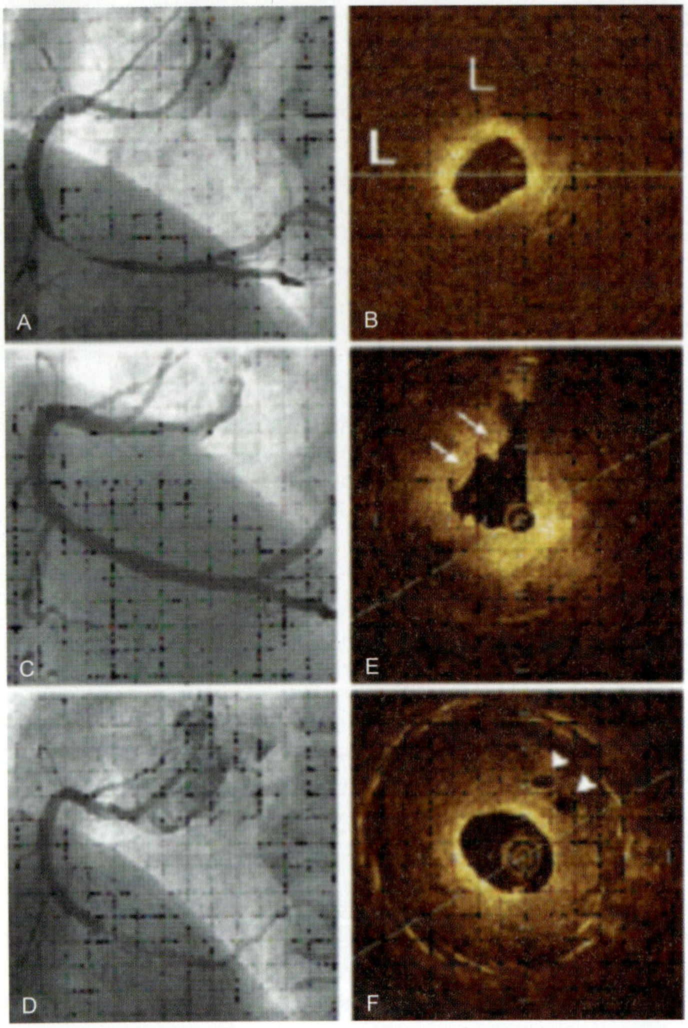

Fig. 34.44: *Left panels (A, C and D) showing angiographic views of coronary arteries with variable disease process, Right panels (B, D and F) showing pictures of corressponding arteries analysed with OCT*

rupture. Clear OCT images of the suspicious lesions were obtained for 20 heart attack patients, 20 with ACS and 17 with stable angina. Vulnerable plaques are believed to have three major characteristics—a deposit of lipids (fats), a thin cap of fibrous material covering the lipid pool, and infiltration of the immune cells called macrophages. The OCT images showed that the heart attack and ACS patients had more lipid in their plaques and significantly thinner fibrous caps than did the stable angina patients. Overall, vulnerable plaques were identified in 72% of the heart attack patients, 50% of those with ACS and only 20% of stable angina patients. "This is the first technique that allows us to study the structural changes underlying vulnerable plaques in living patients, and it supports the conclusions of previously reported postmortem studies", says Jang. "We still need to gather more data to confirm these characteristics, and our group will carry out further studies of how plaques develop and rupture. Someday OCT may provide information that will guide treatments to prevent plaque rupture and its disastrous consequences.

First-in-Human Evaluation of a Novel Robotic-Assisted Coronary Angioplasty System

The main aim **of a Novel Robotic-Assisted Coronary Angioplasty is** to evaluate the safety and feasibility of a robotic angioplasty system in delivery and manipulation of coronary guidewires, balloons, and stents in patients undergoing elective percutaneous coronary intervention (PCI).

Background: A remote-control, robotic-assisted angioplasty system is under development to address some of the procedural challenges and occupational hazards associated with traditional PCI.

Clinical Utility of Robotic Systems (Fig. 34.45)

Robotic systems have been suggested to enhance the precision of cardiovascular procedures with increased accuracy. One of the technical features of the robotic system is the capability to control and accurately position (1 mm steps) the stent delivery system. The recent STLLR (Stent Deployment Techniques on clinical outcomes of patients treated with the cypheRstent) trial highlighted the impact on clinical outcomes of geographic miss and stent misplacement . Although endovascular imaging guidance is likely necessary to improve the precision of stent placement, the robotically assisted system facilitates the positioning of the stent delivery system with a high degree of accuracy. In addition, robotic systems have been suggested to reduce radiation exposure.

Despite the significant evolution in interventional device technologies, the actual procedural methodology and workflow in the catheterization laboratory has remained unchanged in the last 25 years. As the current practice of interventional cardiology evolves into more complex PCI procedures, interventional cardiologists, the professional societies U.S. Food and Drug Administration, and International atomic energy agency called for enhanced catheterization laboratory safety by reducing radiation exposure to both patients and operators and making the overall catheterization laboratory environment more ergonomically friendly through technological innovations. Incorporating a remote-control, robotic-assisted PCI system into the catheterization laboratory might address some of the procedural deficiencies and occupational hazards associated with traditional PCI in addition to contributing to a higher degree of precision and control for the interventional procedure.

Technique

Patients with coronary artery disease and clinical indication for elective PCI were enrolled. The coronary angioplasty procedure was performed with the CorPath 200 robotic system (Corindus, Inc. Natick, Massachusetts). The system consists of a remote interventional cockpit and a multi-component bedside unit that enables the operator to advance, retract, and rotate guidewires and rapid exchange catheters. The primary endpoint was device clinical success (30% residual stenosis) without in-hospital major adverse cardiac events. Technical success was defined as the ability of the system to complete all the planned angioplasty steps on the basis of procedural segments. Patients were followed up to 30 days after angioplasty procedure.

The retrospective evaluation study of lens injuries and dose (RELID) study revealed that interventional cardiologists have cataract-type eye opacities 3 times more often than age-matched controlled group. The mean fluoroscopy time from this study compares favorably with the results of the study of 9,650 patients undergoing single-vessel PCI (11.5 min vs. 18.3 min) and with a sub-group of 7,242 patients whose fluoroscopy time was 23 min (11.5 min vs. 12.7 min). Shorter fluoroscopy time translated into reduced radiation exposure for the patient and the operator and reduced contrast fluid usage. In our study, 1 of the most important findings was the significant (97.1%) reduction in radiation exposure to the operator performing the robotic PCI procedure. The patient radiation exposure was within the normal reported limits: 2.1 Gy versus 1.9 Gy. Also, although the study was not designed to show differences in contrast volume usage, the total volume of

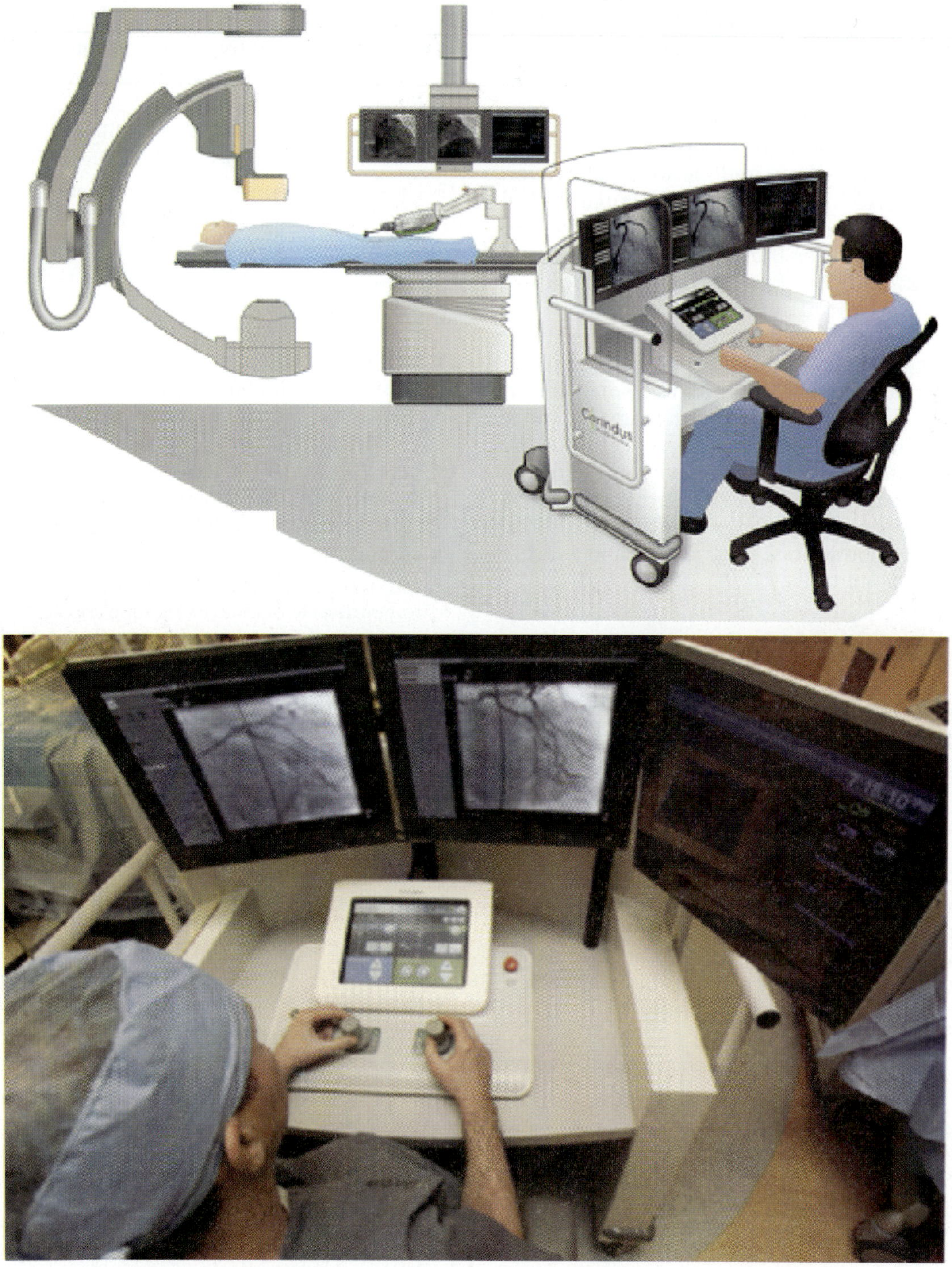

Fig. 34.45: *The method of performing robot-assisted coronary angioplasty*

contrast agents used in this study seemed to be less, compared with what has been reported in other clinical series. The lower contrast usage might be attributed to the complete procedure control enabled by the interventional cockpit environment. Another subjective but still important finding was the level of technical "comfort" expressed by the operators. Although no specific measurement of this variable was used in this study, both operators perceived this system to be more comfortable compared with the typical technique used for coronary intervention. Most of the cases were performed under a controlled environment, in which the operator had the opportunity to focus on the performance of the procedure, having a close proximity of the monitors and not distracted by the physical strain of the lead apron and standing position.

In early clinical experience, the use of the robotic system seems not to reduce the overall periprocedural times compared with manual PCI of single lesions . However, we believe that, as this technology underwent initial clinical evaluation, the rigor of the study procedure in addition to the time required to register the data added additional procedural time. In addition, from the operator point of view, there was an initial learning and technology adaptation curve that we believe will improve over time, leading to shorter procedural times. However, this study still represents an early feasibility study in a small cohort of patients, and the use of this technology in more challenging anatomies including the presence of severe tortuosity, severe calcification, or interventions requiring multiple wires and balloons needs to be further studied. A larger, prospective, multicenter pivotal clinical trial designed to test the robotic angioplasty system in a larger number of patients is underway.

BIBLIOGRAPHY

1. Stroupe KT, Morrison DA, Hlatky MA, Barnett PG, Cao L, Lyttle C, Hynes DM, Henderson WG. "Cost-effectiveness of coronary artery bypass grafts versus percutaneous coronary intervention for revascularization of high-risk patients". Circulation 2006;114 (12): 1251–1257.
2. Meier B, Bachmann D, Lüscher T. "25 years of coronary angioplasty: almost a fairy tale". Lancet 2003;361 (9356): 527.
3. Dotter CT, Judkins MP. "Transluminal treatment of arteriosclerotic obstruction". Circulation 1964;30 (5): 654–70.
4. SoS Investigators. "Coronary artery bypass surgery versus percutaneous coronary intervention with stent implantation in patients with multivessel coronary artery disease (the Stent or Surgery trial): a randomised controlled trial". Lancet 2002;360 (9338): 965–70.
5. Boden WE, RA O'Rourke, et al. ["Optimal medical therapy with or without PCI for stable coronary disease." N Engl J Med 2007;356(15): 1503–16.
6. Hannan EL, Wu C, Walford G, *et al.* "Drug-eluting stents vs. coronary-artery bypass grafting in multivessel coronary disease". N. Engl. J. Med. 2008;358 (4): 331–41.
7. Weintraub WS, Spertus JA, Kolm P, et al. "Effect of PCI on quality of life in patients with stable coronary disease". The New England Journal of Medicine 2008;359 (7): 677–87.
8. Kolata, Gina. "New Heart Studies Question the Value Of Opening Arteries" *The New York Times*, March 21, 2004. Retrieved January 29, 2011.
9. Michaels AD, Chatterjee K. "Cardiology patient pages. Angioplasty versus bypass surgery for coronary artery disease". Circulation 2002;106 (23): e187–90.
10. Mercado, N, Flather, MD, Boersna, E, et al., on Behalf of the Trial Investigators CABG vs Stenting for Multivessel Disease: a Meta-analysis of ARTS-1, SoS, ERACI-2, and MASS-2, Presentation at European Society of Cardiology Congress 2003 (23): 2093–8.
11. Mauri L, Hsieh WH, Massaro JM, Ho KK, D'Agostino R, Cutlip DE. "Stent thrombosis in randomized clinical trials of drug-eluting stents". The New England Journal of Medicine 2007;356 (10): 1020–9.
12. European Society of Cardiology Science News, 2007 Thrombosis is the price for the success of drug-eluting stents
13. UK's NHS endorsed 'Best Treatments' advice on 'clinical evidence for patients from the BMJ' on Coronary angioplasty and its risks.
14. Yang EH, Gumina RJ, Lennon RJ, Holmes DR, Rihal CS, Singh (2005). "to 2003". Journal of the American College of Cardiology *46* (11): 2004–2009.
15. Duran AD, Duran GD, Ramirez RR, et al. Cataracts in interventional cardiology personnel. Retrospective evaluation study of lens injuries and dose (RELID Study). Eur Heart J 2009;30:872.
16. Kline LW, Miller DL, Balter S, et al. Occupational hazards in the interventional laboratory: time for a safer environment Catheter Cardiovasc Interv 2009;73:432–438.
17. Di Biase L, Wang Y, Horton R, et al. Ablation of atrial fibrillation utilizing robotic catheter navigation in comparison to manual navigation and ablation: single-center experience J Cardiovasc Electrophysiol 2009;20:1328–1335.
18. Beyar R, Wenderow T, Lindner D, Kumar G, Shofti R. Concept, design and pre-clinical studies for remote control percutaneous coronary interventions EuroIntervention 2005;1:340–345.
19. Beyar R, Gruberg L, Delleanu D, et al. Remote-control percutaneous coronary interventions. Concept, validation, and first-in-humans clinical trial. J Am Coll Cardiol 2006;47:296–300.
20. Solomon SB, Patriciu A, Bohlman ME, Kavoussi LR, Stoianovici D. Robotically driven interventions: a method of using CT fluoroscopy without radiation exposure to the physician Radiology 2002;225:277–282.
21. Marescaux J, Leroy J, Gagner M, et al. Transatlantic robot-assisted telesurgery Nature 2001;413:379–380.
22. Argenziano M, Katz M, Bonatti J, et al. Results of the prospective multicenter trial of robotically assisted totally endoscopic coronary artery bypass grafting Ann Thorac Surg 2006;81:1666–1674.
23. Subramanian VA, Patel NU, Patel NC, Loulmet DF. Robotic assisted multivessel minimally invasive direct coronary artery bypass with port-access stabilization and cardiac positioning: paving the way for outpatient coronary surgery? Ann Thorac Surg 2005;79:1590–1596.

35 Percutaneous Transcatheter Management of Valvular Heart Diseases

The field of percutaneous valve replacement and repair is currently developing at a rapid pace: percutaneous treatment of valvular heart disease is now one of the fastest developing areas of cardiology. Transcatheter aortic and pulmonary valve replacement and a variety of mitral valve therapy approaches have been successfully performed in hundreds of patients (*see* the table below). A number of problems related to operator technique or specific devices have been encountered and solved (Fig. 35.1).

Efforts to develop and refine percutaneous catheter-based approaches to cardiac valve repair and replacement have advanced rapidly over the past several years. Such clinical strategies were initiated as early as the 1950s with the introduction of simple catheter devices for treating pulmonic stenosis.

Treatment of stenotic lesions matured in the early 1980s with the advent of balloon valvuloplasty, which has become the predominant therapy for primary pulmonic and mitral stenosis lesions. Percutaneous aortic balloon valvuloplasty, however, has yielded largely unfavorable results and is now seldom performed because of its substantial risks and short-lived benefits.

New innovations have been directed toward the two most frequent forms of valvular heart disease in the industrialized West: (1) aortic stenosis and (2) mitral regurgitation, which account for more than 70% of the cases of acquired valve disease in the United States and Europe.

As the populations of the United States and other industrialized countries continue to age, the need for less invasive and safer methods of treating valvular disease (particularly calcific aortic stenosis) will continue to grow. Careful evaluations comparing percutaneous approaches with conventional surgical approaches are likely to serve as an impetus for extending the use of the new, less invasive techniques from high-risk patients to other, lower-risk patient groups.

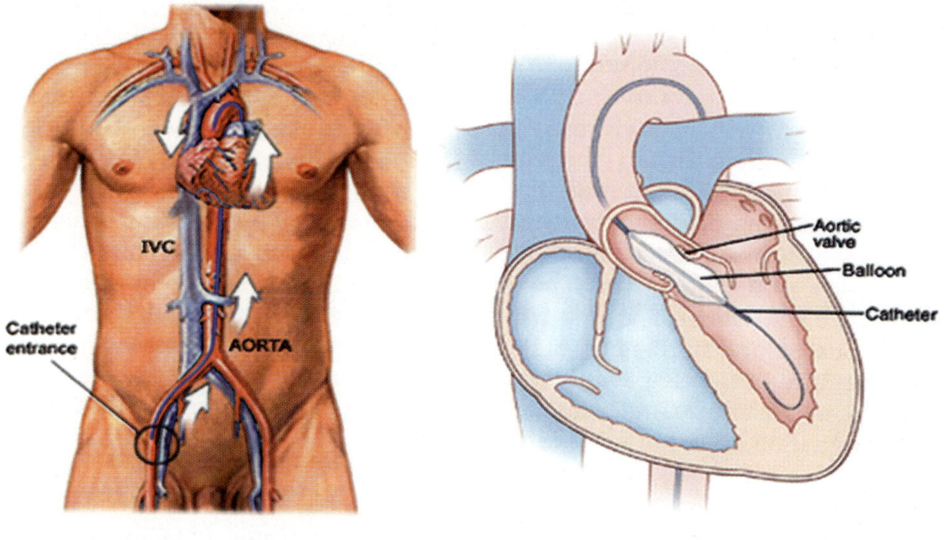

Fig. 35.1: *Method of delivery of balloon in ballon valvoplasty of stenosed aortic valve*

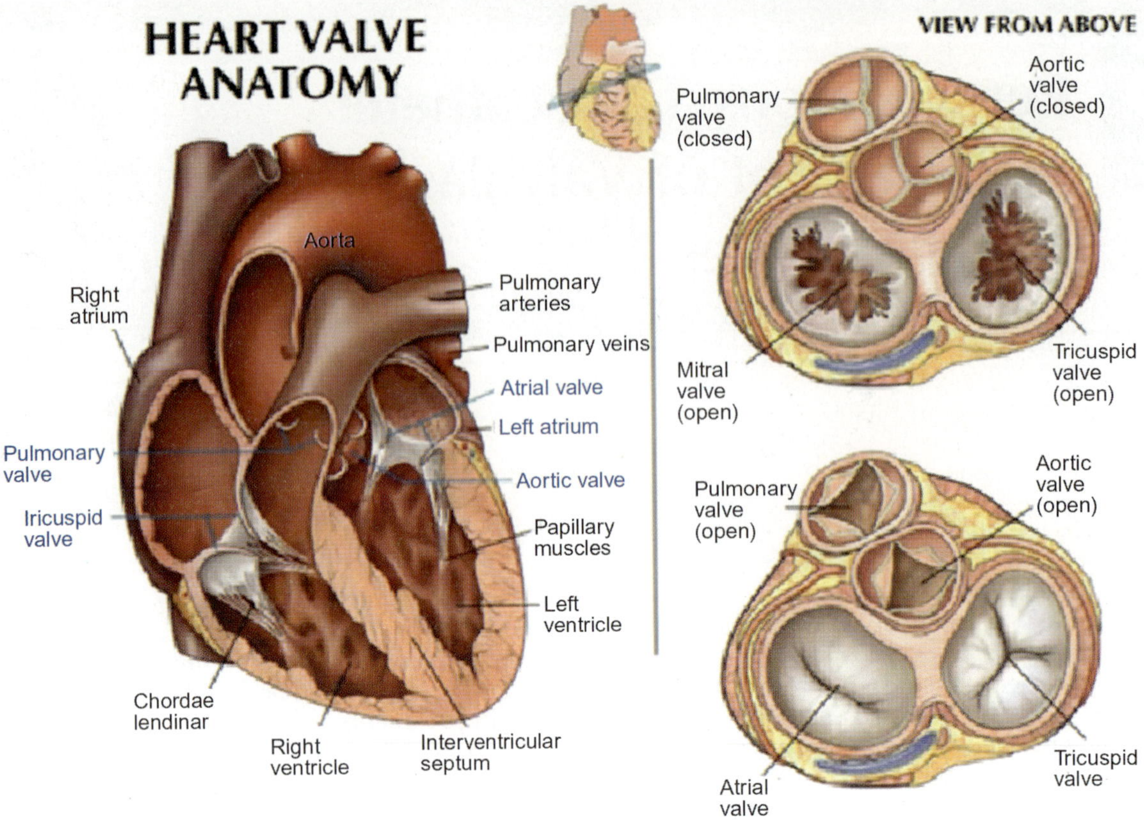

Fig. 35.2: *Showing the four valves in the heart that allow blood to move only in 1 direction are the aortic, mitral, tricuspid, and pulmonic valves. The aortic and pulmonic valves, when open, allow the blood to leave the heart and, when closed, prevent the blood from returning to the heart. The mitral and tricuspid valves, when open, allow the blood to move from the atria to the ventricles and, when closed, prevent the blood from moving backward into the atria*

BASIC CONCEPTS IN PERCUTANEOUS APPROACHES

The incidence of valvular heart disease is expected to increase over the next several decades as the "baby boomer" generation passes into advanced decades of life. Treatment of heart disease—primarily valvular heart disease (as medical treatments for atherosclerosis improve—is expected to represent one of the main arenas for maintaining good health in this aging population.

With the increasing availability of cardiopulmonary bypass, surgical expertise, and intensive care facilities, valve repair and replacement are widely performed to relieve symptoms and improve prognosis of valvular heart disease, despite the associated morbidity and mortality. However, many patients with major comorbidities, particularly elderly patients, still do not undergo potentially beneficial interventions because of the high surgical risk. Investigations into the current management of patients with valvular heart disease in Europe and the United States showed that as many as one-third of elderly patients with severe symptomatic aortic stenosis, and a similar number of patients with mitral regurgitation, were not referred for surgical management by the attending practitioner. The percentage of nonreferrals from the cardiologist's office is likely to be even higher, and that from the general practitioner's office may be higher still.

A catheter-based alternative to surgery could significantly reduce morbidity and mortality, thus making treatment available to patients not currently considered surgical candidates. In addition, a less invasive therapy might permit treatment of valvular heart disease at an earlier stage and thereby prevent the onset of progressive ventricular dysfunction.

Moreover, patients show a strong preference for minimally invasive therapies in general, especially those patients who have undergone many operations. Finally, successful use of percutaneous approaches to valve replacement and repair could have a substantial positive economic impact by virtue of the associated reductions in intensive care unit (ICU) and hospital stays.

Realization of the potential benefits of these innovations may result in a paradigm shift, challenging long-standing traditional principles in the evaluation and treatment of valvular heart disease. Both short-term and long-term data are probably needed to assess percutaneous approaches against conventional surgical approaches with respect to superiority in safety and noninferiority in efficacy.

Patient Selection of Patients in Percutaneous Approaches

The excellent results of contemporary surgical approaches to valvular heart disease have set a high standard for any

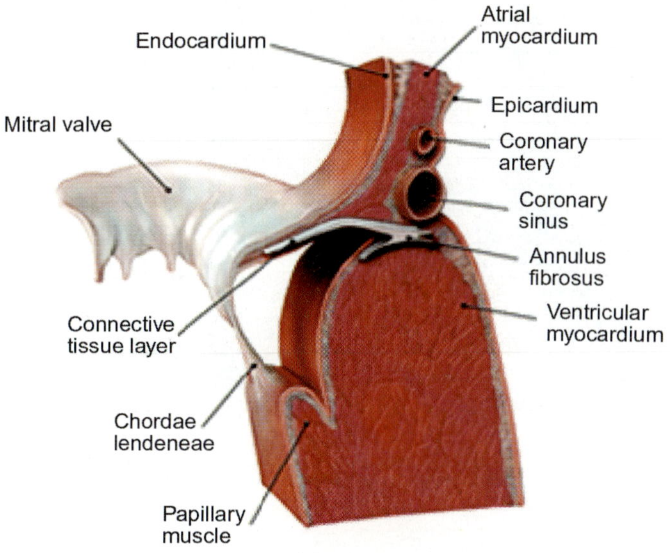

Fig. 35.3: *Showing mitral valve and its surrounding structures*

new treatment strategies being considered. However, patients who are considered candidates for less invasive procedures may present a different risk profile than patients who are currently referred for surgery (at both the high end and the low end of the risk spectrum); therefore, comparisons with current outcome standards may not be appropriate.

Thus, it is essential to keep in mind that patients referred for valvular interventions today tend to be elderly and to have increased surgical risk associated with congestive heart failure, the emergency nature of the operation, left ventricular dysfunction, coronary disease, previous operations, and (most important) severe comorbidities. Measures of invasiveness and effectiveness will also have to be weighed against the realities of patient expectations in potential patient candidate pools (those who currently may or may not be referred for surgery).

In the context of the outstanding track record achieved for surgical aortic valve replacement, for example, large trials with extremely large sample sizes will be required to prove equivalent hemodynamic and clinical results with the new nonsurgical devices in good (low-risk) surgical candidates. Such trials will require close collaboration between interventional cardiologists, echocardiographers, engineers, and surgeons.

Although significant challenges in patient selection and clinical trial design remain to be solved, the patient populations who may ultimately benefit most from treatment with these new technologies should become better defined over the course of the clinical trial process. These creative new transcatheter approaches may change the face of valve therapy and extend treatment to a larger proportion of the valve disease population. Hybrid procedures combining percutaneous techniques with minimally invasive surgery may also become more popular.

For the near term, percutaneous techniques in central mitral regurgitation and percutaneous aortic valve replacement in particular remain investigational and should be restricted to patients considered to be at high risk or patients who are not candidates for conventional surgical treatment (Table 35.1).

Knowledge of Anatomical Location of AV and Semilunar Valves Prior to Valvuloplasty (Figs 35.2, 35.3 and 35.7)

The normal human heart contains four valves that regulate blood flow into and out of the heart. The aortic and pulmonic valves are known as the semilunar valves whereas the tricuspid and mitral valves are referred to as the atrioventricular valves. All the valves are trileaflet, with the exception of the mitral valve, which has two leaflets. All four cardiac valves are surrounded by fibrous tissue forming partial or complete valvular rings, or annuli. These annuli join the fibrous skeleton of the heart to anchor and support the valvular structures.

Table 35.1: *Wilkins score*

Grade	*Mobility*	*Thickening*	*Calcification*	*Subvalvular thickening*
1	Highly mobile with only leaflets tips restricted	Leaflets near normal in thickness (4–5 mm)	A single area of increased echo brightness	Minimal thickening just below the mitral leaflets
2	Leaflet mid portions have normal mobility	Midleaflets normal, considerable thickening of margins (5–8 mm)	Scattered areas of brightness confined to leaflet margins	Thickening of chordal structures extending to one of the chordal length
3	Valve continues to move forward in diastole	Thickening extending through the entire leaflets (5–8 mm)	Brightness extending into the mid portion of the leaflets	Thickening extended to distal third of the chords
4	No or minimal forward movement of the leaflets in diastole	Considerable thickening of all leaflet tissue (>8–10 mm)	Extensive brightness throughout much of the leaflet tissue	Extensive thickening and shortening of all chordal structures extending down to the papillary muscle

Adapted from Wilkins et al with permission from BMJ Publishing Group Ltd. Copyright 1988 BMJ Publishighn Group Ltd and British Cardiovascular Society.

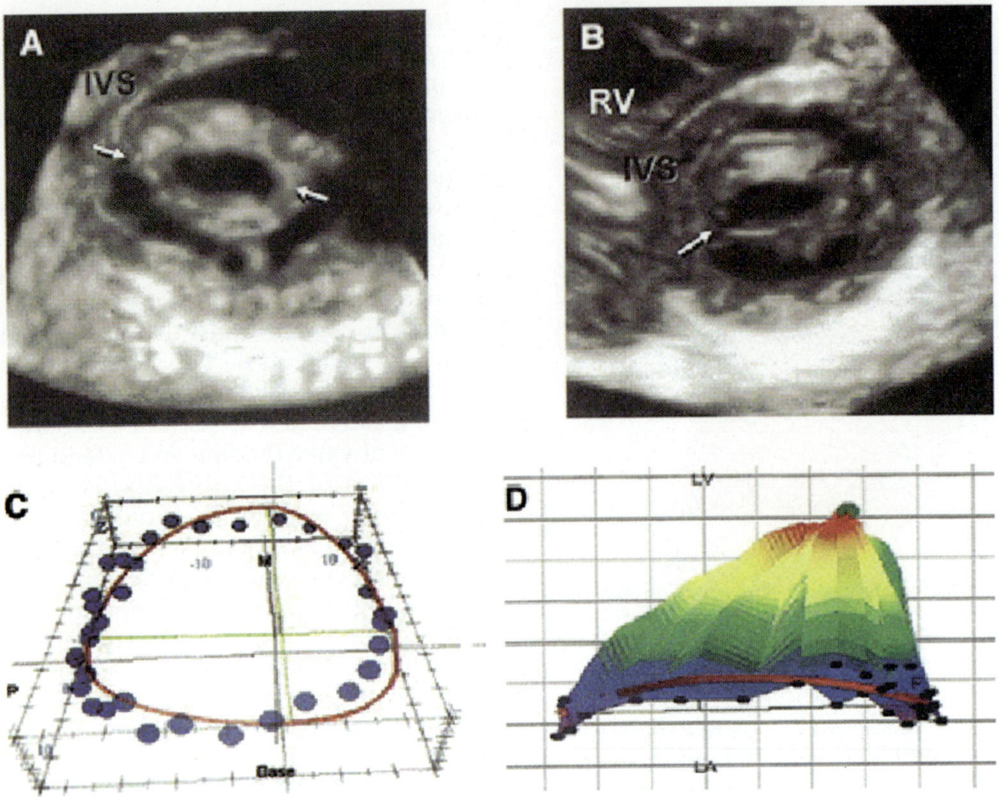

Fig. 35.4: *Real-time volumetric imaging and analysis of the mitral valve. (Top) Baseline image before mitral balloon valvuloplasty (A) shows a restricted mitral valve opening with bicommissural fusion. After valvuloplasty, splitting of the medial commissure and posterior leaflet tear can be seen (B). (Bottom) Example of 3-dimensional reconstruction of the mitral annulus (C) and leaflets (D) obtained in a patient with dilated cardiomyopathy, showing the saddle shape of the annulus and increased leaflet tenting volume. IVS = interventricular septum; LA, left atrium; LV, left ventricle; M, medial; P, posterior; RV, right ventricle.*

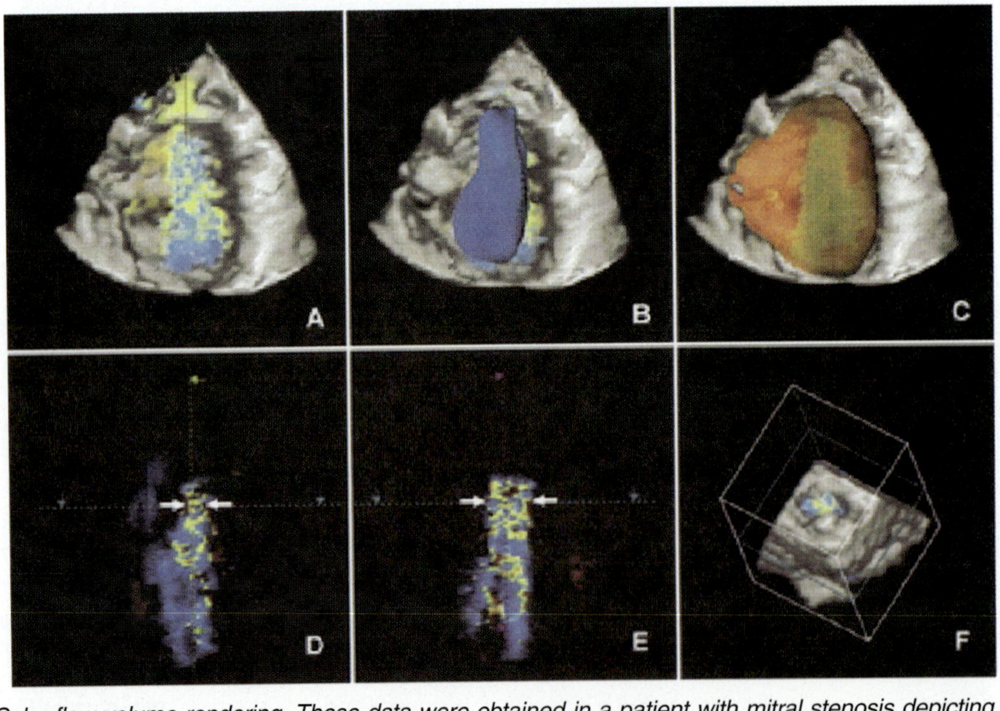

Figs 35.5A to F: *Color flow volume rendering. These data were obtained in a patient with mitral stenosis depicting a three-dimensional (3D) mitral regurgitant (MR) jet in systole (A). Both regurgitant jet and left atrium (LA) could be manually traced to estimate the MR and LA volume, displayed as a surface-rendered images superimposed on the 3D image (B and C). The vena contracta (arrows) of the regurgitant jet is shown in two orthogonal views (D and E). The level of the vena contracta is visualized along with the gray-scale*

The aortic valve is located between the left ventricular outflow tract and the ascending aorta. It forms the centerpiece of the heart and closely approximates many other important cardiac structures; specifically, the pulmonic valve anteriorly, mitral valve posterolaterally, and tricuspid valve posteromedially.

The mitral valve connects the left atrium and the left ventricle. The mitral valve opens during diastole to allow the blood flow from the left atrium to the left ventricle. During ventricular systole, the mitral valve closes and prevents backflow to the left atrium. The normal function of the mitral valve depends on its six components, which are:

1. The left atrial wall
2. The annulus
3. The leaflets
4. The chordae tendineae
5. The papillary muscles
6. The left ventricular wall.

COMPONENTS OF THE MITRAL VALVE APPARATUS

The pulmonic valve divides the right ventricular outflow tract from the pulmonary artery. In normal conditions, the pulmonic valve prevents regurgitation of deoxygenated blood from the pulmonary artery back to the right ventricle. It is a semilunar valve with three cusps, and it is located anterior, superior, and slightly to the left of the aortic valve.

The right atrioventricular valve complex (the tricuspid valve) is made up of the three valve leaflets, the annulus, the supporting chordae tendineae, and the papillary muscles. The atrial and ventricular masses, conduction system tissue, and support structure of the fibroelastic cardiac skeleton allow coordinated actions of the tricuspid valve (Figs 35.4A–D, 35.7).

PERCUTANEOUS BALLOON AORTIC VALVULOPLASTY

Percutaneous balloon aortic valvuloplasty was developed after the successes achieved with mitral and pulmonary valvuloplasties in the 1980s. This procedure provides only modest hemodynamic improvement and is associated with a high incidence of restenosis. Long-term survival after this procedure is not significantly different from the natural history of aortic stenosis (Figs 35.8–35.14).

At present, percutaneous balloon aortic valvuloplasty is done primarily in inoperable patients for the purpose of achieving temporary improvement in quality of life or buying time before more definitive treatment can be

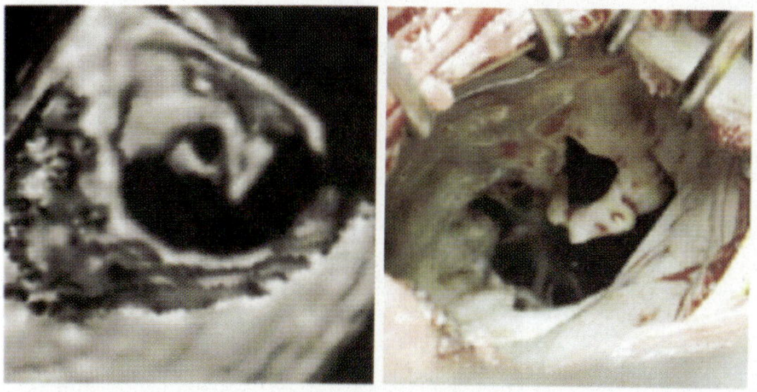

Fig. 35.6: *Volume rendering of the mitral valve obtained from real-time 3-dimensional data. The data set on the left was obtained in a patient with a perforated anterior mitral leaflet, which was confirmed by an intraoperative image (right). Reproduced, with permission, from Schwalm et al. J Am Soc Echocardiogr 2004;17:919–22*

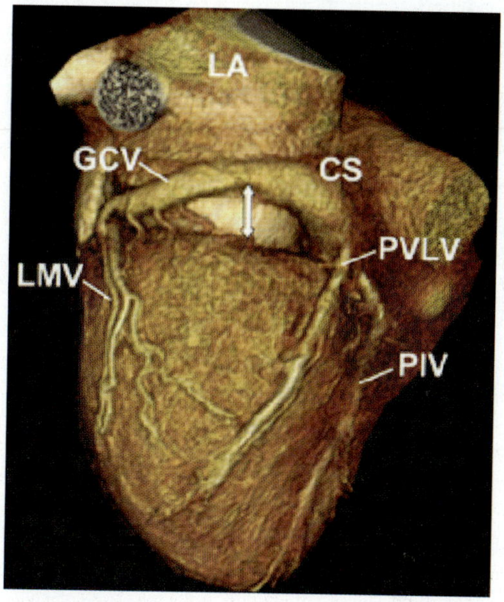

Fig. 35.7: *Coronary venous anatomy and relation between coronary sinus and mitral annulus with the use of 3D volume rendered reconstructions, the anatomy of the coronary venous system and the relation between the coronary sinus (CS) and the mitral valve annulus can be assessed. In this patient, the CS courses along the posterior wall of the left atrium (LA), rather than along the mitral valve annulus. In patients with a large distance between the CS and the mitral annulus (indicated by the white arrow), a percutaneous mitral annuloplasty may not be feasible. GCV, great cardiac vein; LMV, left marginal vein; PIV, posterior interventricular vein; PVLV, posterior vein of the left ventricle*

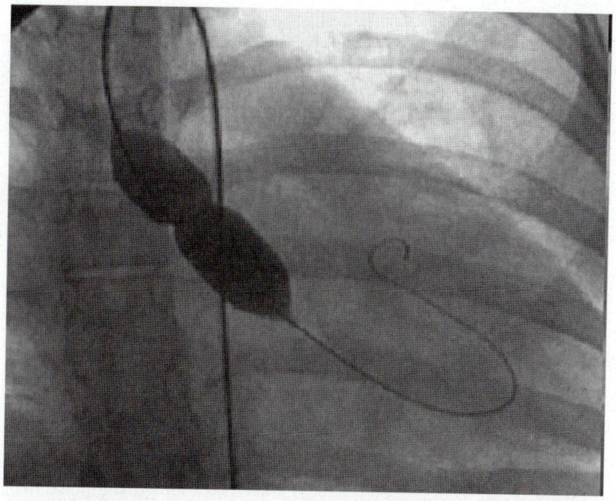

Fig. 35.8: *Percutaneous aortic balloon valvuloplasty. The valvuloplasty balloon is inserted across the aortic valve over a stiff wire into the left ventricle. The fluid-filled balloon is inflated for a few seconds to dilate the stenotic valve*

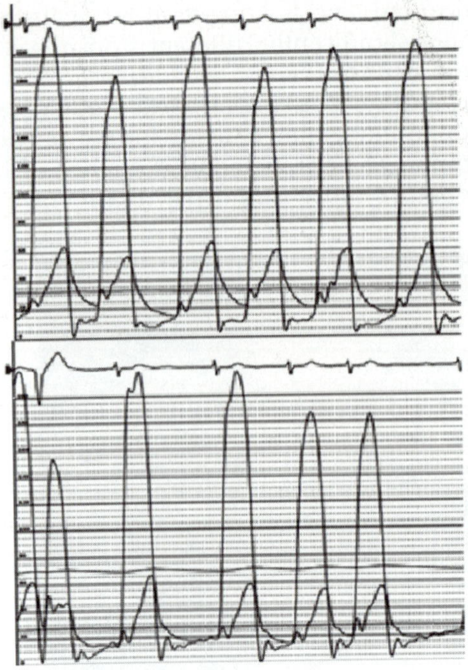

Fig. 35.9: *Left atrial and ventricular pressure measurements and significant reduction has been observed in the transvalvular mitral gradient after mitral valvuplasty*

performed. The current focus of scientific interest has shifted from balloon aortic valvuloplasty to percutaneous aortic valve replacement.

Percutaneous Aortic Valve Replacement

The current design requirements for a permanent catheter-based aortic valve system are formidable and have evolved over the past few years since the first successful percutaneous aortic valve implant by Cribier et al. Design engineers currently favor the use of biologic trileaflet tissue valves, and pericardium has been the valve material of choice.

Percutaneous aortic valve replacement is indicated for high-risk patients with a predicted EuroSCORE greater than 30% and an actual 30 days mortality lower than 10%. It is contraindicated in patients with severe calcification of the aortic valve and severe peripheral vascular disease.

Technical Aspects of Procedure

The trileaflet valve is sewn or affixed to a stent (or cage) and mounted on a catheter system for deployment. The earliest percutaneous aortic stent valves were large (24 to 26 French), stiff devices, but successive iterations have reduced the system profiles of some devices to 18 French. The following is a summary of the different types of aortic valves that are currently available:

Cribier-Edwards Valve (Edwards Life sciences, Irvine, CA)—stainless steel stent; equine pericardial valve; currently available in 23 and 26 mm diameters.

CoreValve (CoreValve, Inc, Irvine, CA)—self-expanding nitinol stent; porcine pericardial tissue valve; repositionable and retrievable.

Direct flow percutaneous aortic valve (Direct Flow Medical, Inc, Santa Rosa, CA)—stentless, inflatable, fabric-cuff; equine pericardial tissue valve.

Lotus Valve System (Sadra Medical, Campbell, CA)—self-expanding nitinol braid-frame; bovine pericardial tissue valve; repositionable and retrievable.

AorTx percutaneous aortic valve (Hansen Medical, Mountain View, CA)—low-profile, folded, metallic frame; pericardial tissue valve; repositionable and retrievable.

The stent valve is deployed either by expansion of the balloon on a balloon-expandable stent or by withdrawal of a sheath that releases a self-expanding stent. The deployed stent valve must remain securely implanted with displacement of the diseased native valve so that the new tissue valve can begin to function immediately.

The hemodynamic performance of catheter-based aortic valves should be similar to that of their surgical counterparts, with minimal transvalvular gradients (< 10 mmHg) and measured aortic valve areas of 1.5–2.0 cm^2. No component

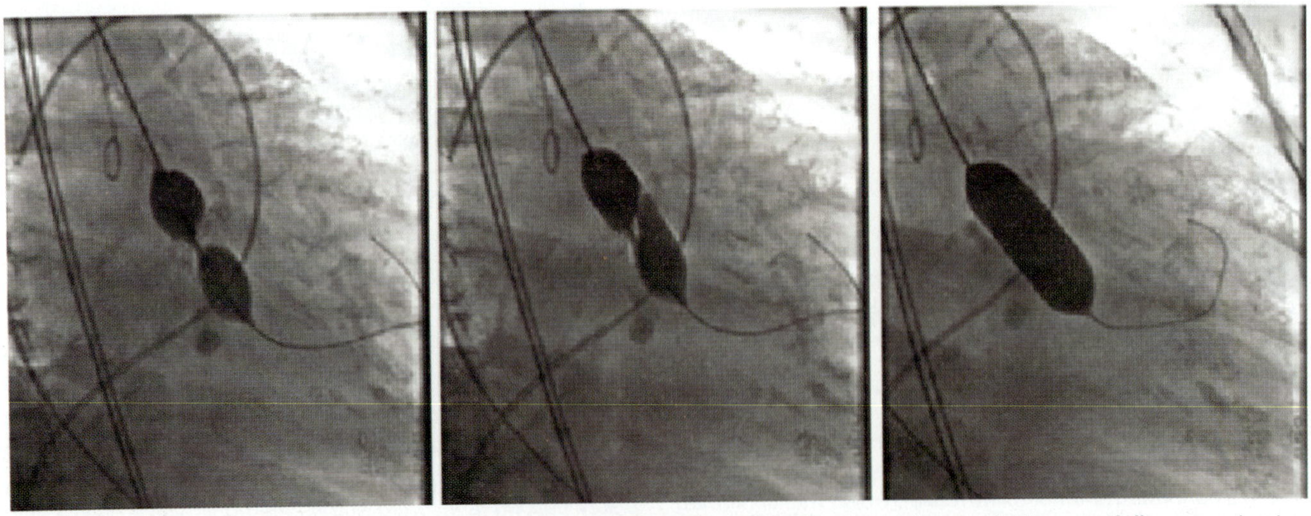

Fig. 35.10: *Left shows full waist after ballon position at aortic valve level. Middle shows less waist in a partially opened valve and complete disappreance of the waist after the valve has been fully dilated (right)*

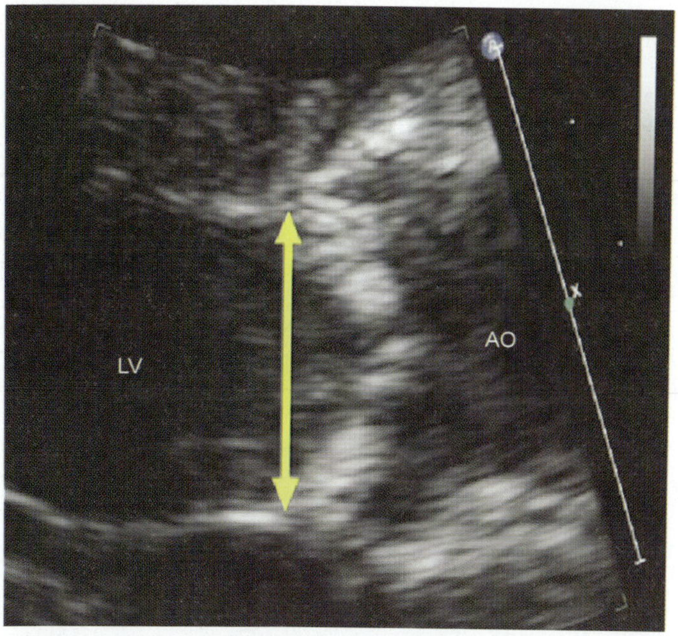

Fig. 35.11: *Measurement of aortic annulus by transthoracic echocardiography. AO, aorta; LV, left ventricle*

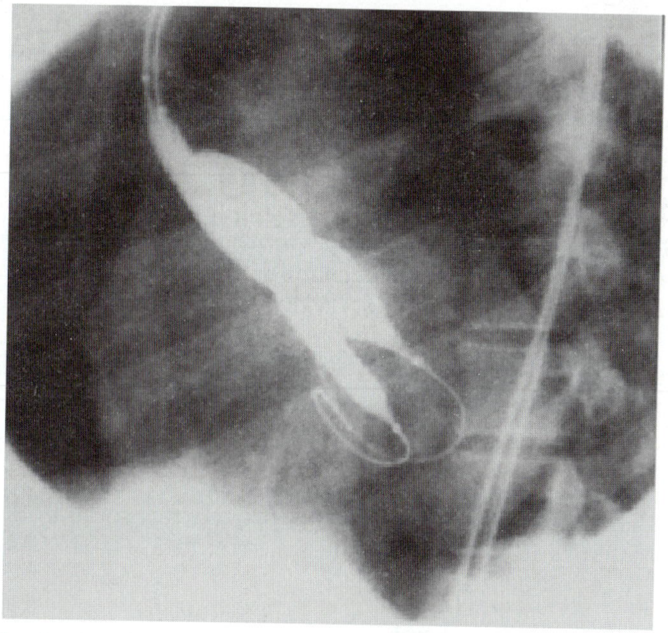

Fig. 35.13: *Showing double balloon for management of aortic valvular stenosis*

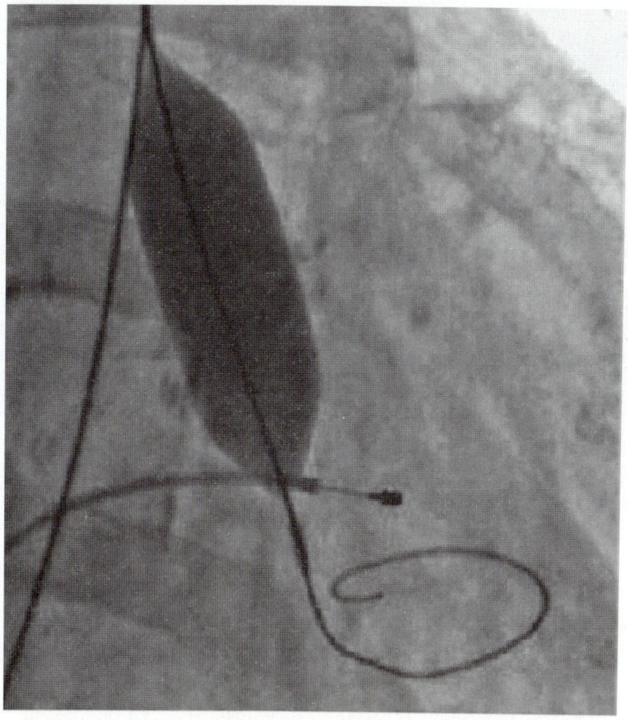

Fig. 35.12: *Balloon aortic valvuloplasty (BAV) via the retrograde approach. After correctly positioning across the stenotic valve the balloon is inflated with dilute contrast material. Note the temporary pacing wire in the right ventricle and the pigtail shaping of the left ventricular wire*

of the stent valve can obstruct the native coronary arteries or interfere with the function of the mitral valve apparatus. In addition, the stent valve must be circumferentially apposed to the aortic annulus to prevent paravalvular aortic regurgitation.

Successful application of catheter-based aortic valve technology is highly dependent on careful attention to operator technique and procedural methodology. All current catheter-based aortic stent valve procedures begin with conventional balloon aortic valvuloplasty to provide an enlarged passageway for the insertion of the larger stent-valve device. Careful patient screening for vascular access and accurate assessment of aortic annulus dimensions for correct valve sizing are critical.

Delivery can be accomplished either via an antegrade approach, requiring transseptal puncture and negotiation of the mitral valve, or via a retrograde approach from the femoral artery. The transapical approach is a relatively

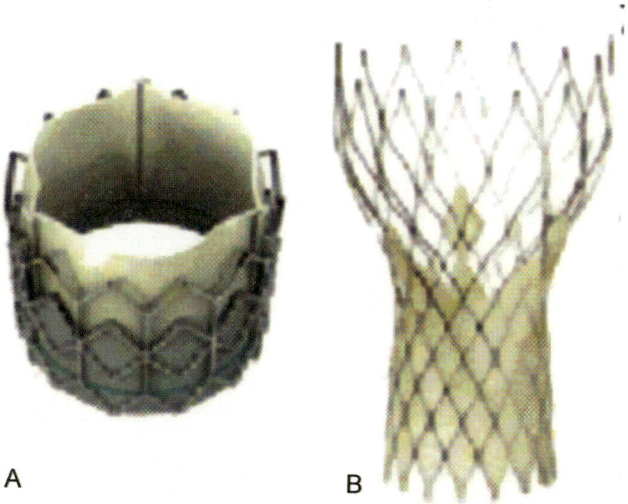

Fig. 35.14: *Current generation transcatheter aortic valve therapies (A) balloon-expandable, stainless steel support structure, bovine pericardial valve; (B) self-expanding, nitinol support structure, porcine pericardial valve*

recent development that is applicable only to a very limited patient population in which the retrograde approach fails. The choice of approach depends on operator experience and the individual case, although lately the retrograde approach has become more popular.

Antegrade Approach

The antegrade implantation technique originally described by Cribier et al is extremely complex, involving transseptal puncture; flotation of a balloon-tipped catheter through the left atrium, left ventricle, and aortic valve to the descending aorta; and arterial exteriorization of the intravascular guide wire. Although this approach combines the lower risk of femoral venous access with the ability to cross more heavily calcified valves, it may jeopardize the anterior leaflet of the mitral valve.

The antegrade technique has proved too complex for widespread dissemination, particularly with first-generation devices.

Retrograde Approach

Because of increased periprocedural complications associated with the transvenous antegrade approach, the transarterial retrograde approach is now preferred. This approach involves femoral artery access (and, usually, surgical arterial repair for closure); negotiation of the femoral, iliac, and aortic vasculature; and retrograde crossing of the calcified aortic valve. In general, the implanted catheter-based aortic valves are oversized relative to the annulus to ensure stability and immobility of the implanted stent and minimize paravalvular regurgitation.

During valve deployment (*see* the image below), additional hemodynamic support devices or temporary rapid right ventricular pacing (to heart rates of 200–220 beats/min) may be necessary to ensure hemodynamic stability and minimize the movement effects of pulsatile aortic flow on stent-valve positioning. After implantation of the stent valve, dilatation with a slightly larger balloon catheter may be needed to reduce paravalvular regurgitation.

Percutaneous Aortic Valve Placement via Retrograde Approach

The retrograde approach, although less technically demanding than the antegrade approach, may be difficult in patients with heavily diseased descending aortas.

Transapical Approach

Transapical aortic valve replacement via a thoracotomy has been described in animal studies and clinical reports.

Access to the cardiac apex during this procedure is achieved through a left anterolateral thoracotomy along the sixth interspace. The transapical access site is gradually dilated, and the crimped valve is introduced inside the diseased native aortic valve. Drawbacks of the procedure include dealing with issues such as pericardial tamponade and having to suture a large puncture wound in the apex of the heart.

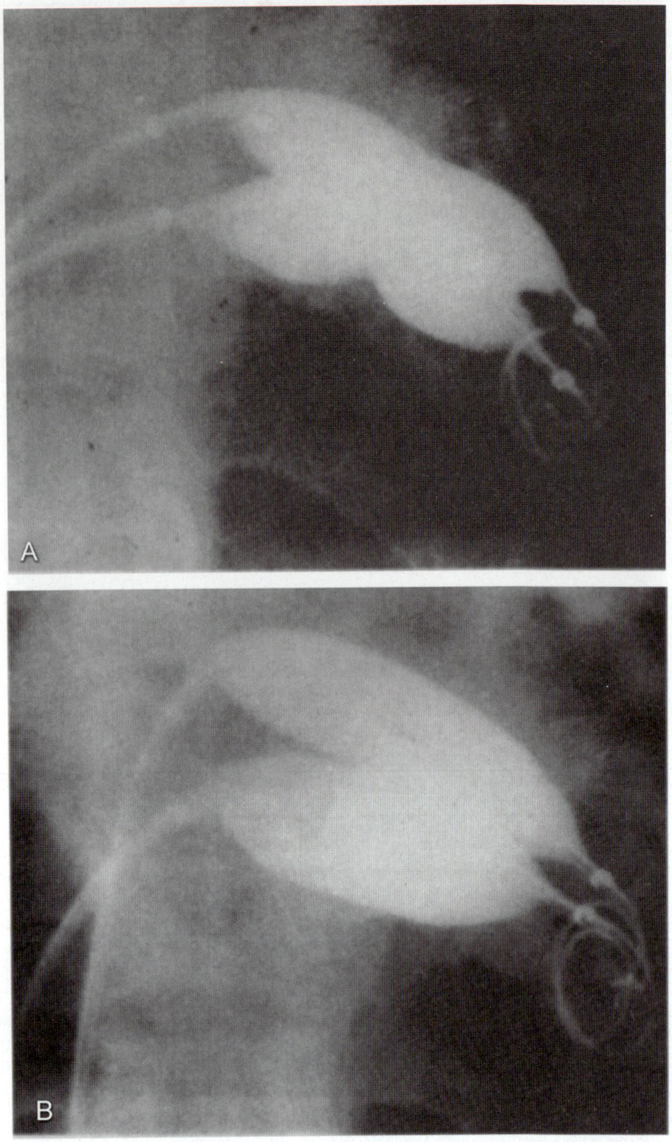

Fig. 35.15: *(A) showing double balloon across the mitral valve indicating the waist found by the stenotic valve. (B) Fully inflated balloon with disappearance of the waist as seen in upper panel*

Table 35.2: *Cinical factors in selection criteria for percutaneous balloon mitral valvuloplasty (PMV)*

I. Factors favour for PMV
1. Echocardiograph score of 8 or less
2. Young age
3. Presence of opening snap
4. No calcification of valve
II. Factors unfavourable for PMV
1. Echocardiographic score 11 or more
2. Age greater than 70
3. No opening snap
4. Atrial fibrillation (long standing)
5. Calcification of valve
6. Subvavular fibrosis
7. Thickened atrial septum (greater than 3 mm)

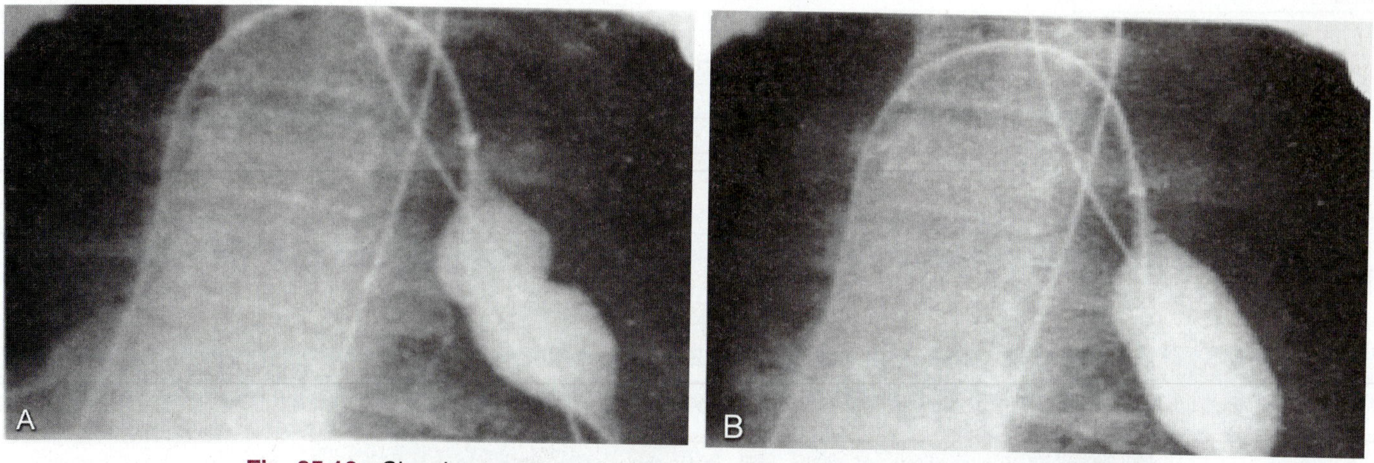

Fig. 35.16: *Showing transseptal dilatation of stenosed MV by balloon valvoplasty*

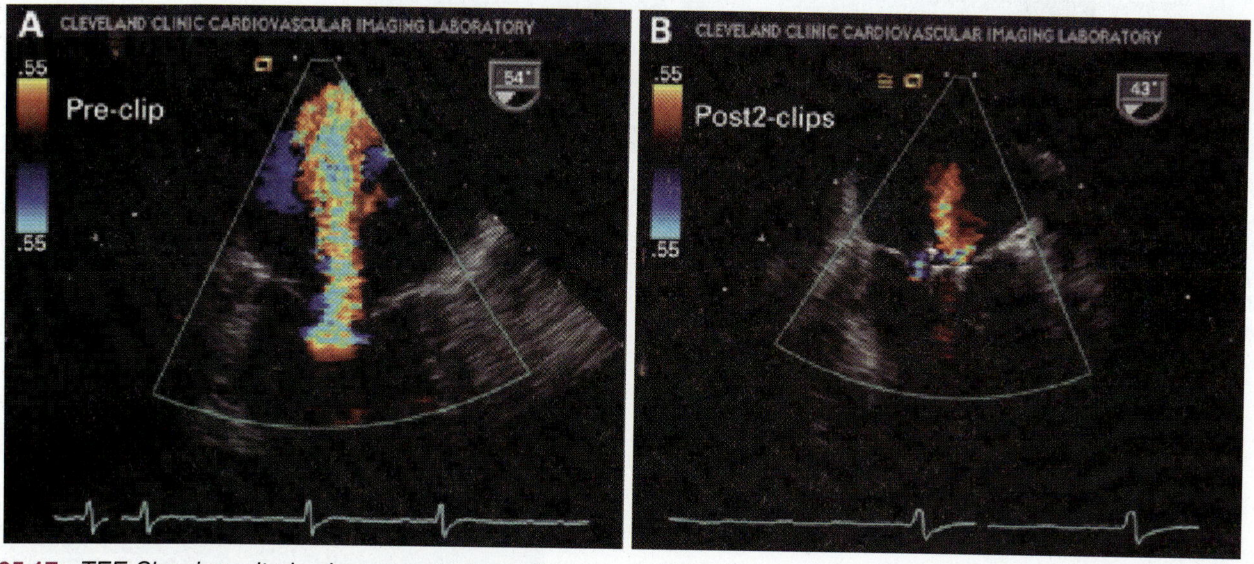

Fig. 35.17: *TEE Showing mitral valve regurgitation before repair (A) and disappearance of mitral regurgitation after repair (B)*

In a retrospective observational comparative study, high-risk elderly patients who underwent conventional aortic valve replacement or transcatheter aortic valve implantation after prior coronary artery bypass grafting had favorable clinical outcomes.

Unbehaun et al performed transapical aortic valve implantation in 300 high-risk patients. The procedure was successful in 99.7% of patients, with a 30 day mortality rate of 4.7% overall. Cumulative survival was reported to be 83% at 1 year, 76% at 1.5 years, and 65% at 2 years and beyond.

Limitations of Procedures

Although enormous enthusiasm for percutaneous aortic valve replacement is noted, this technology is still in its infancy. The following issues remain to be resolved:

Complications such as device migration, compression of the left main artery, mitral valve laceration, paravalvular leak, and thromboembolism must be reduced.

Technical issues related to optimization of access, reduction of delivery system and prosthesis profiles, balloon-expandable stents, repositionable and retrievable devices, and different sizes of devices must be addressed Adequate imaging [e.g. transesophageal echocardiography (TEE), computed tomography (CT), and intracardiac echocardiography (ICE)] must be incorporated into the procedure for accurate determination of prosthesis size so as to reduce the incidence of paravalvular insufficiency and future prosthetic mismatch.

PERCUTANEOUS MITRAL VALVULOPLASTY (COMMISSUROTOMY)

Of the percutaneous valve procedures, percutaneous mitral valvuloplasty has by far the longest track record; it has also been the subject of extensive clinical evaluation. In properly selected patients, the rate of success—defined as a doubling of the baseline mitral valve area or an increase to at least 1.5 cm^2 without causing more than moderate mitral regurgitation or other significant complications—appears to be in the range of 85–99%. Possible complications include mitral regurgitation, atrial septal defect, and left ventricular dysfunction (Figs 35.15A and B, 35.24A–D).

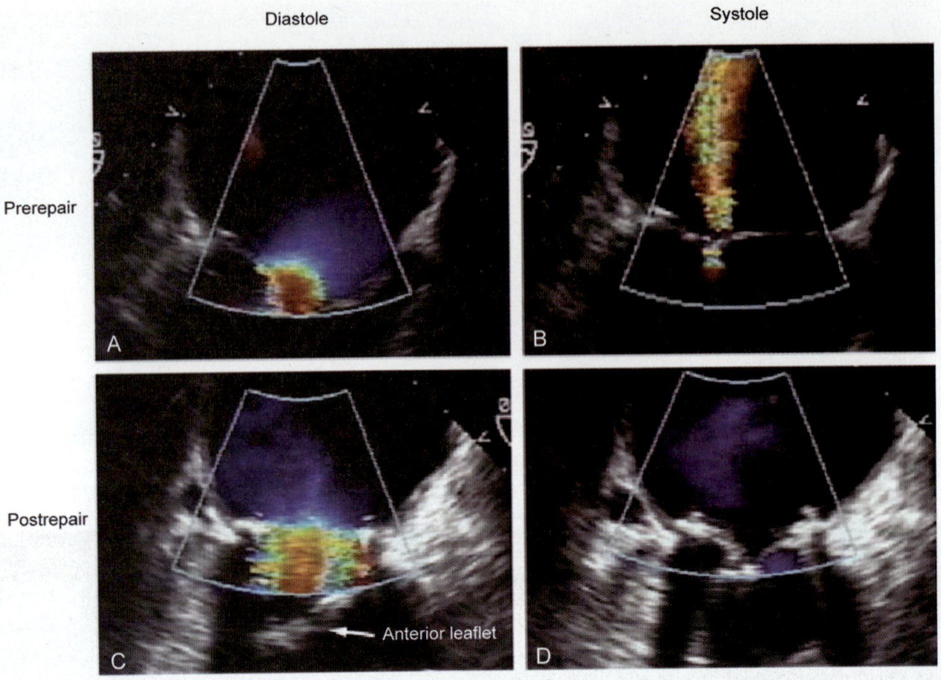

Fig. 35.18: *A patient with long-standing rheumatic mitral stenosis and regurgitation undergoing a rheumatic repair. (A and B): On pre-bypass echo, the stenotic and insufficient mitral valve is demonstrated. (C and D): After insertion of an autologous pericardial patch into the posterior leaflet, decalcifying commissurotomy, resection of the submitral apparatus to the anterior leaflet, and reattachment of the mobile anterior leaflet to both papillary muscles with adjustable ACR, the valve is fully competent with insignificant gradient. A full rigid ring also is placed (AnnuloFlow, Sorin Group). These types of more comprehensive ACR repairs for rheumatic valves have been quite stable in the intermediate-term*

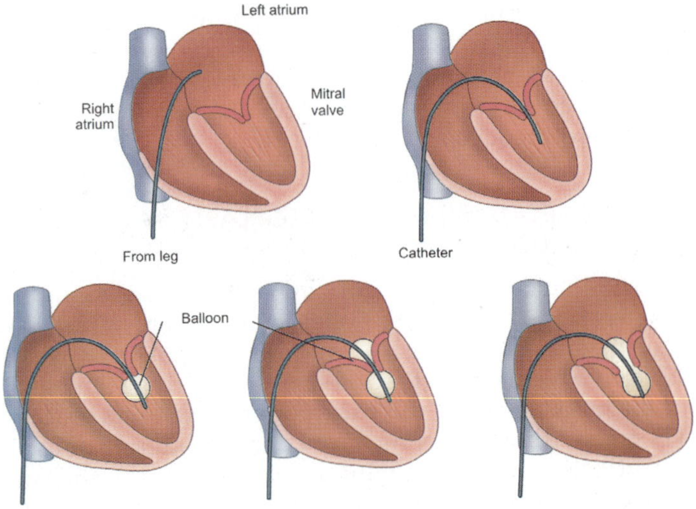

Fig. 35.19: *Diagram showing transcatheter management of mitral valve*

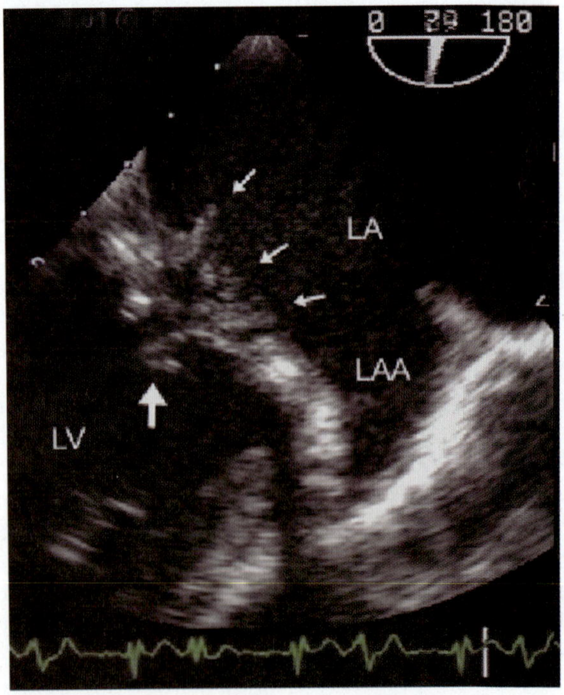

Fig. 35.20: *Lower esophageal two chamber view a massive endocarditis on mitral valvuloplasty*

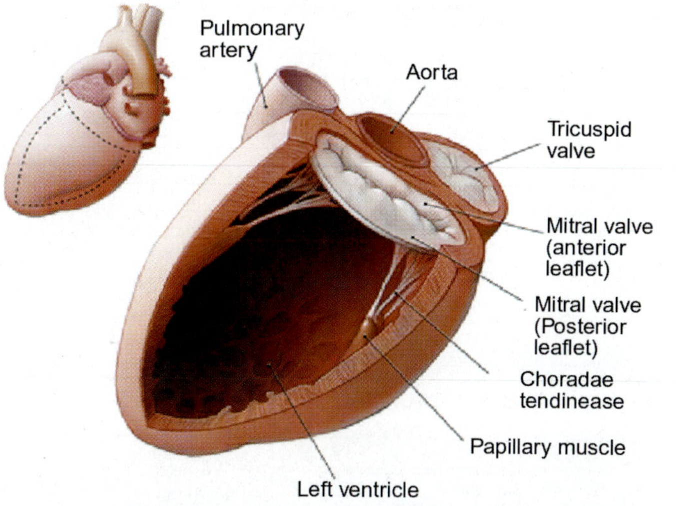

Fig. 35.21: *Anatomy showing components of mitral valve apparatus*

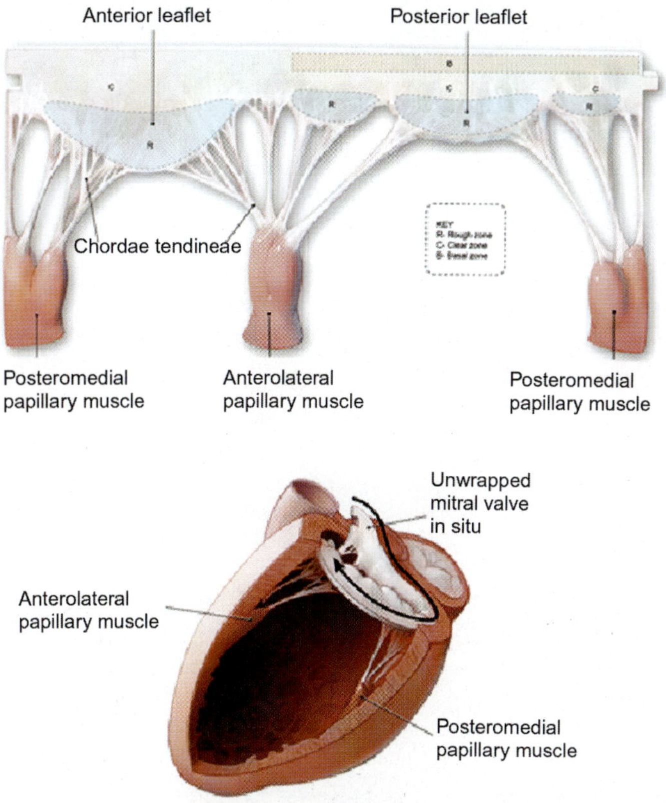

Fig. 35.22: *Anatomy showing components of mitral valve leaflets*

Technical Aspects of Procedure

Percutaneous mitral valvuloplasty is widely practiced in the United States. It is effective in patients with commissural fusion secondary to rheumatic disease; however, it is not applicable to mitral stenosis secondary to mitral annular calcification. The procedure is typically performed under TEE or ICE with a single Inoue balloon, a double balloon, or a rigid mechanical device.

Percutaneous mitral valvuloplasty is performed via an antegrade approach involving transseptal puncture

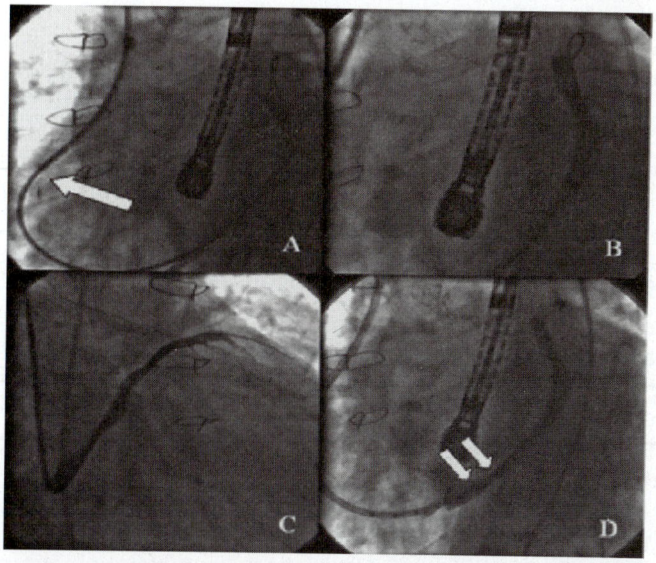

Fig. 35.23: *Procedural steps of percutaneous mitral valvuloplasty using Carillon system-coronary venous cannulation. (A) Coronary artery angiography in LAO30 CRAN20 view. A 6F multipurpose catheter is advanced over a wire and a 9F guiding catheter is advanced over the multipurpose catheter-the arrow indicated tip of the guiding catheter; (B) venous outflow after coronary artery angiography with guiding catheter LAO 30 view; (C) RAO 30 view; (D) marker catheter introduced into the guiding catheter. The arrow indicates 1 cm markers.*

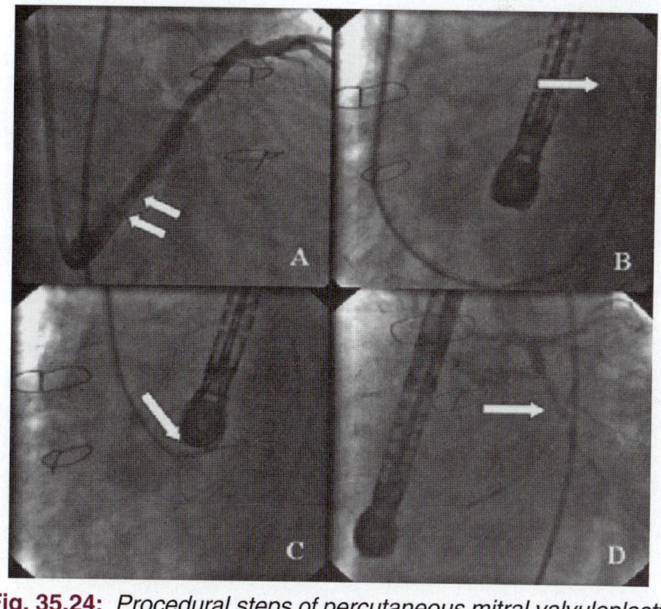

Fig. 35.24: *Procedural steps of percutaneous mitral valvuloplasty using Carillon system—venous calibration and implantation of the device. (A) 9F guiding catheter was introduced into coronary venous system over the diagnostic catheter, which was later replaced with a calibration catheter, having 1 cm marks (arrows) and coronary venography was performed in RAO 30 projection allowing assessment of the vein length; (B) implantation of the distal anchor (arrow) in LAO 30 CAUD 20 view; (C) implantation of the proximal anchor (arrow); (D) after assessment of coronary arteries and transesophageal echocardiography for evaluation the efficacy, the device is released. Coronary angiography in RAO 35 CAUD 20 after device implantation shows normal flow in the circumflex artery despite crossing the artery with the device within vein (arrow)*

followed by flotation of a balloon-tipped catheter through the left atrium to the mitral valve level. The most distal part of the balloon is placed against the subvalvular apparatus and inflated first to secure the position. This step is followed by inflation of the proximal part of the balloon, which helps anchor the balloon to the mitral position. If the balloon position looks optimal, the middle part is inflated, thus increasing the mitral valve area.

Percutaneous Mitral Valve Repair

For stenotic mitral valves, catheter-based balloon valvuloplasty is now the primary therapeutic option whereas until relatively recently, regurgitant valves have been amenable only to surgical treatment. Valve repair is increasingly preferred because it is associated with better survival and avoids the need for anticoagulation; moreover, it conserves the papillary muscle architecture and its vital role in overall ventricular function.

Myxomatous disease and functional regurgitation, which are the most common mechanisms of mitral valve

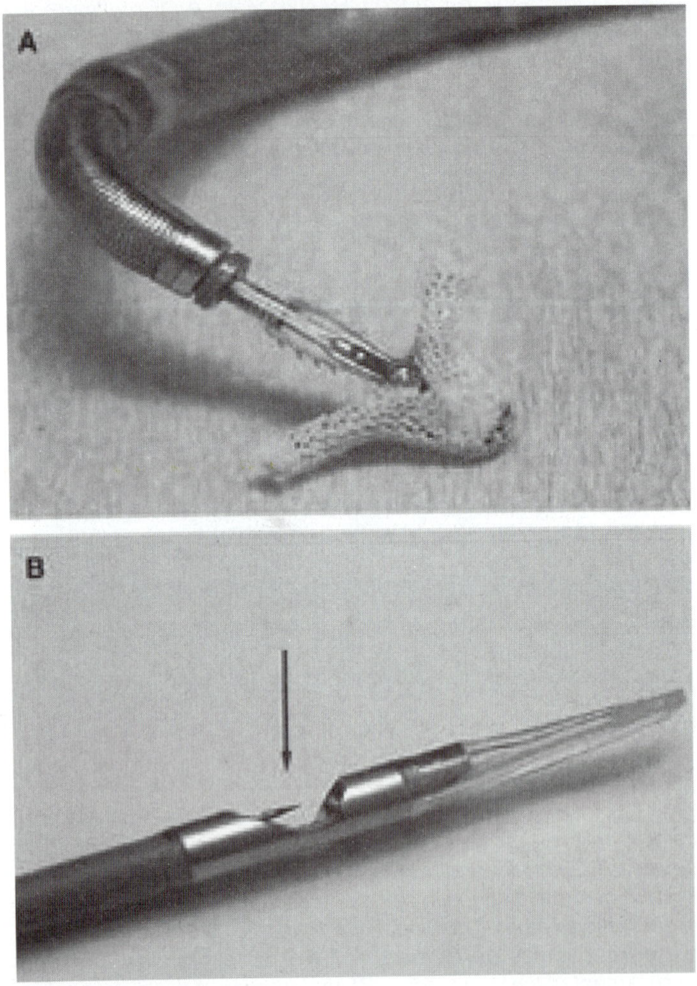

Fig. 35.25: *Two devices that reproduce the Alfieri edge-to-edge mitral valve repair method (A) A delivery system, in which the distal clip is used for leaflet coaptation (MitraClip®). Picture supplied by and reproduced with permission of Evalve, Menlo Park, CA. (B) Guide catheter with vacuum port (arrow) and internal needle and suture system*

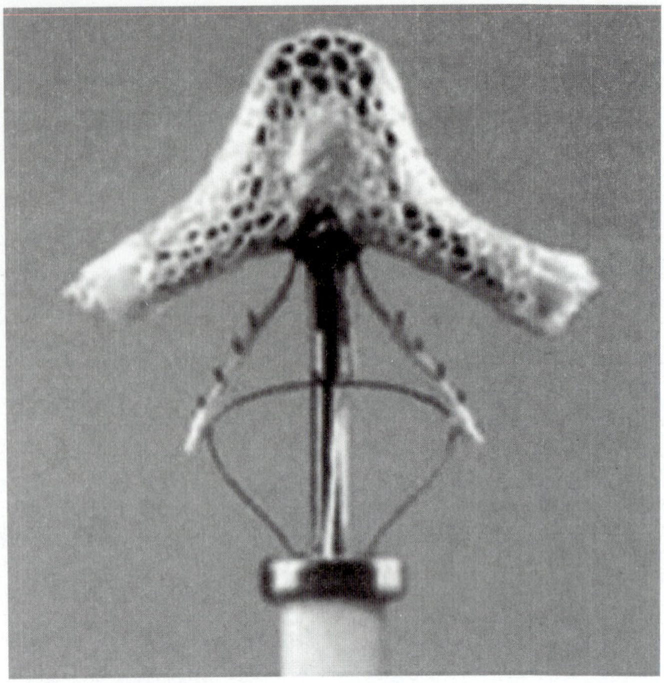

Fig. 35.26: *MitraClip mitral valve repair system mounted over the guiding catheter*

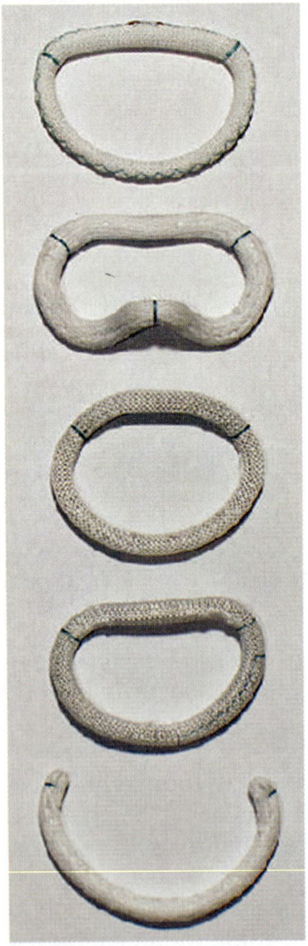

Fig. 35.27: *Examples of commercially available annuloplasty rings. From top: St. Judes Rigid Saddle Shaped Ring, Edwards Geoform, Edwards Physio, Edwards ETlogix, Edwards Cosgrove*

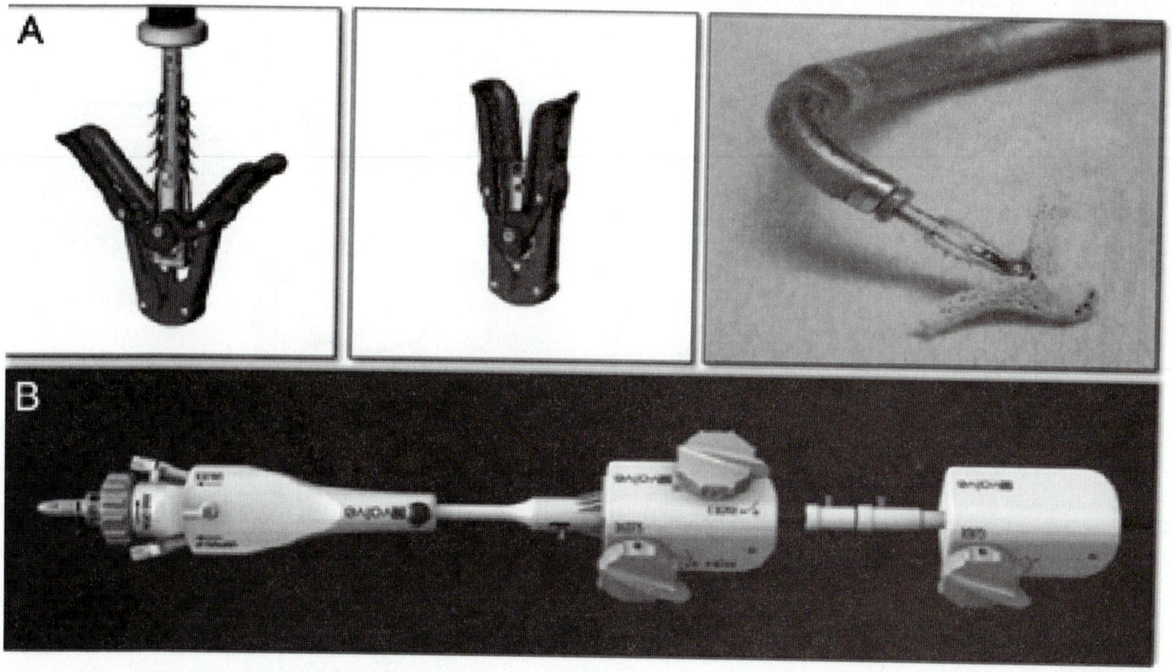

Fig. 35.28: *The evalve MitraClip (A) The evalve MitraClip. The clip arms are open (left) when the device is passed across the mitral leaflets from the left atrium into the left ventricle. The gripper is the barbed piece seen in the upper left panel, parallel to the shaft of the delivery system. When the leaflets are grasped, the gripper helps to fix the leaflets within the clip arms (middle). The clip is covered with polyester fabric (right). (B) The steering knobs are shown on the right-hand side of the device for maneuvering the clip within the left atrial cavity. At the far left of the picture is the knob that is used to open and close the clip, and the release mechanism*

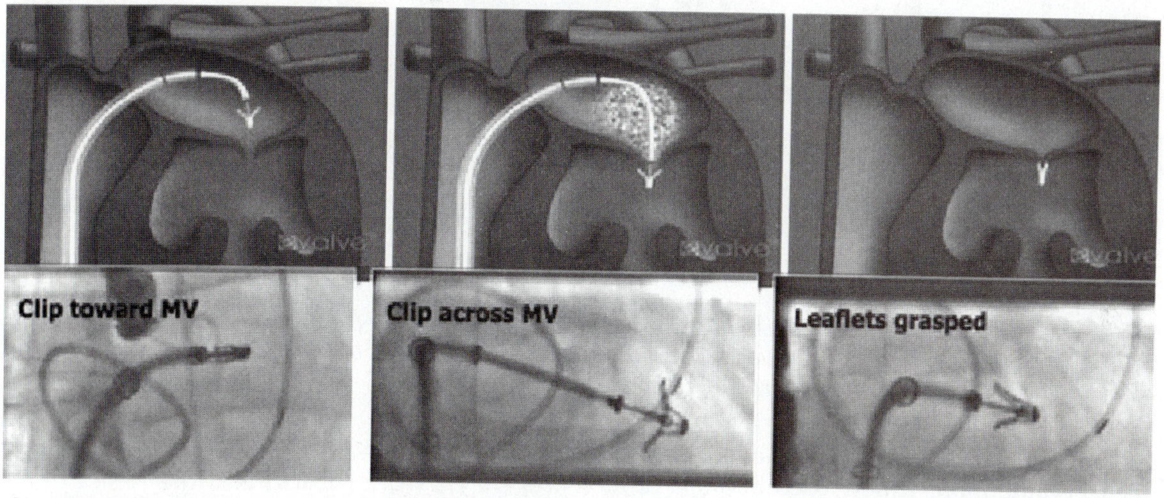

Fig. 35.29: *Showing basic steps of the evalve MitraClip procedure (Top) The left panel shows the clip being steered through the left atrium toward the center of the mitral orifice. The middle panel illustrates the device across the mitral valve (MV) with the clip arms open, before the clip has been pulled back to grasp the mitral leaflets. The right panel shows, in the cartoon, the clip has been released. (Bottom) In the fluoroscopic figure, the leaflets have been grasped and clipped closed partially, before full closure and release of the clip*

dysfunction, are also the most amenable to valve repair. Various techniques have now been developed for reducing mitral regurgitation via a catheter-based approach in these circumstances (Figs 35.25–35.34).

Technical Aspects of Procedure

The following are potential components of percutaneous mitral valve repair.

Edge-to-Edge Repair

The concept of edge-to-edge repair was developed as a surgical strategy for treating mitral regurgitation caused by anterior leaflet prolapse. The technique, first described by Alfieri (and consequently referred to as the Alfieri stitch), opposes the central portions of the anterior and posterior mitral valve leaflets to create a double-orifice valve with reduced leaflet excursion and less regurgitation.

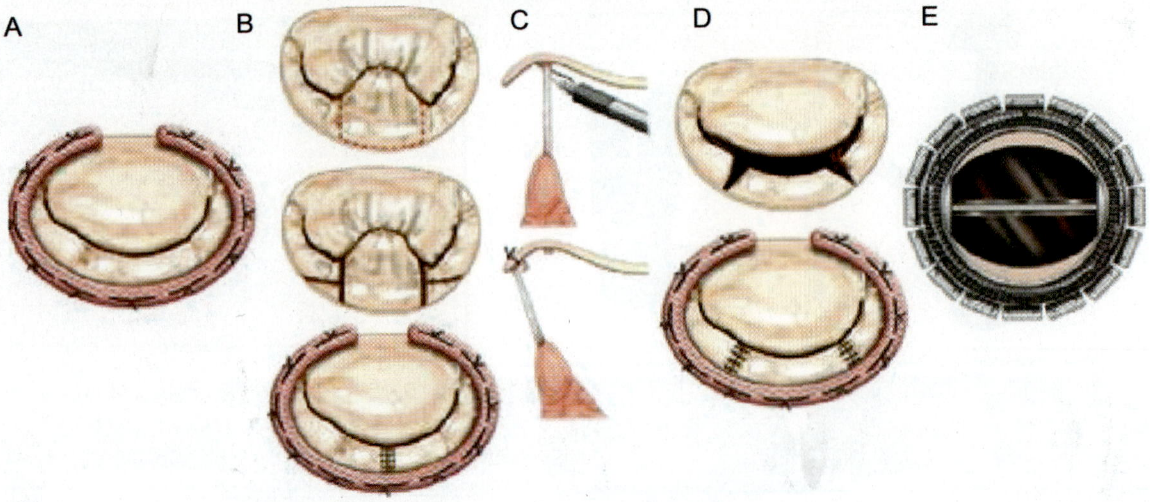

Figs 35.30A to E: *Common established surgical techniques used to correct mitral regurgitation (A) Ring annuloplasty. (B) Quadrangular resection and sliding leaflet plasty. (C) Chordal transfer. (D) Cleft closure. (E) Mitral replacement. Illustration by Craig Skaggs with permission*

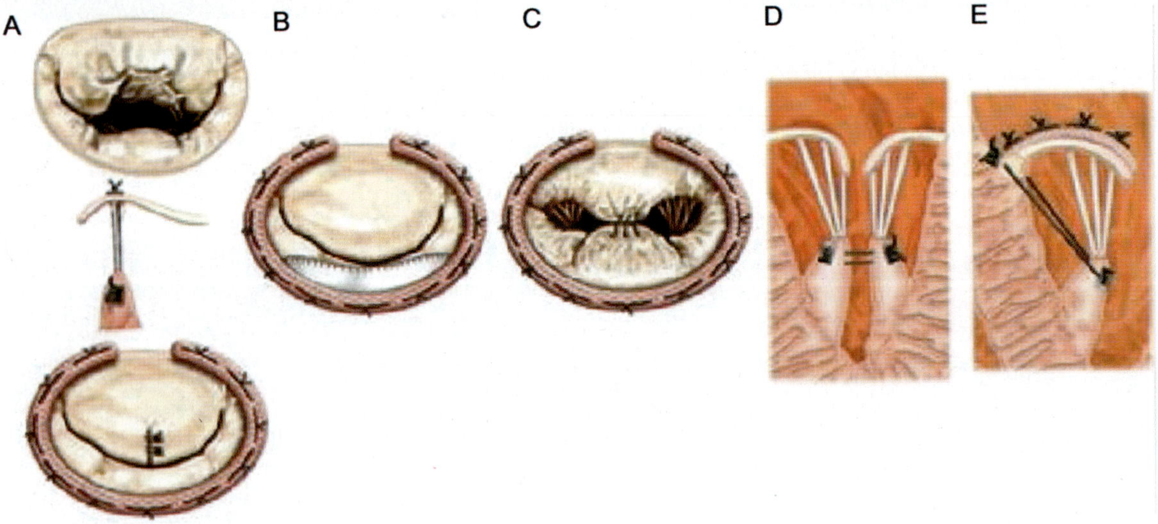

Figs 35.31A to E: *Newer surgical techniques used to repair regurgitant mitral valve (A) chordal replacement. (B) Posterior leaflet augmentation. (C) Edge-to-edge Alfieri stitch (valve shown in diastole with double orifice). (D) Papillary muscle approximation. (E) Posterior wall reduction. (Figure illustration by Craig Skaggs with permission)*

The edge-to-edge repair, initially performed as a rescue operation, later became more widely used because of its simplicity and encouraging results. Furthermore, its uncomplicated nature encouraged interventionalists to develop an analogous transcatheter-based technique. In the surgical procedure, however, the repair is usually combined with an annuloplasty, which is not currently the case in the corresponding catheter-based procedure.

Two devices are now available that can be used for percutaneous mitral valve repair: the MitraClip (Evalve, Inc, Menlo Park, CA) and the Mobius II (Edwards Lifesciences, Irvine, CA). Delivery requires a transseptal puncture (see the image below) followed by deployment of a clip or suture to create a bridge between the anterior and posterior valve leaflets. To date, the largest clinical experience has been with the MitraClip.

Percutaneous Mitral Valve Repair via Transseptal Puncture

If the location of the clip is suboptimal, the clip can be reopened and repositioned; only after the final position is confirmed is the delivery system detached. In some cases, deployment of two devices has been necessary to achieve adequate reduction of mitral regurgitation. At 6 months, the device is completely incorporated into the tissue bridge, mimicking the result of surgery. The procedure is performed with general anesthesia under the guidance of fluoroscopy and TEE.

The procedure is technically demanding and is likely to be limited to specialist centers with experienced interventionalists and echocardiologists who work closely together.

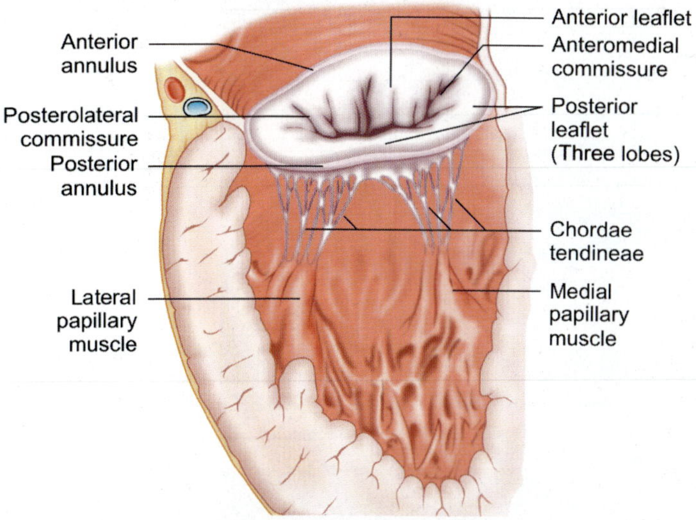

Fig. 35.32: *Showing anatomical features of mitral valve apparatus*

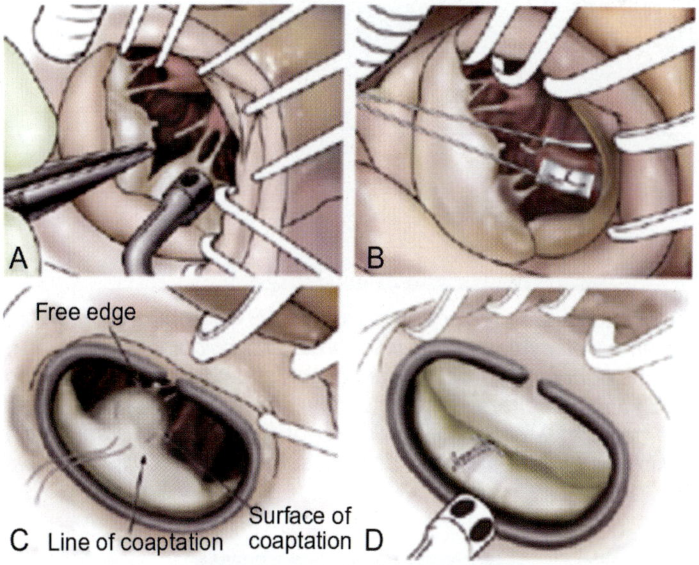

Fig. 35.33: *Showing sequential steps in "adjustable artificial chordal replacement. (A) A ruptured chordi tendine from the posterior papillary muscle to the posterior leaflet is evident. (B) A pledgetted anchor suture is placed longitudinally in the papillary muscle, and a 2-0 Gore-Tex artificial chord is passed through the anchor pledget and left untied. (C) After Carpentier ring placement (AnnuloFlow, Sorin Group), the chord is retrieved and woven as a loop into the leaflet in three full-thickness bites: free edge, flaring laterally through the surface of coaptation, and then angling back medially through the line of coaptation, emerging onto the atrial surface of the leaflet. (D) The chordal slip knot is adjusted during valve testing to produce good anterior-posterior and left to right leaflet symmetry, and no residual leak. The knot is then tied tightly and completed*

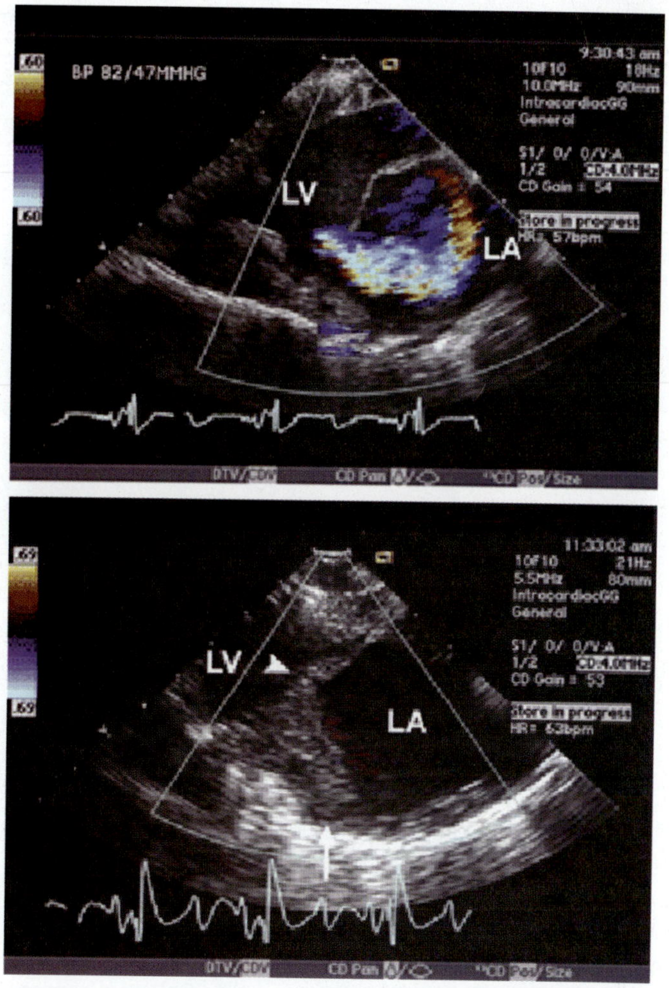

Fig. 35.34: *Reduction of ischemic mitral regurgitation with Percutaneous Device Implantation (Top) Parasternal long-axis view with color-flow echocardiography showing moderately severe mitral regurgitation (grade 3+) present 4 months after surgical ligation of obtuse marginal arteries. (Bottom) Parasternal long-axis view with color-flow echocardiography showing elimination of mitral regurgitation following device implantation. With device implantation, there is reduction in the anterior-posterior dimension of the mitral annulus (arrow) and increased leaflet coaptation (arrowhead)*

Annuloplasty

Annuloplasty is a fundamental component of most mitral valve surgery and can sometimes be used alone to treat functional mitral regurgitation. The goal is to rectify annular dilatation while reducing the anteroposterior diameter of the valve to promote better leaflet coaptation and reduce regurgitation.

Optimal surgical results are usually achieved with insertion of a prosthetic band or ring, though other techniques using pericardium, Dacron, or sutures alone are described. The central role of annular dilatation in the progression of mitral regurgitation makes it an important target for catheter-based treatments.

The coronary sinus, which has already been the target for interventions such as biventricular pacing, has been considered for this procedure because of its close relation with the atrioventricular groove. Shortening or reshaping the annulus by inserting a device into the coronary sinus has the potential to mimic a surgical annuloplasty. Experi-

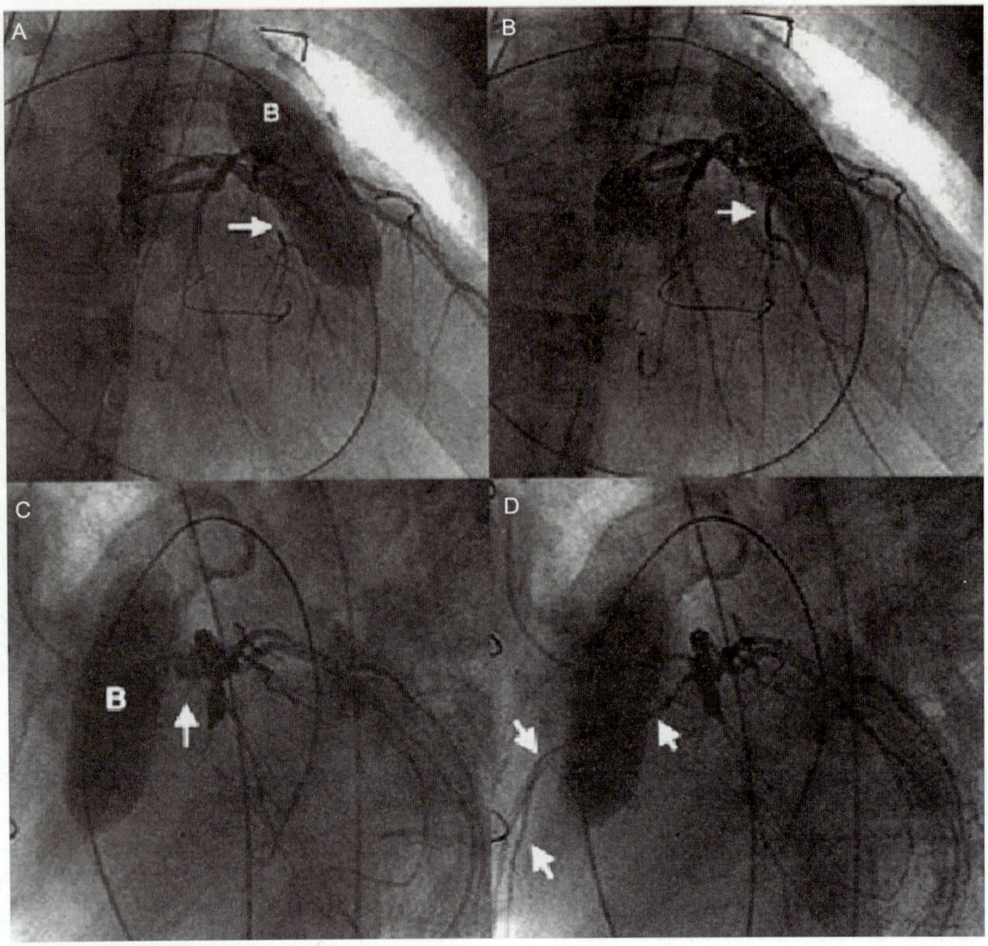

Fig. 35.35: *A patient with tetralogy of Fallot and pulmonary atresia, the conduit passed over a large anterior RV coronary branch that arose from the proximal left coronary artery. Selective coronary angiograms with simultaneous inflation of an angioplasty balloon (B) in the conduit demonstrate occlusion of this RV branch. Angiography from a right anterior oblique projection shows (A) early occlusion of the anomalous coronary (arrow), with persistent distal contrast, and (B) subsequent resumption of flow as the balloon was deflated (arrow). (C and D) Subsequent angiography in a lateral projection demonstrates complete occlusion of the coronary branch with balloon inflation to higher pressure. In C, the arrow indicates the proximal stump of the occluded vessel, which then fills (multiple arrows) as the balloon is deflated in D*

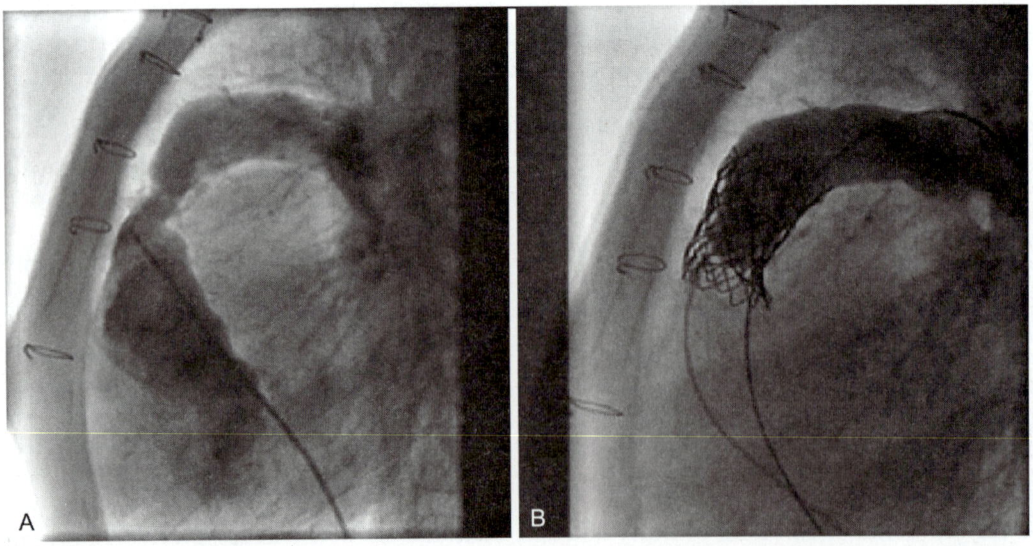

Fig. 35.36: *The implantation of the percutaneous pulmonary valve was performed with excellent results (A) severe stenosis of the homograft. (B) resolution of the stenosis, no regurgitation*

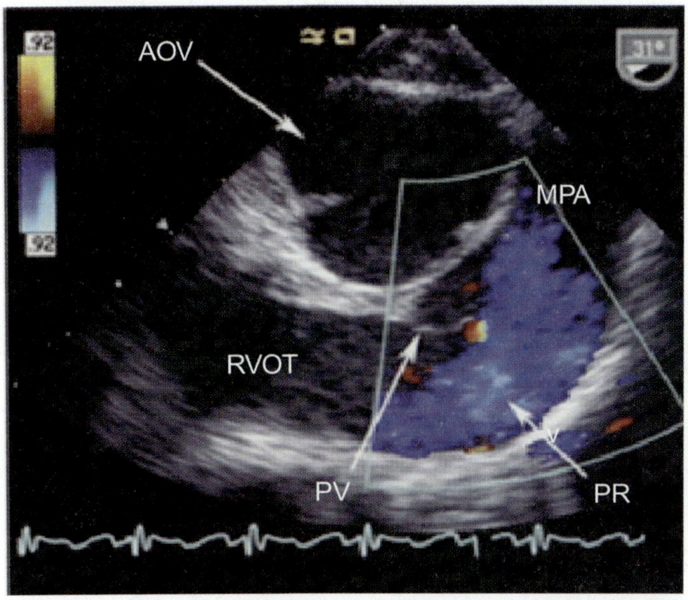

Fig. 35.37: *Preoperative echocardiogram demonstrating severe pulmonary valve regurgitation located anteriorly through the gap created by the transannular patch. (AOV, aortic valve; MPA, main pulmonary artery; PR, pulmonary regurgitation; PV, pulmonary valve; RVOT, right ventricular outflow tract.)*

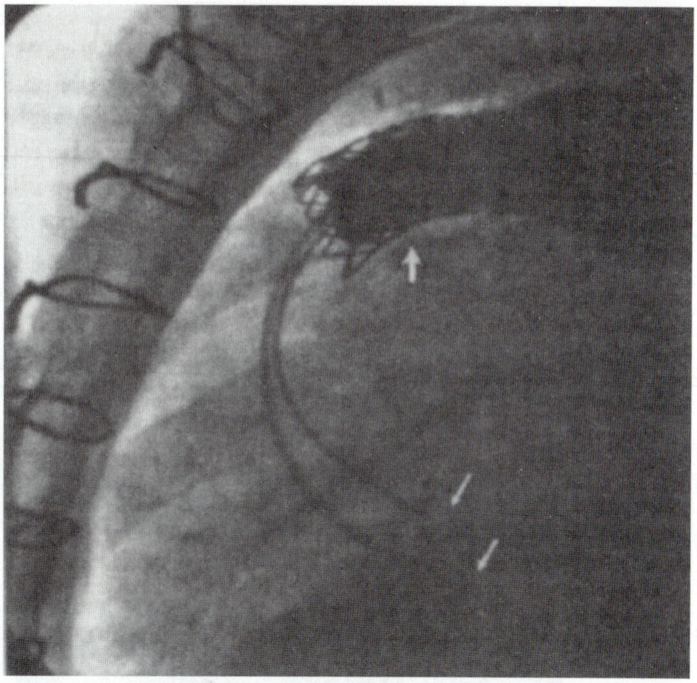

Fig. 35.38: *Showing double balloon (arrows) across PV for dilatation of valve in patient with pulmonic stenosis*

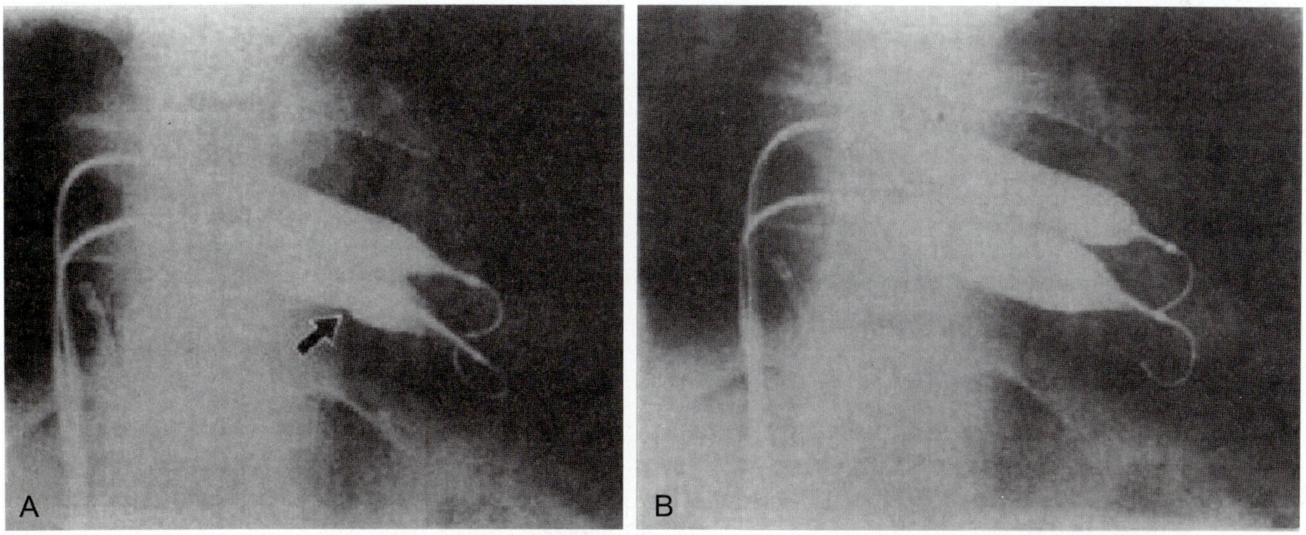

Fig. 35.39: *The Inoue double balloon was used for dilatation of tricuspid stenosis in an adolescent*

mental proof-of-concept was supplied by the publication of an initial human feasibility study using the Viking device (Edwards Lifesciences, Irving, CA).

A catheter is advanced into the coronary sinus via a transjugular access site, and the anchoring device is placed in the distal coronary sinus with a tensioning element (a wire or spring surrounded by absorbable material) that attaches the device to the proximal coronary sinus anchor.

This approach is suitable for degenerative prolapse, functional congestive heart failure, and ischemic mitral regurgitation. However, it is limited by the substantial variations in normal coronary sinus anatomy, the varying distance between the coronary sinus and mitral valve annulus, and the possibility of circumflex artery compromise. It also does not address the anterior annulus problems.

Detailed imaging including angiography and venography, form an important aspect of the "decision to proceed" algorithm. Other concerns include late dilatation of the anterior annulus, leaflet tethering due to papillary muscle displacement, and annular calcification. Finally, the long-term consequences of leaving such an implant in the coronary sinus are unknown though experience obtained with pacing wires is reassuring.

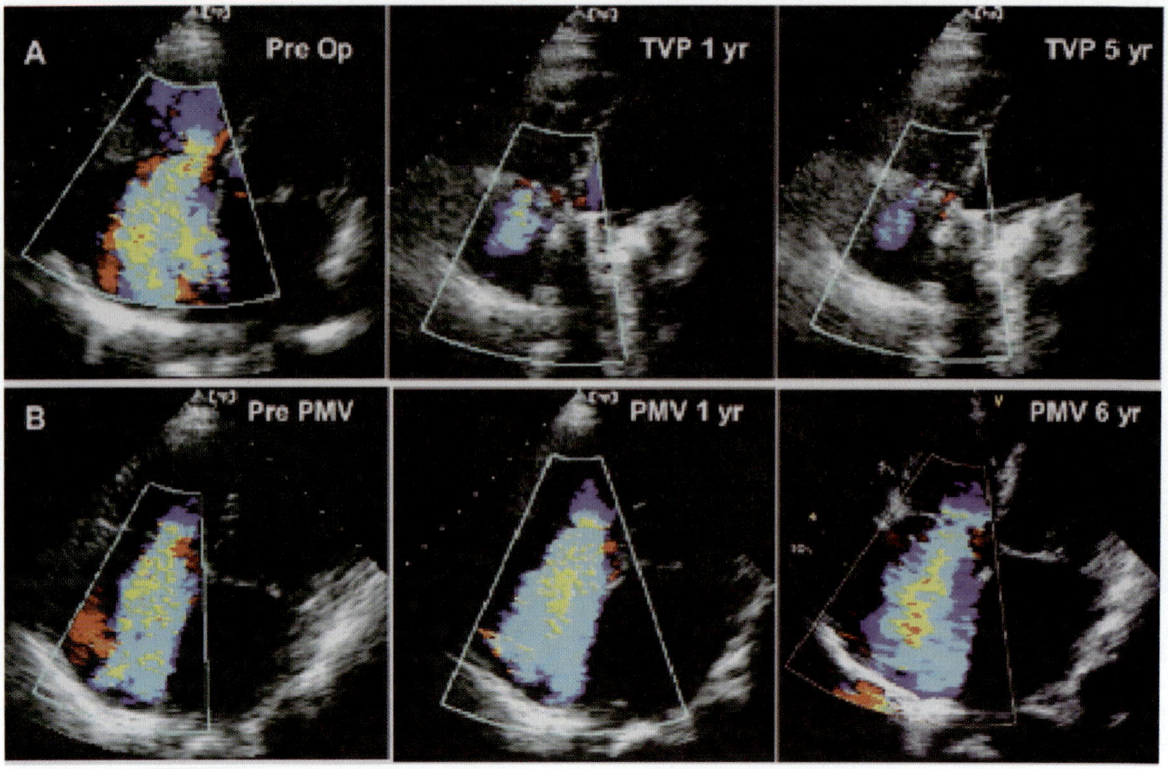

Figs 35.40A and B: *Severe functional TR and RV enlargement were significantly decreased by TV repair on postoperative 1-year and 5-year follow-up echocardiography (A). Severe TR and RV size were unchanged after PMV alone (B).*

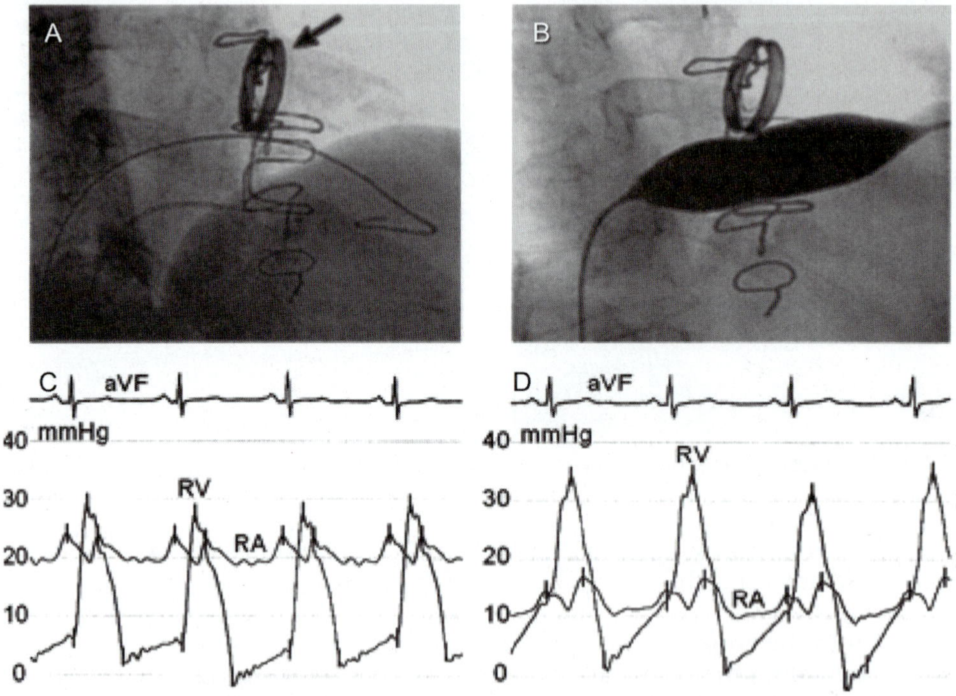

Fig. 35.41: *(A) Fluoroscopic image in the right anterior oblique/cranial view demonstrates the guidewire that was passed through the center of the stenotic bioprosthetic valve. Mechanical mitral valve (black arrow) and bioprosthetic tricuspid valve (yellow arrow) are shown. (B) Balloon valvuloplasty was performed with the use of a balloon with a maximum diameter of 25 × 40 mm and an inflation pressure of 16 atm. (C) Before the procedure, the mean right atrial pressure was 21 mmHg and the right ventricular end-diastolic pressure was 5 mmHg. The mean diastolic gradient across the tricuspid valve was 13 mmHg. (D) After the procedure, the mean right atrial pressure was 12 mmHg and the right ventricular end-diastolic pressure was 10 mmHg. The mean diastolic gradient across the tricuspid valve was improved to 6 mmHg*

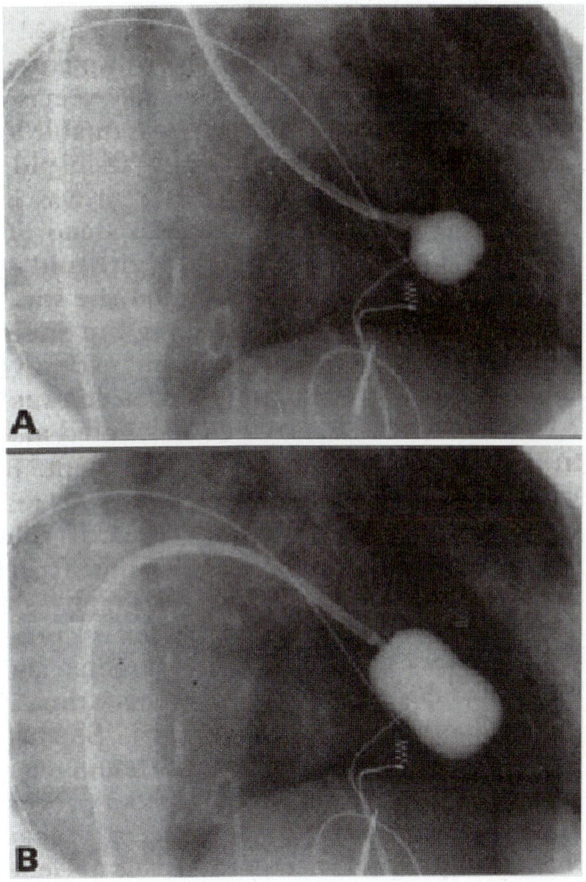

Figs 35.42A and B: *The Inoue balloon was used for dilatation of tricuspid stenosis in an adolescent . The valve was reached by an over-the-wire approach with a 0.025 exchange length guidewire. The Inoue stylet would not reach the tricuspid orifice because the right atrium was so large. The Inoue balloon's special dilatation characteristics allowed good positioning at the tricuspid orifice. After dilatation to 27.5 mm, the pressure drop across the valve was reduced from 12 to 5 mmHg. Further dilatation at 30 mm, however, created moderately severe tricuspid reflux without a further reduction of gradient. The Inoue balloon is suitable for dilatation of tricuspid stenosis but small increments in dilatation size may be required for optimal reduction in gradient without creating significant reflux*

Combined Mitral and Left Ventricular Remodeling

A novel off-pump surgical transventricular repair that involves placement of a tensioning cable directly through the left ventricular chamber (Coapsys; Myocor, Inc, Maple Grove, MN) has been developed to address mitral annular and ventricular dimensional corrections associated with mitral repair strategies. In this technique, anchoring pads on either side of the ventricle are used to allow the cable to apply tension across the chamber. This shortens the septal lateral dimension and remodels the left ventricular chamber. Surgical approach to mitral valve repair using external pads and transventricular cord. This technique has been adapted to transpericardial percutaneous use in animal models. Tether places tension on septal-lateral dimension of mitral valve and also remodels basal left ventricle with reorientation of papillary muscles.

This approach is unique in that it is the only mitral repair that directly remodels the left ventricular chamber, which gives it certain potential advantages in cases of functional mitral regurgitation.

A transpericardial percutaneous (subxiphoid) method that can reproduce the effects of the surgical approach (I-Coapsys) is in development in early clinical trials.

Percutaneous Pulmonary Valve Replacement

Of the valve replacement procedures, percutaneous pulmonary valve replacement actually represents the largest clinical experience. Acquired pulmonary valve disease in adults is rare with regurgitation in the setting of pulmonary hypertension being the most frequent cause.

In individuals with complex congenital heart disease, however, pulmonary valve dysfunction is common and often the principle reason for late complications. Pulmonary regurgitation commonly occurs following tetralogy of Fallot repair (Figs 35.35–35.38).

Thus, for the rapidly growing population of survivors with repaired congenital heart disease, a percutaneous approach to pulmonary valve replacement could avoid the morbidity and discomfort attendant on repeated open-heart surgery.

Percutaneous pulmonary valve replacement is indicated for congenital pulmonary stenosis and pulmonary stenosis and regurgitation in a patient with congenital heart disease who has previously undergone right ventricular outflow tract surgery.

Technical Aspects of Procedure

Implantation of a transcatheter pulmonary valve was first reported by the authors in 2000 in a 12-year-old boy with a stenosed and regurgitant prosthetic conduit. This procedure has since been performed in more than 125 patients with repaired congenital heart disease (aged 7–58 years).

Drawbacks of Procedure

The main limitation of percutaneous pulmonary valve replacement is the meager selection of device sizes. A much wider selection of sizes must be developed for optimal treatment of young children and patients with dilated right ventricular outflow tracts. Positioning of the devices also remains a challenge but is not as critical as it is for aortic valve procedures; preprocedural imaging may assist in identifying the optimal position for deployment.

PERCUTANEOUS TRICUSPID VALVE REPAIR

Percutaneous tricuspid valve devices remain in the pre-clinical stages of development. Tricuspid annular devices must be correctly positioned to avoid obstruction of the coronary sinus ostium or damage to the atrioventricular node (Figs 35.39–35.42).

An advantage of these devices is that they can be deployed under significantly tighter time constraints than other valve devices because right chamber pressures are lower and rapid pacing will not be required. Their disadvantages include the greater fragility of tricuspid valve leaflets, the lack of firm surrounding tissue in the tricuspid annulus, and the frequent annular dilatation in patients with tricuspid regurgitation. Percutaneous tricuspid valves also will not prevent further annular dilation and may therefore be susceptible to future dehiscence or embolization.

However, the greatest limitations facing tricuspid valve therapies are not the valve-related factors but, rather, the disease-related factors in this population, including right ventricular failure and advanced pulmonary hypertension.

BIBLIOGRAPHY

1. Sharma S, Mehra A, Rahimtoola SH. Valvular heart disease: a century of progress. Am J Med. Aug 2008;121(8):664–73.
2. Cribier A, Eltchaninoff H, Bash A, Borenstein N, Tron C, Bauer F. Percutaneous transcatheter implantation of an aortic valve prosthesis for calcific aortic stenosis: first human case description. Circulation. Dec 10 2002;106(24):3006–8.
3. Rosengart TK, Feldman T, Borger MA, Vassiliades TA Jr, Gillinov AM, Hoercher KJ. Percutaneous and minimally invasive valve procedures: a scientific statement from the American heart association council on cardiovascular surgery and anesthesia, Council on clinical cardiology, Functional Genomics and translational biology interdisciplinary Working group, and Quality of care and outcomes research interdisciplinary working group. Circulation. Apr 1 2008; 117(13):1750–67.
4. Feldman T, Leon MB. Prospects for percutaneous valve therapies. Circulation. Dec 11 2007;116(24):2866–77.
5. Webb JG, Chandavimol M, Thompson CR, Ricci DR, Carere RG, Munt BI, et al. Percutaneous aortic valve implantation retrograde from the femoral artery. Circulation. Feb 14 2006;113(6):842–50.
6. Coats L, Bonhoeffer P. New percutaneous treatments for valve disease. Heart. May 2007;93(5):639–44.
7. Munt B, Webb J. Percutaneous valve repair and replacement techniques. Heart. Oct 2006;92(10):1369–72.
8. Walther T, Dewey T, Wimmer-Greinecker G, Doss M, Hambrecht R, Schuler G, et al. Transapical approach for sutureless stent-fixed aortic valve implantation: experimental results. Eur J Cardiothorac Surg. May 2006;29(5):703–8.
9. Lichtenstein SV, Cheung A, Ye J, Thompson CR, Carere RG, Pasupati S. Transapical transcatheter aortic valve implantation in humans: initial clinical experience. Circulation. Aug 8 2006;114(6):591–6.
10. Huber CH, Cohn LH, von Segesser LK. Direct-access valve replacement a novel approach for off-pump valve implantation using valved stents. J Am Coll Cardiol. Jul 19 2005;46(2):366–70.
11. Kodali SK, O'Neill W, Moses JW, Kapadia S, Williams M, Hanzel G, et al. Preliminary Results from the Percutaneous Endovascular Implantation of Valves Trial in High Risk Patients with Critical Aortic Stenosis. Am J Cardiol. 2006;98 (Suppl 1):48M.
12. Kodali SK, O'Neill WW, Moses JW, Williams M, Smith CR, Tuzcu M, et al. Early and late (1 year) outcomes following transcatheter aortic valve implantation in patients with severe aortic stenosis (from the United States REVIVAL trial). Am J Cardiol. Apr 1 2011;107(7):1058–64.
13. Stortecky S, Brinks H, Wenaweser P, Huber C, Pilgrim T, Windecker S, et al. Transcatheter aortic valve implantation or surgical aortic valve replacement as redo procedure after prior coronary artery bypass grafting. Ann Thorac Surg. Oct 2011;92(4):1324–31.
14. Unbehaun A, Pasic M, Drews T, Dreysse S, Kukucka M, Hetzer R, et al. Analysis of Survival in 300 High-Risk Patients up to 2.5 Years After Transapical Aortic Valve Implantation. Ann Thorac Surg. Oct 2011;92(4):1315–23.
15. Vassiliades TA Jr, Block PC, Cohn LH, Adams DH, Borer JS, Feldman T. The clinical development of percutaneous heart valve technology: a position statement of the Society of Thoracic Surgeons (STS), the American Association for Thoracic Surgery (AATS), and the Society for Cardiovascular Angiography and Interventions (SCAI) Endorsed by the American College of Cardiology Foundation (ACCF) and the American Heart Association (AHA). J Am Coll Cardiol. May 3 2005;45(9):1554–60.
16. Webb JG, Harnek J, Munt BI, Kimblad PO, Chandavimol M, Thompson CR, et al. Percutaneous transvenous mitral annuloplasty: initial human experience with device implantation in the coronary sinus. Circulation. Feb 14 2006;113(6):851–5.
17. Feldman T, Wasserman HS, Herrmann HC, Gray W, Block PC, Whitlow P, et al. Percutaneous mitral valve repair using the edge-to-edge technique: six-month results of the EVEREST Phase I Clinical Trial. J Am Coll Cardiol. Dec 6 2005;46(11):2134–40.
18. Feldman T, Wasserman HS, Herrmann HC, Whitlow PL, Block PC, Gray WA, et al. Edge-to-edge mitral valve repair using the Evalve MitraClip: One year results of the EVEREST phase I clinical trial. Am J Cardiol. 2005;96(Suppl):49H.
19. Feldman T, Foster E, Glower DD, Kar S, Rinaldi MJ, Fail PS, et al. Percutaneous repair or surgery for mitral regurgitation. N Engl J Med. Apr 14 2011;364(15):1395–406.
20. Grossi EA, Patel N, Woo YJ, Goldberg JD, Schwartz CF, Subramanian V, et al. Outcomes of the RESTOR-MV Trial (Randomized Evaluation of a Surgical Treatment for Off-Pump Repair of the Mitral Valve). J Am Coll Cardiol. Dec 7 2010;56(24):1984–93.
21. Lutter G, Ardehali R, Cremer J, Bonhoeffer P. Percutaneous valve replacement: current state and future prospects. Ann Thorac Surg. Dec 2004;78(6):2199–206.

36 Percutaneous Transcatheter Management of Congenital Heart Diseases

Although the first balloon angioplasty performed by Andreas Gruentzig was a milestone, it does not mark the birth of interventional cardiology or transcatheter cardiac procedures. These date back to the 1950s with Rubio-Alvarez's pulmonary valve wire valvuloplasty and the 1960s when William Rashkind first performed balloon septostomy for transposition of the great arteries. The first transcatheter closure of a congenital defect was then reported by Werner Porstmann in 1967, describing the use of his Ivalon plug for the closure of patent ductus arteriosus (PDA). Throughout the following years, transcatheter

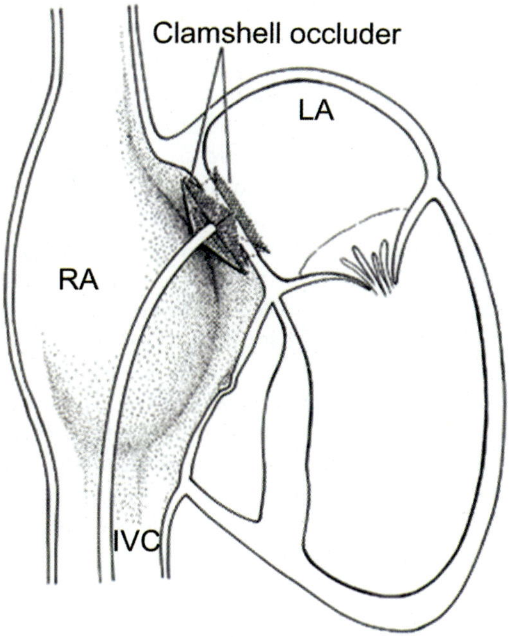

Fig. 36.1: *Transvenous catheter technique have been devised to cross the open secundum septal defect and release a variously-shaped expandable framework to seal the opening. One of the requirements however is that the defect have sufficient tissue to act as an anchorable "lip" so that the device remains stable and does not migrate over time*

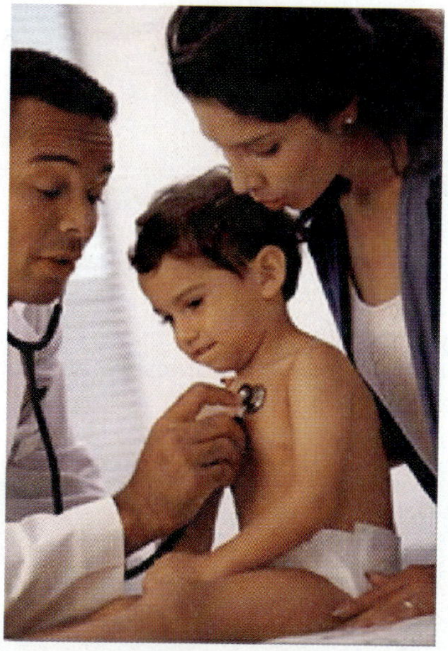

Fig. 36.2: *A young child being examined by an interventional cardiologist prior to percutaneous transcatheter management of L-R shunt*

closure of atrial septal defects (ASDs) in the mid-1970s and ventricular septal defects (VSDs) in the late 1980s became possible. The Rashkind PDA occluder with its double-umbrella design was the prototype of occluder devices and had been used to close a variety of congenital and acquired defects. Several other devices have been developed over the years based on similar concept of using two umbrellas wedging the defect in between. Most of these early devices are no longer available as their use was rather cumbersome and associated with higher complication rates than conventional surgical alternatives. The development of the Amplatzer family of closure devices in the mid-1990s marked another important milestone for interventional cardiology. The design allows the use of relatively small delivery catheters. The inherent self-centring mechanism and the ability to retrieve the device if needed prior to release were among the features that have led to their wide spread use. However, for PDA closure, coils have been used that allow closure of smaller defects; although with the development of detachable coils, larger PDAs can be closed with coils as well (Figs 36.1–36.4).

Percutaneous transluminal angioplasty (PTA) is effective in relieving vascular obstructive lesions in most cases. However, in some cases elastic recoil of the vessel wall and intimal dissection may result in ineffective relief of the obstruction. Stents provide a more effective relief of obstruction by exerting radial forces, preventing elastic recoil of the vessel wall and compressing dissection flaps against the vessel wall. While describing PTA in 1964, Dotter and Judkins anticipated the need for an endovascular splint to keep the vessel lumen open. Later in the same decade, Dotter implanted a spiral coil spring prosthesis in experimentally created vascular stenotic lesions. The concept and technology of stents remained dormant until the early 1980s when self-expanding double helical spiral stents were implanted in animal models. Further developments followed, as reviewed elsewhere. In the mid-1980s. Palmaz et al designed stainless steel mesh stents and implanted them in rabbit aortas, the hepatobiliary circulation and canine coronary arteries, thus demonstrating the feasibility of the stent concept. Clinical studies in the late 1980s and early 1990s showed that stents are useful in the management of obstructive lesions of the coronary, iliac and renal arteries in adult subjects. Pediatric application of stent technology followed later. The usefulness of stents are as follows:

1. Teating obstructive lesions of the branch pulmonary arteries, systemic, pulmonary veins, and aorta and right ventricular outflow conduits
2. Keeping the ductus arteriosus open in patients with pulmonary atresia and hypoplastic left heart syndrome
3. Maintaining the patency of stenosed aortopulmonary collateral vessels or surgically created but obstructed shunts have been well demonstrated.

Types of stents: Stents may be classified on the basis of their delivery mechanism, the material with which they are made up of (composition) and their configuration.

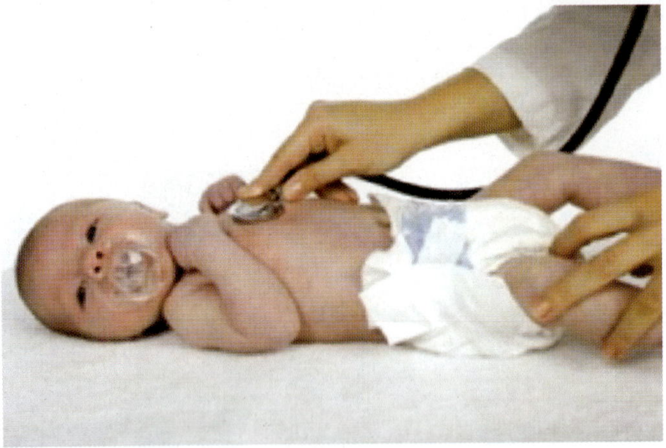

Fig. 36.3: *A young child in being examined by the doctor before he is taken up for percutaneous transcatheter management of congenital heart disease*

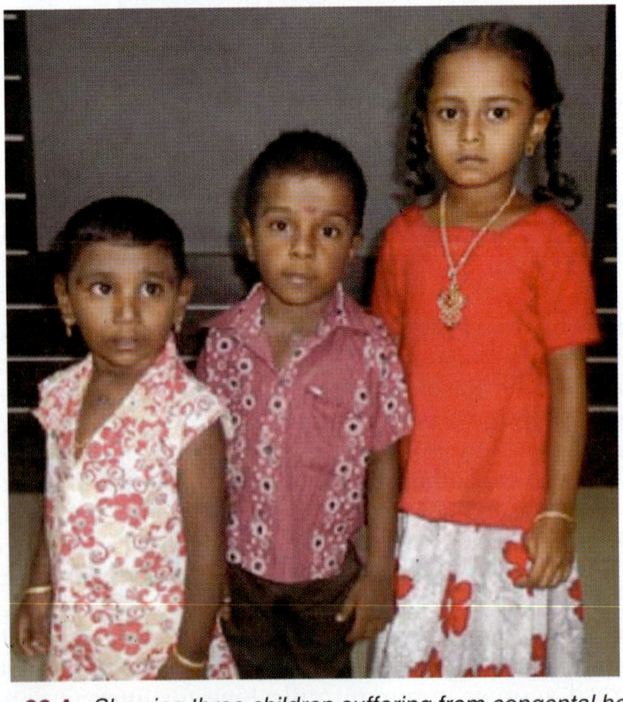

Fig. 36.4: *Showing three children suffering from congental heart disease. From left (ASD secundum), middle (VSD) and right (PDA) who have been registered for transcatheter management*

Delivery Mechanism (Figs 36.5–36.7)

Stents may be balloon-expandable or self-expandable. Balloon-expandable stents are mounted on balloons, positioned across the site of the obstruction and implanted by inflating the balloon. The diameter of the balloon determines the expanded diameter of the stent; to date, these are the most commonly used stents. The Palmaz stent, which was the first stent available for pediatric use and the more recently used stents, namely Bridge, NuMed CP, IntraStent double strut and corinthian, are also balloon-expandable stents. Self-expandable stents are restrained within a covering sheath. After positioning the stent in the desired location, withdrawal of the sheath uncovers the stent which then assumes its original shape. In growing children, the use of self-expandable stents is limited Balloon-expandable stents can be further dilated at a later date, but self-expandable stents cannot be further enlarged. Also, there is some evidence to suggest that there is a greater degree of intimal proliferation with self-expandable stents. For these reasons, balloon-expandable stents are usually selected for implantation in children.

Composition: Stents are most commonly made up of metals to impart radial strength. Stainless steel (316 L) is used most often as in the Palmaz, Bridge and IntraStents. Platinum-iridium, nitinol, cobalt-based alloys, titanium and tantalum have also been used. Stents made up of these metals remain within and get incorporated into the vessel wall. Due to the lack of growth of stented segments, biodegradable materials may offer an advantage and several biodegradable

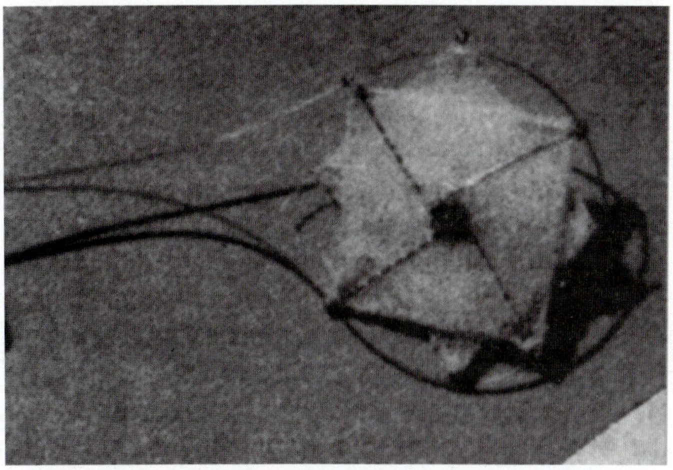

Fig. 36.5: *Rashkind double disk umbrella device*

polymers have been used to construct stents. The ideal characteristics of biodegradable stents are:

i. Sufficient radial strength to prevent vessel recoil.
ii. Should not produce thrombotic or inflammatory response nor intimal proliferation.
iii. The stent material should be resorbed within weeks to months of implantation.
iv. The breakdown products should not be toxic. Several types of materials and designs have been tested in animal models but there is limited experience in the use of biodegradable stents in human coronary arteries.

Configuration: A number of stent designs have been used including a slotted tube, mesh, coil-loop and ring. The slotted tube designs or their variations are used in the majority of stents in clinical practice.

Method of implantation: Before implantation of the stents, informed consent from the patient/parents as appropriate, is obtained. Some of the stents are used on an off-label basis which should also be communicated to the patient. It is performed under conscious sedation, some cardiologists do so under general anesthesia. Cardiac catheterization is performed to confirm the clinical and echocardiographic diagnosis and to exclude other cardiac defects. Pressure gradients across the obstructive lesion are determined and selective cineangiography in multiple angiographic projections is performed initially to demonstrate the stenotic lesions. The following measurements are made:

i. Diameters of the stenotic lesion and of the vessel proximal and distal to the obstructive lesion
ii. The diameter of the contralateral pulmonary artery in patients with branch pulmonary artery stenosis (BPS)
iii. "Stentable" length of the vessel.

All the measurements are taken in two orthogonal views and averaged. Foreshortening of the vessel length is taken into account when the anatomy is deemed to indicate this. These measurements are utilized in the selection of the expanded diameter and length of the stent. An arterial line is placed to monitor blood pressure and oxygen saturation during the procedure. Heparin (100 units/kg) is administered and activated clotting time monitored and maintained between 200 and 250 s by giving additional doses of heparin if needed.

An end-hole catheter [5 F multi-A2 (Cordis, Miami, FL)] or 7 F balloon wedge (Arrows International. Reading, PA) catheter] is positioned across the stenotic lesion with the help of a soft-tipped 0.035" Benston (Cook, Bloomington, IN) guidewire. The guidewire and catheter are advanced as distally as possible. The catheter is left in place while the guidewire is removed and replaced with either an extra-stiff exchange length 0.035" Amplatz (Cook) or a super-stiff, short-tip Amplatz (Meditech, Nautik, MA) guidewire. The catheter is then removed. If the approach to the lesion is tortuous or difficult to reach, we select a 0.038" super-stiff Amplatz wire (Meditech). An appropriate-sized long blue Cook sheath (Cook) with a multipurpose curve and a radioopaque marker at the tip is introduced over the stiff wire. Once the tip of the sheath is past the site intended to be stented, the dilator is removed and the sheath flushed.

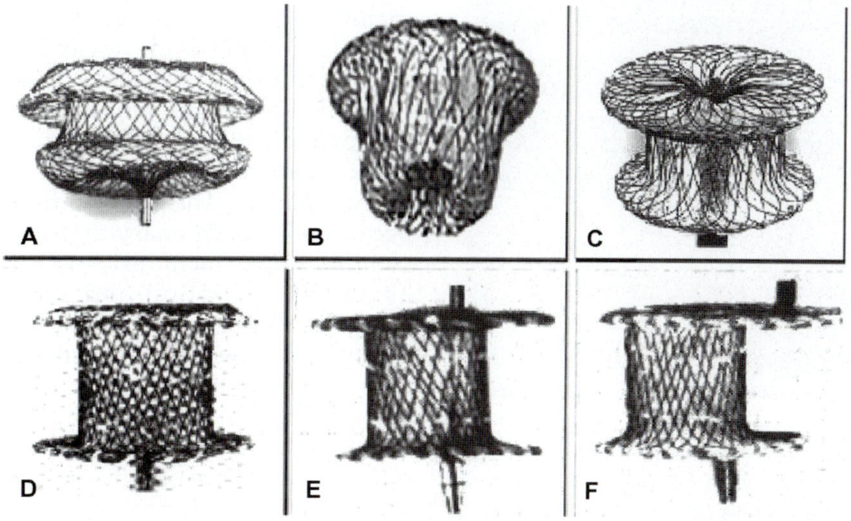

Figs 36.6A to F: *The amplatzer devices used for transcatheter closure of ventricular septal defects. (A) Amplatzer septal occluder; (B) Amplatzer PDA occluder; (C) Amplatzer muscular VSD occluder; (D) new concentric amplatzer VSD occluder; (E and F) new eccentric amplatzer VSD occluders*

Sometimes, the dilator has to be withdrawn slightly to position the tip of the sheath at the desired location.

The selection of the diameter of the sheath is obviously dependent upon the size of the stent delivery catheter. It is always better to select a balloon delivery system that would allow the smallest possible diameter of the sheath. Most recently, IntraStent doubleStrut stents [ParaMount and DoubleStrut ill (IntraTherapeutics, St Paul. MN)] have been used. The later stents are mounted on balloon-in-balloon (BIB) catheters (NuMed Inc., Hopkinton, NY) and the size of the sheath used is 1 F larger than that needed for the BIB catheter.

The balloon catheter, with the stent mounted on it, is advanced over the stiff guidewire within the sheath and positioned across the obstructive lesion; the tip of the sheath is withdrawn proximal (or distal in aortic coarctation) to the site of obstruction, based on bony landmarks. Contrast is also injected via the side-arm of the blue Cook sheath and the position of the stent adjusted as necessary. In cases in which the BIB catheter is used, the inner balloon is inflated to the pressure recommended by the manufacturer and the position of the stent adjusted, if needed, followed by inflation of the outer balloon, thus implanting the stent. The balloon catheter is then advanced slightly, centering the balloon across the distal (or proximal in aortic coarctation) end of the stent and the outer balloon reinflated to ensure apposition of the stent against the vessel wall. The balloon catheter is then centered over the proximal (distal in coarctation of the aorta) end of the stent by advancing the tip of the sheath over the deflated balloon into the stent, thus preventing inadvertent displacement of the latter. The outer balloon is then reinflated to ensure apposition of the proximal (distal) stent against the vessel wall. If the diameter of the outer balloon is not as large as the desired diameter of the stent. Additional balloon expansion with balloons of a larger diameter is performed.

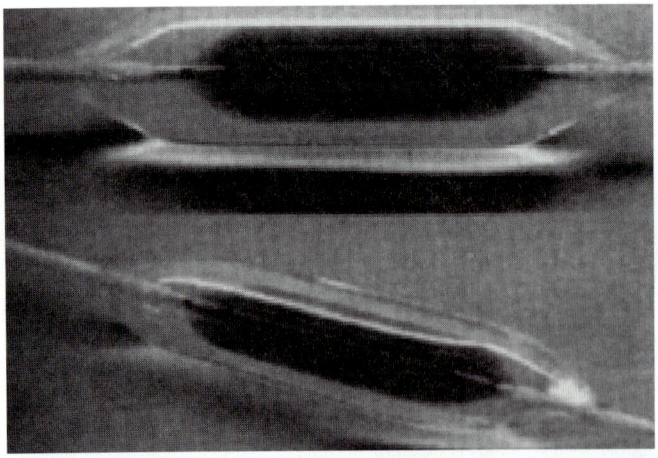

Fig. 36.7: *The BIB balloon has an inner balloon, constructed from the same material as the so-called "Tyshak II" balloon, whereas the outer balloon is constructed from a heavier gauge material as used in the Z-Med higher pressure balloon. The BIB balloon allows controlled delivery of stents and adjustment of stent position after inflation of the inner balloon. This prevents stent migration and the balloon design prevents flaring of the stent*

Following removal of the balloon catheter, a multitrack catheter (Braun, Bethlehem, PA) is positioned over the wire and pressure pullback tracings and angiogram performed to assess the results of stent implantation.

The effect of heparin is not reversed nor any additional doses administered. Intravenous cefazolin 25 mg/kg/dose (maximum of 1.0 g) is started in the catheterization laboratory and two additional doses at 6–8 h intervals administered. Aspirin in platelet-inhibiting doses (5–10 mg/kg/day) is started on the day following the procedure and continued for 6 weeks. Use of heparin overnight on the day of the procedure and more potent platelet-inhibiting drugs or anticoagulation with coumadin have been undertaken in the past. At present, the data do not indicate a need for intensive anticoagulation; aspirin alone appears to suffice. However, in Fontan circulations, anticoagulation with coumadin may be advisable.

Chest X-ray two dimensional and Doppler echocardiographic studies, and quantitative pulmonary perfusion scans (in patients with BPS) are performed on the morning following the procedure. Chest X-ray and echocardiographic studies are carried out 1, 6 and 12 months after the procedure and yearly thereafter. Repeat hemodynamic and angiographic evaluation, with an intent to redilate the stent, if necessary, 1–2 years after stent deployment may be a good idea, especially in a growing child.

ATRIAL SEPTAL DEFECTS

Definition and Indications for Closure

An ASD is a persistent communication between the two atria caused by a hole in the inter atrial septum. Atrial septal defects present the most common congenital heart defect diagnosed in adults and occurs in approximately 4 of 100,000 newborns. The most common type is the secundum ASD, which occurs in the region of the fossa ovalis and represents ≥ 75% of all cases. Primum ASDs, coronary sinus, and sinus venosus defects are less common. Transcatheter closure is possible only for the secundum type. This is mainly because of the lack of sufficient rims surrounding the defect to anchor the device or due to associated defects such cleft atrioventricular valves or anomalous drainage of pulmonary veins requiring open surgical repair. An unrepaired ASD can lead to left-to-right shunt, secondary right ventricular volume overload, and pulmonary overcirculation. This leads to right-sided heart failure and occasionally pulmonary arterial hypertension. Patients' symptoms may include dyspnoea, fatigue, or palpitations, as atrial fibrillation and atrial flutter are common consequences of long-standing untreated ASD. Symptoms commonly get worse with increasing age, even with smaller defects, due to an increase in left-to-right shunt caused by changes in ventricular compliance with age.

Transcatheter or surgical closure of an ASD is indicated if there is evidence of right-sided volume overload as seen by echocardiography irrespective of the patient's symptoms. Other indications for ASD closure include the presence of significant left-to-right shunt, defined as a pulmonary-to-systemic flow (Qp/Qs) ratio of >1.5:1, and

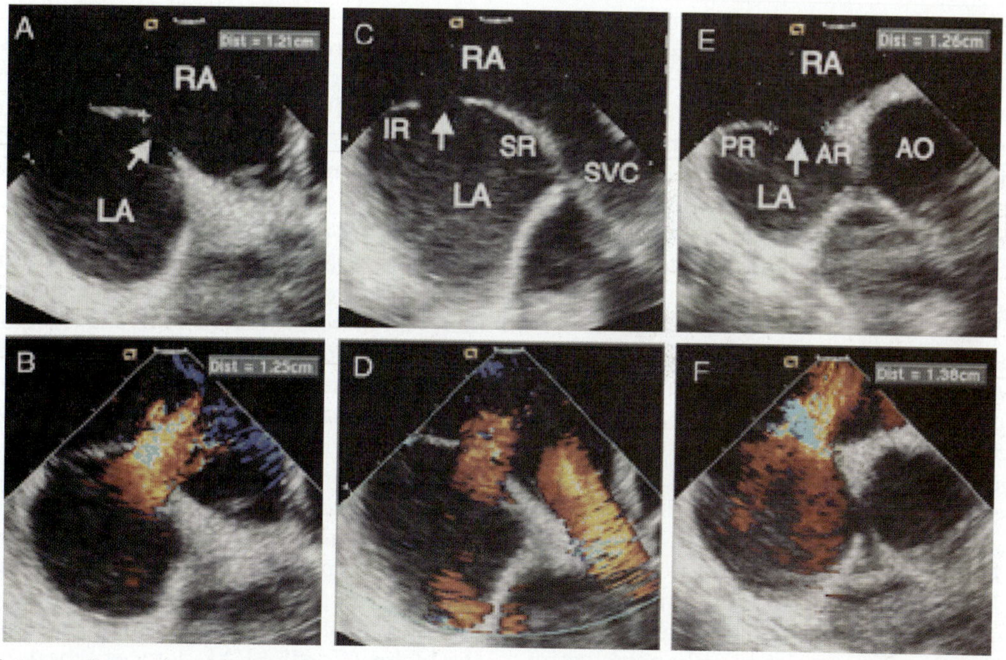

Figs 36.8A to F: *Intracardiac echocardiographic images in secundum ASD. (A, B) Septal view without and with color Doppler demonstrating moderate size ASD measuring about l2.5 mm defect (arrow). (C, D) Long axis view without and with color Doppler demonstrating the defect (arrow) and the superior rim (SR), inferior rim (IR). (E, F) Short axis view without and with color Doppler demonstrating very short anterior rim (AR) and posterior rim (PR) and the defect (arrow). RA, right atrium; LA, left atrium; SVC, superior vena cava; AO, aortic valve*

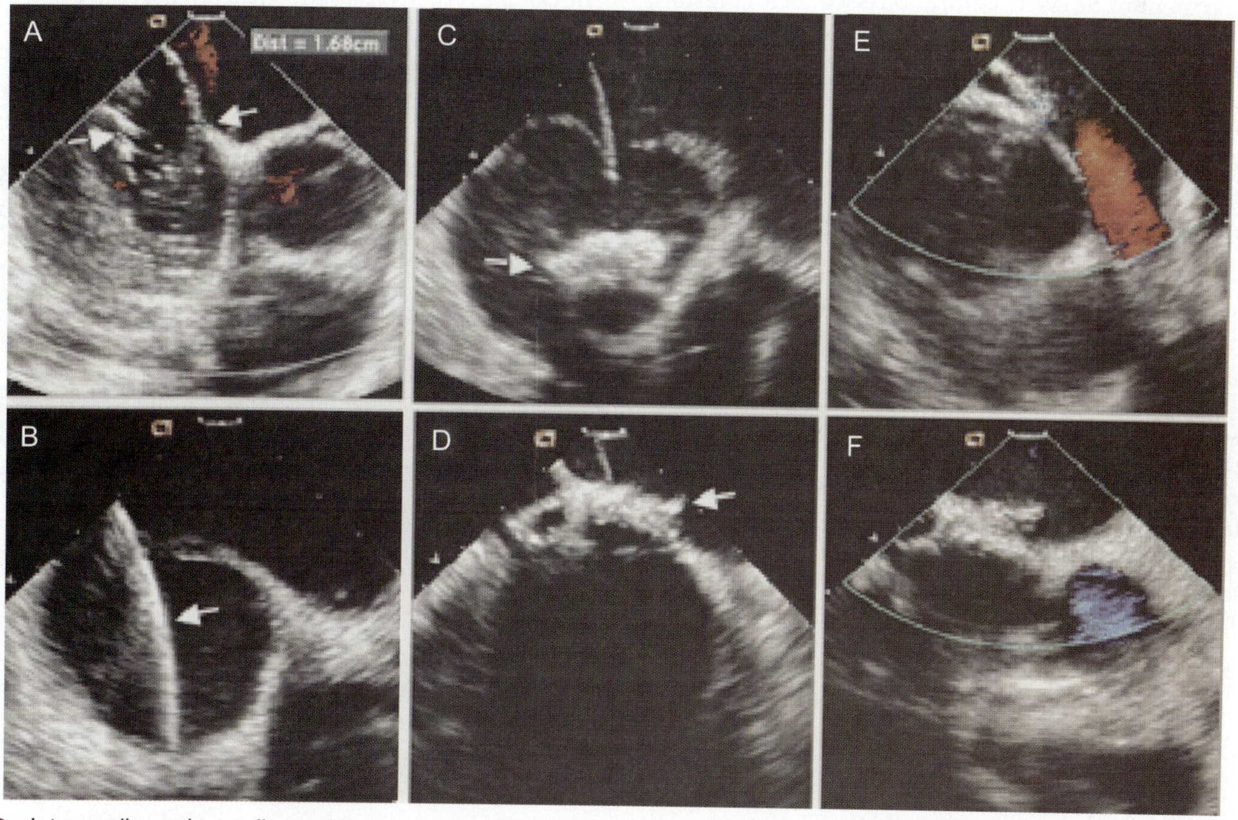

Fig. 36.9: *Intracardiac echocardiographic images during deployment of a 30 mm Helex device (A) Balloon sizing of the defect using "stop flow" technique. Arrows indicate size of the balloon. (B) Passage of the guidewire (arrow) into the left upper pulmonary vein, over which the delivery sheath was passed. (C) Deployment of the left atrial desk (arrow). (D) Deployment of the right atrial desk (arrow). (E, F) Assessment of final result by color Doppler in long (E) and short axis (F), both demonstrating good device position and no residual shunt in a patient with ASD*

the occurrence of paradoxical embolism or documented orthodeoxia-platypnoea syndrome. Surgical closure is preferred for nonsecundum ASDs or if surgical repair for associated defects is needed. Important prerequisites for ASD closure are pulmonary arterial pressures less than two-thirds systemic and a pulmonary vascular resistance < 7 Woods units. Atrial septal defect closure in patients with severe irreversible pulmonary arterial hypertension is contraindicated as it may shorten their life-expectancy.

Atrial Septal Defect Closure Devices

The Amplatzer septal occluder (ASO) (AGA Medical, Plymouth, MN, USA) is a double-disc device with a self-centring mechanism. In the multicentre, nonrandomized pivotal trial including 442 patients comparing transcatheter closure using the ASO with surgical closure revealed equivalent success rates. However, complication rates and the length of hospital stay were better than for surgical closure. The ASO is the most widely used device for the closure of ASDs. Defects up to 40 mm in diameter can be closed with this occluder. Dacron patches are embedded into the discs and connecting waist to enhance closure. Complete endothelialization occurs between 6 and 12 months from closure.

The Helex occluder is a nonself-centring double-disc device that consists of one single nitinol wire frame in the shape of a coil that is covered by polytetrafluoroethylene (Gore-Tex) membrane (W.L. Gore and Associates, Flagstaff, AZ, USA). The nitinol wire is spun as two opposing spirals that configure themselves as two separate discs once advanced outside the delivery sheath. Following the first human implant in 1999, the device has gained popularity worldwide. Only defects as large as 18 mm by balloon stretch diameter can be closed effectively with this device. The CardioSEAL and its self-centring successor named STARFlex are double-disc occluders, which were modifications to the early clamshell device (NMT Medical, Boston, MA, USA). The device itself consists of two square-shaped umbrellas made of Dacron, mounted on spring coils allowing flexible positioning of each arm. Similar to the Helex device, only defects up 20 mm by balloon stretching can be closed effectively with these devices. The CardioSEAL device is approved only for VSD closure in the USA; however, many use this device for the closure of ASDs and patent foramen ovale (PFO). A niche device for the multifenestrated atrial septum is the Amplatzer cribriform occluder. This device is similar in design to the Amplatzer PFO device, but with two equal-sized discs.

Closure Technique (Figs 36.8A-F, 36.10A-D)

For the most part, transcatheter ASD closure is performed in a similar fashion with the different devices available to date. The procedure can be performed under fluoroscopic guidance with either simultaneous transoesophageal (TEE) or intracardiac echocardiography (ICE) monitoring. The atrial septum and surrounding structures need to be evaluated carefully by means of echocardiography. Sufficient rims, defined as at least 5 mm distance from the defect to the structure, allow for safe anchoring of the device. A deficient anterior rim is no contraindication for the placement of an ASO as the device wraps around the posterior aortic wall. Prior to actual device deployment, most manufacturers recommend balloon sizing of the defect. Alternatively, the size of the device can be chosen based on the measurement of the defect by echocardiography only.

Following determination of the defect size, the ASD can be closed with the device of choice. For the ASO, a device 0–2 mm larger than the "stop flow diameter" of the defect using a balloon is chosen. For the STARFlex/CardioSEAL or Helex occluder, a device twice the diameter of the balloon occluding the defect is chosen. This limits the size of defects that can be closed with these devices to 18–20 mm in diameter.

The device is loaded onto the delivery system and the left atrial disc/umbrella is deployed inside the left atrium. The disc/umbrella assembly is then withdrawn until it is very close to the septum, then the connecting waist is deployed to "stent" the defect in the case of the ASO or until the disc is flushed against the septum in the case of the Helex/CardioSEAL devices. Then, the right atrial disc is deployed by further retraction of the delivery sheath over the cable. Prior to release, a safe and good position of the device has to be confirmed. Echocardiography (TEE or ICE) is of paramount importance to determine device position and that surrounding structures are not interfered with. The device is then released. After release, the device is again evaluated by echocardiography to ensure proper position and to assess closure result.

Patients are placed on acetyl salicylic acid 2 days prior to procedure, and continue for 6–12 months after

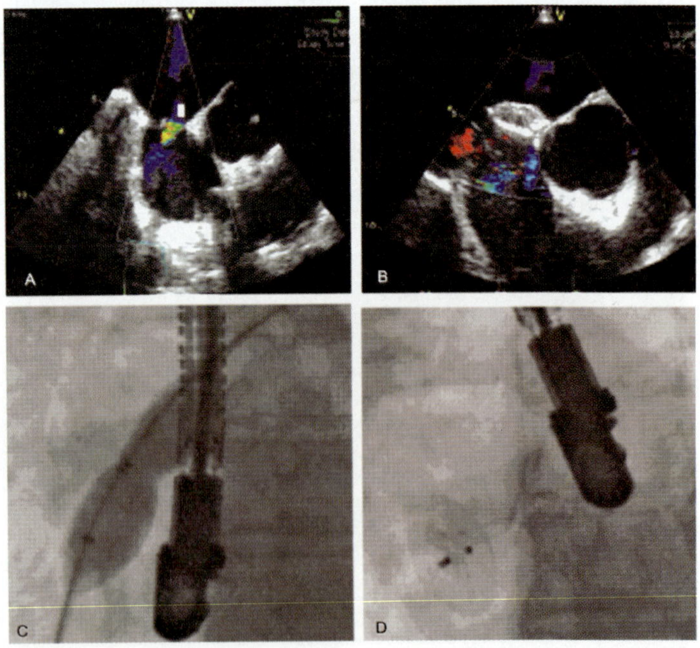

Fig. 36.10: *Percutaneous atrial septal defect (ASD) closure (A and B) TEE image of an ASD before and after the deployment of an Amplazer septal occluder (ASO). (C) Fluoroscopic image of the sizing balloon across the interatrial septum. (D) Fluoroscopic image of the ASO after deployment*

procedure. Owing to migraine headaches in ≥ 10% of patients, the addition of 75 mg per day of clopidogrel for 1–3 months has been a practice over the last 5 years. Patients undergoing uncomplicated transcatheter ASD closure can be discharged home the following day. Transthoracic echocardiogram is done the day following closure to establish a new baseline for future surveillance evaluations. Patients are recommended to follow-up at least annually following device closure and repeat echocardiography is recommended between 3 months and 1 year after device closure and periodically thereafter.

Periprocedural complications such as device embolization, thrombus formation, stroke, perforation, and tamponade are rare with near-zero procedural mortality. Early postprocedurally, transient atrial fibrillation may occur. Long-term complications are rare, with the erosion of the device into surrounding structures being the most serious and feared one. The overall incidence is estimated at <0.1% for the ASO. Patients at higher risk for device erosion are those with defects associated with deficient anterior-superior rims and an oversized device. Thrombus formation on the closure device if occurring on the left atrial side, can have catastrophic consequences. Occurrence of device-related thrombus formation seems to be related to the design of the device and appears to be the lowest with the Amplatzer and Helex occluders. If thrombus formation occurs, treatment with warfarin usually results in resolution of thrombi.

VENTRICULAR SEPTAL DEFECTS

Definition and Indications for Closure

A VSD is a persistent communication between the right and the left ventricles. It can occur as a congenital defect or can be acquired in the setting of an acute myocardial infarction, trauma or iatrogenic following aortic valve replacement or myomyectomy surgeries.

Congenital Ventricular Septal Defects

Ventricular septal defects are the most common form of congenital heart defects in children. The most common type of VSD is the perimembranous type that accounts for ≥ 80% of all cases. The remaining 20% are muscular VSDs. Those can be further subdivided into inlet, trabecular, and infundibular defects, depending on their locations. Large, unrestricted VSDs lead to a large left-to-right shunt and congestive heart failure, which may become evident in the very first few weeks of life. If left untreated, shunting will eventually lead to pulmonary arterial hypertension with increased pulmonary vascular resistance and Eisenmenger's physiology, at which point the shunt reverses to a predominant right-to-left shunt. Small or restrictive VSDs are usually diagnosed early in life, as they create significant murmurs. There is a good chance that both perimembranous and muscular VSDs would close spontaneously in the first few years of life. Closure of symptomatic, nonrestrictive VSDs is indicated in infancy. Patients commonly present with signs and symptoms of heart failure including poor growth, tachypnoea, tachycardia and diaphoresis. Timing of closure, however, needs to be individualized. Infants with asymptomatic, restrictive VSDs can usually be closely followed. If the defect closes spontaneously, no further intervention is warranted.

Congenital Ventricular Septal Defects in Adults

Large, unrestrictive VSDs are rarely diagnosed in adulthood. If a small VSD persists into adulthood, closure,

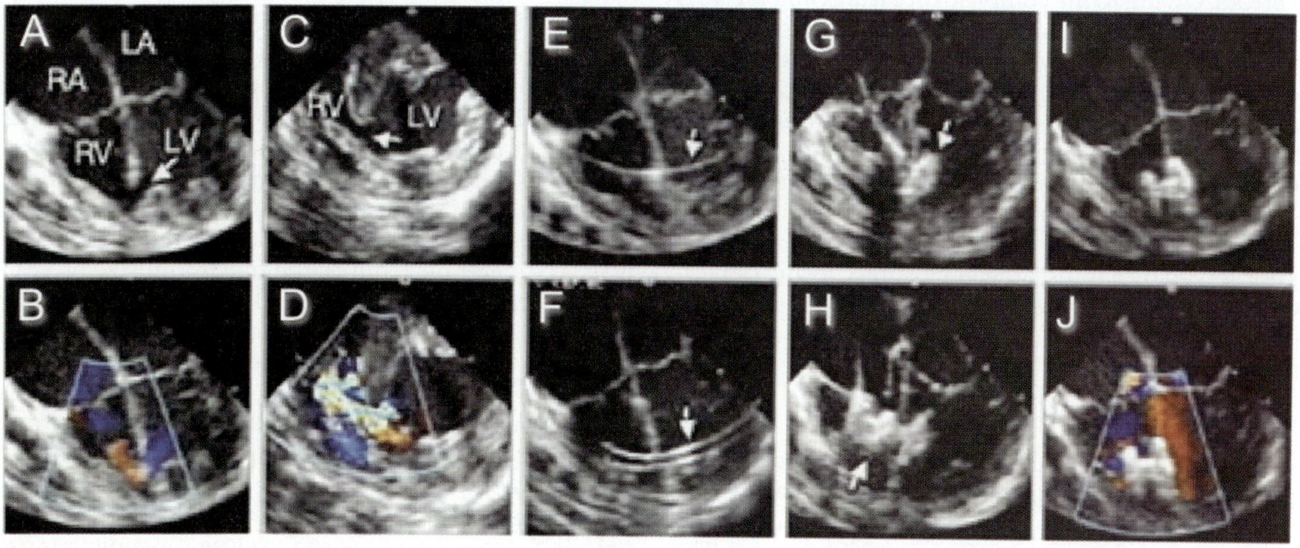

Fig. 36.11: *TEE images of muscular ventricular septal defect closure with an Amplatzer muscular VSD device. (A) Apical four-chamber view of a muscular VSD; (B) Color Doppler flow across the VSD; (C) The muscular VSD in the short-axis view; (D) Color Doppler flow across the muscular VSD in the short-axis view; (E) Wire across the VSD; (F) Sheath across the VSD; (G) The left ventricular disc is deployed in the left ventricle; (H) The right ventricular disc is deployed in the right ventricle; (I) The device is released from the delivery cable; (J) There is no residual shunt across the VSD by color Doppler. RA, Right atrium; RV, Right ventricle; LA, left atrium; LV, left ventricle*

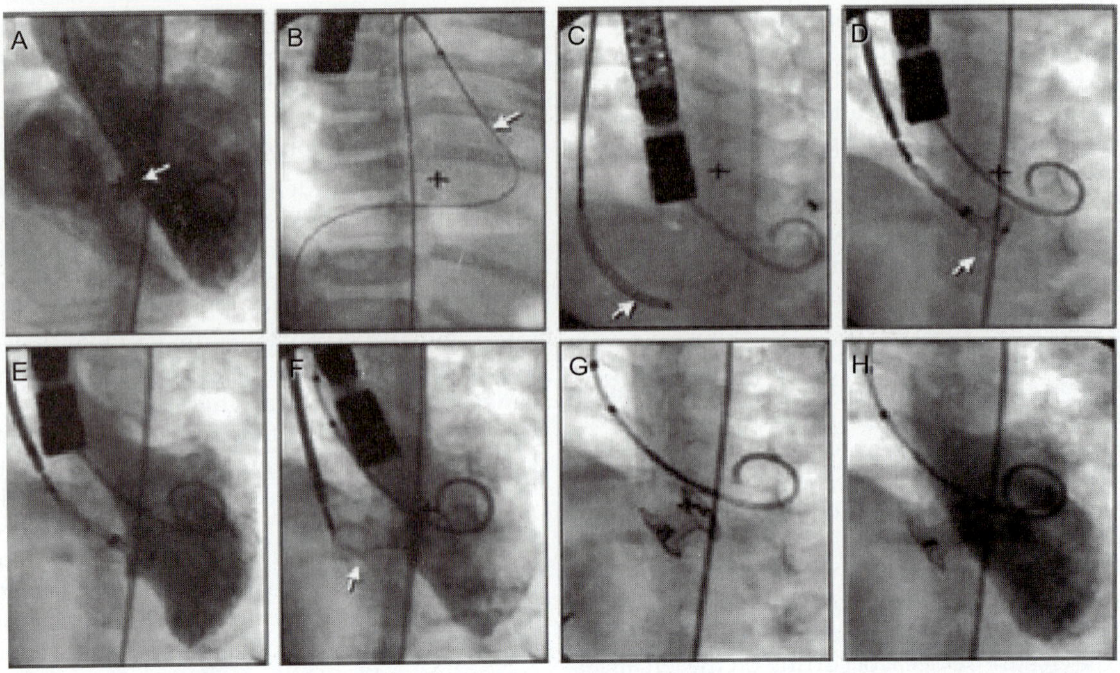

Fig. 36.12: *Fluoroscopic and angiographic steps in the closure of a muscular VSD. (A) LV angiogram demonstrates the presence of a single mid-muscular VSD; (B) The wire is across the VSD from the left ventricle; (C) The delivery sheath is in the left ventricle from the right internal jugular and the device is being advanced; (D) The left-sided disc is advanced into the left ventricle. (E) LV angiogram to confirm the position of the left ventricular disc; (F) The right disc is deployed in the right ventricle; (G) The device is released from the delivery cable; (H) LV angiogram shows complete closure of the muscular VSD with the Amplatzer muscular VSD device*

however, is necessary for the following indications: left ventricular and/or left atrial volume overload; history of infective endocarditis or development of aortic valve insufficiency caused by the VSD. Transthoracic echocardiography is the best diagnostic tool to assess the size of the left atrium and ventricle. We do not recommend to rely on the calculation of the Qp/Qs ratio since it is flawed with many errors. Owing to the complexity of transcatheter VSD closure and the higher incidence of complications, surgical VSD closure remains the gold standard for the treatment of most VSDs. Transcatheter VSD closure, as opposed to surgical closure, can be considered in patients with muscular defects, especially if the VSD is remote from the tricuspid and aortic valves. Patients with residual defects after surgical closure or patients with iatrogenic defects after aortic valve replacement surgery or myomyectomy are better served by a transcatheter closure. Closure of perimembranous VSDs is possible with the Amplatzer perimembranous VSD occluder; however, the risk of complete heart block is high, at 5–6%.

Acquired Ventricular Septal Defect

The second group of VSDs consist of acquired defects occurring after myocardial infarction or residual defects after surgical repair. Postmyocardial infarction VSDs nowadays occur relatively rarely in <0.2% of cases. The mortality and morbidity of this condition if left untreated, is extremely high, estimated to be >90%. Owing to the high operative mortality (≥ 50%), transcatheter closure is an attractive alternative. Patient selection and timing of transcatheter VSD closure are critical and highly determine the outcome. The procedure is complicated by the patient's haemodynamic instability and the nature of the VSDs, which are rather irregular and large with surrounding tissue necrosis, making stable device positioning difficult. Mortality after transcatheter postmyocardial infarction VSD closure is probably in the range of 25–35% and may be even higher in patients with frank cardiogenic shock.

Ventricular Septal Defect Closure Devices

The Amplatzer muscular VSD occluder (AGA Medical, Plymouth, MN, USA) is the only device specifically designed for congenital muscular VSDs. Since its initial use in 1998, it has become the most popular device to close muscular VSDs worldwide. Similar to the ASO for ASDs, the muscular VSD occluder is made of nitinol wire mesh in the form of a self-expandable double-disc device. The waist diameter determines the maximum size of VSD that can be treated. The largest available device for congenital defects is 18 mm in diameter and that for postinfarct VSDs is 24 mm in diameter. The mechanism of closure, again similar to the ASO, involves stenting of the actual defect by the waist and subsequent thrombus formation within the device and eventual complete endothelialization. Common contraindication to the use of this device includes a distance of <4 mm between the VSD to any of the four valves. A second device used to close congenital, muscular VSDs, and postmyocardial infarction VSDs is the aforementioned CardioSEAL occluder.

Transcatheter closure of perimembranous VSD has been difficult due to its close proximity to surrounding valves. Specifically designed for perimembranous VSDs, the

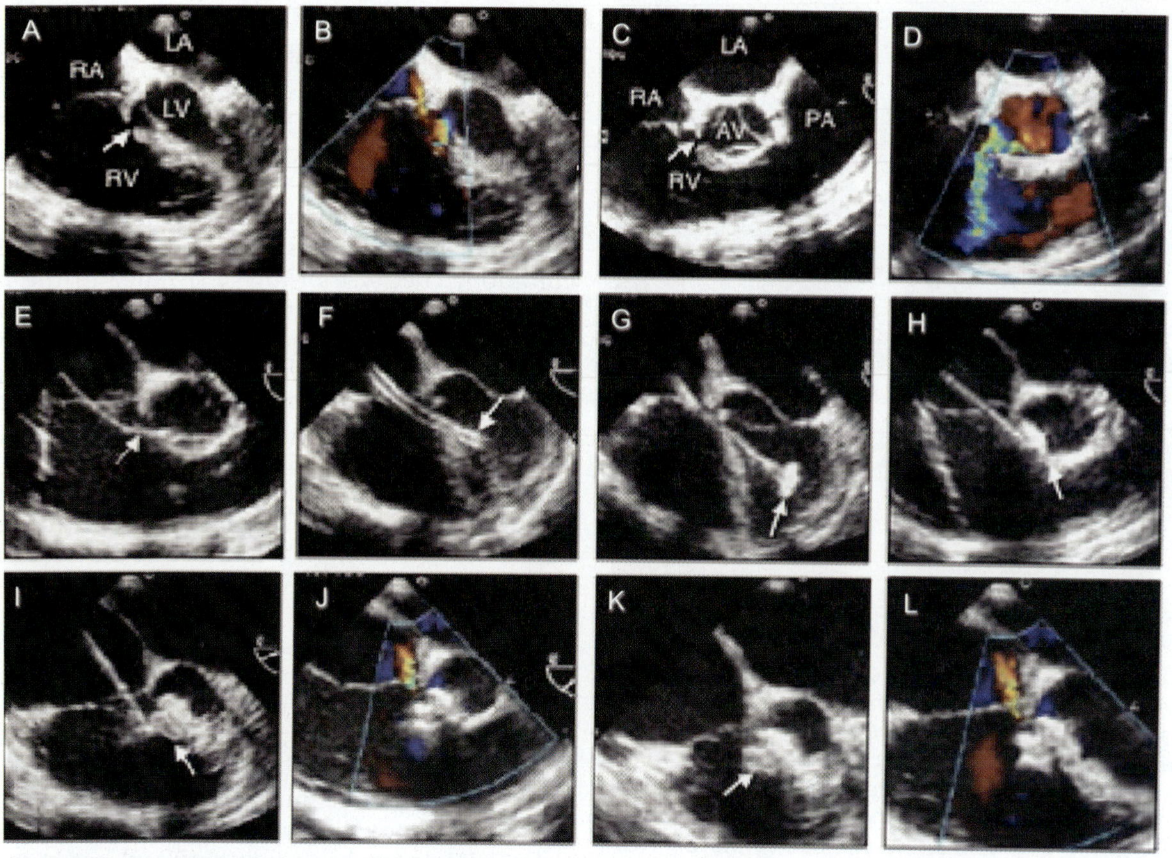

Fig. 36.13: *TEE images of perimembranous VSD closure with an Amplatzer membranous VSD device. (A–D) 2-D and color images of a perimembranous VSD. (E) Wire across the perimembranous VSD. (F) Sheath through the perimembranous VSD. (G–I) Steps of device deployment. (J–L) The device is released with no residual shunt. RA, Right atrium; RV, Right ventricle; LA, left atrium; LV, left ventricle*

Amplatzer membranous VSD occluder was first implanted in 2002. Owing to its unique design, it overcame several obstacles and problems of prior devices used for this indication. It is designed differently from the muscular VSD occluder from AGA. However, similar to Amplatzer family of devices, it is made of nitinol wire and is self-expandable. The waist length is only 1.5 mm, accommodating the defect located in the thin-walled membranous septum. The left ventricular disc is asymmetric with a shorter aortic end of the left ventricular disc. This allows stable positioning, yet minimal encroachment on the aortic valve region. Following device placement, conduction abnormalities to the degree of complete atrioventricular block may occur and remain a concern with this device.

The Amplatzer postinfarct VSD device is very similar to the congenital muscular VSD device. However, the length of the waist is 10 mm to accommodate the thick septum in adult patients and the disks are 5 mm larger than the waist. As mentioned above, the largest size available is 24 mm.

Owing to the higher incidence of complete heart block after membranous VSD closure with the Amplatzer membranous VSD device, some operators prefer to use coil devices to close such defects.

Closure Technique (Figs 36.11A-J, 36.15A and B)

Transcatheter VSD closure is technically more challenging than ASD closure. Nevertheless, success rates for transcatheter VSD closure is >90% in experienced hands. Closing acquired VSDs is even more complex due to co-morbidities as well as local factors such as surrounding necrotic myocardial tissue and resulting difficulties in safely anchoring a device. To exemplify VSD closure technique in general, we briefly describe the steps of transcatheter VSD closure using the Amplatzer muscular VSD occluder. Prior echocardiographic assessment of the size, number, and location of the VSDs is of paramount importance. The procedure is preferentially performed under general anaesthesia with continuous TEE and fluoroscopic guidance. For single muscular VSD, one can perform the closure under fluoroscopic guidance alone with or without transthoracic echocardiography. Echocardiography is essential to evaluate the relationship of the device to the atrioventricular valves. Access is obtained in the femoral artery and vein. If the VSD, however, is located in the mid-ventricular septum, or in the posterior or apical septum, the right internal jugular vein should be used as the venous access for better device deployment. Left ventriculography is performed to define the location, size, and number of VSDs. For membranous defects, the best projection is the

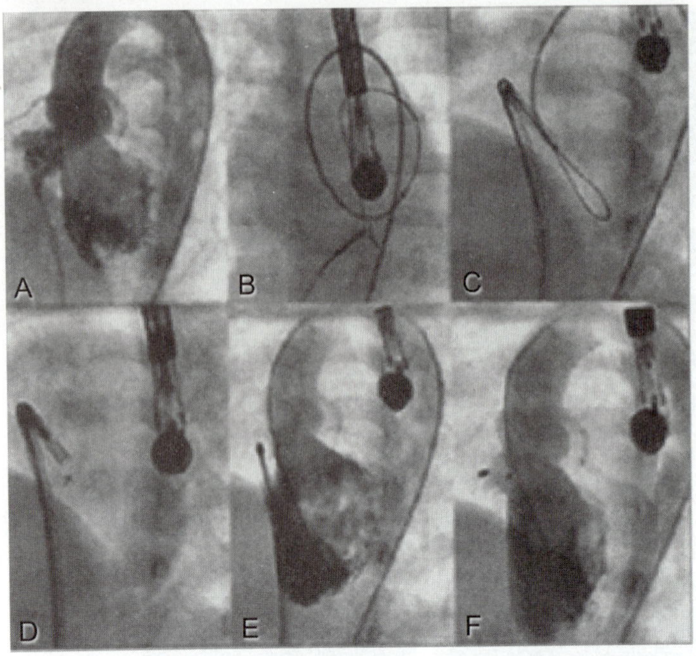

Fig. 36.14: *Steps in transcatheter closure of PMVSD with AAVSDO: (A) Left ventricular angiogram in long axial oblique view showing perimembranous VSD, (B) Cine-radiographic frame showing the 0,032" exchange length wire being snared from the pulmonary artery to form an arteriovenous wire loop, (C) Cine-radiographic frame showing the sheath directed into left ventricle with a wire loop formed by introducing the SF RCA catheter into the left ventricle from the aorta, (D) LV disc deployed with the marker toward the apex, (E) Angiogram in long axial oblique view showing the device in position before release, (F) LV angiogram in long axial oblique view showing the device in position after release, PMVSD, perimembranous ventricular septal defect; AAVSDO, asymmetrical Amplatzer membranous VSD occluder; VSD, ventricular septal defect; RCA, right coronary artery; LV, left ventricle*

long axial oblique (60° left anterior oblique/20° cranial), and for mid-muscular defects, the best projection is the four-chamber view (35° left anterior oblique/35° cranial). Defect sizes are measured by either TEE or left ventriculography at end-diastole. Following device selection, the defect is crossed, usually from the left ventricular side using a Judkins right catheter, a wire is passed and exteriorized from the venous side (jugular for muscular defects/femoral for membranous defect), and the delivery sheath is advanced over this wire to the left ventricle. Placement of the amplatzer VSD occluders is comparable with the ASO with a sequential deployment of the left-sided disc, followed by the waist and the right-sided disc. Prior to release, a stable position is confirmed by echocardiography and/or angiography. The surrounding valves are interrogated confirming normal function.

Potential major complications include device embolization, arrhythmias, air embolism, haemolysis, valvular regurgitation, or higher degree heart blocks. In the initial US multicentre trial for muscular VSD closure, peri-procedural major complication rate was 10.7%. In more recent studies, this complication rate has decreased to 2.8%

PATENT DUCTUS ARTERIOSUS

Definition and Indications for Closure

A PDA is a persistent communication between the descending aorta and the pulmonary artery. This critical component of the foetal circulation usually closes within 72 h after birth. It is a common congenital heart defect, comprising approximately 10% of all defects. Owing to the loud murmur, diagnosis is usually made in infancy or childhood. Because of low resistance in the pulmonary vasculature, this lesion results in left-to-right shunt. If small, it usually does not lead to symptoms. However, larger PDAs are associated with significant left-to-right shunt, usually resulting in symptoms of heart failure, frequent chest infections, and failure to thrive early in life.

Owing to systemic hypertension, small-to-moderate PDAs can present with new symptoms of heart failure in adulthood. This is due to an increase in the left-to-right shunt. Another complication associated with PDAs is the risk for endarteritis. Although no data are available directly comparing closure of small, haemodynamically non-significant PDAs in asymptomatic patients vs. dental prophylaxis for the prevention of endarteritis, it is commonly accepted to close all audible PDAs to prevent the risk of endarteritis, occurrence of heart failure, and irreversible pulmonary arterial hypertension. It is controversial to close small silent PDAs that are incidentally found on echocardiography.

Surgical closure has largely been replaced by transcatheter closure. Particularly in adults, surgical closure carries greater risks due to the calcifications of the PDA and surrounding friable tissue. However, if the PDA is associated with other congenital abnormalities that require surgical correction, it can be ligated during the same procedure.

Patent Ductus Arteriosus Closure Devices

Small PDAs, measuring <2–3 mm in diameter, can usually be closed using coils. Commonly used coils are Gianturco coils or Flipper coils, which are detachable. Another coil device is the Nit-Occlud PDA occluder, which is available outside the USA Aside from the minimal diameter of the communication, the anatomy of the PDA is important to

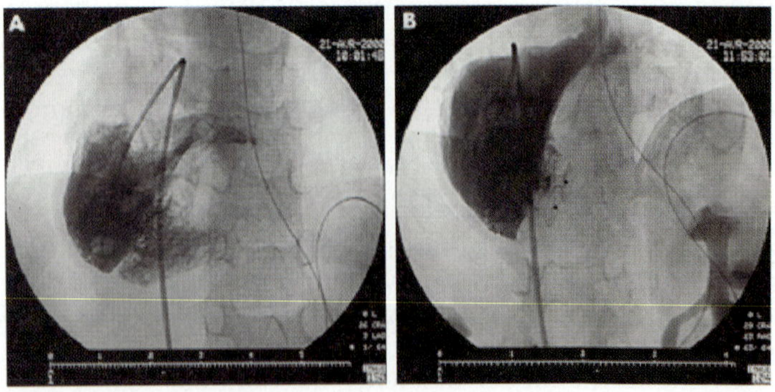

Fig. 36.15: *Multiple ventricular septal defect (VSD) closure. (A) Complex heart disease with "Swiss cheese" VSD. (B) Quite complete closure with two amplatzer VSD devices*

allow successful closure with coils. Commonly, the PDA has the shape of a funnel, with an ampulla on the aortic aspect of the duct and narrowest point usually close to the pulmonary arterial insertion. Those duct morphologies, if small in diameter, can be closed effectively with coils. Owing to the lack of discrete constriction, tubular ducts without a distinct ampulla are more difficult to close with coils; they carry a higher risk of coil migration. Although it is technically possible to close larger PDAs with multiple coils, most operators prefer to close PDAs larger than 3 mm in diameter with the Amplatzer duct occluder.

The Amplatzer duct occluder consists of an aortic retention disc and a plug which is 4 mm smaller in diameter than the retention disc. The largest device can close PDAs measuring up to 11–12 mm in diameter at the pulmonic end. PDAs larger than 12 mm in diameter can be closed with Amplatzer VSD or ASD occluders.

Closure Technique (Figs 36.16A and B, 36.19)

Careful procedural planning is necessary, considering several aspects of the PDA morphology such as duct size at its narrowest portion, size, and shape of the ampulla, and height and weight of the patient. Smaller PDAs, defined as <2–3 mm, are usually coiled; whereas larger PDAs are closed using the Amplatzer duct occluder. In the case of coil closure, a coil diameter of at least twice the diameter of the measured minimal duct diameter is chosen. The length of the coil is determined by the size of the ampulla. Several turns of the coil are placed in the ampulla, with less than half a turn of the coil being placed in the pulmonary arterial end of the PDA. If incomplete closure is found, a second coil should be deployed in a similar fashion. Success rate is high, with complete closure of the PDA being accomplished in nearly all cases when the device was placed successfully Inability to deliver the coils especially in small infants is one of the scenarios when surgical closure may be necessary. Periprocedural complications are rare, coil embolization in the pulmonary artery or descending thoracic aorta may occur, although with controlled release, detachable coils, this complication is much less. Haemolysis is a rare complication of PDA closure and is caused by excessive shear stress destroying red blood cells. It is usually seen only in patients with large

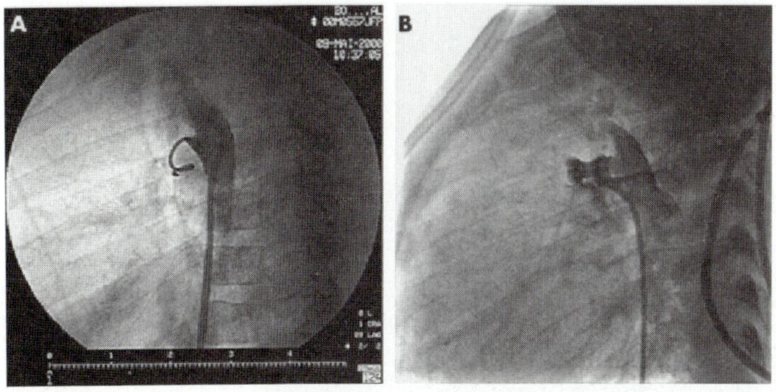

Fig. 36.16: Patent ductus closure. (A) Small ductus closed with a single coil. (B) Larger ductus with an Amplatzer PDA device. Note the immediate residual flow. It will close within a few hours

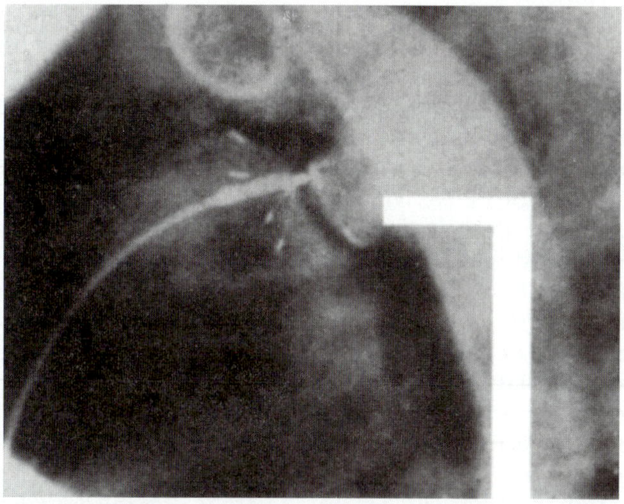

Fig. 36.17: Aortogram after opening of both the disks of RUD shows no flow across the ductus

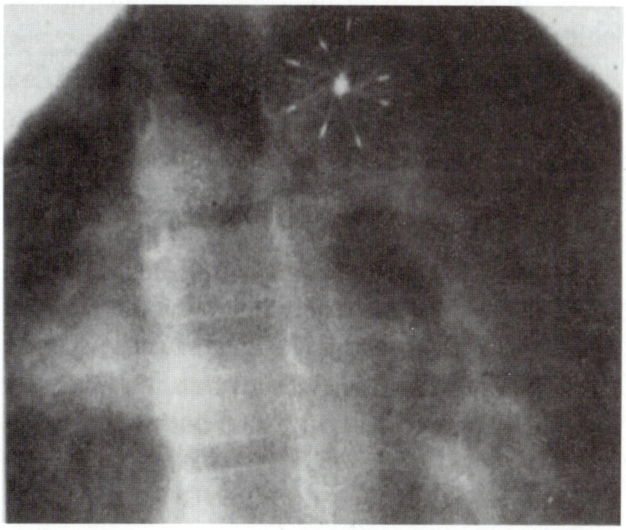

Fig. 36.18: RD after implantation as seen in the AP view

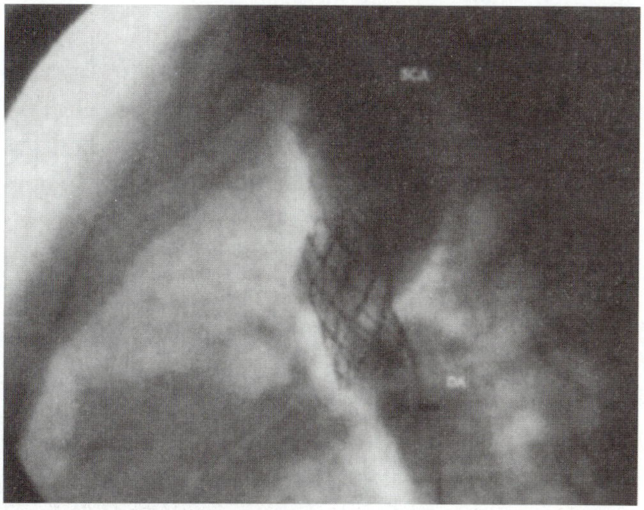

Fig. 36.19: Descending aortogram in lateral view after deployment of stent. PDA is completely closed and coarct segment is dilated. PDA, patent ductus arteriosus

PDAs and residual flow after the procedure. Incidence is <1%. The approach for coil deployment can be either retrograde from the aortic side or antegrade from the venous side. We prefer to use the antegrade route, since the arterial catheter is used for angiography to verify coil position prior to release.

Closure of PDAs with the Amplatzer duct occluder is carried out after aortography and delineation of the exact duct morphology. A device at least 2 mm larger than the narrowest PDA diameter is chosen. The delivery sheath is placed from the venous side into the descending thoracic aorta. The device is deployed in a similar fashion as the other Amplatzer occluder. Angiography in the descending aorta is performed to verify device position prior to release. If position is not optimal, the device can be recaptured and the steps are repeated. Commonly, small residual shunt through the device is seen immediately after the device has been released. This shunt disappears within few days in most patients. Most common PDA morphologies are amenable to closure with the Amplatzer duct occluder. However long, tubular ducts are difficult to close with the Amplatzer duct occluder. In such cases, Amplatzer Vascular Plug-II can be used. Complications occur rarely with the Amplatzer duct occluder embolization and haemolysis are described sporadically. In some patients with pulmonary arterial hypertension (mean pulmonary artery pressure >30 mmHg), it is better and safer to use the Amplatzer muscular VSD device. The risk of device migration with Amplatzer muscular VSD device in this position is less than the conventional PDA device.

COARCTATION OF THE AORTA

Since the introduction of surgical therapy by Crafoord and Nylin. and Gross and Hufnagal in the mid-1940s, surgical correction has become the standard treatment for aortic coarctation. Following adaptation of the balloon angioplasty technique of Gruntzig et al to aortic coarctation. it was applied in the clinical management of this condition in the early 1980s. Despite initial controversies reviewed elsewhere, balloon angioplasty was eventually adopted as a treatment mode of choice to manage both native and post-surgical coarctation in children. adolescents and adults. although its use remains controversial in neonates and infants. Despite reasonably good short- and long-term results with remain which include restenosis, probability of aortic rupture. formation of aneurysm and the inability to effectively treat long-segment tubular narrowing. Because of these and other reasons. endovascular stenting of aortic coarctationhas gained acceptance over the last decade. The perceived advantages of stents over balloon angioplasty are:

i. Ability to expand a tubular long-segment coarctation. hypoplastic isthmus and distal transverse aortic arch.
ii. Increase the diameter of the coarcted segment independent of the intimal tear.
iii. Decrease prevalence of restenosis.
iv. Prevent dissection of the torn intimal flap by facilitating apposition of the intima against the media.
v. Prevention of aneurysms because of support of the weakened aortic wall with the stent and neointima. Furthermore, experimental work in animal models has demonstrated immediate and short-term relief of aortic obstruction. prevention of restenosis and aneurysms, and feasibility of redilatation at follow-up. Based on these studies, it may be concluded that stents serve as useful adjuncts to balloon angioplasty in the management of aortic coarctation. O'Laughlin et al were the first to report the use of a stent for treatment of aortic coarctation although the results in a 12-year-old child were marginal. Subsequently number of other workers reported the use of stents in aortic coarctation with encouraging results.

Indications: The indications for employing stents are:

i. Long-segment coarctation
ii. Associated hypoplasia of the isthmus or aortic arch
iii. Tortuous coarctation with malalignment of the proximal with the distal aortic segment.
iv. Recurrent aortic coarctation or an aneurysm following prior surgical or balloon therapy.

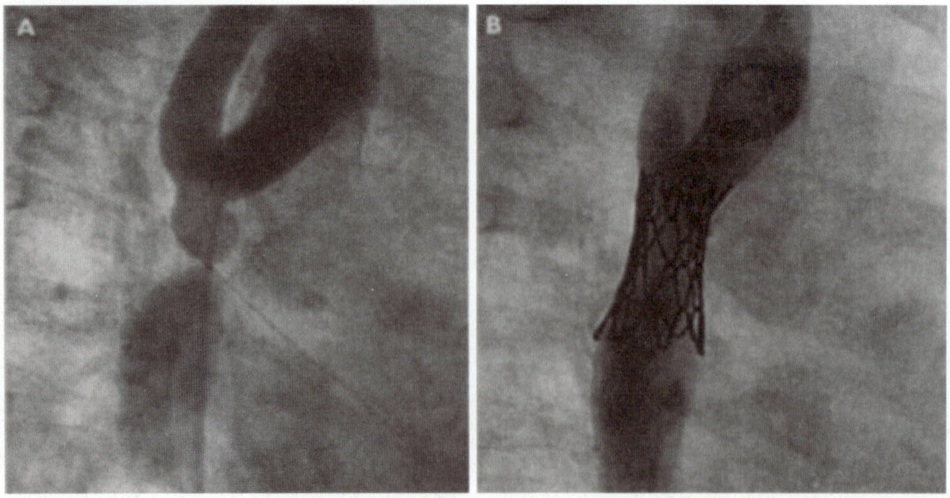

Fig. 36.20: *Showing balloon catheter across coarctation of aorta (left) and complete disappreance of aortic constriction after successful dialatation with stent implantation*

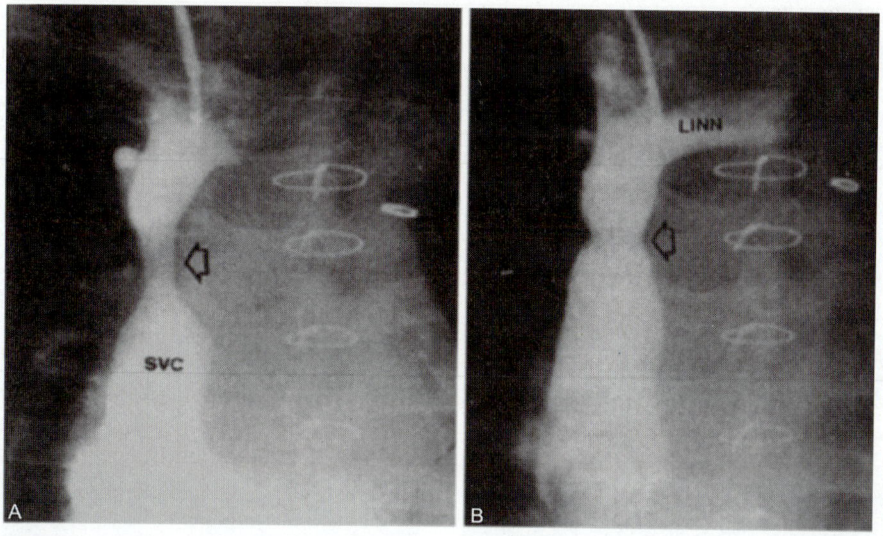

Fig. 36.21: *Selected superior vena caval (SVC) cineangiographic frames demonstrating long-segment stenosis (unfilled arrow) of the SVC 1 year following cardiac transplantation (A). Following stent placement, there was improvement in the angiographic appearance with complete disappearance of gradient (B)*

Because of issues related to growth and the need for large sheaths for implantation. Most cardiologists limit stent usage to adolescents and adults.

Technique (Figs 36.20A and B)

The technique is as described previously. To avoid potential balloon rupture, the tip of the guidewire is placed in the right subclavian artery instead of the ascending aorta, the usual practice for balloon angioplasty. The stent should not be positioned across the origins of the left common carotid and left subclavian arteries. However, on occasion, it is not possible to avoid the subclavian artery. In such situations, one may carefully traverse the stent cells (in between the struts) with a soft guidewire followed by a multi-Az catheter (Cordis). The stent cell is then dilated with an angioplasty balloon of a diameter equal to the proximal left subclavian artery; uncompromised flow to the left subclavian artery was found in these patients. Predilatation of the coarcted segment by balloon angioplasty prior to stenting is no longer recommended.

Immediate results: Reduction of the peak systolic pressure gradients and increase in diameter of the coarcted segment have been demonstrated following: stent implantation. Stenting was effective in postsurgical and postballoon recoarctations as well as in native coarctations. The ratio of the diameters of the coarctated segment to the descending aorta at the level of the diaphragm increased to unity in many of the patients undergoing aortic stenting. Improvement in the size of the hypoplastic isthmus or transverse aortic arch and exclusion of the aneurysm if such is present also occurred after stent placement.

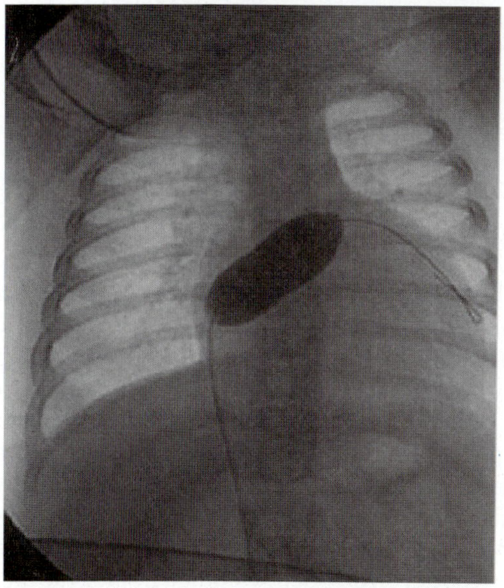

Fig. 36.22: *Pulmonary artery stenting in TOF*

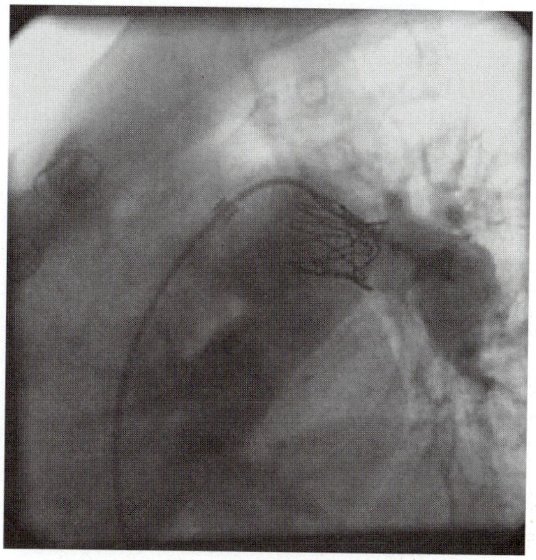

Fig. 36.23: *TOF MAPCA dilatation*

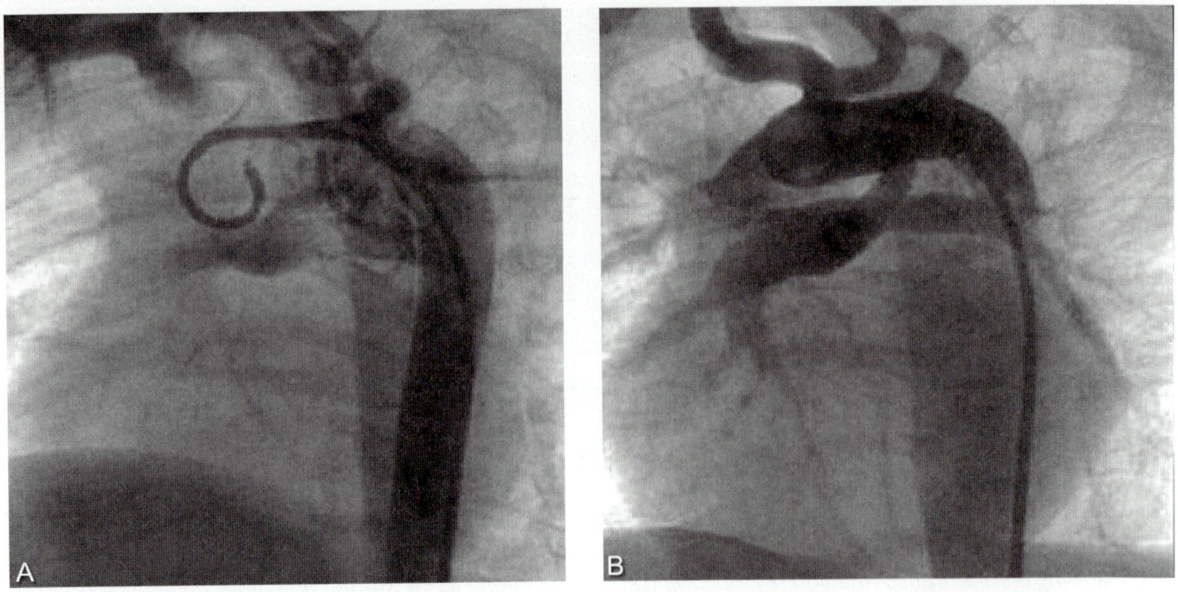

Figs 36.24A and B: *(A) Multiple aorto pulmonary collateral; (B) T shunt catheter coil closure*

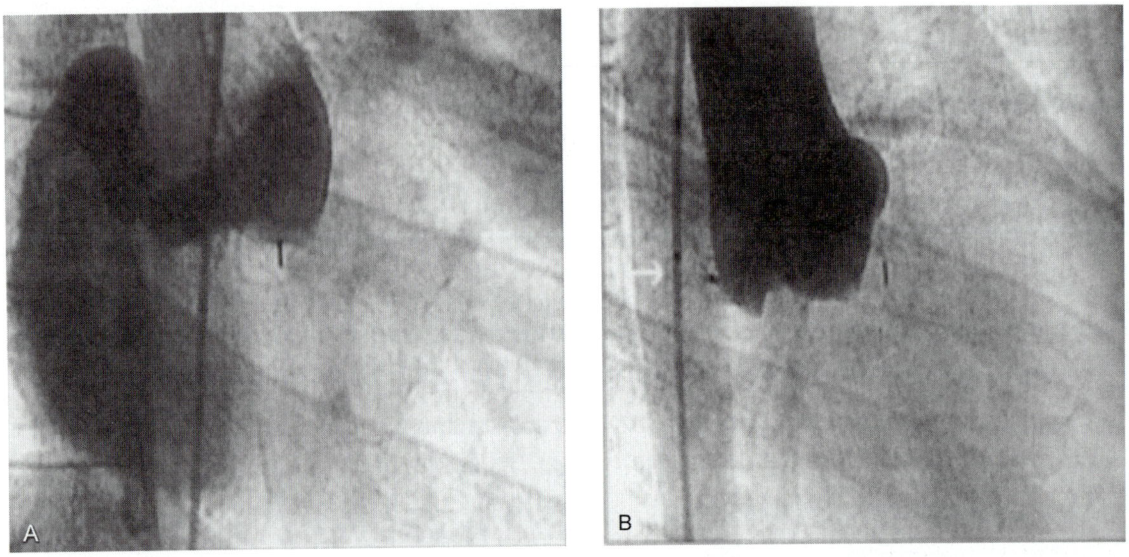

Figs 36.25A and B: *(A) Aortic root angiogram (right anterior obliquc projection) showing the markedly dilated proximal RCA and the large. densely opacified fistula connected to the RA; (B) Aortic root angiogram (right anterior oblique projection) after deployment of the ADO (arrow) showing complete occlusion of the fistula*

Complications: Vessel disruption, displacement of the stent and aneurysms may occur but are infrequent. Balloon rupture, which results in inadequate stent expansion and stent migration has been reported, but may be prevented by avoiding curvature of the balloon/stent assembly, by the use of newer stents with less injurious ends and by the use of BIB catheters. Because of the large size of the sheath required, loss of pulse and bleeding from the puncture site may occur. The use of vascular closure devices may help circumvent this problem. Rare complications include myocardial infarction and retroperitoneal hemorrhage.

Follow-up results: In most studies, there was only a short-term and incomplete follow-up in a limited number of patients. However, three studies examined the results of more than 20 patients at a mean follow-up of 2 years or more. The pressure gradients across the coarctation site (blood pressure, Doppler or catheterization) remained low and systemic hypertension decreased both in degree and frequency with a consequent decrease in the need for antihypertensive medications. No evidence of fracture/displacement was observed, although no systematic or complete follow-up was achieved in the majority of studies. Residual or recurrent obstruction was present in a few patients and in these, successful redilatation with larger balloons was accomplished. Detailed angiographic studies by Suarez de Lezo et al revealed no detectable neointimal

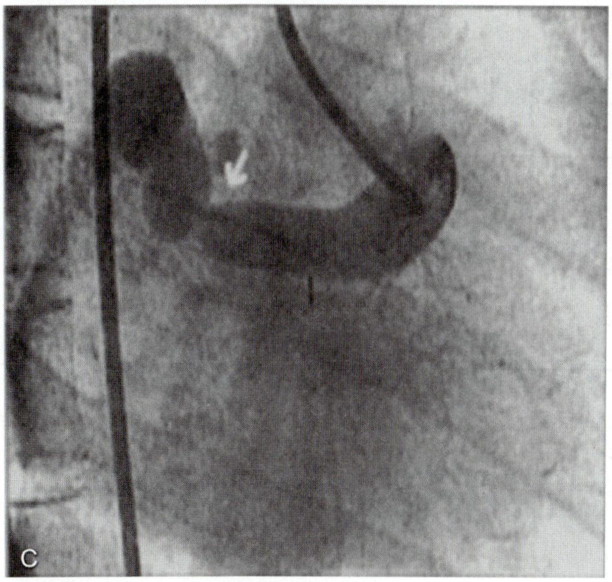

Fig. 36.25C: *Selective right coronary arteriography (right anterior oblique projection) shows the large fistula opening into the RA. The mid-segment shows a stenosis (arrow) with an aneurysmal pouch distal to it*

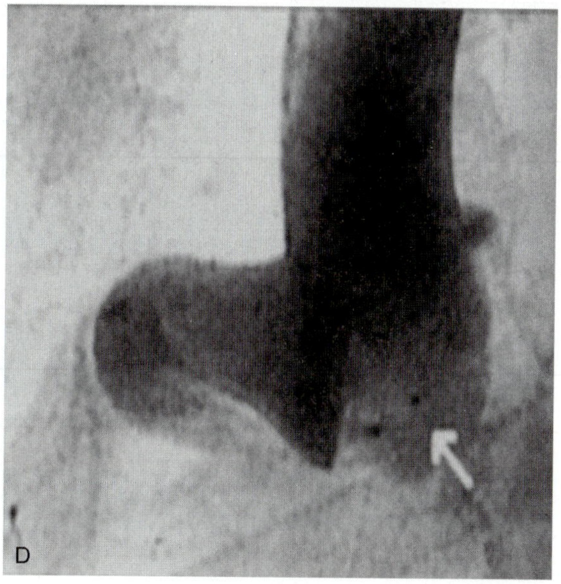

Fig. 36.25D: *Aortic root angiogram (left anterior oblique projection) after deployment of the ADO (arrow). The fistula is occluded and there is improved filling of the distal branches of the RCA*

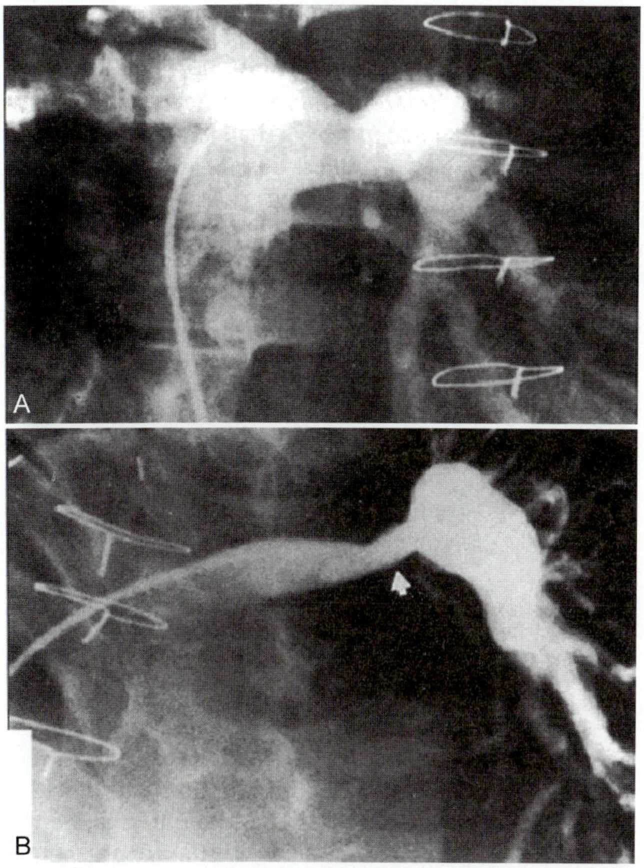

Figs 36.26A and B: *Selected cineangiographic frames from a pulmonary arteriogram in sitting up (A) and left anterior oblique (B) views. In "A", the left pulmonary artery stenosis is not well visualized while in "B", it is clearly defined (arrow). These cineframes illustrate the importance of obtaining multiple views to demonstrate branch pulmonary artery stenosis*

proliferation in 75% of the patients; in the remaining patients, focal neointimal ridge formation was observed at the ends of the stent, causing minimal restenosis. Segmental analysis of the aorta revealed an increase in the nonstented segments of the aorta, consistent with normal growth. Two (7%) young patients developed small new aneurysms which were obliterated by coil placement following angiographic detection. However, the overall follow-up.

TRANSCATHETER MANAGEMENT OF CYANOTIC CONGENITAL HEART DEFECTS

In this review, the role of transcatheter methods in the management of cyanotic congenital heart defects is discussed. In patients with interventricular right-to-left shunting secondary to pulmonary outflow tract obstruction (most commonly tetralogy of Fallot), balloon dilatation may be an effective palliative procedure in a substantial proportion of patients, obviating the need for a palliative shunt. It is recommend this if the patient's size or cardiac anatomy makes that patient an unsuitable candidate for safe total surgical correction. Infundibular myectomy with atherectomy catheter in tetralogy of Fallot patients may become a useful adjunct in the management of these infants. Cyanotic children with interatrial right-to-left shunt secondary to severe valvular pulmonary stenosis respond to balloon pulmonary valvuloplasty in a manner similar to that seen with isolated pulmonary valve stenosis. In these patients, balloon valvuloplasty is the treatment of choice and may be corrective in most cases. In patients with a narrowed Blalock-Taussig shunt, balloon angioplasty may improve pulmonary oligemia and systemic arterial hypoxemia and may obviate the need for a second systemic-to-pulmonary artery shunt. Balloon angioplasty is

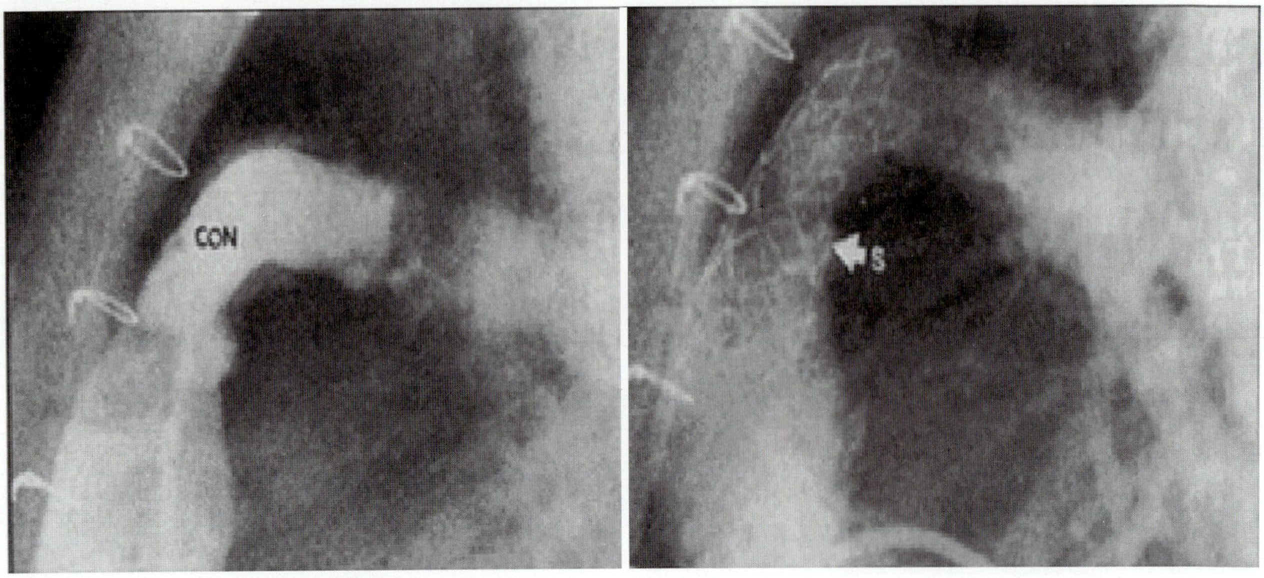

Fig. 36.27: *Selected cineangiographic frames from a lateral view of the patient showing stenotic conduit (CON) prior to and following implantation of a stent (S). Note that the lower end of the stent was dilated with a larger balloon*

recommended if the patient's cardiac defect is not amenable to surgical correction at a low risk either because of the size of the patient or because of the complexity of the cyanotic heart defect. In patients with pulmonary valve atresia, initial opening of the atretic pulmonary valve by either laser or surgery with subsequent balloon dilatation is potentially beneficial in reducing the total number of surgical procedures that these children are likely to require.

PARAVALVULAR LEAKS (Figs 36.22, 36,23–36.30)

In certain relatively frequent though seldom treated cases, a paravalvular leak is observed. Though transcatheter closure can be attempted, it remains nevertheless one of the most difficult interventions of its kind if not the most difficult. Appropriate assessment of the leak can only be performed by transoesophageal echocardiography. Small jets cause severe haemolysis, and large leaks result in cardiac insufficiency. In some instances, the defect may involve more than half of the valve circumference. As far as the mitral valve is concerned, implantation of a device is carried out by means of an arteriovenous loop formed through the atrial septum following transseptal puncture. The results achieved so far have been rather disappointing, mainly for lack of an appropriate device with an adapted shape. Crossing the leak is easier at the aortic valve level, and, as it is often small, the results are better.

Vascular Embolisation

The principle of embolisation consists of positioning a device at the origin or at the distal extremity of the vessel in order to achieve complete or partial mechanical occlusion. Thrombotic occlusion of the vessel is brought about by slowing down the blood flow and by the device characteristics. Various devices are available.

Detachable Balloons

These are deflated balloons inserted through a guiding catheter and pushed to the implantation site. They are inflated by means of a microcatheter containing a contrast solution. Upon withdrawal of the microcatheter, the balloon is closed by a valve.

This complex method requires relatively large catheters, and the balloons used have been reported to deflate prematurely. Detachable balloons are best used in medium sized vessels.

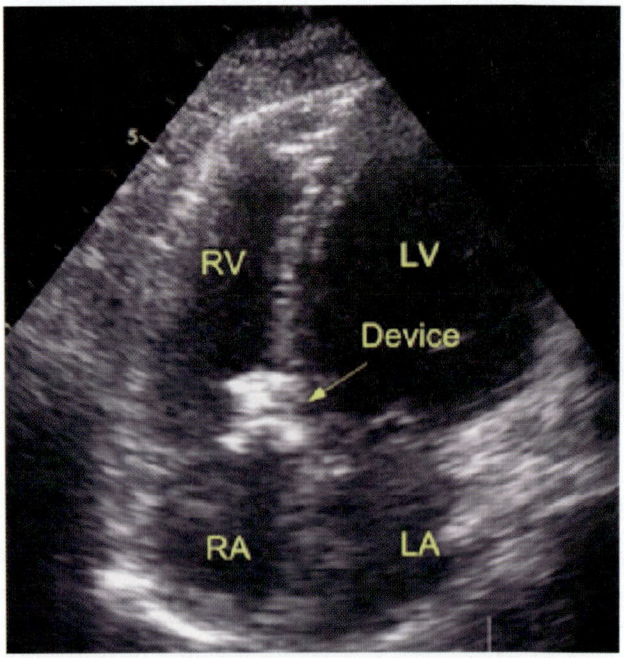

Fig. 36.28: *Echocardiogram in apical five chamber view showing a device closing a ruptured sinus of valsalva aneurysm (RSOV)*

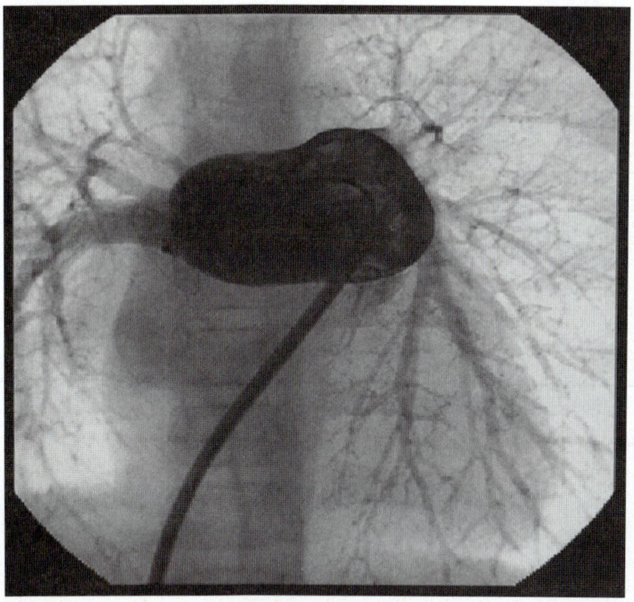

Fig. 36.29: *Transcatheter closure of direct communication between right pulmonary artery and left atrium using Amplatzer device*

Coils

These are metallic wires of variable shape, length, and rigidity. They can be either bare or with strands and can be either pushed and delivered or detachable. Implantation of detachable coils can be controlled and delivery is performed only when the positioning is judged acceptable. Various mechanisms for detachment have been developed.

Prostheses

Any device initially designed for occlusion of arterial ducts and atrial or ventricular septal defects can be used. These types of devices include the CardioSEAL/STARFlex and Amplatzer devices.

In addition, the new Amplatzer "Plug" made of very thin Nitinol wire mesh and very easy to position is worth mentioning (Figs 36.27–36.29).

Indications

Coronary Artery Fistulae (Figs 36.24a-d)

Treatment of fistulae between the coronary artery and the cardiac chambers has been carried out via the surgical approach for many years. Such fistulae may involve the right or the left coronary artery and sometimes both. The fistula may drain into any of the cardiac chambers though most often into the right chambers. Accurate diagnosis of the lesion by means of selective contrast injection into each coronary artery using conventional angiographic views is essential. The normal coronary branches must be carefully studied to ensure that they are not occluded and potential multiple feeding to the fistula must be identified. The fistula flow, which is often very significant, may hinder visibility of the native coronary flow. It is crucial that vital coronary arteries should not be occluded by the procedure; contrast injections should be made (if necessary beyond a balloon inflated in the main vessel) in order to visualise all branches while looking for ECG changes. The feeding coronary artery may have a large diameter allowing easy advancement of the closure equipment to the fistula. Its opening into the cardiac chamber may be very large or very narrow. Successive narrowings may be observed. Except for the very small ones, these fistulae do not close or become reduced of their own accord. The occlusion method (coils or occluding device) is selected according to the angiographic aspects. Only a few teams have had the opportunity to perform such procedures because of the relative rarity of this pathology. The indication may be the presence of significant flow in the fistula, creating a left-to-right shunt or less often a left-to-left shunt, and also cardiac insufficiency caused by coronary steal.

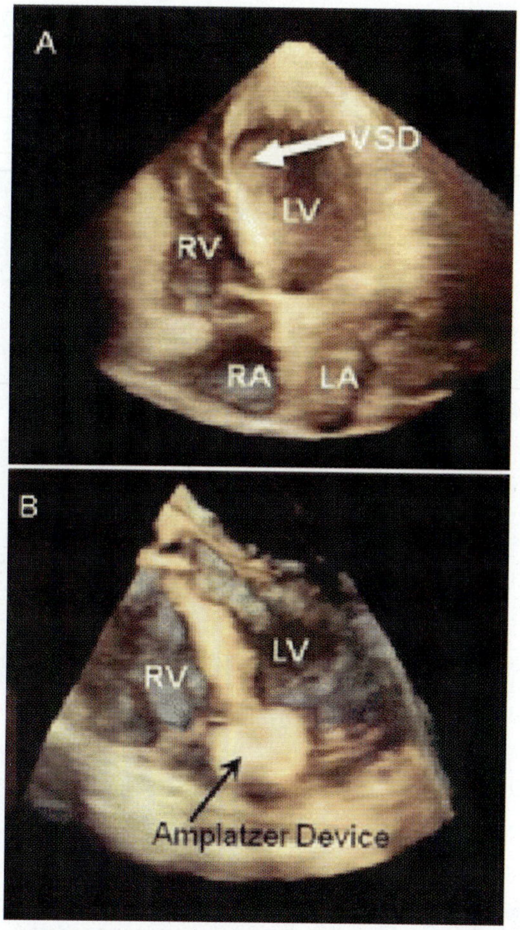

Fig. 36.30: *Transcatheter closure of muscular ventricular septal defects. Real-time 3D transthoracic echocardiography demonstrates the apical septal thinning and ventricular septal defect (A) After the transcatheter closure, real-time 3D transoesophageal echocardiography demonstrates the final position of the deployed occluder device. (B) LA, left atrium; LV, left ventricle; RA, right atrium; RV, right ventricle; VSD, ventricular septal defect; Adapted with permission from Halpern et al).*

Surgical Systemic Pulmonary Shunts

Most surgical shunts are amenable to transcatheter closure. Indication for closure may be the presence of excessive flow

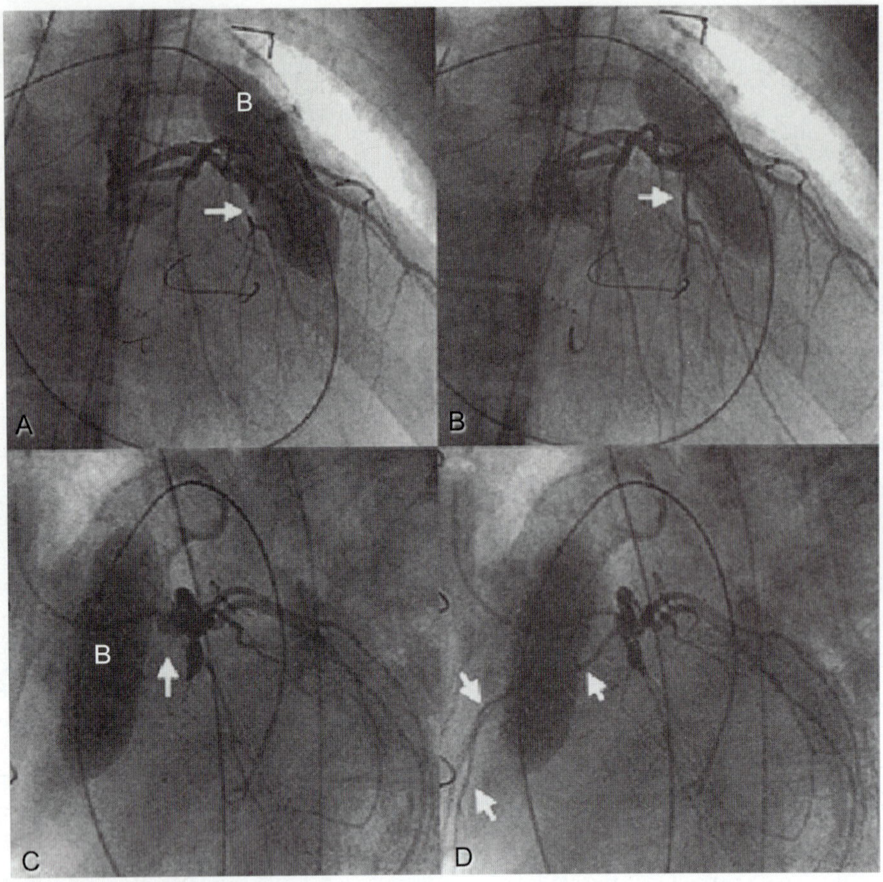

Figs 36.31A to D: *A patient with tetralogy of fallot and pulmonary atresia, the conduit passed over a large anterior RV coronary branch that arose from the proximal left coronary artery. Selective coronary angiograms with simultaneous inflation of an angioplasty balloon (B) in the conduit demonstrate occlusion of this RV branch. Angiography from a right anterior oblique projection shows (A) early occlusion of the anomalous coronary (arrow) with persistent distal contrast and (B) subsequent resumption of flow as the balloon was deflated (arrow). (C and D) Subsequent angiography in a lateral projection demonstrates complete occlusion of the coronary branch with balloon inflation to higher pressure. In C, the arrow indicates the proximal stump of the occluded vessel which then fills (multiple arrows) as the balloon is deflated in D*

or the fact that the shunt has become superfluous. Transcatheter closure may also be performed in some specific situations at the time of complete repair, just before surgery due to its simplicity and to the potential surgical difficulties. Devices used include pushed or detachable coils inserted via the arterial approach, especially for Blalock-Taussig shunts. As coil migration is not a rare occurrence, closure can be performed by placing a balloon in the pulmonary branch in order to stop the flow. Potts or Waterston shunts closure should only be performed, if pulmonary resistance allows it, with double-disk devices such as the CardioSEAL/STARFlex device or PDA, ASD, or VSD Amplatz occluders.

Aortopulmonary Collateral Vessels

It is necessary to identify clearly which vessels should be occluded and when. These major aortopulmonary collateral arteries (MAPCAs), originating in the aorta or its branches and feeding pulmonary segments, may or may not be connected to the central pulmonary artery. Prior diagnostic catheterisation plays a crucial role by allowing visualisation of the central pulmonary artery through direct or indirect contrast injection (aortography, MAPCA, or venous pulmonary wedge injections). Selective injections in MAPCAs visualise those connected to the central pulmonary artery and amenable to closure, though the other collateral vessels should be unifocalised or surgically connected to the central pulmonary artery. Transcatheter closure can be performed before the complete repair operation. Indeed, the considerable flow of the MAPCAs results in a very significant venous pulmonary return which may hinder the performance of surgery. Closure can also be undertaken after the operation, in particular after "unifocalisation". Transcatheter closure can be carried out with various devices described earlier, and especially with coils or Amplatzer occluding devices.

Device selection is made according to size, anatomy, and presence of tapering segments. The arterial approach is used; however, when the procedure is performed before complete surgical repair, antegrade closure can be achieved by crossing the ventricular septal communication. Approach selection should be made according to the implantation angle of the vessels.

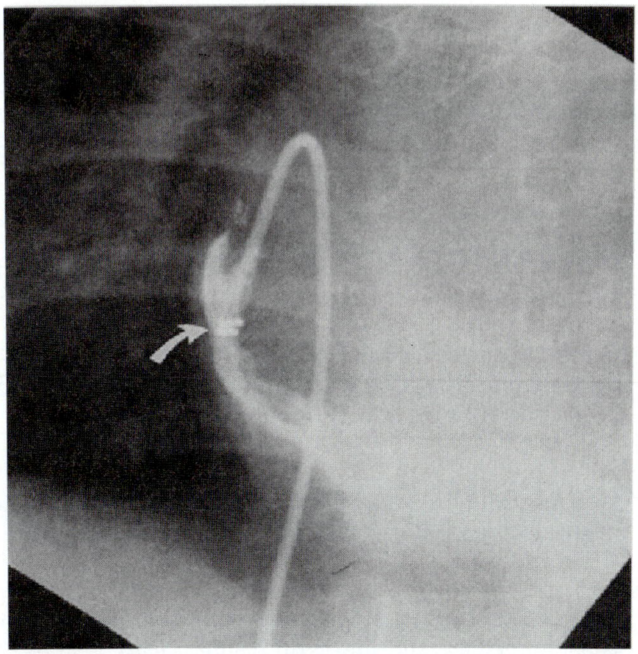

Fig. 36.32: *Frontal projection shows the end-hole catheter engaged in the systemic venous side of the fenestration. Contrast can be seen entering the pulmonary venous atrium. The curved arrow marks the Weck clips. The previously placed Wallstent can be seen in the pulmonary artery*

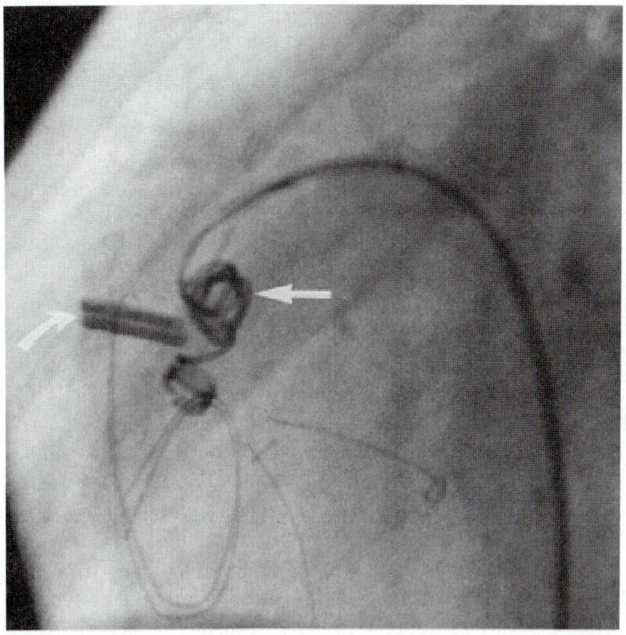

Fig. 36.33: *Lateral projection showing the first coil astride the narrowing demarcated by Weck clips (curved arrow). A second coil (straight arrow) is being placed on the systemic venous side of the graft fenestration. Note the residual external pacemaker wires from previous operations*

Pulmonary Sequestrations

Sequestrations are vascularised pulmonary territories without bronchi for ventilation. Due to the flow volume and risk of infection, occlusion is often considered. This is

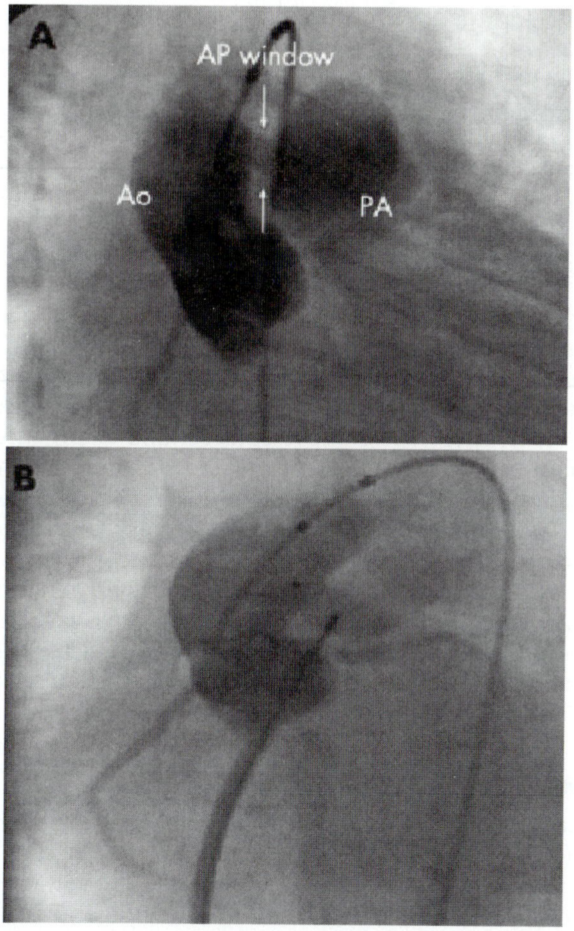

Fig. 36.34: *(A) Showing APW by angiography and transcatheter closure of the aortopulmonary window in a symptomatic infant using the Amplatzer ductal occluder (B)*

typically observed in patients with scimitar syndrome. In most cases, occlusion can be performed with pushed coils; however, the size of the feeding artery may require use of an occluding device.

Pulmonary Arteriovenous Fistulae

Fistulae between the pulmonary artery and the pulmonary vein are of congenital origin in most cases, they are often single and voluminous. They cause cyanosis and in some instances embolic accidents. Acquired fistulae such as those observed at long-term follow-up after a surgically created cavopulmonary shunt are mostly small and multiple. All kinds of devices, and especially coils, can be used (Fig. 36.28).

Left Superior Vena Cava and SVC Stenosis

The persistent superior left vena cava generally drains into the right atrium through the coronary sinus, and the innominate vein is often absent. Conversely, the left superior vena cava may drain into the left atrium, directly or through an unroofed coronary sinus. In this setting, closure of the vena cava is recommended because of the resulting right-to-left shunt. Occlusion can be performed percutaneously, especially via the left jugular approach with occluding devices rather than coils, placed just above the heart. In the presence of multiple perforations in the coronary sinus, occlusion of the vena cava may paradoxically induce left to right shunting. In such instances, even if transcatheter perforation closure may be considered, surgical management is probably the most appropriate option (Figs 36.21A and B).

Superior Vena Cava to Inferior Vena Cava or Pulmonary Vein Shunts

Following the performance of a superior cavopulmonary connection, pulmonary resistance may become significant. In such settings, shunts to vessels with less resistance can appear. In most cases these connections drain into the inferior vena cava, but may also connect with the pulmonary veins. They arise from normal vessels, such as the azygos vein if not ligated during surgery, or a forgotten left superior vena cava draining into the coronary sinus, or other natural vessels which become enlarged. When these shunts are large and not numerous, closure can be performed with several kinds of occluding devices. Though occlusion of multiple, small size vessels can be successfully performed, other new collateral connections appear.

Potential Complications

Potential risks associated with these interventional procedures have always been considered as higher than those of previously used techniques. These risks are especially related to the use of voluminous and complex devices through large lumen catheters. However, the theoretical risks should not be overestimated compared to the risks of surgical treatment.

Vessel Embolisation

- Various native vessels or surgically created ones may be closed by transcatheter technique
- In some instances, such closures have to be performed just before or after another surgical procedure
- Various devices can be used depending on the length, size and shape of the vessels.

These procedures can generate immediate and acute complications due to device embolisation induced by incorrect placement or inaccurate assessment of the orifice or the vessel size. Such a potential occurrence should always be anticipated, and consequently the operator should be familiar with the retrieval techniques and ensure that the equipment required for such manoeuvres is readily available, or arrange for easy access to surgical facilities. The retrieval equipment consists of large size guiding catheters and various snares or forceps.

However, such a dramatic complication is neither the most frequent nor the most difficult to deal with. There is another potential and much more hazardous complication, namely air or clot embolism caused by inadequate anticoagulation. Appropriate heparin treatment is essential to prevent its occurrence. It can be treated in most cases with general or local fibrinolysis.

Finally, mid to long-term complications have been reported. Instances of device fracture have been described, generally without clinical consequences, as well as rare cases of cardiac embolism and perforations. Persistence of a residual shunt has caused haemolysis in some cases.

BIBLIOGRAPHY

1. Gibbs JL. Interventional catheterisation. Opening up I: the ventricular outflow tracts and great arteries. Heart 2000;83: 111–15.
2. Gibbs JL. Interventional catheterisation. Opening up II: venous return, the atrial septum, the arterial duct, aorto-pulmonary shunts, and aortopulmonary collaterals, Heart 2000;83:237–40.
3. Rashkind WJ, Mullins CE, Hellenbrand WE, et al. Nonsurgical closure of patent ductus arteriosus: clinical application of the Rashkind PDA occluder system. Circulation 1987;75:583–92.
4. Hijazi ZM, Geggel RL. Transcatheter closure of large patent ductus arteriosus (> or = 4 mm) with multiple Gianturco coils: immediate and mid-term results. Heart 1996;76:536–40.
5. Masura J, Walsh KP, Thanopoulous B, et al. Catheter closure of moderate- to large-sized patent ductus arteriosus using the new Amplatzer duct occluder: immediate and short-term results. J Am Coll Cardiol 1998;31:878–82.
6. Carminati M, Giusti S, Hausdorf G, et al. A European multicentric experience using the CardioSeal and Starflex double umbrella devices to close interatrial communications holes within the oval fossa. Cardiol Young 2000;10:519–26.
7. Carminati M, Chessa M, Butera G, et al. Transcatheter closure of atrial septal defects with the STARFlex device: early results and follow-up. J Interv Cardiol 2001;14:319–24.
8. Masura J, Gavora P, Formanek A, et al. Transcatheter closure of secundum atrial septal defects using the new self-centering Amplatzer septal occluder: initial human experience. Cathet Cardiovasc Diagn 1997;42:388–93.
9. Zahn EM, Wilson N, Cutright W, et al. Development and testing of the Helex septal occluder, a new expanded polytetrafluoroethylene atrial septal defect occlusion system. Circulation 2001;104:711–6.
10. Sideris EB, Sideris CE, Stamatelopoulos SF, et al. Transcatheter patch occlusion of experimental atrial septal defects. Catheter Cardiovasc Interv 2002;57:404–7.
11. Omeish A, Hijazi ZM. Transcatheter closure of atrial septal defects in children & adults using the Amplatzer septal occluder. J Interv Cardiol 2001;14:37–44.
12. Harper RW, Mottram PM, McGaw DJ. Closure of secundum atrial septal defects with the Amplatzer septal occluder device: techniques and problems. Catheter Cardiovasc Interv 2002;57:508–24.
13. Chessa M, Carminati M, Butera G, et al. Early and late complications associated with transcatheter occlusion of secundum atrial septal defect. J Am Coll Cardiol 2002;39: 1061–5.
14. Meier B, Lock JE. Contemporary management of patent foramen ovale. Circulation 2003;107:5–9.
15. This paper summarises the clinical implications of the patent foramen ovale and the indications for closure, with many important references quoted.

16. Piechaud JF. Hypoxemia related to right-to-left shunting through a patent foramen ovale: successful percutaneous treatment with the CardioSeal device. J Interv Cardiol 2001; 14:57–60.
17. Morandi E, Anzola GP, Angeli S, et al. Transcatheter closure of patent foramen ovale: a new migraine treatment? J Interv Cardiol 2003;16:39–42.
18. Lock JE, Block PC, McKay RG, et al. Transcatheter closure of ventricular septal defects. Circulation 1988;78:361–8.
19. Thanopoulos BD, Tsaousis GS, Konstadopoulou GN, et al. Transcatheter closure of muscular ventricular septal defects with the Amplatzer ventricular septal defect occluder: initial clinical applications in children. J Am Coll Cardiol 1999;33: 1395–9.
20. Hijazi ZM, Hakim F, Haweleh AA, et al. Catheter closure of perimembranous ventricular septal defects using the new Amplatzer membranous VSD occluder: initial clinical experience. Catheter Cardiovasc Interv 2002;56:508.

37 Management of Valvular Heart Diseases with Prosthetic Valves

Replacing defective heart valves with prostheses in newborns is a difficult task, which is compounded by the fact that the new valves need to grow along with the children's hearts. Two surgeons at Boston Children's Hospital were faced with infants, one with severe mitral regurgitation and one with mitral stenosis, who required their mitral valves replaced. To solve the problem, the physicians modified. **Medtronic**'s melody transcatheter valve, that's normally indicated for replacement of the pulmonary valve. The valves will be made to expand as the kids grow via catheterization with balloon dilatation, hopefully reducing the need for further surgeries.

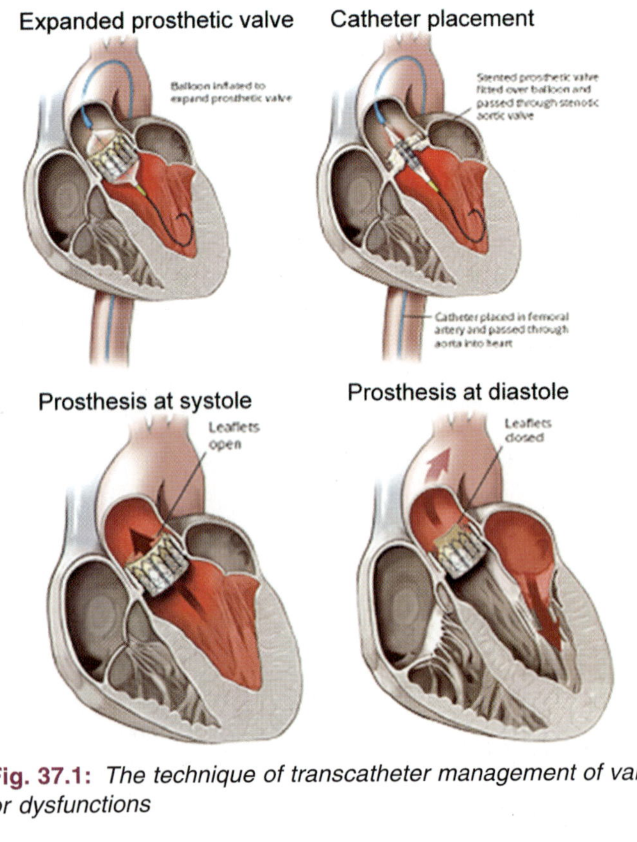

Fig. 37.1: *The technique of transcatheter management of valve or dysfunctions*

Chronic rheumatic valvular dysfunctions lead to very high morbidity and mortality among patients unless they are helped with either reconstructive surgery or replacement of an artificial valve. Two types of artificial valves which are available to-day have their own limitations and till date there is no ideal valve which could closely resemble with natural valve in terms of cost and postoperative long-term outcome. Synthetic valve do give rise to bleeding disorders due to anticoagulants and predispose to thromboembolic phenomenon and infection leading.

Surgical replacement of the tricuspid valve using a pericardial patch to avoid injury to the conduction system to vital organ dysfunctions. Although tissue valves do not need anticoagulants but still it could be the seat of infections and are often rejected in mismatched cases. Undoubtedly, tissue valve is preferable in pregnant women and younger children where anticoagulants may pose life-threatening

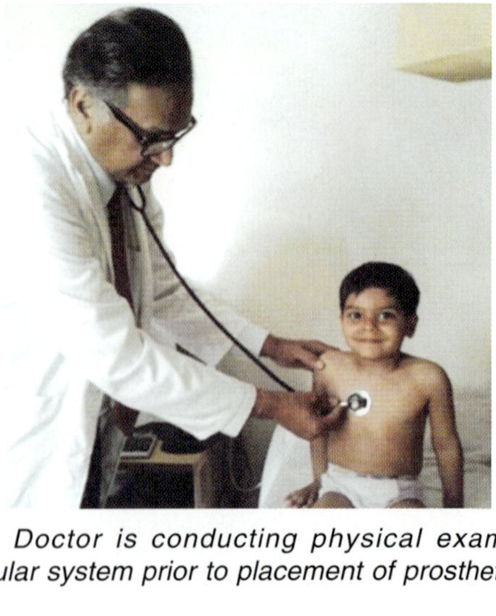

Fig. 37.2: *Doctor is conducting physical examination of cardiovascular system prior to placement of prosthetic valve*

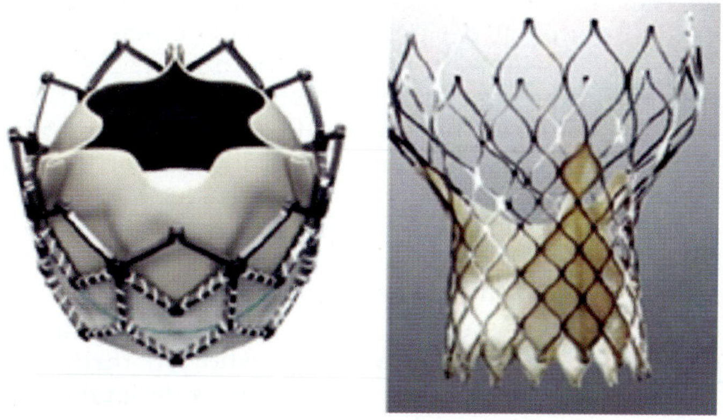

Fig. 37.3: *Biological aortic valve prothesis with stent. Left: SAPIEN XT™, Edwards make. Right: CoreValve™, Medtronic make*

complications. The lifespan of this valve, is shorter than the synthetic valve due to its rapid degeneration. In developing countries, rheumatic process is so extensive that often more'than one valves (multivalvular) are affected which further complicates the final management of the patients besides the cost implications among poor patients. Sincere efforts are still continued to manufacture such a valve which could satisfy all the properties of an ideal valve and come within the reach of low socioeconomic strata of people where a large segment of population is affected every year particularly in developing countries of South-East Asia.

The search for the ideal therapy for valve replacement continues. The major options include mechanical or tissue valves with an increasing variety of tissue valves becoming available. The key factor continues to be thrombogenicity versus durability. Aortic valve surgery primarily consists of replacement. This is aided by the increased variety of options allowing tailoring of the procedure to the patient's native valve disease. Mitral valve surgery has greater potential for repair which affords preservation of the native valve, optimizing function and reducing long-term complications. An increasingly popular concept is treatment of secondary or functional mitral valve regurgitation in the setting of depressed left ventricular function. The routine use of intraoperative transesophageal echocardiography and a trend toward the use of minimally invasive procedures are altering the conduct of valve operations. The field of valvular surgery continues to be an evolving and challenging one for the cardiac surgeon. The growing number of options for valve replacement therapy is testament to the probe of finding the perfect answer for valve replacement. These options do, however, allow for improved tailoring of the operation for a given patient (Figs 37.1 and 37.2).

VALVE REPLACEMENT OPTIONS

The major dichotomy in valve replacement therapy continues to be between mechanical and bioprosthetic (tissue) valves. Given the ridors of regulation surrounding such materials, the current available valves largely

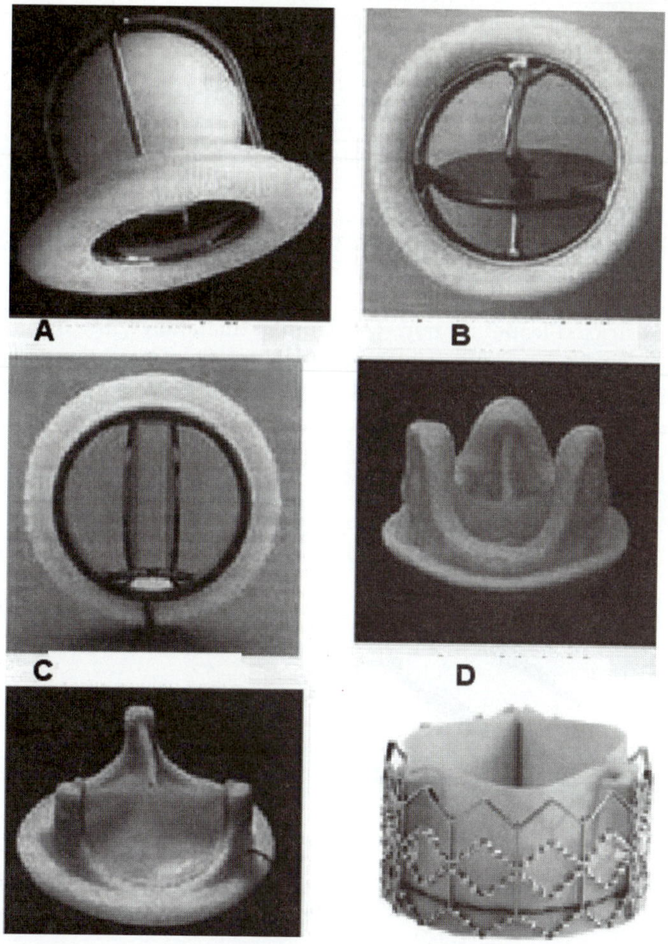

Fig. 37.4: *Showing six types of prosthetic heart valves: (A) Starr-Edwards mitral caged ball valve. (Courtesy of Baxter Edwards CVS.) (B) Medtronic Hall tilting disk valve. (Courtesy of Medtronic Heart Valve Division.) (C) St. Jude bileaflet valve. (Courtesy of St. Jude Medical, Inc.) (D) Hancock porcine valve (Courtesy of Medtronic Heart Valve Division.) E. Carpentier-Edwards bovine pericardial valve. (F) The Edwards-SAPIEN valve for percutaneous application (Courtesy of Baxter Edwards CVS)*

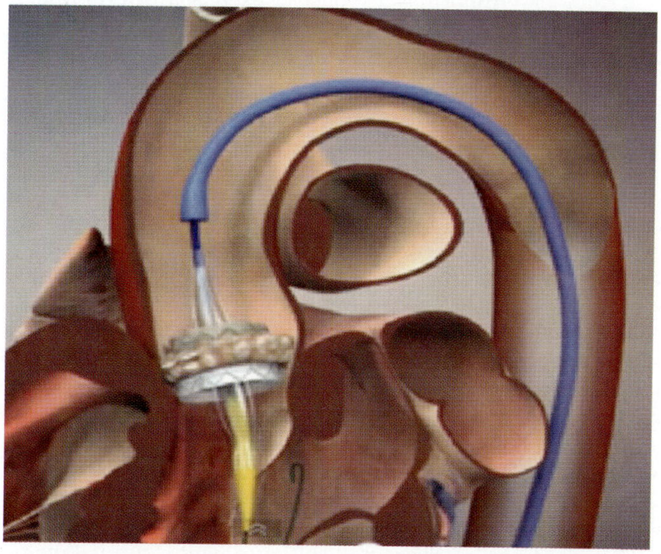

Fig. 37.5: *Transcatheter aortic valve replacement*

Table 37.1: *Characteristics favoring valve repair versus replacement*

Favoring valve replacement	*Favoring valve repair*
Rheumatic valve disease	Mitral prolapse
Endocarditis	
Inexperienced surgeon	Excessive leaflet mobility
Complex mitral valve morphology	Ischemic mitral valve regurgitation
Calcified and fibrosed valve	Bicuspid aortic valve with prolapse
Restricted leaflet motion	Annular dilatation with normal
Extensive leaflet destruction	leaflets

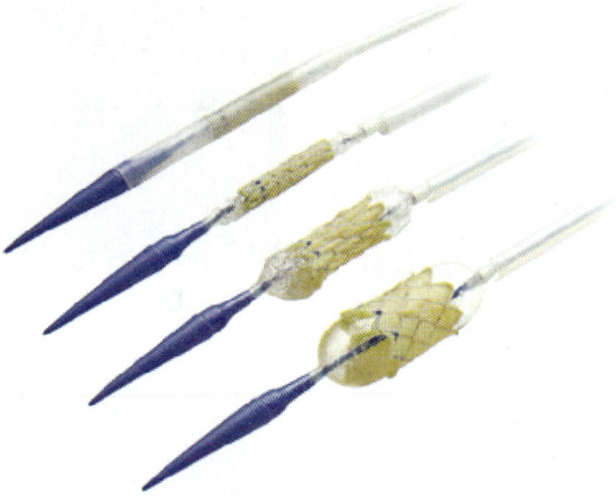

Fig. 37.6: *Medtronic's transcatheter pulmonary heart valve used for mitral calve replacement in infants*

represent variations on well proven prostheses as opposed to radically different designs. Although there were a variety of mechanical valves in the past, the most widely used mechanical valves in recent years have utilized the bileaflet valve popularized by the St. Jude's (St. Paul, MN) prosthesis. The basic material is pyrolite carbon and the design includes two-hinged semicircular leaflets. Several manufactures have developed variations on this design, but none has been proven dearly superior. Based primarily on historic data, all continue to share a propensity to possible thrombosis and embolism. A recent meta-analysis of two popular mechanical valves showed thromboembolism, valve thrombosis, and bleeding rates in the 0.5% to 2% per year range. Therefore, the need for long-term warfarin anticoagulation of the mechanical valve still exists. The tendency for thrombosis continues to be higher in

Table 37.2: *Clinical factors leading to selection of a bioprosthetic versus a mechanical valve*

Factors favoring Age > 70 yr	*Factors favoring Age < 50 yr*	*Factors favoring Age <60 yr*
Bleeding diathesis	Endocarditis	Combined multi-valvular placement
High risk for trauma	Female considering pregnancy	Patients with other indications for chronic anticoagulation
Poor compliance	Female considering pregnancy	

Table 37.3: *Management of severe asymptomatic aortic stenosis (AS): current ACC/AHA guidelines*

Indication	*Class*
1. Symptomatic patients with severe AS	I
2. Patients with severe AS before undergoing coronary artery bypass surgery	I
3. Patients with severe AS undergoing surgery on the aorta or other hand valves	I
4. Patients with moderate AS undergoing coronary artery bypass surgery or surgery on the aorta or other heart valves	IIa
5. Asymptomatic patients with servere AS and	
• Left ventricular (LV) systolic dysfunction	IIa
• Abnormal response to exercise (for example, hypotension)	IIa
• Ventricular techycardia	IIb
• Pronounced or excessive LV hypertrophy (≥ 15 mm)	IIb
• Valve area <0.6 cm²	IIb
6. Prevention of sudden death in asymptomatic patients with none of the findings listed under indication 5	III

Box 37.1: *The following questions should be systematically answered when examining a prosthesis by echocardiography*

- Does the history or clinical presentation of the patient suggest a prosthesis related disorder (for example, new onset of severe dyspnoea, fever, etc)?
- Is the prosthesis firmly implanted as a whole (absence of rocking)?
- In a bioprosthesis, are there morphologic signs of degeneration (thickened, immobile or pathologically mobile leaflets or leaflet segments)?
- In a mechanical prosthesis, do the occluder discs move normally?
- How much regurgitation is there, and is it transprosthetic or paraprosthetic?
- What are the mean and maximal transprosthetic gradients, are they in the normal range, and have they changed substantially from baseline?
- Are there fixed or mobile mass lesions attached to the prosthesis (thrombus, vegetation, pannus)?
- Are there other signs of endocarditis, in particular abscess formation at the prosthetic ring, fistulae, or a pericardial effusion?
- The first routine postoperative assessment is particularly important, since it serves as baseline for later comparison, especially with regard to transprosthetic gradients, prosthetic regurgitation, right ventricular peak pressure, left ventricular function, and other aspects.

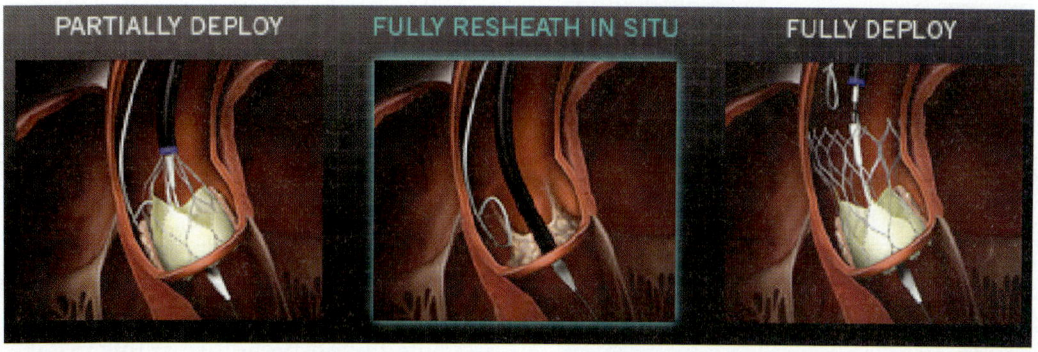

Fig. 37.7: *Jude medical has received European CE Mark approval for its 23 mm portico transcatheter aortic heart valve and transfemoral delivery system. Transcatheter aortic valve implantation (TAVI) is used in patients with severe aortic stenosis who are at very high surgical risk or with contraindications to surgical aortic valve replacement. The Portico is the first transcatheter aortic valve implantation system with a fully resheathable valve, allowing for easy repositioning and fine-tuning of valve placement at the implant site. It can even be retrieved at all times until the moment it is fully deployed*

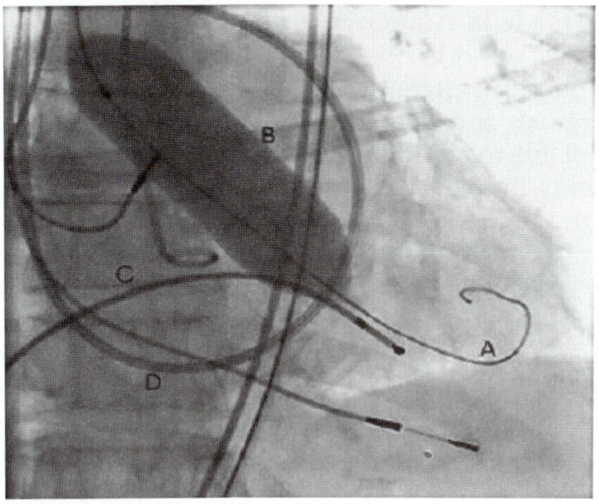

Fig. 37.8A: *Balloon aortic valvuloplasty is typically performed with a Tyshak balloon. An angiogram is performed to confirm proper positioning of the balloon, and during a short period of rapid ventricular pacing, the balloon is inflated. This frequently causes aortic insufficiency, and therefore, intense monitoring is required during this period*

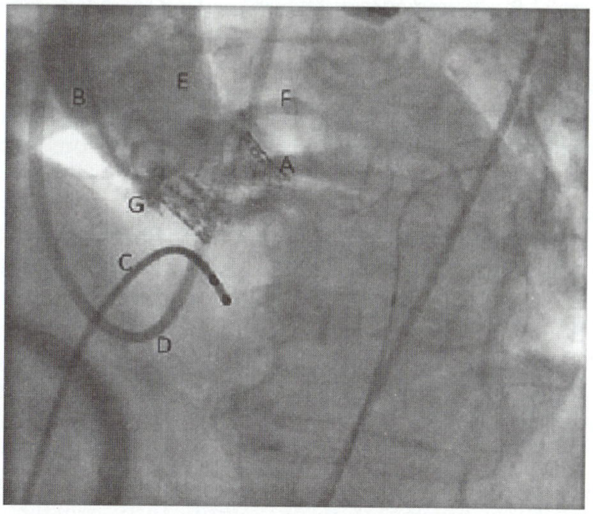

Fig. 37.8C: *Transcatheter transfemoral approach—completion angiogram of the implanted aortic valve is shown. Note that the contrast filled aortic root and ascending aorta are clearly seen, along with the take-off of the right and left coronary arteries*

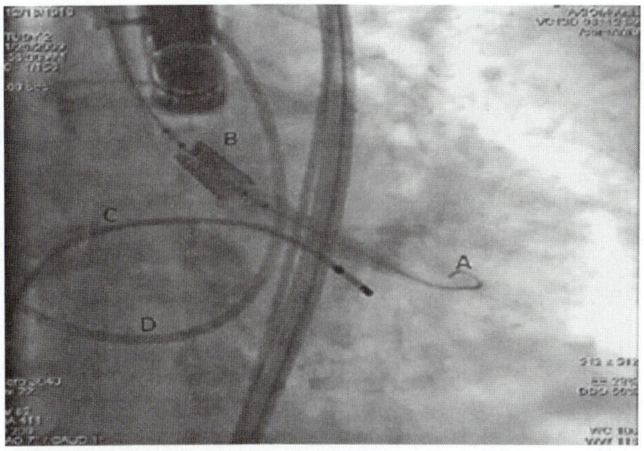

Fig. 37.8B: *Transcatheter transfemoral retrogradeapproach. The valve is advanced over a stiff guidewire into the aortic position in a retrograde manner. It is positioned such that 60% of the valve is on the ventricular side, and 40% of the valve is on the aortic side of the annulus. An angiographic image of the positioned valve in the retrograde position is shown*

mechanical prosthesis in the mitral position as compared with the aortic position. Overall improved valve design has allowed generally lower levels of anticoagulation.

Bioprosthetic (tissue) valves are known to be less thrombogenic but also less durable. Though most consensus guidelines still recommend short-term (4–12 weeks) warfarin therapy (often with aspirin) for the newly implanted tissue valve, long-term therapy usually consists of daily aspirin use only. A variety of bioprosthetic valves exist that differ in types of tissue used, preparation of the tissue leaflets, and construction of the valve leading to different implantation techniques. The three major tissue types are human, porcine valves that use porcine aortic valve leaflets, and bovine valves in which leaflets are constructed of bovine pericardium stamped out and sewn into a stent. The two manufacturers of the most widely used stented tissue valves, Medtronic (Min-neapolis, MN; porcine) and Edwards (Irvine, CA; bovine pericardium) tout these as "third generation" valves with average

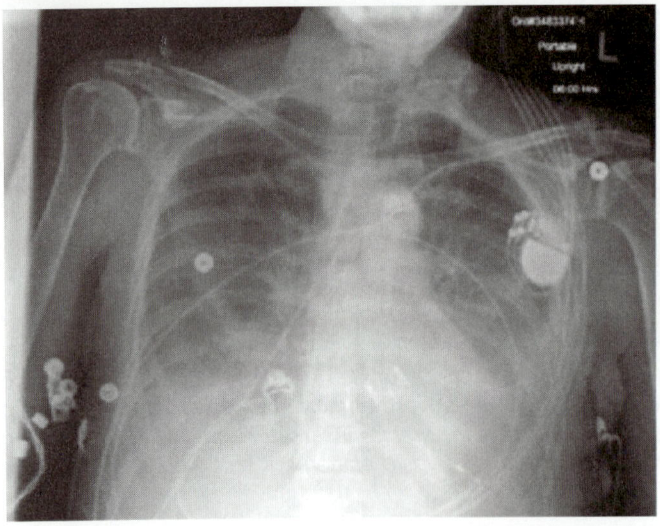

Fig. 37.9: *AP radiograph showing valve prosthesis in situ*

durability of 10–15 years. It is also of interest that durability appears to increase with age of the patient at the time of implantation. The major types of tissue valve construction are stented, stentless, homograft and autograft. Stented valves are self-contained and are placed with fairly routine and reproducible techniques involving suturing the sewing ring to the annulus of the valve to be replaced. The bulk of the stent results in an effective orifice area that is commonly less than that of the original (Fig. 37.12).

Stentless valves are currently applicable for aortic valve replacement. They are typically porcine aortic roots that have been modified with a sewing cuff. They may be implanted within the native aortic root or some versions may be placed as a "mini-root" replacement. In general, the technical demands for implantation are significantly greater with increased potential for variable results such as postoperative aortic regurgitation. The advantage is that in most cases, the effective orifice area is maintained to a greater degree, than with stented versions. Durability, however, appears to be similar. Homografts are similar to stentless valves with regard to implant techniques. They are human valves that are harvested from cadavers and treated to maintain tissue flexibility and reduce antigenicity. The most common treatment is cryopreservation. They typically have no attached artificial material. In most cases of aortic valve homografts, they consist of a generous amount of ascending aorta and the attached anterior leaflet of the mitral valve. This may be advantageous in selected cases in which additional reconstruction of the aorta or patching of the mitral valve is required. Pulmonary homografts are also available although their durability is less than that of aortic homografts. In general, they are reserved for reconstruction of the right ventricular outflow tract in infants, children, and young adults. The major drawback for all homografts is availability in numbers and sizes (Figs 37.3–37.7).

Autografts imply the transfer of the pulmonary valve to the aortic position, typically as a root replacement with replacement of pulmonary valve with a homograft. Commonly referred to as the *Ross procedure* and named for the surgeon who first developed it, this represents the most technically demanding of the procedures for aortic valve replacement. Its use is generally reserved for aortic valve disease in the pediatric or young adult population in whom there is a desire to avoid long-term anticoagulation with the hope of increased durability when compared with most other tissue valve replacements (Tables 37.1–37.3, 37.5, 37.6 and Boxes 37.1–37.3).

Homografts for mitral valve replacement have been described by selected centers but the technical demands, short- and medium-term reliability concerns have prevented widespread use at this point.

AORTIC VALVE DISEASE

Most aortic valve disease in young adults continues to be treated with leaflet excision followed by replacement. At this point, the wide variety of options comes into play with choices made in relation to a number of factors including patient age, comorbidities, need for concomitant procedures, availability of a given replacement, technical expertise of the surgeon, and patient compliance. Numerous articles are available to aid in iliis choice. A mechanical prosthesis represents the most durable, technically easiest valve to implant, with ready availability in a variety of sizes. This is usually considered the valve of choice for adults up to approximately age 65. The two major drawbacks are the need for long-term anticoagulation with warfarin and the potential for so-called valve mismatch, which results in a valve that is too small for a given patient, leading to a residual pressure gradient that is too high. Though an enlargement procedure can be done to accommodate a larger valve if a small annulus is encountered, this adds to potential for perioperative complications. The problems of long-term warfarin use are well documented, and include inadequate monitoring leading to under or over anticoagulation, and tetragenic considerations.

The next most popular choice in replacement is stented tissue valves. They share with mechanical valves the

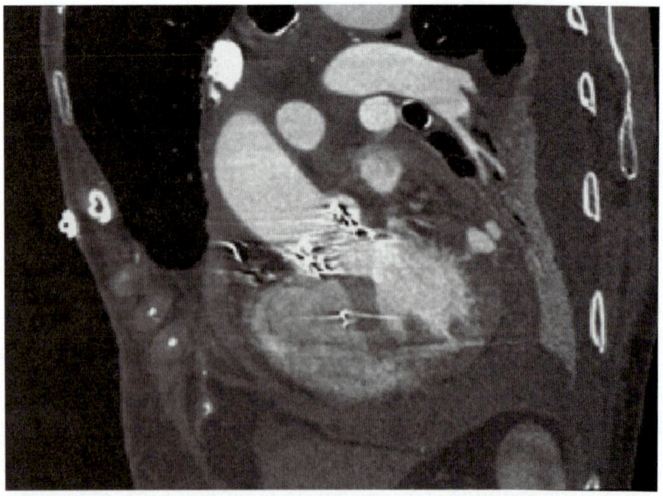

Fig. 37.10: *Sagittal CT reconstruction of the thorax showing the implanted aortic valve. The left ventricle free wall defect with small pseudoaneurysm is also again noted*

properties of implantation and ready availability in a variety of sizes. There is less thrombogenicity with no need for long-term anticoagulation. Durability remains a problem as noted above. They are considered the valve of choice for elderly patients. The cutoff age may also be influenced by factors that may affect expected life expectancy, such as associated coronary artery disease. They may also be a consideration in younger patients in whom anticoagulation may be relatively contraindicated. Continued improvements in technique and perioperative care have resulted in improved results for reoperations to the extent that limited durability of a valve should not completely preclude its use.

Stentless valves are RELATIVELY new, implying that long-term data in large numbers are yet to be determined. In terms of availability and durability, they should still be considered equivalent to the stented tissue valves. The major advantage over a stented valve is the improvement in effective orifice size for any given annulus. At least one form of this group of valves has the added ability to be implanted as an aortic root with subsequent reimplantation of the coronary arteries. This is at the cost of increased technical requirements and associated increased perioperative complications such as bleeding, heart block, and valve dysfunction. The possible need for associated cardiac procedures such as concomitant coronary artery bypass may also be a factor. At this point, indications seem to be similar to those of stented tissue valves with the addition of use when the annulus size is smaller, leading to increased potential for mismatch if a stented or mechanical valve is

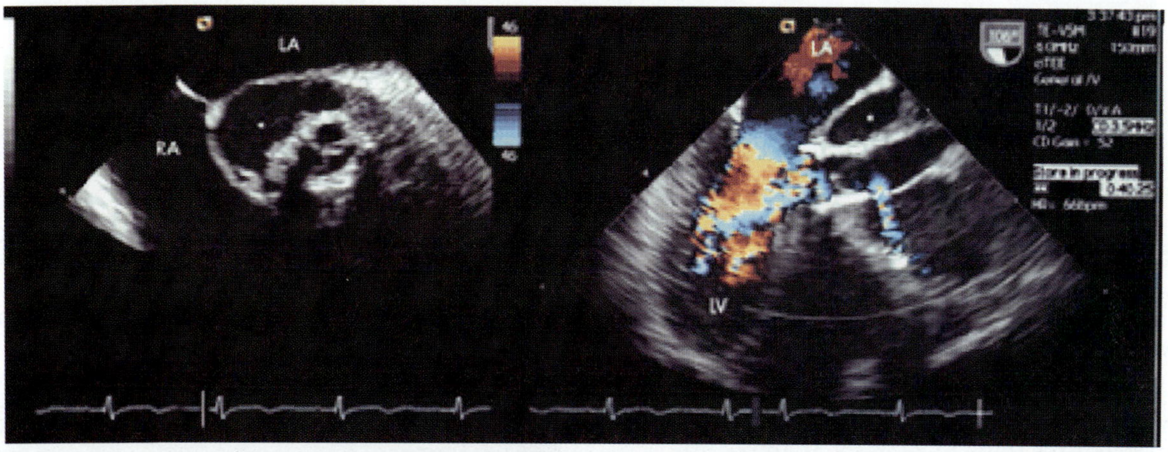

Fig. 37.11: *Composite xenograft failure. A transoesophageal two dimensional image in the short-axis (left panel) and the long-axis projection (right panel, colour Doppler image) shows an extended echo-free space (*) around the aortic composite graft with a bioprosthesis (Shelhigh porcine stentless aortic prosthesis 21). In the short-axis view, the left atrium (LA) and right atrium (RA) are depicted as well as the three cusp valve in the centre of the composite graft wall which itself is surrounded by haematoma (*). Both images are obtained during diastole (white lines on the ECG). There is moderately severe aortic insufficiency. Additionally, there is a leak at the right coronary artery reimplantation site. Intraoperatively, a dehiscence was also detected at the distal suture line of the composite graft. Both the distal and the right coronary cusp leakage caused the periaortic haematoma. It was suspected that a low grade endocarditis caused this situation. LV, left ventricle*

Table 37.4: *Indications for echocardiography in interventions for valvular heart disease and prosthetic valves*

Indication	*Class*
1. Assessment of the timing of valvular intervention based on ventricular compension, function, and/or severity of primary and secondary lesions	1
2. Selection of alternative therapies for mitral valve disease such as balloon valvuloplasty, operative valve repair, valve replacement	1
3. Use of echocardiography (especially TEE) in guiding the performance of interventional techniques and surgery (e.g. balloon valvotomy and valve repair) for valvular disease	
4. Postintervention baseline studies for valve function (early) and ventricular remodelling (late)	1
5. Reevaluation of patients with valve replacement with changing clinical signs and symptoms, suspected prosthetic dysfunction (stenosis, regurgitation) or thrombosis	11
6. Routine reevaluation study after baseline studies of patients with valve replacements with mild to moderate ventricular dysfunction without changing clinical signs or symptoms	11a
7. Routine reevaluation at the time of increased failure rate of a bioprosthesis without clinical evidence of prosthetic dysfunction	11b
8. Routine reevaluation of patients with valve replacements without suspicion of valvular dysfunction and unchanged clinical signs and symptoms	111
9. Patients whose clinical status precludes therapeutic interventions	111

Type of valve	Aortic prosthesis		Mitral prosthesis	
	Normal findings	Abnormal findings	Normal findings	Abnormal findings
Caged-ball (Starr-Edwards)	OC S_1 CC P_2 SEM	Aortic diastolic murmur Decreased intensity of opening or closing click	CC OC S_2 SEM	Low-frequency apical diastolic murmur high-frequency holosystolic murmur
Single tilting-disk (Bjŏrk-Shiley or Medtronic-Hall)	OC CC S_1 P_2 SEM OM	Decreased intensity of closing click	CC S_2 OC DM	High-frequency holosystolic murmur Decreased intensity of closing click
Bileaflet-tilting-disk (St.Jude medical)	OC CC S_1 P_2 SEM	Aortic diastolic murmur Decreased intensity of closing click	CC S_2 OC DM	High-frequency holosystolic murmur Decreased intensity of closing click
Heterograft bioprosthesis (Hancock or Carpentier-Edwards)	S_1 AC P_2 SEM	Aortic diastolic murmur	MC S_2 MO SEM DM	High-frequency holosystolic murmur

Fig. 37.12: *Acoustic characteristics of various mechanical and bioprosthetic valves. (From Vongpatanasin W, Hillis LD, et al. Prosthetic heart valves. N Engl J Med 1996;355:410)*

used. They would be considered an alternative to annular enlarging procedures (Figs 37.7–37.13, 37.16, 37.18).

As mentioned, homografts are human aortic valves that are typically cryopreserved and usually come as an entire aortic root. Currently, they are considered much in the way stentless valves are, with very similar modes of implantation, the preferred being root replacement. The major drawbacks are limited durability and limited availability. Pulmonary homografts are also now available but used primarily for replacement in the right ventricular outflow tract Autografts as used in the Ross procedure represent the most technically demanding of the aortic replacement procedures. This procedure is rather uniquely suited for the pediatric population in that growth of the autograft has been noted, there is no need for warfarin anticoagulation, and durability is rather good though also limited (Table 37.4).

Aortic valve repair may be possible in selected circumstances. Isolated perforation of the leaflet may be patched. Leaflets may be intact and the pathology may lie in dilation of the sinotubular junction. Appropriate-sized graft replacement of the ascending aorta may correct the insufficiency. Aortic valve repair is limited in part by the technical demands but more commonly by the lack of appropriate pathology.

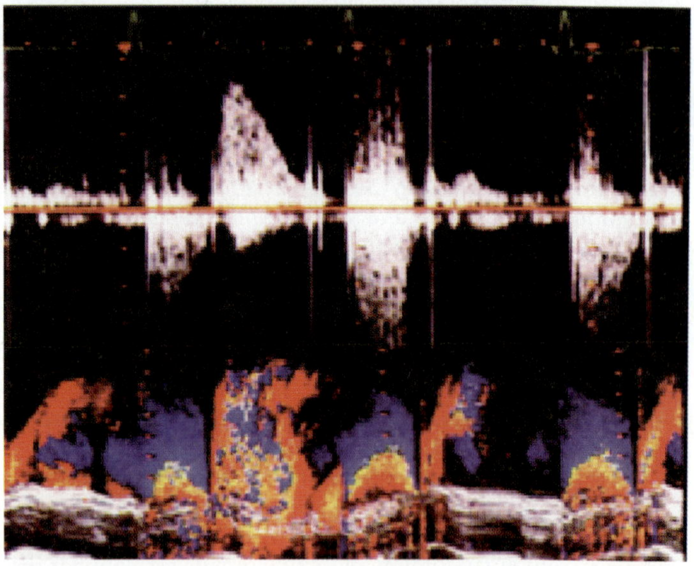

Fig. 37.13: *Doppler color flow through malfunctioning Carpenter-Edward prosthetic aortic valve showing a cyclic (every 30–60 beats) failure in closure of leaflet resulting in acute massive aortic regurgitation. In these sporodic cycles contineous wave Doppler (upper panel showed the abscence of closing click followed by signal of acute massive regurgitation (slope of the diastolic regurgitant jet >3 m/s) with an increase in the velocity of forward aortic flow in subsequent systole. Color flow showed a two dimensional display of the aortic regurgitation jet (mid-panel) in patient with acute severe breathlessness and intermittent syncopal episodes*

MITRAL VALVE DISEASE

Replacement therapy for mitral valve disease follows much the same guidelines as for aortic valve disease, although

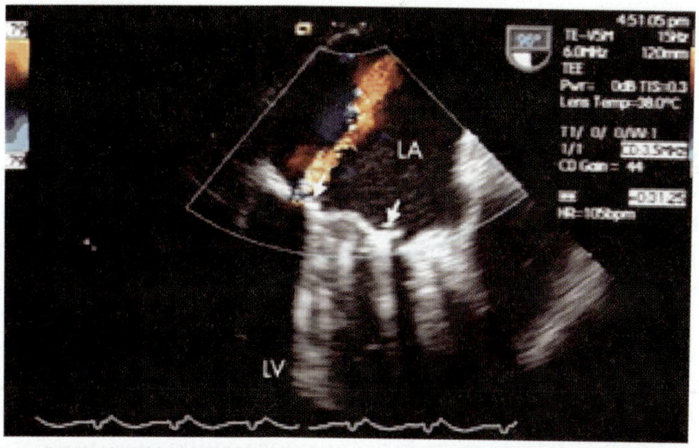

Fig. 37.14: *Paravalvar leak. Transoesophageal, two dimensional, colour Doppler image (longitudinal section) of the left atrium (LA) and left ventricle (LV) showing a bileaflet mitral prosthesis with the sewing ring marked by arrows and a posteriorly located paravalvar leak causing mild mitral regurgitation*

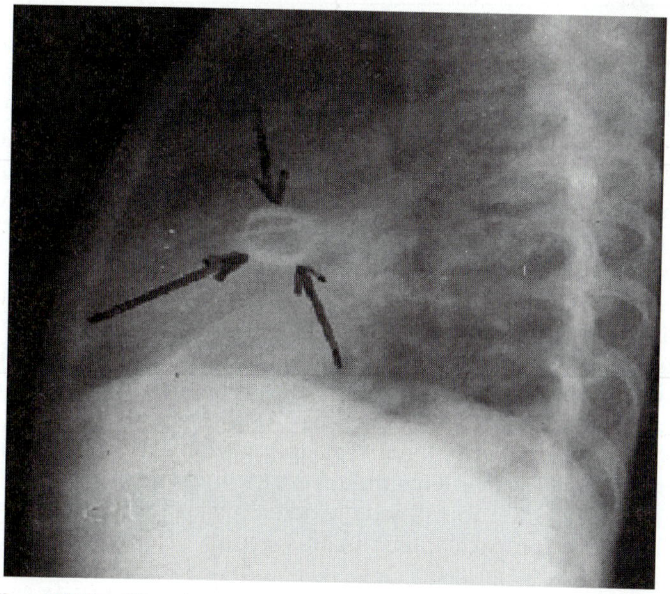

Fig. 37.15: *Showing anatomical location of Björk Shilley mitral valve visualised in lateral position of X-ray chest PA view with mitral valve replacement in a patient with calcified native mitral valve*

the options are commonly limited to stented tissue valves or mechanical prosthesis. In the course of mitral valve replacement, the concept of chordal preservation is now generally accepted. Maintaining a connection between the valves, usually the annulus, and the papillary muscle has been felt to improve long-term left ventricular (LV) function. A variety of techniques have been described, including imbrication of portions of the leaflet with the chorda still attached to the papillary muscle, or placement of artificial chordae from the annulus to the muscle.

Repair of the mitral valve, however, has much greater applicability compared with aortic valve surgery and should be considered the first choice when possible. Many more variables are involved including the exact nature of the valve pathology, the experience of the surgeon and the availability of methods to assess the immediate results, such as intraoperative transesophageal echocardiography (TEE). Many of the techniques of valve repair are well described. A major trend in mitral valve surgery in recent years has been the treatment of what may be thought of as secondary mitral valve disease. Advancements in mitral valve repair techniques and myocardial protection have prompted reconsideration of the concept of correcting mitral regurgitation (MR) in the setting of severe ventricular dysfunction. Specifically, the group of patients under discussion here are those felt to have MR secondary to changes in the ventricle with relatively normal appearing leaflets (Box 37.2).

Radio-opaque marker studies of components of the mitral valve in vivo demonstrate the dynamic nature of each component and suggest that the valve may have a role other than just maintaining one way flow from the atria to the ventricle. In this specific subset of patients, the regurgitation is a result of and not the cause of the cardiomyopathy. Selected subsets of cardiomyopathic hearts regardless of the etiology (idiopathic, ischemic) remodel toward a dilated state. The two major effects of the cardiomyopathy on the mitral valve are dilation of the annulus (primarily posterior) and tethering of the leaflets by the chordae and papillary muscle toward the apex. The leaflets and chordae themselves are generally not altered. The effect is malcoaptation of the leaflets resulting in progressive regurgitation. This corresponds to a type I and III defect in the Carpentier classification. In years past, conventional wisdom was that correction of MR (typically via replacement) in the setting of severe LV dysfunction was contraindicated because of

Box 37.2: *Management of prosthetic valves: key points*

- Management of valve prostheses (particularly in patients with valve regurgitation) begins with selection of the optimal time point for valve replacement
- Aortic prosthesis—patient mismatch (effective orifice area < 0.85 cm^2/m^2) is prevented by choosing a properly sized prosthesis ring diameter
- Generally, anticoagulation in patients with aortic bileaflet prostheses should be kept at an INR 2.0–3.0; other mechanical valves and bioprostheses 3 months postoperatively at 2.5–3.5
- Bleeding in patients with valve prostheses is more frequent than valve thrombosis
- Prosthetic valve thrombosis in haemodynamically stable patients should be primarily treated with thrombolytics
- Oral anticoagulation throughout pregnancy is related to a 6–7% rate of embryopathy
- Intravenous heparin during the first trimester of pregnancy eliminates the risk of embryopathy, but is related to a 9% risk of valve thrombosis

the poor results. The theory was that the "pop-off" mechanism of the regurgitant mitral valve was disrupted leading to overt cardiac failure (Figs 37.14, 37.15, 37.19, 37.24, 37.25).

In 1995, Bolling et al. reported surgical results on 16 patients with LV ejection fraction (LVEF) 9–25% in functional New York Heart Association (NYHA) class IV with severe MR. All underwent ring mitral annuloplasty and, where indicated, tricuspid valve annuloplasty and coronary artery bypass. There were no perioperative deaths and the 1-year actuarial survival was 75%. On medium-term follow-up, the survivors were in NYHA class I or II with a mean LVEF of 25% and overall reduction in hospitalization when compared with their preoperative status. Subsequent longer-term follow-up as well as reports by others have shown similar results. In general, operative morbidity and mortality have been low and there has been functional improvement in this group of chronically ill patients.

The typical patient under consideration for this type of therapy is in NYHA class III-IV under poor control, with LVEF generally less than 30%; there is severe MR with normal appearing leaflets, no evidence of perforation, significant thickening, or prolapse. One caveat concerns the assessment of the MR, and generally it has been a combination of catheterization, TEE and transthoracic echocardiography. Optimization of the patient's congestive failure is recommended prior to surgery.

The primary procedure involves an undersized annuloplasty with one of the many commercially available rings or bands. Undersizing means the usual methods of determining ring size by the intracommissural distance or the area of the anterior leaflet are replaced by taking the ring one to two sizes smaller than that determined by the above methods, or by simply using the smallest of the commercial rings available.

Intraoperative use of TEE is essential to evaluate the procedure although one is cautioned regarding the intraoperative assessment of MR prior to annuloplasty. As the MR can be very dynamic in nature in these patients, the conditions of general anesthesia including alterations in preload and afterload may reduce the severity of the regurgitation. Provocative maneuvers such as aggressively increasing the afterload may help in this assessment. More important is the knowledge of the status of the valve in the awake, ambulatory setting.

Subsequent mitral stenosis has been rare, in part because the rings or bands used are still within a reasonable size range and the leaflets themselves usually are normal. The incidence of systolic anterior motion is also very low even though the smaller rings are used. This is related to the altered ventricular geometry in these patients, which increases the angle between the aortic and the mitral valve.

There is evidence that annuloplasty or other valve repair is superior to replacement in a variety of ways including improved short- and long-term function. Further support lies in the historic reports of the poor results of mitral valve replacement in the setting of severely depressed function. However, it is believed some of this was related to the then traditional method of total excision of the valve and subvalvar apparatus. Improved perioperative management and replacement with chordal preservation has prompted some to revisit this issue. A recent report assessed 44 patients with MR and LV dysfunction (EF < 35%) over a 9-year period; 27 (61%) were in NYHA class III-IV. The etiology was ischemia (30%), valvar (40%), or dilated cardiomyopathy (30%). Mitral valve repair was performed in 80%; the remainder underwent mitral valve replacement. Of the replacement group, most were done for primary valve pathology, all with chordal preservation. In this study, mitral valve replacement was not demonstrated to increase mortality over repair. The experience of other centers appears to confirm this. Improved recognition of the role the mitral valve plays in overall ventricular function has led some to adopt a more aggressive approach to moderate mitral valve regurgitation in those patients with coronary artery disease undergoing coronary artery bypass. Experience and improved perioperative care, together with the ability to correct the regurgitation without replacement, has resulted in significant reductions in short- and long-term morbidity and mortality. As always, these studies suggest trends that ultimately may require randomized studies to confirm. These should be considered early data in the growing options for surgery in the treatment *of* cardiomyopathy and heart failure.

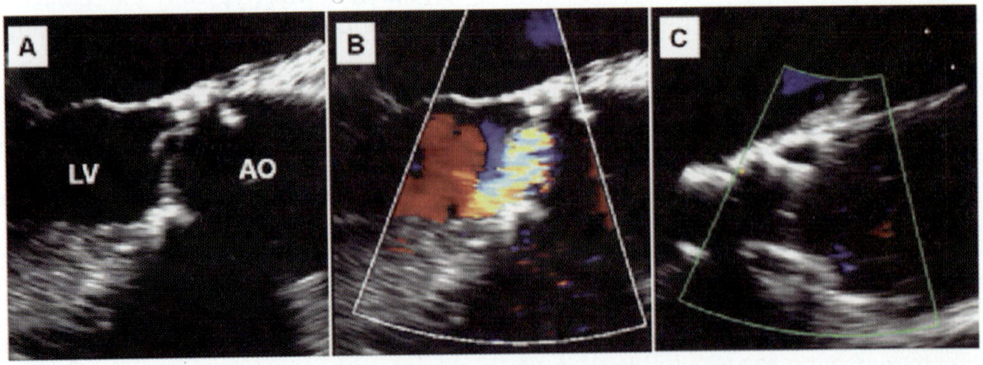

Fig. 37.16: *Echocardiographic results of "valve-in-valve" implantation in a patient with degenerated aortic bioprosthesis. (A and B) Carpentier-Edwards bioprosthesis with severe aortic regurgitation. (C) absence of residuel regurgitation after Medtronic CoreValve implantation. AO, aorta; LV, left ventricle*

Table 37.5: *Normal Doppler values of prosthetic valves*

Prosthetic valve	*Peak velocity (m/sec)*	*Mean gradient (mmHg)*
Aortic position		
Starr-Edwards	3.1 ± 0.5	24 ± 4
Björk-Shiley	2.5 ± 0.6	14 ± 5
St. Jude	3.0 ± 0.8	11 ± 6
Medtronic-Hall	2.6 ± 0.3	12 ± 3
Aortic hormograft	0.8 ± 0.4	7 ± 3
Hancock	2.4 ± 0.4	11 ± 2
Carpentier-Edwards	2.4 ± 0.5	14 ± 6
Mitral position		
Starr-Edwards	1.8 ± 0.4	5 ± 2
Blöck-Shiley	1.6 ± 0.3	5 ± 2
St. Jude	1.6 ± 0.3	5 ± 2
Medtronic-Hall	1.7 ± 0.3	3 ± 1
Hancock	1.5 ± 0.3	4 ± 2
Carpentier-Edwards	1.8 ± 0.2	7 ± 2

Modified from Notlestad SY, Zabalgoritia M. In: Otto CM. The practice of clinical echocardiography, 1997, p. 803.

Table 37.6: *Recommended anticoagulation therapy for patients with mechanical prosthetic valves*

Level of risk	*Prosthesis type*	*Recommended INR*
Low	Single-tilting disk	3.0–4.0
	Double-tilting disk	2.5–3.0
High	Caged disk	3.0–4.5
	Caged ball	3.0–4.5
	Multiple prostheses	3.0–4.5

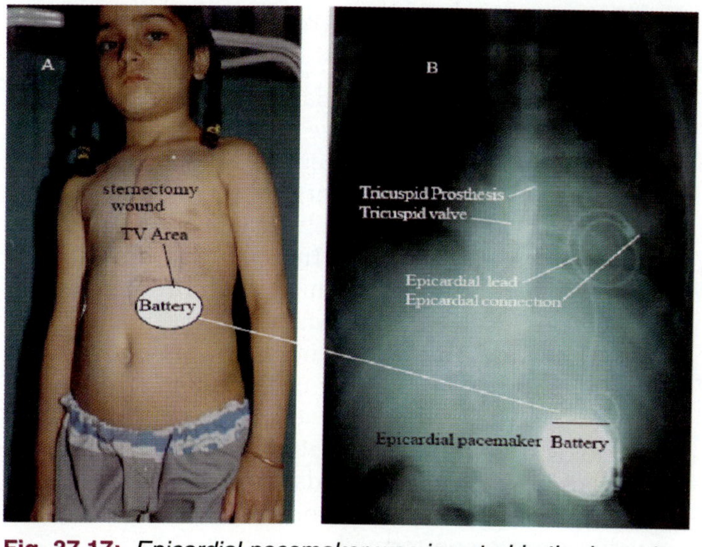

Fig. 37.17: *Epicardial pacemaker was inserted in the heart in a 6-years-old child with primary tricuspid regurgitation while during fixing the prosthetic tricuspid valve she developed complete heart block and life was saved by selectively implanting the pacer (A). (B) shows the X-ray of chest visualising tricupid prosthesis and epicardial lead has been shown connected with the battery placed into the abdominal region*

TRICUSPID VALVE DISEASE

In many cases of MR secondary to cardiomyopathy, associated tricuspid regurgitation may also be seen as a consequence of ventricular dilation and elevated pulmonary artery pressures. Aggressive concomitant therapy for tricuspid valve regurgitation is recommended. It has been felt in the past that with correction of the MR, the pulmonary pressures should fall resulting in the improvement of the tricuspid insufficiency. This is not immediate, and in some cases does not occur. Therefore, a tricuspid annuloplasty should be performed if moderate to severe regurgitation exists (Figs 37.17, 37.26 and 37.27).

In other cases of tricuspid disease, many of the same principles apply as with mitral disease. Often, annular dilation leading to regurgitation is amenable to one of several annuloplasty techniques. Replacement, if needed, is usually limited to either a mechanical or stented tissue valve. In general, the preference is for tissue valves. The lower pressure involved as well as the lower flow for a given area create increased risk for thrombosis with a mechanical valve. These factors may also contribute to less stress and increased durability for the tissue valves.

Transesophageal Echocardiography

A key to the discussion of current valve surgery is the use of intraoperative TEE. In many centers, its use has become routine for cardiac surgical procedures. Specific for valve surgery, it can provide an improved visualization of the valves in the functioning state as an aid to assessing pathology. Following any valve procedure, repair or replacement, it can provide immediate feedback on the functioning of the new or repaired valve prior to completion of the operation. It can also be an aid in assessing the amount of retained intracardiac air to help guide appropriate measures (Figs 37.21–37.23).

One caveat for the use of TEE is the need for experienced operators. In selected cases, cardiologists are called on to assist in interpretation in the operating room. With increasing frequency, cardiac anesthesiologists are being trained in many aspects of TEE use. One also needs to be cognizant of the changes in hemodynamics in the anesthetized patient that may alter the appearance of valve function. The most common example is in the subset of patients with functional MR. In some cases, decreased afterload may lead to apparent improvement in the degree of regurgitation. Maneuvers such as volume loading or pharmacologically increased afterload may allow better assessment of the pathology.

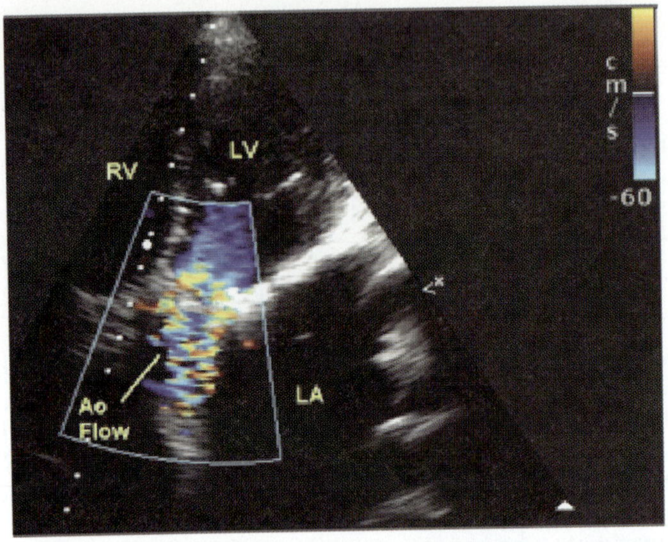

Fig. 37.18: *Turbulent aortic flow in prosthetic aortic valve. Some turbulence can occur even without prosthetic valve dysfunction. Basically, a prosthetic valve in the aortic position is always partially obstructive, more so when a small prosthesis is placed as in aortic stenosis with a small aortic annulus. This is often called patient-prosthesis mismatch. Hence, it is worthwhile documenting gradients serially so that any significant rise can alert the possibility of new obstruction developing like thrombus or pannus formation*

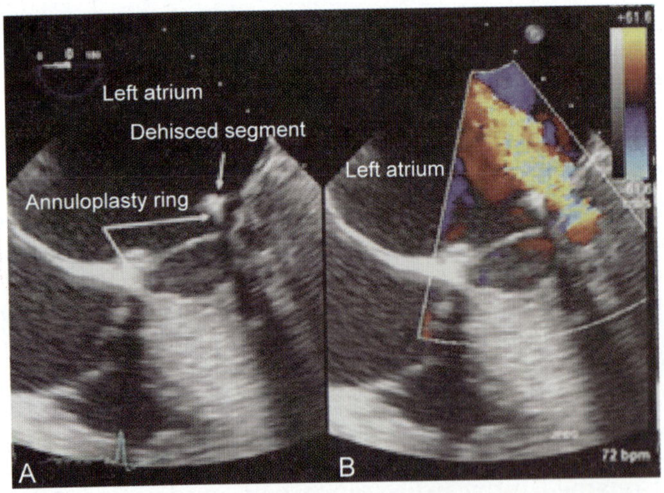

Fig. 37.19: *Dehisced Colvin-Galloway Ring, 2D Imaging (A) A two dimensional (2D) transesophageal echocardiography (TEE) image showing a dehiscence of the posterior aspect of the mitral annuloplasty ring. The exact ring type cannot be delineated, and the correct assessment of the dehiscence characteristics cannot be depicted. (B) A 2D TEE color Doppler image showing that the mitral regurgitation is para-ring (outside the annuloplasty ring but within the original mitral valve annulus)*

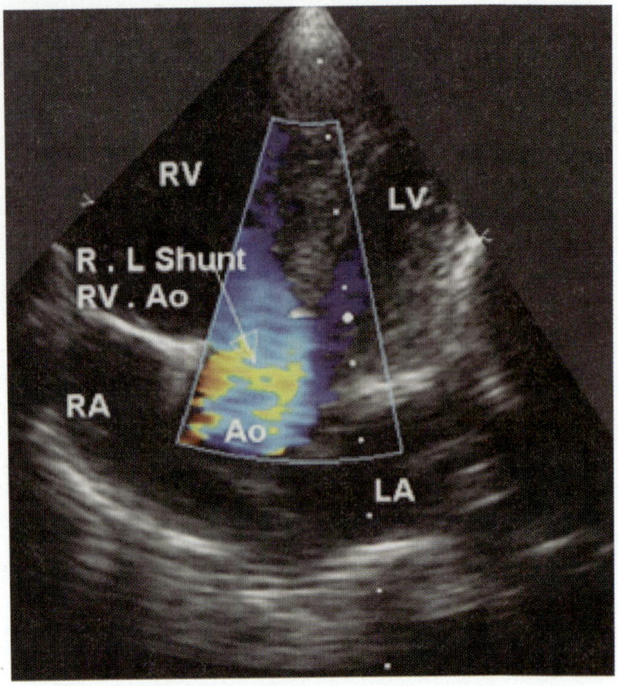

Fig. 37.20: *Apical five chamber view in tetralogy of Fallot with colour flow mapping (Colour Doppler imaging) in systole with right to left shunt across the VSD. Blue stream moving from right ventricle across the VSD to the aorta is clearly visualised in this frame. There is also a blue stream from the left ventricle to the aorta*

MINIMALLY INVASIVE SURGERY

Another issue that has gathered increasing interest in cardiac surgery and in particular, valve procedures, has been that of minimally invasive surgery. In general, this refers to techniques that are intended to reduce the short- and long-term effects of the surgical procedure. In most cases of valve surgery, this involves smaller or alternative incisions or approaches to the valve coupled with additional technology. Examples include a partial sternotomy for aortic or mitral valve surgery, limited right thoracotomy aided by video/endoscopic assistance with alternative means of providing cardiopulmonary bypass, and robotic assistance in mitral valve surgery as the pinacle of technologic assistance. Limitations to this trend include the increased technical demands; increased costs related to the technology and limitations on what concomitant procedures can be performed.

VALVE DYSFUNCTION AND COMPLICATIONS RELATED TO PROSTHETIC VALVES

A. Atrial fibrillation

Up to 50% of patients undergoing valve surgery experience postoperative atrial fibrillation. Management of atrial fibrillation:

1. In patients without a previous history of atrial fibrillation, the arrhythmia is often self-limited.

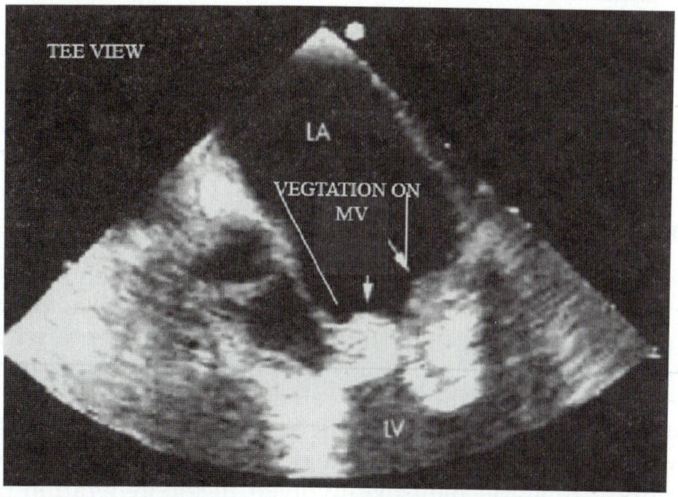

Fig. 37.21: *TEE view showing large vegetation (arrow) in the mitral valve secondary to fungal endocarditis*

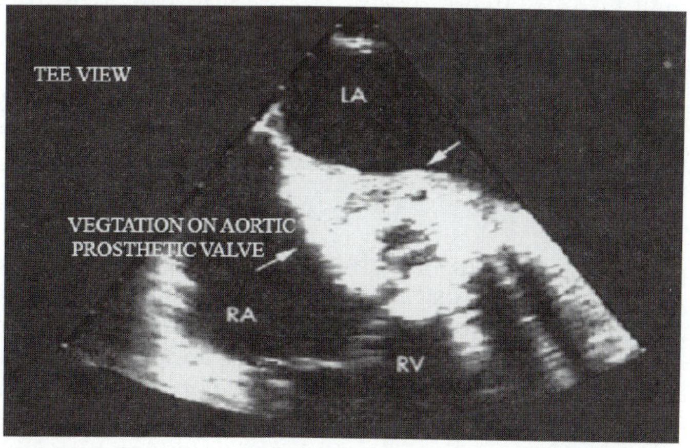

Fig. 37.22: *TEE view showing periannular abscess arrows in a prosthetic valve endocarditis*

2. For patients with persistent atrial fibrillation beyond 24 hours, anticoagulation, direct current cardioversion, and a short course of antiarrhythmic therapy are warranted.
3. Beta blockade or amiodarone prophylaxis has been found to reduce the incidence of postsurgical atrial fibrillation.

B. Conduction Disturbances

High-grade heart block requiring permanent pacemaker implantation has been described in 2–3% of patients after valve replacement and 8% following repeat valve surgery. It is caused by trauma to the bundle of His or from postoperative edema of the periannular tissue. Aortic or mitral annular calcification, preoperative conduction disturbance, advanced age, infectious endocarditis, and tricuspid valve surgery are associated with higher rates of postoperative conduction abnormalities leading to permanent pacemaker implantation.

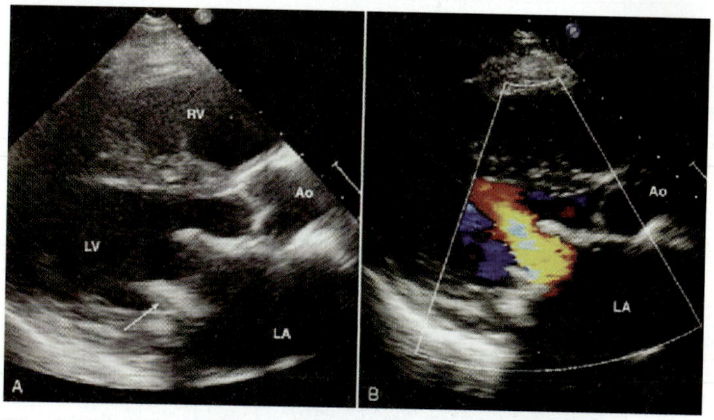

Fig. 37.23: *Bioprosthetic mitral valve, parasternal long-axis view of a stented mitral bioprosthetic valve. (A) The valve struts (arrow) Protrude the ventricular chamber, with antegrade flow seen with color Doppler (B) Directed toward the ventricular septum*

C. Endocarditis

Approximately 3–6% of patients with prosthetic heart valves will experience prosthetic valve endocarditis. Prosthetic valve endocarditis is typically associated with large vegetations since microorganisms are sheltered from the host defense mechanisms (Figs 37.21 and 37.22).

1. Early prosthetic valve endocarditis <60 days following implantation) is typically caused by *Staphylococcus epidermidis*. The clinical course is often fulminant, with high mortality rates ranging from 20–70%.
2. Late prosthetic valve endocarditis occurs most commonly in patients with multiple prostheses and bioprosthetic valves, especially in the aortic position. Its clinical course resembles that of native valve endocarditis. Streptococci are the most common infectious agents, followed by Gram-negative bacteria, enterococci, and *S. epidermidis*.

Box 37.3: *Follow-up in prosthetic valves: key points*

- Immediately after valve surgery, Doppler echocardiography should be obtained in all patients
- The first outpatient workup should include the patient's history, physical examination, ECG, chest X-ray, complete blood count, creatinine, electrolytes, lactase dehydrogenase, INR and Doppler echocardiography
- Follow-up visits in asymptomatic patients without complications or new murmurs can be performed at yearly intervals and without Doppler echocardiography
- Complications after valve replacement: thromboembolic bleeding, ventricular failure, pulmonary hypertension, sudden death, arrhythmias, conduction abnormalities, mechanical complications and infective endocarditis
- Transvalvar or paravalvar regurgitation is detected by Doppler echocardiography; the latter may be harmless, but may represent a haemodynamic problem or may be a sign of prosthetic endocarditis
- Infections of prosthetic heart valves are a very serious complication (0.1–2.3% per patient year). In suspected endocarditis, the threshold for transoesophageal echocardiography should be low

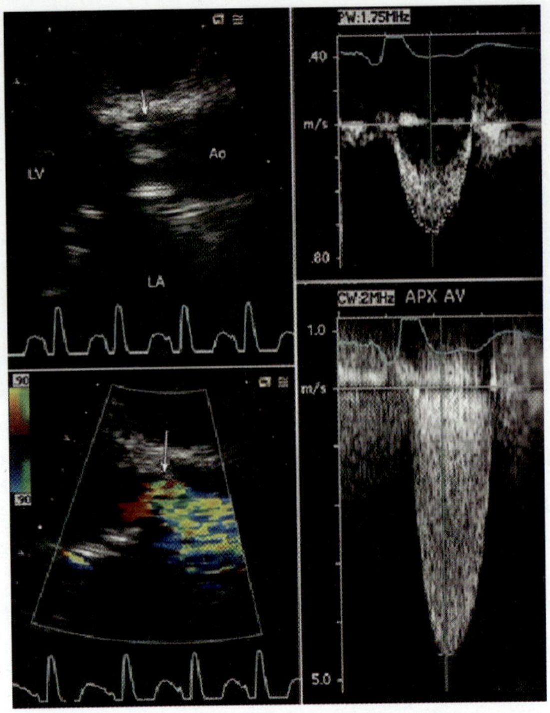

Fig. 37.24: *Bioprosthetic aortic valve stenosis. LV outflow diameter is measured in a parasternal long-axis view in mid-systole (2.7 cm) (upper left) with color Doppler (lower left) demonstrating increased flow velocity at the valve level even though the leaflets are not well seen. LV outflow tract velocity (0.6 m/sec) is recorded with pulsed Doppler from an apical approach (upper right). The highest CW Doppler signal of flow across the valve (4.6 m/s) was recorded from the apical the valve (4.6 m/s) was recorded from the apical window (lower right). In this example, the velocity of 4.6 m/s, velocity ratio of 0.13, and calculated valve area of 0.75 cm², all are consistent with severe prosthetic stenosis*

3. TEE is the imaging modality of choice with sensitivity of 95% and specificity of 90% in diagnosis. It is useful also in detecting complications including abscess, tissue invasion, dehiscence, and fistula formation; and monitoring the efficacy of medical therapy.

Medical therapy: Medical cure of prosthetic valve endocarditis caused by staphylococci, Gram-negative organisms, or fungi is rare. Streptococcal prosthetic valve endocarditis responds to medical therapy alone in 50% of cases. Patients with mechanical prosthetic valve endocarditis should continue to receive anticoagulation. In the absence of anticoagulation, prosthetic valve endocarditis is associated with an up to 50% incidence of stroke. Continuing anticoagulation for patients with prosthetic valve endocarditis is associated with a 10% incidence of cerebral embolization. There is no conclusive evidence for increased hemorrhage with warfarin in patients with prosthetic valve endocarditis.

Surgical therapy: Valve replacement surgery is indicated in the setting of:

1. Persistent bacteremia despite intravenous antibiotics
2. Tissue invasion or fistula formation
3. Recurrent embolization
4. Fungal infection
5. Prosthesis dehiscence or obstruction
6. New or worsening heart block
7. Congestive heart failure.

D. Hemolysis

Subclinical hemolysis is present in many patients with mechanical valves but rarely results in significant anemia.

Clinical hemolysis occurs in 6–15% of patients with caged ball valves but is uncommon with normal bioprosthetic or tilting disk valves. Clinical hemolysis is also associated with multiple prosthetic valves, small prostheses, periprosthetic leaks and prosthetic valve endocarditis. Mechanisms involved in the generation of hemolysis.

Laboratory examination and diagnostic testing: TEE is the most widely used diagnostic technique although cinefluoroscopy can be used to document restriction in occluder mobility. No imaging modality, however, can clearly differentiate thrombus from pannus. Frequently they coexist. Echocardiographic features suggestive of thrombus include soft, irregular or mobile mass.

Medical Therapy

1. Fibrinolytic therapy is considered the treatment of choice for right-sided prosthetic valve thrombosis because the consequences of distal embolization are less severe than in left-sided prosthesis. Streptokinase and urokinase are the most commonly used agents. Fibrinolytic therapy has an initial success rate of 82%, overall thromboembolism rate of 12%, and a 5% incidence of major bleeding episodes. Similar rates of success (80–86%) and complications (10% cerebrovascular accident) have been described for left-sided prosthetic valve thrombosis. Thrombolysis may be a reasonable alternative to surgery for mitral or aortic prosthetic valve thrombosis in patients with a small thrombus burden, particularly if there is hemodynamic compromise.
   a. The recommended dosage for streptokinase is a 250,000-U bolus given over 30 minutes, followed by an infusion of 100,000 U/h.
   b. Urokinase is given as an infusion of 4,400 U/kg per hour.
   c. Duration of thrombolytic therapy has varied between 2 hours and 120 hours; however, thrombolysis should be stopped if there is no hemodynamic improvement after 24–72 hours. TEE is useful in assessment of progress.
   d. Following successful thrombolysis, close follow-up of anticoagulation along with serial Doppler echocardiography on an individual basis is recommended.
2. Anticoagulation with heparin and warfarin is generally recommended for small thrombus (<5 mm). The regimen consists of intravenous heparin followed by subcutaneous heparin 17,000 U twice a day and warfarin (INR 2.5–3.5) for up to 3 months.

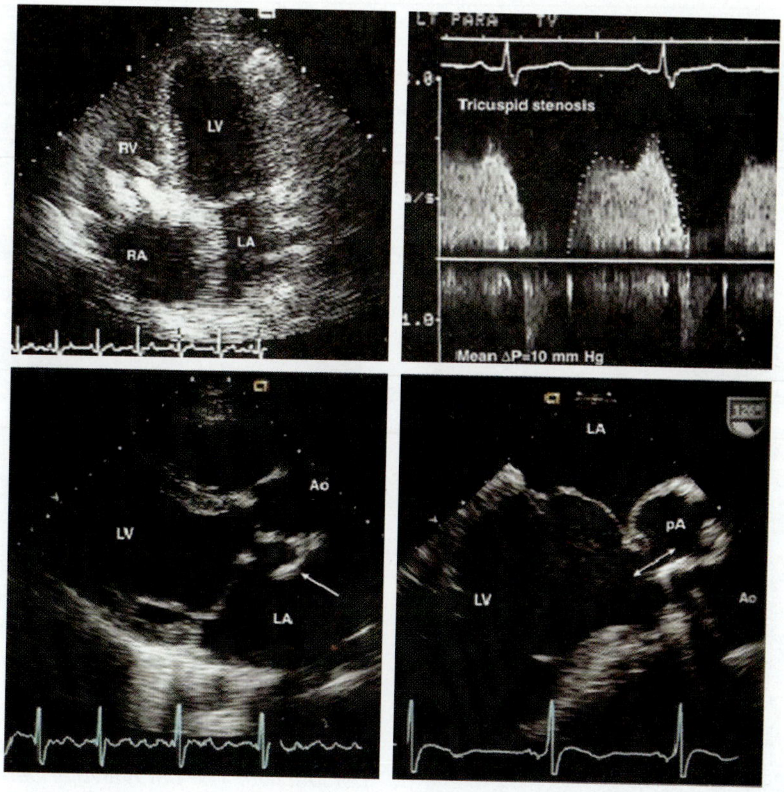

Fig. 37.25: *Aneurysm of the mitral aortic intravalvular fibrosa. In a 20-year-old adolescent with a mechanical aortic valve replacement, the TTE longer image (left) shows a pseudoaneurysm between the posterior aspect of the aortic prosthesis and the base of the anterior mitral leaflet (arrow). The TEE image (right) shows the narrow neck of the pseudoanurysm (double arrow). Doppler color flow imaging showed flow into the pseudoaneurysm the LV systole (with flow back into the LV), and the associated collapse of the pseudoaneurysm in diastole*

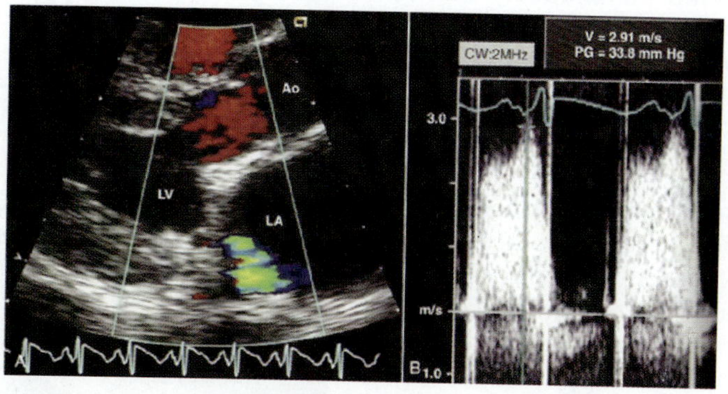

Fig. 37.26: *Mechanical mitral valve thrombosis. Mechanical mitral valve, inadequate anticoagulation, and pulmonary edema, the TTE parasternal long-axis view (A) shows only mild regurgitation. However, CW Doppler from the apex. (B) shows a very antegrade velocity with a maximum pressure gradient (PG) of 34 mmHg and mean gradient of 25 mmHg. Pressure half-time is difficult to estimate because the a-wave is superimposed on the diastolic deceleration slope. (From Stout KK, Otto CM: Pregnancy in women with valvular heart disease)*

Surgical approach: The lowest surgical mortality reported has been approximately 5%. The risk profile of the individual patient must be balanced against the expertise and experience at each center.

1. Valve replacement and debridement is generally performed for left-sided prosthetic valve thrombosis unless the thrombus is small or the patient has a prohibitive surgical risk.
2. Surgery is also indicated in the case of unsuccessful thrombolysis 24 hours following discontinuation of the infusion.

E. Dehiscence

Detachment of the sewing ring from the annulus may occur in the early postoperative period because of poor surgical techniques, excessive annular calcification, chronic steroid

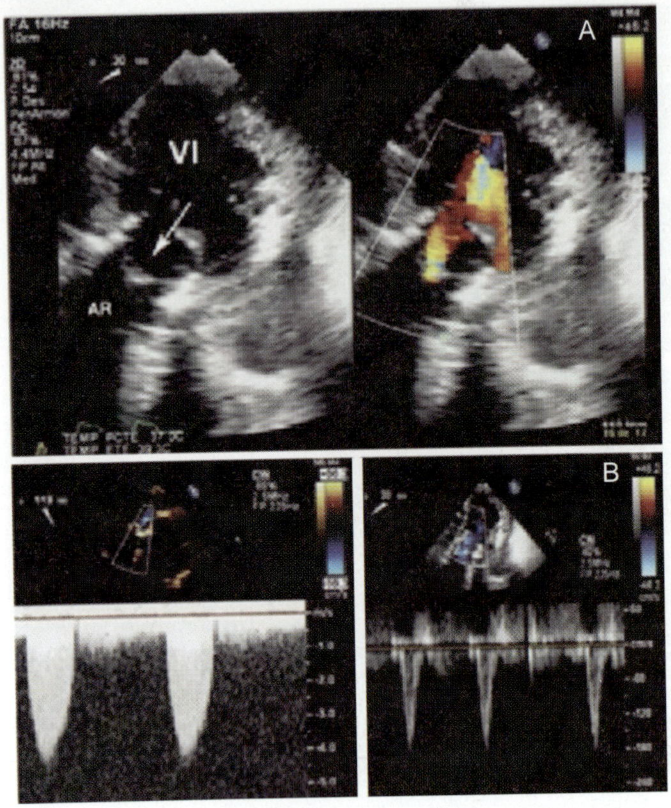

Fig. 37.27: *Aortic valve hemodynamic assessment before and after transthoracic implantation of the aortic valve prosthesis. (A) two dimensional deep transgastric transesophageal view (left) and color Doppler (right); the prosthesis is well positioned, the leaflets show coaptation, and there is mild central regurgitation. (B) spectral Doppler data obtained continuously during intraoperative transesophageal echocardiography before (left) and after (right) transthoracic implantation of the aortic valve prosthesis; note the normalization of the transvalvular flow velocity. AR, aortic root; LV, left ventricle*

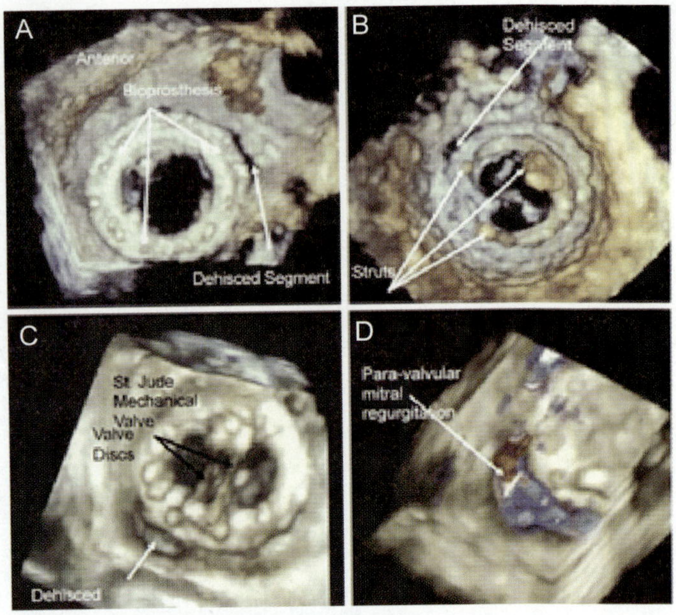

Fig. 37.28: *Dehisced Mitral Prostheses (A) En-face view from the left atrium. A bioprosthesis ring is seen, as well as the dehisced portion at the lateral aspect. (B) En-face view from the left ventricle; the bioprosthesis struts are noted. (C) Diastolic frame of a St. Jude mechanical prosthesis, seen from the left atrial perspective. The paravalvular dehisced portion can be seen. (D) Using full-volume color Doppler acquisition, the mitral regurgitation can be clearly seen originating at the dehisced portion*

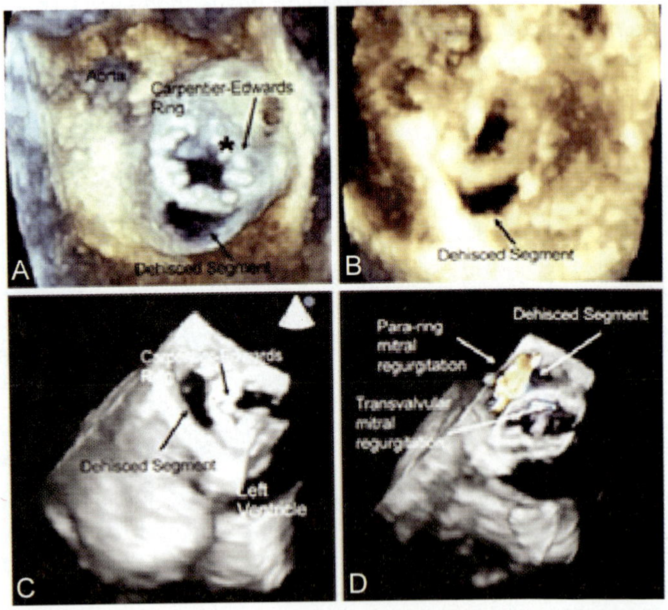

Fig. 37.29: *Dehisced Carpentier-Edwards ring, real-time three dimensional transesophageal echocardiography (A) En face view from the left atrium showing a dehisced Carpentier-Edwards ring. The typical characteristics of this ring can clearly be seen: a closed ring with a straightened superior segment (*). (B) En-face view from the left ventricular perspective. (C) Cropped image obtained from the full-volume image, clearly showing the mitral ring in place and the dehisced portion. (D) Full-volume color Doppler image showing two origins of the mitral regurgitation: para-ring mitral regurgitation through a dehisced segment and transvalvular mitral regurgitation from malcoaptation of the valve leaflets*

use, fragility of the annular tissue (particularly following prior valve operations), or infection. Late dehiscence.occurs mainly from infectious endocarditis. Abnormal rocking of the prosthesis on echocardiography or cinefluoroscopy is an indication for urgent surgery. (Some rocking may occur with preservation of the mitral valve apparatus.) (Fig. 37.25).

F. Patient-Prosthesis Mismatch

All prosthetic valves with the exception of stentless aortic homografts have effective orifices that are smaller than that of native valves. There is an inherent pressure gradient and relative stenosis with each prosthesis. Occasionally, when an inappropriately small prosthesis is placed, the ensuing low output may cause symptoms. This mismatch occurs most frequently after valve placement for aortic stenosis.

1. In a patient with a small annulus, a hemodynamically favorable prosthesis like the aortic homograft or the tilting disk valve is preferred. Alternatively, the annulus may be enlarged surgically in order to accommodate a prosthesis of acceptable size.

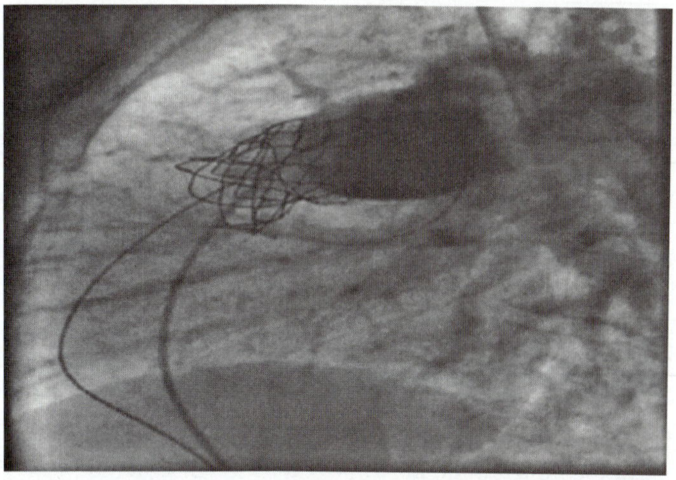

Fig. 37.30: *The melody pulmonary valve (medtronic) angiogram (lateral projection) of the main pulmonary artery after implantation of the melody valve*

2. Aortic prostheses less then 21 mm in diameter are not recommended for a large or physically active patient.
3. Surgery generally consists of replacement with a larger prosthesis and annular reconstruction.

G. Pannus Formation

Valve obstruction occurs in up to 5% of mechanical valves per year. Valve thrombosis and pannus formation are responsible for the majority of mechanical prosthesis obstructions. Little is known about the causes of fibroblastic proliferation in pannus formation. Foreign body reactions to the prosthesis, inadequate anticoagulation, endocarditis, and blood flow turbulence in the mitral position have been implicated as potential causes. TEE is generally required to identify the cause of prosthetic valve obstruction.

H. Embolic Stroke

Following an embolic stroke, the risk of recurrent stroke is approximately 1% per day for the first 2 weeks.

1. If no evidence of hemorrhage is detected on CT scan at 24–48 hours, intravenous heparin should be administered after a small to moderate embolic stroke. Maintaining anticoagulation reduces this risk of recurrent stroke to one-third but carries an increased risk of hemorrhagic transformation of 8–24%, particularly during the first 48 hours.
2. In patients with larger infarcts, anticoagulation should be withheld for 5–7 days.
3. Anticoagulation is withheld for 1–2 weeks in the setting of hemorrhagic transformation.
4. Aspirin or clopidogrel may be needed in the event of recurrent strokes despite adequate anticoagulation.
5. Rarely, reoperation with placement of a tissue valve is needed for recurrent embolization.

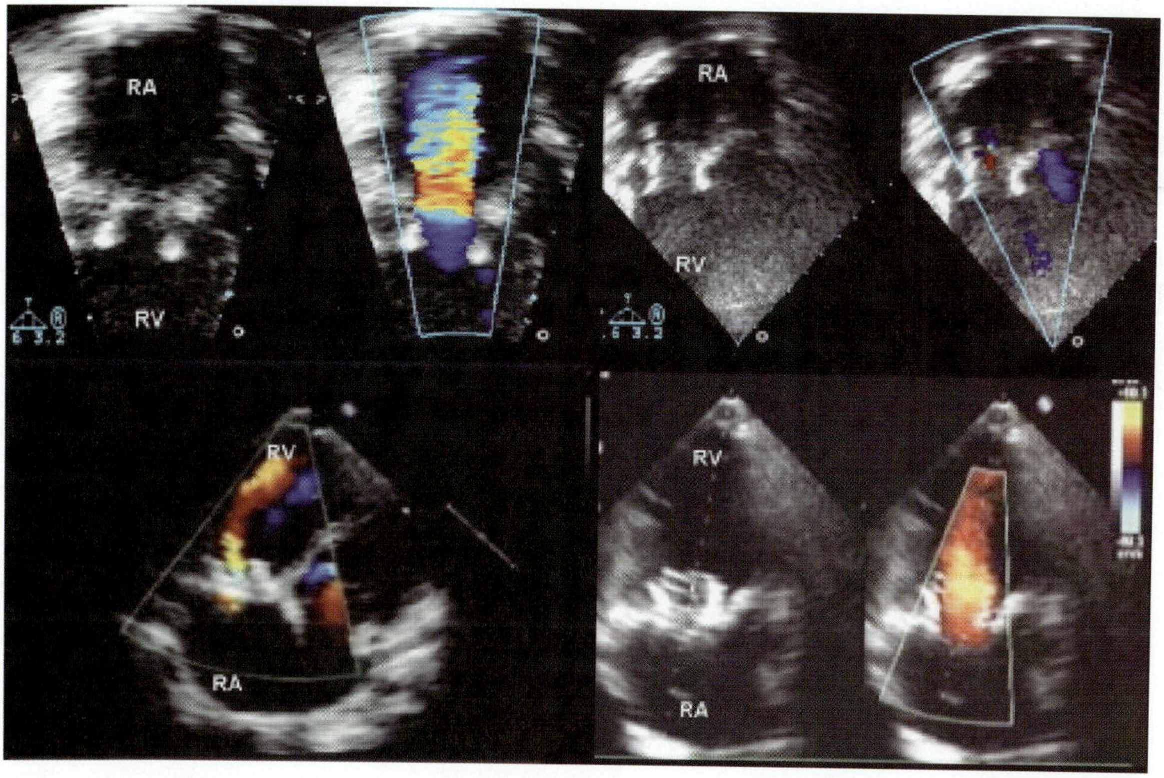

Fig. 37.31: *Before and after 2D and color Doppler transthoracic echocardiograms (Top). The severe regurgitation of the bioprosthesis in the orthotopic TV position (top left) is abolished after Melody valve insertion (top right). (Bottom) The bottom left image shows a narrow stenotic jet of color flow that is relieved after melody valve deployment (bottom right). 2D, two dimensional; RA, right atrium; RV, right ventricle*

Conclusion

There continues to be a growing number of options available for the treatment of valvular heart disease. Although the search for the ideal replacement continues, the variety currently available has improved the options. There is an increasing appreciation of the interrelationship between the mitral valve and the ventricle that go beyond the issues of stenosis or regurgitation alone. The increasing use and value of intraoperative TEE makes this modality almost mandatory. Finally, improvements are being sought to alter the approach to the operation with the hope of improving patient comfort and outcome.

BIBLIOGRAPHY

1. Grunkemeier GL, Wu Y: Our complication rates are lower than theirs: statistical critique of heart valve comparisons. J *Thome Cardio Sc Surg* 2003, 125:290–300.
2. Starr A, Fessler CL, Grunkemeier G: Heart valve replacement surgery: past, present and future. *Clin Exp Pharmaco Physiol* 2002,29:735–738.
3. Schoen FI: Future directions in tissue heart valves: impact of recent insights from biology and pathology. *J Heart Valve Dis* 1999,8:350–358.
4. Wemley lA, Crawford MH: Choosing a prosthetic heart valve. *Cardiol Clin* 1998, 16:491–504.
5. Fann II, Burdon TA: Are the indications for tissue valves different in 2001 and how do we communicate these changes to our cardiology colleagues? *Curr Opin Cardiol* 2001, 16: 126–135.
6. David TE: Aortic valve replacement with stentless pordne bioprostheses. *J Card Surg* 1998,13:344–351.
   Westaby S: Stentless bioprostheses in aortic root disease. *Semin Thomc Cardio Sc Surg* 2001,13:273–282.
7. Park SZ, Reardon MI: Current status of stentless aortic xenografts. *Curr Opin Cardiol* 2000, 15:74–81.
8. Kouchoukos NT: Aortic allografts and pulmonary autografts for replacement of tile aortic valve and aortic root. *Ann Thome Surg* 1999,67: 1846–1848.
9. Dacey L: Pulmonary homografts: current status. *Curr Opin Cardiol* 2000, 15:86–90.
10. Staab ME, Nishimura RA, Dearani IA: Aortic valve homo grafts inadults: a clinical perspective. *Mayo Clin Physiol* 1998,73: 231–238.
11. Elkins RC, Lane MM, McCue C: Ross operation in children: late results. *J Heart Valve Dis* 2001, 10:736–741.
12. Gatzoulis MA: Ross procedure: tile treatment of choice for aortic valve disease? *Int J Cardiol* 1999, 71:205–206.
13. Reardon MJ, Oury IH: Evolving experience witll cryopreserved mitral valve allografts. *Curr Opin Cardiol* 1998, 13:85–90.
14. Thamilarasan M, Griffin B: Choosing tile most appropriate valve operation and prosthesis. *Curr Clin J Med* 2002, 69:688–690.
15. Sapirstein IS, Smith PK: The "ideal" replacement heart valve. *Am Heart J* 2001, 141:856–860.
16. Chatterjee S, Gardner TI: Factors determining selection of valve prosthesis-tissue or mechanical: current status. *Adv Cardiol* 2002.39:189–194.
17. Birkmeyer NI, O'Connor GT, Baldwin IC: Aortic valve replacement: current clinical practice and opportunities for quality improvement. *Curr Opin Cardiol* 2001,16:152–157.
18. Braunwald E: Aortic valve replacement: an update at the turn of the millennium. *Ellr Heart J* 2000, 21:1032–1033.
19. David TE: Aortic valve repair for management of aortic insufficiency. *Adll Card Surg* 1999, 11:129–159.
20. Espada R, Westaby S: New developments in mitral valve repair. *Om Opin Cardiol* 1998, 13:80–84.
21. Lawrie GM: Mitral valve repair vs replacement. Current recommendations and long-term results. *Cardiol Clin* 1998,16:437–448.
22. Bolling SF, Deeb M, Brunsting LA, Bach OS: Surgery for acquired heart disease: early outcome of mitral valve reconstruction in patients with end stage cardiomyopathy. *J Thome Cardiol Surg* 1995, 109:676–683.
23. Bolling SF, Pagani FD, Deeb GM, Bach OS: Intermediate-term outcome of mitral reconstruction in cardiomyopathey. *J Thome Cardio Sc Surg* 1998, 115:381–388.
24. Bishay ES, McCartlly PM, Cosgrove OM, et al.: Mitralvalve surgery in patients with severe left ventricular dysfunction. *Ellr J Cardio Thome Surg* 2000,17:213–221.
25. Bolling SF: Mitral reconstruction in cardiomyopathy. J *Heart Vallie Disease* 2002 (Suppl l):S26–S31.
26. Byrne IG, Aranki SF, Cohn LH: Repair versus replacement of mitral valve for treating severe ischemic mitral regurgitation. *Coron Artery Dis* 2000, 11:31–33.
27. Adams DH, Filsoufi F, Aklog L: Surgical treatment of the ischemic mitral valve. ! *Heart Vallie Disease* 2002, II (Suppl 1): S21–S25.
28. Dreyfus G, Milaiheanu S: Mitral valve repair in cardiomyopathy. *Heart Lung Tramplant* 2000, 19(5uppl 8):S73–S76.
29. Lachmann L, Shirani L, Plestis KA: Mitral ring annuloplasty: an incomplete correction of functional mitral regurgitation associated with left ventricular remodeling. *Curr Cardio Rep* 2001,3:241–246.

38 Diagnosis and Management of Cardiac Arrhythmia in Fetus and Newborn

Arrhythmias are potentially life-threatening problems in the fetus and newborn. Appropriate management depends on accurate diagnosis. Atrioventricular reentry is the most common type of supraventricular tachycardia in both the fetus and newborn. It should be distinguished from other types of tachycardia such as atrial flutter, atrial ectopic tachycardia, permanent junctional reentry tachycardia, and ventricular tachycardia. Neonatal and fetal bradycardias are less common clinical problems. Sustained bradycardia is most often caused by complete atrioventricular block. It can be mimicked by the more common but benign occurrence of nonconducted atrial premature beats.

Fetal and neonatal arrhythmias are diverse in type and severity. They include both tachycardias and bradycardias. The innate physiological properties of the fetal and neonatal myocardiums make them more vulnerable to these high or low ventricular rates. Irregularities of fetal and neonatal cardiac rhythm commonly occur, and rarely have serious consequences; however, it is important to realize that sustained tachycardias and bradycardias can lead to heart failure and hydrops fetalis (Fig. 38.1).

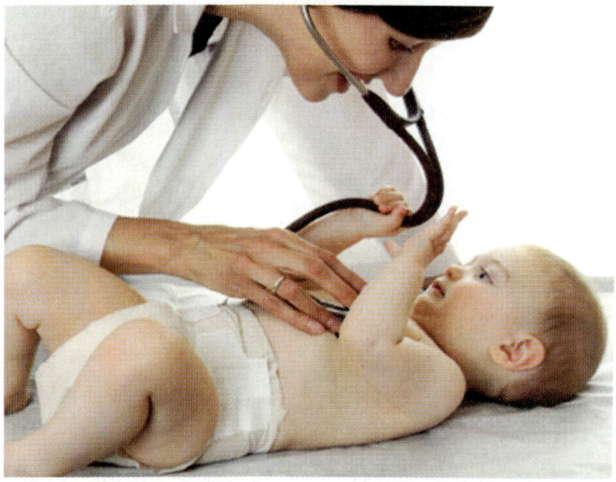

Fig. 38.1: *Showing attending doctor examining the newborn for cardiac arrhythmia*

Historical Background in Fetal Arrhythmia

Prenatal recognition and treatment of fetal tachycardia began in the 1970s. After the first report of prenatal diagnosis using M-mode echocardiography was published in 1980 by Kleinman et al. many reports of prenatal treatment of fetal tachycardia using various types of antiarrhythmic drugs were published in the 1980s. In the 1990s, researchers were more focused on refractory cases. To enable a more detailed prenatal diagnosis, measurement of the ventriculoatrial (VA) interval was reported in 1998, and the magnetocardiogram was introduced as a useful modality. In the 21st century, researches began to focus on better strategies to manage fetal arrhythmia by conducting multicenter trials with larger numbers of patients.

Fetal Arrhythmia: Prenatal Diagnosis and Perinatal Management

Arrhythmias are discovered in about 1% of fetuses. Of these arrhythmias, 10% are considered potential sources of morbidity. Most disturbances of fetal cardiac rhythm are isolated extrasystoles that are of little clinical importance. Sustained arrhythmias may be associated with heart failure, however, manifesting as nonimmune hydrops fetalis. One of the most remarkable examples of successful fetal therapy resulting in intact fetal survival is the conversion of sustained tachycardia in the hydropic fetus. The treatment of fetal cardiac arrhythmias requires a clear understanding of the mechanism of the arrhythmia, a search for structural cardiac and extracardiac anomalies, and an understanding of the pharmacology and pharmacokinetics of potent antiarrhythmic agents in the mother and fetus.

Normal Fetal Cardiac Rhythm

The sinoatrial (SA) node has characteristics that allow depolarization to occur faster than it does in other myocardial cells, initiating the contraction sequence. When the SA node depolarizes, the atrial myocardium contracts in a synchronous fashion with the lateral walls moving toward the interatrial septum, forcing blood into the ventricular chambers. The electrical impulse generated at the SA node is conducted through the atrial myocardium to the atrioventricular (AV) node. From the AV node, the signal is propagated to the right and left ventricular chambers through the Purkinje fibers and causes ventricular mechanical systole. During diastole, the atrial and ventricular chambers relax, allowing filling to occur. This relaxation phase of the heart is also very important in the human fetus because it is during this portion of the repolarization of the heart that abnormalities in electrical conduction can produce serious arrhythmias.

The fetal heart functions in many ways similar to the adult heart. It is important to understand some of the distinguishing features, however, the fetal heart rate is significantly higher (120–160 beats/min) than the adult heart rate (50–70 beats/min). The fetal myocardium is less compliant than the infant or adult heart. In addition, sometimes there are aberrant pathways connecting the atrial and ventricular chambers, providing an accessory route for AV depolarization.

Methods of Assessment (Figs 38.2–38.7)

In the newborn or adult patient, a 12-lead electrocardiogram (ECG) is used to establish the type of arrhythmia.

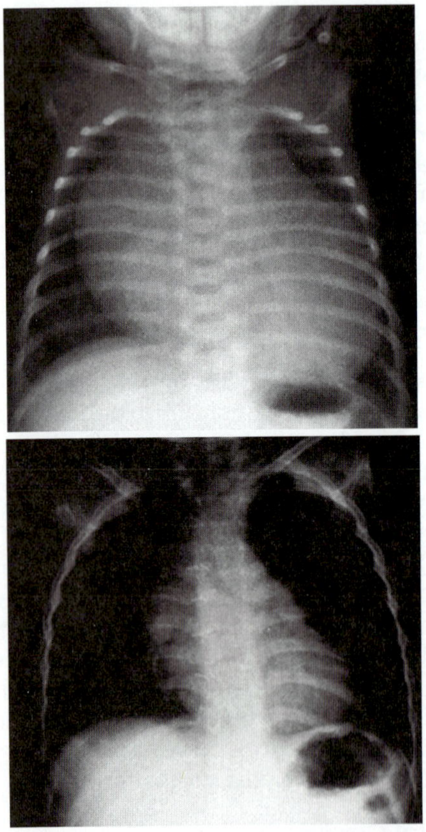
A
B

Fig. 38.2: *(A) Preoperative chest roentgenogram of neonate undergoing repair of Ebstein's anomaly associated with multiple ventricular septal defects and SVT. (B) Recent postoperative chest roentgenogram of neonate undergoing repair of Ebstein's anomaly associated with multiple ventricular septal defects.There is reduction of cardiac size due to arrest of cardiac arrhythmias*

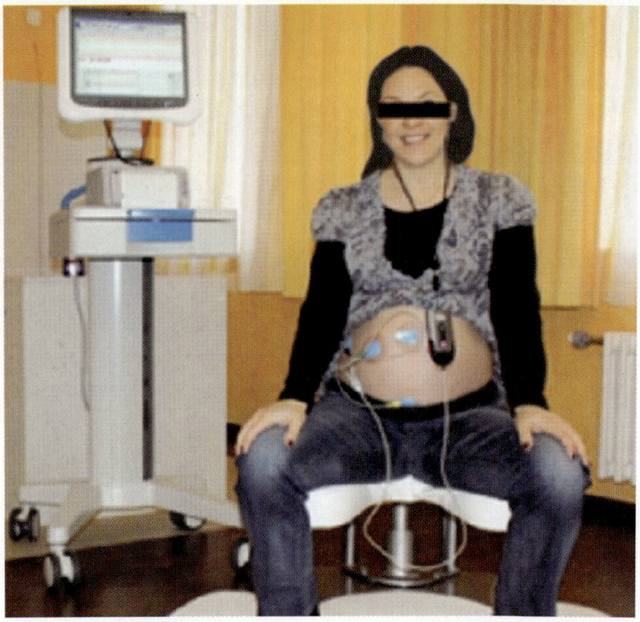

Fig. 38.3: *Portable transabdominal fetal ECG monitoring device with 5 electrodes attached to the maternal abdomen. Continuous telemetric trans-abdominal fetal ECG monitoring of ambulatory women undergoing labour induction is feasible and acceptable to women*

The prenatal diagnosis cannot rely on an ECG through the maternal abdominal wall because the fetal P waves are rarely seen, and the fetal QRS complex is dwarfed by the signals from the maternal abdominal ECG, and insulating properties of the vernix caseosa. Investigators rely primarily on ultrasound.

Fetal studies usually begin with an examination of fetal and cardiac anatomy by the use of two dimensional ultrasound. The fetus is also examined for collections of fluid in the pericardial sac, the pleural spaces, the abdomen, and the skin. The amount of amniotic fluid is recorded. Cardiac size and wall thickness are evaluated.

M-mode ultrasound traditionally has been used to establish the type of arrhythmia. The M-mode cursor is positioned so that it crosses one structure that moves with atrial contraction (atrium, AV valves) and one structure that moves with ventricular contraction (ventricle, semilunar valves). In this manner, the relative timing of events can be established.

- Fetal magnetocardiography
- Fetal echocardiography
- Fetal electrocardiography
- Skiagram of the chest
- Fetal kinetocardiography
- Tansesophageal electrophysiologic procedure
- 24-hour ambulatory electrocardiography
- Fetal kinetocardigraphy.

Maternal SS-A Antibody

Fetal bradycardia is diagnosed when the fetal ventricular heart rate is slower than 100 bpm, mainly due to AV block. Approximately half of all cases are caused by associated

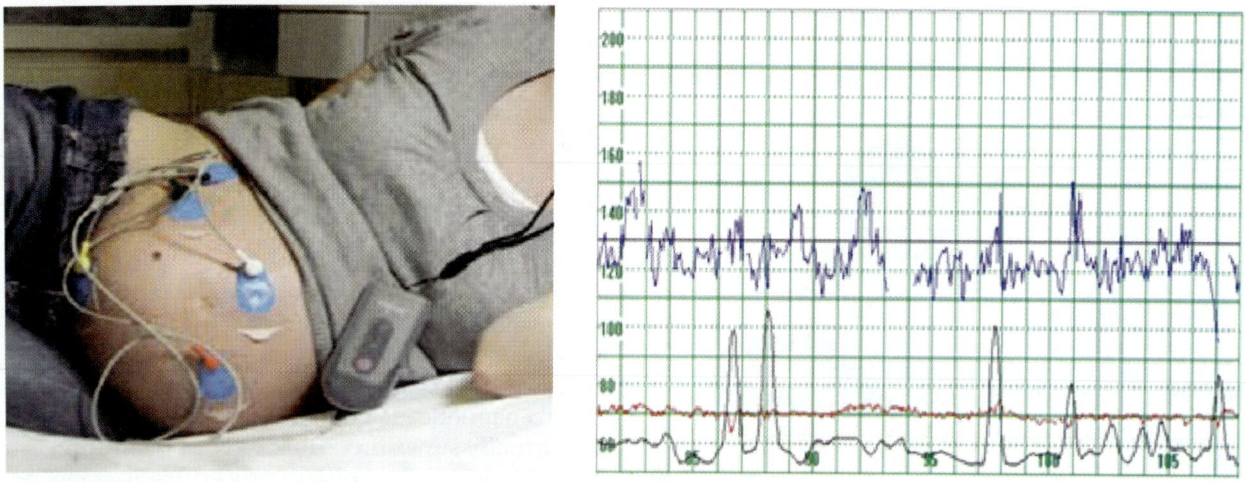

Fig. 38.4: *Continuous fetal and maternal heart rate electrocardiogram (ECG) monitoring was evaluated using the Monica AN24™ System, which showed a fetal heart rate trace with little signal loss*

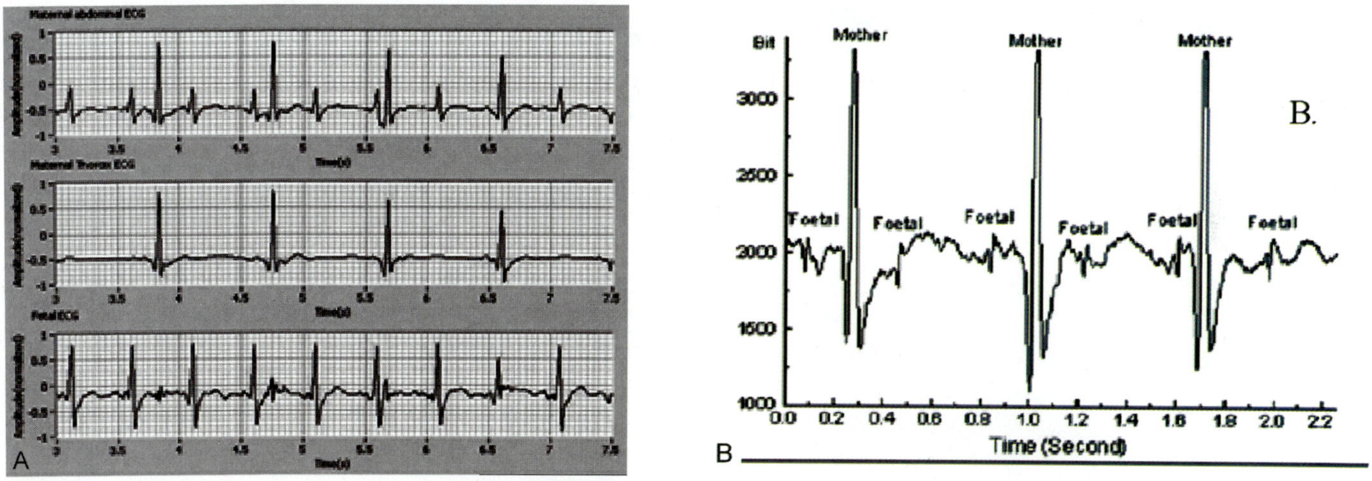

Fig. 38.5: *(A and B) Monitoring the fetal electrocardiogram (fECG) is currently one of the most promising methods to assess fetal heart health. However, the main problem associated with this method is that signals recorded from maternal abdomen are affected by noise and interferences: the maternal electrocardiogram (mECG) being the dominant interference*

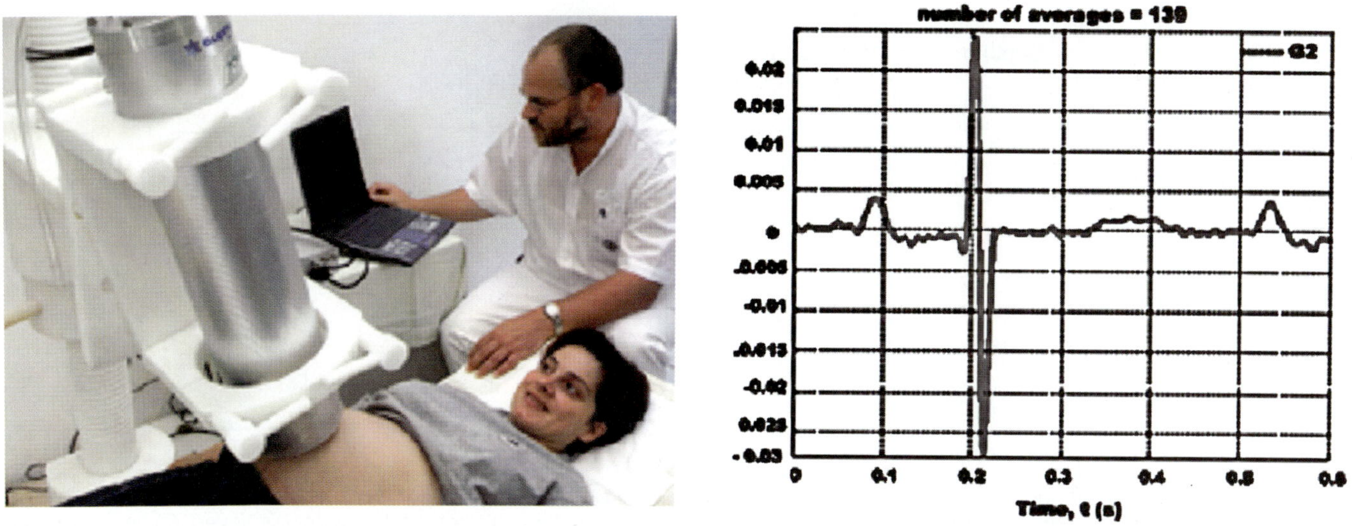

Fig. 38.6: *Fetal MCG showing SQUID system from the IPHT in use (left); unshielded recording of a fetal magnetocardiogram (right)*

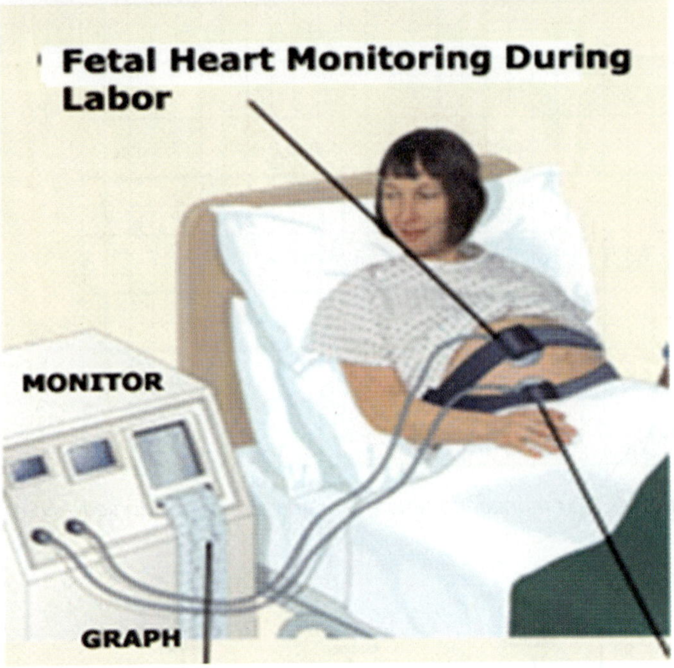

Fig. 38.7: *Electronic fetal heart monitoring during uterine contractions*

congenital heart disease (CHD), and the remaining cases that have normal cardiac structure are often caused by **maternal SS-A antibody.** The two most common CHD associated with AV block are left atrial isomerism and discordant AV connection. Maternal SS-A antibody to AV block is usually that for 52 kd SS-A, and many mothers are rarely diagnosed with collagen disease when the fetus develops AV block. Although rare, the other important cause of fetal bradycardia is long QT syndrome, which can cause 2:1 AV block or sinus bradycardia-blocked paroxysmal atrial contraction (PAC) with bigeminy also mimics 2:1 AV block and causes fetal bradycardia.

Magnetocardiography is similar to ECG since the electromagnetic currents of the heart display patterns that are virtually superimposable. At our institution, a transesophageal electrophysiologic procedure is often performed in infants with sustained fetal tachyarrhythmias. For bradyarrhythmias and fetal ectopy, an ECG and 24 hour ambulatory recording are usually sufficient to define the rhythm.

Fetal Magnetocardiography

The fetal magnetocardiogram (MCG) is a more recent addition to the noninvasive tools used to diagnose fetal

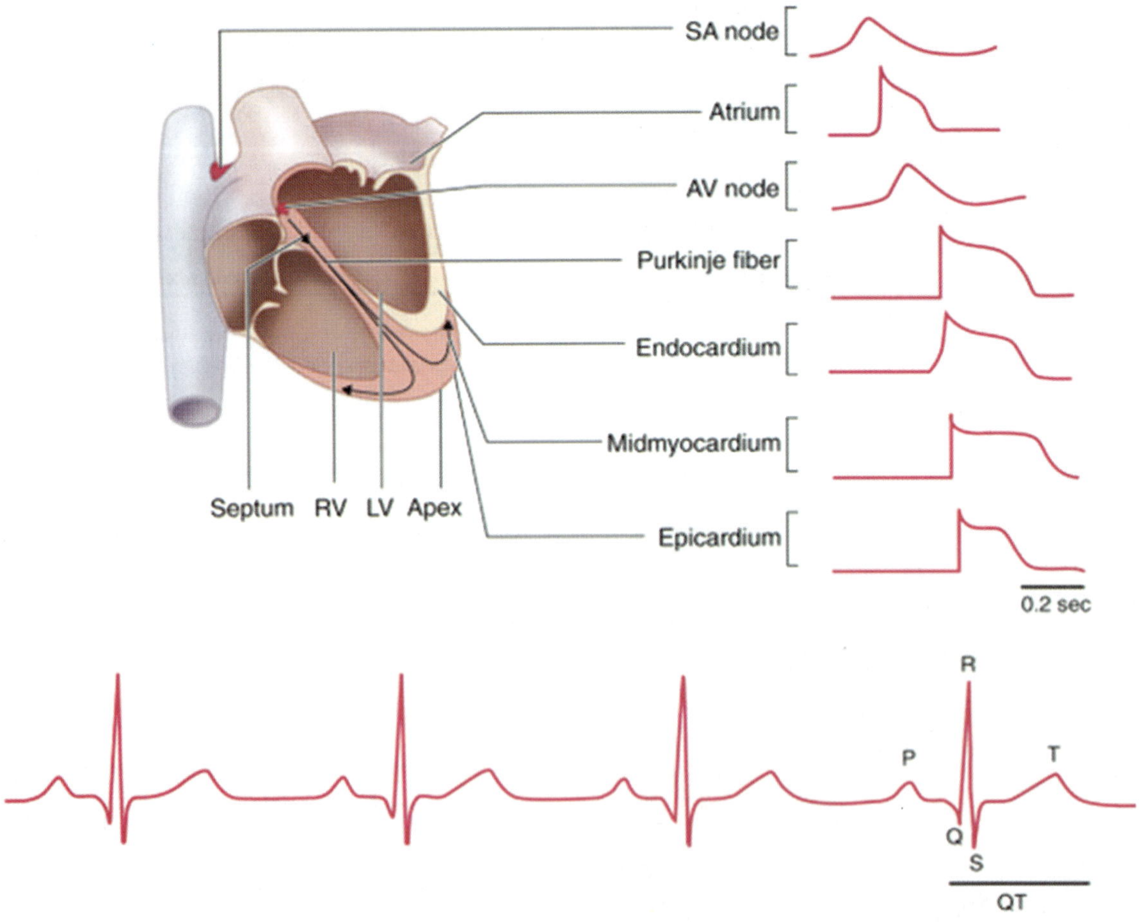

Fig. 38.8: *Electrical activity in the myocardium. Top, schematic of a human heart with illustration of typical action potential waveforms recorded in different regions. Bottom, schematic of a surface electrocardiogram; three sequential beats are displayed. (From Nerbonne J, Kass R: Molecular physiology of cardiac repolarization. Physiol Rev 2005;85:1206.)*

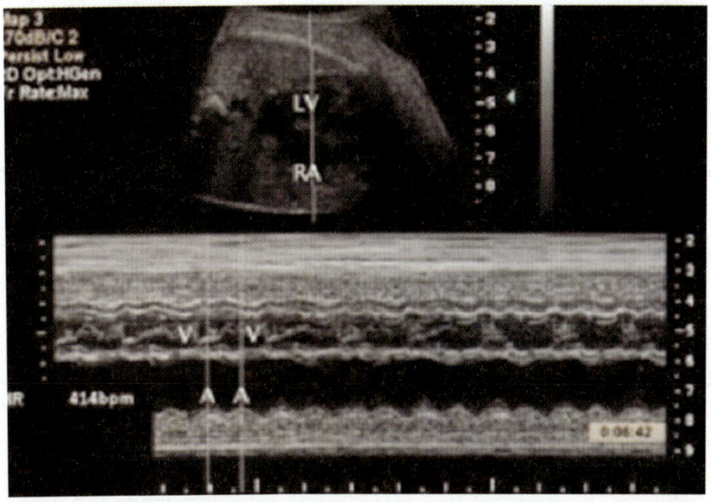

Fig. 38.9: *M-mode tracing using a four chamber view to demonstrate atrial (A) and ventricular (V) wall motions. The M-mode is directed simultaneously through the left ventricle (LV) and right atrium (RA). There is atrial flutter with an atrial rate of 414 beats/min (bpm), functional 2:1 atrioventricular block, and a regular ventricular rate of 207 bpm*

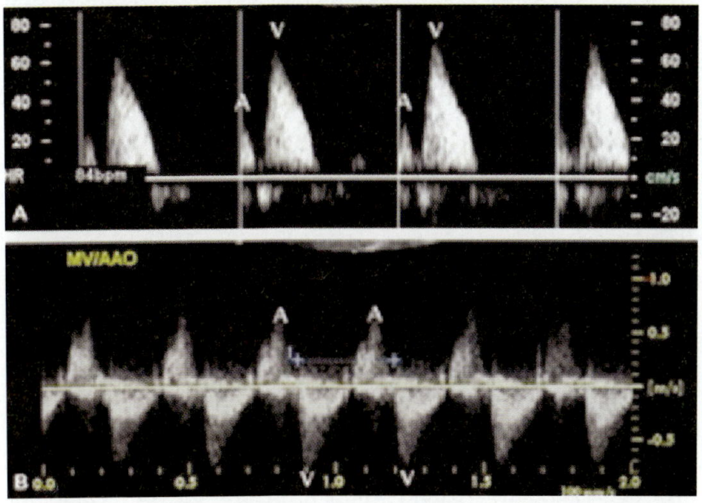

Fig. 38.10: *Pulsed Doppler flow modalities. (A) Simultaneous ascending aorta (V) and superior vena cava (A). Doppler flow recording at 20 weeks of gestation showing sinus bradycardia with normal 1:1 atrioventricular conduction. (B) Simultaneous inflow/outflow Doppler of a 19-week fetus with long ventriculo-atrial tachycardia of 190 beats/min due to fetal thyrotoxicosis. The mother had a medical history of Graves' disease for which she had been treated with propylthiouracil and radioactive iodine*

arrhythmias. The fetal MCG is an alternative signal source for fetal heart rate monitoring that seems to offer significant advantages over other methods. The fetal MCG is the magnetic analog of the fetal ECG but exhibits superior signal quality because of the favorable transmission properties of magnetic signals. Fetal MCG typically has a much greater signal-to-noise ratio and is free of maternal interference compared with fetal ECG monitoring. Because of the expense and sophistication of the instrumentation,

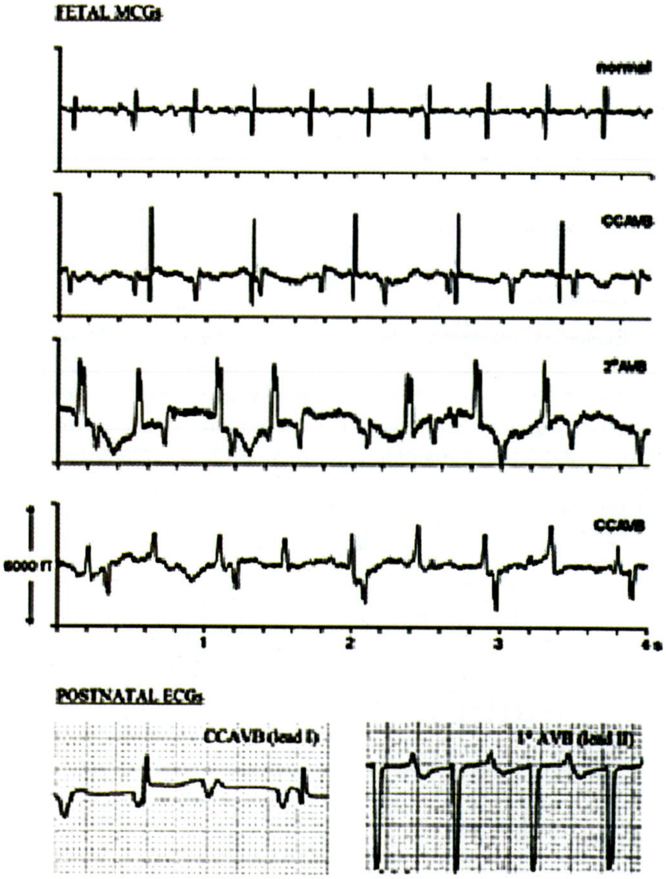

Fig. 38.11: *Representative tracings depicting P-wave amplitudes in normal subjects and subjects with CCAVB and 2°AVB. Gestational ages of subjects in the top three tracings are 32 to 33 weeks. The fourth tracing, taken from a subject with CCAVB at 36 weeks' gestation, shows an example in which the P wave was transiently larger than the QRS complex. Postnatal ECGs (bottom) are from subjects in the second and third tracings above. In the left tracing, note atrial situs inversus in a subject with complex congenital heart disease; in the right tracing, note first-degree AV block with left QRS axis deviation. Both tracings show prominent P waves*

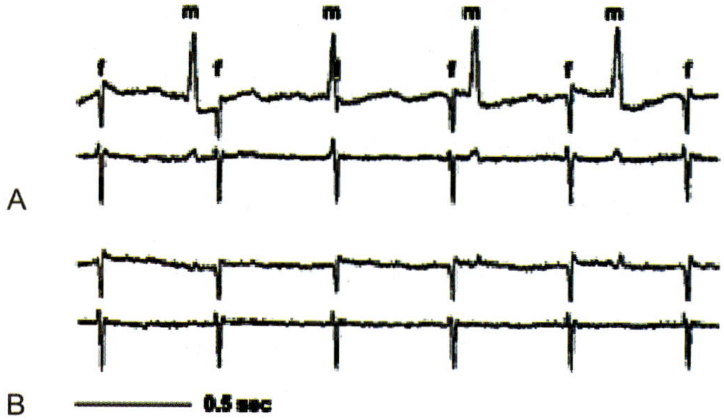

Fig. 38.12: *Fetal magnetocardiogram in the 29th week of gestation. Two selected channels, one with a strong and one with a weak maternal artefact, before (A) and after (B) digital subtraction of the maternal signal (m, maternal R wave; f, fetal R wave)*

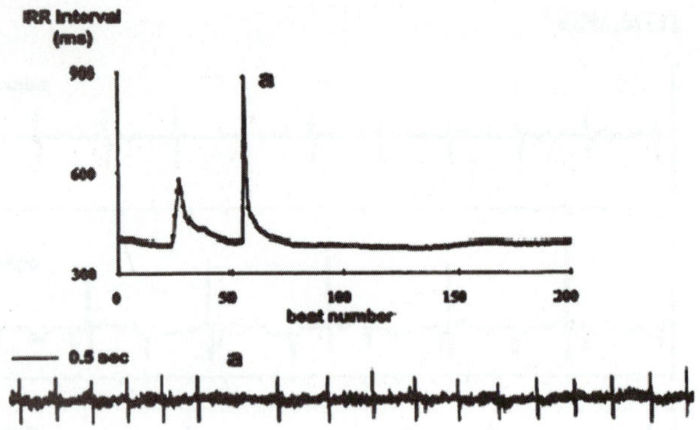

Fig. 38.13: *Episode of fetal bradycardia in the 20th week of gestation: a sudden lengthening of the RR interval to 881 ms (a) is shown in the time series of the RR intervals and in the signal trace*

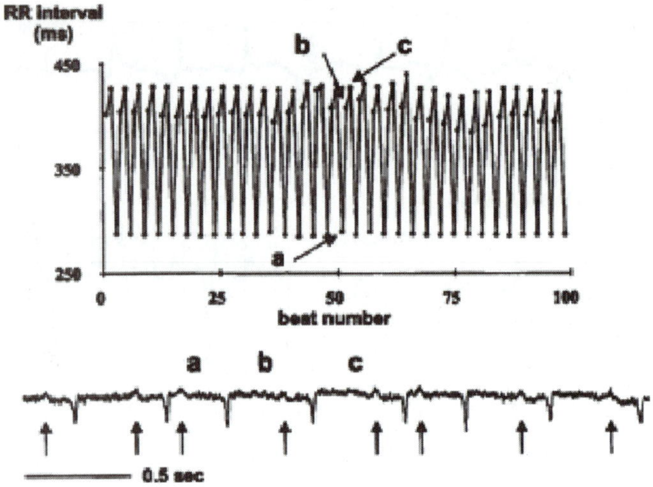

Fig. 38.14: *Time series and signal trace of a fetus in the 31st week of gestation: (a) extrasystolic beat followed by two beats, (b and c), of normal duration. Note the timing of the P waves (?)*

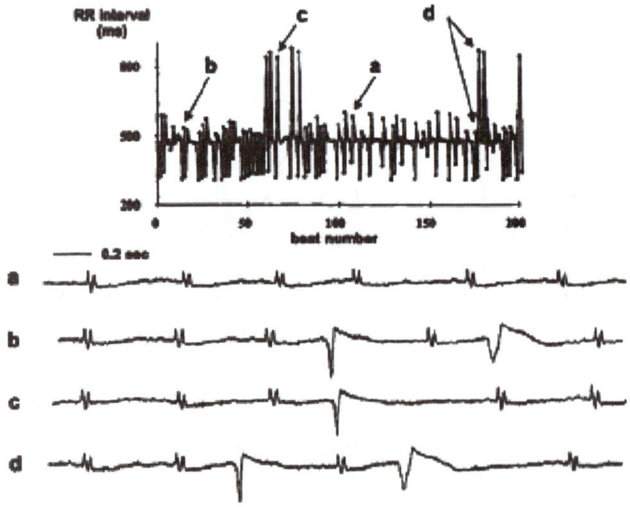

Fig. 38.15: *Time series and signal trace of a fetus in the 35th week of gestation. The signal traces show premature beats (a) with QRS morphology similar to normal complexes (supra-ventricular extrasystoles), (b) with differing QRS morphology, (c and d) with a prolonged pause*

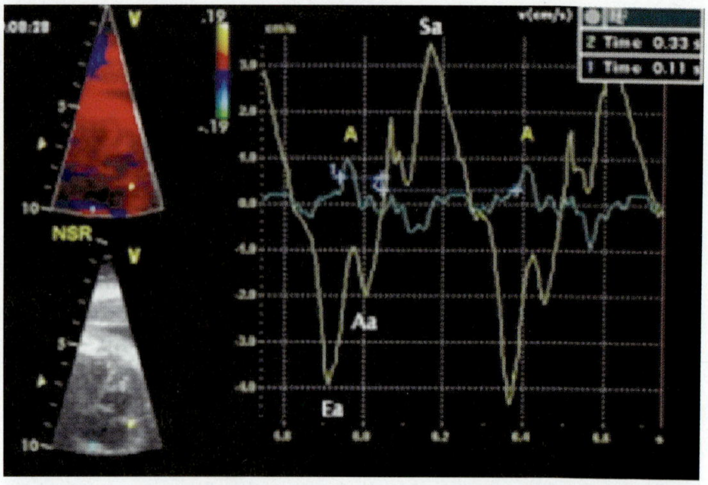

Fig. 38.16: *Normal tissue Doppler imaging from the right atrioventricular (AV) groove and the right atrial wall. Sequential analysis of regional tissue motion at the AV groove results in two diastolic [early diastolic filling phase (Ea) and atrial contraction (Aa)] waves and one systolic (Sa) wave*

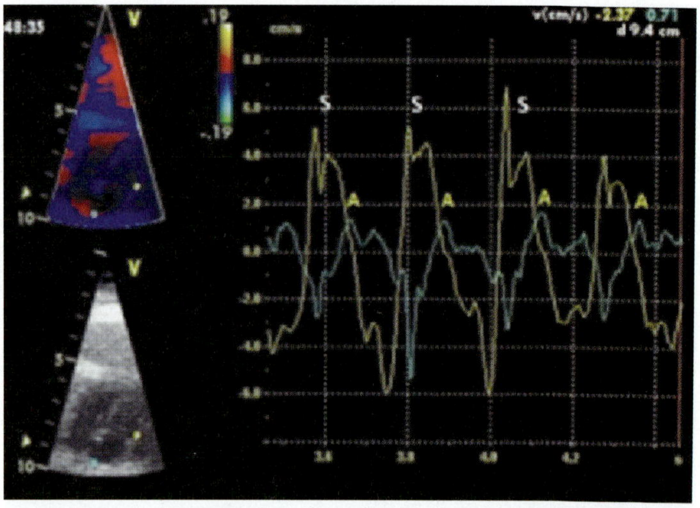

Fig. 38.17: *Tissue velocity imaging of a short-ventriculoatrial tachyarrhythmia with a heart rate of 230 beats/min. Right atrial systole (A) occurs at the very end of ventricular systole (S). Atrioventricular reentry as supraventricular tachycardia mechanism was confirmed by postnatal transoesophageal electrophysiological study*

only a few groups in the world are working in this area, however, impressive progress has been made. A database of normative fetal conduction findings in several hundred fetuses has been validated against ECG. The heart rate and the waveform obtained by the fetal MCG are particularly useful for the diagnosis of specific types of fetal arrhythmias, such as Wolff-Parkinson-White syndrome and long QT syndrome.

Fetal Electrocardiography (Figs 38.8–38.55)

Several groups have published ECG data in the fetus during stable sinus rhythm. The signal-to-noise ratio for fECG is

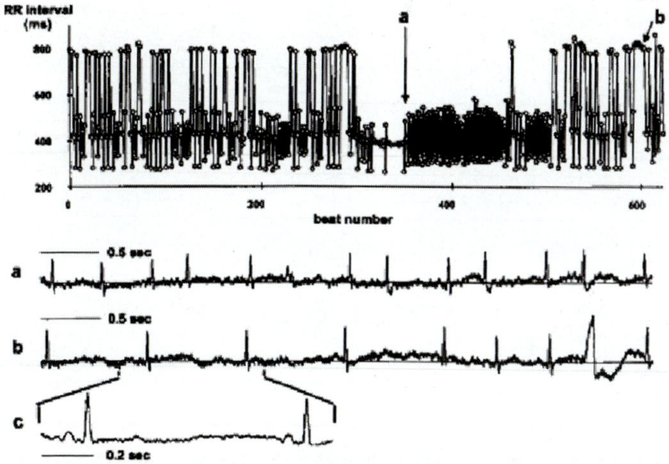

Fig. 38.18: *Time series and signal trace of a fetus in the 34th week of gestation with complex arrhythmias. Traces show (a) transition from sinus rhythm to bigeminy with narrow and wide QRS complexes, (b) several beats with period doubling followed by a return to sinus rhythm interrupted by an ectopic beat, and (c) averaged signal of the bradycardia beats showing lack of a P wave suggesting a sino-atrial block*

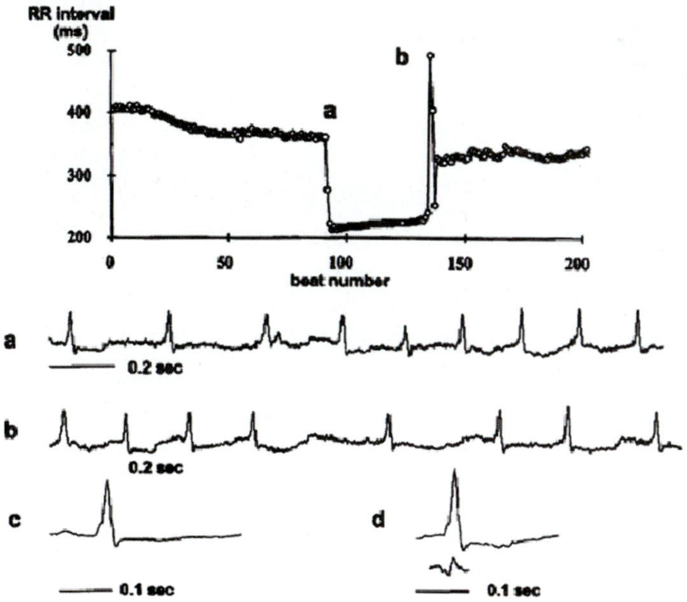

Fig. 38.19: *Time series and signal trace of a fetus in the 37th week of gestation with an episode of tachycardia. The signal traces show (a) the beginning and (b) the termination of the episode; (c) is the signal-averaged normal sinus beat showing the P wave and (d) is the signal averaged tachycardia beat showing the embedded P wave*

generally not as good as with fMCG as averaging of multiple beats during a 20 second period is usually needed. This also limits its capabilities during frequently changing arrhythmias. Near term, and in some cases prior to 25 weeks' gestation, recordings have been possible. Because of the high rate of fetal demise in the third trimester, particularly in older mothers, additional studies using fECG or fMCG should be performed to

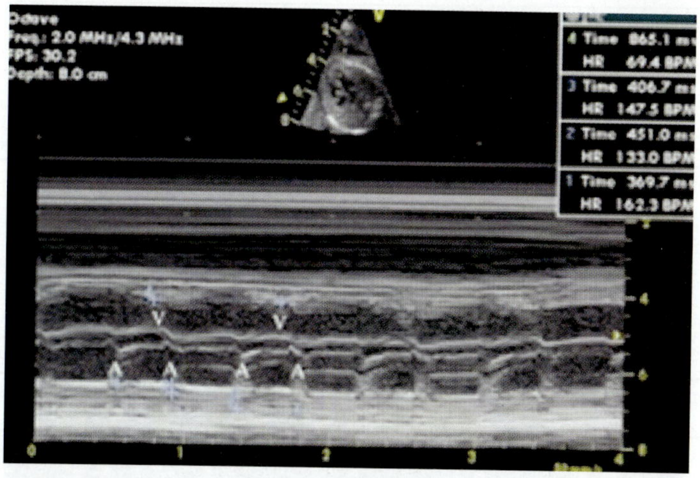

Fig. 38.20: *M-mode echocardiography at 20 weeks showing significant fetal bradycardia (V-V: 67 beats/min) related to atrial bigeminy. There is atrial beat-to-beat variation with the premature atrial beats (A-A interval: 370 ms) being blocked and the normal atrial impulses (450 ms) being conducted. A repeat echocardiogram showed normal cardiac rhythm 1 week later*

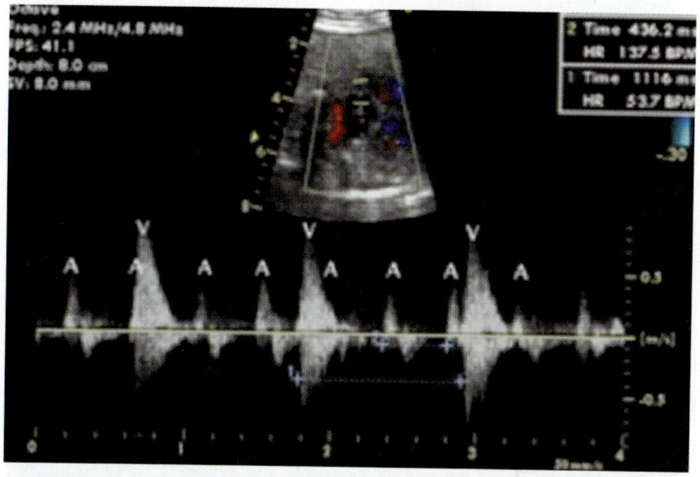

Fig. 38.21: *Simultaneous Doppler of the aorta and superior vena cava showing complete atrioventricular block. The atrial (A-A) rate was 138 beats/min (bpm) and the ventricular (V-V) rate was 54 bpm with complete atrioventricular dissociation*

evaluate these techniques in detecting fetal ischemia prior to the onset of labor.

Fetal Kinetocardiography

Recent advances in echocardiography allow assessment of the kinetic movement of myocardium. The cursor can be displayed from various locations from atrium or ventricle giving the timing sequence of cardiac events. Other new modalities, such as velocity vector imaging, tissue Doppler imaging, and combined fMCG/Doppler imaging may also add to arrhythmia analysis, but are so new that their importance is difficult to judge at this time.

Fetal Echocardiography

Pulsed Doppler ultrasound for rhythm assessment and detection of flow disturbances (regurgitation, stenosis).

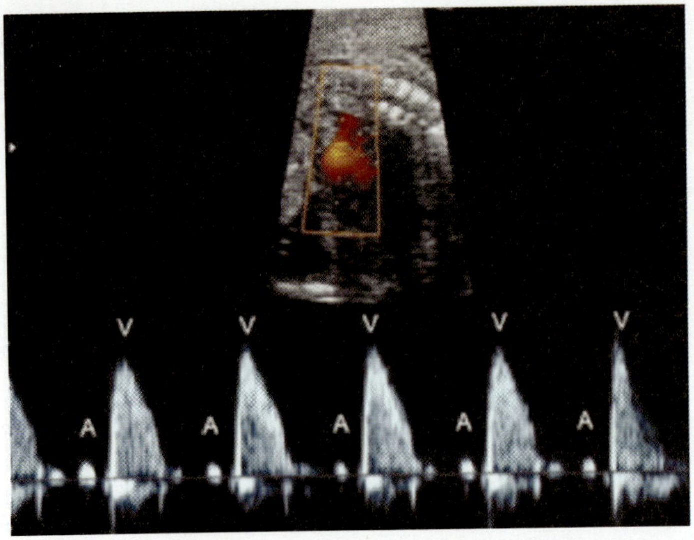

Fig. 38.22: *Example of a normal Doppler tracing obtained by simultaneous pulse wave Doppler of the aorta and the SVC. The Doppler sample volume is simultaneously placed within the aorta and the SVC*

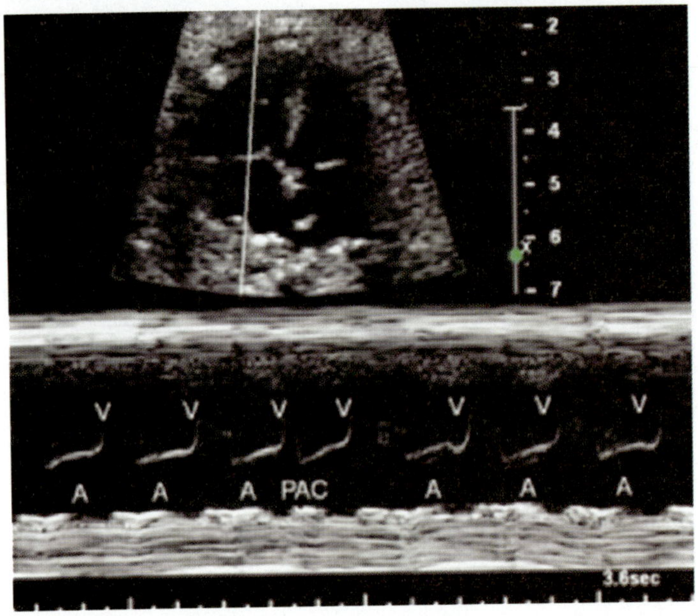

Fig. 38.23: *Example of a normal Doppler tracing obtained by simultaneous pulse wave Doppler of the aorta and the SVC. The Doppler sample volume is simultaneously placed within the aorta and the SVC*

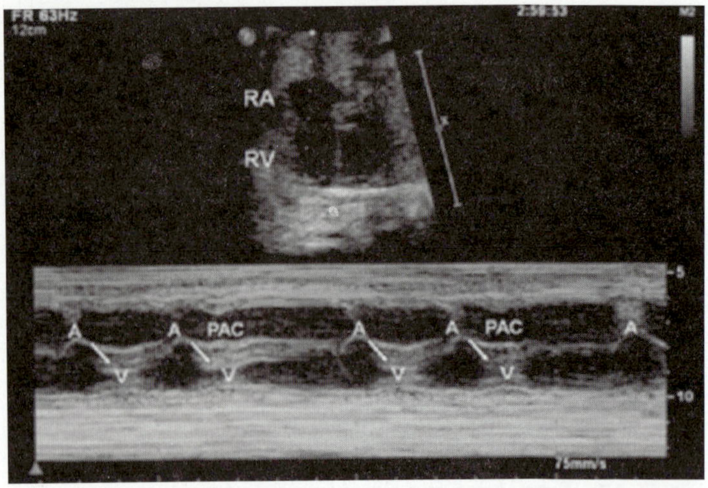

Fig. 38.24: *Blocked PAC. M-mode tracing from a four chamber view with the transducer beam through the RA and the RV. There are blocked PAC's in a trigeminy pattern. Only the normal atrial contractions (A) are followed by a ventricular contraction (V)*

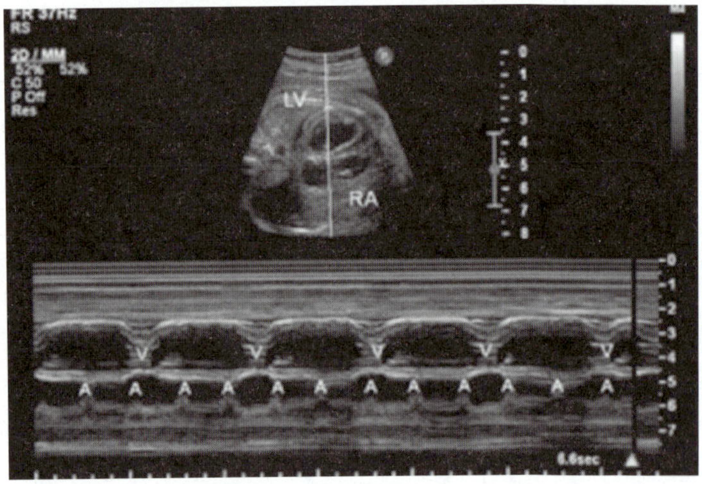

Fig. 38.25: *Complete heart block. M-mode tracing from a four chamber view with the transducer beam through the RA and the LV. There are regular atrial contractions (A) with a normal heart rate of 125 bpm and independent ventricular contractions (V) with a heart rate of 50 bpm*

The rhythm assessment begins with measurement of the heart rate and its variability. The atrial rate and ventricular rate should be assessed independently because they may not have an one-to-one association.

The next phase of the fetal rhythm assessment is determination of atrial and ventricular activation. Our laboratory has used many fetal Doppler interrogation sites for rhythm interpretation. The venous sampling sites (superior and inferior vena cavae) are useful for determination of atrial rates and rhythm, and the inflow–outflow region of either ventricle is useful for determining the association between ventricular diastolic events and ventricular systolic flow events. Normal sinus rhythm is determined on the basis of a normal rate, a stable sequence of atrial to ventricular contractions, and accelerations in heart rate with fetal activity or uterine contractions. Tricuspid or mitral inflow Doppler shows a stable A wave caused by atrial contraction. There should be little (<20%) or no reflux of flow into the systemic veins.

Abnormal atrial activation associated with atrial premature contractions, supraventricular tachycardia (SVT), junctional rhythm with retrograde conduction, or AV dissociation is identified by intermittent or continuous systemic venous reflux noted by Doppler. The so-called cannon A wave is caused by atrial contractions against a closed AV valve. This reversal of flow also is noted when

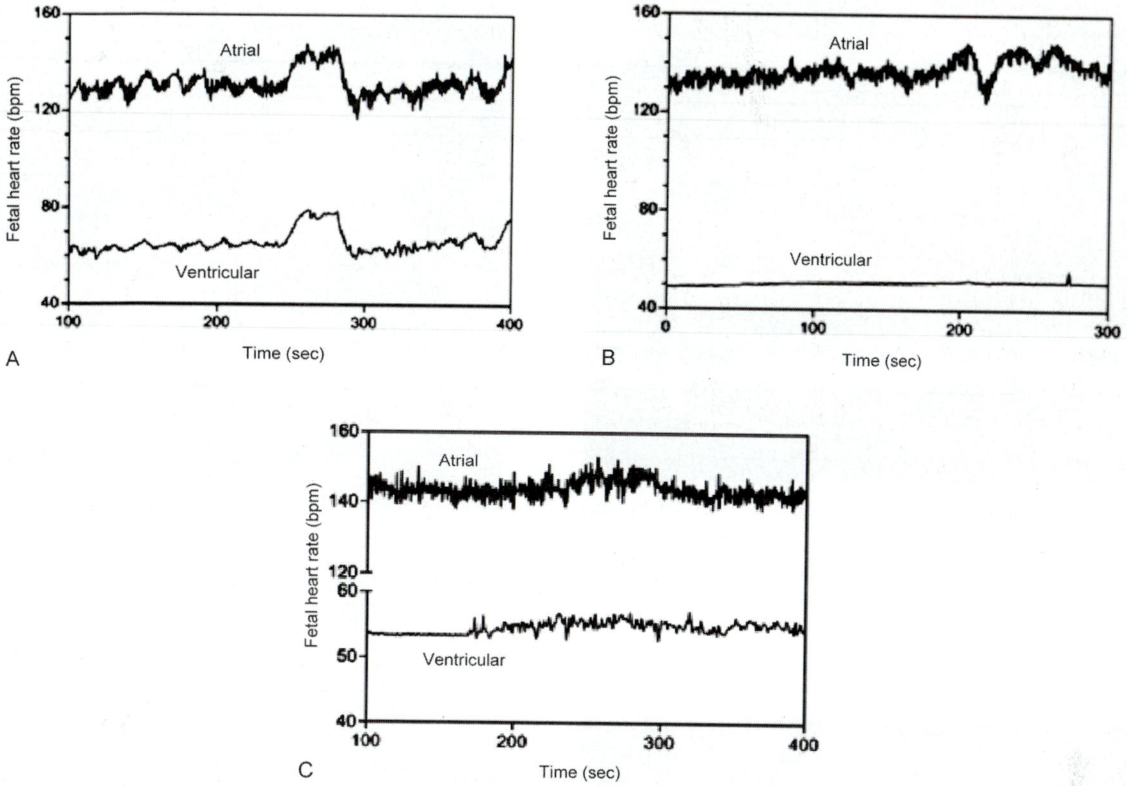

Fig. 38.26: *Fetal heart rate patterns in fetal AVB atrial and ventricular fetal heart rate tracings from fetus showing (A) reactive pattern at 28 weeks' gestation and (B) nonreactive pattern at 32 weeks' gestation. In the reactive pattern, the atrial and ventricular tracings were highly correlated; even variations as small as 3 beats/min (bpm) were often correlated. The degree of ventricular reactivity and the amplitude of the beat-to-beat fetal heart rate variability varied strongly with mean ventricular rate. At rates >70 beats/min, ventricular reactivity was exaggerated and the amplitude of the ventricular accelerations actually exceeded that of the atrial accelerations. As mean ventricular rate declined, the amplitude of the ventricular accelerations and the beat-to-beat fetal heart rate variability progressively decreased. Notice that atrial reactivity is present in the nonreactive pattern. Both patterns showed prominent atrial beat-to-beat variability due to the presence of ventriculophasic sinus arrhythmia. Unlike normal beat-to-beat variability, its amplitude does not diminish during heart rate acceleration. (C) Atrial and ventricular fetal heart rate tracings from fetus at 30 weeks' gestation showing abrupt transition from the nonreactive to the reactive pattern. AVB, atrioventricular block*

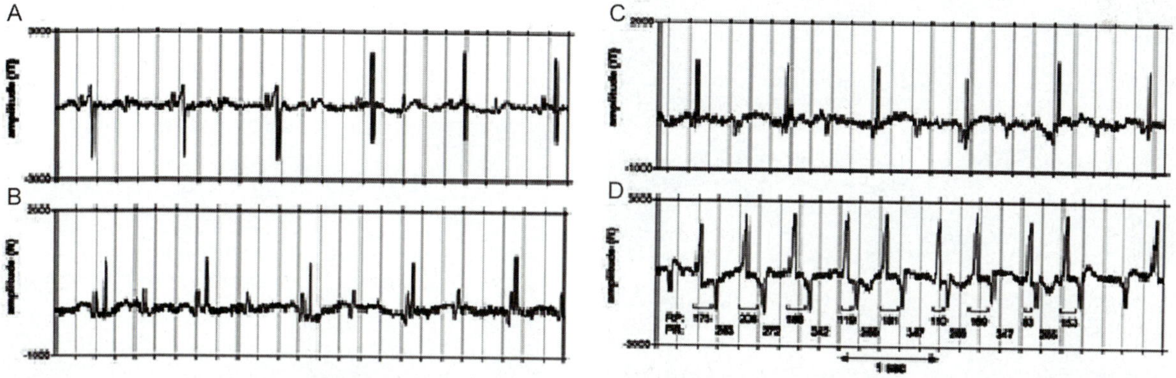

Fig. 38.27: *Rhythm strips from second-degree (2°) atrioventricular block (AVB) subjects showing: (A) intermittent preexcitation with QRS normalization in fetus at 32 weeks' gestation; (B) varying PR interval due to transient atrioventricular dissociation in fetus two at 37 weeks' gestation; (C) period of low atrial rhythm (PR = 55 ms) in fetus with 2 atrial rhythms at 24 weeks' gestation; in the high rhythm (not shown), PR interval was approximately 107 ms; and (D) transition of sinus rhythm (1:1 conduction) from stable RP/PR to alternating RP/PR in fetus at 33 weeks' gestation. After several beats with relatively constant RP/PR, the fourth atrial beat conducts slowly, shortening RP of the succeeding beat. Rather than blocking, the fifth atrial beat not only conducts, it does so more rapidly than the prior beat, prolonging RP of the succeeding beat. The alternating (short-long) RP intervals of the ensuing beats continue to show PR prolongation during the "long" phase of the cycle and conduction at short RP during the "short" phase until block occurs, notably, during the "long" phase. The tracings were processed to remove maternal interference but were not signal averaged*

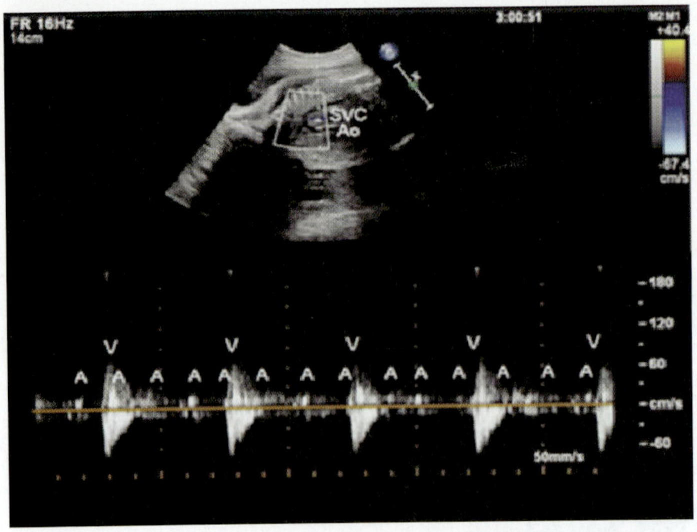

Fig. 38.28: *Simultaneous pulse wave Doppler of the aorta and vena cava superior of a fetus with complete heart block showing backflow following atrial contractions (A) in the superior vena cava with an atrial rate of 140/min (A) and in the same direction aortic outflow following ventricular contractions (V) which are independent with a regular rate of 60/min*

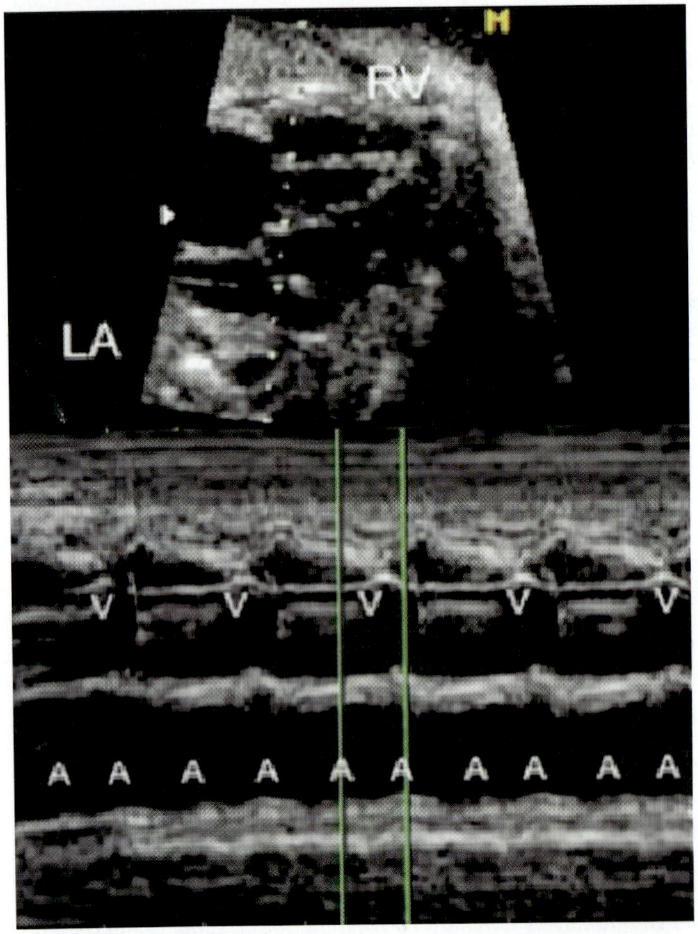

Fig. 38.29: *Atrial flutter. Simultaneous M-mode tracing to record the RV and LA freewall movements during the cardiac cycles. The atrial rate is very fast and regular at 462 bpm while the ventricular rate is 231 bpm suggesting 2:1 AV conduction*

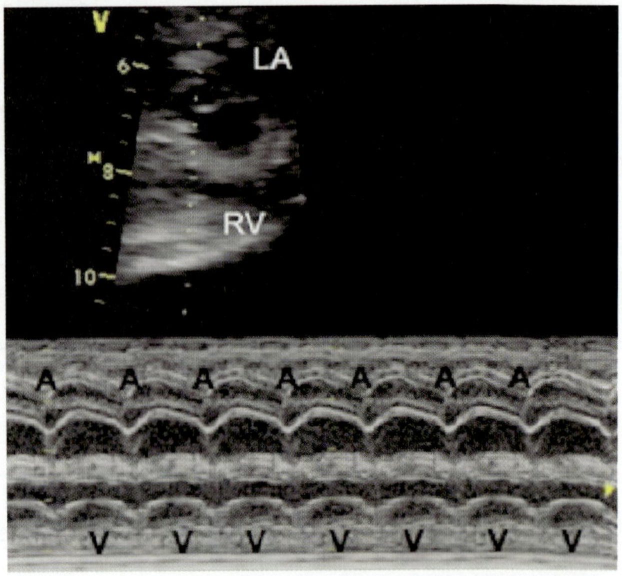

Fig. 38.30: *SVT with a heart rate of 240 bpm. M-mode tracing through the right atrium (bottom) and the right ventricle (top). There is 1:1 AV-conduction with a short AV-interval*

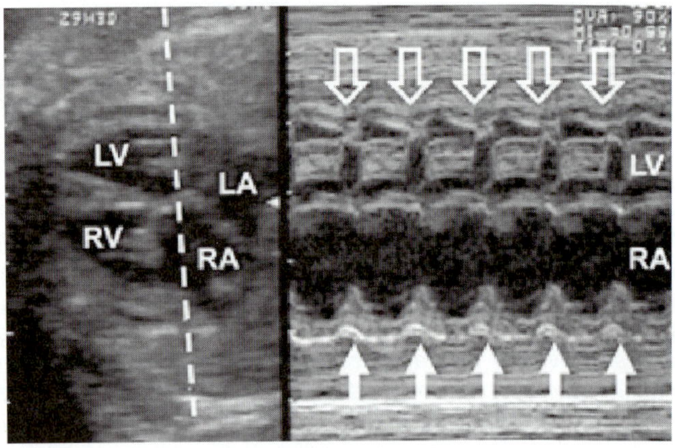

Fig. 38.31: *Simultaneous M-mode recording of both ventricles and atria. M-mode recording in a fetus with supraventricular tachycardia reveals 1:1 relation of atrial (closed arrow) and ventricular contraction (open arrow) with a ventricular rate of 210 bpm. LA, left atrium; LV, left ventricle; RA, right atrium; RV, right ventricle*

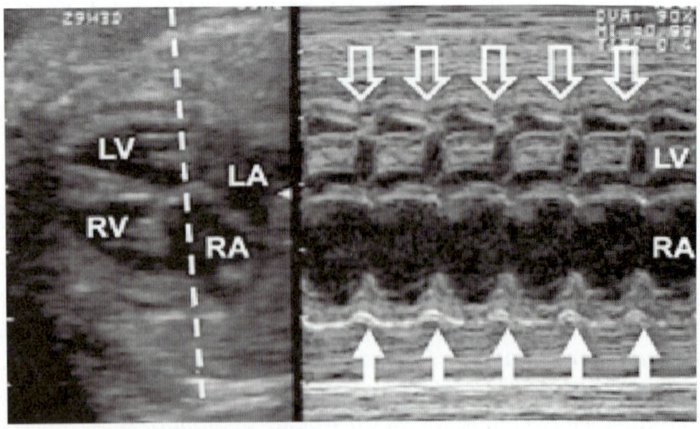

Fig. 38.32: *M-mode recording in a fetus with atrial flutter and 2:1 atrioventricular conduction, with an atrial (closed arrow) rate of 510 bpm and a ventricular (open arrow) rate of 255 bpm. LA, left atrium; LV, left ventricle; RA, right atrium; RV, right ventricle*

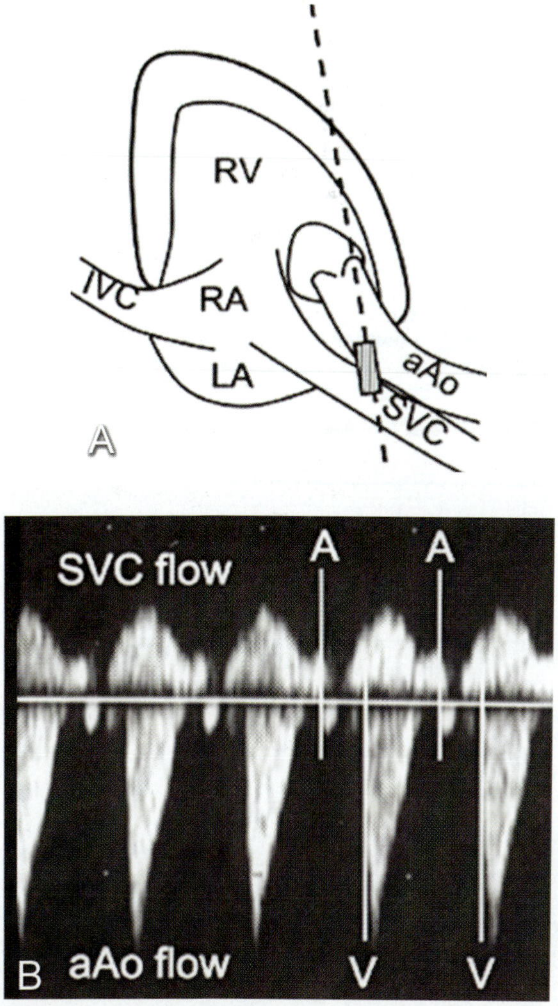

Fig. 38.33: *Simultaneous Doppler trace of the ascending aorta (aAo) and the superior vena cava (SVC). Beginning of reverse flow at SVC (A) and forward flow at aAo (V) represent the timing of atrial and ventricular contraction, respectively. IVC, inferior vena cava; LA, left atrium; RA, right atrium; RV, right ventricle*

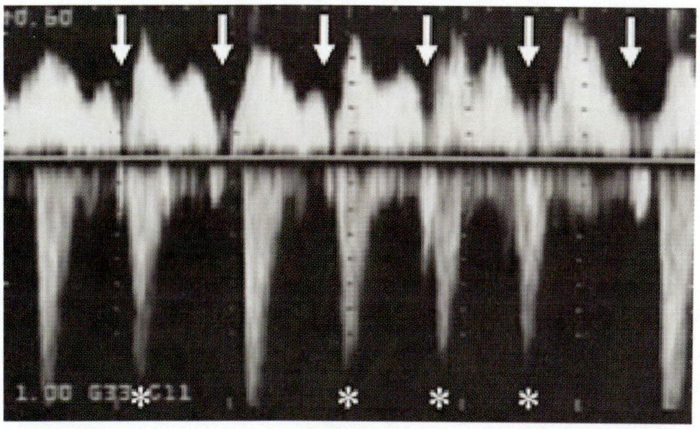

Fig. 38.34: *Simultaneous Doppler trace of the ascending aorta and the superior vena cava in a fetus with ventricular or junctional tachycardia reveals regular atrial contraction with reversal flow at the superior vena cava (arrows) and faster ventricular contraction (asterisk)*

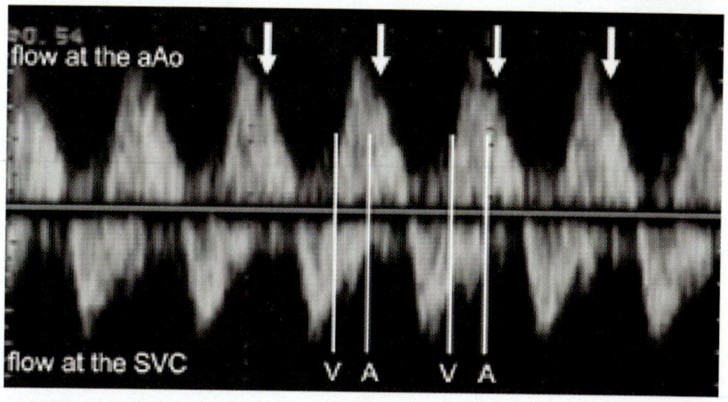

Fig. 38.35: *Simultaneous Doppler trace of the ascending aorta (aAo) and the superior vena cava (SVC) in a fetus with supraventricular tachycardia with short-ventriculoatrial interval. Although high-velocity reversal flows of SVC is almost over-wrapped to the flow of aAo, the starting point of the reversal flow can be detected from the interrupted forward flow of SVC*

ventricular compliance is abnormal, which can be seen in fetal acidosis and intrauterine growth restriction.

If the sample volume size is increased and the transducer is positioned in the inflow–outflow region of the ventricle, the noninvasive P-R interval can be determined during sinus rhythm. This measurement tends to overestimate P–R interval, and recently Bergman[6] suggested that using the mitral valve closure may be more closely predictive of actual P-R interval. It should be noted that the measurement represents activation mechanically, so that any disease slowing electromechanical activation of either the atrium or the ventricle, may lengthen this interval, and it is not specific for AV nodal disease. In addition, the inflow-outflow view may not be as predictive of the P-R interval during tachycardia, however, because of changes in diastolic timing.

The third aspect of fetal rhythm assessment is determination of the mechanism of arrhythmia. Important issues include the following:

1. Are atrial and ventricular contraction rates normal or abnormal?
2. If the contraction rates are abnormal, is there a regular or stable pattern of contraction in the atrium and ventricle?
3. If the pattern of contraction is irregular, is the irregularity repetitions or irregularly irregular?
4. What is the association between the atrial and ventricular contractions?

Answering these questions defines the rhythm, and electrophysiologic texts can be used to specify further the diagnosis or differential diagnosis. A full description of the arrhythmia usually cannot occur, however, until the postnatal period. In a select few institutions worldwide, fetal magnetocardiography may be available for prenatal rhythm assessment.

Types of Arrhythmias

Isolated Extrasystole

Isolated extrasystoles are the most commonly noted fetal arrhythmia. They often are detected during routine

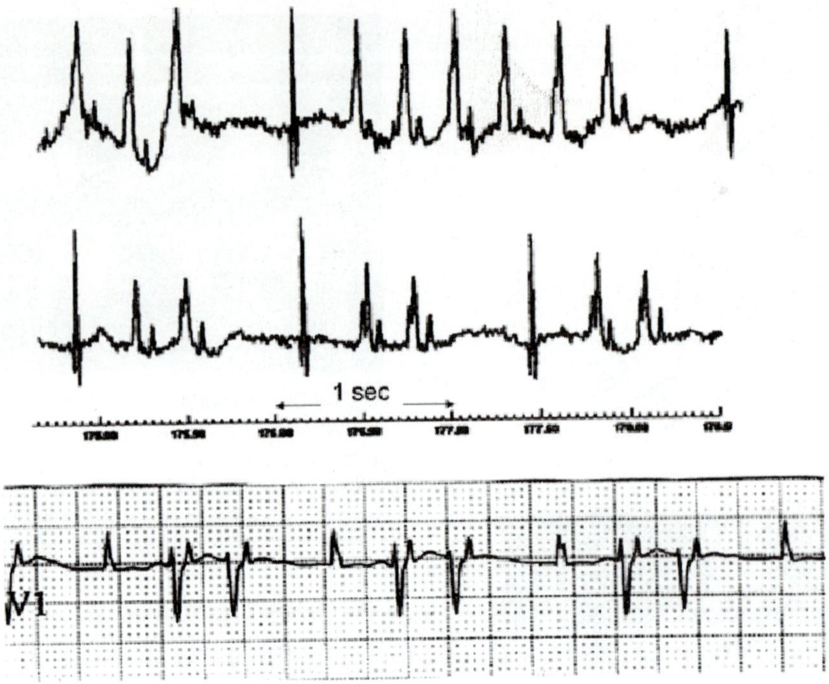

Fig. 38.36: *The top two tracings of fMCG show nonsustained ventricular tachycardia and ventricular couplets due to myocarditis in a 29 weeks fetus. After delivery, only couplets were noted (bottom tracing)*

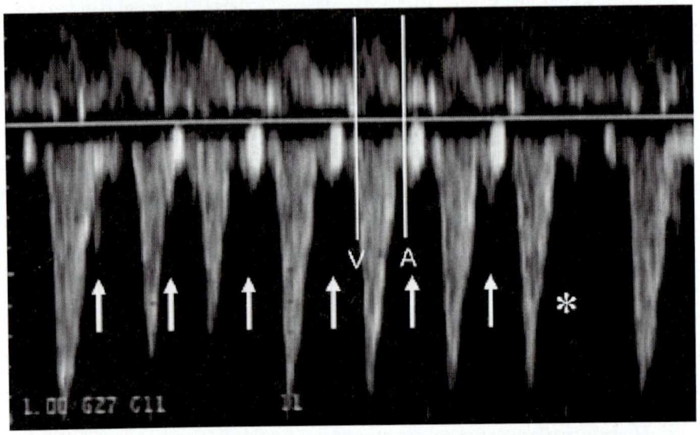

Fig. 38.37: *Simultaneous Doppler trace of the ascending aorta and the superior vena cava in a fetus with 1:1 atrioventricular conducted tachycardia with long ventriculoatrial interval. Tachycardic atrial contraction (A, arrows) disappears after the seventh ventricular contraction (asterisk), and the tachycardia is stopped*

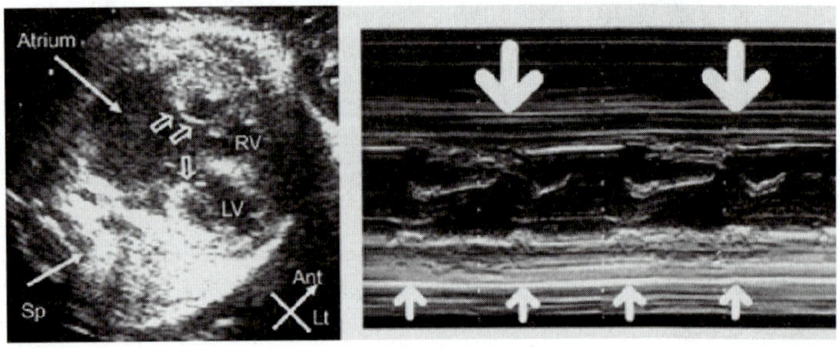

Fig. 38.38: *Left panel reveals four chamber view of polysplenia with the single atrium, the common atrioventricular valve (open arrows) and cardiomegaly. Right panel reveals simultaneous M-mode recording of ventricles (large arrows) and atria (small arrows) in this case, which demonstrates 2:1 atrioventricular block. Ant, anterior; Lt, left; LV, left ventricle; RV, right ventricle; Sp, spine*

auscultation at a prenatal visit. These arrhythmias almost always are supraventricular in origin and constitute about 85% of the fetal arrhythmias encountered. Occasionally, these extrasystoles are junctional or ventricular in origin. Isolated ectopy seems to be a self-limited process, resolving completely before or immediately after delivery. Of fetuses with premature atrial contractions, however, 1% have concomitant structural heart disease. Of such patients, 0.5–1% develop a reentrant tachycardia later in gestation All such fetuses should undergo a targeted ultrasound, including an echocardiographic evaluation, to rule out structural anomalies, and weekly auscultations should be done throughout pregnancy to rule out a sustained tachyarrhythmia.

Supraventricular Tachycardia

(Figs 38.56–38.65, 38.69–38.80)

SVT is the most common serious arrhythmia detected prenatally. It accounts for about 6% of referrals. The rate of SVT is characteristically between 240 and 260 beats/min,

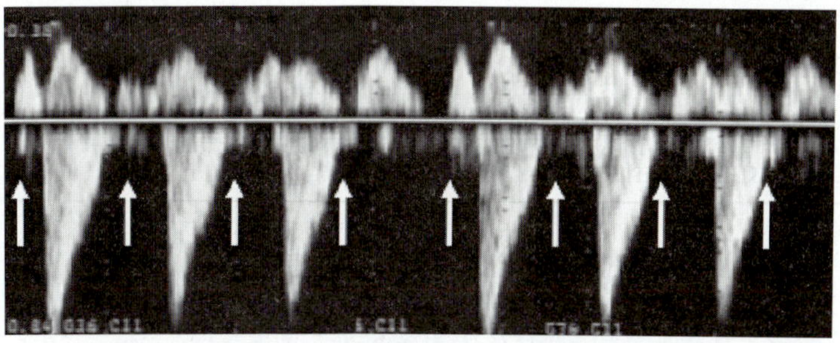

Fig. 38.39: *Wenckebach type atrioventricular block. Simultaneous Doppler trace of the ascending aorta and the superior vena cava reveals atrial contraction with regular rhythm (arrows), atrioventricular conducting time of gradual prolongation, and block with pose of ventricular contraction*

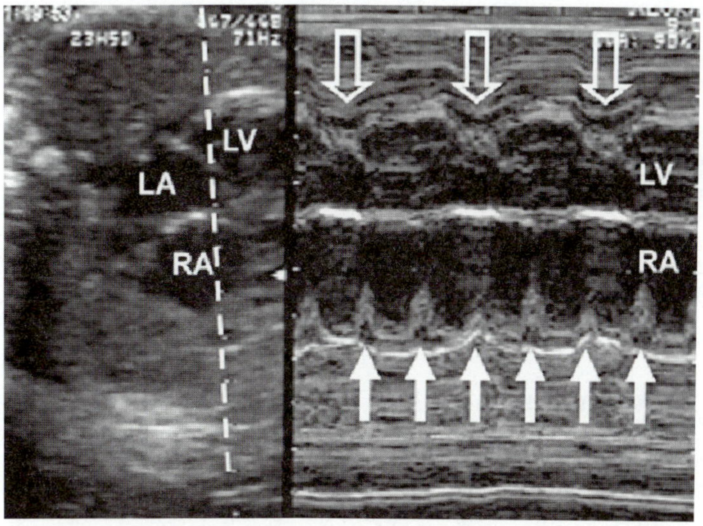

Fig. 38.40: *Simultaneous M-mode recording of both ventricles and atria in a fetus with complete atrioventricular block reveals complete dissociation of atrial and ventricular contraction with a ventricular rate of 65 bpm. Large arrows, ventricular contractions; small arrows, atrial contractions; LA, left atrium; LV, left ventricle; RA, right atrium*

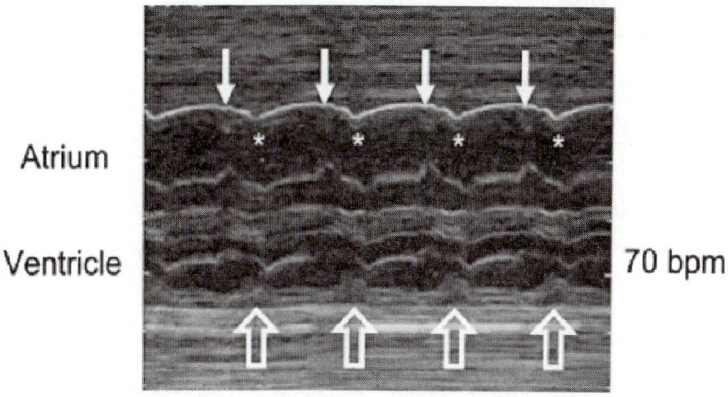

Fig. 38.41: *Simultaneous M-mode recording of ventricles and atria in a fetus with blocked paroxysmal atrial contraction (PAC) with bigeminy. The PAC (asterisk) shortly after regular atrial conduction (small arrows) does not conduct to the ventricle causing bradycardia with a ventricular rate of 70 bpm*

with 1:1 AV concordance. Most tachyarrhythmias noted in the fetus are supraventricular in origin and can result from one of three mechanisms. Supraventricular tachyarrhythmias can be reentrant (reciprocating, related to a circular, or "circus", movement of electrical activity), automatic (arising in an irritable ectopic focus above the bundle of His), or a manifestation of atrial flutter or fibrillation.

The most common mechanism of SVT in the fetus and neonate involves an electrical impulse that reenters the atrium from the ventricle, resulting in a circular movement of repeated electrical stimulation that is faster than, and independent of, the normal sinus nodal pacemaker. Such a circus movement can occur within the AV node because of dissociation of the conduction tissue, resulting in a fast and slow limb, as in the adult. In the fetus, reentrant SVT is almost always due to a discrete accessory conduction pathway outside of the AV node, however, that directly connects the atrial and ventricular myocardium (Kent's bundle in Wolff-Parkinson-White syndrome) and serves as the fast limb that bypasses the delayed conduction of the AV nodal tissue (Table 38.3).

To establish AV reentrant tachycardia, a premature atrial contraction occurs at a pivotal time during the cardiac cycle when the accessory connection is still refractory in the antegrade direction. The impulse encounters the AV node after its shorter refractory period. The impulse conducts slowly through the AV node and the ventricular muscle, then encounters the accessory conduction pathway in the retrograde direction, after a significant time delay. After retrograde reentry of the electrical impulse into the atrial muscle through the accessory pathway, a circular (circus) movement of electrical activity that incorporates the AV node in the antegrade direction is established. The wave of depolarization stimulates atrial and ventricular contraction at a rate regulated by the properties of the electrical circuit—the conduction rate and the refractory period. The heart beats at the rate of the fastest pacemaker; this electrical stimulus drives the heart at a tachycardiac rate that is independent of the SA node.

Antiarrhythmic agents that depress conduction and prolong refractory periods in the AV nodal or accessory conduction tissue can disturb the reentrant circuit and may be useful for the termination and prevention of reentrant tachycardia. These agents include the cardiac glycosides (digoxin), α-blockers (propranolol), type Ia antiarrhythmics (quinidine), type Ic antiarrhythmics (flecainide) and type III antiarrhythmics (amiodarone, sotalol).

Ectopic or automatic tachycardias occur when there is spontaneous depolarization of a pacemaker focus within the atrium. In contrast to the sudden-onset, sudden cessation pattern of reentrant tachycardias, these tachycardias are usually incessant with varying degrees of AV block.

Fetuses with a tachyarrhythmia have decreased cardiac output and are at risk for hydrops. Protracted SVT can lead to cardiac failure in a matter of days. The exact mechanism for the development of heart failure and hydrops fetalis is unclear. The progression to hydrops *in utero* seems to follow right heart failure, with tricuspid regurgitation and

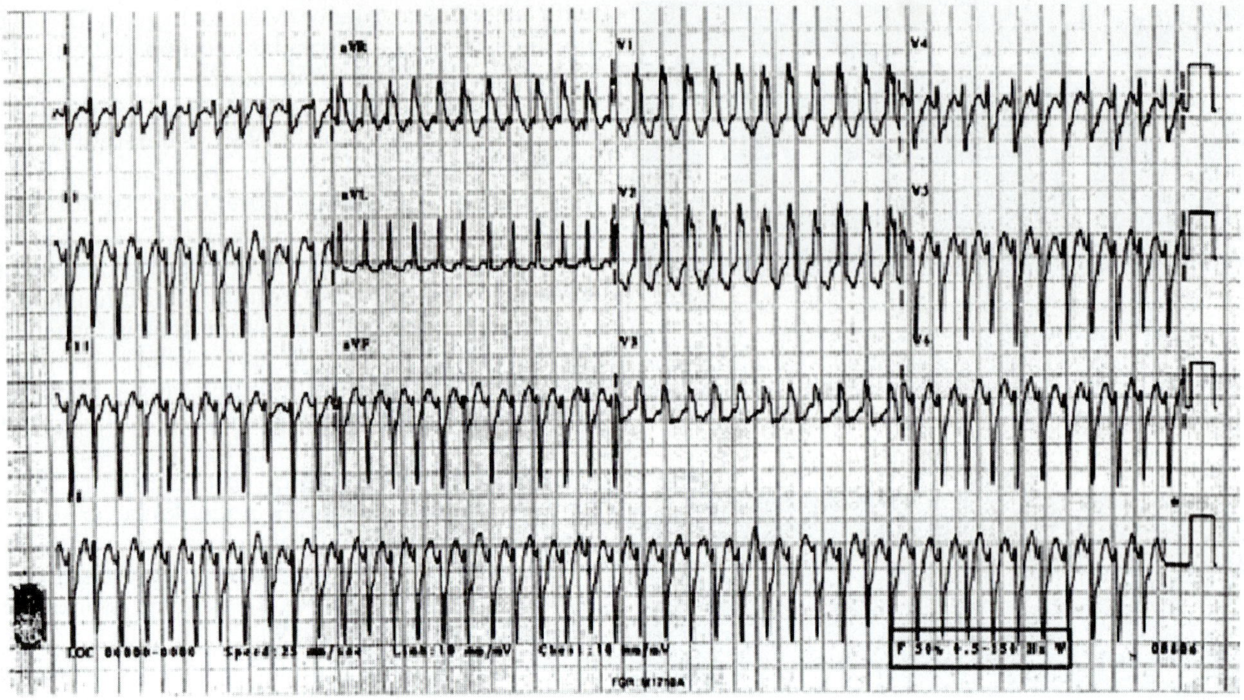

Fig. 38.42: *Incessant idiopathic ventricular tachycardia of infancy. A rapid, wide QRS tachycardia with a right bundle-branch block pattern and a QRS axis of around 90°. The shorter secondary R wave in V1 suggests VT. Ventricular dissociation is not easy to see but the rhythm strip at the bottom does suggest irregular P waves superimposed on the T waves. The origin of the VT is presumably from the posterior left ventricle*

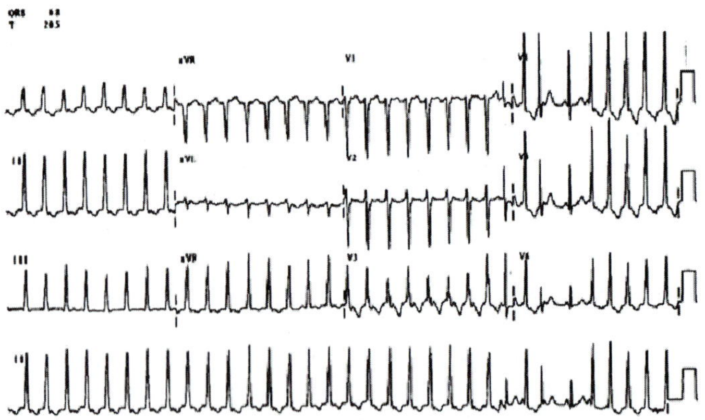

Fig. 38.43: *Complete atrioventricular block. A recording from a neonate whose mother has Sjögren's syndrome. The atrial rate is normal at 140 beats/min. The ventricular rate is 65 beats/min and there is complete AV dissociation. The QRS complexes are normal. The baby had a structurally normal heart and there was no immediate indication for pacemaker implantation*

right ventricular dilation signifying impending decompensation. Gembruch and colleagues showed that in the human fetus with SVT, pulsatile venous flow velocity waveforms in the inferior vena cava, ductus venosus, and left hepatic vein show a normal biphasic forward pattern below a "critical" heart rate of about 210 beats/min, whereas pulsatile reversal of blood flow with monophasic forward flow during systole and reversed flow in diastole was noted when the heart rate was greater than 210 beats/min. It has

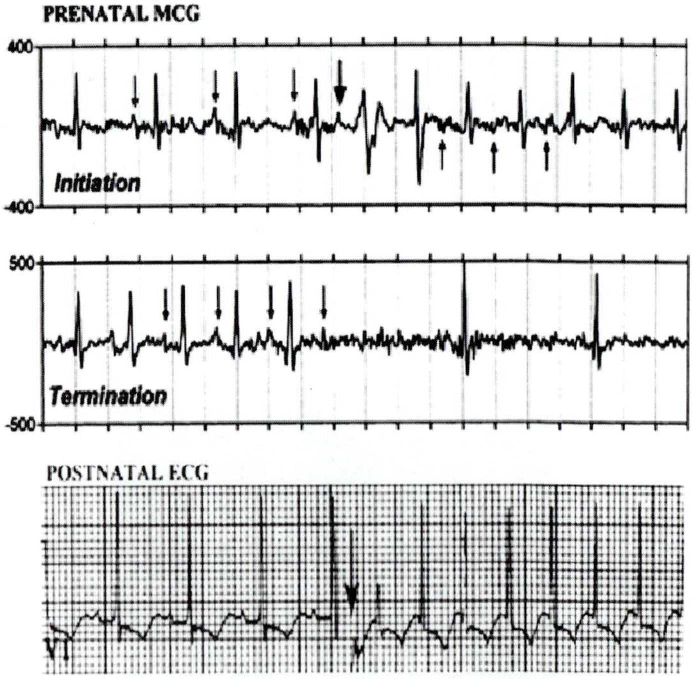

Fig. 38.44: *The top two panels are 4-second fMCG tracings showing initiation and termination of SVT in subject 1. SVT initiates with a spontaneous PAC (thick arrow). Thin arrows indicate P waves. The first few beats of SVT are aberrantly conducted. Termination is attributable to antegrade block in the AV node and is followed by marked transient bradycardia. The bottom panel shows postnatal initiation of SVT in lead V1 by a single extrastimulus, indicated by the arrow, during transesophageal pacing procedure*

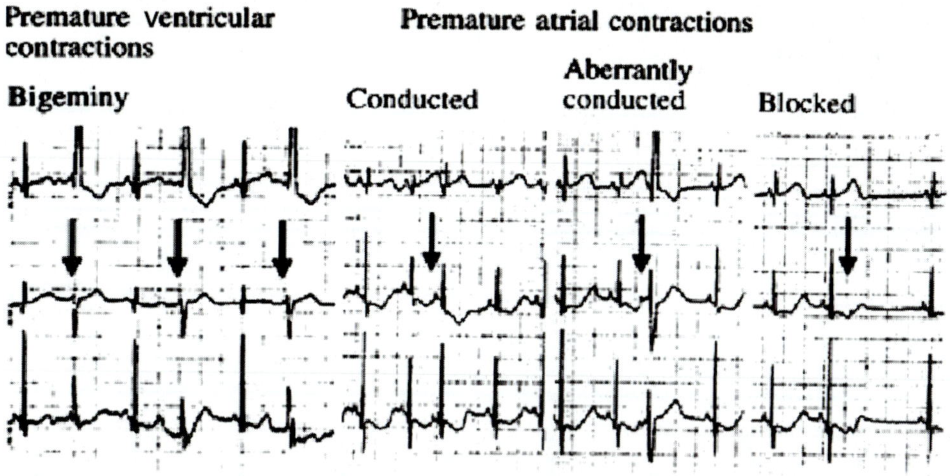

Fig. 38.45: *Ectopy. The left panel shows a three-lead rhythm strip of PVCs marked by arrows. Note that no early P wave precedes these beats. The three subsequent panels show PACs conducted with a normal-appearing QRS and an aberrant QRS and not conducted through the AV node (arrows) (note the P waves)*

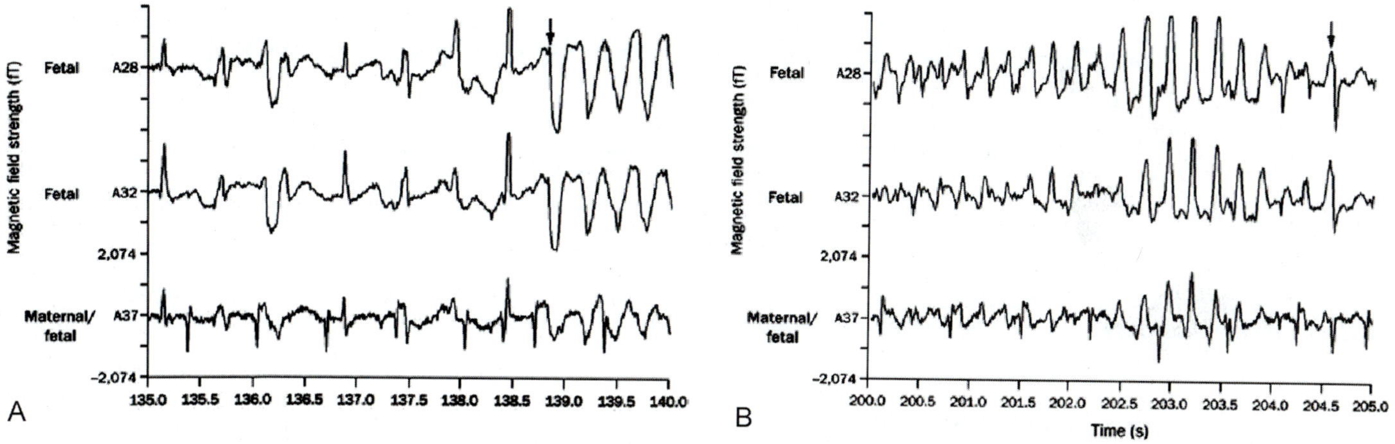

Fig. 38.46: *(A) Onset of torsades de pointes ventricular tachycardia occurs after 138.5 s (arrow). (B) Termination of torsades de pointes occurs at 204.5 s (arrow). Arrhythmia was triggered by use of amiodarone to treat what was initially considered, on the basis of findings from echocardiography, to be drug-refractory fetal ventricular tachycardia. (Permission obtained from Elsevier Ltd. © Cuneo, B. F. et al. Am J Cardiol. 2003; 91, 1395–1398)*

been postulated that either passive liver congestion associated with cardiac failure or decreased hepatic perfusion from decreased cardiac output may result in hypoalbuminemia, leading to decreased oncotic pressure and transudation of fluid into interstitial spaces.

Atrial Flutter and Fibrillation (Figs 38.63 and 38.75)

Atrial flutter and fibrillation are infrequent causes of SVT in the fetus. Atrial flutter seems to result from a circus movement of electrical activity within the body of the atrium. The atrial rate postnatally is typically 300 beats/min. In the fetus, rates of 400–460 beats/min are the rule, with varying degrees of AV block. Atrial flutter has been associated with a poor prognosis, which may be due to its association with structural heart disease in 20% of cases and the development of hydrops fetalis. In contrast to postnatal therapy of atrial flutter, in which increasing the degree of AV block with a resultant decrease in the ventricular rate may lead to a decrease in heart failure, control of the ventricular response rate in fetuses with severe hydrops secondary to atrial flutter has not resulted in an improvement in the fetal hemodynamic status. Kleinman and Copel suggested that this lack of improvement is probably due to the unique cardiovascular dynamics of the fetus—its relatively restrictive ventricular myocardium and its relatively volume—loaded right heart. They concluded that much of the decompensation accompanying tachyarrhythmias reflects diastolic rather than systolic dysfunction. Specifically, unless the atrial flutter is controlled with resumption of a 1:1 AV contraction sequence, there will continue to be atrial contractions against a closed or partially closed AV valve, resulting in atrial pressure waves that keep mean systolic venous pressure high, retarding the resolution of fetal edema and effusions. This condition may require an agent such as sotolol after control of the ventricular response rate with digoxin. Atrial fibrillation seems to be even rarer than flutter; however, the same principles apply to therapy.

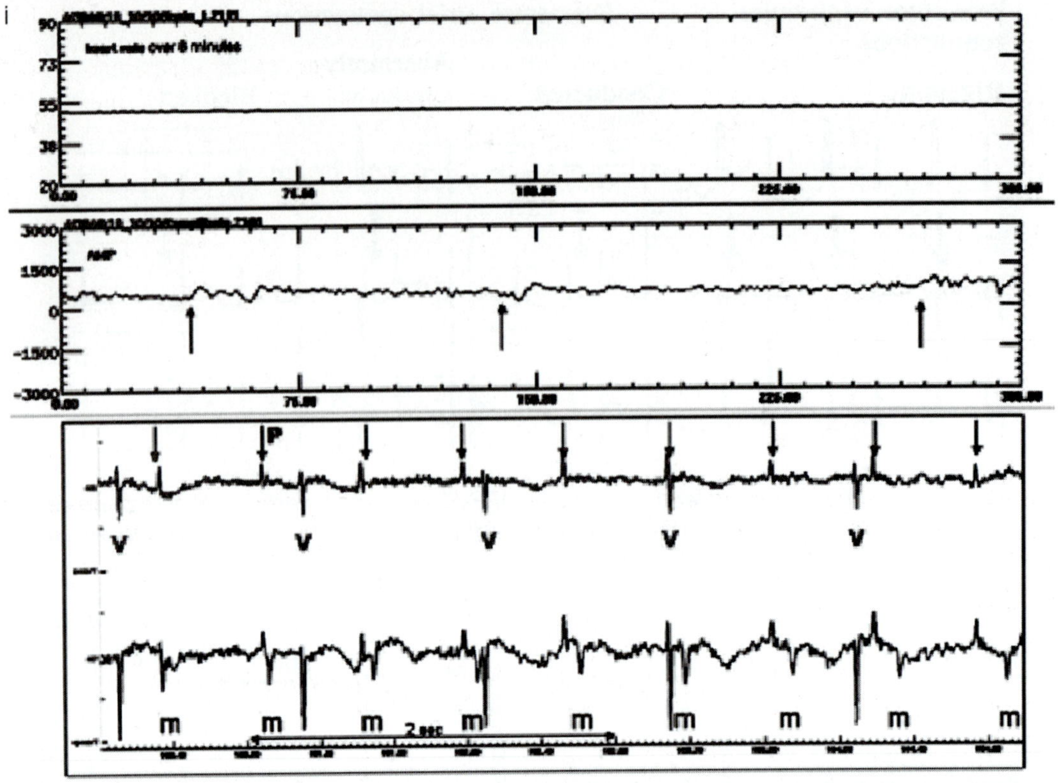

Fig. 38.47: *FMCG recording from a 24-week GA fetus with complete heart block. Note in the top two tracings that the rate is stable at about 52 beats/minute during 5 minutes. There is no reactivity of the ventricular rate with the fetal movement, denoted by the upward-facing arrows in the actogram tracing. In the lower tracing, the maternal QRS is marked "m", fetal QRS "V", and the fetal P waves with the downward-facing arrows. Note complete atrioventricular dissociation. The QRS duration is not prolonged in this case, but due to the non-reactivity and low rate, this fetus will require pacing after birth*

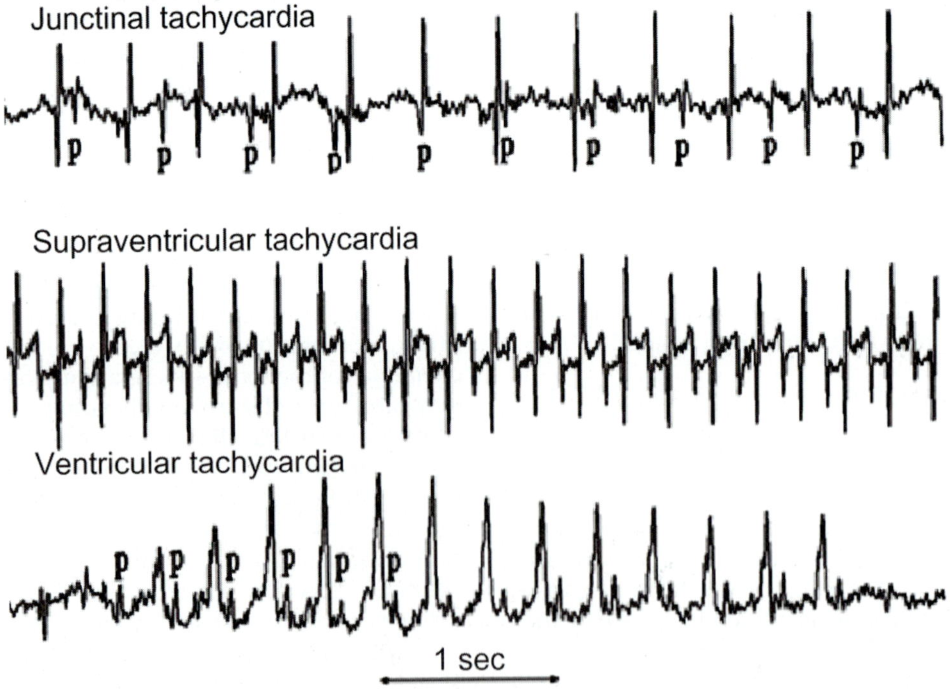

Fig. 38.48: *Three different forms of fetal tachycardia are shown using fMCG. P waves are denoted in the top and bottom tracings with a "p". Note AV dissociation during junctional and ventricular tachycardia, but 1:1 association during SVT. JET and VT are distinguished by the narrow QRS of JET and the wide QRS of VT*

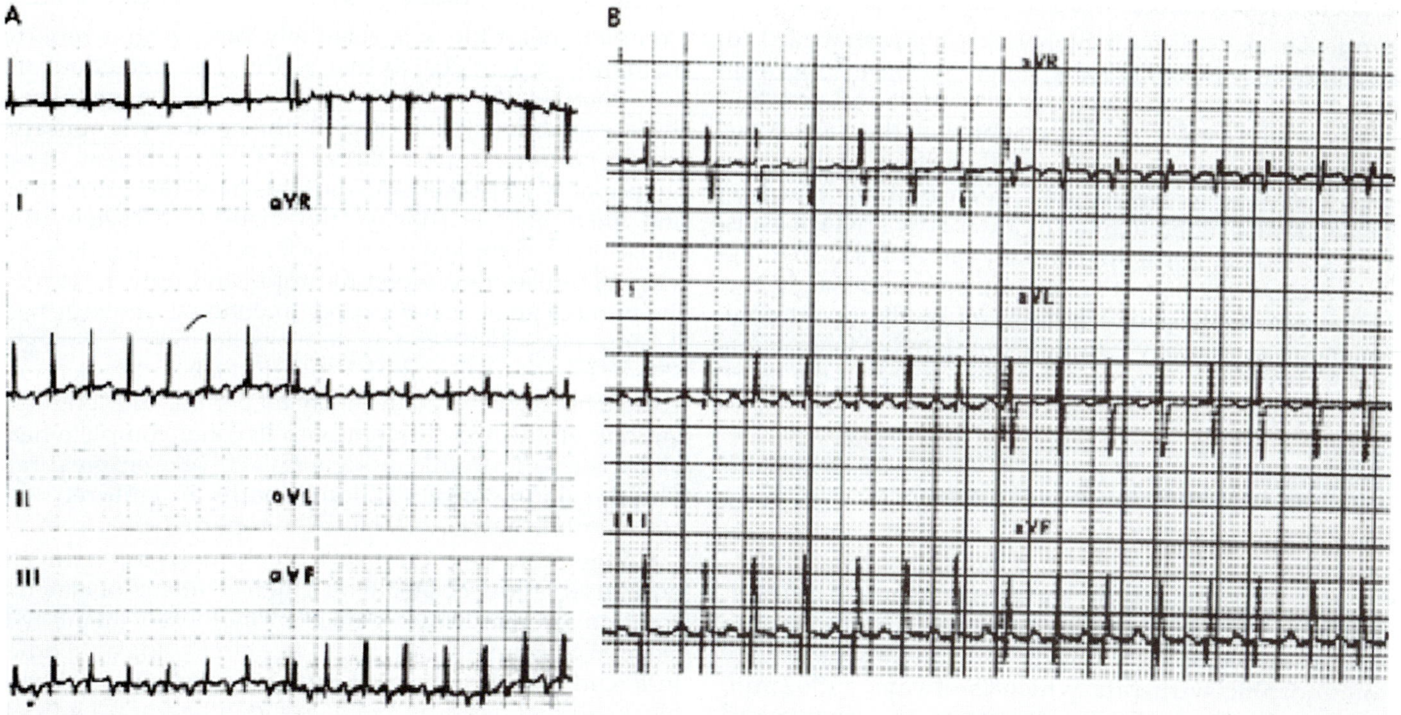

Fig. 38.49: *Fetal supraventricular tachycardia (A) shows form of junctional reciprocating tachycardia and (B) shows atrial ectopic tachycardia*

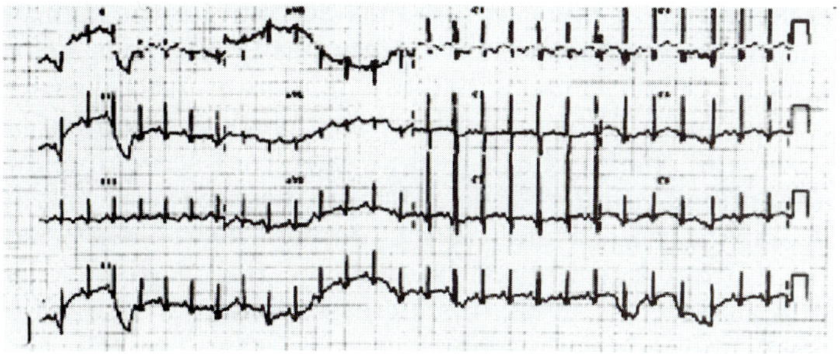

Fig. 38.50: *Supraventricular tachycardia has one-to-one AV conduction, and fetal heart rate is between 200 and 300 beats per minute*

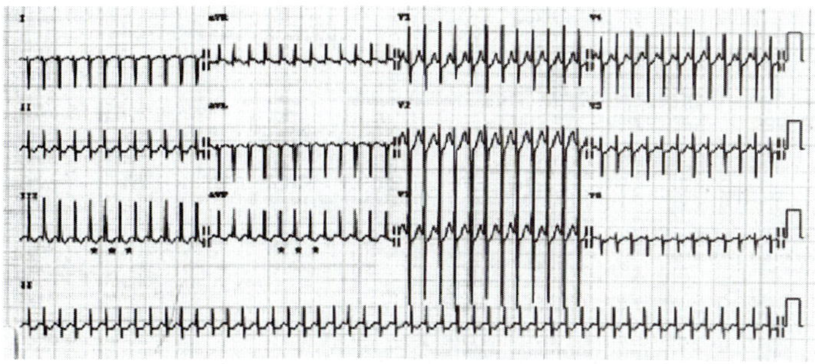

Fig. 38.51: *This neonate with cardiac arrhythmias due to umbilical venous catheterisation who had a supraventricular tachycardia requiring treatment with intravenous adenosine administration*

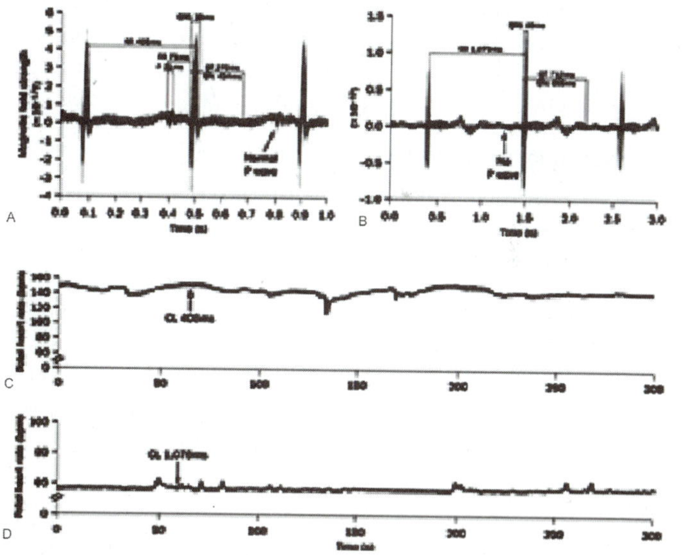

Fig. 38.52: *Signal-averaged electrograms of fetal magnetocardiography recordings from a fetus with maternal SSA/Ro autoantibody isoimmunization. (A) Sinus rhythm is present at 19 weeks of gestation. (B) At 20 weeks, complete atrioventricular block had developed with a prolonged QTUc interval of 686 ms. The P wave appears absent because it is signal-averaged away when not stably associated with the QRS interval. (C) At 19 weeks, the fetal heart rate trend over 5 min (arrow) documents stable sinus rhythm at ≥ 145 bpm. (D) At 20 weeks, the fetal heart rate trend over 5 min (arrow) shows third-degree atrioventricular block at 55 bpm. Abbreviation: CL, cycle length*

Ventricular Tachycardia (Figs 38.65, 38.84, 38.86 and 38.87)

Ventricular tachycardia is highly variable with regard to rate. Rates vary from 400 beats/min to 170 beats/min. The diagnosis is made with M-mode or Doppler echocardiography, which shows AV dissociation with the ventricular chamber contracting at a faster pace than the atrial chamber. Not all of these fetuses require antiarrhythmic therapy. Misdiagnosing ventricular tachycardia as SVT, which leads to the administration of digoxin, may cause life-threatening ventricular fibrillation. It is imperative to understand the mechanism of the tachyarrhythmia so that a rational management strategy can be formulated. Most of the workers believe that therapy should be started if the heart rate is sustained at greater than 200 beats/min or if there is associated hydrops fetalis (Figs 38.95 and 38.96).

Treatment of Ventricular Tachycardia

Treatment of ventricular tachycardia is rare and poorly understood in the neonate. The electrocardiographic criteria of ventricular tachycardia (wide QRS complexes of different morphology to the sinus QRS complexes, atrioventricular dissociation) should be fulfilled. The arrhythmia is usually monomorphic with rate which is always >150/min. Intravenous magnesium sulphate in the severe and permanent forms, oral beta-blockers in forms triggered by acceleration of the sinus rhythm, oral amiodarone alone or associated with propranolol are prescribed. It is advocated that isolated, idiopathic ventricular tachycardia of the neonate usually carry a good prognosis which is not dependent on the tachycardia of the permanence of the arrhythmia. Simple treatment (beta-blocker or amiodarone) is usually associate with restoration of sinus rhythm and definitive cure during the first year of life.

Bradyarrhythmias (Figs 38.56 and 38.60)

Bradyarrhythmias may be the result of blocked premature contractions, sinus bradycardia, or AV block. About 5% of all fetal arrhythmias are classified as slow. The most common cause of fetal bradyarrhythmias with ventricular rates less than 60 beats/min is complete heart block. These fetuses can be divided into two groups: (1) fetuses with complex congenital heart disease and (2) fetuses with immune complex-related damage to the fetal conduction tissue secondary to maternal autoantibodies.

Complete Heart Block (Figs 38.47, 38. 54 and 38.82)

Complete heart block is relatively rare, with a reported incidence of 1 in 20,000 live births. The detection of *in utero* complete AV block is associated with congenital heart disease in about 50% of cases. If the anatomy is abnormal (most commonly AV canal defect, outflow vessel abnormality, or isomerism), the fetus may develop hydrops and die *in utero* or shortly after birth. In a review of 26 fetuses with complete heart block and AV canal defect, at least 18 fetuses developed hydrops, and only 1 survived the immediate neonatal period. In contrast, the prognosis is more favorable if the anatomy is normal. In a review, 85% of fetuses with complete heart block and structurally normal hearts survived the neonatal period. The long-term outlook of affected children with isolated complete heart block is also favorable, with a 95% 20-year survival rate. The development of cardiomyopathy in children with autoimmune heart block has been reported.

Congenital complete heart block in an anatomically normal fetus is associated with a high incidence of maternal connective tissue disease. Almost all mothers of infants with isolated congenital heart block have circulating antibodies. In a study of 54 mothers of infants with congenital heart block, all had anti-Ro (SS-A) and 76% had anti-La (SS-B) antibodies. Immunofluorescent stains show selective binding of immune complexes to His-Purkinje tissue and fetal myocardium, which causes inflammation and fibrosis in the region of the AV node and bundle of His. The immune-complex binding and inflammatory infiltration of fetal ventricular myocardium may account for the clinical finding of congestive cardiomyopathy that has been reported. Most women with these circulating antibodies are asymptomatic. When complete heart block is identified *in utero* or in the newborn period, maternal screening for autoantibodies and collagen vascular disease is warranted. Overall the risk of a fetus having complete heart block when the mother has known connective tissue disease is estimated to be 1 in 60; this increases to 1 in 20 if anti-Ro (SS-A) antibody is present.

Some have proposed that the mechanical P-R interval can be used to evaluate for P-R prolongation in SSA-positive mothers, however, it is unclear that this would effectively screen those at risk, since repolarization abnormalities (prolongation of QT) can not be detected with this method,

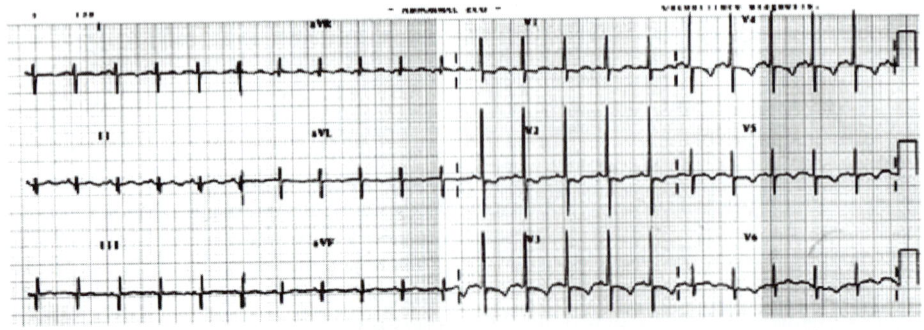

Fig. 38.53: *Newborn with birth asphyxia and myocardial damage with ECG changes (T wave inversion in all the V leads with narrow q waves in the inferior leads). There was myocardial dysfunction and an increased troponin T level*

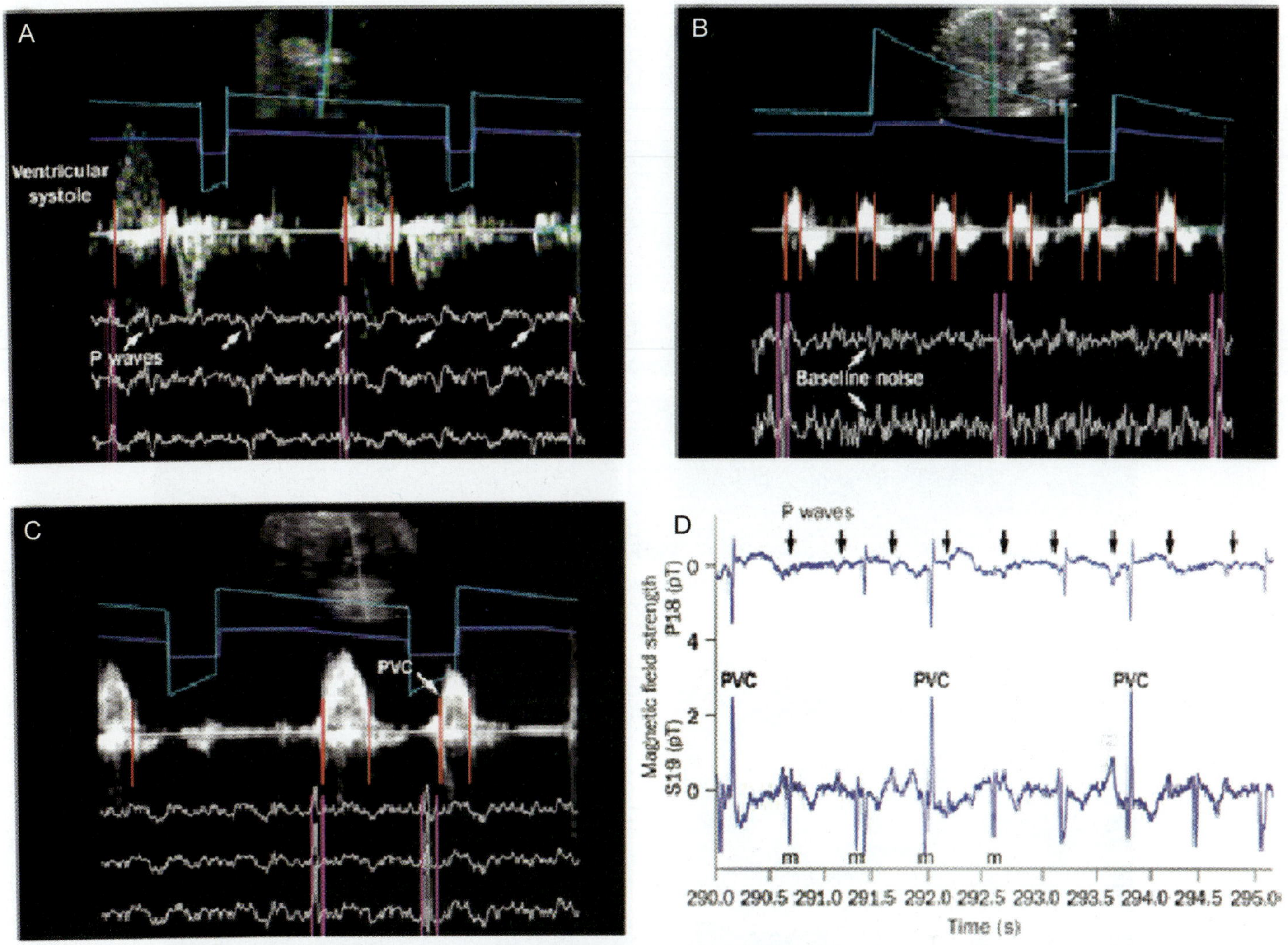

Fig. 38.54: *Simultaneous fetal magnetocardiography and Doppler echocardiography recordings from a fetus with isoimmune third-degree atrioventricular block at 23 weeks and 4 days of gestation. The two data types (echocardiographic and magnetocardiographic) were superimposed using timing marker channels (gray and turquoise lines) to provide a single image during postprocessing. QRS complexes (pink vertical lines) precede mechanical atrial wall and ventricular systolic velocities (red vertical lines), which enables interpretation of the electromechanics of the fetal heart. (A) P waves are indicated by arrows and are not conducting. (B) Baseline noise (arrows) results from Doppler echocardiography frequencies that must be removed during signal processing. Atrial wall velocities (red lines) and QRS complexes indicate atrioventricular dissociation. (C) Ventricular systolic Doppler events including a PVC (arrow). (D) A fetal magnetocardiography recording from this fetus shows third-degree atrioventricular block and a narrow QRS duration with frequent ventricular ectopy. P waves (arrows) are not conducting. Abbreviations: m, maternal; PVC, premature ventricular contraction*

and the onset of AV block appears to be very rapid. This technique has shown that fetuses with PR prolongation can have other pathologies, however, including incomplete AV block, atrial flutter and long QT syndrome. The mechanical PR interval overestimates the actual P-R interval.

Effective prenatal treatment for complete heart block has not been established. Maternal administration of α-agonists such as terbutaline has not been associated with improved hemodynamic status (resolution of hydrops), despite increasing the heart rate. This situation is probably similar to atrial flutter/fibrillation in that cannon A waves associated with atrial contractions against a closed AV valve need to be reduced to decrease the systemic venous pressure that should result in resolution of the hydrops. Recently, some authors have associated the use of α-sympathomimetics with better outcomes. Attempts to reduce the circulating maternal antibodies have included the use of plasmapheresis and the administration of prednisone. Prednisone is a poor choice for fetal immunosuppression because it is largely inactivated by the placenta. Maternal dexamethasone or betamethasone therapy may hold more promise. Two attempts at fetal pacemaker placement have been reported. Neither attempt resulted in fetal survival. In general, the prognosis for congenital heart block is good when the ventricular rate is greater than 55 beats/min in the structurally normal fetus. When complete heart block is identified in a fetus, close echocardiographic follow-up is necessary to look for the development of hydrops fetalis.

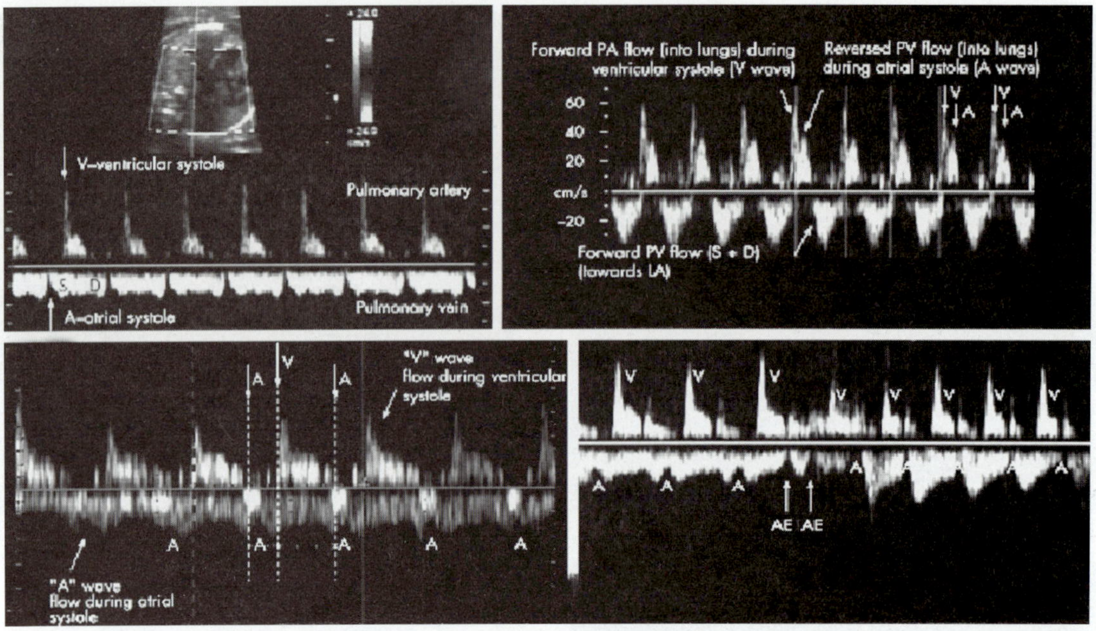

Fig. 38.55: *Evaluation of fetal arrhythmias from simultaneous pulsed wave Doppler in pulmonary artery and vein*

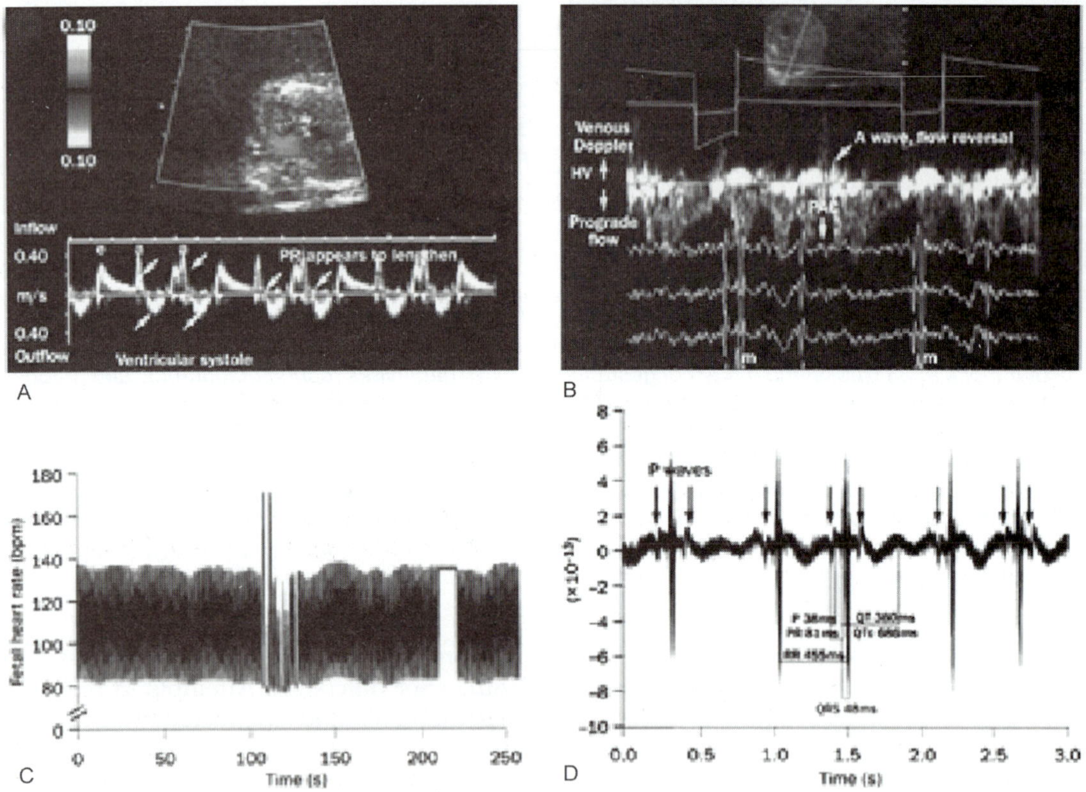

Fig. 38.56: *Fetal magnetocardiography and Doppler echocardiography tracings from a fetus with a rhythm pattern that simulated Mobitz type I second-degree atrioventricular block at 18 weeks and 1 day of gestation. This fetus presented with tachyarrhythmia (not shown) of 260 bpm. (A) Doppler echocardiography of the left ventricular inflow and outflow shows that atrioventricular conduction appears prolonged and followed by dropped ventricular events (upward arrows) and hidden atrial events (downward arrows). (B) Simultaneous fetal magnetocardiography and Doppler echocardiography demonstrates venous flow reversal (diagonal arrow) consistent with cannon A waves after alternate QRS complexes that are caused by blocked PACs (down-facing arrows). (C) The fetal heart rate trends show persistence of this alternating rhythm over most of the 5 min recording. (D) A 20 s signal-averaged trace of the QRS interval before the pause led to a final diagnosis of blocked atrial trigeminy. Abbreviations: a, atrial; e, passive inflow; HV, hepatic vein; PAC, premature atrial contraction*

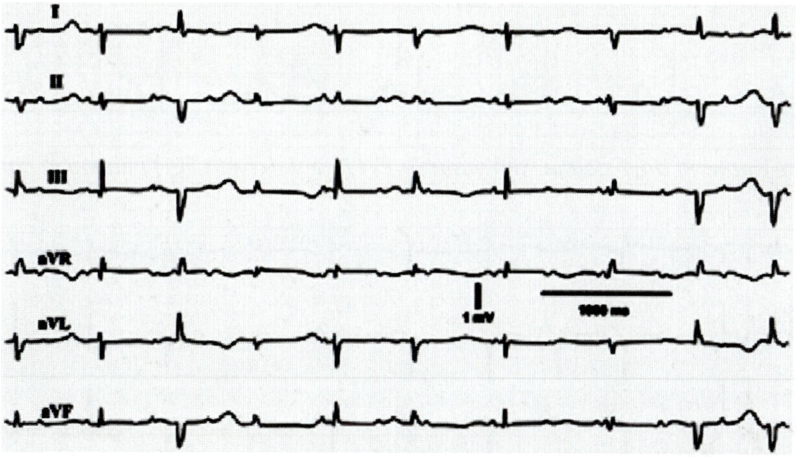

Fig. 38.57: *Six-lead ECG during a bradycardic episode in which extreme prolongation of QT interval (as long as 760 ms1/2) is detectable. The third-grade AV block (HR 78 bpm, atrial rate 135 bpm) is due to the ventricular refractoriness. Polymorphic QRS complexes resulting from variant intraventricular conduction delays lead to different QRS durations up to 90 ms*

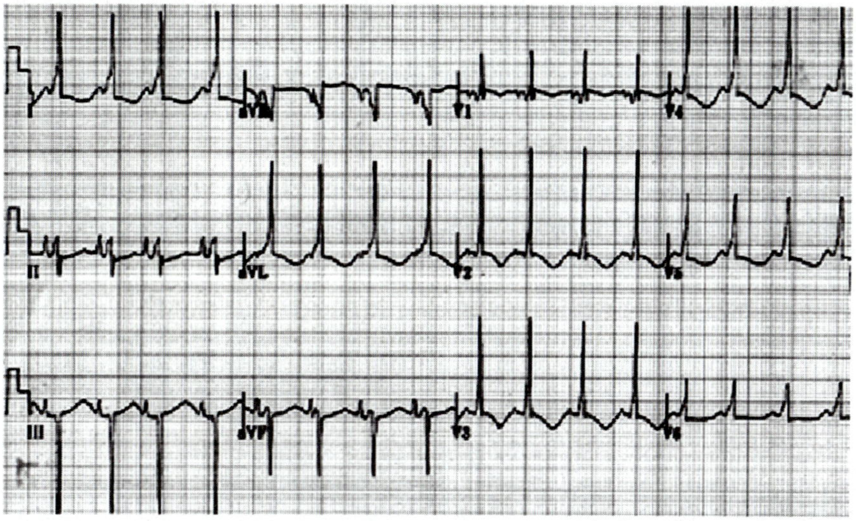

Fig. 38.58: *A 12-lead ECG demonstrates preexcitation (Wolff-Parkinson-White syndrome) during sinus rhythm. The precordial delta wave transitions from negative in V1 to positive between leads V2 and V3, consistent with a septal accessory pathway. Although a net positive QRS polarity in V1 suggests a left-sided accessory pathway in older patients, its significance is unclear in neonates who have predominant right-sided forces*

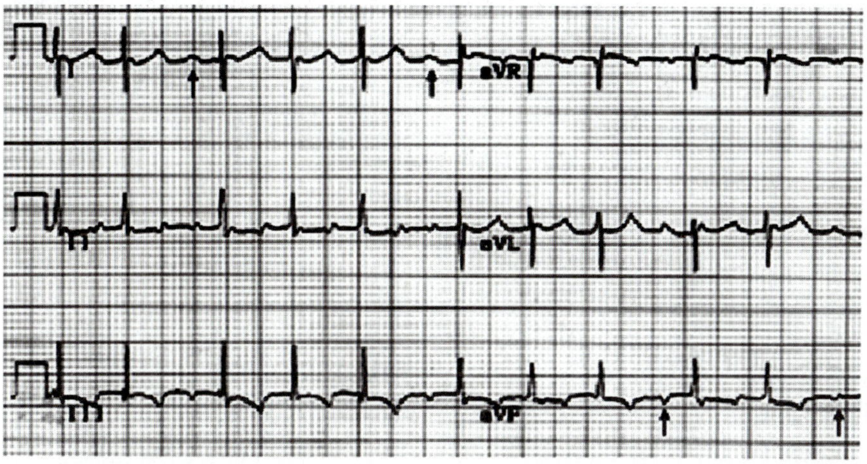

Fig. 38.59: *A limb-lead ECG (at half standard; 5 mm/mV) demonstrating ectopic atrial tachycardia with an atrial cycle length of 220 ms and variable atrioventricular conduction. The P-wave morphology (arrows) suggests a lateral right atrial origin with a positive P-wave in lead I and a biphasic P-wave in lead AVF. A narrow-complex QRS is seen with 2:1 and 3:1 atrioventricular conduction*

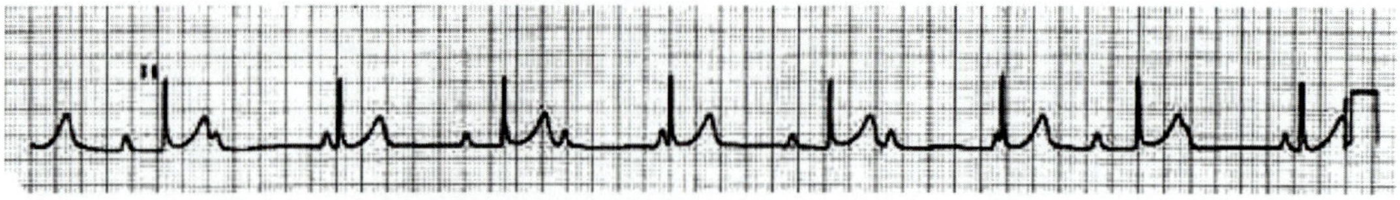

Fig. 38.60: *ECG of a neonate showing bradycardia with variable PR interval, fixed R-R interval in congenital complete heart block*

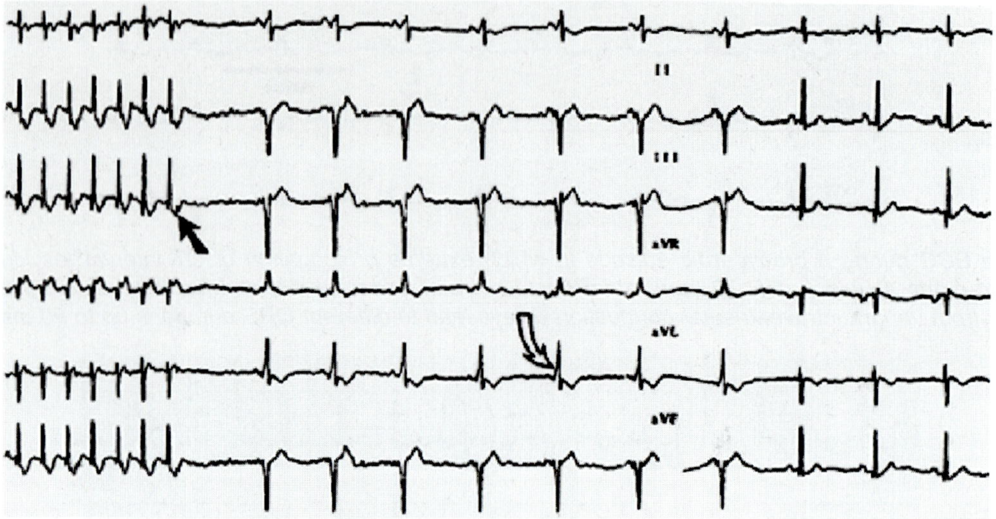

Fig. 38.61: *Adenosine in atrioventricular (AV) reentry tachycardia. Administration of intravenous adenosine to a neonate with orthodromic AV reentry tachycardia. Note that tachycardia terminates with a nonconducted P wave (solid arrow). There is then a sinus bradycardia with obvious ventricular preexcitation (open arrow). As the sinus rate accelerates the delta wave disappears and the QRS returns to normal*

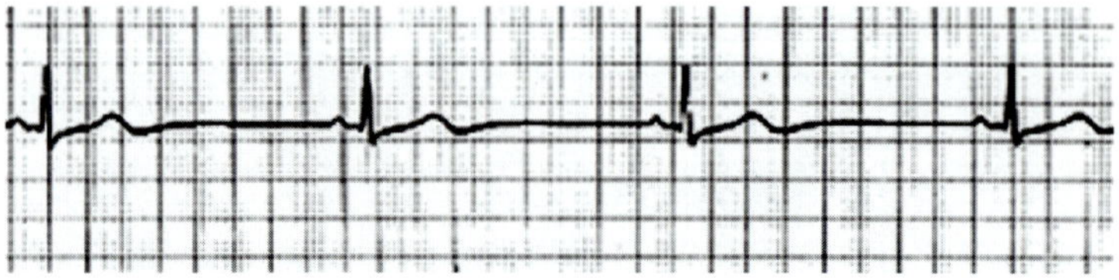

Fig. 38.62: *ECG showing sinus bradycardia in neonate*

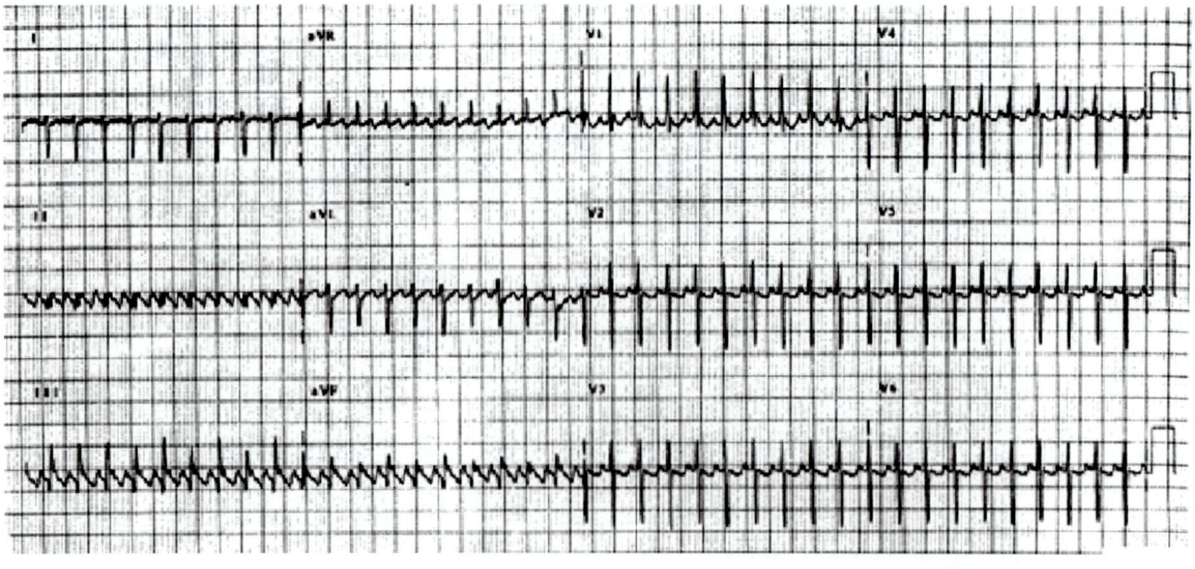

Fig. 38.63: *Atrial flutter. A recording from a neonate with idiopathic atrial flutter. The flutter rate is 460 beats/min with 2:1 conduction giving a ventricular rate of 230 beats/min. "Saw tooth" flutter waves are best seen in leads II, III and aVF*

Table 38.1: *Differential diagnosis of fetal arrhythmias*

Atrial rate	*Atrial rhythm*	*Ventricular rate*	*Ventricular rhythm*	*AV or VA association*	*Differential diagnosis*
Normal	Regular	> Atrial rate 180–200/min	Regular	Dissociated or intermittent 1:1	Accelerated ventricular or junctional rhythm
Normal	Regular	> Atrial rate 210–400/min	Regular or minimally irregular	Dissociated or 1:1	Ventricular tachycardia, junctional tachycardia
Normal	Regular	< Atrial rate 40–110/min	Regular	Dissociated	3rd-degree AV block
Normal	Regular	< Atrial rate 70–110/min	Irregular	Intermittent dissociated	2nd-degree AV block
High 200–300/min	Regular	Same as atrial rate	Regular	1:1	AV reentrant SVT, AV node reentrant SVT
High 180–300/min	Regular but varying	Same as atrial rate	Same as atrial rhythm	1:1	Permanent junctional reciprocating tachycardia
High 300–450/min	Regular	< Atrial rate 150–225/min	Regular or irregular	1:1, 2:1, 3:1, or variable	Atrial flutter
High 180–220/min	Regular but varying	Same as atrial rate	Same as atrial rhythm	1:1	Sinus tachycardia
High	Irregular "chaotic"	Same as atrial rate	Irregular	Variable	Chaotic atrial tachycardia, atrial flutter/fibrillation
Low 80–110/min	Regular	Same as atrial rate	Regular	1:1	Sinus bradycardia, junctional rhythm

AV, atrioventricular; VA, ventriculoatrial; SVT, supraventricular tachycardia.

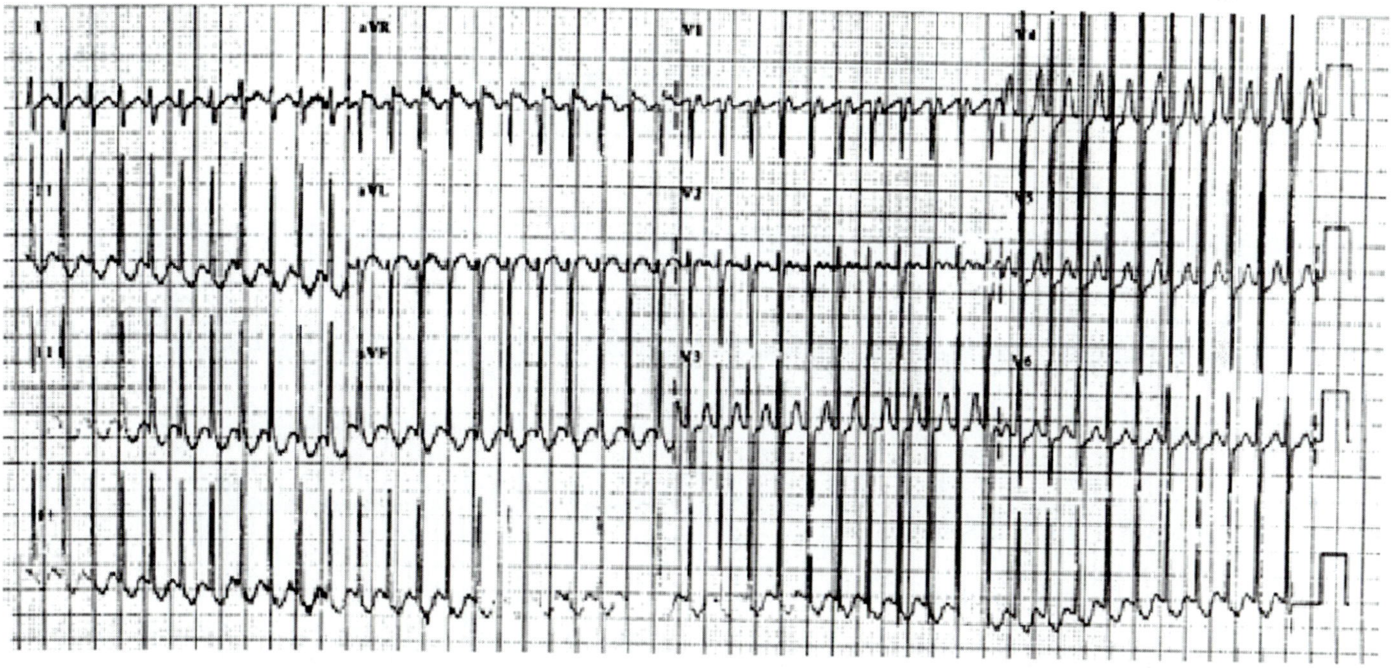

Fig. 38.64: *ECG atrial ectopic tachycardia. The PR interval is prolonged and P waves are in the terminal portion of the previous QRS (best seen in lead V1). The presentation was with apparent "dilated cardiomyopathy" but myocardial impairment was secondary and improved once the arrhythmia was controlled*

The presence of hydrops fetalis is a poor prognostic sign, and when it is associated with structural heart disease, it almost always is fatal. Our experience with fetal MCG in the evaluation of 29 fetuses with congenital heart block has documented junctional or ventricular tachycardia in 30% of fetuses, both in the structural and isoimmune groups. This may explain the high mortality seen prenatally. In addition, repolarization abnormalities (QT prolongation, T wave alternans) and myocardial hypertrophy may also increase risk of sudden fetal demise.

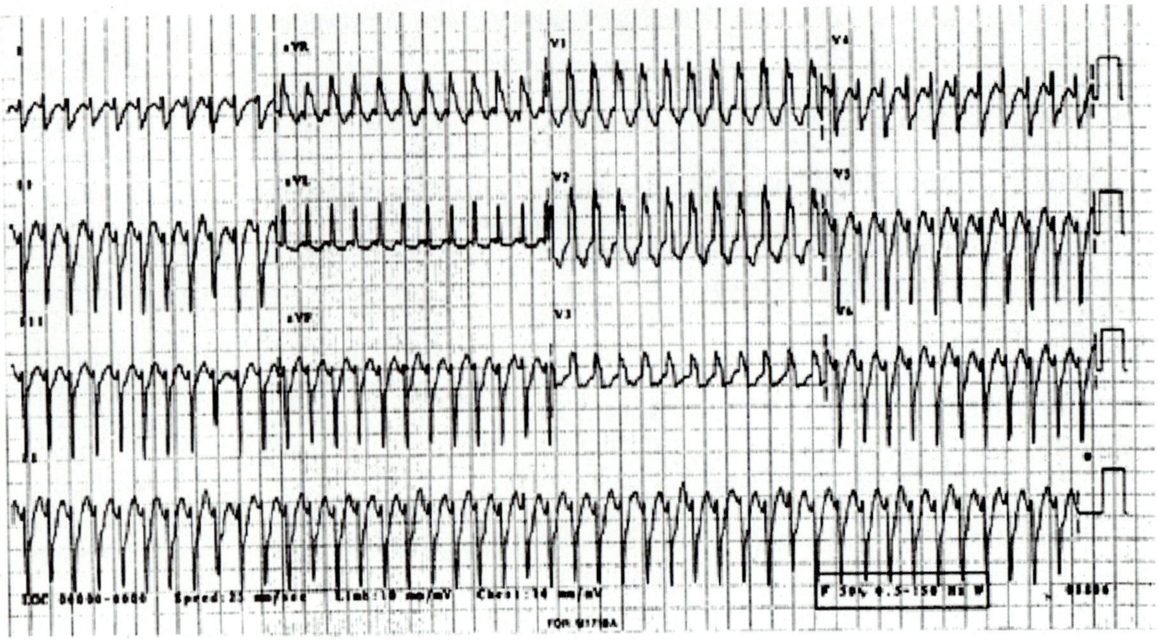

Fig. 38.65: *Incessant idiopathic ventricular tachycardia of infancy. A rapid, wide QRS tachycardia with a right bundle-branch block pattern and a QRS axis of around –90°. The shorter secondary R wave in V1 suggests VT. Ventricular dissociation is not easy to see but the rhythm strip at the bottom does suggest irregular P waves superimposed on the T waves. The origin of the VT is presumably from the posterior left ventricle*

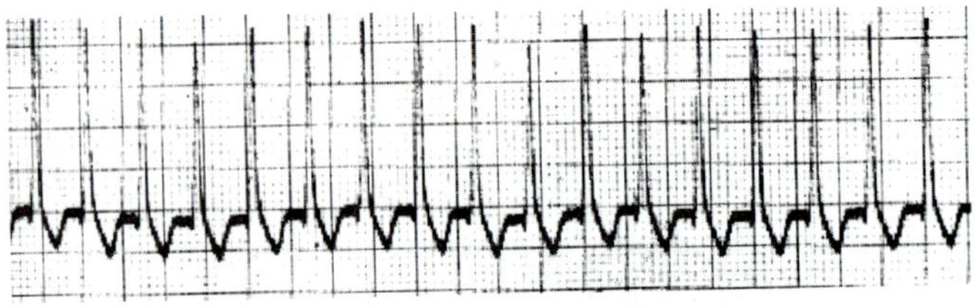

Fig. 38.66: *Supraventricular tachycardia in a newborn baby*

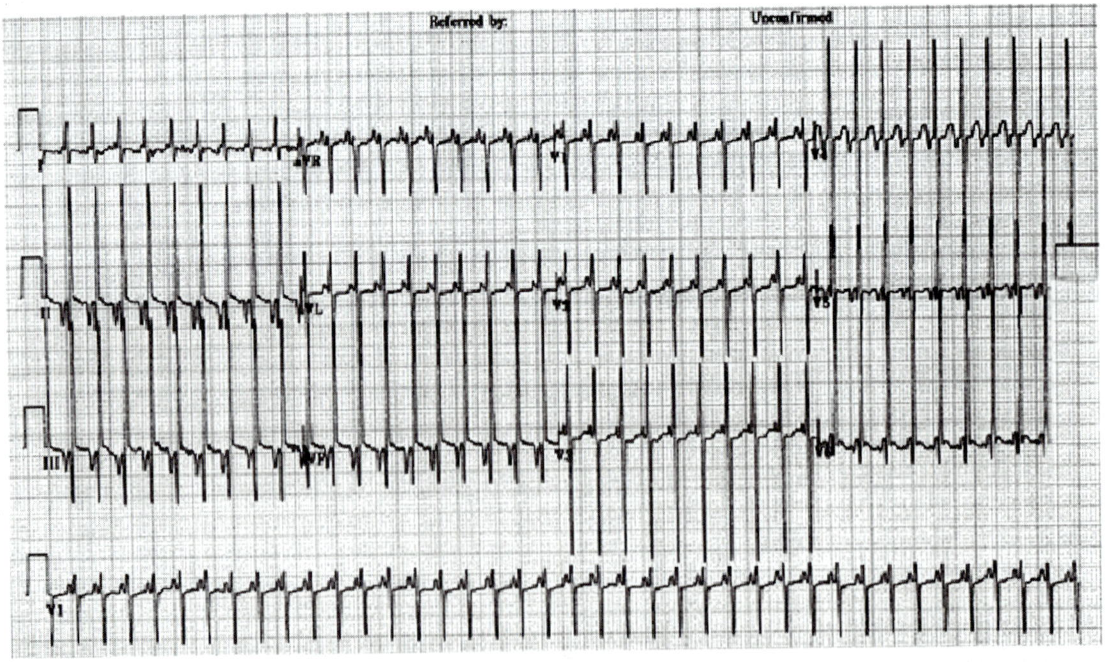

Fig. 38.67: *Permanent junctional reciprocating tachycardia. An incessant arrhythmia with a characteristic appearance. Note the very long RP interval and the deeply inverted P waves in leads II, III and aVF. This is a type of orthodromic atrioventricular (AV) reentry over a relatively slowly conducting concealed right posteroseptal pathway*

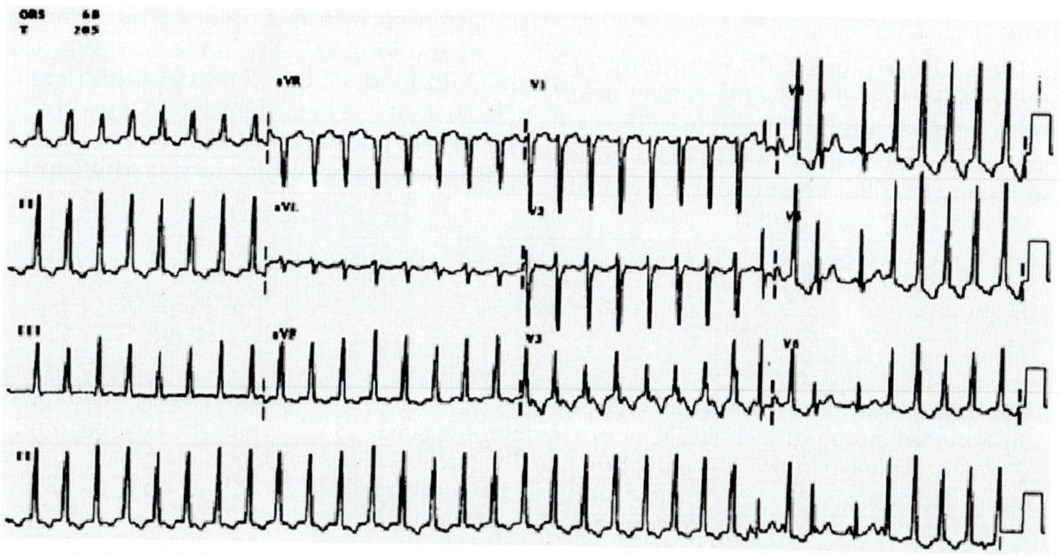

Fig. 38.68: *Ventricular tachycardia in infancy. The QRS is relatively narrow but is obviously wide compared with the sinus beat seen in leads V4-6. There is 1:1 VA conduction in the first ¾th of the recording but slower dissociated P waves are seen after the sinus beats in the last ¼th*

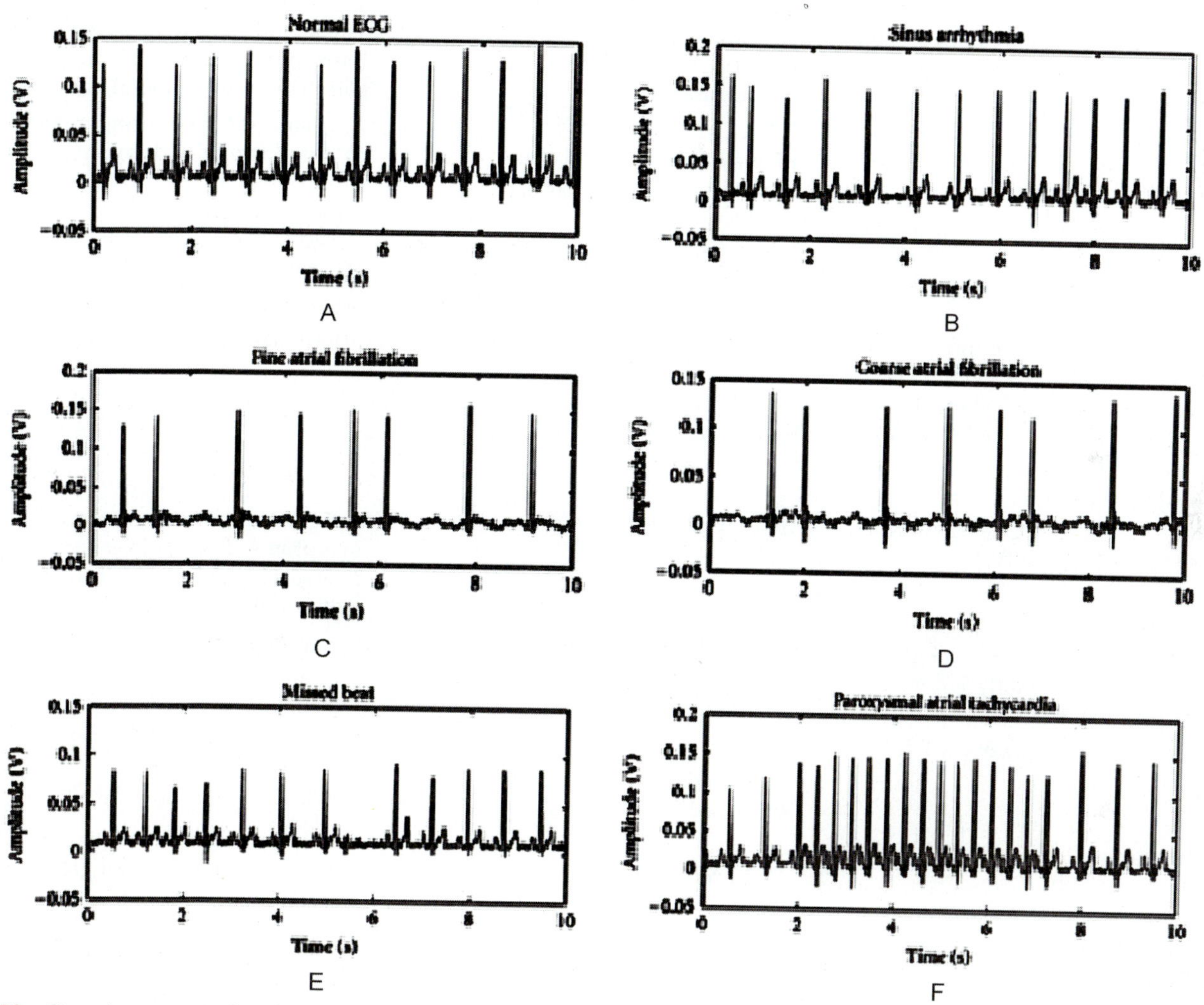

Fig. 38.69: *Signals representing five common and well-known supraventricular arrhythmias were gathered, using a Fluke MPS450 patient simulator. The signals were processed using the same methodology as for real patient data. Respiration simulation was programmed, in order to mimic utterly the behavior of a sick patient. The five conditions were fine and coarse atrial fibrillation, paroxysmal atrial tachycardia, sinus arrhythmia and missed beat. These signals were recorded for different heart rates*

Long QT Syndrome (Fig. 38.60)

Evidence in the literature suggests that the long QT syndrome accounts for a fraction of the sudden infant death syndrome. Newborn infants with prolongation of the Q-T interval often show sinus bradycardia, which led a group of investigators to review the fetal heart rate tracings of 18 children born from singleton pregnancies at or near term in whom long QT syndrome was diagnosed after birth or in childhood. Of the 17 fetuses with long QT syndrome, 12 (71%) showed persistent fetal sinus bradycardia (baseline heart rate permanently <120 beats/min). Two fetuses had additional intermittent tachyarrhythmias. These investi-

Table 38.2: *Therapies for fetal tachyarrhythmias*

Condition and drug	*Dose range*	*Therapeutic level and effect*	*Adverse effects*
Atrial flutter			
Digoxin	LD 1,200 µg per 24 h IV in 3 divided doses; MD 375750 ìg daily PO in two equal daily doses	0.7–2.0 ng/mL Mild nausea, fatigue and sinus bradycardia, first-degree atrioventricular block, rare nocturnal Wenchebach atrioventricular block	Severe nausea and/or vomiting, severe sinus bradycardia or atrioventricular block, maternal and fetal proarrhythmia
Sotalol	160–480 mg daily in two equal daily doses or every 8 h PO	NA Improved survival, bradycardia, first-degree atrioventricular block, P and QRS widening, QT prolongation	Nausea and/or vomiting, dizziness, fatigue, bundle-branch block, maternal and/or fetal proarrhythmia
Supraventicular tachycardia*			
Flecainide‡	100–300 mg daily in equal doses given every 8 h PO	0.2–1.0 µg/mL Mild IVCD, headachem QT prolongation	Visual and central nervous system symptoms, bundle branch block, QT prolongation, fetal or neonatal proarrhythmia
Amiodarone‡	LD 1,800–2,400 mg daily in equal doses given every 6 h for 48 h; MD 200–600 mg daily PO	0.7–2.8 mg/mL Maternal and/or fetal sinus bradycardia, first-degree atrioventricular block, P and QRS widening, QT prolongation	Nausea and/or vomiting, maternal and/or fetal thyroid dysfunction, photosensitivity rash, thrombocytopenia, bundle-branch block, proarrhythmia, torsades de pointes in fetuses with long QT syndrome
Procainamide‡	LD 500–600 mg over 20 min IV; MD 2–6 mg/min IV Initially 1,250 mg, followed in 1 h by 750 mg, then 250–1,000 mg every 3–6 h PO	4–10 µg/mL uterine irritability, QT prolongation	Nausea and/or vomiting, hypotension, proarrhythmia, blood dyscrasias
Ventricular tachycardia			
Magnesium sulfate[81]	LD 2–4 g IV followed by 1–2 g/h IV	1.5–3.0 mmol/L	Fatigue, central nervous system symptoms, stop for loss of patellar reflex at levels of 3.5–5.0 mmol/L, cardiac arrhythmias at high levels
Lidocaine	LD 1.0–1.5 mg/kg IV followed by 1–3 mg/min IV	1.5 5.0 µg/mL	Central nervous system symptoms
Propranolol	40–80 mg every 8 h PO	NA Increased uterine tone, bronchoconstriction	Fatigue, bradycardia, hypotension
Dexamethasone	LD 4–8 mg PO; MD 4 mg daily	NA Fluid retention	Similar to other corticosteroids. Short-term use preferred, fetal growth restriction
Sotalol	160–480 mg daily in two equal daily doses or every 8 h PO	NA Bradycardia, first-degree atrioventricular block, P and QRS widening, QT prolongation	Nausea and/or vomiting, dizziness, fatigue, bundle-branch block, maternal and/or fetal proarrhythmia

*Sotalol or digoxin dosed as for atrial flutter are also commonly used to treat supraventricular tachycardia. ‡These doses of amlodarone, flecalninde and procalnamide can be used to treat either ventricular or supraventricular tachycardias. Abbreviations: IV, intravenous; IVCD, intraventricular conduction delay; LD, loading dose; MD, maintenance dose; PO, oral gators concluded that sinus bradycardia in the fetal heart rate tracing during delivery or pregnancy may indicate long QT syndrome in the fetus and that these fetuses should undergo postnatal ECG to rule out or confirm a prolongation of the Q-T interval. The prenatal diagnosis of long QT syndrome has been reported using fetal MCG. Fetal treatment using magnesium and lidocaine has also been reported.

Treatment of Supraventricular Tachycardia (Table 38.2)

At our institution, the perinatologist and pediatric cardiologist in consultation formulate a treatment plan. When SVT is diagnosed in the fetus, a detailed ultrasound is performed to determine fetal growth; to exclude any associated structural anomalies; and to look for the presence of pericardial, pleural, or ascitic fluid. The pediatric cardiologist determines the atrial and ventricular rates of contraction, atrial and ventricular size and function, and presence and magnitude of AV valve regurgitation. Immediate pharmacologic therapy is undertaken if there is evidence of hydrops fetalis or hemodynamic compromise. Otherwise, the patient is admitted for continuous electronic fetal heart rate monitoring to ascertain the proportion of time spent in tachycardia. Our practice has been to manage patients expectantly if the arrhythmia is not sustained (<50%) and there is no evidence of fetal hemodynamic compromise.

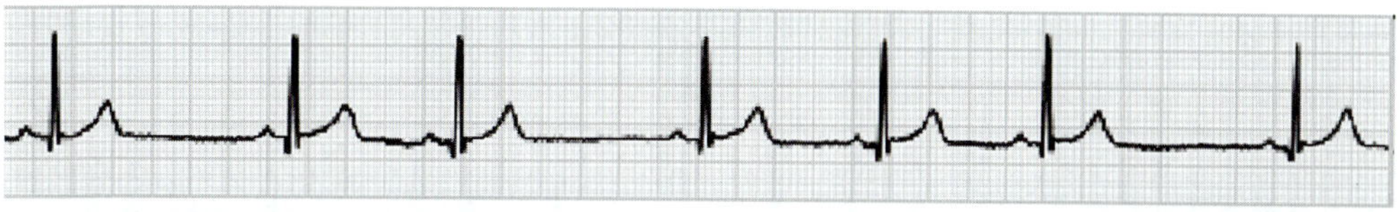

Fig. 38.70: *Electrocardiogram from 3-day-old boy showing marked sinus arrhythmia, a common finding in paediatric traces*

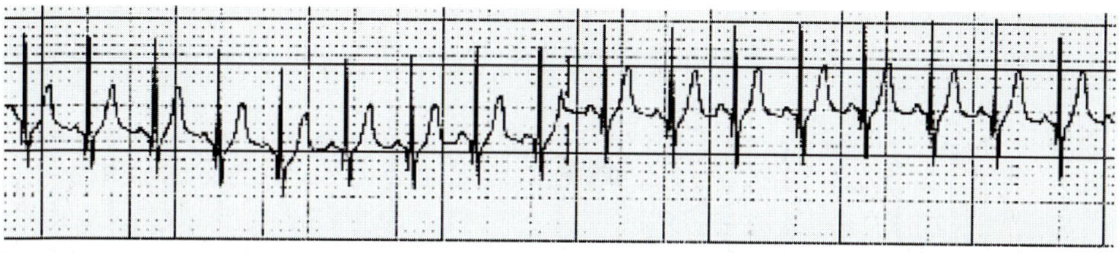

Fig. 38.71: *Electrocardiogram from 2-month-old child with sinus tachycardia*

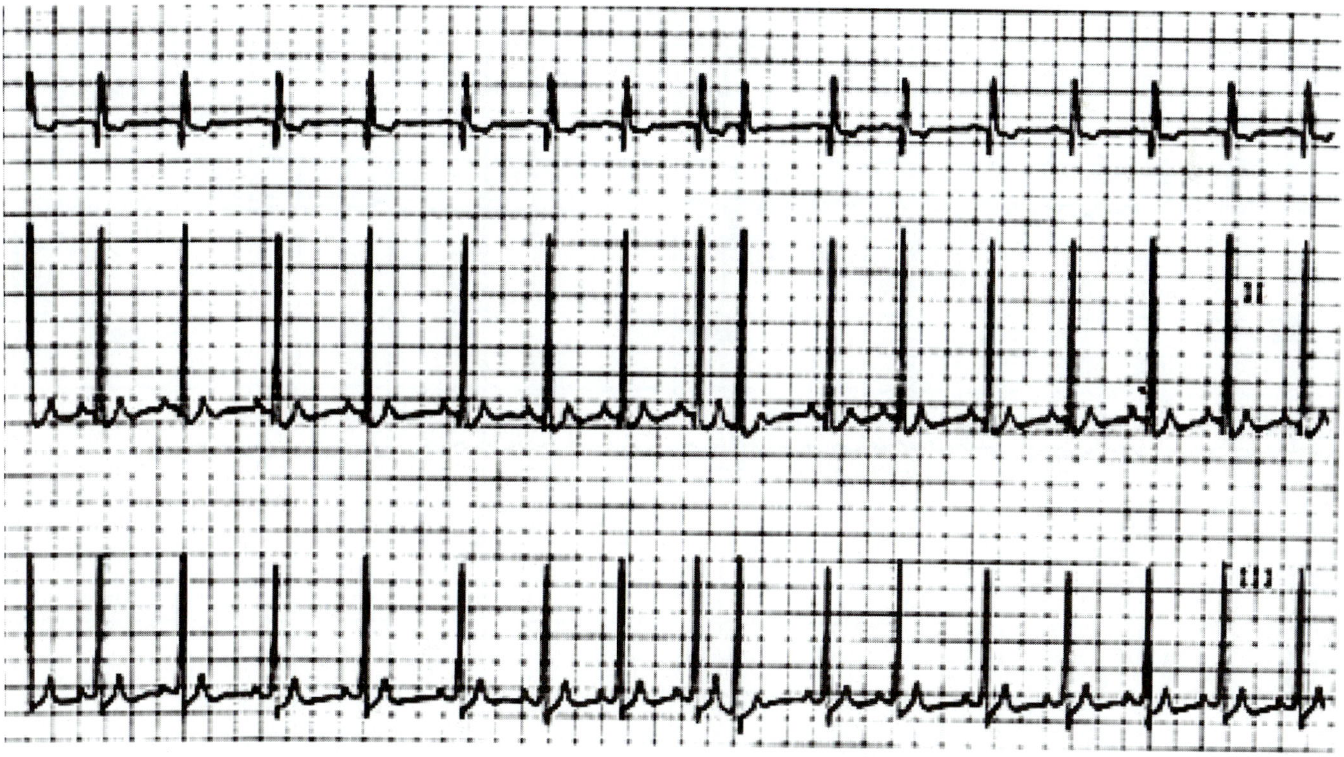

Fig. 38.72: *Electrocardiogram from 7-day-old child with supraventricular premature beats*

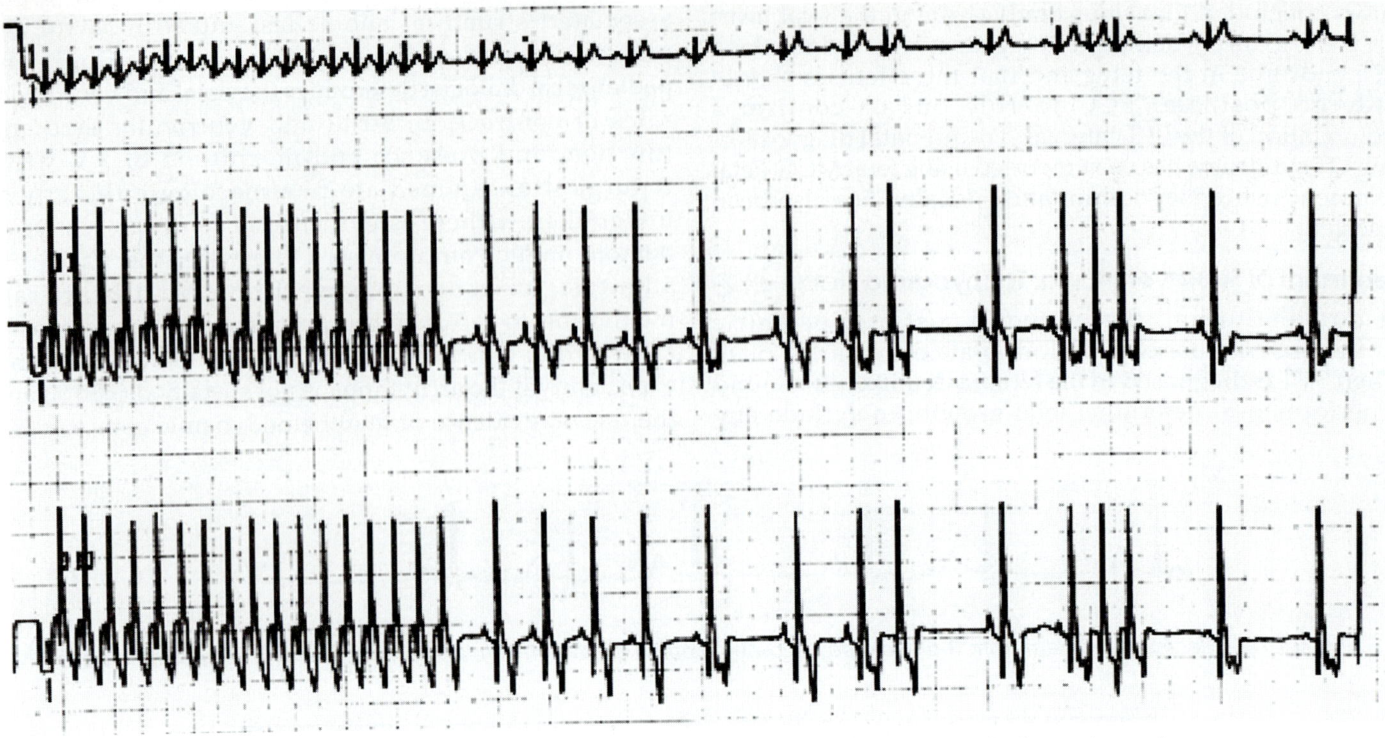

Fig. 38.73: *Electrocardiogram from 3-months-old child with supraventricular tachycardia*

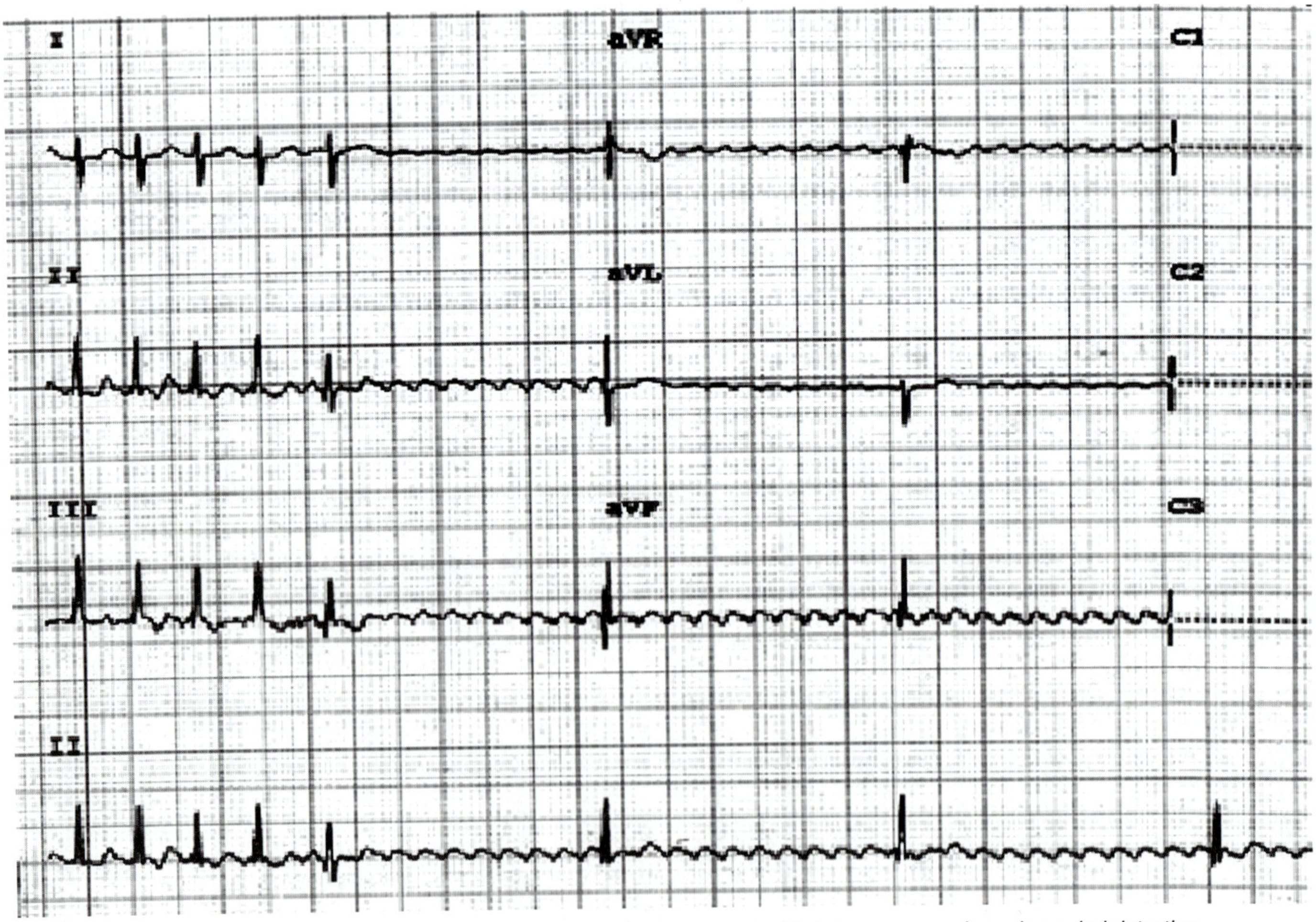

Fig. 38.74: *Supraventricular tachycardia requiring treatment with intravenous adenosine administration*

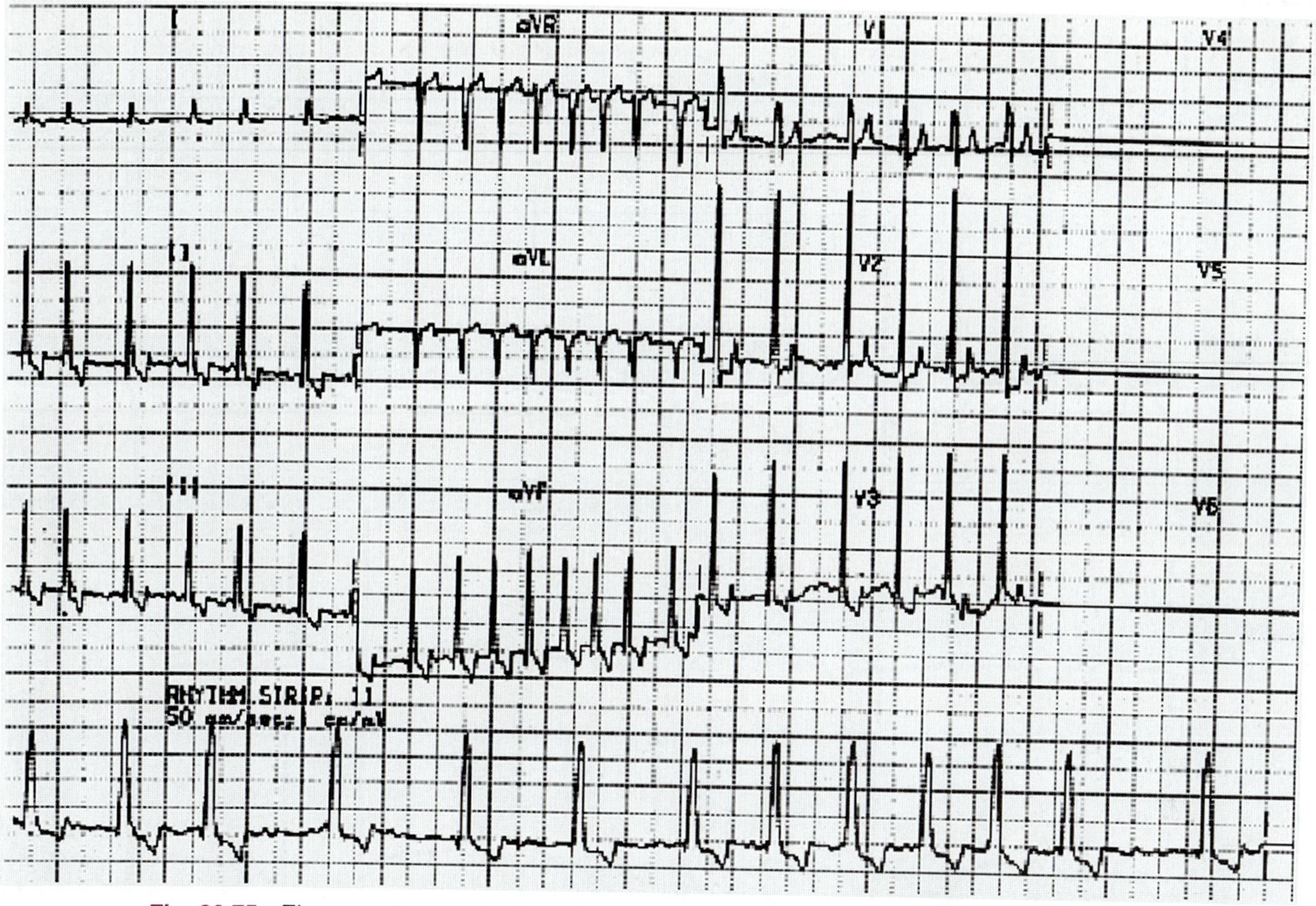

Fig. 38.75: *Electrocardiogram from newborn baby with atrial fibrillation with fast ventricular rate*

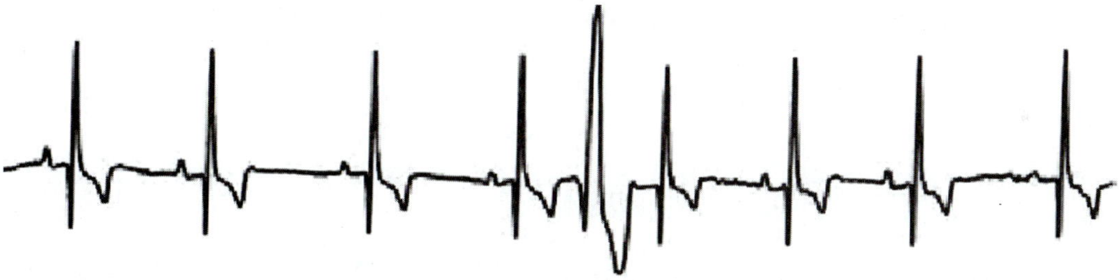

Fig. 38.76: *Electrocardiogram from 2-months-child with interpolated ventricular ectipic*

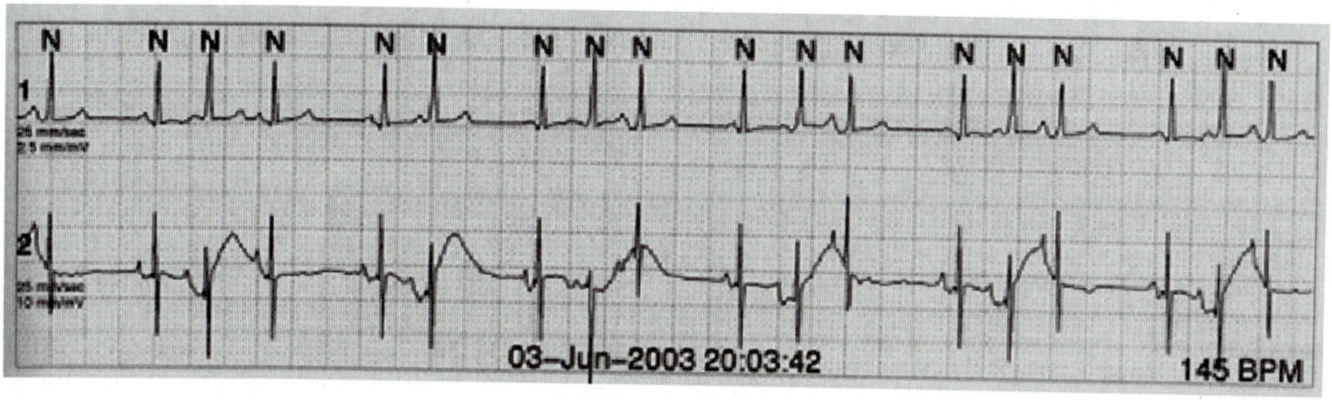

Fig. 38.77: *A 24-hour Holter on a child a month after birth shows preexcitation and premature atrial beats in one of the patients with cardiac tumor*

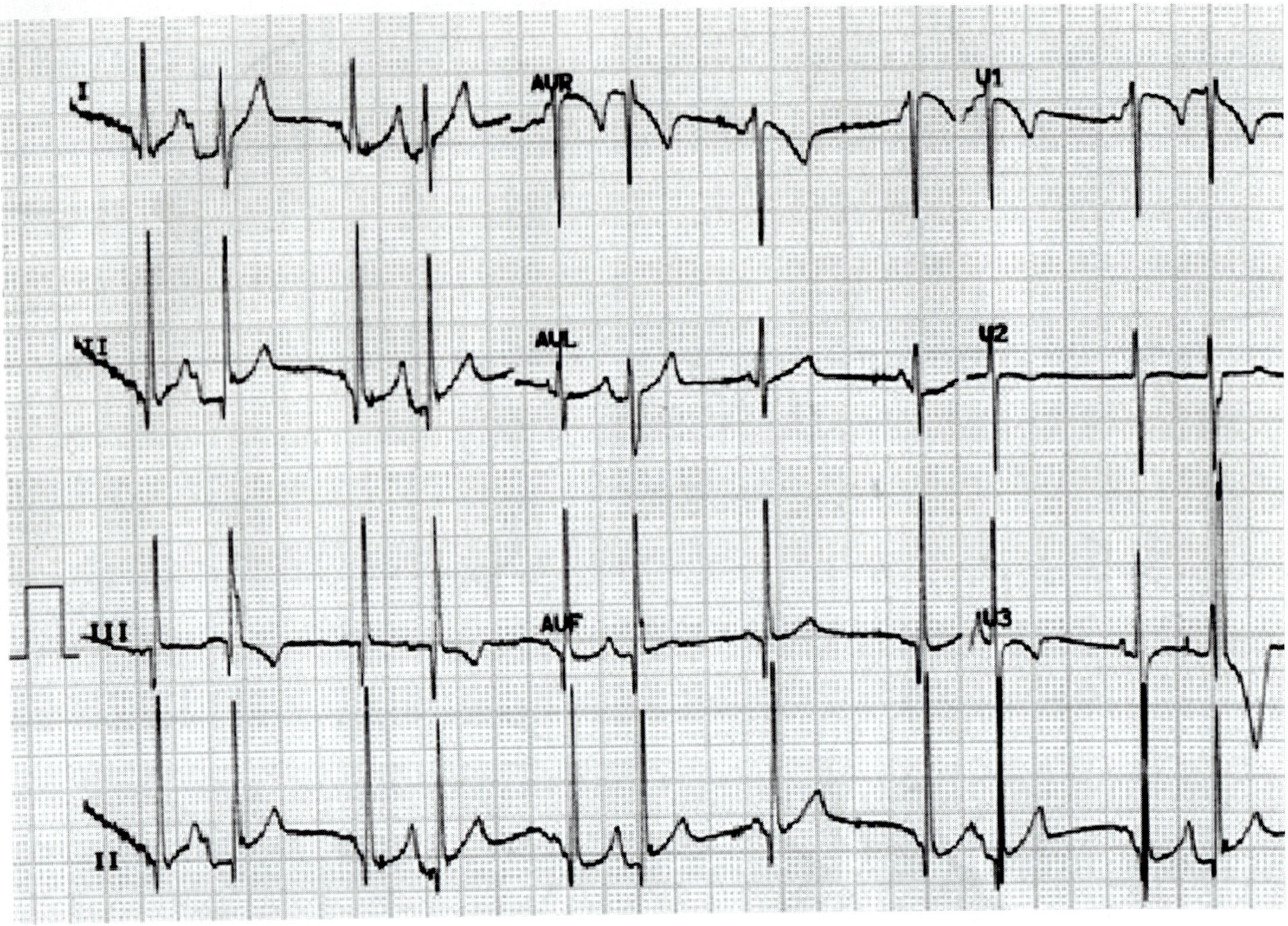

Fig. 38.78: *In 3-years-old child with intracardiac neoplasm, 12-lead ECG reveals loss of pre-excitation but ongoing premature atrial complexes*

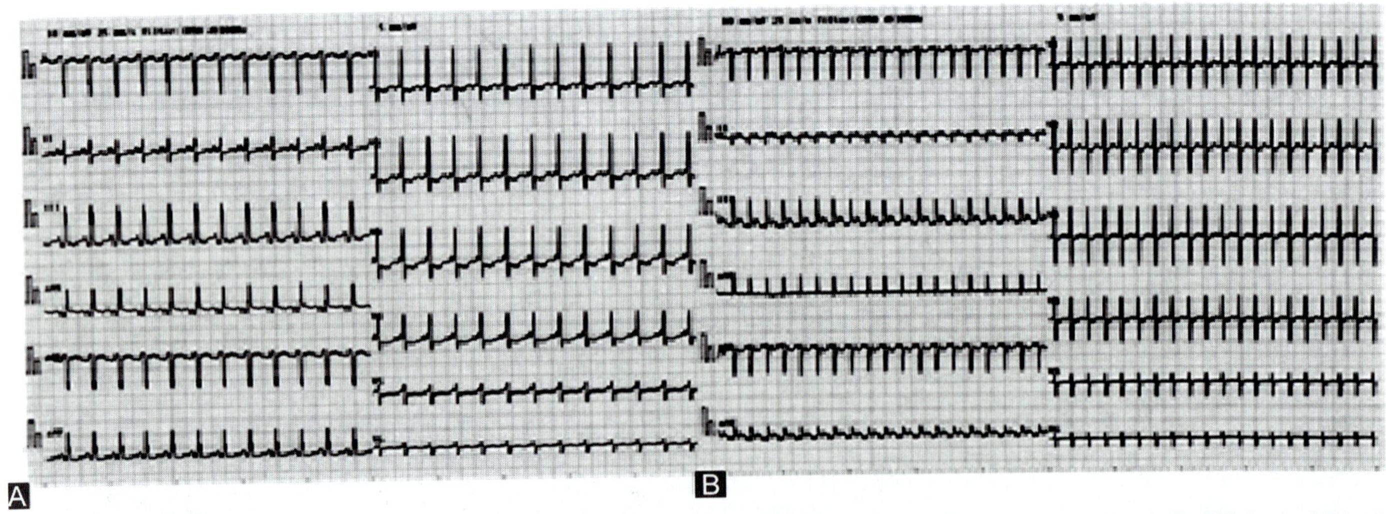

Fig. 38.79: *Electrocardiogram of the sinus rhythm showed preexcitation (A) and supraventricular tachycardia (B) in a child with cardiac tumor*

Increasingly, fetal magnetocardiography (fMCG) is being used to determine mechanism-specific treatment (or nontreatment). In some circumstances, when the characteristics of the tachycardia suggest that it may be ventricular or junctional, when tachycardia is seen in combination with bradycardia, or when it is intermittent

Table 38.3: *Distinguishing tachyarrhythmias in infants*

	Sinus tachycardia	*SVT*	*Atrial flutter*	*VT*
History	Sepsis, fever, hypervolemia, etc.	Usually otherwise normal	Most have a normal heart	Many with abnormal heart
Rate	Almost always <230 b/min	Most often 260–300 b/min	Atrial 300–500 b/min Vent. 1:1 to 4:1 conduction	200–500 b/min
R-R interval variation	Over several seconds may get faster and slower	After first 10–20 beats, extremely regular	May have variable block (1:1, 2:1, 3:1) giving different ventricular rates	Slight variation over several beats
P wave axis	Same as sinus almost always visible P waves	60% visible P waves	Flutter waves (best seein in LII, LIII, aVF, V_1)	May have sinus P waves continuing unrelated to VT (AV dissociation) retrograde P waves, or no visible P waves
QRS	Almost always same as slower sinus rhythm	After first 10–20 beats, almost always same as sinus	Usually same as sinus, may have occasional beats different from sinus	Different from sinus (not necessarily "wide")

SVT, supraventricular tachyeardia
VT, ventricular tachycardia

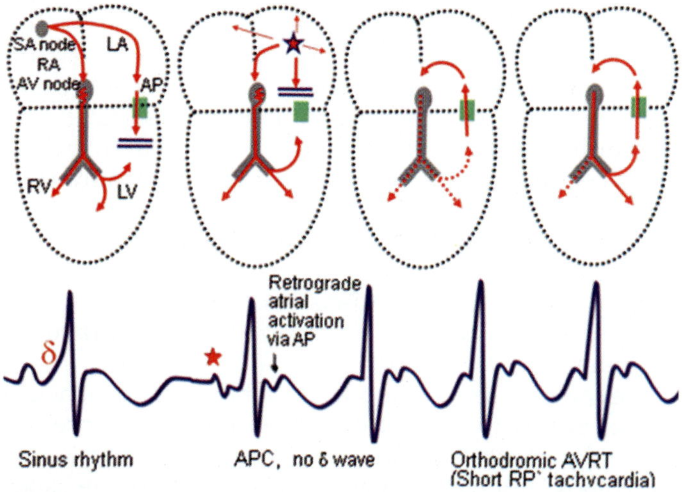

Fig. 38.80: *Illustrations showing conduction of cardiac impulse through aberrant pathways*

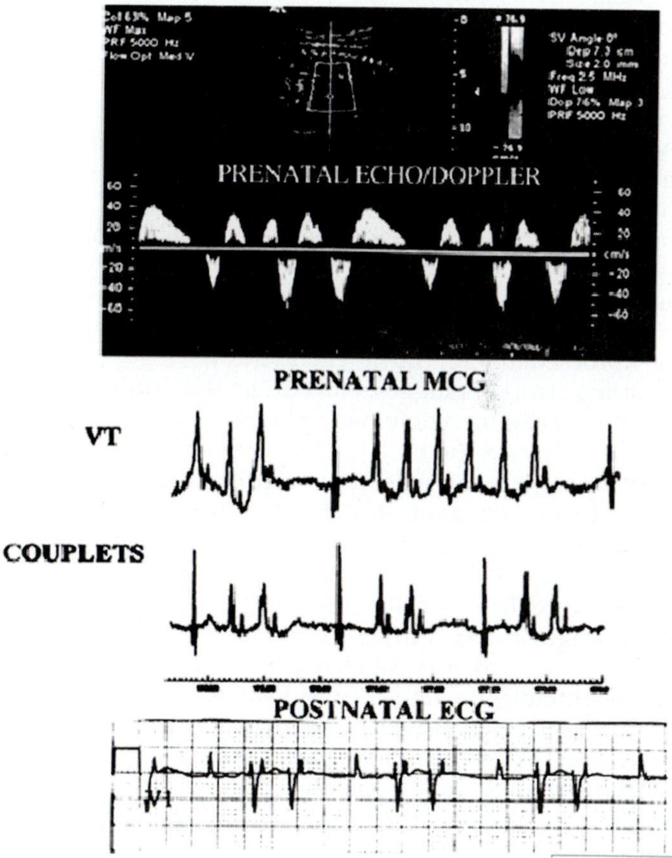

Fig. 38.81: *Complex ventricular arrhythmias related to myocarditis including couplets and nonsustained VT first noted by echo/Doppler (top tracing), in a 32-week gestation fetus evaluated by fMCG (middle tracing) and confirmed by postnatal monitoring (lower tracing)*

and does not require immediate therapy, fMCG can be obtained prior to initiation of therapies.

Although spontaneous resolution of sustained fetal SVT has been reported, about 60% of such fetuses show hemodynamic compromise. Van Engelen and associates noted hydrops fetalis in 22 of 48 fetuses that presented with SVT. The development of hydrops fetalis can be rapid, with progression in 24–48 hours. In addition, when there is hydrops fetalis, conversion of the tachyarrhythmia with medical therapy is more difficult. For all of the aforementioned reasons, we institute pharmacologic therapy in almost all cases of sustained fetal SVT remote from term. If

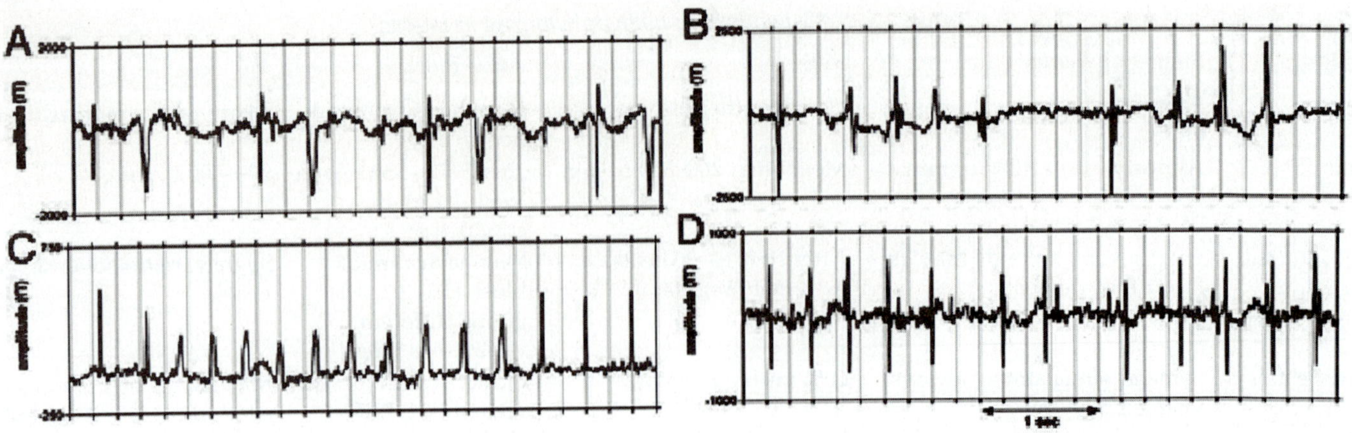

Fig. 38.82: *Ectopy and tachycardia in 3° fetal AVB rhythm strips from 3° atrioventricular block (AVB) fetuses showing: (A) ventricular bigeminy with wide ectopic complexes; (B and C) episodes of nonsustained VT in fetuses, respectively; and (D) junctional ectopic tachycardia in fetus with highly irregular ventricular rhythm at 19 weeks' gestation*

the fetus is at term, we recommend delivery with postnatal management.

Digoxin

Digoxin is considered the first-line drug in the treatment of fetal SVT, and maternally administered digoxin is usually successful in converting the tachyarrhythmia in the nonhydropic fetus. As mentioned previously, it has become increasingly apparent, however, that when hydrops develops, fetal tachyarrhythmia is more difficult to convert with the use of maternally administered drugs. This is likely the result of poor placental transfer of antiarrhythmic drugs in the hydropic fetus. Van Engelen and coworkers showed that the median number of drugs and the number of days to conversion were higher in the hydropic fetus than they were in the nonhydropic fetus with SVT. At least four separate groups reported subtherapeutic levels of digoxin in the hydropic fetus after transplacental therapy before they proceeded with direct fetal therapy.

Various workers suggests that direct fetal intramuscular injection of digoxin combined with transplacental therapy seems to shorten the time to cardioversion and sustained sinus rhythm. Because delays in cardioversion can lead to intrauterine or neonatal death, we start with the intravenous route for maternal digoxin loading over the first 24 hours (1–1.5 mg), followed by large oral maintenance doses (0.5–0.75 mg/day) to maintain maternal serum digoxin levels in the high therapeutic range (1.5–2 ng/mL). If there is no sinus rhythm after maternal levels are therapeutic, the fetus can be loaded with digoxin at a dose of 88 mg/kg (estimated nonhydropic fetal weight for gestational age) into the fetal buttock under direct ultrasound guidance. Repeat injections can be performed at 12 hour intervals (not to exceed three injections) to maintain sinus rhythm more than 50% of the time.

Cordocentesis enables direct access to the fetal circulation and may allow a quicker response to therapy. The fetal intramuscular route provides a more sustained release of the medication and poses less risk to the fetus than cordocentesis. Thirteen cases of SVT complicated by hydrops were treated with intravenous therapy by way of the umbilical vein by Hansmann and colleagues when transplacental therapy failed. There were five deaths, and a mean of 7 injections (range 2–25) was required to achieve a sustained sinus rhythm.

The first intramuscular injection of digoxin is not always sufficient to sustain a normal sinus rhythm; fetuses may require a second or third injection. Presumably, on the basis of predicted pharmacokinetics, the supraventricular tachycardia recurs when the fetal digoxin level becomes subtherapeutic. The decrease in hydrops associated with conversion of the arrhythmia may lead to higher (therapeutic) fetal drug concentrations secondary to increased placental transfer or a decrease in the fetal volume of distribution of maternally administered drugs. If maternal intravenous and direct fetal intramuscular therapy with digoxin fails to sustain a normal sinus rhythm in the hydropic fetus, a second transplacental antiarrhythmic drug should be instituted.

The choice of second-line agents for the treatment of fetal SVT depends to a large extent on the experience and regional preference of the cardiology community; a strict "cookbook" approach is naive. The most important aspect in choosing antiarrhythmic agents is a clear understanding of the mechanism of the tachycardia and knowledge of the mode of action and possible toxicities of the agents for both mother and fetus. All antiarrhythmic agents are proarrhythmic to some degree. Even digoxin, the drug of choice in the initial treatment of in *utero* SVT, can lead to a fatal arrhythmia. Digoxin may shorten the effective refractory period within the accessory conduction pathway in Wolff-Parkinson-White syndrome, allowing potentially rapid conduction in the fetus if cardiac rhythm deteriorates into atrial fibrillation. Digoxin may cause a rapid conduction of the fibrillatory waves, leading to ventricular tachycardia. Presently, it is not possible to diagnose Wolff-Parkinson-White (WPW) syndrome *in utero* with conventional methods. Although the risks of antiarrhythmic therapy seem small given the infrequency of atrial fibrillation in the fetus, it is imperative to receive informed

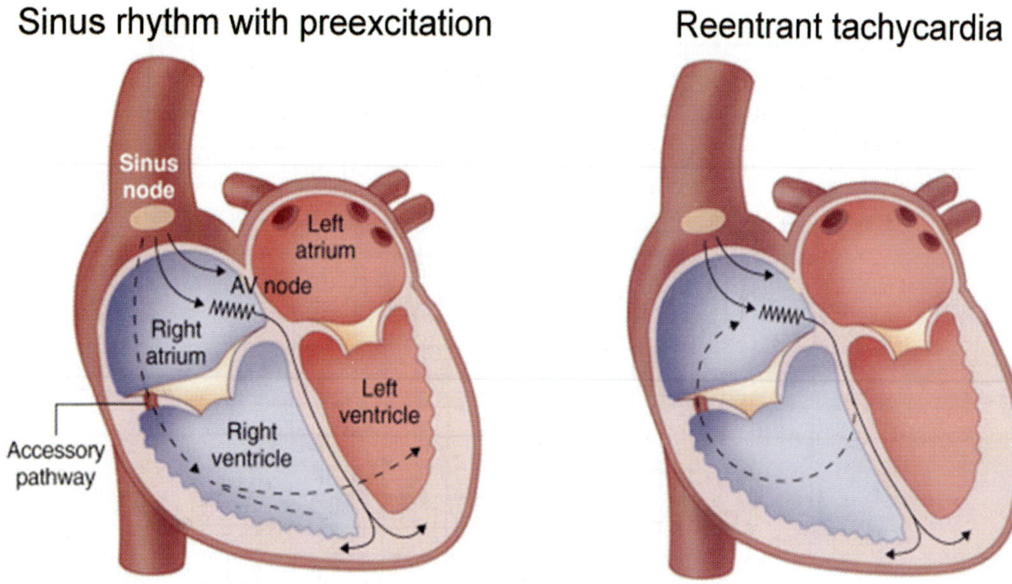

Fig. 38.83: *Accessory pathway in sinus rhythm and in orthodromic reentrant tachycardia. (From Basson CT: A molecular basis for Wolff-Parkinson-White syndrome with courtesy N Engl J Med 2001;344:1861)*

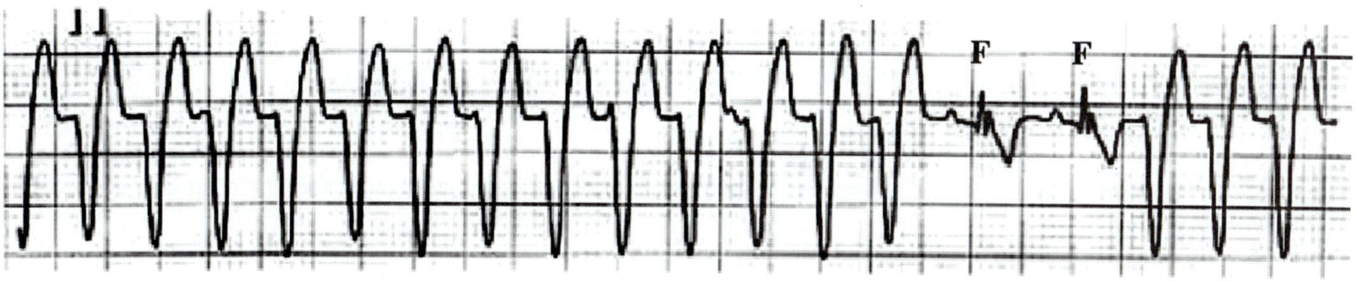

Fig. 38.84: *Electrocardiogram from in infant with ventricular tachycardia and fusion beats (F)*

consent from the parents of these fetuses before administering such agents. WPW may be suspected if the echocardiographic mechanical P-R interval is quite short (less than 70 ms). In those centers where fMCG is available, this method can confirm the presence of WPW. To date, we have not altered therapy, even when fMCG has shown WPW because the evidence base for its danger is not clear in the fetal period.

β-Blockers

Propranolol or esmolol may be effective in slowing the rapid ventricular rate associated with atrial tachycardia. β-blockers are commonly prescribed in pregnancy to treat hypertension and generally are well tolerated and considered relatively safe. There are reports of intrauterine growth restriction with their use, however, which may be due primarily to the underlying pathophysiology of the disease. Although the favorable maternal profile makes β-blockers an attractive second-line agent, their efficacy in treating fetal SVT in the setting of hydrops is modest at best. This class of drugs generally is contraindicated in patients with asthma and diabetes.

Quinidine

Quinidine is a type I antiarrhythmic that blocks the sodium current responsible for the rapid phase 0 of the action potential and is a reasonable choice as a second-line agent. It also decreases conduction velocity and prolongs the refractory period in atrial, ventricular, His-Purkinje, and accessory conduction tissue. Quinidine is effective for reentrant tachycardias that use these pathways. Quinidine also is one of the drugs of choice for control of rapid ventricular response to atrial fibrillation/flutter. For flutter or fibrillation, digoxin should be administered before quinidine to prevent the rapid ventricular response that may occur if quinidine's vagolytic action enhances AV nodal conduction at the outset of therapy. Quinidine may prolong P-R, QRS, and PT intervals and may precipitate ventricular tachycardia associated with excessive Q-T interval prolongation. This effect seems to be idiosyncratic rather than dose related. This proarrhythmic potential affects about 2–5% of adult patients taking this medication. Quinidine also can result in noncardiac side effects in a substantial percentage of users including gastrointestinal upset (up to 50%), and less commonly fever, skin rash,

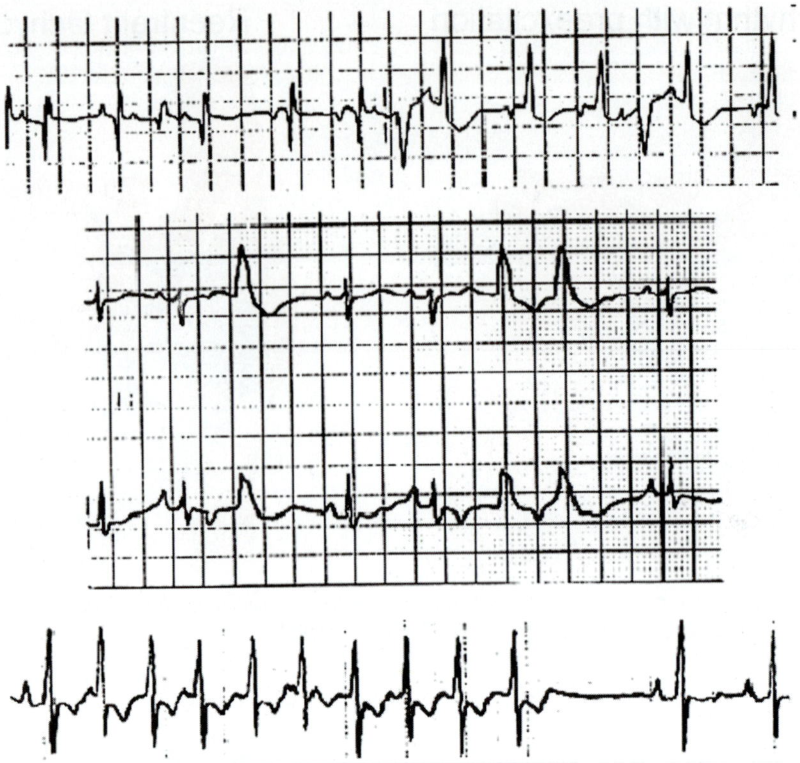

Fig. 38.85: *Arrhythmias and conduction anomalies in a newborn infant with glutaric aciduria type II. This 1-day-old child was referred for neonatal cardiac control because fetal echocardiography diagnosed atrial bigeminy during routine follow-up. Echocardiography was normal, and 12-lead ECG showed premature atrial and ventricular beats (top). During his first month of life, the patient experienced many episodes of atrial tachycardia (bottom). The diagnosis of fatty acid oxidation disorder was suspected because of neonatal recurrent hypoglycemia. At 4 months of age, hypertrophic hypokinetic cardiomyopathy was diagnosed; the child died at 7 months of age during cardiogenic shock*

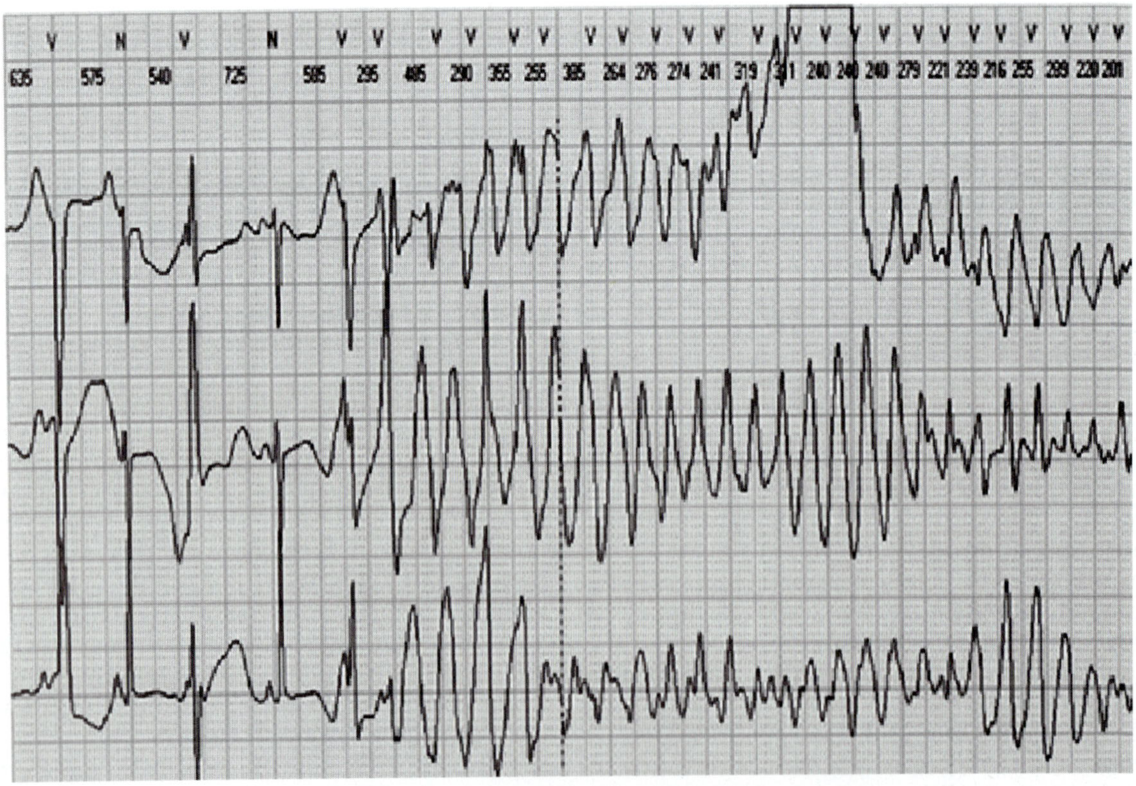

Fig. 38.86: *Polymorphic neonatal ventricular tachycardia (torsade de pointes) recorded on Holter 24-hour monitoring*

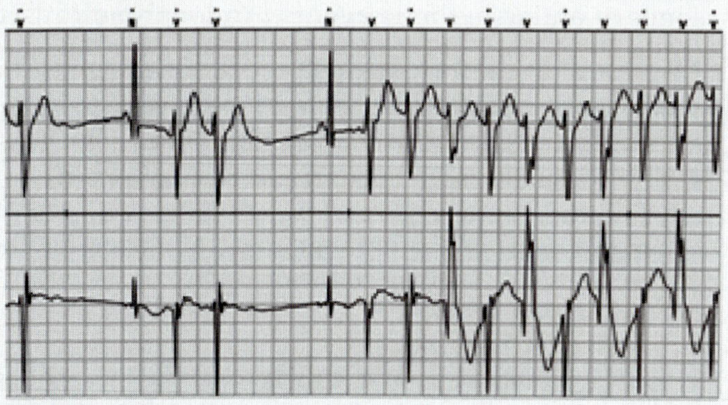

Fig. 38.87: *Holter recording showing simultaneous ECG channels demonstrating an episode of bidirectional VT in a patient with history of syncope. Alternating different morphologies of ventricular complex are seen during tachycardia. This is diagnostic of catecholaminergic polymorphic VT*

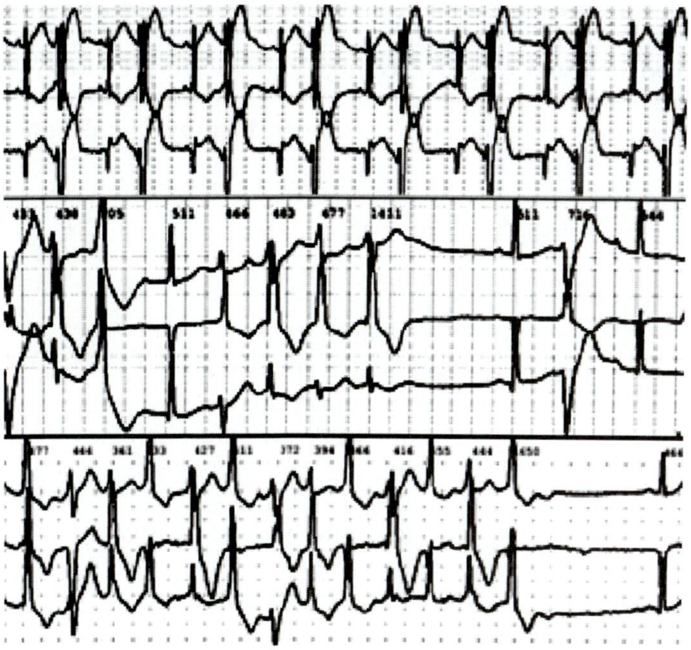

Fig. 38.88: *Ambulatory ECG tracings of ventricular arrhythmias in Andersen-Tawil Syndrome. The top panel recorded in a newborn boy with the G144S mutation in KCNJ2 shows sinus rhythm with premature ventricular beats in a bigeminal pattern. The middle and bottom panels recorded in the boy's mother with the same mutation show runs of polymorphic and bidirectional ventricular tachycardia*

cinchonism, autoimmune thrombocytopenia, and hemolytic anemia. In addition, quinidine can lead to a twofold or greater increase in the serum digoxin level. We empirically decrease the digoxin dose by 50% before quinidine administration.

Procainamide

A few investigators have used oral procainamide, a type I antiarrhythmic agent, as second-line therapy, although reports of its use are largely anecdotal. It is probably no more effective than quinidine, and intravenous administration, at least, has been associated with onset of uterine contractions.

Flecainide

Many institutions have found success using flecainide as a second or third agent when digoxin alone has not converted the arrhythmia. Flecainide is a class IC agent. In addition to its more potent antiarrhythmia properties, flecainide has been found to have greater placental crossing ability than digoxin. It has been shown to be 59% successful in cases where digoxin has failed in the hydropic fetus. Flecainide has a narrow therapeutic range. Careful monitoring of the maternal ECG for undue QRS prolongation and prolongation of the P-T interval is neccessary. Fetal and maternal MCG has been reported during flecainide therapy for fetal SVT in hydropic fetuses.

Verapamil

Our experience with verapamil has been disappointing. Verapamil has been associated with profound cardiac depression and cardiac arrest after intravenous administration in the fetus and neonate and has fallen out of favor. In older series, it had been used effectively in the absence of hydrops, when frequent breaks in tachycardia were noted. Presently, we rarely treat such cases.

Amiodarone

We have had good success with amiodarone in patients who fail digoxin therapy in the setting of hydrops fetalis. Amiodarone is a class III antiarrhythmic agent that profoundly affects action potential duration and refractoriness within the atrium, AV node, accessory pathways and ventricle. It also is useful for the treatment of ventricular tachycardia and a variety of SVTs. We have treated several patients with SVT complicated by hydrops fetalis with amiodarone when they were unresponsive to multiple agents including digoxin, procainamide,

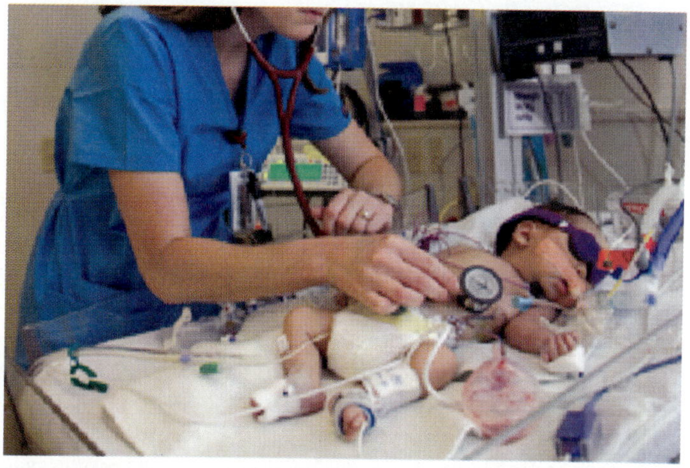

Fig. 38.89: *Doctor is examining a sick neonate physically and resting ECG is being taken for the type of cardiac arrhythmia*

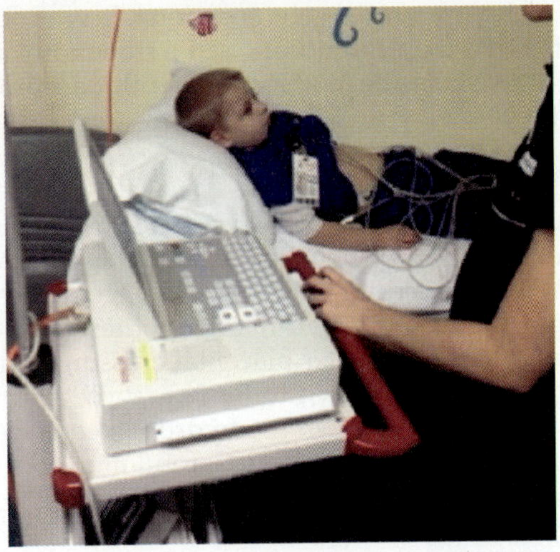

Fig. 38.90: *Electrocardiogram is being obtained in the assessment of cardiac arrhythmia in a younger child*

verapamil, and quinidine. All cases resulted in cardioversion with no untoward effects. We reported our experience with amiodarone in 25 fetuses with incessant tachycardia and either hydrops fetalis (*n* = 23) or ventricular dysfunction (*n* = 2) who failed digoxin monotherapy and secondary antiarrhythmic agents. Amiodarone caused progressive slowing of the tachycardia rate over time and promoted more sustained periods in sinus rhythm. Fewer than 50% of fetuses with atrial flutter showed a sustained cardioversion, however. In the remaining cases, the heart rate control alone allowed maintenance of the pregnancy. These findings strongly support the use of amiodarone as the transplacental antiarrhythmic drug of choice for the hydropic fetus with digoxin-refractory tachycardia with 1:1 concordance. Sotolol may be more successful in sustained conversion of atrial flutter.

Hyperthyroidism and hypothyroidism have been reported as a result of amiodarone's molecular similarity to thyroxine. Biochemical hypothyroidism was detected in five infants but progressed to require treatment in only one infant who received chronic postnatal amiodarone treatment. This agent, similar to all the other antiarrhythmic agents, can have a proarrhythmic effect that may result from Q-T interval prolongation. In addition, amiodarone has an extraordinarily prolonged half-life (25–110 days). The life-threatening toxicities do not seem to be a major risk in the pediatric and reproductive age groups. Nevertheless, we do not recommend its use as a first-line agent, but it can be used in cases refractory to traditional therapy. The low rates

Table 38.4: *Supraventricular tachycardias*

	R-R regularity	*P wave morphology*
Atrial tachycardias		
Sinus tachycardia	Regular	Positive in II, III, aVF
Sinus node re-entry	Regular	Positive in II, III, aVF
Atrial tachycardia, unifocal	Regular	P different from sinus
Atrial tachycardia, multifocal	Irregular	≥3 different P wave morphologies
Atrial flutter, common, counterclockwise	Regular, irregular if variable AV block	
Atrial flutter, uncommon, clockwise AV block	Regular, irregular if variable waveform II, III, aVF	Upright flutter waves; positive
Atrial fibrillation	Irregularly irregular	Irregular fibrillation waves
AV junctional tachycardias		
AV reentry (using accessory pathways)		
Orthodromic	Regular	Retrograde P in ST-T wave
Antidromic	Regular preexcited	Retrograde P, short RP
Slow conducting	Regular	Retrograde P at end of T wave or later (long RP)
Atriofascicular (antidromic)	Regular preexcited	Retrograde P, short RP
AV nodal reentry		
Common (slow-fast)	Regular	Retrograde P obscured by QRS or alters the end of QRS (short RP)
Uncommon (fast-slow)	Regular	PR-RP approximately equal
Nonparoxysmal junctional tachycardia*	Regular, slow rate	AV dissociation
Automatic junctional tachycardia*	Regular	AV dissociation

* Site of origin usually infranodal. AV, atrioventricular

of serious maternal and fetal side effects in our experience rival other antiarrhythmic agents, such as flecainide and sotolol, which have been associated with fetal death. We have not had a fetal death with amiodarone therapy in our patients.

Sotolol

Sotolol is the most recent addition to *in utero* antiarrhythmic agents and is reported to be effective in 80% of fetuses with atrial flutter and 60% with SVT. Sotolol is a nonselective α-blocker that also prolongs the Q-T interval. It is used widely outside the United States for the treatment of supraventricular and ventricular arrhythmias. Two of our patients with AV reciprocating SVT failed sotalol therapy at 400 mg/day and responded to amiodarone. Sotolol has shown a 25–30% mortality rate for 1:1 reciprocating tachycardia when administered to hydropic fetuses. It seems to be an excellent choice for digoxin-refractory atrial flutter. Major adverse effects are related to β-blockade and prolongation of the Q-T interval. The occurrence of torsades de pointers is dose related, in contrast to quinidine.

Intrapartum Management

Electronic fetal heart rate monitoring is the mainstay in modern obstetrics for obtaining reassurance of normal acid-base status of the fetus during labor. It relies on interpretation of fetal heart rate, variability, and periodic changes. Such reassurance is not possible in fetuses with sustained arrhythmias. Biophysical profiles are of limited benefit in the intrapartum period, and serial fetal scalp blood sampling is not a very palatable option. Therefore,

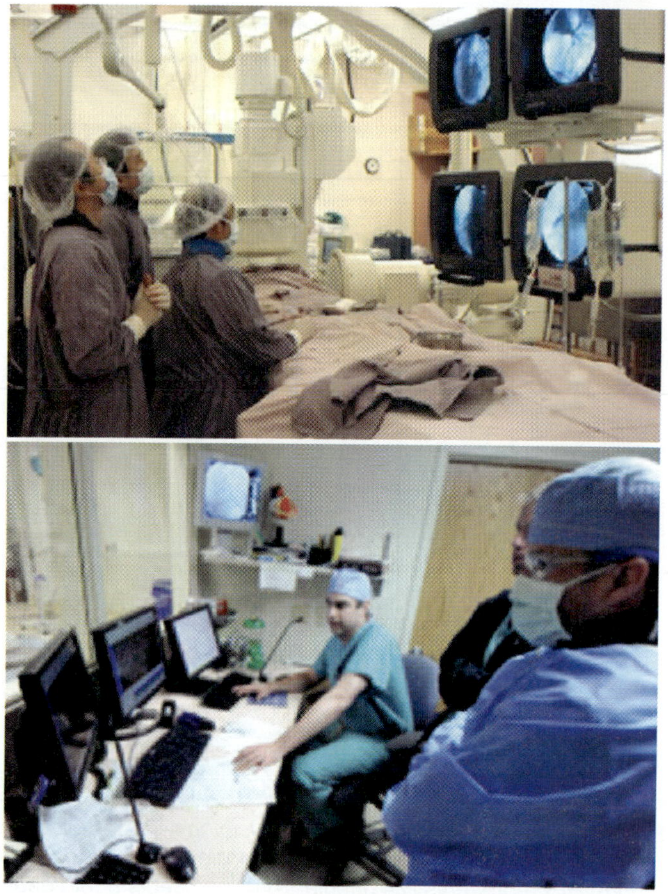

Fig. 38.91: *(Upper) Patient is undergoing electrophysiological study and ablation procedure for cardiac arrhythmia. The record is being analysed for the effectiveness of the procedure (bottom)*

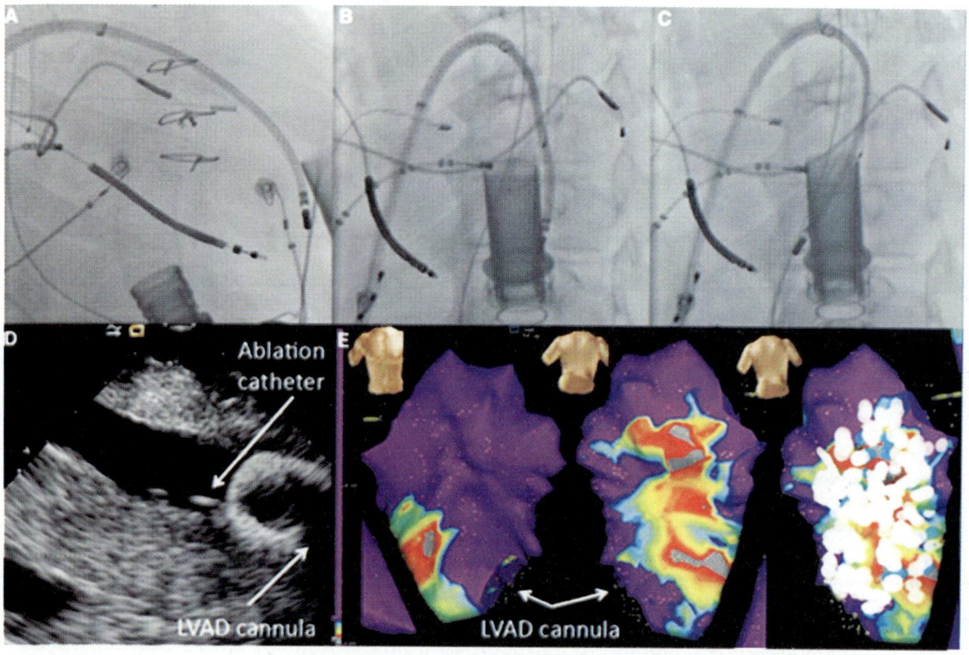

Fig. 38.92: *Mapping and ablation of an inferior wall scar in the presence of a left ventricular assist device (LVAD). (A–C) Robotic catheter position in the right (A) and left (B, C) anterior oblique fluoroscopic views with the catheter tip around the LVAD inflow cannula. (D) Intracardiac echocardiographic image of the LVAD cannula and the ablation catheter. (E) Three dimensional scar maps and ablation lesions*

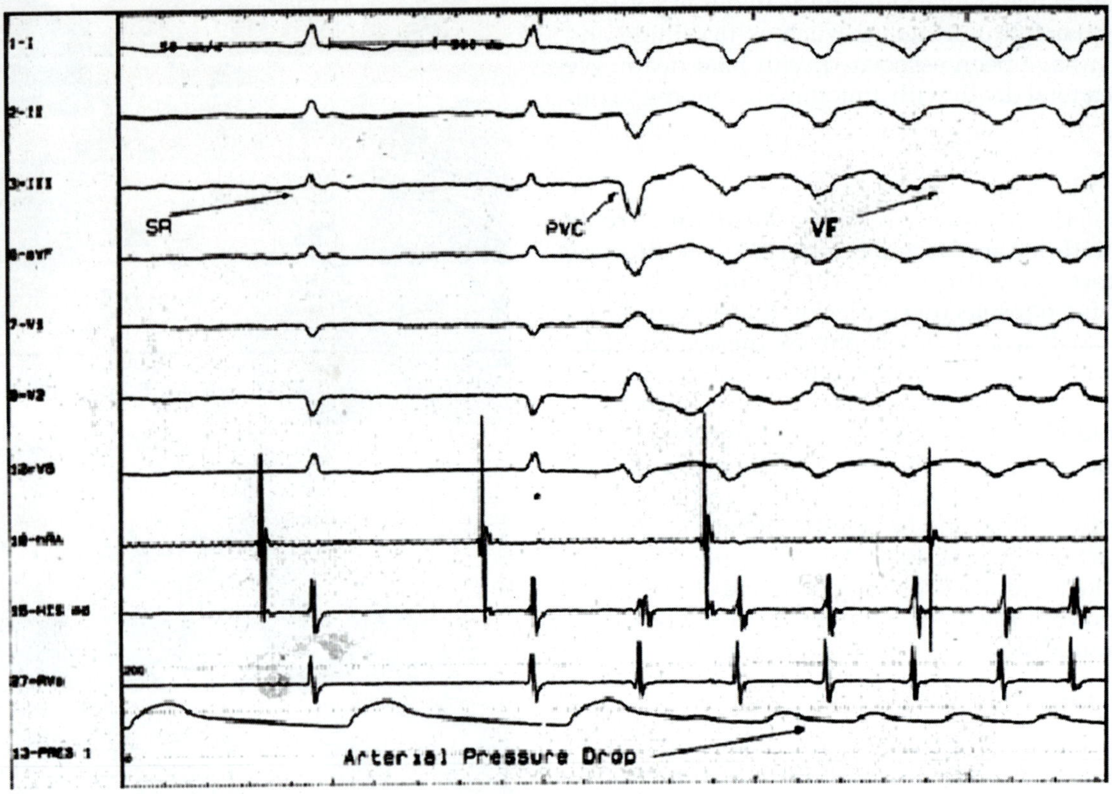

Fig. 38.93: *Tracing from the electrophysiology study showing initiation of ventricular fibrillation by characteristic premature ventricular contraction noticed in surface electrocardiographic leads (I, II, III, aVF, VI, V2, V6), intracardiac leads (hRA represents high right atrium, HIS represents His bundle, RVa represents right ventricle), and the arterial pressure line (PRES) showing the blood pressure drop following the arrhythmia*

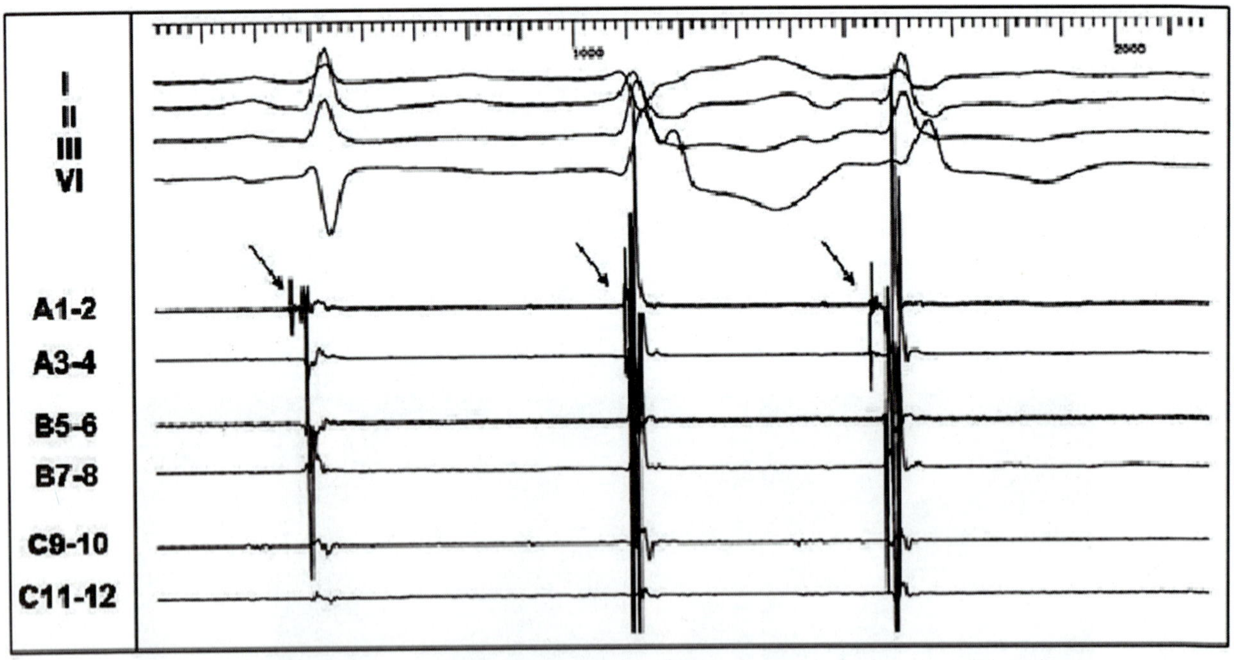

Fig. 38.94: *Intracardiac electrograms during spontaneous ventricular ectopy in a patient with Andersen-Tawil syndrome. Displayed are surface leads I, II, III, V1, and intracardiac electrograms recorded from the anterior left ventricle. The first sinus beat is followed by two successive ventricular ectopic beats, each with a different morphology. The arrows indicate Purkinje potentials preceding the local ventricular electrograms in sinus rhythm and the ectopic beats. The first ectopic beat is from an adjacent Purkinje site—hence the late Purkinje relative to the QRS. (Courtesy of Dr Prashanthan Sanders, Dr Frederic Sacher, and Dr Michel Haissaguerre, Hôpital Cardiologique du Haut-Lévêque)*

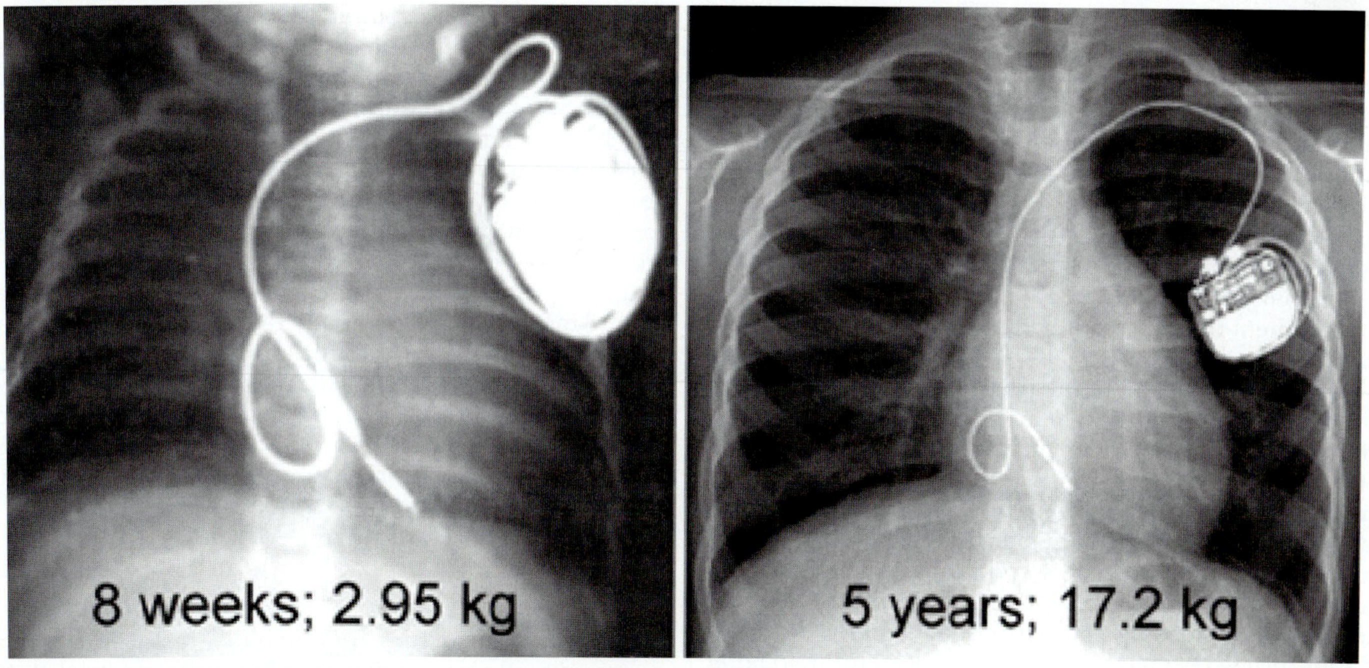

Fig. 38.95: *Left panel shows lead position in a baby with congenital complete heart block who was born prematurely with hydrops. A transvenous endocardial pacemaker was implanted at the age of 8 weeks when she weighed 2.95 kg. At 5 years of age (weight 17.2 kg), she still has the initial lead and generator (right panel). The redundant loop of lead formed in the right atrium has not yet been taken up and will allow generator replacement without the need for lead advancement*

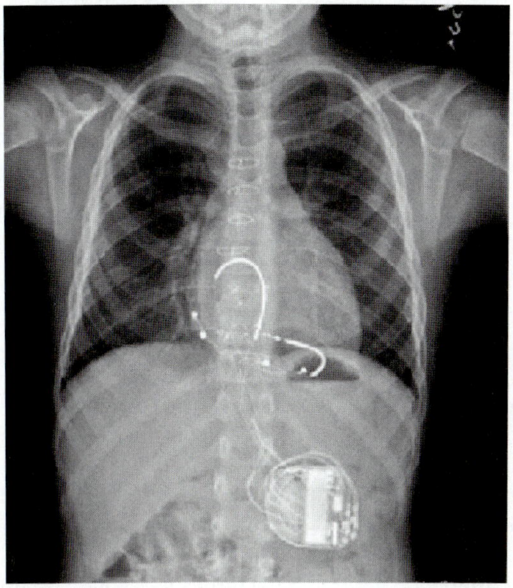

Fig. 38.96: *Skiagram of cheast PA view showing pacing and implantable cardioverter defibrillators in a new born child with prolonged QT-interval*

these pregnancies are usually delivered by cesarean section because of the inability to assess fetal well being.

Pulse oximetry has proved to be a most useful tool for assessing oxygenation in both adults and children. New technology has been developed for intrapartum fetal pulse oximetry. The devise consists of a sensor that is placed transvaginally alongside the fetal face. Currently, there is no evidence in the literature that fetal pulse oximetry (FPO) as an adjunct to electronic fetal heart rate monitoring improves neonatal outcome. However, in pregnancies complicated by sustained fetal arrhythmias, this may be one of the few instances where this technology may be useful for reassurance of normal acid-base status of the fetus during labor.

The importance of managing fetal arrhythmia has increased over the past three decades. Although most fetal arrhythmias are benign, some types cause fetal hydrops and can lead to fetal death. With the aim of improving the outcome in such cases, various studies for prenatal diagnosis and perinatal management have been published. Detailed analysis of the type of arrhythmia *in utero* is possible using M-mode and Doppler echocardiography. In particular, a simultaneous record of Doppler waveform at the superior venous cava and the ascending aorta has become an important and useful method of assessing the interval between atrial and ventricular contractions. Common causes of fetal tachycardia (ventricular heart rate faster than 180 bpm), are paroxysmal supraventricular tachycardia (SVT) with 1:1 atrioventricular (AV) relation and atrial flutter with 2:1 AV relation. Of fetal SVT, short ventriculoatrial (VA) interval tachycardia due to atrioventricular reentrant tachycardia is more common than long VA interval. Most fetuses with tachycardia are successfully treated *in utero* by transplacental administration of antiarrhythmic drugs. Digoxin is widely accepted as a first-line antiarrhythmic drug. Sotalol, flecainide and amiodarone are used as second-line drugs when digoxin fails to achieve conversion to sinus rhythm. Fetal bradycardia is diagnosed when the fetal ventricular heart rate is slower than 100 bpm, mainly due to AV block. Approximately half of all cases are caused by associated congenital heart disease, and the remaining cases that have normal cardiac structure are often caused by maternal SS-A antibody. The efficacy of prenatal treatment for fetal AV block is limited compared with treatment for fetal tachycardia. Beta-stimulants and steroids have been reported as effective transplacental treatments for fetal AV block. Perinatal management based on prospective clinical study protocol rather than individual experience is crucial for further improvement of outcome in fetuses with tachycardia and bradycardia.

The importance of managing fetal arrhythmia has increased over the past three decades. Fetal arrhythmia is often found during fetal heart monitoring or routine prenatal ultrasound examination. Although most fetal arrhythmias are benign, some cause fetal hydrops and can lead to fetal death. To improve the outcome in such cases, various studies of prenatal diagnosis and perinatal management have been published. Up-to-date knowledge of effective methods of diagnosing fetal arrhythmia and the selection of appropriate perinatal treatment is crucial for managing affected fetuses. In the present paper, we summarize the current method of prenatal diagnosis and perinatal management of fetal arrhythmia based on recent publications.

Conclusion

Echocardiography remains the dominant modality for prenatal diagnosis of arrhythmias, although fetal ECG and magnetocardiography provide additional important information in selected groups of patients. With regard to fetal tachycardias, refinements in the echocardiographic assessment can provide helpful additional information regarding the mechanism of tachycardias and so guide optimal prenatal therapy. The treatment of fetuses with immune-mediated heart block remains contentious and robust multicenter trial data will be required to examine fetal cardiac outcome and potential adverse effects of therapy on both the fetus and the mother. Venous and arterial Doppler flow profiles must take account of the mechanism of arrhythmia and may not always be a valid marker of cardiac compromise.

Perinatal management of fetal arrhythmia is important to improve the outcome of affected fetus. Accurate prenatal diagnosis is crucial to the selection of the appropriate prenatal and postnatal treatments. However, there are still many issues regarding the management of both fetal tachycardia and bradycardia, and more useful strategies must be investigated. Perinatal management based on prospective clinical study protocol, rather than on individual conditions is crucial for further improvement of the outcome of affected fetuses.

Refractory SVT

Flecainide and sotolol have a proven effect on refractory SVT as single agents and with other antiarrhythmic agents in children and adults. There must be concern about the proarrhythmic potential of these drugs in combination, but Price et al found the combination of the two drugs to be safe and effective in refractory SVT in infants. It is important to note that flecainide solution currently has to be made up each week by the pharmacy. It precipitates in the cold, which can lead to dangerous overdosing, and therefore must not be refrigerated. Furthermore, milk interferes with absorption of flecainide, and thus a high serum concentration of flecainide can develop when milk feeds are stopped—for example, during diarrhoeal illness. Radiofrequency ablation can be performed in infants less than 18 months old. It is usually reserved for drug resistant or life-threatening arrhythmias, often in the presence of structural heart disease. The most common associated congenital heart diseases subjected to this procedure are Ebstein's malformation of tricuspid valve, single ventricle/corrected transposition of the great arteries complex, tetralogy of Fallot, and hypertrophic cardiomyopathy.

Fetal Tachycardias and Management of the Hydropic Infant

Persistent or recurrent SVT usually in the form of an accessory pathway mediated tachycardia or atrial flutter can lead to hydrops or fetal death. Simpson et al showed that 65% of the tachycardias in the fetus were persistent and that the incidence of hydrops was 41%. The incidence of congenital heart defects was 4% in the same study and 12% in another study by Boldt et al of the defects, a ventricular septal defect was the most common.

Summary of Important Dos and Don'ts for Antiarrhythmic Medication

- DO monitor flecainide and digoxin concentrations
- DO NOT use β-blocker with calcium channel blocker
- DO NOT use intravenous verapamil below 1 year of age
- DO monitor QT intervals with sotalol
- DO halve the dose of digoxin when given with amiodarone

BIBLIOGRAPHY

1. Simpson J. Fetal arrhythmia. In: Snider AR, Serwer GA, Ritter SB (eds). Echocardiography in Pediatric Heart Disease. St. Louis: Mosby Year Book, 1997;93–8.
2. Simpson J. Fetal arrhythmias. In: Allan L, Hornberger LK, Sharland G (eds). Textbook of Fetal Cardiology. London: Greenwich Medical Media, 2000;423–37.
3. Kleinman CS, Hobbins JC, Jaffe CC, Lynch DC, Talner NS. Echocardiographic studies of the human fetus: prenatal diagnosis of congenital heart disease and cardiac dysrhythmias. Pediatrics 1980;65:1059–67.
4. Gembruch U, Redel DA, Bald R, Hansmann M. Longitudinal study in 18 cases of fetal supraventricular tachycardia: Doppler echocardiographic findings and pathophysiologic implications. Am Heart J 1993;125:1290–1301.
5. Van Engelen AD, Weijtens O, Brenner JI, et al. Management outcome and follow-up of fetal tachycardia. J Am Coll Cardiol 1994; 24:371–75.
6. Simpson JM, Sharland GK. Fetal tachycardias: management and outcome of 127 consecutive cases. Heart 1998; 79:576–81.

7. Jaeggi E, Fouron JC, Fournier A, et al. Ventriculo-atrial time interval measured on M-mode echocardiography: a determining element in diagnosis, treatment, and prognosis of fetal supraventricular tachycardia. Heart 1998; 79:582–7.
8. Wakai RT, Strasburger JF, Li Z, Deal BJ, Gotteiner NL. Magnetocardiographic rhythm patterns at initiation and termination of fetal supraventricular tachycardia. Circulation 2003; 107:307–12.
9. Krapp M, Kohl T, Simpson JM, Sharland GK, Katalinic A, Gembruch U. Review of diagnosis, treatment, and outcome of fetal atrial flutter compared with supraventricular tachycardia. Heart 2003; 89:913–17.
10. Fouron JC, Fournier A, Proulx F, et al. Management of fetal tachyarrhythmia based on superior vena cava/aorta Doppler flow recordings. Heart 2003; 89:1211–16.
11. Jaeggi ET, Nii M. Fetal brady- and tachyarrhythmias: new and accepted diagnostic and treatment methods. Semin Fetal Neonatal Med 2005; 10:504–14.
12. Dancea A, Fouron JC, Miro J, et al. Correlation between electrocardiographic and ultrasonographic time-interval measurements in fetal lamb heart. Pediatr Res 2000; 47:324–28.
13. Nii M, Hamilton RM, Fenwick L, Kingdom JC, Roman KS, Jaeggi ET. Assessment of fetal atrioventricular time intervals by tissue Doppler and pulse Doppler echocardiography: normal values and correlation with fetal electrocardiography. Heart 2006; 92:1831–37.
14. Carvalho JS, Prefumo F, Ciardelli V, Sairam S, Bhide A, Shinebourne E. Evaluation of fetal arrhythmias from simultaneous pulsed wave Doppler in pulmonary artery and vein. Heart 2007; 93:1448–53.
15. Cotton JL. Identification of fetal atrial flutter by Doppler tissue imaging. Circulation 2001; 104:1206–07.
16. Jaeggi E, Fouron JC, Drblik SP. Fetal atrial flutter: diagnosis, clinical features, treatment, and outcome. J Pediatr 1998; 132:335–39.
17. Lisowski LA, Verheijin PM, Benatar AA et al. Atrial flutter in the perinatal age group: diagnosis, management and outcome. J Am Coll Cardiol 2000; 35:771–77.
18. Ebenroth ES, Cordes TM, Darragh RK. Second-line treatment of fetal supraventricular tachycardia using flecainide acetate. Pediatr Cardiol 2001; 22:483–87.
19. The treatment of fetal dysrhythmias. Circulation 2000; 101: 2721–26.
20. Cuneo BF, Strasburger JF. Management strategy for fetal tachycardia. Obstet Gynecol 2000; 96:575–81.
21. Strasburger JF, Cuneo BF, Michon MM, et al. Amiodarone therapy for drug-refractory fetal tachycardia. Circulation 2004; 109:375–79.
22. Krapp M, Gembruch U, Baumann P. Venous blood flow pattern suggesting tachycardia-induced 'cardiomyopathy' in the fetus. Ultrasound Obstet Gynecol 1997; 10:32–40.
23. Naheed ZJ, Strasburger JF, Deal BJ, Benson DW, Gidding SS. Fetal tachycardia: mechanisms and predictors of hydrops fetalis. J Am Coll Cardiol 1996; 27:1736–40.
24. Simpson JM, Milburn A, Yates RW, et al. Outcome of intermittent tachyarrhythmias in the fetus. Pediatr Cardiol 1997; 18:78–82.
25. Rosenthal E. Fetal heart block. In: AllanL, HornbergerLK, SharlandG (eds). Textbook of Fetal Cardiology. London: Greenwich Medical Media, 2000; 438–52.
26. Schmidt KG, Ulmer HE, Silverman NH, Kleinman CS, Copel JA. Perinatal outcome of fetal complete atrioventricular block: a multicenter experience. J Am Coll Cardiol 1991; 91:1360–66.
27. Maeno Y, Himeno W, Saito A, et al. Clinical course of fetal congenital atrioventricular block in the Japanese population: a multicenter experience. Heart 2005; 91:1075–79.
28. Lopes LM, Tavares GMP, Damiano AP et al. Perinatal outcome of fetal atrioventricular block. One-hundred-sixteen cases from a single institution. Circulation 2008; 118: 1268–75.
29. Frohn-Mulder IM, Meilof JF, Szatmari A, Stewart PA, Swaak TJ, Hess J. Clinical significance of maternal anti-Ro/SS-A antibodies in children with isolated heart block. J Am Coll Cardiol 1994; 23:1677–81.
30. Groves AM, Allan LD, Rosenthal E. Outcome of isolated congenital complete heart block diagnosed in utero. Heart 1996; 75:190–94.
31. Buyon JP, Hiebert R, Copel J, et al. Autoimmune-associated congenital heart block: demographics, mortality and recurrence rates obtained from national neonatal lupus registry. J Am Coll Cardiol 1998; 31:1658–66.
32. Jaeggi ET, Hamilton RM, Silverman ED, Zamora SA, Hornberger LK. Outcome of children with fetal, neonatal or childhood diagnosis of isolated congenital atrioventricular block. J Am Coll Cardiol 2002; 39:130–37.
33. Hofbeck M, Ulmer H, Beinder E, Sieber E, Singer H. Prenatal findings in patients with prolonged QT interval in the neonatal period. Heart 1997; 77:198–204.
34. Friedman DM, Kim MY, Copel JA, et al. Utility of cardiac monitoring in fetuses at risk for congenital heart block. The PR interval and dexamethasone evaluation (PRIDE) prospective study. Circulation 2008; 117:485–93.
35. Zhao H, Cuneo BF, Strasburger JF, et al. Electrophysiological characteristics of fetal atrioventricular block. J Am Coll Cardiol 2008; 51:77–84.
36. Nield LE, Silverman ED, Taylor GP, et al. Maternal anti-Ro and anti-La antibody-associated endocardial fibroelastosis. Circulation 2002; 105:843–48.
37. Groves AM, Allan LD, Rosenthal E. Therapeutic trial of sympathomimetics in three cases of complete heart block in the fetus. Circulation 1995; 92:3394–96.
38. Hayashi T, Kaneko M, Kim KS, et al. Outcome of prenatally diagnosed isolated congenital complete atrioventricular block treated with transplacental betamethasone or ritodrine therapy. Pediatr Cardiol 2009; 30:35–40.
39. Copel JA, Buyon JP, Kleinman CS. Successful in utero therapy of fetal heart block. Am J Obstet Gynecol 1995; 173: 1384–90.
40. Rosenthal D, Druzin M, Chin C, et al. A new therapeutic approach to the fetus with congenital complete heart block: Preemptive, targeted therapy with dexamethasone. Obstet Gynecol 1998; 92:689–91.
41. Shinohara K, Miyagawa S, Fujita T, Aono T, Kidoguchi K. Neonatal lupus erythematosus: results of maternal corticosteroid therapy. Obstet Gynecol 1999; 93:952–57.
42. Sonesson SE, Salomonsson S, Jacobsson LA, et al. Signs of first-degree heart block occur in one-third of fetuses of pregnant women with anti-SSA/Ro 52-kd antibodies. Arthritis Rheum 2004; 50:1253–61.

43. Moak JP, Barron KS, Hougen TH, et al. Congenital heart block: Development of late-onset cardiomyopathy, a previous underappreciated sequela. J Am Coll Cardiol 2001; 37:238–42.
44. Udink ten Cate FEA, Breur JMPJ, Cohen MI, et al. Dilated cardiomyopathy in isolated congenital complete atrioventricular block: Early and long-term risk in children. J Am Coll Cardiol 2001; 37:1129–34.
45. Sreeram N, Wren C. Supraventricular tachycardia in infants: response to initial treatment. Arch Dis Child 1990; 65127–129–29.
46. Rhodes L A, Walsh E P, Saul J P. Conversion of atrial flutter in paediatric patients by transesophageal atrial pacing: a safe, effective, minimally invasive procedure. Am Heart J 1995;130:323–27.
47. Peng CC, Chen MR, Hou CJ, et al. Atrial flutter in the neonate and early infancy. Jpn Heart J 1998;39:287–95.
48. Pagis B, Villain E, Hidden Lucet F, Frank R, Sidi D. Wolff Parkinson-White syndrome in the child. A case report with associated atrial fibrillation. Arch Pediatr 2003;1038–41.
49. Szumowski L, Walczak F, Urbanek P, et al. Risk factors of atrial fibrillation in patients with Wolff Parkinson White syndrome. Kardiol Pol 2004;60:206–16.
50. Skinner JR, Chung SK, Montgomery D, et al Near miss SIDS due to Brugada syndrome. Arch Dis Child 2005;90:528–29.
51. Perry JC. Ventricular tachycardia in neonates. Pacing Clin Electrophysiol 1997;20:2061–64.
52. Walsh EP. Clinical approach to diagnosis and acute management of tachycardias in children. In: Walsh EP, Saul JP, Triedman JK, eds. Cardiac arrhythmias in children and young adults with congenital heart disease. Philadelphia: Lippincott Williams and Williams, 2001;103–104..
53. Dixon J, Foster K, Wyllie J, et al. Guidelines and adenosine dosing in supraventricular tachycardia.Arch Dis Child 2005. 901190–1191.1191.
54. Van Engelen AD, Weijtens O, Brenner J I, *et al.* Management, outcome and follow-up of fetal tachycardia. J Am Coll Cardiol 1994;24:1371–75.
55. Benson DW, Dunnigan A, Bendit D G. Follow up evaluation of infant paroxysmal atrial tachycardia: transesophageal study. Circulation 1987;75:542–549.
56. Boldt T, Eronen M, Andersson S. Long term outcome in fetuses with cardiac arrhythmias. Obstet Gynecol 2003;102 1372–79.
57. Simpson JM, Yates RW, Sharland GK. Irregular heart rate in the fetus: not always benign. Cardiol Young 1996;628–31.
58. Ito S, Gow R, Verjee Z, et al. Intravenous and oral propafenone for treatment of tachycardia in infants and children: pharmacokinetics and clinical response. J Clin Pharmacol 1998;38:496–501.
59. Perry JC, Garson A. Supraventricular tachycardia due to Wolff-Parkinson-White syndrome in children: early disappearance and late recurrence. J Am Coll Cardiol 1991;16:1215–20.
60. Deal BJ, Keane JF, Gillette PC, Garson A. Wolff-Parkinson-White syndrome and supraventricular tachycardia during infancy: management and follow up. J Am Coll Cardiol 1985;5:130–135.
61. Mehta AV, Sanchez G R, Sacks E J, *et al.* Ectopic automatic atrial tachycardia in children: clinical characteristics, management and follow up. J Am Coll Cardiol 1988;11:379–85.
62. Gillette PC, Garson A. Electrophysiologic and pharmacologic characteristics of automatic atrial tachycardia. Circulation 1977;56:571–75.
63. Klersy C, Chimienta M, Marangoni E, et al Factors that predict spontaneous remission of ectopic atrial tachycardia. Eur Heart J 1993;14:1654–56.
64. Baursfeld U, Gow RM, Hamilton RM, *et al.* Treatment of atrial ectopic tachycardia in infants less than 6 months old. Am Heart J 1995;129:1145–48.
65. Strasburger JF, Huhta JC, Carpenter RJ, et al: Doppler echo cardiography in the diagnosis and management of persistent fetal arrhythmias. J Am Coll Cardiol 1986;7:1386.
66. Huisman TWA, Stewart PA, Wladimiroff JW: Ductus venosus blood flow velocity waveforms in the human fetus: A Doppler study. Ultrasound Med Biol 1992;18:33.
67. Tulzer G, Khowsathit P, Gudmundsson S, et al: Diastolic function of the fetal heart during second and third trimester: A prospective longitudinal Doppler-echocardiographic study. Eur J Pediatr 1994;153:151.
68. Rizzo G, Arduini D, Romanini C: Inferior vena cava flow velocity waveforms in appropriate and small for gestational age fetuses. Am J Obstet Gynecol 1992;166:1271.
69. Hecher K, Campbell S, Doyle P, et al: Assessment of fetal compromise by Doppler ultrasound investigation of the fetal circulation: arterial, intracardiac, and venous blood flow velocity studies. Circulation 1995;91:129.
70. Bergman G, Jacobsson LA, Wahren-Herlenius M et al: Doppler echocardiographic and electrocardiographic atrioventricular timeintervals in newborn infants: evaluation of techniques for surveillance offetuses at risk for congenital heart block. Ultrasound Obstet Gynecol 2006;28(1):57–62.
71. Ko JK, Deal BJ, Strasburger JF, et al: Supraventricular tachycardia mechanisms and their age distribution in pediatric patients. Am J Cardiol 1992;69:1028.
72. Benson DW, Dunnigan A, Benditt DG: Follow-up evaluation of paroxysmal atrial tachycardia: Transeso-phageal study. Circulation 1987;75:542.
73. Deal BJ, Keane JF, Gilette PC, Garson A Jr: Wolff-Parkinson-White syndrome and supraventricular tachycardia during infancy: Management and follow-up. J Am Coll Cardiol 1985;5:130.
74. Garson A Jr. Systematic interpretation of cardiac arrhythmias. In Gilette PC, Garson A Jr (eds): Pediatric Arrhythmias: Electrophysiology and Pacing. Philadelphia, WB Saunders, 1990.
75. Garson A Jr, Gillette PC, McNamara DG. A Guide to Cardiac Dysrhythmias in Children. Houston, TX, Baylor College of Medicine Press, 1979.
76. Menendez T: Usefulness of magnetocardiography for the investigation of fetal arrhythmias. Am J Cardiol 2001;88:334.
77. Van Leeuwen P: Fetal magnetocardiography in the diagnosis of fetal arrhythmia. Br J Obstet Gynaecol 1999; 106:1200.
78. Strasburger JF, Wakai RT, Zhimin Li, et al: Prenatal Preexcitation: Magnetocardiographic Assessment of Wolff-

Parkinson White Syndrome in the Fetus. North American Society of Pacing and Electrophysiology. San Diego, May 8, 2002.

79. Hamada H, Horigome H, Asaka M, et al. Prenatal diagnosis of long QT syndrome using fetal magnetocardiography. Prenatal Diagn 1999;19:677.
80. Kleinman CS, Copel JA, Weinstein EM, et al: In utero diagnosis and treatment of fetal supraventricular tachycardia. Semin Perinatol 1985;9:113.
81. Gembruch U, Krapp M, Baumann P: Changes of venous blood flow velocity waveforms in fetuses with supraventricular tachycardia. Ultrasound Obstet Gynecol 1995;5:394.
82. Johnson P, Sharland G, Allan L, et al: Umbilical venous pressure in nonimmune hydrops fetalis: Correlation with cardiac size. Am J Obstet Gynecol 1992;167:1309.
83. Kleinman C, Copel J: Fetal cardiac arrhythmias: Diagnosis and therapy. In Creasy RK, Resnik R (eds): Maternal-Fetal Medicine. Philadelphia, WB Saunders, 1994.
84. Michaelsson M, Engle MA: Congenital complete heart block: An international study of the natural history. Cardiovasc Clin 1972;4:85.
85. Schmidt KG, Ulmer HE, Silverman NH, et al: Perinatal outcome of fetal complete atrioventricular block: A multicenter experience. J Am Coll Cardiol 1991;91:1360.
86. Shenker L, Reed KL, Anderson CF, et al. Congenital heart block and cardiac anomalies in the absence of maternal connective tissue disease. Am J Obstet Gynecol 1987;157:248.
87. Vetter LV, Rashkind WJ: Congenital complete heart block and connective tissue disease. N Engl J Med 1983;309:236.
88. Buyon JP, Winchester RJ, Slade SG, et al. Identification of mothers at risk for congenital heart block and other neonatal lupus syndromes in their children. Arthritis Rheum 1993; 36:1263.
89. Moak JP, Barron KS, Hougen TJ, et al. Congenital heart block: development of late-onset cardiomyopathy, a previouslyunderappreciated sequela. J Am Coll Cardiol 2001;37(1):238–42.
90. Litsey SE, Noonan JA, O'Connor WN, et al: Maternal connective tissue disease in congenital heart block: Demonstration of immunoglobulin in cardiac tissue. N Engl J Med 1985;312:98.
91. Ramsey-Goldman R, Hom D, Deng JS, et al: Anti-SS-A antibodies and fetal outcome in maternal systemic lupus erythematosis. Arthritis Rheum 1986;29:1269.
92. Cuneo BF, Strasburger JF, Wakai RT et al: Conduction system disease in fetuses evaluated for irregular cardiac rhythm. Fetal Diagn Ther 2006;21(3):307–13.
93. Groves AM, Allan LD, Rosenthal E: Therapeutic trial of sympathomimetics in three cases of complete heart block inthe fetus. Circulation 1995;92(12):3394–6.
94. Jaeggi ET, Fouron JC, Silverman ED, et al. Transplacental fetal treatment improves the outcome of prenatally diagnosedcomplete atrioventricular block without structural heart disease. Circulation 2004;21;110(12):1542–8.
95. Cuneo BF, Zhao H, Strasburger JF et al: Atrial and ventricular rate response and patterns of heart rate acceleration Am J Cardiol. 2007;100(4):661–5.
96. Buyon JP, Swersky SH, Fox HE, et al: Intrauterine therapy for presumptive fetal myocarditis with acquired heart block due to systemic lupus erythematosis. Arthritis Rheum 1987; 30:44.
97. Bierman FZ, Baxi L, Jaffe I, Driscoll J: Fetal hydrops and congenital complete heart block: Response to maternal steroid therapy. J Pediatr 1988;112:646.
98. Watson WJ, Katz VL: Steroid therapy for hydrops associated with antibody-mediated congenital heart block. Am J Obstet Gynecol 1991;165:553.
99. Blanford AT, Pearson-Murphy BE: In vitro metabolism of prednisolone, dexamethasone, betamethasone, and cortisol by the human placenta. Am J Obstet Gynecol 1977;127:264.
100. Copel JA, Buyon JP, Kleinman CS: Successful in utero therapy of fetal heart block. Am J Obstet Gynecol 1995; 173:1384.
101. Carpenter RJ, Strasburger JF, Garson A, et al: Fetal ventricular pacing for hydrops secondary to complete atrioventricular block. J Am Coll Cardiol 1986;8:1434.
102. Walkinshaw SA, Welch CR, McCormack J, Walsh K: In utero pacing for hydrops secondary to complete atrioventricular block. J Am Coll Cardiol 1986;8:1434.
103. Zhao H, Cuneo BF, Strasburger JF, Huhta JC et al: Electrophysiological characteristics of fetal atrioventricular block. J Am Coll Cardiol. 2008;51(1):77–84.
104. Zhao H, Strasburger JF, Cuneo BF, et al. Fetal cardiac repolarization abnormalities. Am J Cardiol. 2006;98(4):491–6.
105. Li Z, Strasburger JF, Cuneo BF et al: Giant fetal magnetocardiogram P waves in congenital atrioventricular block: a marker of cardiovascular compensation? Circulation 2004, 110(15):2097–101.
106. Beinder E, Grancay T, Menendez T, Singer H, Hofbeck M: Fetal sinus bradycardia and the long QT syndrome. Am J Obstet Gynecol 2001;185:743.
107. Cuneo BF, Ovadia M, Strasburger JF et al: Prenatal diagnosis and in utero treatment of torsades de pointes associated withcongenital long QT syndrome. Am J Cardiol 2003;1;91(11):1395–8.
108. Garite, TJ, Dildy, GA, McNamara, H, et al. A multicenter controlled trial of fetal pulse oximetry in the intrapartum management of nonreassuring fetal heart rate patterns. Am J Obstet Gynecol 2000;183:1049.
109. Klauser, CK, Christensen, EE, Chauhan, SP, et al. Use of fetal pulse oximetry among high-risk women in labor: A randomized clinical trial. Am J Obstet Gynecol 2005; 192:1810.
110. East, CE, Brennecke, SP, King, JF, et al. The effect of intrapartum fetal pulse oximetry, in the presence of a nonreassuring fetal heart rate pattern, on operative delivery rates: a multicenter, randomized, controlled trial (the FOREMOST trial). Am J Obstet Gynecol 2006;194:606.
111. Bloom, SL, Spong, CY, Thom, E, et al. Fetal pulse oximetry and cesarean delivery. N Engl J Med 2006;355:2195.
112. Cuneo BF, Strasburger JF: Management strategy for fetal tachycardia. Obstet Gynecol 2000;96:575.
113. Naheed ZJ, Strasburger JF, Deal BJ, et al: Fetal tachycardia: Mechanisms and predictors of hydrops fetalis. J Am Coll Cardiol 1996;27:1736.
114. Perry JC, Garson A Jr: Supraventricular tachycardia due to Wolff-Parkinson-White syndrome in children: Early disappearance and late recurrence. J Am Coll Cardiol 1990; 16:1215.

115. Lundberg A: Paroxysmal atrial tachycardia in infancy: Long-term follow-up study of 49 subjects. Pediatrics 1982; 70:638.
116. Leuthold A, Wakai RT, Martin CB: Noninvasive in utero assessment of PR and QRS intervals from the fetal magnetocardiogram. Early Hum Dev 1999;54:235.
117. Zhao H, Chen M, Van Veen BD et al: Simultaneous fetal magnetocardiography and ultrasound/Doppler imaging. IEEE Trans Biomed Eng. 2007;54(6 Pt 2):1167–71.
118. Zhao H, Wakai RT: Simultaneity of foetal heart rate acceleration and foetal trunk movement determined by foetal magnetocardiogram actocardiography. Phys Med Biol 2002;47:839.
119. Cuneo BF, Ovadia M, Strasburger JF, et al: Prenatal diagnosis and in utero treatment of torsades de pointes associated with congenital long QT syndrome. Am J Cardiol 2003;91:1395.
120. Zhao H, Cuneo BF, Strasburger JF, Huhta JC et al: Electrophysiological characteristics of fetal atrioventricular block. J Am Coll Cardiol. 2008;1;51(1):77–84.
121. Nii M, Hamilton RM, Fenwick L, et al: Assessment of fetal atrioventricular time intervals by tissue Doppler and pulse Doppler echocardiography: normal values and correlation with fetal electrocardiography. Heart 2006;92:1831.
122. Pasquini L, Seale AN, Belmar C et al PR interval: a comparison of electrical and mechanical methods in the fetus. Early Hum Dev. 2006;83(4):231–7.
123. Garite, TJ, Dildy, GA, McNamara, H, et al. A multicenter controlled trial of fetal pulse oximetry in the intrapartum management of nonreassuring fetal heart rate patterns. Am J Obstet Gynecol 2000;183:1049.
124. Klauser, CK, Christensen, EE, Chauhan, SP, et al. Use of fetal pulse oximetry among high-risk women in labor: A randomized clinical trial. Am J Obstet Gynecol 2005; 192:1810.
125. East, CE, Brennecke, SP, King, JF, et al. The effect of intrapartum fetal pulse oximetry, in the presence of a nonreassuring fetal heart rate pattern, on operative delivery rates: a multicenter, randomized, controlled trial (the FOREMOST trial). Am J Obstet Gynecol 2006;194:606.
126. Bloom, SL, Spong, CY, Thom, E, et al. Fetal pulse oximetry and cesarean delivery. N Engl J Med 2006;355:2195.
127. Cuneo BF, Strasburger JF, Wakai RT et al: Conduction system disease in fetuses evaluated for irregular cardiac rhythm. Fetal Diagn Ther 2006;21(3):307–13.
128. Naheed ZJ, Strasburger JF, Deal BJ, et al: Fetal tachycardia: Mechanisms and predictors of hydrops fetalis. J Am Coll Cardiol 1996;27:1736.
129. Perry JC, Garson A Jr: Supraventricular tachycardia due to Wolff-Parkinson-White syndrome in children: Early disappearance and late recurrence. J Am Coll Cardiol 1990; 16:1215.
130. Lundberg A: Paroxysmal atrial tachycardia in infancy: Long-term follow-up study of 49 subjects. Pediatrics 1982; 70:638.
131. Leuthold A, Wakai RT, Martin CB: Noninvasive in utero assessment of PR and QRS intervals from the fetal magnetocardiogram. Early Hum Dev 1999;54:235.
132. Zhao H, Wakai RT: Simultaneity of foetal heart rate acceleration and foetal trunk movement determined by foetal magnetocardiogram actocardiography. Phys Med Biol 2002;47:839.
133. Zhao H, Wakai RT: Simultaneity of foetal heart rate acceleration and foetal trunk movement determined by foetal magnetocardiogram actocardiography. Phys Med Biol 2002;47:839.
134. Cuneo BF, Ovadia M, Strasburger JF et al: Prenatal diagnosis and in utero treatment of torsades de pointes associated withcongenital long QT syndrome. Am J Cardiol 2003;1;91(11):1395–8.
135. Nii M, Hamilton RM, Fenwick L, et al: Assessment of fetal atrioventricular time intervals by tissue Doppler and pulse Doppler echocardiography: normal values and correlation with fetal electrocardiography. Heart 2006;92:1831.
136. Pasquini L, Seale AN, Belmar C et al: PR interval: a comparison of electrical and mechanical methods in the fetus. Early Hum Dev. 2006;83(4):231–7.
137. Smith GC, Fleming JE: Prolonged fetal pre-ejection period corrected for PR interval associated withcerebral palsy. Eur J Obstet Gynecol Reprod Biol 1997;71(1):95–7.
138. Gardiner HM: Keeping abreast of advances in fetal cardiology. Early Hum Dev 2006;82:415.
139. Reddy UM, Ko CW, Willinger M: Maternal age and the risk of stillbirth throughout pregnancy in the United States. Am J Obstet Gynecol 2006;195:764.
140. Strasburger JF, Cuneo BF, Michon MM et al: Amiodarone therapy for drug-refractory fetal tachycardia. Circulation 2004;109(3):375–9.

39 Management of Heart Failure in Children and Adolescents

The most likely causes of pediatric congestive heart failure depend on the age of the child. Congestive heart failure in the fetus, or hydrops, can be detected by performing fetal echocardiography. In this case, congestive heart failure may represent underlying anemia (e.g. Rh sensitization, fetal-maternal transfusion), arrhythmias (usually supraventricular tachycardia), or myocardial dysfunction (myocarditis or cardiomyopathy). Curiously, structural heart disease is rarely a cause of congestive heart failure in the fetus although it does occur. Atrioventricular valve regurgitation in the fetus is a particularly troubling sign with respect to the prognosis (Fig. 39.2).

Neonates and infants younger than age 2 months are the most likely group to present with congestive heart failure related to structural heart disease. The systemic or pulmonary circulation may depend on the patency of the ductus arteriosus, especially in patients presenting in the first few days of life. In these patients, prompt cardiac evaluation is mandatory. Myocardial disease due to primary myopathic abnormalities or inborn errors of metabolism must be investigated. Respiratory illnesses, anemia, and known or suspected infection must be considered and appropriately managed.

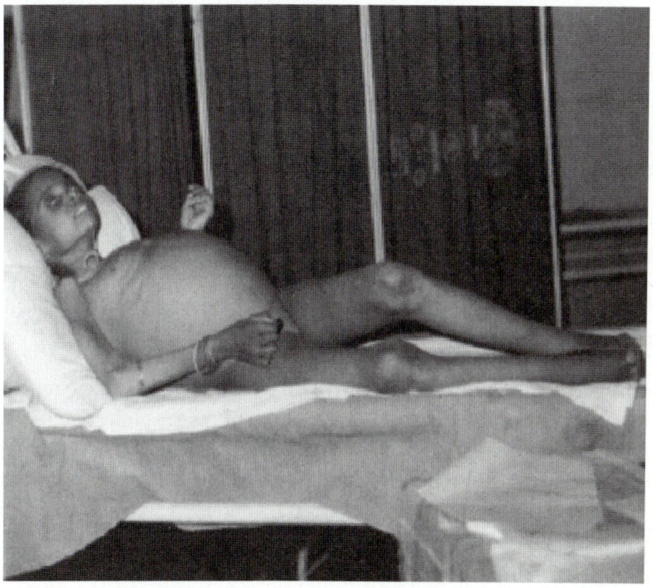

Fig. 39.1: *Photograph of a young patient showing generalized edema of the body, ascites and semiconcious state of mind in severe form of heart failure*

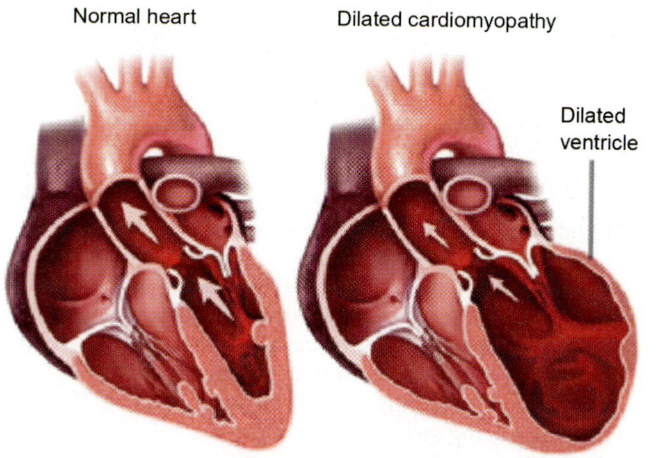

Fig. 39.2: *Showing normal heart (left) and dilated cardiomyopathy as one of the causes of heart failure (right)*

In older children, congestive heart failure may be caused by left-sided obstructive disease (valvar or subvalvar aortic stenosis or coarctation), myocardial dysfunction (myocarditis or cardiomyopathy), hypertension, renal failure, or, more rarely, arrhythmias or myocardial ischemia. Illicit drugs such as inhaled cocaine and other stimulants are increasingly precipitating causes of congestive heart failure in adolescents; therefore, an increased suspicion of drug use is warranted in unexplained congestive heart failure.

Although congestive heart failure in adolescents can be related to structural heart disease (including complications

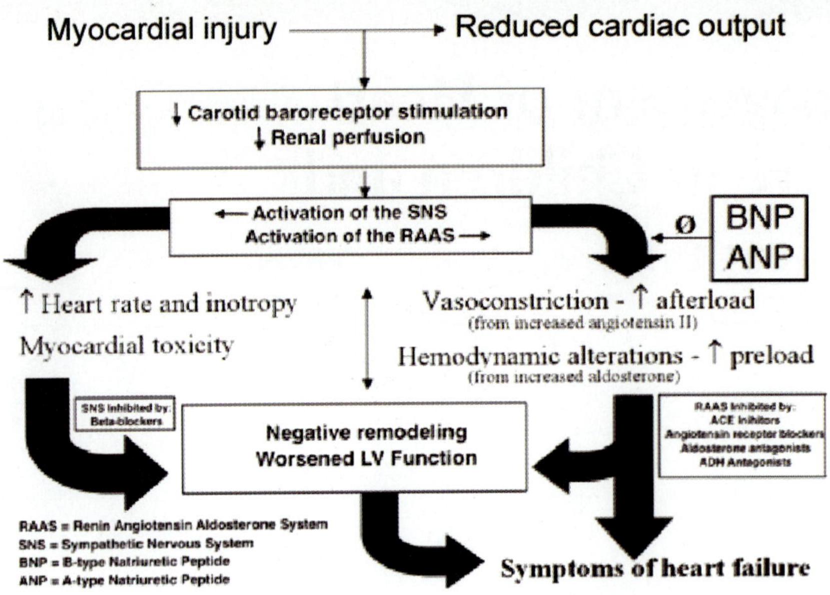

Fig. 39.3: *Diagram explaining various steps in the pathophysiology of heart failure*

Table 39.1: *Stages of heart failure*

A. Patients at high risk of developing HF because of the presence of conditions that are strongly associated with the development of HF (such patients have no identified structural or functional abnormalities of the pericardium, myocardium, or cardiac valves and have never shown signs or symptoms of HE)	Systemic hypertension; coronary artery disease; diabetes mellitus; history of cardiotoxic drug therapy or alcohol abuse; personal history of rheumatic fever; family history of cardiomyopathy
B. Patients who have developed structural heart disease that is strongly associated with the development of HF but who have never shown signs or symptoms of HF	LV hypertrophy or fibrosis; LV dilatation or hypocontractility; asymptomatic valvular heart disease; previous myocardial infarction
C. Patients who have current or prior symptoms of HF associated with underlying structural heart disease	Dyspnea or fatigue caused by LV systolic dysfunction; asymptomatic patients who are undergoing treatment for symptoms of HF
D. Patients with advanced structural heart disease and marked symptoms of HF at rest despite maximal medical therapy and who require specialized interventions	Patients who are frequently hospitalized for HF or cannot be safely discharged from the hospital; patients in the hospital awaiting heart transplantation; patients at home receiving continuous intravenous support for symptom relief or being supported with a mechanical circulatory assist device; patients in a hospice setting for the management of HF

HF indicates heart failure.

after surgical palliation or repair), it is usually associated with chronic arrhythmia or acquired heart disease, such as cardiomyopathy.

Pathophysiology in Heart Failure (Figs 39.2 and 39.3)

Heart failure may be defined as that pathophysiological state in which an abnormality of cardiac function is responsible for the failure of the heart to pump blood at a rate commensurate with the metabolic requirements of the body. The heart may fail if it is confronted with:

1. An excessive preload, i.e. increase in tension in ventricular cardiac muscle fibers leading to excessive expansion of ventricles in diastole as seen in left to right shunt, mitral regurgitation and complete heart block;
2. Abnormally high afterload as in hypertension, coarctation of the aorta and aortic stenosis
3. Impaired myocardial contractility as in myopathy, myocarditis
4. Inadequate diastolic filling as in hypertrophic or restrictive cardiomyopathy, constrictive pericarditis and tachyarrhythmias. Chronic heart failure is a clinical syndrome in which heart disease reduces cardiac output, increases venous pressures, and is accompanied by molecular abnormalities that cause progressive deterioration of the failing heart and premature death of myocardial cells.

At the onset of heart failure various compensatory mechanisms with salutary effects come into play. But, the same compensatory mechanisms if pressed into play indefinitely potentiate heart failure, the possible mechanisms of which are described below:

1. **The compensatory increase in sympathetic tone** increases the heart rate, augments myocardial contractility and causes systemic vasoconstriction which help to maintain tissue perfusion pressure. But when sympathetic action is undeterred, tachycardia and peripheral vasoconstriction (increased afterload) leads to substantial increase in cardiac work and myocardial oxygen consumption. Furthermore, at the cellular level, compensatory gain in cardiac excitation-contraction coupling mediated by sympathetic stimulation ultimately become unsuccessful as evidenced by unwanted diastolic leak of sarcoplasmic reticulum calcium leading to depletion of intracellular calcium and loss of contractility.
2. **The compensatory stimulation of renin-angiotensin-aldosterone system** causes vasoconstriction and renal retention of salt and water which increases diastolic filling pressure and increase myocardial contractility through Frank-Starling mechanism. But when these effects are excessive, it causes systemic and pulmonary venous congestion and increases afterload. In addition, renin-angiotensin-aldosterone system is responsible in mediating renal hyporesponsiveness to the natriuretic peptides, which facilitates progression of heart failure. The compensatory ventricular hypertrophy initiated and regulated by many of the signaling molecules that mediate the neurohormonal responses in the failing heart provides more contractile elements. However, maladaptive hypertrophy ultimately results in myocardial cell death and fibrosis.
3. **An inflammatory response secondary to increased wall stress and stretching of myocardial fibers** results in production of cytokines and free radicals leading to apoptosis. If uninterrupted, apoptosis will lead to necrosis, fibrosis and further dysfunction. The extracellular matrix remodeling is promoted by neurohormonal activation and activation of pro-inflammatory cytokines. Increase plasma levels of matrix metalloproteinases are associated with severe heart failure and probably reflect progressive remodeling. There is up-regulation of myocardial matrix metalloproteinases associated with decreased fibrillar collagen cross-link formation in patients with chronic systolic heart failure with cardiomyopathic ventricles.

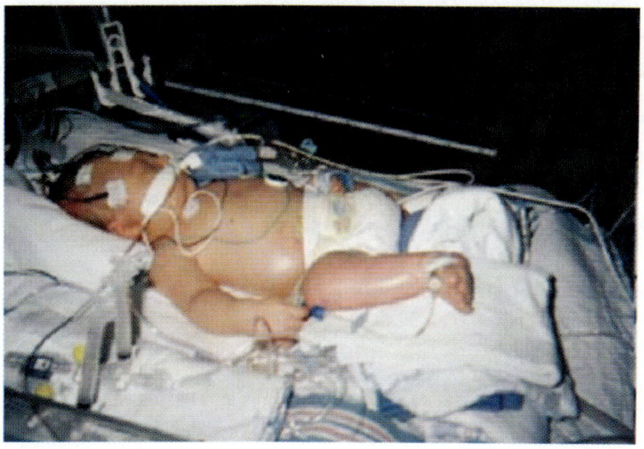

Fig. 39.4: *Showing generalised edema of the body in an infant with heart failure*

Classification in Heart Failure (Table 39.1)

Heart failure can be classified according to a variety of factors (*see* heart failure criteria and classification). The New York Heart Association (NYHA) classification for heart failure comprises four classes, based on the relationship between symptoms and the amount of effort required to provoke them as follows:

Class I patients have no limitation of physical activity
Class II patients have slight limitation of physical activity
Class III patients have marked limitation of physical activity
Class IV patients have symptoms even at rest and are unable to carry on any physical activity without discomfort.

The American College of Cardiology/American Heart Association (ACC/AHA) heart failure guidelines complement the NYHA classification to reflect the progression of disease and are divided into four stages as follows (Table 39.3):

Stage A: Patients are at high risk for heart failure but have no structural heart disease or symptoms of heart failure.

Stage B: Patients have structural heart disease but have no symptoms of heart failure

Stage C: Patients have structural heart disease and have symptoms of heart failure

Stage D: Patients have refractory heart failure requiring specialized interventions.

Etiology in Pediatric Heart Failure (Table 39.2)

Despite advancement in surgical management, chronic heart failure in children is frequently associated with congenital heart disease. Chronic heart failure occurs most commonly in these patients as a result of excessive ventricular volume overload, pressure overload, post-operative cardiac sequelae with residual lesions or myocardial damage, pulmonary vascular disease, or consequence of chronic hypoxia. Other causes of chronic heart failure in children are cardiomyopathy (hypertrophic, dilated, restrictive, or noncompaction), congenital or acquired coronary artery abnormalities, endocarditis, Eisenmenger syndrome, primary pulmonary hypertension, cor pulmonale, incessant tachyarrhythmias, chronic anemias and rheumatic heart diseases. Among the cardiomyopathy, dilated cardiomyopathy accounts for most cases of chronic heart failure in children. The underlying cause of dilated cardiomyopathy includes a wide variety of etiologies: idiopathic, inherited, infective, infiltrative, nutritional, iatrogenic or toxic, and cardiomyopathy associated with generalized muscle disease or

Table 39.2: *Leading causes of CHF in relation to age*

Birth to 1st week
- Aortic atresia
- Transposition of great vessels
- Coarctation of aorta

1 week to 1 month
- Coarctation of aorta
- TGA
- Endocardial fibroelastosis

1 month to 2 months
- TGA
- Endocardial fibroelastosis

2 months to 3 months
- Coarctation of aorta
- Total anomalous pulmonary venous return
- VSD

3 months to 6 months
- VSD

6 months to 12 months
- VSD
- ASD (ostium primum)
- CHF is rarely present in utero with exception of paroxysmal supraventricular tachycardia and anemia due to Rh incompatibility. It is often interpreted as intrauterine asphyxia and mother is subjected to cesarean section.

After first year of life, CHF is much less frequent and it is due to variety of causes:
- Arrhythmias
- Viral myocarditis
- Acute rheumatic carditis
- Cardiomyopathy.

mitochondrial disorders. Generally, 30% of cases of myocarditis result in chronic heart failure. Mason et al found evidence of myocarditis in 10% of adults with new-onset heart failure who did not have coronary heart disease. It is likely that this figure is much higher in children without structural heart disease.

Aetiological Factors According to Different Ages of Development

CHF in the Fetus

Disorders that are fatal in the immediate neonatal period are often well tolerated in the fetus due to the pattern of fetal blood flow (e.g. transposition of great vessels). Supraventricular tachycardia, severe bradycardia due to complete heart block, anaemia, severe tricuspid regurgitation due to Ebstein's anomaly of the tricuspid valve or mitral regurgitation from atrioventricular canal defect, myocarditis etc. may cause CHF in the fetus. Most of these are recognised by fetal echocardiography. Severe CHF in the fetus produces hydrops fetalis with ascites, pleural and pericardial effusions and anasarca. Digoxin or sympathomimetics to the mother may be helpful in cases of fetal tachyarrhythmia or complete heart block, respectively.

CHF on First Day of Life

Most structural heart defects do not cause CHF within hours of birth. Instead, myocardial dysfunction secondary to asphyxia, hypoglycemia, hypocalcemia or sepsis are

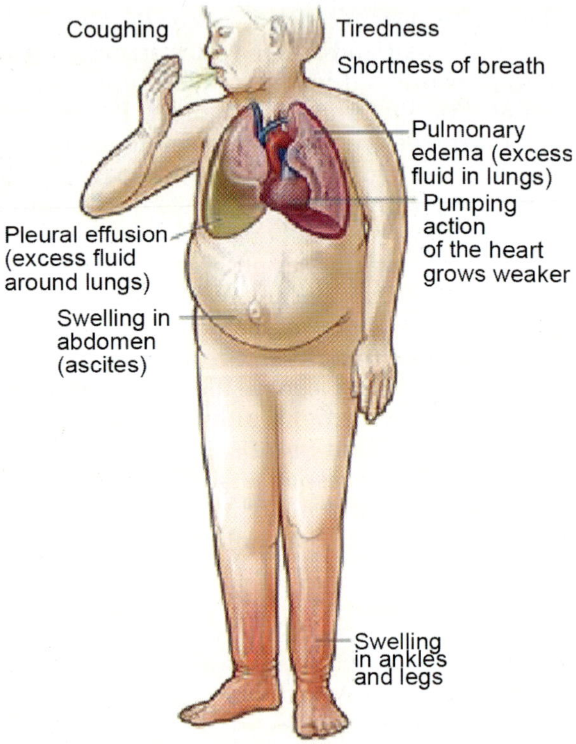

Fig. 39.5: *Diagram showing various signs and symptoms in heart failure*

Table 39.3: *NYHA functional classification of heart failure*

Class	*Functional capacity*
I	Patient without limitation of physical activity
II	Patients with sight limiations of physical activity, in which ordinary physical activity leads to fatigue, palpitation, dyspnea, or anginal pain; they are comfortable at rest.
III	Patients with marked limitations of physical activity, in which less than ordinary activity results in fatigue, palpitation, dyspnea, or anginal pain; they are comfortable at rest.
IV	Patients who are not only unable to carry on any physical activity without discomfort but who also have symptoms of heart failure or the anginal syndrome even at rest; the patient's discomfort increases if any physical activity is undertaken

Source: American Heart Association. Classes of heart failure. Available at:http://www.heart.org/HEARTORG/Conditions/HeartFailure AboutHeartFailure/Classes-of-Heart-Failure_UCM_306328_Article.jsp. Assessed: September 6,2011.

usually responsible for CHF on the first day. Tricuspid regurgitation secondary to hypoxia induced papillary muscle dysfunction or Ebstein's anomaly of the valve is also recognised. This improves as the pulmonary artery pressure falls over the next few days.

CHF in First Week of Life

Serious cardiac disorders which are potentially curable but carry a high mortality if untreated, often present with CHF in the first week of life. Accordingly, a sense of urgency should always accompany evaluation of the patient with CHF in the first week. The closure of the ductus arteriosus is often the precipitating event leading to catastrophic deterioration in a seemingly healthy neonate. It follows that prostaglandins E1 (now available in India) should be utilised in such babies.

Regarding CHF in this age group a few points need to be emphasised:

i. Peripheral pulses and oxygen saturation (by a pulse oximeter) should be checked in both the upper and lower extremities. A lower saturation in the lower limbs means right to left ductal shunting and occurs due to pulmonary hypertension, coarctation of aorta or aortic arch interruption.
ii. An atrial or ventricular septal defect (ASD/VSD) does not lead to CHF in the first two weeks of life. Therefore, an additional cause must be sought (e.g. coarctation of aorta or TAPVC).
iii. Premature infants have a poor myocardial reserve and a patent ductus arteriosus (PDA) may result in CHF in the first week in them.
iv. Adrenal insufficiency due to enzyme deficiencies or neonatal thyrotoxicosis could present with CHF in the first few days of life.

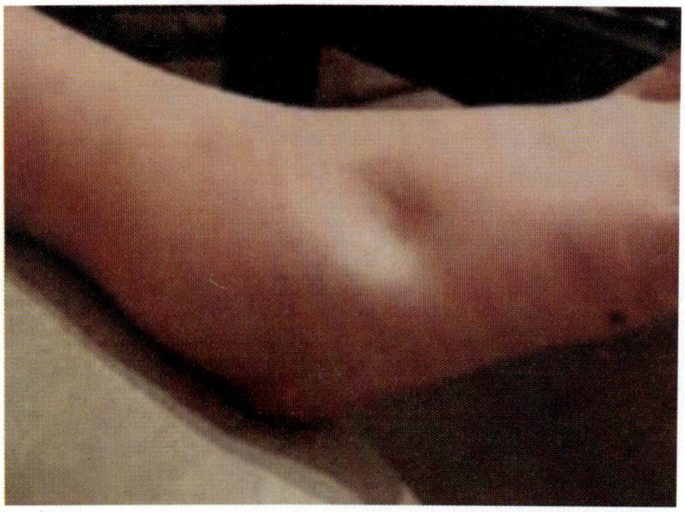

Fig. 39.6: *Pitting edema over foot in a patient with heart failure*

CHF Beyond Second Week of Life (Fig. 39.4)

The most common cause of CHF in infants is a ventricular septal defect that presents around 6–8 weeks of age. This is because the volume of the left to right shunt increases as the pulmonary resistance falls. Although a murmur of VSD is apparent by 1 week, the full blown picture of CHF occurs around 6–8 weeks.

Other left to right shunts like PDA present similarly. The fall in pulmonary vascular resistance is delayed in presence of hypoxic lung disease and at high altitude and could somewhat alter the time course accordingly.

Medical management of CHF is perhaps most important in this age group, since the VSD may close on follow-up. It is equally important to understand that spontaneous improvement in CHF could result from development of obstructive pulmonary arterial hypertension, even in early childhood.

Left coronary artery arising from the pulmonary artery (LCAPA), a rare disease in this age group merits separate mention, since it is curable and often missed. As the pulmonary artery pressure decreases in the neonatal period, these babies suffer from episodes of excessive crying with sweating (angina) and myocardial infarction.

The electrocardiogram shows pathologic q waves or left ventricular hypertrophy. These infants are often misdiagnosed as having "dilated cardiomyopathy".

Table 39.4: *Prevalence of signs and symptoms in systolic and diastolic heart failure*

Symptoms	*Diastolic HF (LVEF >50%)*	*Systolic HF (LVEF <50%)*
Dyspnea on exertion	85%	96%
Paroxysmal nocturnal dyspnea	55%	50%
Orthopnea	60%	73%
Physical examination		
Jugular venous distension	35%	46%
Rales	72%	70%
Displaced apical impulse	50%	60%
S3	45%	65%
S4	45%	66%
Hepatomegaly	15%	16%
E dema	30%	40%
Chest film		
Cardiomegaly	90%	96%
Pulmonary venous hypertension	75%	80%

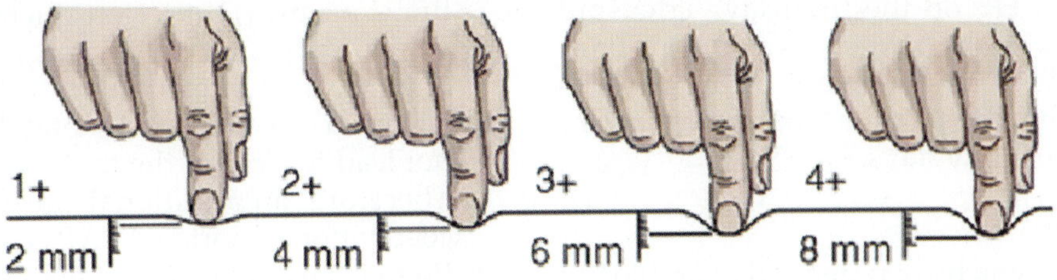

Fig. 39.7: *Assessment of the severity of peripheral edema*

Table 39.5: *Clinical manifestations of CHF*
Cardiomegaly
Failure to thrive
Tachycardia
Wheezing
Tachypnea
Dyspnea
Gallop rhythm
Peripheral edema (Figs 39.6 and 39.7)
Rales
Hepatomegaly
Peripheral cyanosis
Sweating
Poor pulses

CHF Beyond Infancy (Fig. 39.1 and 39.5)

Onset of CHF beyond infancy is unusual in patients with congenital heart disease and suggests a complicating factor like valvular regurgitation, infective endocarditis.

Types of Heart Failure (Table 39.4)

Systolic Heart Failure

Diminished cardiac output is caused by a complex interaction of various factors. Systolic dysfunction is characterized by diminished ventricular contractility that results in an impaired ability to increase the stroke volume

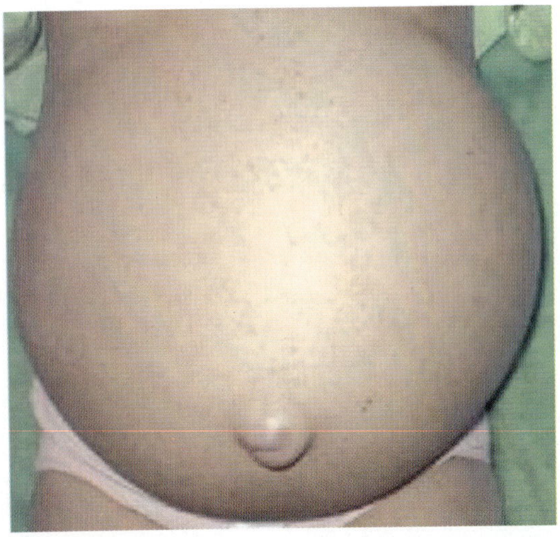

Fig. 39.8: *Ascites in a patient with congestive heart failure*

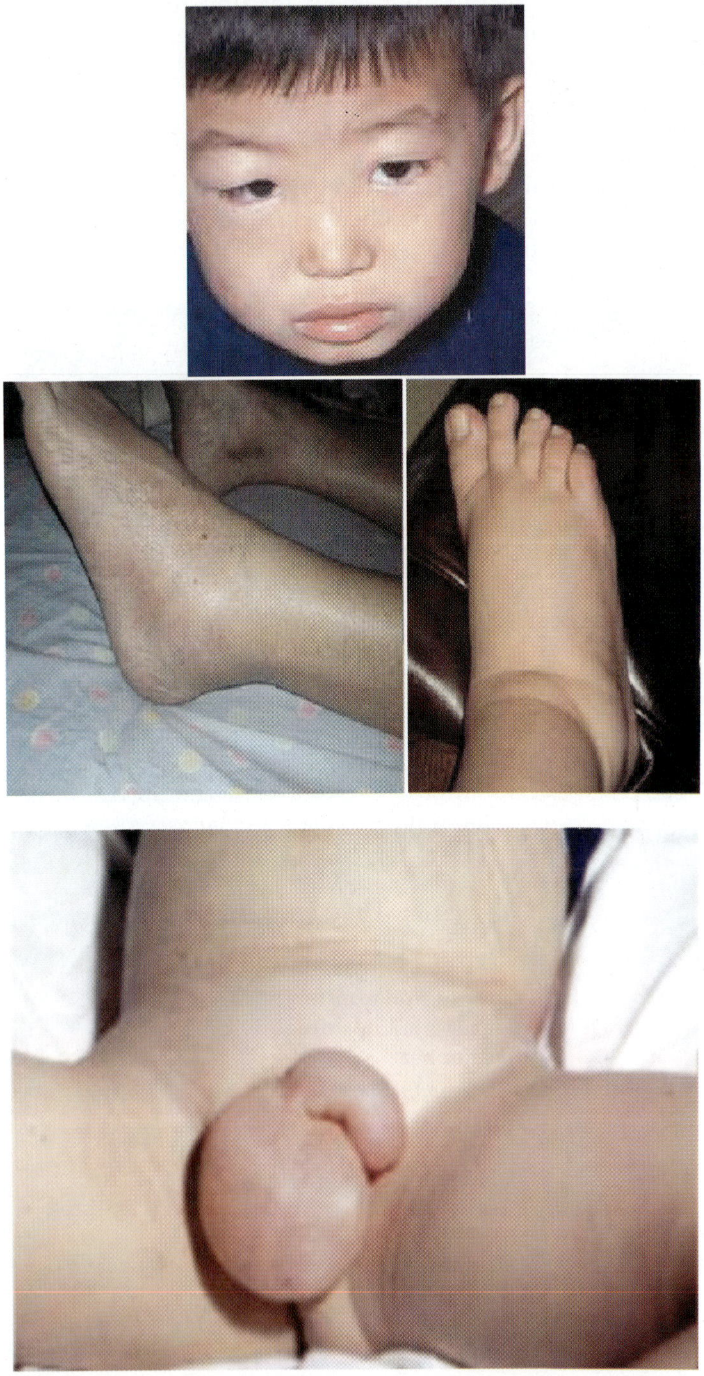

Fig. 39.9: *Edema of various parts of the body in heart failure*

Table 39.6: *Criteria for diagnosis of diastolic heart failure*

European study group:
1. Evidence of CHF
2. Normal or mildly abnormal LV systolic function
3. Evidence of abnormal LV relaxation, filling, distensibility or stiffness

Framingham heart study:
1. Definitive diagnosis of CHF (signs and symptoms S; CXR; response to diuretics)
2. LVEF greater than or equal to 50% within 72 hours of episodes
3. Objective evidence of LV diastolic dysfunction (abnormal LV relaxation/filling! distensibility indices by catheterization)

to meet systemic demands. Factors such as anatomic stresses (e.g. coarctation of the aorta) that contribute to an increased afterload (end-systolic wall stress), as well as neurohormonal factors that increase systemic vascular resistance, also lead to systolic dysfunction.

Diastolic Heart Failure

Diastolic dysfunction results from decreased ventricular compliance, necessitating an increase in venous pressure to maintain adequate ventricular filling. Causes of primary diastolic dysfunction include an anatomic obstruction that prevents ventricular filling (e.g. pulmonary venous obstruction), a primary reduction in ventricular compliance (e.g. cardiomyopathy, transplant rejection), external constraints (e.g. pericardial effusion), and poor hemodynamics after the Fontan procedure (e.g. elevated pulmonary vascular resistance).

Chronic Heart Failure

In chronic heart failure, myocardial cells die from energy starvation, from cytotoxic mechanisms leading to necrosis, or from the acceleration of apoptosis or programmed cell death. Necrosis stimulates fibroblast proliferation, which results in the replacement of myocardial cells with collagen. The loss of myocytes leads to cardiac dilation and an increased afterload and wall tension, which results in further systolic dysfunction. In addition, the loss of mitochondrial mass leads to increased energy starvation.

Acute Heart Failure

During acute congestive heart failure, the sympathetic nervous system and renin-angiotensin system act to maintain blood flow and pressure to the vital organs. Increased neurohormonal activity results in increased myocardial contractility, selective peripheral vasoconstriction, salt and fluid retention, and blood pressure maintenance. As a chronic state of failure ensues, these same mechanisms cause adverse effects.

The myocardial oxygen demand, which exceeds the supply, increases because of an increase in the heart rate, in contractility, and in wall stress. Alterations in calcium homeostasis and changes in contractile proteins occur, resulting in a hypertrophic response of the myocytes. Neurohormonal factors may lead to direct cardiotoxicity and necrosis.

Clinical History in Heart Failure

Thorough history taking and physical examination including an assessment of the upper-extremity and lower-extremity blood pressures, are crucial in the evaluation of an infant or child with congestive heart failure (Fig. 39.10).

Regardless of the etiology, the first manifestation of congestive heart failure is usually tachycardia. An obvious exception to this finding occurs in congestive heart failure due to a primary bradyarrhythmia or complete heart block. As the severity of congestive heart failure increases, signs of venous congestion usually ensue. Left-sided heart failure

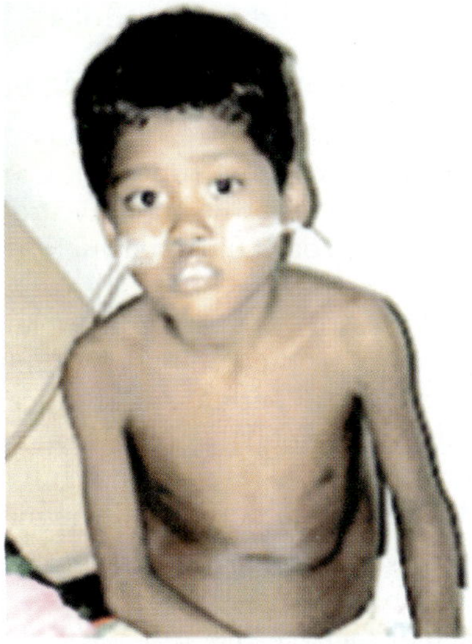

Fig. 39.10: *Showing treatment of heart failure with administration of intranasal oxygen in an older child with ASD septum primum defect*

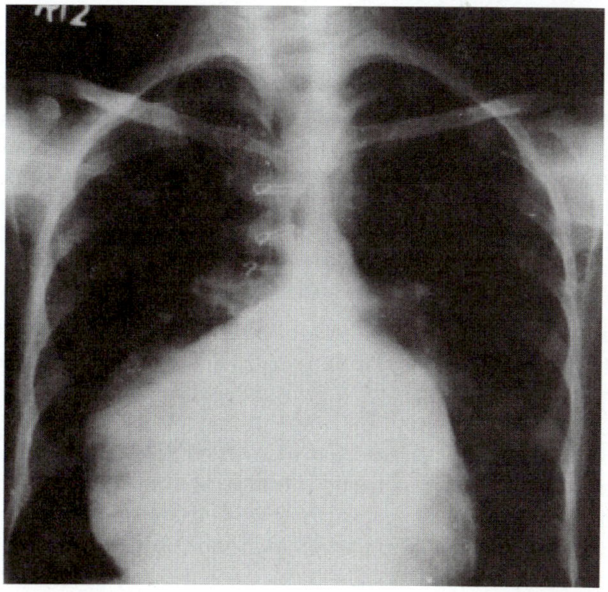

Fig. 39.11: *Chest X-ray PA view showing globular heart in in patient with biventricular failure*

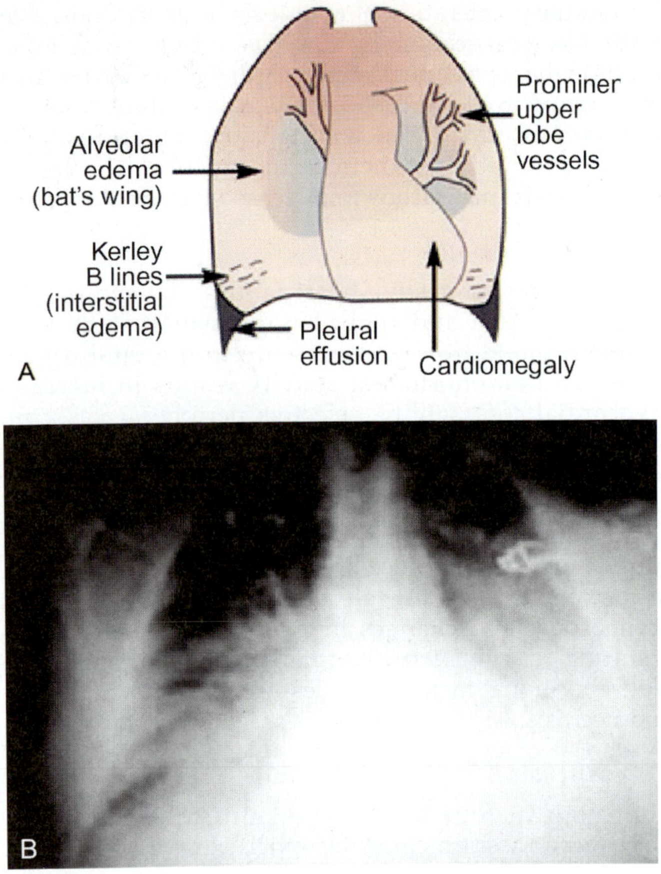

Fig. 39.12: *(A) Classic signs of acute heart failure that can be seen on a chest X-ray of left ventricular failure. (B) Pleural effusion on a chest X-ray*

is generally associated with signs of pulmonary venous congestion, whereas right-sided heart failure is associated with signs of systemic venous congestion. Marked failure of either ventricle, however, can affect the function of the other, leading to systemic and pulmonary venous congestion.

Later stages of congestive heart failure are characterized by signs and symptoms of low cardiac output. Generally, congestive heart failure with normal cardiac output is called compensated congestive heart failure, and congestive heart failure with inadequate cardiac output is considered decompensated.

Symptoms and Signs in Heart Failure (Table 39.5)

Clinical findings may include hypotension, cool extremities with poor peripheral perfusion, a thready pulse, and decreased urine output. Chemical evidence of renal and liver dysfunction may be present, as well as a diminished level of consciousness. Children with uncompensated congestive heart failure, particularly older children, generally have a lower cardiac output than that which most experienced clinicians would estimate on the basis of the clinical signs.

Symptoms and signs due to venous congestion: Right-sided (hepatomegaly, ascites, abdominal pain, pleural effusion, edema, jugular venous distention); left-sided (tachypnea, retractions, nasal flaring or grunting, rales, pulmonary edema).

Symptoms and signs due to low cardiac output: Fatigue or low energy, pallor, sweating, cool extremities, nausea/vomiting, poor growth, dizziness, altered consciousness, and syncope.

Heart failure is a clinical syndrome consisting of signs and symptoms that arise from congested organs and hypoperfused tissues. Impaired myocardial function results in cardiomegaly, tachycardia, gallop rhythm, poor peripheral perfusion and growth retardation.

Cardiomegaly occurs in most patients with heart failure except in pulmonary venous obstruction and constrictive pericarditis. A sleeping heart rate above 160 per minute in infants and above 100 per minute in children is usually present in heart failure (Figs 39.11 and 39.12).

A protodiastolic gallop at the time of rapid ventricular filling is a sign of impaired ventricular function.

Poor peripheral perfusion manifests itself by cold extremities, weak pulses and low blood pressure associated with skin mottling.

Growth retardation is noted in infants with chronic heart failure.

Dyspnea and tachypnea are the typical signs of increased pulmonary venous pressure.

Respiratory rates may be as high as 80–100 per minute and are associated with retraction, grunting and poor feeding. Wheezing may be the earliest and occasionally the only evidence of pulmonary edema.

Rales are relatively uncommon sign of pulmonary edema in the pediatric age group.

Cyanosis, in the absence of intracardiac right to left shunt, may be present and is secondary to impaired pulmonary gas exchange as well as due to sluggish peripheral circulation.

Exercise intolerance is an important feature of heart failure in older children and young adults.

Characteristic Findings in Children with Heart Failure

Many classes of disorders can result in increased cardiac demand or impaired cardiac function. Cardiac causes include arrhythmias (tachycardia or bradycardia), structural heart disease, and myocardial dysfunction (systolic or diastolic).

Noncardiac causes of congestive heart failure include processes that increase the preload (volume overload), increase the afterload (hypertension), reduce the oxygen-carrying capacity of the blood (anemia), or increase demand (sepsis). For example, renal failure can result in congestive heart failure due to fluid retention and anemia.

Cardiac rhythm disorders may be caused by the following:

- Complete heart block (Figs 39.13–39.21)
- Supraventricular tachycardia
- Ventricular tachycardia
- Sinus node dysfunction

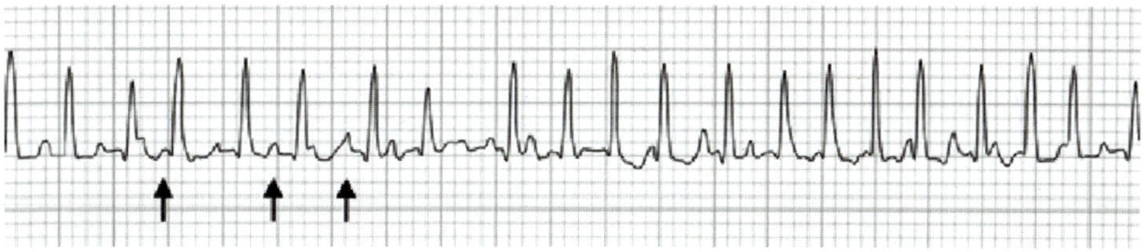

Fig. 39.13: *Multifocal atrial tachycardia with decompensated heart in a 15-year-adolescent male showed; heart rate >100 bpm (usually 100–150 bpm; may be as high as 250 bpm). Irregularly irregular rhythm with varying PP, PR and RR intervals. At least three distinct P-wave morphologies in the same lead. Isoelectric baseline between P-waves (i.e. no flutter waves). Absence of a single dominant atrial pacemaker (i.e. not just sinus rhythm with frequent PACs). Some P waves may be nonconducted; others may be aberrantly conducted to the ventricles*

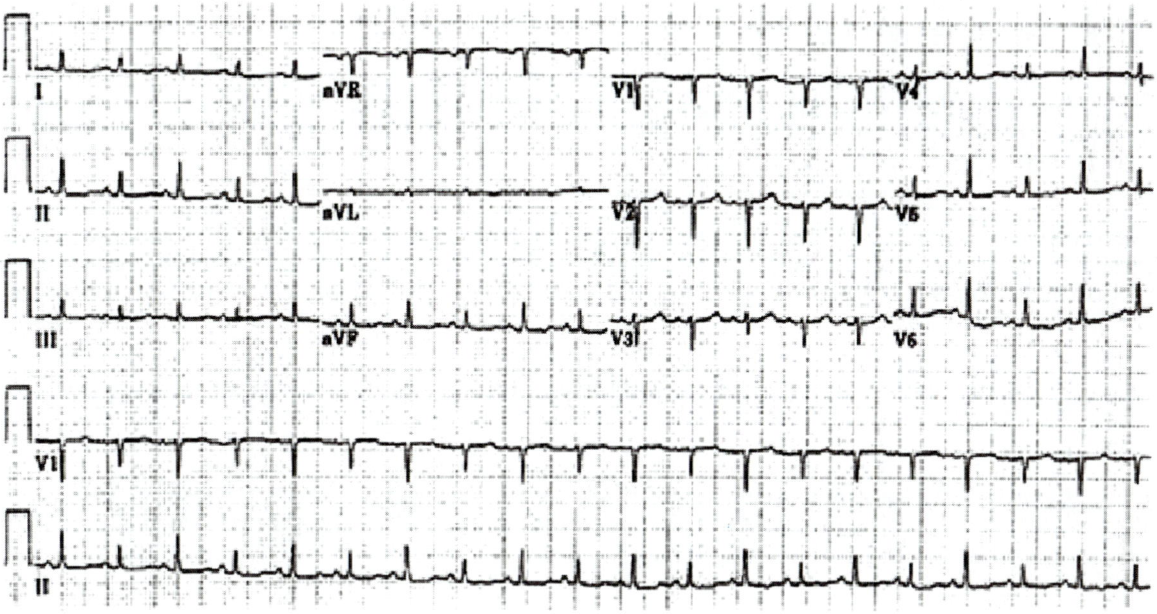

Fig. 39.14: *Massive pericardial effusion (tamponade) in a 9-year-old boy showed a triad of: low voltage, tachycardia and electrical alternans*

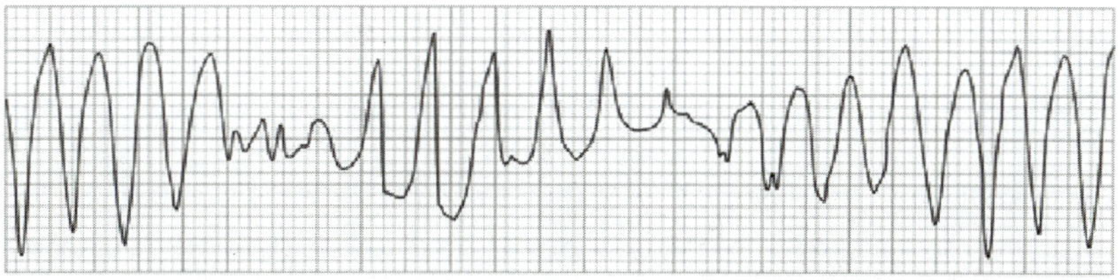

Fig. 39.15: *ECG in 10-year-old male child shows polymorphic VT and torsades de pointes during short runs of TdP or single lead recording the characteristic "twisting" morphology may not be apparent. Bigeminy in a patient with a known long QT syndrome may herald imminent TdP. TdP with heart rates > 220 beats/min are of longer duration and more likely to degenerate into VF. Presence of abnormal ("giant") T-U waves may precede TdP in a patient with heart failure*

Volume overload may be caused by the following:
- Structural heart disease (e.g. ventricular septal defect, patent ductus arteriosus, aortic or mitral valve regurgitation, complex cardiac lesions)
- Anemia
- Sepsis.

Pressure overload may be caused by the following:
- Structural heart disease (e.g. aortic or pulmonary stenosis, aortic coarctation)
- Hypertension

Systolic ventricular dysfunction or failure may be caused by the following:
- Myocarditis
- Dilated cardiomyopathy
- Malnutrition
- Ischemia

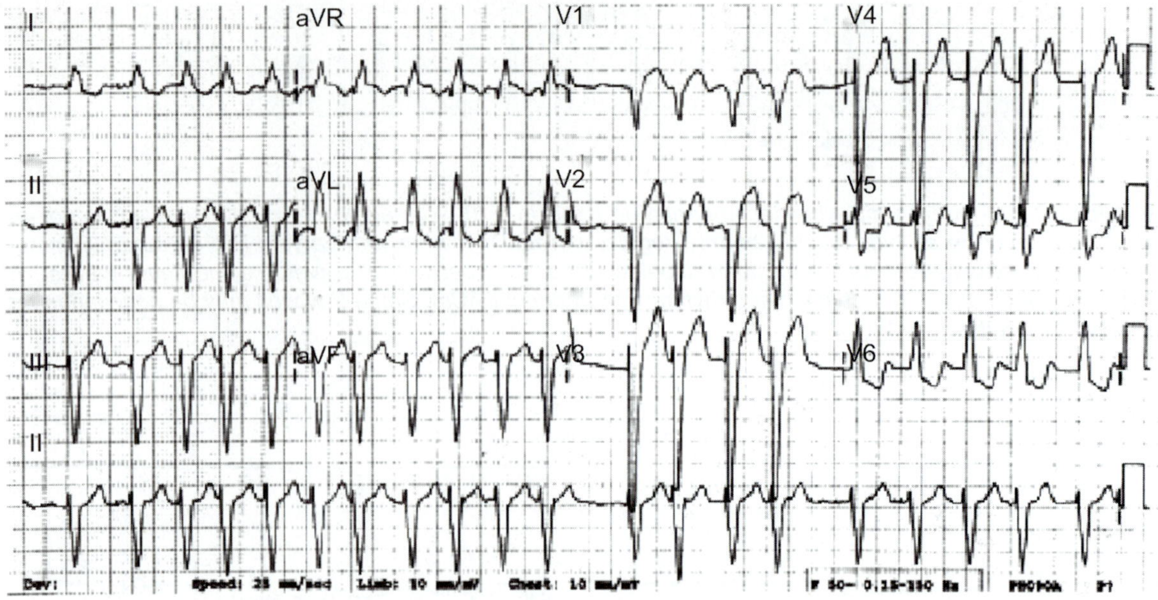

Fig. 39.16: *Dilated cardiomyopathy in a 12-year-old male child. ECG showing interventricular conduction delays (e.g. LBBB) occur due to cardiac dilatation. Diffuse myocardial fibrosis may lead to reduced voltage QRS complexes, particularly in the limb leads. There may be a discrepancy of QRS voltages with signs of hypertrophy in V4–6 and relatively low voltages in the limb leads. Abnormal Q waves are most often seen in leads V1 to V4 and may mimic the appearance of a myocardial infarction ("pseudoinfarction" pattern)*

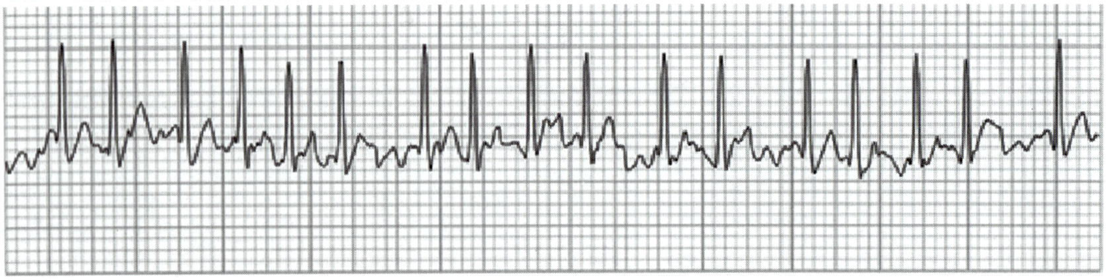

Fig. 39.17: *Atrial fibrillation in a 7-year-old female child. ECG showing irregularly irregular rhythm. No P waves. Absence of an isoelectric baseline. Variable ventricular rate. QRS complexes usually < 120 ms unless preexisting bundle-branch block, accessory pathway, or rate-related aberrant conduction. Fibrillatory waves may be present and can be either fine (amplitude < 0.5 mm) or coarse (amplitude >0.5 mm). Fibrillatory waves may mimic P waves leading to misdiagnosis*

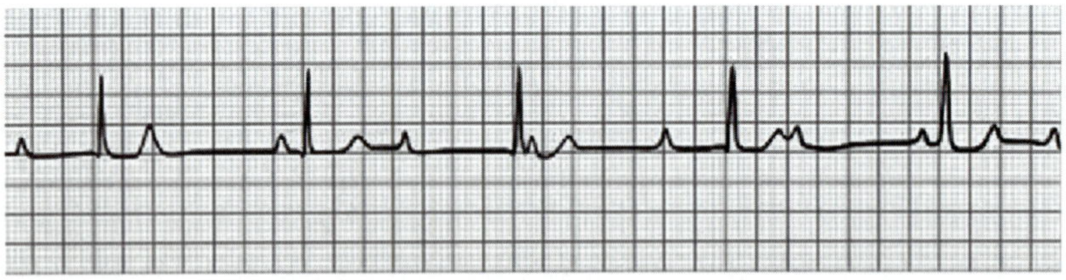

Fig. 39.18: *Complete heart block in a 10-year-old boy ECG showing complete heart block, there is complete absence of AV conduction—none of the supraventricular impulses are conducted to the ventricles. Perfusing rhythm is maintained by a junctional or ventricular escape rhythm. Alternatively, the patient may suffer ventricular standstill leading to syncope (if self-terminating) or sudden cardiac death (if prolonged). Typically, the patient will have severe bradycardia with independent atrial and ventricular rates, i.e. AV dissociation*

Diastolic ventricular dysfunction or failure may be caused by the following:
- Hypertrophic cardiomyopathy
- Restrictive cardiomyopathy
- Pericarditis
- Cardiac tamponade (pericardial effusion)

Laboratory Investigations

It is to be remembered that heart failure is a clinical syndrome and for the most part is not associated with a diagnostic laboratory test.

Appropriate laboratory testing includes assessment of the following: Oxygen saturation, complete blood count (CBC),

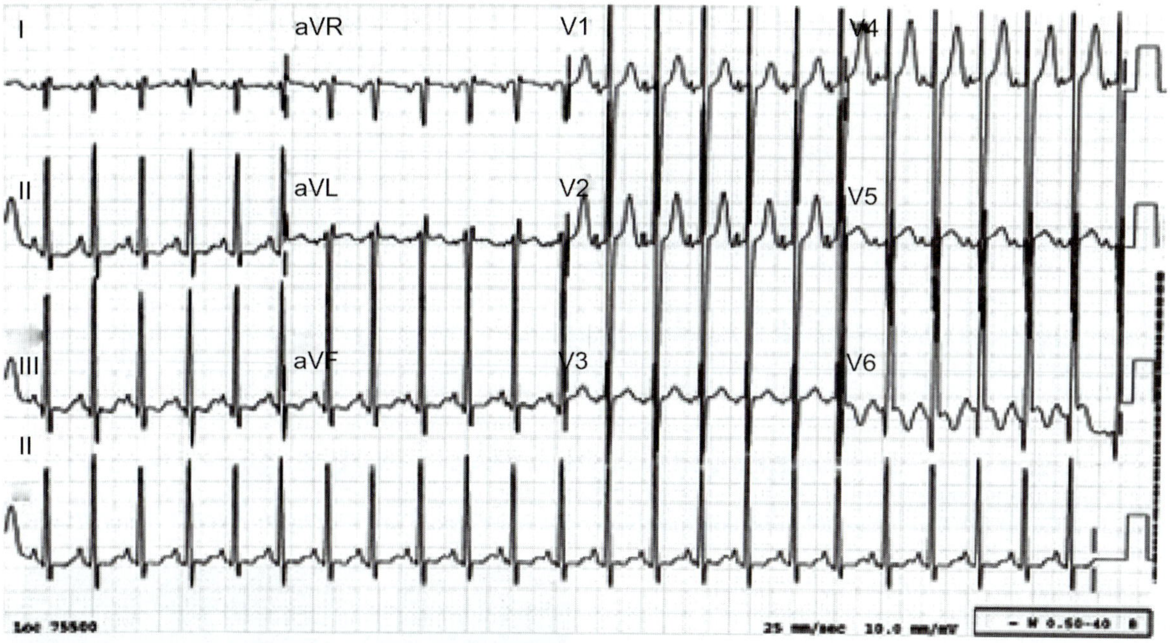

Fig. 39.19: *ECG of a young child from day 1 of presentation in patient with ALCAPA. Typical prominent Q waves are present in lead V6. Conversely, typical abrupt loss of R waves in mid-precordial leads and prominent Q waves in leads I and aVL associated with ALCAPA are not present*

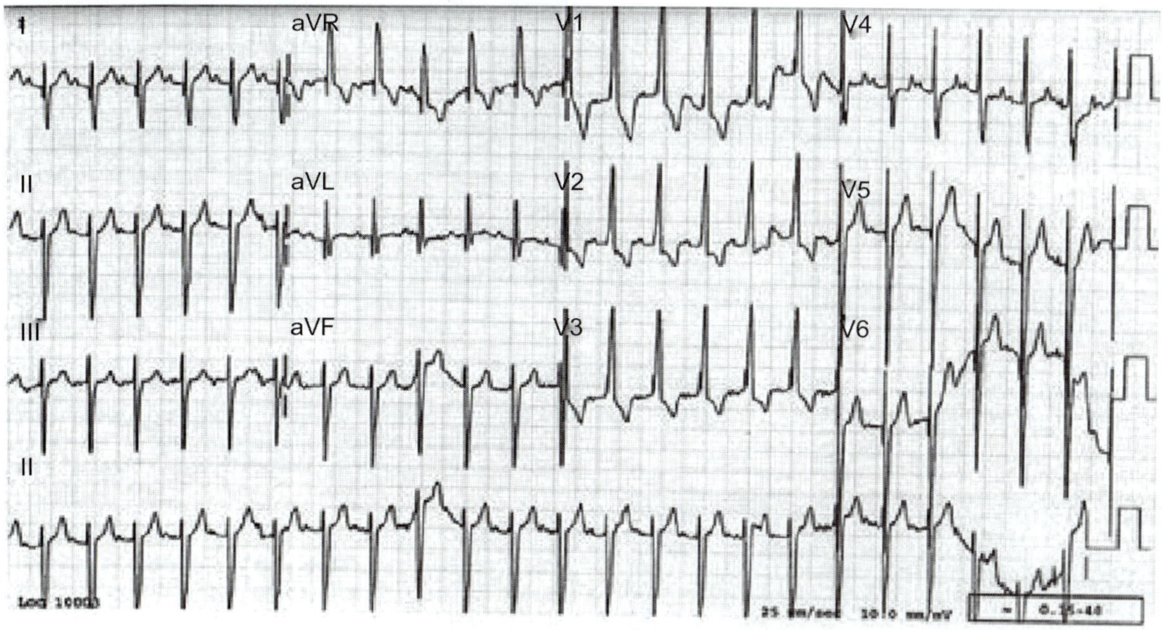

Fig. 39.20: *ECG of CAVC (common AV canal) or endocardial cushion defect with superior QRS axis in a young child who presented with heart failure*

hemoglobin concentration, electrolyte levels, calcium level, cardiac biomarkers, blood urea nitrogen (BUN) level, creatinine level, and renal and hepatic function.

The CBC count can reveal signs of anemia or infection. Brain natriuretic peptide (BNP) or N -terminal prohormone **BNP (NT-proBNP)** levels are elevated as a result of ventricular dilation. Elevation of serum BNP level is particularly useful in distinguishing patients with congestive heart failure from those with a primary respiratory process. BNP levels of more than 100 pg/mL are associated with congestive heart failure in adults and children. Normal levels may be slightly higher in neonates. **Cardiac troponin** may be elevated in cases of myocarditis or after ischemic injury due to coronary anomaly or cardiomyopathy, as well as in noncardiac conditions in which cardiac perfusion may be compromised (sepsis).

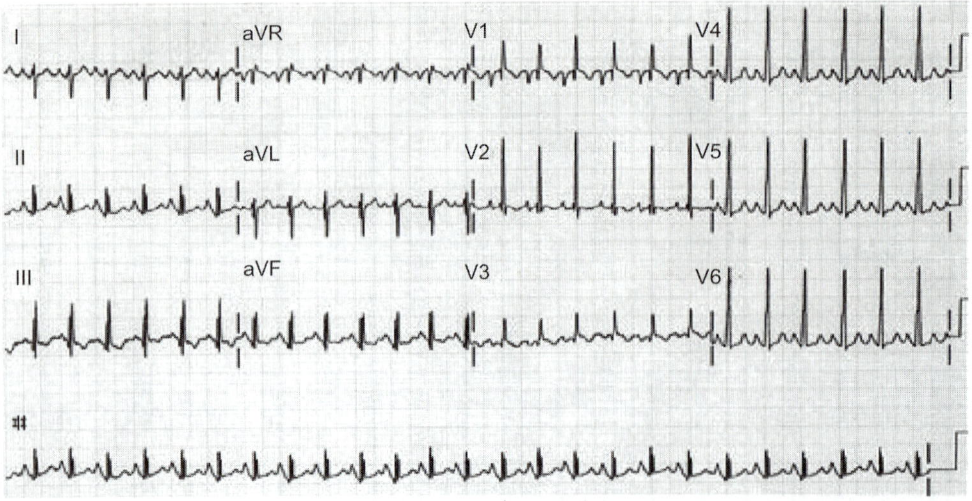

Fig. 39.21: *ECG of TAPVR with right atrial enlargement, right ventricular hypertrophy-in 5 years old child with CCF*

Table 39.7: *Abnormalities resulting in systolic dysfunction*

Myocyte compartment
- Myocyte loss (necrosis, apoptosis, aging)
- Abnormal force transduction (e.g. dystrophin mutations)
- Abnormal force generation (calcium release, substrate deficiency)
- Abnormal relaxation (abnormal calcium reuptake)
- Excessive myocyte hypertrophy

Myocardial load
- Volume overload (mitral or aortic regurgitation, renal or hepatic failure)
- Pressure overload (hypertension, increased arterial stiffness)

Heart rate and conduction
- Excessive tachycardia (weeks)
- Discoordinate contraction (right ventricular pacing)

Extracellular matrix compartment
- Fibrosis
- Altered metabolism (cardiofibroblast function, protein synthesis and degradation, paracrine/autocrine signaling)

Cardiac structure
- Abnonnal myocardial fiber "wrapping" or alignment
- Focal infarction or aneurysm.
- Advanced remodeling (increased sphericity)

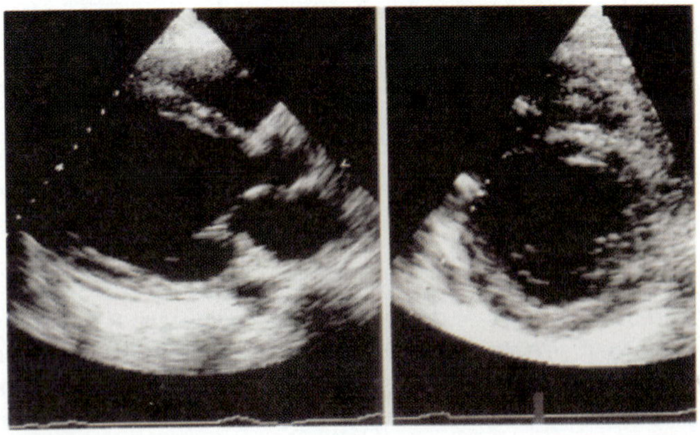

Fig. 39.22: *Long-axis and short-axis 2D views of LV showing posterior wall infarction and hypokinetic anterior wall with cavity dilatation and poor LVEF =<15% in patient with breathlessness and effort angia*

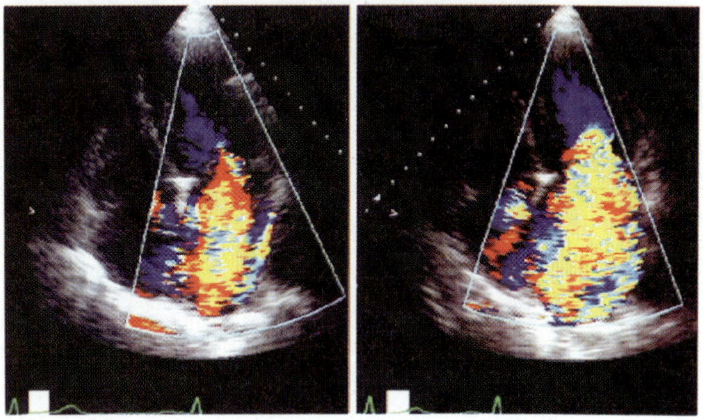

Fig. 39.23: *Apical four chamber view from a patient with ischemic cardiomyopathy and significant functional mitral regurgitation at rest (left). Note the increase in MR severity with stress, indicating development of severe ischemic dysfunction with stress*

The evaluation of serum electrolyte levels in the patient with congestive heart failure may demonstrate hyponatremia secondary to water retention. Elevated potassium levels may represent renal compromise or even tissue destruction due to low cardiac output. Significant tissue hypoxia increases serum lactate concentration and depletes the serum bicarbonate level. In more chronic congestive heart failure states, reduced renal blood flow may be expressed as increased BUN and creatinine levels.

Pulse oximetry, as well as a **hyperoxia test** in newborns, may be useful. The systemic saturation on room air is a more reliable measure of oxygenation than are observations for cyanosis alone, which are often misleading. The partial pressure of arterial oxygen (PaO_2) when the patient is receiving 100% oxygen (hyperoxia test) may help in distinguishing intracardiac mixing malformations from pulmonary disease in the setting of hypoxia. Blood gas abnormalities may show respiratory alkalosis in mild forms of congestive heart failure or metabolic acidosis in patients with evidence of low cardiac output or ductal-dependent congenital heart disease.

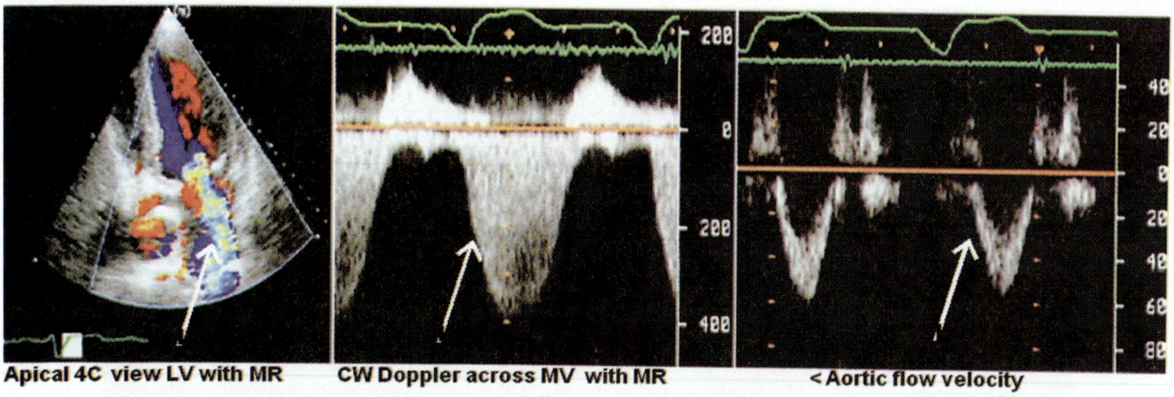

Fig. 39.24: *Apical four chamber view of LV showing gross MR in color Doppler mode (left) and continuous wave Doppler (middle) Note the peak left ventricular—left atrial pressure drop is 60 mmHg indicating severely raised LA pressure and low cardiac output state as shown with low aortic flow velocity (right) in patient with ischemic cardiomyopathy (LVEF = <15%)*

Chest Radiography

It shows cardiomegaly and increased pulmonary vascular markings (Fig. 39.11).

Electrocardiography

It is not helpful in the diagnosis of heart failure except when secondary to tachyarrhythmias, heart block ormyocardial ischaemia (Figs 39.13–39.21).

Serum Brain Type Natriuretic Peptide

It is a relatively new biochemical marker which has proven to be very useful in the diagnosis of heart failure, especially in patients with acute dyspnea In such a setting, brain type natriuretic peptide levels more than 500 picogram per milliliter have a 90% predictive value for the presence of heart failure and levels less than 100 picogram per milliliter have a 90% predictive value for the absence of heart failure. Brain type natriuretic peptide levels between 100 and 500 picogram per milliliter are somewhat less helpful, and other tests may be needed for diagnosis. Serum brain type natriuretic peptide level in heart failure patients helps to guide and monitor therapy, detects preclinical disease, and possibly reduces the need for cardiac imaging.

Echocardiography (Figs 39.22–39.33)

It is perhaps the most useful test in understanding the mechanism and cause of heart failure in children and young adults. Decreased shortening fraction and ejection fraction, and low velocity of circumferential fibre shortening are direct evidence of left ventricle systolic dysfunction.

Doppler-derived indices that are useful in the evaluation of heart failure include change in left ventricular systolic pressure, stress-velocity index and strain rate imaging. Assessment of left ventricle diastolic function include spectral Doppler imaging of the mitral inflow, pulmonary venous Doppler, tissue Doppler imaging and flow-propagation velocities by color M-mode echocardiography (Figs 39.24–39.26, 39.31–39.33).

Myocardial Performance Index (Tei Index)

It is a new echocardiographic parameter in global assessment of left or right ventricular function, although the value of

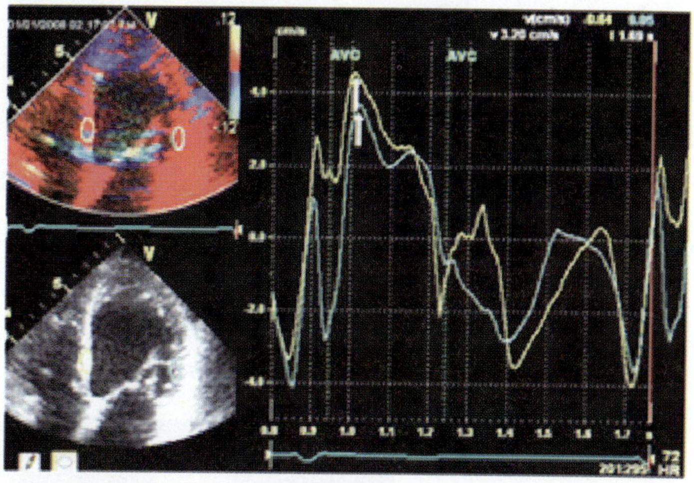

Fig. 39.25: *Shows colour-coded tissue Doppler image using the apical four chamber view from a heart failure patient with widened QRS, but no significant mechanical dyssynchrony before cardiac resynchronization therapy. There was similar timing in peak velocities (arrows) from septal to lateral wall, determined between aortic valve opening (AVO) and aortic valve closure (AVC). This patient did not have a favourable clinical nor ventricular function response to resynchronization therapy*

Tei index is age dependent. In children, the normal Tei Index values for left ventricle and right ventricle are reported to be 0.35 plus or minus 0.03 and 0.32 plus or minus 0.03, respectively.

Metabolic Exercise Testing

It allows determination of peak oxygen consumption, anaerobic threshold, oxygen pulse, and ventilatory equivalent for carbon dioxide, which are useful to quantitate cardiovascular functional capacity.

CT Scanning and MRI (Fig. 39.35)

Computed tomography (CT) scanning or magnetic resonance imaging (MRI) may be useful in evaluating chamber size and ventricular mass, cardiac function, and wall motion; delineating congenital and valvular

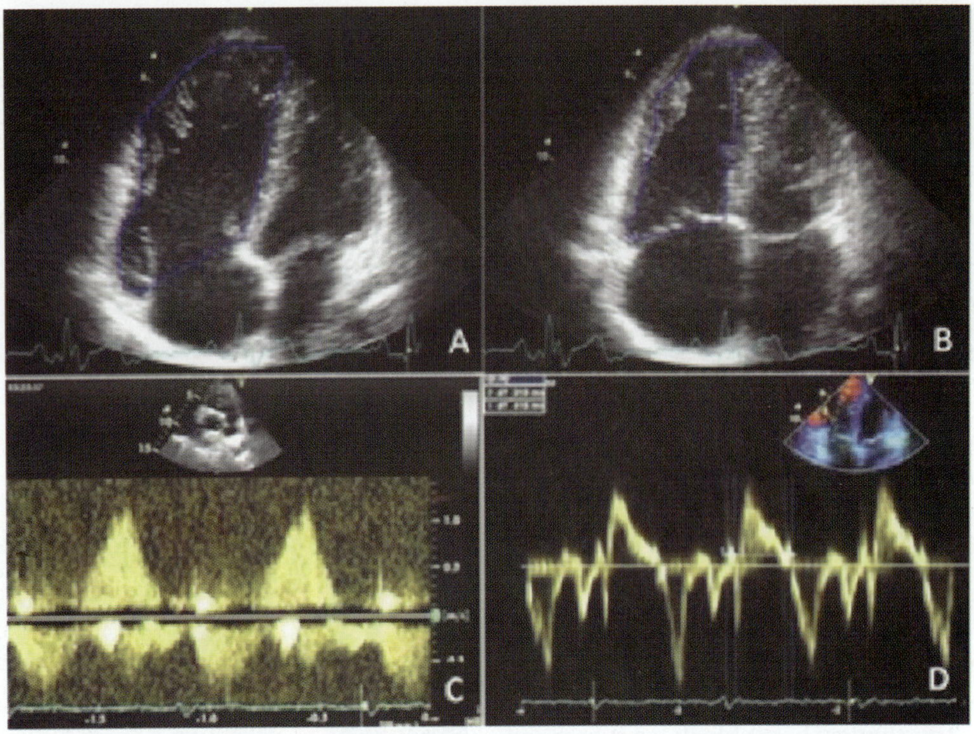

Fig. 39.26: *Echocardiographic measurements in a patient with tetralogy of Fallot repair. (A and B) Moderate right ventricular (RV) dilatation: RV areas were measured, including trabeculation in cavity area; indexed end-diastolic RV (EDRV) area was 23.3 cm/m²; indexed end-systolic RV (ESRV) area was 11.5 cm²/m². Cardiac magnetic resonance (CMR) confirmed these results: EDRV volume was 114 mL/m²; ESRV volume was 72 mL/m². (C) Severe pulmonary regurgitation (PR) (grade 3) with pulmonary diastolic retrograde flow detected from the left pulmonary artery; CMR PR fraction was 52%. (D) Tei index calculated from tissue Doppler imaging measurements was 0.32; CMR RV ejection fraction was 42%*

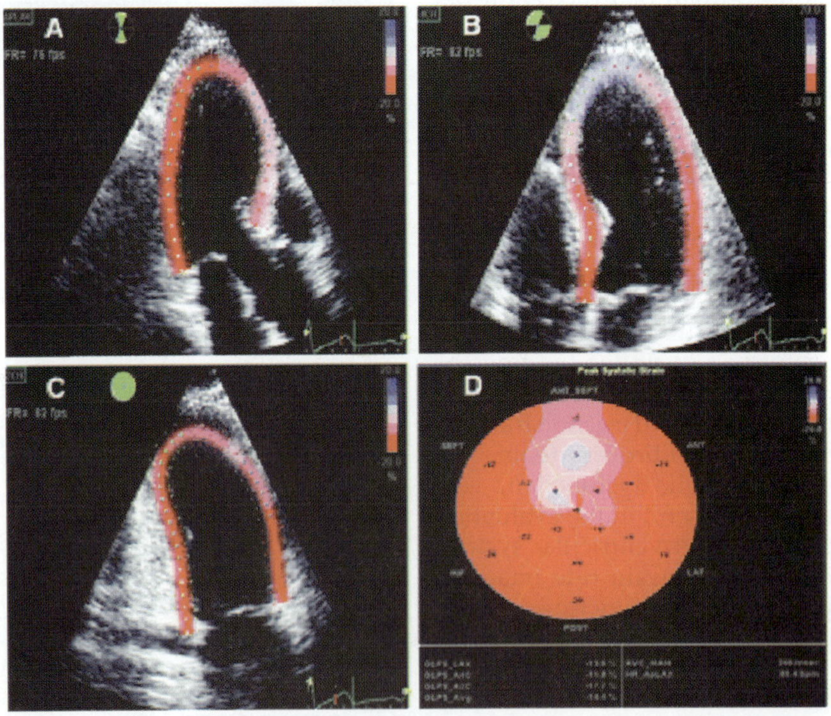

Fig. 39.27: *Apical long-axis (A), four chamber (B), and two chamber views (C) with a bull's-eye summary (D) and corresponding global strain of a patient after acute anteroseptal myocardial infarction. The bull's-eye view provides an overview of strain of all individual LV segments and a value for global LV strain. Normal strain is represented in red; decreased (less negative) strain is represented in blue. In this example, the amount of strain is clearly decreased in the anteroseptal LV segments consistent with the region of infarction. In addition, global LV strain is decreased (GLPS Avg –14.4%; normal values range from –20.3% to –24.1%)*

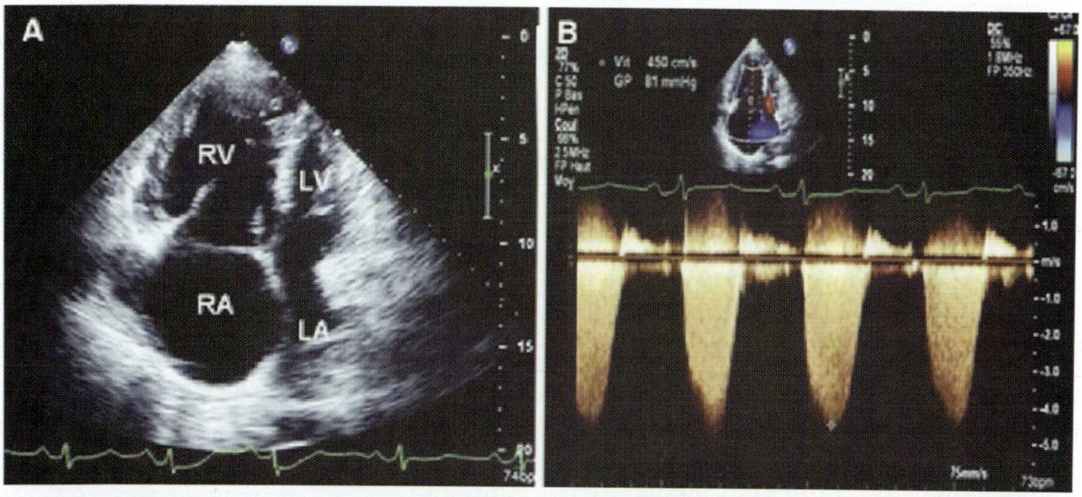

Fig. 39.28: *(A) Apical four chamber view showing gross dilatation of RA and RV, (B) Color Doppler view at tricuspid valve showing gross tricuspid regurgitation with gradient of more than 100 mmHg in a patient with primary pulmonary hypertension with CCF*

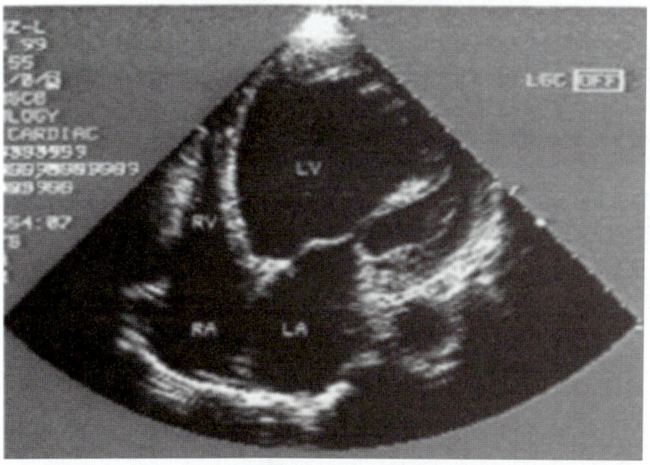

Fig. 39.29: *Two dimensional echocardiogram showing a four chambers view of the heart in a patient with systolic dysfunction. Note dilated LV. (LV, left ventricle; RV, right ventricle; RA, right atrium; LA, left atrium)*

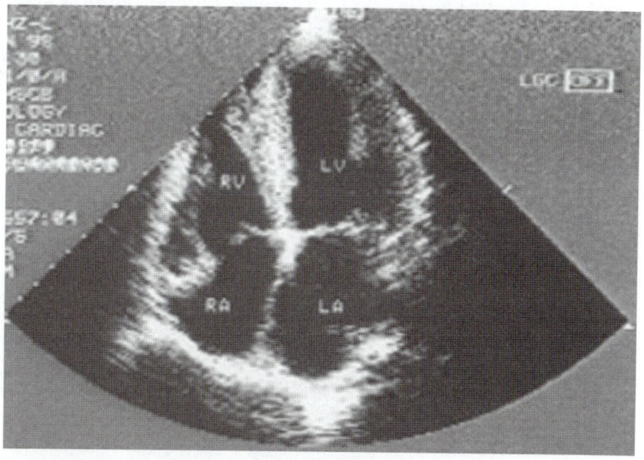

Fig. 39.30: *Two dimensional echocardiogram showing a four chambers view of the heart in a patient with diastolic dysfunction. Note the normal LV size with hypertrophy*

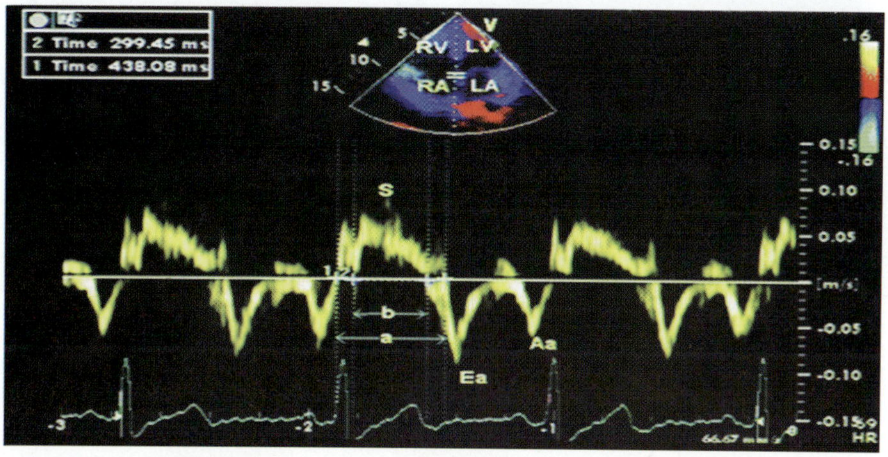

Fig. 39.31: *Myocardial performance index (MPI). Normal doppler tissue-imaging wave form obtained at the septal mitral valve annulus in an apical four chamber view from a healthy patient. The spetral doppler profile is characterized by single positive waveform (S) above the baseline and negative waveforms in early (Ea) and late (Aa) diastole. The Doppler-dervied MPI, (a–b)/b, is calculated by measuring two intervals in the same cardiac cycle from Doppler tissue recordings: (1) a is the interval between cessation of the late diastolic annular velocity (Aa) and onset of the early diastolic annular velocity (Ea); and (2) b is the duration of the systolic annular velocity (S). LA, left atrium; LV, left ventricle; RA, right atrium; RV, right ventricle*

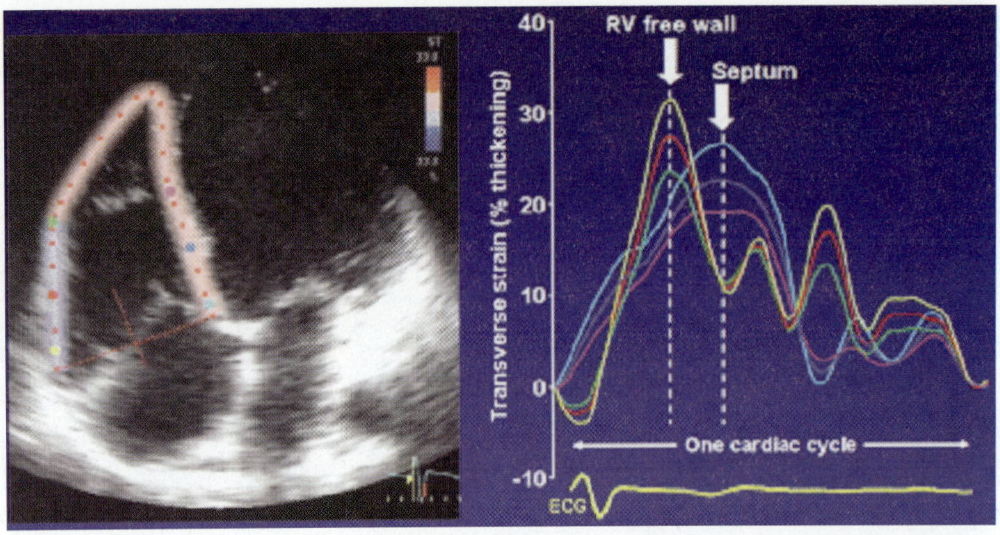

Fig. 39.32: *RV failure. (A) Showing speckle tracking of 2D echocardgraphic image of the right ventricle. (B) Strain vs time plotted for various regions of the RV. It shows delay in time to peak strain in the septum compared to the RV free wall*

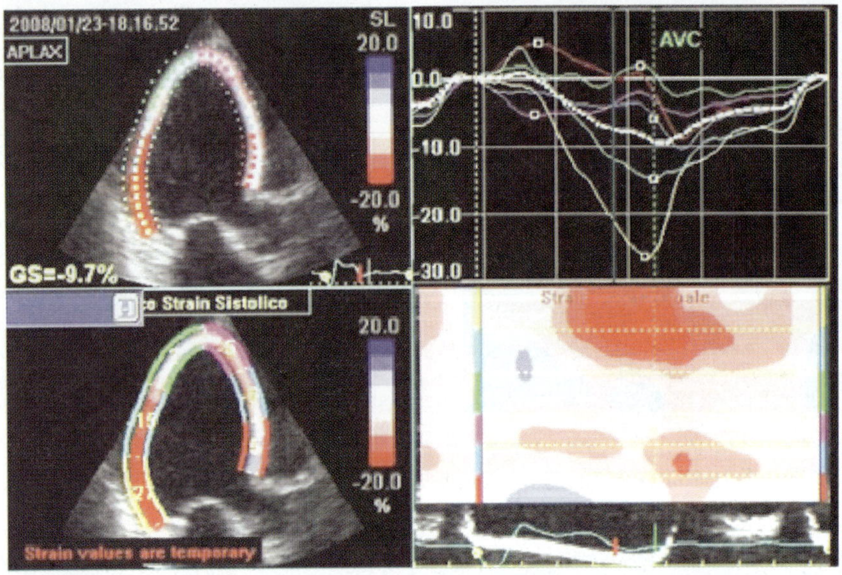

Fig. 39.33: *Representation of 2D-strain (speckle tracking) of the left ventricle in the apical long-axis view in a patient with systolic heart failure. The upper right panel depicts the strain curves sampled in each of the analyzed myocardial segments. It is also possible to calculate a global strain index (GS), which in this case is clearly diminished (GS = 9,7%; see upper left panel). The lower left panel shows peak systolic strain for each segment while the lower right panel shows longitudinal strain processed according to a color map of curvilinear anatomical M-mode. From top to bottom: the basal, mid, and apical posterolateral wall, followed by the apical, mid, and basal interventricular anterior septum wall; in red the segments with higher contractility*

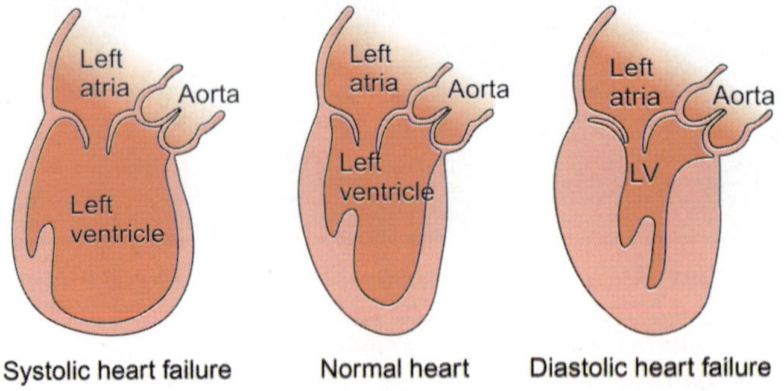

Fig. 39.34: *Diagrams showing structural morphology of myocardium and intracavitory dimensions in systolic and diastolic types of heart failure when compared to normal heart (middle)*

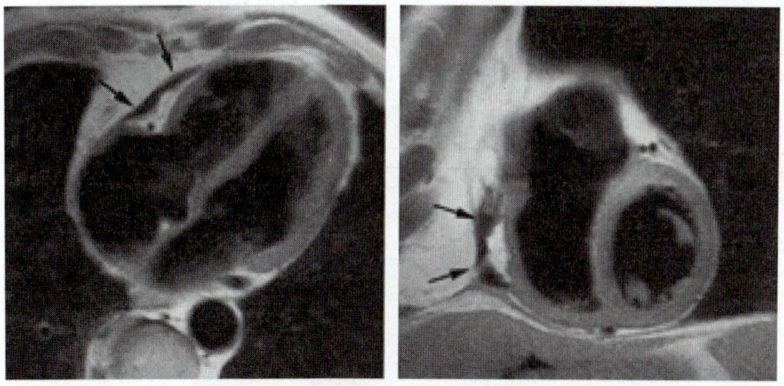

Fig. 39.35: *Constrictive pericarditis in a 18-year-adolescent presenting with right heart failure showing pericardial calcifications on chest X-ray and computed tomography. Axial (left) and short-axis (right) T1-weighted FSE shows low-signal irregular thickening of the pericardium along the basal part of the right ventricle (RV) free wall and right atrioventricular groove*

abnormalities; and demonstrating the presence of pericardial disease. However, cardiac CT scanning is usually not required in the routine diagnosis and management of heart failure, and echocardiography and MRI may provide similar information without exposing the patient to ionizing radiation.

The benefits of cardiac MRI (cMRI) include the ability to obtain a great deal of information with a noninvasive test. This modality provides detailed functional and morphologic information; can be used to assess ischemic versus nonischemic disease, infiltrative disease, and hypertrophic disease; and can be employed to determine viability. It is used principally for the delineation of congenital cardiac abnormalities and for the assessment of valvular heart disease, and it is the gold standard for evaluating RV function.

MRI has become particularly useful for evaluating abnormalities in wall motion and viable myocardium, and MRI results can help to predict the success of revascularization in patients with low ejection fractions. However, the detailed information obtained by MRI must be balanced by its high costs and the fact that this imaging modality cannot be performed in patients with implantable defibrillators.

Nuclear Imaging

Radionuclide Multiple-gated Acquisition Scanning

Radionuclide multiple-gated acquisition (MUGA) scan is a reliable imaging technique for evaluation of LV and RV function and wall motion abnormalities. Because of its reliability, LV ejection fraction (LVEF), as determined by MUGA scanning, is often used for serial assessment of postchemotherapy LV function (Fig. 39.36).

Electrocardiogram-gated Myocardial Perfusion Imaging

The high-photon flux of compounds labeled with technetium-99m (99mTC) makes it feasible to acquire myocardial perfusion images in an ECG-gated mode. ECG-gated single-photon emission CT (SPECT) images allow for assessment of global LVEF, regional wall motion, and regional wall thickening at rest in patients with documented stress-induced wall motion and perfusion abnormalities.

In general, LVEF from gated SPECT agrees well with resting LVEF determined by other modalities. Quality assurance is important, however, because determinations of LVEF with gated SPECT may be less accurate, even invalidated, in the presence of an irregular heart rate, low count density, intense extracardiac radiotracer uptake adjacent to the LV, or a small LV (Fig. 39.37).

Combined interpretation of perfusion and function on ECG-gated images substantially increases the confidence of interpretation. Taillefer and associates reported that the interpretation of stress and rest end-diastolic section, rather than summed ungated sections, may enhance the overall sensitivity for the detection of mild coronary artery disease. ECG-gated images are useful for recognizing artifactual defects caused by attenuation (breast and diaphragm) and thus are useful in the quality control of SPECT imaging. ECG-gated SPECT imaging is currently considered the state of the art of radionuclide myocardial perfusion imaging. There are three important practical issues that need to be addressed in the evaluation of patients with presumed ischemic dysfunction as follows:

Assessment of the relative regional myocardial uptake of thallium-201 (201 Tl; often after rest reinjection), 99mTc-

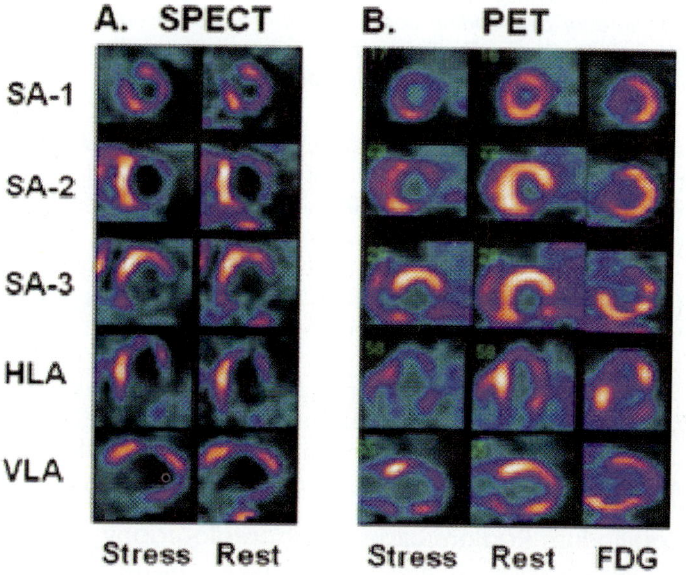

Fig. 39.36: *(A) 99mTc sestamibi (MIBI) exercise stress and rest images in a 20-year-old adolescent with known CAD and congestive heart failure. The MIBI images show severe apical, anterior, lateral, and inferior defects with no improvement on the resting images. (B) The dipyridamole stress 82Rb images show severe apical, anterior, lateral and inferior-basal defects, and a moderate-to-severe septal defect. The resting 82Rb images show marked anterior, septal and anterolateral improvement, and mid-inferior improvement. The FDG-PET images showed preserved or increased activity in the anterolateral, lateral, inferior and inferior-basal walls, demonstrating a classical mismatch pattern in these regions*

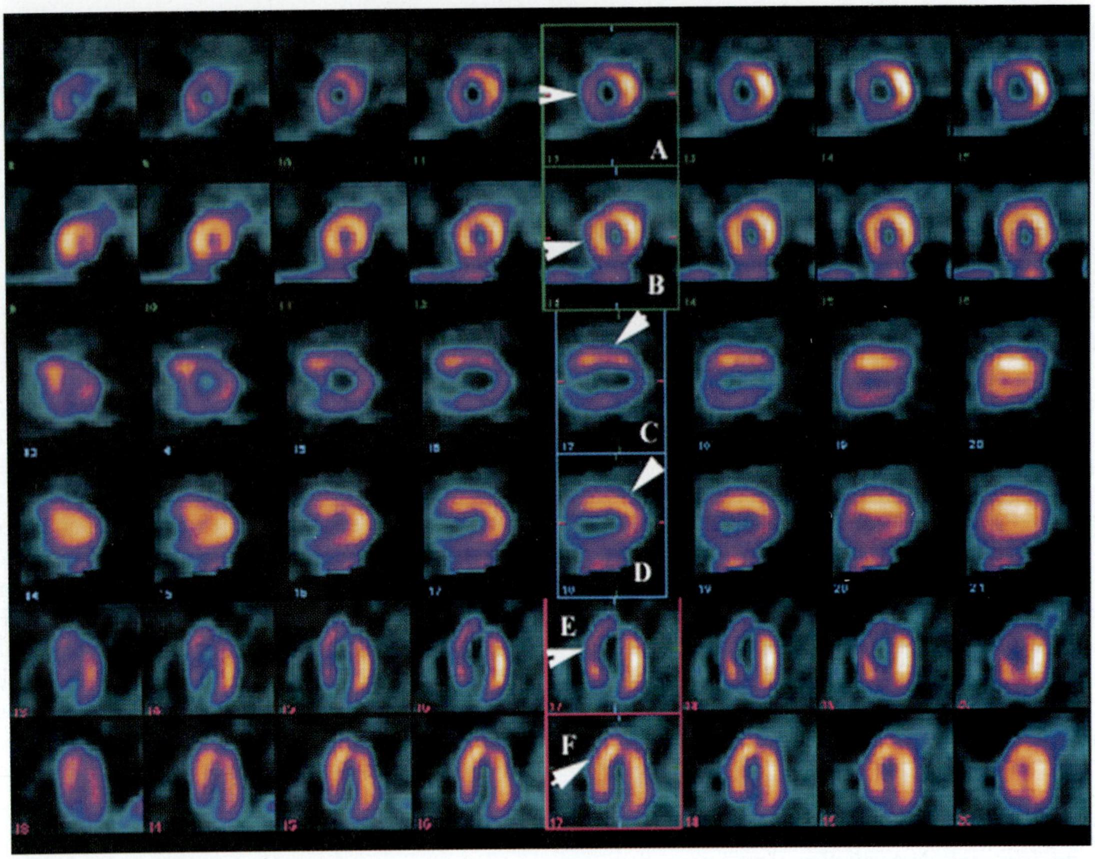

Fig. 39.37: *These images represent a typical appearance of reduced relative myocardial isotope uptake in the region supplied by the left anterior descending coronary artery (arrows) during stress (frames A, C and E) with normalization of relative uptake at rest (frames B, D and F). This pattern is consistent with a high-grade proximal LAD lesion supplying a bed of viable (noninfarcted) myocardium in a patient with diastolic heart failure*

sestamibi, or 99mTc-tetrofosmin (often after rest administration of nitroglycerin); when the resting uptake of radiotracer is greater than 50% of normal, expect recovery of function after revascularization.

Assessment of the presence of demonstrable ischemia (e.g. partially reversible defect) in a myocardial segment with decreased uptake, even if the resting uptake is less than 50%.

Data reported in 2011 from a STICH viability substudy failed to demonstrate a significant impact on survival based on the extent of viable myocardium in patients with CAD and LV dysfunction treated surgically or medically.

Equilibrium Radionuclide Angiocardiography

Equilibrium radionuclide angiocardiography (ERNA) uses ECG events to define the temporal relationship between the acquisition of nuclear data and the volumetric components of the cardiac cycle. Sampling is performed repetitively over several hundred heartbeats, with physiologic segregation of nuclear data in accordance with their occurrence within the cardiac cycle.

Data are quantified and displayed in an endless-loop, cinegraphic format for additional qualitative visual interpretation and analysis. Equilibrium blood-pool labeling is achieved by use of 99mTc. Data are analyzed by use of a computer, generally with some operator interaction.

Analysis may be obtained in either the frame or list mode. Radionuclide data are collected and segregated temporally. The process generally requires 3–10 minutes for completion of each view. Following data acquisition, data from the several hundred individual beats are summed, processed, and displayed as a single representative cardiac cycle.

Data from the left anterior oblique (LAO) view are also used for qualitative analysis of global LV function. On this view, overlap of the two ventricles is minimal. In a count-based approach, LVEF and other indices of filling and ejection are calculated from the LV radioactivity preset at various points throughout the cardiac cycle.

RV function is best evaluated by first-pass techniques. The LAO view provides qualitative information concerning contraction of the septal, inferoapical and lateral walls. The anterior view provides data concerning regional motion of the anterior and apical segments. The left lateral or left posterior oblique view provides optimal qualitative information concerning contraction of the inferior wall and posterobasal segment.

ERNA may easily be combined with additional physiologic stress testing or provocation, which may be in the form of either physiologic stress, such as exercise; pharmacologic stress, with the use of positive inotropic agents, such as dobutamine or isoproterenol; or psychological stress. The degree of confidence with ERNA is moderately high. False-positive and false-negative findings are infrequent.

Radionuclide Ventriculography (Fig. 39.37)

Radionuclide ventriculography is most often performed as part of a myocardial perfusion scan to obtain accurate measurements of LV function and right ventricular EF, but it is unable to directly assess valvular abnormalities or cardiac hypertrophy and has limited value for assessing volumes or more subtle indices of systolic or diastolic function.

Catheterization and Angiography (Fig. 39.39)

In patients with a nonischemic cardiomyopathy, perfusion deficits and segmental wall-motion abnormalities suggestive of coronary artery disease are commonly present on noninvasive imaging. Only coronary angiography, however, can reliably demonstrate or exclude the presence of obstructed coronary vessels.

According to the American College of Cardiology/American Heart Association (ACC/AHA), Heart Failure Society of America (HFSA) and European Society of Cardiology (ESC), cardiac catheterization and coronary angiography should be considered for patients with heart failure in the following situations:

- When symptoms worsen without a clear cause in patients with heart failure, no angina, and known coronary artery disease.
- In heart failure caused by systolic dysfunction in association with angina or regional wall-motion abnormalities and/or scintigraphic evidence of reversible myocardial ischemia when revascularization is being considered.
- When pretest probability of underlying ischemic cardiomyopathy is high and surgical coronary procedures are being considered.
- Before cardiac transplantation or left ventricular assist device placement.
- In cases of heart failure secondary to postinfarction ventricular aneurysm or other mechanical complications of myocardial infarction.
- For these patients, the procedures are frequently indicated when systolic dysfunction of unexplained cause is present on noninvasive testing or when normal systolic function with episodic heart failure suggests ischemically mediated LV dysfunction. However, although coronary angiography may be indicated in young patients to exclude the presence of congenital coronary anomalies, this procedure may not be as useful in older patients, because revascularization has not been shown to improve clinical outcomes in patients without angina. Despite this, because revascularization may improve LV function, some experts suggest that coronary artery disease should be excluded whenever possible, especially in patients with diabetes mellitus or other states associated with silent myocardial ischemia. The degree of confidence is moderately high.

Right-Sided Heart Catheterization

Right heart catheterization is useful in providing important hemodynamic information about filling pressures, vascular resistance, and cardiac output when there is doubt about the patient's fluid status; in heart failure refractory to initial therapy; in the presence of significant hypotension (systolic blood pressure typically < 90 mmHg or symptomatic low

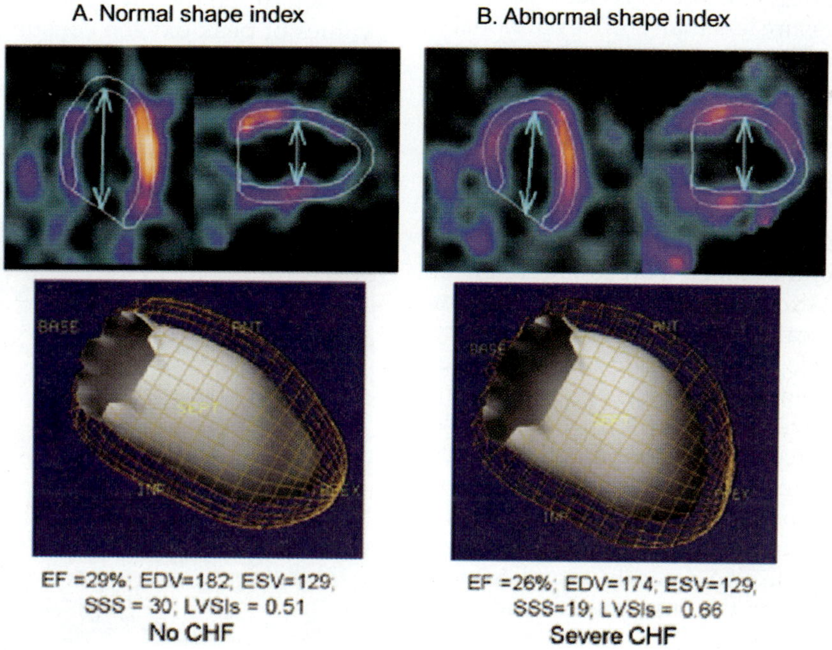

Fig. 39.38: *Illustration of two cases with similar low LVEF but differing LV shape index. (A) The patient with no signs of congestive heart failure (CHF) has a more severe perfusion defect than the other patient but has a normal LV shape index and an elongated LV cavity. (B) The other patient, who has severe congestive heart failure, has an abnormal LV shape index and a more spherical left ventricle. ANT, anterior; SEPT, septal; INF, inferior;LVSIs, systolic LV shape index. (Reproduced with permission)*

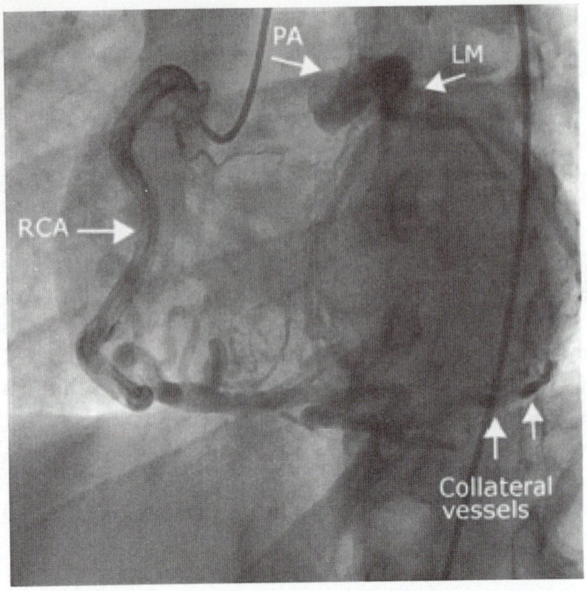

Fig. 39.39: *Coronary angiography showed an anomalous left coronary artery arising from the pulmonary artery (ALCAPA) with retrograde filling through collaterals from an enlarged right coronary artery*

systolic blood pressure) and/or worsening renal function during initial treatment; and when heart transplantation or placement of a mechanical circulatory support device is being considered. However, it plays a limited role in the diagnosis of heart failure, as studies evaluating right heart catheterization and overall improved outcomes have been essentially neutral.

Normal right-sided hemodynamics include right atrial pressure less than 7 mmHg, RV pressure less than 30/7 mmHg, pulmonary pressure less than 30/18, pulmonary capillary wedge pressure (PCWP) less than 18 mmHg, and cardiac index (CI) greater than 2.2 L/min/m^2.

PCWP can be measured by using a pulmonary arterial catheter (Swan-Ganz catheter). This helps to differentiate cardiogenic causes of decompensated heart failure from noncardiogenic causes, such as acute respiratory distress syndrome (ARDS), which occurs secondary to injury to the alveolar-capillary membrane rather than to alteration in Starling forces. A PCWP exceeding 18 mmHg in a patient not known to have chronically elevated left atrial pressure is indicative of cardiogenic decompensated heart failure. In patients with chronic pulmonary capillary hypertension, capillary wedge pressures exceeding 25 mmHg are generally required to overcome the pumping capacity of the lymphatics and produce pulmonary edema.

Large V waves may be observed in the PCWP tracing in patients with significant mitral regurgitation because large volumes of blood regurgitate into a poorly compliant left atrium. This raises pulmonary venous pressure and may cause pulmonary edema.

Left-Sided Heart Catheterization

Left-sided heart catheterization and coronary angiography should be undertaken when the etiology of heart failure cannot be determined by clinical or noninvasive imaging methods or when the etiology is likely to be due to acute myocardial ischemia or infarction. Coronary angiography is particularly helpful in patients with LV systolic dysfunction and known or suspected coronary artery disease in whom myocardial ischemia is thought to play a dominant role in the reduction of LV systolic function and the worsening of heart failure.

Assessment of Functional Capacity (Fig. 39.40)

The European Society of Cardiology (ESC) indicates the 6-minute walk test is a good indicator of functional status and prognosis in patients with heart failure. It evaluates distance walked, dyspnea index on a Borg scale from 0 to 10, oxygen saturation, and heart rate response to exercise. A normal value is walking more than 1,500 feet. Patients who walk less than 600 feet have severe cardiac dysfunction and a worse short- and long-term prognosis.

Cardiopulmonary stress testing (maximal exercise stress testing with measurement of respiratory gas exchange) can help assess a patient's chance of survival within the next year, as well as determine the need for referral for either cardiac transplantation or implantation of mechanical circulatory support. The ACC/AHA and HFSA do not recommend routine maximal exercise stress testing but indicate it may be useful in situations such as the following with measurement of gas exchange:

- To assess the disparity between symptomatic limitation and objective indicators of disease severity.
- To distinguish non-HF-related causes of functional limitation, specifically cardiac versus pulmonary.
- To consider whether patients are candidates for cardiac transplantation or mechanical circulatory support.
- To determine the prescription for cardiac rehabilitation values of peak oxygen consumption of less than 50% of predicted or less than 14 cc/kg/min reflect poor cardiac performance and a likelihood of 1-year survival less than 50%, facilitating referral for cardiac transplantation or mechanical circulatory device placement.

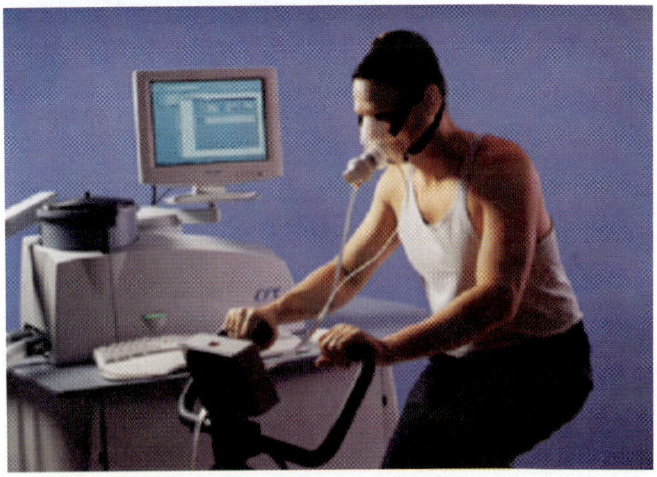

Fig. 39.40: *Cardiopulmonary stress test is simply "stress-testing" with some additional complementary measurements. Stress tests use a bicycle or treadmill to look at heart function at rest and during exercise stress*

Endomyocardial Biopsy (Fig. 39.41)

It is useful in establishing the etiology of heart failure in patients with history of systemic diseases such as collagen vascular disease, infiltrative or storage disease, giant cell myocarditis and with rapidly progressive heart failure despite conventional therapy.

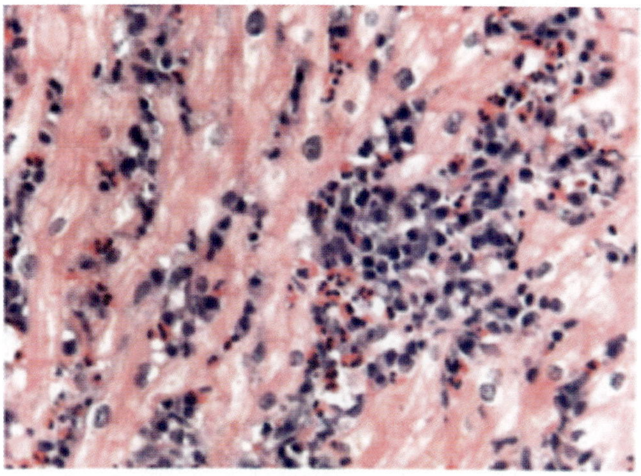

Fig. 39.41: *Eosinophilic myocarditis. The patient had severe heart failure and peripheral eosinophilia. Immunosuppression improved heart failure and probably primary hypereosinophilic syndrome (H&E; original magnification ×400)*

The Management of Congestive Heart Failure (CHF)

It is difficult and sometimes dangerous without knowledge of the underlying cause. Consequently, the first priority is acquiring a good understanding of the etiology. The goals of medical therapy for congestive heart failure include the following:

Reducing the preload
- Enhancing cardiac contractility
- Reducing the afterload
- Improving oxygen delivery
- Enhancing nutrition.

As previously discussed, the causes of congestive heart failure vary, and they appear in different patients to variable degrees. Thus, the medical management of congestive heart failure in children should be tailored to the specific details of each case.

MANAGING ACUTE CONGESTIVE HEART FAILURE IN THE NEONATE OR INFANT

Acute presentation of the ill newborn or infant with congestive heart failure warrants immediate concern regarding potential sepsis or ductal-dependent congenital heart disease. The evaluation and treatment of these patients are often best performed in the neonatal or pediatric intensive care unit (ICU).

The initial management involves the usual assessment of the patient's airway, breathing, and circulation (ABCs); achieving IV access; laboratory testing including a blood culture; and empiric antibiotic therapy. Management of low cardiac output can be initiated by using a dopamine infusion of 5–10 mcg/kg/min; acidosis can be corrected with the administration of fluid and/or bicarbonate.

Calcium should be administered when hypocalcemia is documented. Because ductal-dependent structural heart disease is a common cause of congestive heart failure in early infancy, echocardiography should be considered early in the evaluation if a diagnosis is not immediately forthcoming.

Anatomic lesions that may lead to heart failure are as follows:
1. Coarctation or interruption of the aortic arch
2. Total anomalous pulmonary venous return
3. Hypoplastic left heart syndrome (or variants including severe mitral valve stenosis and/or aortic valve stenosis or atresia)
4. Truncus arteriosus
5. Pulmonary atresia
6. Transposition of the great arteries.

Conditions to consider in young infants with a more protracted congestive heart failure course include those producing significant left-to-right shunts including large ventricular septal defects, aortopulmonary shunts, and arteriovenous malformations.

Prostaglandin

An alprostadil (PGE1) infusion is indicated when ductal-dependent cardiac lesions are diagnosed or when they cannot be ruled out in a timely fashion. Absent femoral pulses or the inability to increase the systemic PaO_2 to above 150 mmHg with a fraction of inspired oxygen (FiO_2) of 1 suggests a ductal-dependent lesion, and treatment with PGE1 is warranted.

PGE1 may theoretically aggravate the condition in some children with total anomalous pulmonary venous connection and obstruction or in children with other etiologies of congestive heart failure, such as sepsis. Whenever possible, echocardiography should be performed before PGE1 treatment is begun. On the other hand, when critical heart disease is present and echocardiography is not immediately available, prostaglandin infusion can be life-saving.

Nonstructural Problems

Nonstructural cardiac problems that occur during this stage include tachyarrhythmias [usually supraventricular tachyarrhythmia (SVT)] and complete heart block. Prompt pharmacologic or electrical cardioversion is warranted in any patient with a tachyarrhythmia who presents with congestive heart failure. Primary cardiomyopathy or myopathic disease secondary to inborn errors of metabolism should be considered in the absence of structural cardiac disease or arrhythmia when cardiac dysfunction is present.

MANAGING ACUTE CONGESTIVE HEART FAILURE IN THE OLDER CHILD

Long-standing but unrecognized congestive heart failure may present acutely; similarly, an acute presentation may represent an acute onset of acquired cardiac disease (myocarditis or arrhythmia). Management of acute decompensation involves treatment of presenting symptoms and adjustment or initiation of long-term therapy.

In older children with acute congestive heart failure, admit to the ICU for diuresis with IV furosemide. For patients with significant hypotension, IV dopamine (5–10 mcg/kg/min) or milrinone (0.3–1 mcg/kg/min) infusion is appropriate until stabilization is achieved. Older children may require the placement of a central venous or pulmonary artery catheter to monitor venous pressure and cardiac output during stabilization.

Nitrates (nitroprusside, nitroglycerin) or nesiritide may be useful in patients with elevated pulmonary capillary wedge pressure and pulmonary congestion due to their venous dilating effects. Nesiritide carries the additional theoretical benefits of reversing deleterious neurohumoral responses and increasing natriuresis. Small studies have been conducted to measure hemodynamic effects of nesiritide in children with dilated cardiomyopathy. However, nesiritide has demonstrated no mortality advantage compared with nitroglycerin for acute decompensated heart failure in a large adult trial.

Managing Chronic or Stable Congestive Heart Failure

If the underlying cause of the congestive heart failure cannot be immediately corrected in a patient who is hemodynamically stable, outpatient management can be initiated by using several agents. Afterload reduction using an ACE inhibitor is indicated in the presence of left ventricular (LV) dysfunction, regardless of symptoms.

Afterload reduction is indicated in patients who have large left-to-right shunts at the ventricular or arterial level (ventricular septal defect or patent ductus arteriosus), left-sided regurgitant lesions (aortic insufficiency or mitral regurgitation), or poor systolic function (myocarditis or dilated cardiomyopathy). ACE inhibitors are the medications of choice. Alternatively, an angiotensin receptor blocker (ARB), such as losartan, may be used in patients in whom ACE adverse effects (particularly cough) may be unacceptable.

In addition to afterload reduction (ACE inhibitor), low-dose furosemide (1 mg/kg/dose PO bid) may be initiated, with or without the addition of another agent for inotropic effect (digoxin), or beta-blockade (carvedilol) to treat mild symptoms of congestive heart failure. The dose of digoxin (0.005–0.010 mg/kg/day PO divided twice daily, not to exceed 0.125–0.250 mg PO qd) is almost never increased, either for effect or according to digoxin levels, which are notoriously unreliable. However, the dose may be decreased in the presence of signs of toxicity. The suspicion of digoxin toxicity should increase if an infant is uninterested in feedings, gags, or vomits frequently. These symptoms are typically due to an overdose or renal failure.

For more severe congestive heart failure, diuretic therapy with oral furosemide may be increased to 2 mg/kg/dose orally 3 times daily or a second agent, such as hydrochlorothiazide or metolazone, can be added. To be most effective, hydrochlorothiazide and metolazone are best administered simultaneously with furosemide to achieve their synergistic effect.

Aldosterone Antagonists

Aldosterone antagonists are potassium-sparing diuretics. Spironolactone or eplerinone have class I indication for use in heart failure in adults including any patient with a left ventricular ejection fraction (LVEF) of less than 40% in the presence of even minimal symptoms. Their mechanism of action in heart failure is unknown. Pediatric studies have not been performed, but these agents have been used in children for a variety of indications including diuretic-induced hypokalemia. The usual dosage for children is spironolactone 1–3.3 mg/kg/day in single or divided doses.

Potassium

For patients taking more than 1 mg/kg of oral furosemide twice daily without ACE inhibitors, spironolactone should be added for its potassium-sparing effect and theoretical beneficial effects on cardiac remodeling. Adult studies have suggested that it prolongs survival in chronic heart failure. Alternatively, serum potassium levels may be monitored, and appropriate supplementation should be provided. Supplemental potassium chloride may be required when high doses of diuretics are used, but most children are extremely averse to the taste of most preparations. Alternatively, aldosterone antagonists may be administered to treat chronic diuretic-induced hypokalemia.

Because ACE inhibitors and aldosterone antagonists cause potassium retention, supplemental potassium should be avoided except in the presence of documented hypokalemia in patients taking these medications.

Sodium

Hyponatremia often accompanies congestive heart failure and is caused by water retention in response to vasopressin (antidiuretic hormone), which is produced as a result of renin-angiotensin activation but may be exacerbated by the use of diuretics and by salt wasting by the kidney.

Sodium supplementation is almost never indicated in infants or children with congestive heart failure except in emergency situations. Severe hyponatremia is generally best managed by reducing the dose of diuretics or by restricting fluid intake although the latter has little use in small children. In any child taking more than 2 mg/kg/d of furosemide, electrolyte levels should be checked every few months, as they should be in any child taking furosemide in conjunction with other diuretics or ACE inhibitors.

Beta-Blockers

Experience with beta-blocker therapy in pediatric patients has increased. The selective beta1-blocker metoprolol and the nonselective beta1-blocker and beta2-blocker carvedilol, used primarily in adults, have generally shown encouraging results in select patients with cardiomyopathy and mild or moderate chronic congestive heart failure. Adults using these beta-blockers (carvedilol) have demonstrated an increased stroke volume and stroke work index during exercise along with a decreased heart rate and LV chamber size.

In addition, carvedilol has been shown to decrease pulmonary artery mean and wedge pressures, decrease cardiac norepinephrine levels, and increase peripheral vasodilation by means of alpha1 blockade. For these reasons, in part, use of carvedilol has increased, particularly in cardiomyopathies.

However, a double-blind, randomized trial (carvedilol vs placebo) in pediatric patients with mild to moderate congestive heart failure failed to demonstrate a benefit in reduction of symptoms or mortality. The power of the study was affected by an unexpectedly high rate of improvement among all patients including those who received placebo. Thus, the exact indications and benefits of carvedilol therapy in children with heart failure remain somewhat unclear.

Anemia

Often overlooked in the management of chronic congestive heart failure is the role of the oxygen-carrying capacity of the blood. Anemia aggravates congestive heart failure by increasing the demands for cardiac output, and careful attention to iron stores or the administration of red cell transfusions often results in a significant improvement.

Nutrition

Nutrition is crucial in the management of chronic congestive heart failure. Particularly during infancy, congestive heart failure increases the metabolic demands while making feeding itself more difficult. Enhanced caloric content feedings and, in some cases, nasogastric or gastrostomy feedings may be necessary to maintain the patient's growth.

Growth

The success of medical therapy of congestive heart failure in infants and small children is judged according to the child's growth. The failure to gain weight in the setting of marked congestive heart failure signifies that the current regimen is not sufficient. A failure to thrive is an indication for increased medical management or, when the option is available, surgical repair of structural heart disease.

DIASTOLIC HEART FAILURE

In last two decades there is a substantial increase in prevalence of diastolic heart failure (DHF) from 38 to 54%. The prognosis of patients suffering from DHF is as ominous as prognosis of patients suffering from systolic heart failure (SHF). The various predisposing factors are old age, female gender, metabolic syndrome, diabetes, arterial hypertension and left ventricular hypertrophy. Elderly patients usually present with DHF in the setting of acute myocardial infarction. As there is epidemiological evolution towards DHF in the population all over the world, a reappraisal of original established set of criteria is necessary for diagnosis of DHF. However, newer modalities of echo-Doppler strain techniques may help in predicting the precursors of DHF. ***These echo variables include left atrial (LA) strain and strain rate, LA stiffness and LA ejection fraction. Segmental left ventricular (LV) deformation analysis for calculating contractile parameters such as strain and strain rate is now possible using noninvasive echo-Doppler techniques.*** It has been reported that LA systolic and diastolic function can also be assessed using these Doppler strain techniques. Although LA enlargement increases with the severity of diastolic dysfunction, the ability of LA volume measurements to discriminate asymptomatic LV diastolic dysfunction from early DHF heart failure has not been possible. However, the concept that an alteration in LA function or stiffness may be the early indicators of occult diastolic dysfunction and is therefore novel and worth exploring.

Pathophysiology in Diastolic Heart Failure

Diastole is the process by which the heart returns to its relaxed state; it is also the time for cardiac perfusion. Drastic changes occur in cardiac pressure-volume relationships during diastole. The diastolic process has four identifiable phases: isovolumetric relaxation time, the time of aortic valve closure to mitral valve opening; early rapid filling after mitral valve opening; diastasis, a period of low flow during mid-diastole and late filling of the ventricles by atrial contraction. Diastole is a complex process that is affected by a number of factors including hypertension, ischemia, heart rate, velocity of relaxation, cardiac compliance (i.e. elastic recoil and stiffness), hypertrophy and segmental wall coordination of the heart muscle. The pathophysiology of diastolic dysfunction includes delayed relaxation, impaired LV filling and/or increased stiffness. These conditions result typically in an upward displacement of the diastolic pressure-volume relationship with increased end-diastolic, left atrial and pulmocapillary wedge pressure leading to DHF. Chronic hypertension is the most common cause of diastolic dysfunction and failure. It leads to left ventricular hypertrophy and increased connective tissue content, both of which decrease cardiac compliance. The hypertrophied ventricle has a steeper diastolic pressure-volume relationship; therefore, a small increase in left ventricular end-diastolic volume causes a marked increase in left ventricular end-diastolic pressure. Another most common cardiac disease associated with abnormal LV diastolic function is myocardial ischemia. Relaxation of the ventricles involves the active transport of calcium ions into the sarcoplasmic reticulum, which allows the dissociation of myosin-actin crossbridges. Myocardial ischemia deprives the system of adequate adenosine triphosphate, which in turn inhibits the dissociation process by altering the balance of the adenosine triphosphate to adenosine diphosphate ratio, which may contribute to diastolic dysfunction. The heart rate determines the time that is available for diastolic filling, coronary perfusion and ventricular relaxation. In DHF, increase in cardiac output relatively depends upon heart rate but a rapid heart rate may further elevate abnormal LV filling pressures. Tachycardia adversely affects diastolic function by several mechanisms: it decreases left ventricular filling and coronary perfusion times, increases myocardial oxygen consumption and causes incomplete relaxation because the stiff heart cannot increase its velocity of relaxation as heart rate increases. In effect, the ventricle may never fully relax to receive blood adequately. Similiarly, atrial fibrillation completely eliminates the late diastolic atrial contribution to LV filling, upon which patients with diastolic dysfunction are dependent, often precipitating pulmonary edema. Diastolic dysfunction is more common in elderly persons, partly because of increased collagen cross-linking, increased smooth muscle content and loss of elastic fibers. These changes tend to decrease ventricular compliance it making more susceptible to the adverse effects of hypertension, tachycardia and atrial fibrillation.

Diagnosis of DHF

The working group for the European Society of Cardiology proposed that diagnosis of DHF requires three obligatory diagnostic criteria to be simultaneously satisfied:

i. Signs and symptoms of congestive heart failure
ii. Normal or mildly abnormal systolic LV systolic function
iii. Evidence of LV diastolic dysfunction (abnormal LV relaxation, filling, diastolic distensibility or diastolic stiffness).

1. **Signs and symptoms of congestive heart failure:** Signs and symptoms of congestive heart failure include lung crepitations, pulmonary oedema, ankle swelling, hepatomegaly, dyspnoea on exertion and fatigue.
2. **Normal or mildly abnormal systolic left ventricular functions:** The presence of normal or mildly abnormal systolic LV function constitutes the second criterion for the diagnosis of heart failure (HF) with normal left ventricular ejection fraction (LVEF) - HFNLVEF. In the present consensus document, an LVEF > 50% is also considered consistent with the presence of normal or mildly abnormal systolic LV function. LVEF needs to be assessed in accordance to the recent recommendations for cardiac chamber quantification of the American Society of Echocardiography and the European Association of Echocardiography. It is of importance to note that in DHF reduced long-axis shortening is frequently compensated for by increased short-axis shortening. As already demonstrated by Frank, Starling, and Wiggers and later re-appraised, LV relaxation depends on endsystolic load and volume. The criterion of presence of normal or mildly abnormal LV function therefore needs to be implemented with measures of LV volumes. To exclude significant LV enlargement, LVEDVI and LV end-systolic volume index cannot exceed 97 mL/m^2 and 49 mL/m^2, respectively.
3. Evidence of LV diastolic dysfunction.

Conventional Doppler Assessment of LV Diastolic Dysfunction

Mitral inflow measurements which included peak early (E) and peak late (A) flow velocities, the E/A ratio, the deceleration time of early mitral flow velocity (DT), the isovolumetric relaxation time (IVRT) at rest and during the valsalva maneuver and the pulmonary venous flow measurements, characterized by peak systolic (S), diastolic (D), and atrial reversal (Ard) velocities; the systolic filling fraction (S/D); and the time difference between A and the duration of atrial reverse flow (Ard-Ad) were originally considered to be indicative of diastolic LV dysfunction if they exceeded specific cut-off values indexed for age group. Because of the absence of pseudonormalization on tissue Doppler imaging (TDI) lengthening velocity measurements, the use of blood flow Doppler measures of diastolic LV function is no longer recommended as a first-line diagnostic approach to diastolic LV dysfunction. Only when TDI lengthening velocities are suggestive but nondiagnostic or when plasma levels of natriuretic peptides are elevated does the simultaneous presence of a low E/A ratio and a prolonged DT or a prolonged Ard-Ad index provide diagnostic evidence of diastolic LV dysfunction.

Tissue Doppler Assessment of LV Diastolic Dysfunctions

Tissue Doppler (TD) echocardiography helps to accurately quantify LV diastolic function. TD may be used to quantify myocardial velocities in multiple segments of the myocardium from different echocardiographic acoustic windows. The most frequently used modality of TD is measurement of LV basal (annular), longitudinal myocardial shortening, or lengthening velocity. Measurements can be obtained either at the septal or at the lateral side of the mitral annulus. The peak systolic (S) shortening velocity and the early diastolic (E2) lengthening velocities are considered to be sensitive measures of LV systolic or diastolic function. Especially, the ratio of early mitral valve flow velocity (E) divided by E2 correlates closely with LV filling pressures. E depends on left atrial driving pressure, LV relaxation kinetics, and age but E′ depends mostly on LV relaxation kinetics and age. Hence, in the ratio E/E2, effects of LV relaxation kinetics and age are eliminated and the ratio becomes a measure of left atrial driving pressure or LV filling pressure. E2 can also be conceptualized as the amount of blood entering the LV during early filling, whereas E represents the gradient necessary to make this blood enter the LV. A high E/E2 thus represents a high gradient for a low shift in volume. Information on LV filling pressures can also be derived from the time interval between the onset of E and the onset of E2 (TE-E2). When the ratio E/E2 exceeds 15, LV filling pressures are elevated and when the ratio is lower than 8, LV filling pressures are low 34. E/E2 is a powerful predictor of survival after myocardial infarction and E/E2 >15 is superior as predictor of prognosis than clinical or other echocardiographic variables. The close correlation between E/E2 and LV filling pressures has been confirmed in heart failure patients with depressed (< 50%) or preserved LV ejection fraction. and in patients with slow relaxation or pseudonormal early mitral valve flow velocity filling patterns. The ratio E/E2 is considered diagnostic evidence of presence of diastolic LV dysfunction if E/E2 > 15, and diagnostic evidence of absence of HFNLVEF if E/E2 < 8. An

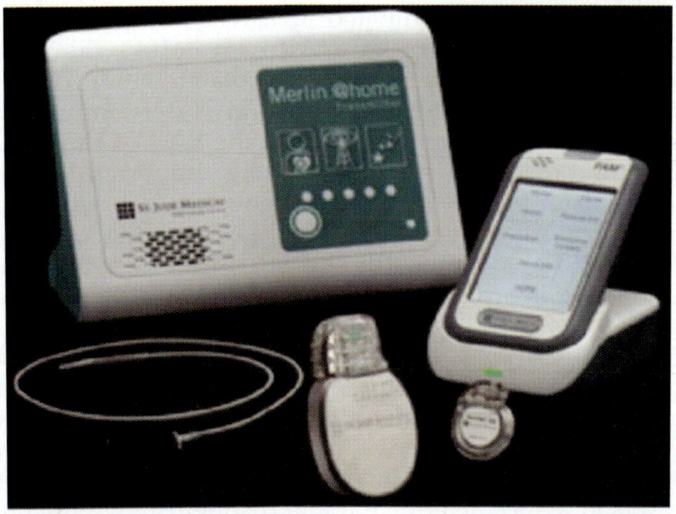

Fig. 39.42: *Showing continuous left atrial pressure monitoring in CHF patients recently published study that analyzed the clinical benefits of frequent and regular left atrial pressure (LAP) monitoring in patients with heart failure, patients wore a special device, called HeartPOD, that monitored their LAP and routed the data wirelessly to their cardiologist*

E/E2 ratio ranging from 8 to 15 is considered suggestive but nondiagnostic evidence of diastolic LV dysfunction and needs to be implemented with other noninvasive investigations.

Invasive Method of Assessment of LV Diastolic Dysfunction (Fig. 39.42)

Definite evidence of abnormal LV relaxation, filling, diastolic distensibility or diastolic stiffness can be acquired invasively during cardiac catheterization. Such evidence consists of a time constant of LV relaxation (ô) >48 ms, an LV end-diastolic pressure >16 mmHg or a mean pulmonary capillary wedge pressure >12 mmHg. A diastolic LV stiffness modulus >0.27 also provides diagnostic evidence of diastolic LV dysfunction. It has been pointed out that mitral flow Doppler alone, with its 40–70% specificity, cannot reliably detect diastolic dysfunction in HFNLVEF TDI including the transmitral flow velocity to annular velocity ratio (E/E2 index), which measures myocardial velocities during the cardiac cycle, is considered more reliable for diagnosing diastolic dysfunction. Oh et al proposed comprehensive Doppler echocardiography with color flow or TDI as the most practical and reproducible method for either confirming or excluding diastolic dysfunction in HFNLVEF. In contrast, Maurer et al recently argued that Doppler-derived diastolic parameters do not provide specific information on intrinsic passive diastolic properties and thus that diastolic dysfunction cannot be diagnosed by Doppler echocardiography. Invasive measurement of pressure-volume (PV) relationships with a conductance catheter system is generally considered most accurate for characterizing diastolic cardiac function. It allows direct detection of LV relaxation abnormalities and passive LV stiffness characterized by a change in diastolic LV pressure relative to diastolic LV volume. A recent study Mario Kasner et al was the first to investigate the accuracy of several echocardiographic Doppler techniques in detecting diastolic dysfunction in HFNLVEF by direct comparison with invasive PV loop data. It was found that no diastolic index of conventional Doppler echocardiography alone was sufficient to make the correct diagnosis. These indices correlated only weakly with diastolic relaxation anomalies and not at all with the degree of LV stiffness. On the other hand, TDI investigations and the LV filling index E/E2 lat were well suited for detecting invasively proven diastolic dysfunction in HFNLVEF patients.

Many studies have shown that atrial function is particularly important when ventricular dysfunction exists. Kurt et al has shown that evaluation of LA systolic and diastolic function using strain Doppler echocardiography has reasonably high accuracy. This study showed that patients with DHF have a significantly reduced LA strain and strain rate during LV systole and increased LA stiffness index. Increased LA stiffness as assessed invasively and noninvasively readily identify patients with DHF from those with LV diastolic dysfunction. On the other hand, LV mass, volumes, and systolic function, LA volumes and atrial pump function were not significantly different in the patients of DHF and LVDD.

LA strain and strain rate (Figs 39.32 and 39.33) are new emerging real-time ultrasound techniques that provide a measure of wall motion or a measure of deformation. Radial and longitudinal atrial or ventricular function can be assessed by the analysis of wall deformation using the rate

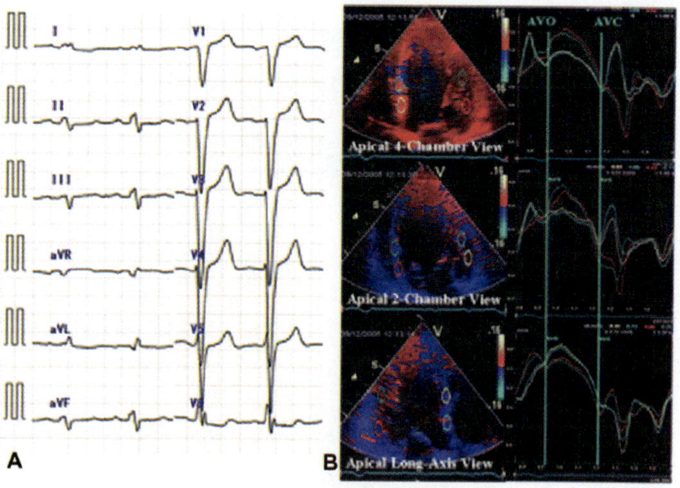

Fig. 39.43: *(A) The 12-lead electrocardiogram before cardiac resynchronization therapy (CRT), demonstrating a QRS width of 160 ms with a left bundle branch block. (B) Longitudinal dyssynchrony by myocardial velocity before cardiac resynchronization therapy was as follows: 23 ms in Yu index and 35 ms in opposing wall delay, indicating no longitudinal dyssynchrony. AVO, aortic valve opening; AVC, aortic valve closure. Apical four chamber view: yellow, basal-interior septum; blue, mid-inferior septum; red, basal-lateral; green, mid-lateral. Apical two chamber view: yellow, basal-anterior; blue, mid-anterior; red, basal-inferior; green, mid-inferior. Apical long-axis view: yellow, basal-anterior septum; blue, mid-anterior septum; red, basal-posterior; green, mid-posterior*

of deformation of a myocardial segment (strain rate) and its deformation over time (strain). A negative strain rate corresponds to myocardial shortening or thickening, whereas a positive strain rate corresponds to myocardial lengthening or thinning. Atrial strain and strain rate measurements are usually obtained during ventricular and atrial systole using sample volumes placed in the atrial myocardium near but clearly superior to the mitral annulus. For LA "diastolic" strain variables (during LV systole) the source of the strain is the ventricle doing external work on the atrium as the LV ejects blood into the aorta. Deformation in the atria is reciprocally related to the deformation of the ventricles, as both apex and the atrial roof are relatively immobile, the ventricle shortens while atria elongates during systole, ventricle elongates and atria shortens during the diastolic phases. In diastasis, there is no deformation. And so the amount and rate of strain measured is determined primarily by ventricular and LV afterload attributes, although it follows that passive atrial tissue properties— on which the LV is also doing work. In addition, because of its thin wall, strain rate imaging in the atria is extra prone to artefacts due to low lateral resolution. Kurt et al has shown that patients with DHF had significantly a lower LA systolic strain and SR as compared to patients with LVDD alone. However, late diastolic strain and SR were similar in patients with DHF and LV diastolic dysfunction.

LA stiffness index: Stiffness is conventionally defined as the force required to displace a passive spring a unit length. Physiologically, it is the change in pressure required to increase the volume of a passive container a unit amount. LA stiffness can be estimated invasively, i.e. by ratio of pulmonary wedge pressure to LA systolic strain and noninvasive. LA stiffness can be calculated by ratio of E/E2 and LA strain. LA systolic strain is determined by averaging values from four sites in the LA myocardium. The units of LA stiffness are mmHg. Importantly, the denominator in this expression, although measured in the LA wall, is determined primarily by longitudinal apically directed displacement of the mitral annulus by the contracting ventricle, whereas the posterior aspect of the LA remains fixed. Hence this index, usually attributed to the LA as a stiffness measure, is very strongly influenced by LV properties. LA stiffness as assessed invasively and noninvasively readily identified patients with DHF from those with LV diastolic dysfunction. Kurt et al has shown that a LA stiffness index of >1.1 mmHg had a sensitivity of 84%, and a specificity of 100% in distinguishing patients with DHF from those with LV diastolic dysfunction. Using E/E2 ratio in lieu of PCWP was also accurate in identifying DHF patients and an index of 0.99 had a sensitivity of 85% and a specificity of 78% in distinguishing patients with DHF from those with LV diastolic dysfunction.

Left atrial volume measurements: A left atrial volume indexed to body surface area (left atrial volume index) >32 mL/m^2 was first recognized in the elderly as a strong predictor ($p = 0.003$) of a cardiovascular event with a higher predictive value than other echocardiographically derived indices such as LV mass index ($p = 0.014$) or LV diastolic dysfunction ($p = 0.029$). In a population-based study, left atrial volume index was also strongly associated with the

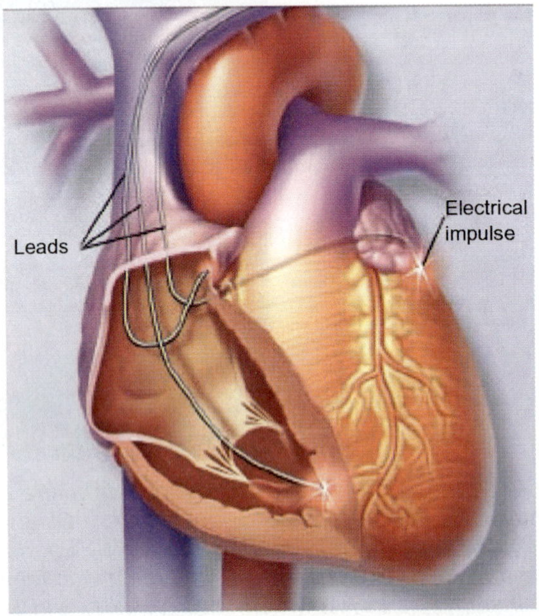

Fig. 39.44: Cardiac resynchronization therapy (CRT), also called biventricular pacing, uses a special kind of pacemaker, called a biventricular pacemaker, designed to help the ventricles contract more normally. It keeps the right and left ventricles pumping together by sending small electrical impulses through the leads. This therapy has been shown to improve the symptoms of heart failure and overall quality of life in certain patients with severe symptoms that aren't controlled with medication

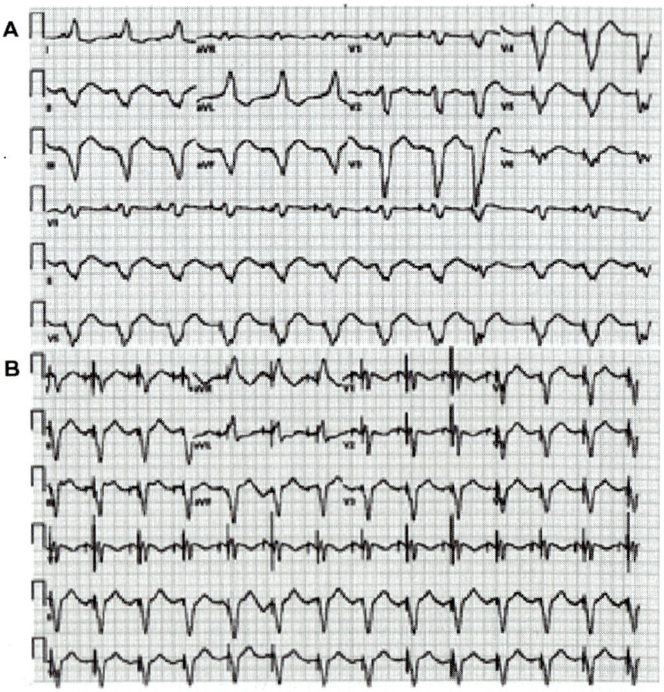

Fig. 39.45: Electrocardiogram (ECG) changes with (A) right ventricular (RV) and biventricular pacing 12-lead ECG from a patient with cardiomyopathy during RV apical pacing, and (B) biventricular (BiV) pacing cardiac resynchronization therapy (CRT) with alteration in the QRS duration and axis

severity and duration of diastolic LV dysfunction: the left atrial volume index progressively increased from a value of 23 + 6 mL/m^2 in normal to 25 + 8 mL/m^2 in mild diastolic LV dysfunction, to 31 + 8 mL/m^2 in moderate diastolic LV dysfunction, and finally to 48 + 12 mL/m^2 in severe diastolic LV dysfunction. Left atrial volume index was therefore proposed as a biomarker of both diastolic LV dysfunction and cardiovascular risk. Left atrial volume index (LAVi) is a more robust marker than left atrial area or left atrial diameter For these reasons, a left atrial volume index >40 mL/m^2 has been taken to provide sufficient evidence of diastolic LV dysfunction when the E/E2 ratio is non-conclusive (i.e. 15>E/ E2 >8) or when plasma levels of natriuretic peptides are elevated. Similarly, a left atrial volume index < 29 mL/m^2 is proposed as a prerequisite to exclude HFNLVEF. Left atrial volume index values of 29 and 40 mL/m^2 correspond, respectively, to the lower cut-off values of mildly abnormal and severely abnormal LA size in the recent recommendations for cardiac chamber quantification of the American Society of Echocardiography and the European Association of Echocardiography.

LV Torsion with 2D Speckle Tracking Echocardiography

Left ventricular torsion (LVtor) and subsequent untwisting play an important role in diastolic filling. Sung-Ji et al has shown that systolic torsion and diastolic untwisting are significantly increased in patients with mild diastolic dysfunction. However, analysis of LVtor with speckle tracking echocardiography needs to be further explored to elucidate the role of torsion in patients with LV diastolic dysfunction (Fig. 39.33).

Device-Based Therapies (Fig. 39.51)

Cardiac Resynchronization Therapy (Fig. 39.43–39.45)

Cardiac resynchronization therapy (CRT) has emerged as a useful therapy in the treatment of chronic congestive heart failure. CRT involves the use of biventricular pacemakers to improve ventricular function by electrically adjusting the timing of right and left ventricular contraction to optimize wall motion and increase filling time. In addition to increasing stroke volume, CRT may allow for reverse remodeling to delay disease progression. Clinical trials in adults with moderate to severe heart failure have demonstrated beneficial effects of CRT use including reduction of symptoms, increased exercise capacity, and decreased morbidity and mortality.

In pediatric practice, resynchronization therapy has been limited; the initial studies described the results for this modality instituted in children with chronic heart failure who required pacemakers for treatment of rhythm disorders. Use of this therapy is more difficult to institute in children, whose small size requires the use of surgically placed epicardial pacemakers rather than percutaneously placed pacemakers. As more registry and retrospective data have accumulated, use of this therapy has increased, and indications based on echocardiographic and electrocardiographic parameters continue to be refined.

Mechanical Support

Mechanical support may be used in the treatment of acute heart failure (i.e. myocarditis or postcardiotomy syndrome) or in chronic heart failure as a bridge to recovery or to a heart transplant. The choice of support therapy depends on the expected duration of use.

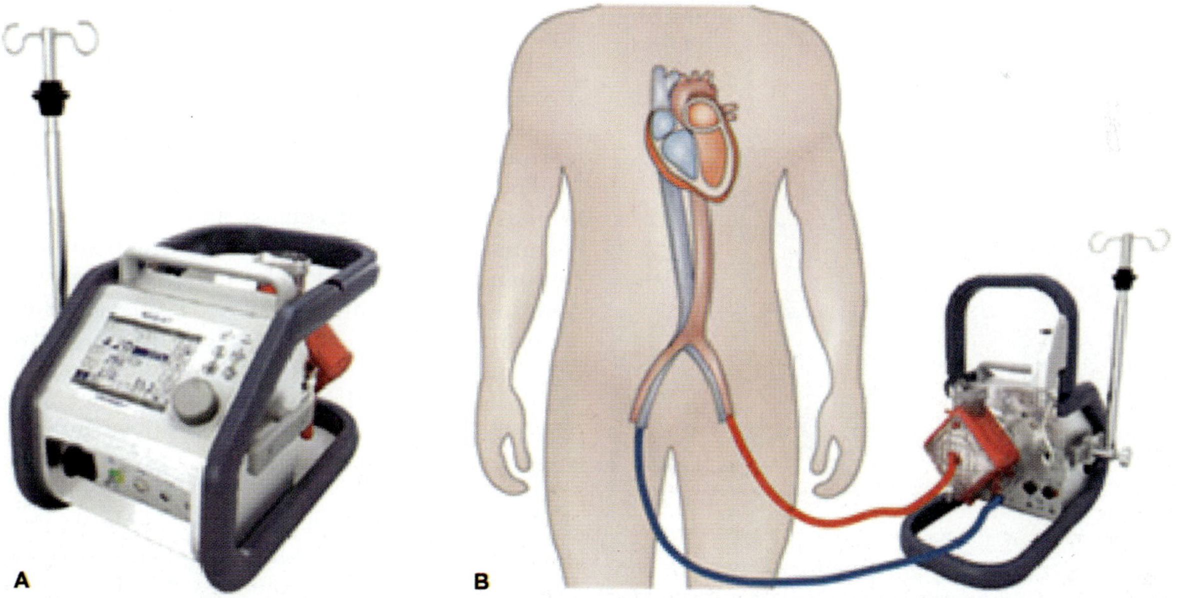

Fig. 39.46: *The device is compact and easily portable, with a total weight of only 9 kg. (A) Venoarterial extracorporeal membrane oxygenation (ECMO) is established by cannulation of a femoral vein and artery using the Seldinger technique. (B) To expedite interhospital transfer these vessels can be located with guidewires before arrival of the outreach team. The cannulas can then be inserted rapidly to begin ECMO before transport by air or ground ambulance. (Images of the Cardiohelp® device courtesy of © Maquet Cardiopulmonary AG)*

Extracorporeal membrane oxygenation (ECMO) therapy may be quickly initiated in unstable patients. Generally, its duration of use is limited to days or weeks because of complications related to infection or anticoagulation. ECMO is used to provide acute temporary support as a bridge to recovery or transplantation.

In a study of ECMO use in 108 patients (73 adults and 35 children), most of whom were suffering from post-cardiotomy cardiac low output, Beiras-Fernandez et al found that pediatric patients who had undergone congenital heart surgery were among the patients who demonstrated the best results from ECMO (Fig. 39.46).

Ventricular assist devices (VADs; e.g. Berlin Heart, EXCOR pediatric system, Thoratec VAD) may be used to provide long-term ventricular support. The EXCOR pediatric system is the first pulsatile mechanical circulatory support device specifically designed for children and was approved by the FDA in December 2011.

The device consists of 1 or 2 external pneumatic blood pumps to support the left ventricle alone or both the left and right ventricles. EXCOR is available in graduated sizes to fit children from newborns to adolescents. Also see FDA approves mechanical cardiac assist device for children with heart failure. Other devices, such as Thoratec HeartMate II, have not received approval for pediatric use but have been used in selected cases for appropriately sized patients. Currently, VADs are not approved for permanent (destination) therapy in pediatric patients and should be considered only as a bridge to transplantation in appropriate candidates (Fig. 39.47).

Cell Replacement Strategy (Fig. 39.48)

Cell replacement strategy is a new era in therapy for patients with myocardial dysfunction. It has been postulated that therapies directly targeted at replacing or regenerating damaged myocardial tissue could prevent progression to heart failure and therefore would be an important contribution to the treatment of ischemic damage to the myocardium. Many cell types have been successfully transplanted into damaged myocardium, including fetal cardiomyocytes, skeletal myoblasts embryonic stem cells, and bone marrow-derived stem cells. The best characterized of these is skeletal myoblast, an immature muscle cell that retains the ability to proliferate. Several studies have used human autologous skeletal myoblasts transplantation to determine if engraftment of these cells leads to long-term improvements in left ventricle function. However, these exciting progresses have many unanswered questions including potential arrhythmic and oncogenic potential of these cells which can only be resolved by larger clinical trials with long-term follow-up.

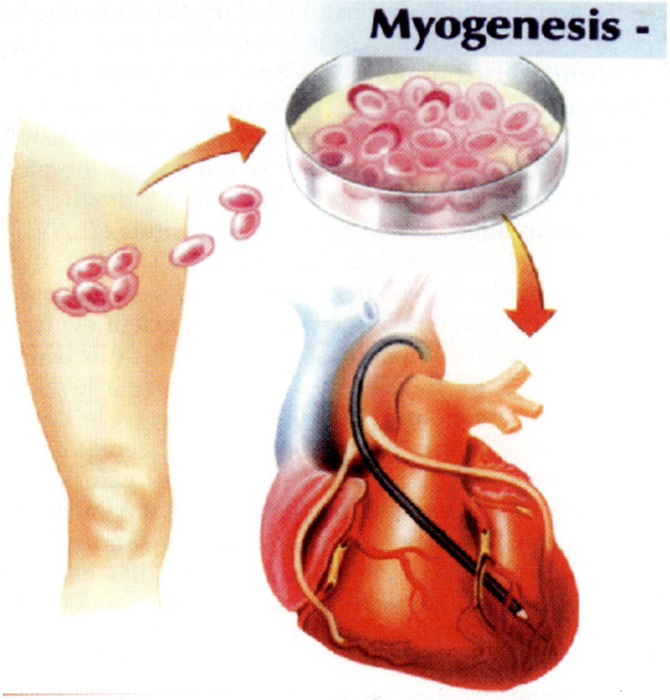

Fig. 39.48: *Diagrammatic depiction of myogenesis in the heart muscle. Myoblasts are super power house cells that originate from human bodys muscle stem cells. These cells have the ability to take on the properties of the other cells such as cardiac muscle cells that make up the heart. Unlike cardiac muscle myoblasts can regenerate and repair themselves. The myoblasts can be transplanted from the skeletal muscles into heart and can stimulate myogenesis. A biopsy of muscle cells from patient thigh is taken and isolated and expanded in culture in a special cell laboratory for 3 weeks. These multiple cells are injected directly into the areas of heart where the muscle is damaged*

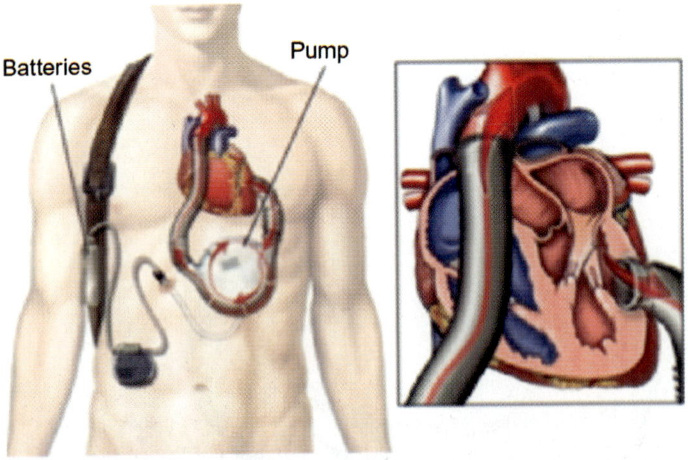

Fig. 39.47: *Showing VADs which are used for people with end-stage refractory congestive heart failure that has not responded to medicine. In the heart, the left ventricle does most of the work. It is usually the chamber that fails first. VADs can be used to support the left ventricle, right ventricle, or both. Getting a VAD is a way to improve the heart's ability to pump without having a heart transplant*

Heart Transplantation (Figs 39.49 and 39.50)

Heart transplant in children of all ages is now accepted as a therapy for end-stage heart failure secondary to cardiomyopathy and palliated congenital heart disease when these diseases are life-threatening or are associated with a poor quality of life. The approach and the criterions of listing for heart transplantation in pediatric age are different than in adults. Role of cardiopulmonary exercise testing is limited by lack of consensus and limited data, the adult value of peak oxygen consumption of 14 milliliter/kilogram/minute guideline does not hold true for children. High pulmonary vascular resistance is another important factor affecting the perioperative mortality and outcome after transplant in pediatric age group. The adult criteria of transpulmonary gradient (pumonary artery mean pressure minus left atrial mean pressure) greater than 15 millimeter of mercury, may not hold true for pediatric age group, as many patients with transpulmonary gradient greater than 15 millimeter of mercury are able to undergo successful transplantation with higher transpulmonary gradient. The most important limitation is availability of donor heart for our growing population of heart failure in pediatric age group and it is important to utilize this presently rare resource to benefit as many children and their families as possible.

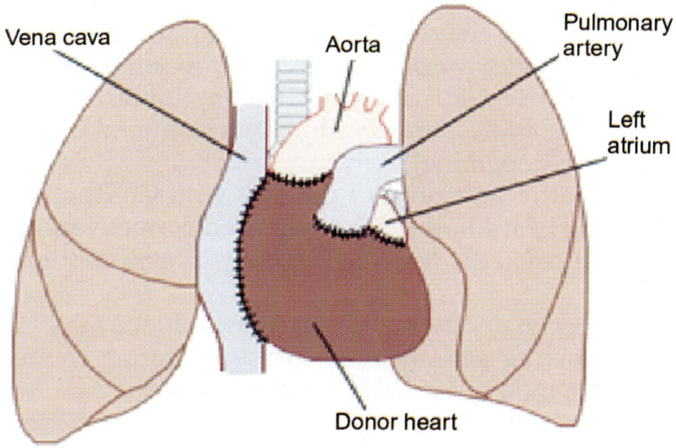

Fig. 39.49: *Diagram illustrating the placement of a donor heart in an orthotopic procedure. Notice how the back of the patient's left atrium and great vessels are left in place*

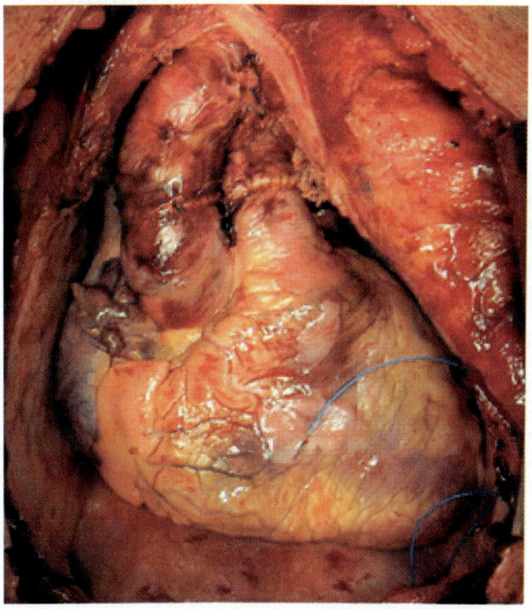

Fig. 39.50: *Transplanted heart in the thorax of recipient*

Other Modes of Management

Maintain infant's temperature in euthermic range. Posture: An infant in CHF has cardiomegaly and congested lungs. Both diminish the volume available for air exchange. In addition, hepatomegaly will limit diaphragmatic excursion in recumbent posture so keep the patient in a suitable chair in inclined posture.

Oxygen administration: If there is respiratory distress, pulmonary venous desaturation is pronounced so increase inspired oxygen concentration will benefit the patient.

Sedation: Restlessness is very common in infants and children with CHF which raises oxygen demands. Sedation with chloral hydrate is useful in infants and children. Morphine is the sedative of choice in acutely ill patient and in postoperative period when pain is an additional factor. **In the second 24 hours,** if the patient has good diuresis, respiratory distress has lessened and heart rate has slowed down, maintenance digoxin and diuretics are switched over to the oral route.

But if inotropics and preload reducers do not produce the desired effect, search for additional problem is made because digoxin has got dynamic action depending upon the pH of blood, electrolyte normality, abnormal blood sugar level and hemoglobin concentration. If child is very anemic, packed blood cells are given which increase oxygen carrying capacity. Attempt is made to maintain electrolyte balance, normal blood sugar and proper blood pH. If child has got pulmonary infection adequate antibiotic treatment is given. If inspite of above variables being normal, after load reducers are considered.

Two more therapeutic principles that can be followed both in the hospital as well as at home are:

- Salt restriction should not interfere with baby's eating.
- Infants should eat enough.
- Restriction of physical activity is not the issue in pediatrics. It may be counter productive because it increases oxygen consumption.
- When the baby improves, can tolerate room air and develops an appetite sufficient to gain weight—maintenance of inotropics and diuretics should be decided and further investigation for proper surgical management should be carried out.

Vasopeptidase Inhibitors

Neutral peptidase is an enzyme that inactivates several of the peptides like atrial natriuretic peptide, brain type natriuretic peptide, bradykinin and adrenomedullin. These peptides have vasodilator, natriuretic and antiproliferative properties. Simultaneous inhibition of neutral peptidase and angiotensin-converting enzyme markedly reduces vasoconstriction, improves sodium and water balance, decrease peripheral vascular resistance and blood pressure and improves local blood flow when compared with angiotensin-converting enzyme inhibition alone.

The only available vasopeptidase inhibitor that has been evaluated in adults with heart failure is omapatrilat, which is not yet recommended for use at this time. Candoxatril and ecadotril are oral forms of neutral peptidase inhibitors which increase levels of natriuretic peptides and are currently in trials in adult patients with heart failure.

Endothelin Receptor Antagonists

Endothelin-1 levels are increased in patients with heart failure and progressively higher plasma concentrations are found in patients with heart failure as their functional class deteriorates. Endothelin-1 plasma level also correlates with pulmonary artery pressure and pulmonary vascular resistance. Although the expression of endothelin-1 within the myocardium may initially represent an adaptive response to stress, over expression of endothelin-1 may eventually be maladaptive by producing focal vasospasm, myocyte necrosis and increased myocardial fibrosis. Non-selective endothelin receptor antagonists such as bosentan, tezosentran and enrasentran are now being evaluated in clinical trials in adults but have yet to demonstrate their clinical utility. Sitaxsentan is a selective endothelin-1A receptor antagonist and a selective pulmonary vasodilator.

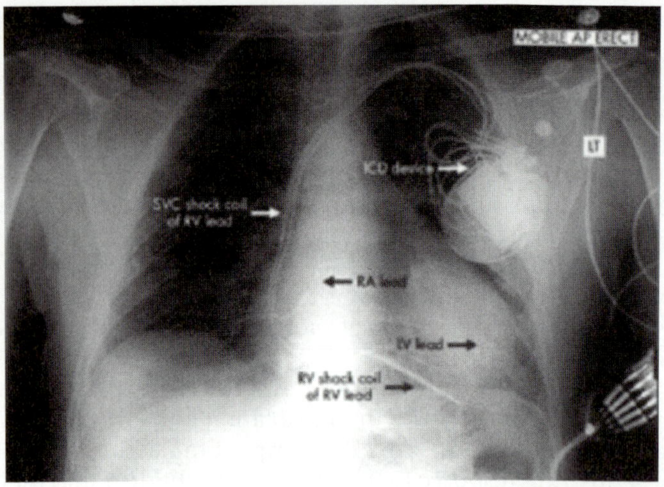

Fig. 39.51: *X-ray chest showing ICD device fitted in a patient with cardiac arrhythmias and heart failure*

Drugs Management of Heart Failure

As a rule, infants first seen in CHF should be hospitalized because CHF is a life-threatening in infants. The administration of therapeutic agents, selection of drugs, determination of appropriate dosage can be done in an inpatient setting. A complete anatomic and physiologic understanding should be obtained as soon as possible to decide about surgery. Once the patient is admitted, a chest film PA view and an electrocardiogram should be taken and blood for blood count, gases, and chemistries should be obtained. A careful history and physical examination and a working diagnosis should be made and treatment is started. If the patient is very ill, two dimensional echocardiography, intravenous line, delivery of oxygen by mask and therapy should be done simultaneously. Once a working diagnosis is made and no emergency surgery is indicated, intravenous diuretic is used, provided serum potassium is normal. Frusemide, a loop diuretic known as high-ceiling diuretic due to the high intensity of its effects is used to improve ventricular function by its preload reduction due to pulmonary vasodilatation. The only contraindication for frusemide is CHF due to tachyarrhythmia. Along with the diuretic, in desperately ill infant-parenteral inotropics (digoxin or dopamine) is given.

In pediatrics, majority of patients with CHF are due to congenital heart disease who will need corrective surgery. The medical treatment of CHF is necessary for three reasons:

1. To correct hemodynamic aberrations due to CHF.
2. To allow the patient to reach the operating room in a better hemodynamic and metabolic state.
3. To give an opportunity for spontaneous improvement of the defect—PDA in premature and VSD closure.

It is reasonable to admit that most treatment strategies used in children with chronic heart failure have been extrapolated from trials in adults. Although there is good rationale for doing this, there are significant differences

Table 39.8: *Use of implantable defibrillators in patients with heart failure*

- Class I
- Cardiac arrest due to ventricular fibrillation (VF) or ventricular tachycardia (VT) not due to transient or reversible cause
- Spontaneous sustained VT in association with structural heart disease
- Syncope of undetermined origin with clinically relevant sustained VT or VF induced at electrophysiological study
- Nonsustained VT with coronary artery disease, prior myocardial infraction and inducible
- Nonsupressible VT
- Class IIa, left ventricular ejection fraction less than or equal to 30%, at least 1 month following myocardial infraction and 3 months after surgical revasculation nb
- Class IIb, cardiac arrest presumed to be due to VF when electrophysiologic testing is precluded by other medical conditions. Severe symptoms, such as syncope, in patients awaiting cardiac transplantation. Nonsustained VT with sustained VT at electrophysiologic study in patients with ischemic heart disease
- Recurrent syncope of undetermined etiology in the presence of ventricular dysfunction.
- Class III-contraindicated
- Increassant VT or VF (ICD may be indicated after arrhythmia control)
- VT or VF due to a transient or reversible condition
- Projected life expectancy less than 6 months
- Significant psychiatric illness that may be aggravated by device implantation or that ma preclude device follow-up
- NYHA class IV heart failure in patients who are not candidates for cardiac transplantation

between the substrate for left ventricle dysfunction between children and adults. In general, pharmacotherapy for chronic compensated heart failure has three goals: (1) the rapid relief of symptoms, (2) slowing of the pathophysiological process involved in left ventricle remodeling and (3) increasing patient survival. Despite the standard pharmacotherapy some children and young adults with heart failure remain in a chronic decompensated state. These patients require intravenous inotropes and vasodilator medications. Some of these patients with end-stage heart failure become inotrope-dependent, and are candidates for newer therapies including but not limited to ventricular assist device as a bridge to transplantation or recovery. Evidence-based medicine for management of pediatric heart failure does not exist at this time. Until large, multicenter trials of children with heart failure are performed, the best course for pediatric cardiologists is to follow the adult literature, cautiously introduce accepted therapies, and follow patients closely.

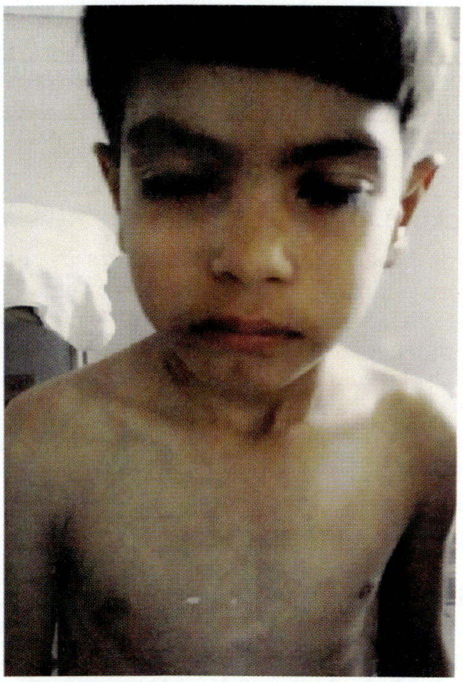

Fig. 39.52: *Photograph of a 7-years-old child who had juvenile rheumatic mitral stenosis (MVA<2.0 cm²) with severe MR (grade 111-1V) enlarged LA with PAH and exertional dyspnoea and showed early signs of heart failure*

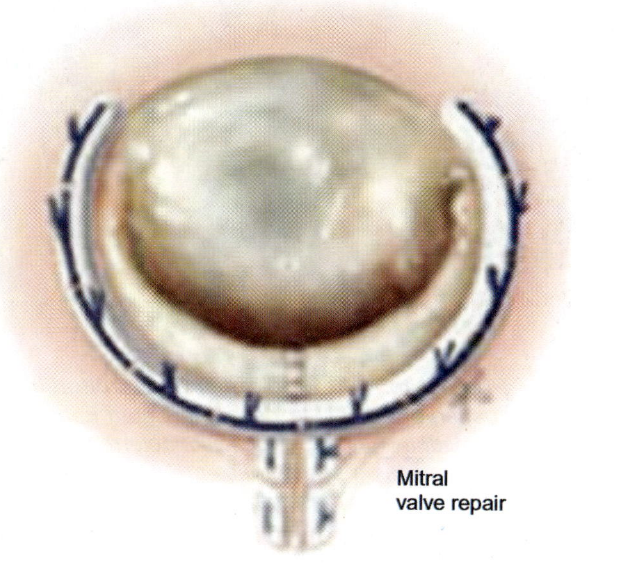

Fig. 39.53: *Showing annuloplasty complete repair of the damaged valve in the mitral valve apparatus*

Diuretics

Diuretics are needed to relieve the volume overload and congestive symptoms, but can activate the renin-angiotensin-aldosterone axis and sympathetic nervous system. Therefore, diuretics except spironolactone have no long-term benefits and do not prevent the disease progression in chronic heart failure. Loop diuretics are preferable to most other diuretics secondary to their effectiveness and potency. Combination therapy has been shown to be more effective than monotherapy with one class at escalating dose because sequential sites in the nephron can be blocked. New diuretics called aquaretic which are vasopressin receptor antagonists are available. Two vasopressin antagonists currently being used in clinical trials are tolvaptan (vasopressin receptor-2 antagonist) and conivaptan (combined vasopressin receptor-1a and -2 antagonists). The potential value of these agents is the fact that they cause elimination of water, without the loss of electrolytes, thus potentially negating the need for frequent follow-up of serum electrolytes levels.

Diuretics relieve congestive symptoms; do not change the long-term outcome. Excess use of diuretics can reduce the preload and cardiac output, resulting in neurohormonal activation and fluid retention—a vicious cycle

1. Furosemide: 1 mg/kg dose BID up to max 6 mg/kg/day
2. Chlorothiazide: 10 mg/kg dose BID up to max 2 gm/day
3. Metolazone: 0.1 mg/kg dose BID up to max 20 mg/day

Aldosterone Antagonist

Aldosterone antagonists (spironolactone and eplerenone) have been shown to reduce mortality in adults with heart failure. Plasma aldosterone levels are elevated in hearfailure, both because of increased production and reduced hepatic clearance. The mechanisms of aldosterone mediated potentiation of heart failure include increased myocardial fibrosis, increased angiotensin-converting enzyme and endothelin activity, increased free radical production, and decreased adrenal nitric oxide. Low dose spironolactone is considered to be an inhibitor of renin-angiotensin-aldosterone axis, rather than diuretic.

Dosage

Spironolactone 1 mg/kg dose BID up to max 200 mg/day
Decreases mortality and morbidity; improves endothelial

vasodilator dysfunction; suppress vascular angiotensin conversion. It should be used with caution in patients with hyponatremia, renal insufficiency, hyperkalemia and hepatic disease.

Digoxin

Digoxin inhibits the sarcolemmal sodium-potassium-adenosine tri-phophatase pump which results in increased intracellular sodium and subsequent increase in intracellular calcium through inhibition of sodium-calcium exchanger. This increase in intracellular calcium results in increased contractility. Other beneficial effects of digoxin include reduction of sympathetic tone and norepinephrine levels. Recent observations suggest that digitalis may have additional effects on cardiac cell function in both the short and long term that include intracellular effects, interactions with specific sodium-potassium-adenosine triphophatase isoforms in different cellular locations, effects on intracellular (including nuclear) signaling, and long-term regulation of intracellular ionic balances through circulating ouabain-like compounds. Digoxin improves symptoms and decreases hospitalization, but there is no evidence that it improves survival in adults. The effect of digoxin on symptoms and /or survival in children with heart failure is unknown.

Dosage: 3–4 mcg/kg dose BID

It increases inotropy; attenuates neurohormonal activation; no effect on mortality, no relationship between serum digoxin level and worsening heart failure, change in left ventricle ejection fraction and exercise tolerance in adults.

Angiotensin-Converting Enzyme Inhibitors and Angiotensin Receptor Blockers

Angiotensin-converting enzyme inhibitors are the mainstay of treatment in all patients with systolic left ventricle dysfunction. The mechanism by which angiotensin-converting enzyme inhibitors benefit patients with heart failure include vasodilation, ventricular remodeling, improved renal function, and blunting the hypertrophic and apoptotic effects of angiotensin II within the myocardium. Angiotensin-converting enzyme inhibitors appear to exhibit a class effect and all members of this class may be equally effective. Potential side effects are hyperkalemia if used concomitantly with spironolactone, cough and angioedema due to decrease degradation of bradykinin, renal dysfunction and azotemia. The low dose angiotensin-converting enzyme inhibitors are recommended in patients receiving spironolactone in order to avoid potential hyperkalemia. It is recommended to start beta-blocker therapy along with angiotensin-converting enzyme inhibitors if there is no contraindication. Angiotensin receptor blockers directly block the effects of angiotensin-II no matter which pathway of production (angiotensin-converting enzyme or chymase). In adults, angiotensin-receptor blockers appear to be as effective as angiotensin-converting enzyme inhibitors in improving symptoms, reducing mortality, reducing wedge pressure, and increasing cardiac output. If patient is intolerant to angiotensin-converting enzyme inhibitors then use angiotensin receptor blockers instead. Currently, angiotensin receptor blockers available are losartan, valsartan and irbesartan. There is little data available on the use of angiotensin receptor blockers in children.

Dosage

It decrease mortality and morbidity; blocks the conversion of angiotensin I to II and activates bradykinin and kallidin; cause vasodilation and natriuresis; reduce afterload >mitigate the process of angiotensin-mediated maladaptation to heart failure; decrease Qp:Qs and improve weight gain in children with left to right shunts.

- Captopril: 0.1 mg/kg dose TID up to max 2 mg/kg/dose
- Enalapril: 0.1 mg/kg dose BID up to max 0.5 mg/kg/day.

Beta-blocker Therapy

The current experience of beta-blockers in children with heart failure is limited, but a number of small trials have shown beneficial effect of carvedilol. Long-term therapy with beta-blockers in adults improves systolic function and energetics and reverses the pathologic remodeling process. The improvement in energetics is by reduction in heart rate, systolic and diastolic wall stress, both of which causes decrease in myocardial oxygen demand, a shift in substrate utilization from free fatty acids to glucose, and shift in the phenotyping of failing heart to more energy-efficient isoforms. Beta-blockade is also associated with a change in the molecular phenotype of the heart. These include up-regulation of the gene expression of the natriuretic peptides and beta-myosin heavy chain, partially prevent down-regulation of beta-2 receptor and angiotensin-2 receptor

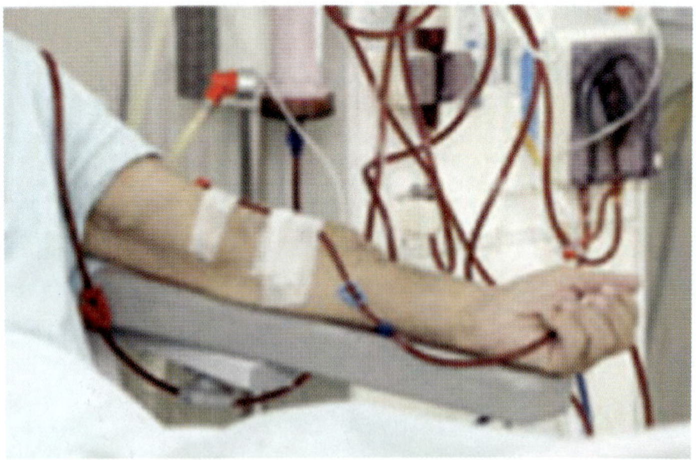

Fig. 39.54: *Photograph showing venovenous ultrafiltration technique, in patients with acute decompensated heart failure with worsening of kidney function, a condition referred to as acute cardiorenal syndrome (type 1). Diuretics are commonly used to treat persistent congestion in these patients, but these drugs might worsen kidney function. An alternative therapeutic approach is venovenous ultrafiltration, which can improve control over the rate and volume of fluid removal, increase net loss of sodium, and reduce neurohormonal activation*

genes, and upregulation of endothelin-A receptor and connective tissue growth factor genes.

Using beta-blockers to manage heart failure is a double-edged sword. The failing heart may be extremely dependent on adrenergic support to maintain circulation, and abrupt adrenergic removal may result in circulatory collapse. Beta-blockers are usually added to angiotensin-converting enzyme inhibitors and other decongestive measures if patient is clinically stable. The purpose of beta-blocker therapy is to slow the progression of the disease. Beta-blockers are not to be added as rescue drugs in patients who are decompensating. The improvement in ventricular function takes 2–3 months to develop. Before therapy is begun, patients should be informed that they may experience some worsening of symptoms for several weeks while the drug is titrated. The worsening of symptoms should be managed by adjusting the diuretics. Uptitration is performed each week and the dose is doubled until a target dosage is reached or until side effects appear.

Most important side effects are bradycardia and if some patients who are sensitive to bradycardia, low dose beta-blockers should be continued. If the patient on beta-blockers developed cardiogenic shock, then a phosphodiesterase type inotrope should be used rather than dobutamine as the beta-receptors are saturated. Beta-blockers reported to be more useful are carvedilol, metoprolol and bisoprolol. Pediatrics studies utilized carvedilol at initial dose of 0.1 milligram per kilogram body weight per day in two divided doses and increase the dose every 1–2 weeks up to a target dose of 0.8 milligram per kilogram body weight per day. Pediatric experience with metoprolol and bisoprolol is very limited.

Dosage

It decrease morbidity and mortality; carvedilol has vasodilatory, antioxidant, antiproliferative and antiapoptotic properties, reversing cardiac remodeling. Dosing is extrapolated from adult data, extreme caution should be used because there could be exacerbation of heart failure.

Metoprolol: 0.1 mg/kg dose BID up to max 1 mg/kg dose, carvedilol: 0.05 mg/kg/dose BID up to max 0.4 mg/kg/dose.

Nesiritide

Brain type natriuretic peptide acts by the guanylate cyclase-coupled natriuretic peptide receptor—a mechanism to produce beneficial, compensatory actions including diuresis, natriuresis, vasodilatation, and inhibition of both be useful in treating heart failure with pulmonary hypertension. In addition to its renal hemodynamic effects, natriuretic peptides have direct renal tubular actions by inhibiting angiotensin II-stimulated sodium and water transport in the proximal-convoluted tubules, and inhibiting water transport in the cortical collecting ducts, through its antagonistic action for vasopressin. Furthermore, brain type natriuretic peptide reduces plasma renin and aldosterone concentrations and inhibits angiotensin II stimulated aldosterone secretion. By these multiple actions brain type natriuretic peptide appears to have a significant role in protecting the heart against myocardial hypertrophy and subsequent interstitial fibrosis. Nesiritide is a recombinant human brain natriuretic peptide manufactured from E. coli with the same amino acid sequence as endogenous peptide. It is indicated for chronic decompensated heart failure. The dosing is currently recommended as a 2 microgram per kilogram bolus followed by a continuous infusion of 0.01–0.03 microgram per kilogram per minute. The dose may be adjusted by giving a 1 microgram per kilogram bolus and increasing the infusion by 0.005–0.01 microgram per kilogram per minute to a maximum of 0.03 microgram per kilogram per minute. Three hours time period is recommended between increasing the dose as 95% of the systemic blood pressure effect will be notable by then. The half life in patients with heart failure is approximately 18–20 minutes with the effect dissipating within 2–4 hours.

Calcium-Sensitizing Agents

Defective myocyte handling of calcium appears to be a central cause of both contractile dysfunction and arrhythmia development in heart failure. Levosimendan is a new class of calcium-sensitizing drug that directly sensitizes troponin C to calcium, thus improving myocardial contractility without causing an increase in myocardial oxygen demand. This sensitization is lost during diastole, allowing normal or improved diastolic function. Levosimendan also leads to vasodilatation through the opening of adenosine triphosphate-sensitive potassium channels. Usually, this is administered as a loading dose of 6–24 microgram per kilogram intravenously over 10 minutes followed by maintenance 0.05–0.2 microgram per kilogram per minute intravenous continuous infusion. Early experience of levosimendan in children after cardiac surgery or dilated cardiomyopathy indicates that it is well tolerated, but prospective studies are needed to evaluate the possible advantages of levosimendan over currently used vasoactive drugs. Pimobendan is another calcium sensitizing agent with higher phosphodiesterase inhibitory action and also inhibits the production of inflammatory cytokines.

Cytokine Antagonists

The current interest in understanding the role tissue necrotizing factor alpha in heart failure, relates to the observation that many aspects of the syndrome of heart failure can be explained by the known biologic effects of this cytokine. When expressed at sufficiently high concentration, tumor necrosis factor alpha mimics some aspects of the so called heart failure phenotype including (but not limited to) progressive left ventricular dysfunction, pulmonary edema, left ventricle remodeling, fetal gene expression and cardiomyopathy. Elevated levels of tumor necrosis factor alpha and other inflammatory cytokines have been associated with heart failure in children with congenital heart disease. Trials with etanercept, a soluble recombinantly produced chimeric tumor necrosis factor alpha antagonist and infliximab, a monoclonal antibody against tumor necrosis factor alpha are underway for treatment of heart failure in adults.

Coenzyme Q 10

Although coenzyme Q 10 (2, 3-dimethoxy-5-methyl-6-decaprenyl-1, 4-benzoquinone) has theoretical benefits to improve the energetics in failing myocardium by helping as an electron carrier in production of adenosine triphosphate, an antioxidant and free radical scavenger with membrane stabilizing properties, no beneficial effects of Coenzyme Q 10 supplementation on the left ventricular ejection fraction, peak oxygen consumption, or exercise duration are found by Khatta and co-workers. Therefore, Coenzyme Q 10 is not recommended at this time until large scale clinical trials have been performed.

Metabolic Therapy

The heart is able to utilize a variety of substrates for energy generation including carbohydrates (glucose and lactate), lipids (free fatty acids and triglycerides) and ketones. This allows a normal heart to maintain its functional performance in a wide range of physiological conditions without experiencing an energy debt. However, an energy deficit has been observed during the development of heart failure that directly relates to patient prognosis. Long-term follow-up studies in patients with idiopathic-dilated cardiomyopathy demonstrate that decreased phosphocreatinine (which is the source of increased phosphocreatinine (which is the source of instant adenosine triphosphate) is an independent predictor of mortality, suggesting that impaired myocardial energetics play an active role in the progression of heart failure. This notion is further supported by consistent observations in clinical trials revealing that energy-costly treatment such as positive inotropic agents (beta-receptor mimetic drugs, phosphodiesterase inhibitors) increase mortality while energy-sparing treatments (e.g. angiotensin-converting enzyme inhibitors, angiotensin II blockers, or beta-blockers) reduce mortality.

Carbohydrates are the primary substrates for fetal hearts, while fatty acids become the predominant fuel in adult hearts, supporting more than two-thirds of the total adenosine triphosphate synthesized. An important change in energy metabolism is observed in hypertrophied and failing heart; increasing reliance on carbohydrates while decreasing fatty acid utilization, an apparent reoccurrence of the fetal metabolic profile. Studies using animal model of heart failure reveal that this shift of substrate preference is associated with the down-regulation of peroxisome proliferator-activated receptor alpha, a transcriptor factor controlling the expression of key enzymes for fatty acid oxidation. Thus, peroxisome proliferator-activated receptor alpha is an attractive candidate for the development of novel and more potent pharmacologic agents that could prove useful in reactivating the normal energy production machinery in failing hearts in the setting of cardiomyopathy.

Ultrafiltration and Refractory Heart Failure (Fig. 39.54)

In ultrafiltration, blood is removed from the body and run through a device that applies hydrostatic pressure across a semipermeable membrane to separate isotonic plasma water. Solutes cross the semipermeable membrane freely, so fluid can be removed without causing significant changes in the concentration of electrolytes and other solutes in serum.

Ultrafiltration was shown to be an effective alternative to intravenous diuretics in the ultrafiltration versus intravenous (IV) diuretics for patients hospitalized for acute decompensated heart failure (UNLOAD) trial. The ACC/AHA and ESC recommend the use of ultrafiltration for fluid reduction for patients with refractory heart failure that is not responsive to medical therapy.

BIBLIOGRAPHY

1. Rajagopal SK, Yarlagadda VV, Thiagarajan RR, Singh TP, Givertz MM, Almond CS. Pediatric heart failure and worsening renal function: Association with outcomes after heart transplantation. J Heart Lung Transplant. Oct 18 2011;
2. Talner N. Heart failure. Heart Disease in Infants, Children, and Adolescents. 1995:1746–73.
3. Kaza AK, Colan SD, Jaggers J, Lu M, Atz AM, Sleeper LA, et al. Surgical interventions for atrioventricular septal defect subtypes: the pediatric heart network experience. Ann Thorac Surg. Oct 2011;92(4):1468–75.
4. Erickson LC. Medical issues for the cardiac patient. Critical Care of Infants and Children. 1996:259–62.
5. [Best Evidence] Frobel AK, Hulpke-Wette M, Schmidt KG, Läer S. Beta-blockers for congestive heart failure in children. Cochrane Database Syst Rev. Jan 21 2009;CD007037.
6. Behera SK, Zuccaro JC, Wetzel GT, Alejos JC. Nesiritide improves hemodynamics in children with dilated cardiomyopathy: a pilot study. Pediatr Cardiol. Jan 2009;30(1):26–34.
7. Jefferies JL, Price JF, Denfield SW, Chang AC, Dreyer WJ, McMahon CJ, et al. Safety and efficacy of nesiritide in pediatric heart failure. J Card Fail. Sep 2007;13(7):541–8.
8. Mehra MR. Optimizing outcomes in the patient with acute decompensated heart failure. Am Heart J. Mar 2006;151(3): 571–9.
9. Konstam MA, Neaton JD, Poole-Wilson PA, Pitt B, Segal R, Sharma D, et al. Comparison of losartan and captopril on heart failure-related outcomes and symptoms from the losartan heart failure survival study (ELITE II). Am Heart J. Jul 2005;150(1):123–31.
10. Rosenthal D, Chrisant MR, Edens E, Mahony L, Canter C, Colan S, et al. International Society for Heart and Lung Transplantation: Practice guidelines for management of heart failure in children. J Heart Lung Transplant. Dec 2004;23(12): 1313–33.
11. Cvelich RG, Roberts SC, Brown JN. Phosphodiesterase type 5 inhibitors as adjunctive therapy in the management of systolic heart failure. Ann Pharmacother. Dec 2011;45(12): 1551–8.
12. Pitt B, Zannad F, Remme WJ, Cody R, et al. The effect of spironolactone on morbidity and mortality in patients with severe heart failure. Randomized aldactone evaluation study investigators. N Engl J Med. Sep 2 1999;341(10):709–17.

13. Pitt B, Remme W, Zannad F, et al. Eplerenone, a selective aldosterone blocker, in patients with left ventricular dysfunction after myocardial infarction. N Engl J Med. Apr 3 2003;348(14):1309–21.
14. Pitt B, Zannad F, Remme WJ, Cody R, Castaigne A, Perez A, et al. The effect of spironolactone on morbidity and mortality in patients with severe heart failure. Randomized Aldactone evaluation study investigators. N Engl J Med. Sep 2 1999; 341(10):709–17.
15. Packer M, Colucci WS, Sackner-Bernstein JD, Liang CS, Goldscher DA, Freeman I, et al. Double-blind, placebo-controlled study of the effects of carvedilol in patients with moderate to severe heart failure. The PRECISE Trial. Prospective Randomized Evaluation of Carvedilol on Symptoms and Exercise. Circulation. Dec 1 1996;94(11):2793–9.
16. Blume ED, Canter CE, Spicer R, Gauvreau K, Colan S, Jenkins KJ. Prospective single-arm protocol of carvedilol in children with ventricular dysfunction. Pediatr Cardiol. May-Jun 2006;27(3):336–42.
17. Shaddy RE, Boucek MM, Hsu DT, Boucek RJ, Canter CE, Mahony L, et al. Carvedilol for children and adolescents with heart failure: a randomized controlled trial. JAMA. Sep 12 2007;298(10):1171–9.
18. [Best Evidence] McAlister FA, Ezekowitz J, Hooton N, Vandermeer B, Spooner C, Dryden DM, et al. Cardiac resynchronization therapy for patients with left ventricular systolic dysfunction: a systematic review. JAMA. Jun 13 2007;297(22):2502–14.
19. Janousek J, Gebauer RA. Cardiac resynchronization therapy in pediatric and congenital heart disease. Pacing Clin Electrophysiol. Feb 2008;31 Suppl 1:S21–3.
20. van der Hulst AE, Delgado V, Blom NA, et al. Cardiac resynchronization therapy in paediatric and congenital heart disease patients. Eur Heart J. Sep 2011;32(18):2236–46.
21. Beiras-Fernandez A, Deutsch MA, Kainzinger S, Kaczmarek I, Sodian R, Ueberfuhr P, et al. Extracorporeal membrane oxygenation in 108 patients with low cardiac output – a single-center experience. Int J Artif Organs. Apr 2011;34(4): 365–73.

40 Cardiac Arrhythmia in Children and Adolescents

The child with arrhythmia, or an irregular fast or slow heart rate, affects approximately 1 in 250–1,000 children and adolescents each year, is a common problem that has numerous etiologies ranging from normal benign variants to malignant arrhythmias. Determining the underlying cause of an irregular rhythm is important, as it may be a life-threatening or serious condition. In the majority of children, the cause of an irregular heart rate is identified by an in-depth history and physical examination, and electrocardiogram, which can be completed by the primary clinician. In some cases, referral to a pediatric cardiologist is required for further diagnostic work-up and if necessary, treatment.

Arrhythmias may be defined as a disturbance in either the formation of impulse or its transmission through various pathways of conduction or through both the combinations. The term sinus arrhythmia is a misnomer as the phenomenon is only an exaggeration of the normal and the impulse arises normally at the S-A node. Similarly, the term nodal rhythm is misleading as this does not mean that

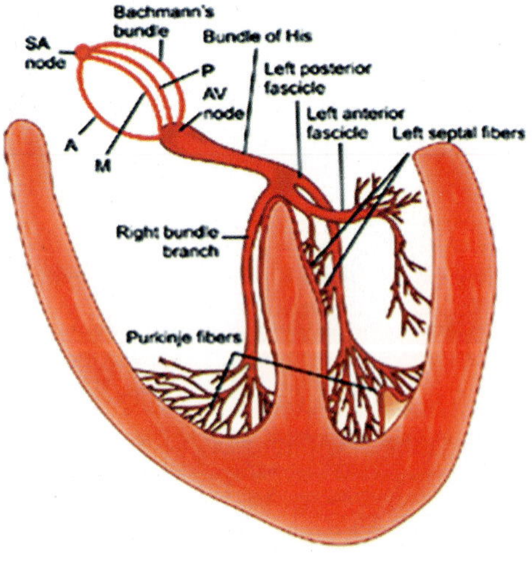

Fig. 40.2: *Diagramatic depiction of different structures of conducting system in human as indicated on the diagram*

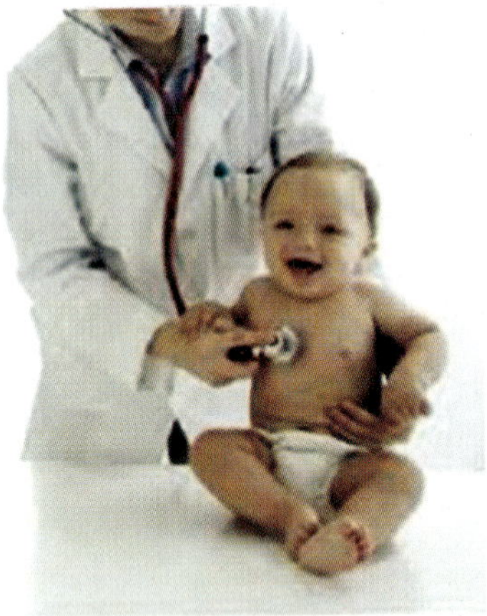

Fig. 40.1: *A doctor is conducting physical examination of a child with cardiac arrhythmia*

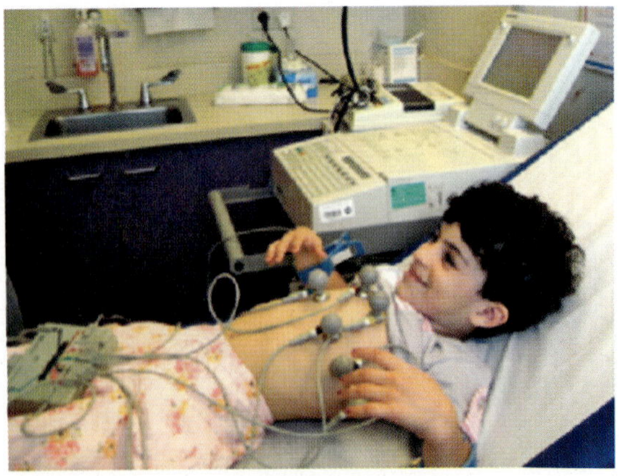

Fig. 40.3: *Electrocardiographic equipment along with precardial leads over the chest of a child prior to obtaining an electrocardiogram*

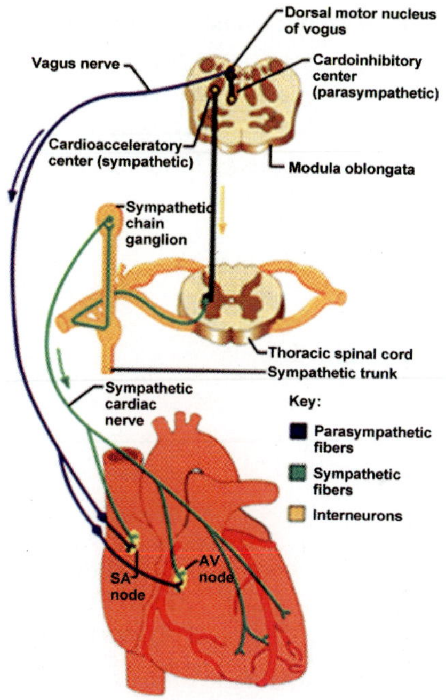

Fig. 40.4: *Autonomic innervation of the heart*

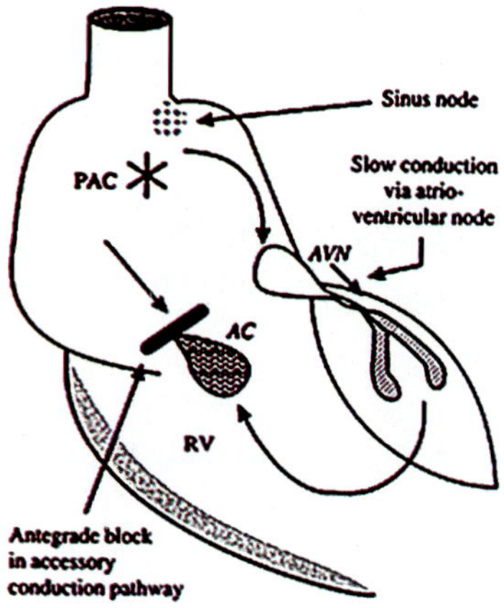

Fig. 40.5: Schematic diagram of the cardiac conduction system in a patient with an accessory conduction (AC) pathway. A premature atrial contraction (PAC) has occurred with a critical coupling interval that is shorter than the antegrade effective refractory period in the accessory connection pathway. The impulse encounters the atrioventricular node (AVN) after its shorter refractory period. The impulse conducts slowly through the AVN and the ventricular muscle, then encounters the accessory conduction pathway in the retrograde direction, after a significant time delay. RV, right ventricle. (Kleinman CS, Copel JC: Electrophysiologic principles and antiarrhythmic therapy. Ultrasound Obstet Gynecol 1:286, 1991.)

Table 40.1: *Differentiate diagnosis in bradyarrhythmias (ventricular rate less than 60)*

Nature of defect	*Ventricular*	*A-V relationship*	*Atrial rate*	*Additional clues*
1. Sinus bradycardia	Less than 60	Normal (1:1)	Less than 60	May be sinus arrhythmia
2. Sinus arrest	Less than 60	May be nodal or ventricular	Less than 60; abrupt halving of atrial rate	none
3. AV-nodal rhythm	Less than 60	Short P-R or P wave buried in QRS or superimposed on S-T segment	Less than 60	Normal QRS complexes-P waves may be hard to see
4. Wenekebach block	Less than atrial rate	P-R interval lengthens with successive beats until QRS is is dropped. The cycle is repeated	Normal; usually over 60	QRS complexes often in pairs or triplets
5. Second degreee block	Usually 30–50; (1/2, 1/3)	2:1 AV block or greater (3:1, 4:1, etc.)	Normal; usually over 60	P waves never occur in QRS complexes
6. Third degree (complete block)	Regular 30–50 (no P-QRS relationship)	A-V dissociation	Normal; usually over 60	P waves from time to time in QRS complexes

Table 40.2: *Initial categorization of tachycardiac rhythms using the 12-lead electrocardiogram*

Rhythm	*Narrow*	*Wide*
Regular	Short-RP Typical (slow-fast) AVNRT Atypical (slow-slow) AVNRT (usually) Orthodromic, AVRT JT AT (less commonly) Long-RP Atypical (fast-slow) AVNRT Orthodromic AVRT (slowly conducting accessory pathway) ST AT (more commonly) PJRT Flutter waves AFI (fixed AV block)	ST, JT, AT, AVNRT, orthodromic AVRT, or AFI with aberrancy Antidromic AVRT Monomorphic ventricular tachycardia
Irregular	AF AFI (variable AV block) MAT	AF, AFI or MAT with aberrancy AF, AFI with preexcitation Polymorphic ventricular tachycardia

Abbreviations: AF, atrial fibrillation: AFI, atrial flutter; AT, atrial tachycardia; AVNRT, antriventricular node reentrant tachycardia; AVRT, atrioventricular reentrant tachycardia; JT, junction tachycardia; MAT, multifocal atrial tachycardia; PJRT, permanent junctinoal reciprocating tachycardia; ST, sinus tachycardia.

Table 40.3: *Characteristics of atrial tachyarrhythmias. A brief guide to help determine the nature of atrial arrhythmias (narrow complex tachycardia, unless there is associated bundle-branch block)*

Cause of atrial arryhthmia	*P-wave characteristics arryhthmia*	*Approximate atrial rate*	*Approximate ventricular rate*	*Ventricular rhythm*
Sinus tachycardia	Normal shape and size; 1:1 correspondance with ventricular complex, normal PR interval, P wave can merge with T waves if very fast	100–200	100–200	Regular
Other atrial tachycardia	P waves likely to be abnormally shaped with PR interval possibly abnormal	100–250	Variable depending on degree of ventricular capture	Usually regular
Atrial flutter	P waves absent; saw-tooth F waves visible at rate of ~300	250–350	Usually ~150 or ~75 (2:1 and 4:1 conduction of atrial impulses respectively	Regular
Atrial fibrillation	No P waves, fibrillating chaotic F waves around the baseline	350–600 (or no regular pattern discernible)	100–180	Irregular; R-R interval constantly varies, as does size of QRS complexes

the impulse arises at the S-A node. It has now been replaced by the term A-V junctional rhythm.

Genesis of Cardiac Dysarrhythmia (Figs 40.2, 40.4–40.6)

It can be caused either by the disturbance of impulse formation or impulse conduction or both.

Disturbance of impulse formation: Disturbance of cardiac impulse formation may lead to the common type of cardiac arrhythmia, called ectopic rhythm. Ectopic rhythms are of two types, either escape beats and escape rhythms or extra systoles and ectopic tachycardias. An escape beat appears when there is a pause in the existing rhythm, and it is, thus always late in appearance and never premature. If the sinus node fails for a long period, repeated escape beats will occur, giving a characteristically slow escape rhythm. The commonest site of escape rhythm is the A-V junction Extrasystoles and ectopic rhythms arise from foci in the specialized conducting tissue, which have been well-defined in the intranodal tracts of the atria. If the extra-systole or tachycardia is above the bifurcation of the bundle of His, it is termed as A-V junctional.

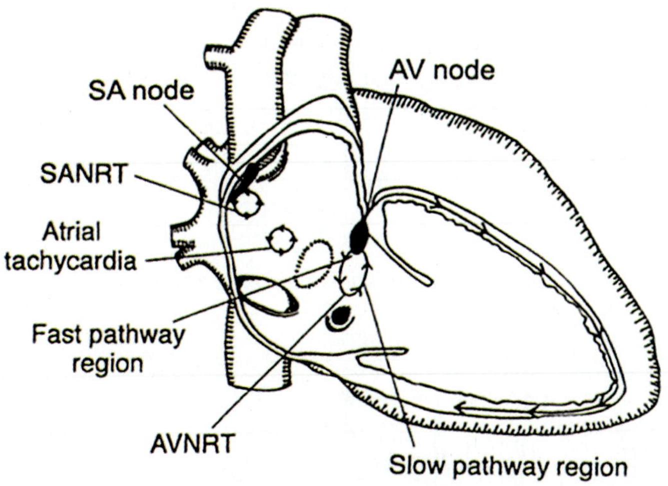

Fig. 40.6: *Diagram possible origins of tachycardia*

Classification of Cardiac Arrhythmias

Anatomically, the dysrhythmias may be classified according to the site of origin of the impulse. Given below given is a simple and workable classification of cardiac arrhythmias:

Site of origin and type of dysrhythmia:

1. **Sinuatrial node** (Figs 40.7–40.21)
   i. Sinus tachycardia
   ii. Sinus bradycardia
   iii. Sinus arrhythmia
   iv. S-A arrest of block
   v. Wandering pacemaker (Fig. 40.14)
   vi. Sinu extrasystoles.
2. **Atria**
   i. Atrial extrasystoles
   ii. Atrial tachycardia
   iii. Atrial flutter (Fig. 40.26)
   iv. Atrial fibrillation (Fig. 40.25)
   v. Chaotic atrial rhythm (Fig. 40.34)
   vi. Atrial standstill
3. **Atrioventricular junction** (Fig. 40.31)
   i. A-V junctional extrasystoles
   ii. A-V junctional tachycardia
   iii. A-V junctional rhythm
   iv. Heart block-first, second and third degree
4. **Ventricles**
   i. Bundle-branch block
   ii. Ventricular extrasystoles
   iii. Ventricular tachycardia
   iv. Ventricular flutter and fibrillation
   v. Ventricular standstill.

It has been, frequently, observed that most of the arrhythmias are transient and may be of only a few seconds duration. It is in that brief period, if the ECG is taken, that a particular type of arrhythmia could be found out, otherwise, in majority of the patients, it could be missed. This problem has been overcome by frequent use of the Holter monitoring system which can detect cardiac arrhythmia, not only being present for a shorter period, but can also provide useful therapeutic guidelines for its final management.

Table 40.4: *P wave morphology in atrial tachycardia–general principles*

Location		*P wave polarity during atrial tachycardia*	
Right atrium	+ or ± in aVL and – in VI	Crista terminalis (CT)	May be +, ±, or – in II, III, aVF in the high, mid and inferior CT, respectively; – or ± in VI; – in aVR
		Tricuspid annulus	– in V1–V2; + in aVL and frequently in 1
		Right atrial appendage	Insufficient data
Left atrium	– in aVL and + in VI	Right pulmonary veins	+ in V1–V6; + in 1: narrow P wave in VI
		Left pulmonary veins	+ in V1–V6; – /isoelectric in aVL; broad or notched P wave in V1
		Mitral annulus	± with initially narrow negative deflection in V1; –/isoelectric in 1 aVL; slightly +/isoelectric in II, III, aVF
		Left atrial appendage	Broadly + in V1–V6; – in 1, aVL; + in II, III, aVF
Interatrial spetum and	Specific to location	Coronary sinus ostium	+ in V1; isoelectric in I: – in II, III, aVF; + in aVL, aVR
		Snteroseptum	–/± in V1; +/± in II, III aVF
		Mid septum	–/± in V1; – in two of three inferior leads (II, III, aVF)
		Left septum	Uncommon; variable findings

Abbreviations: +, positive; –, negative; ±, biphasic

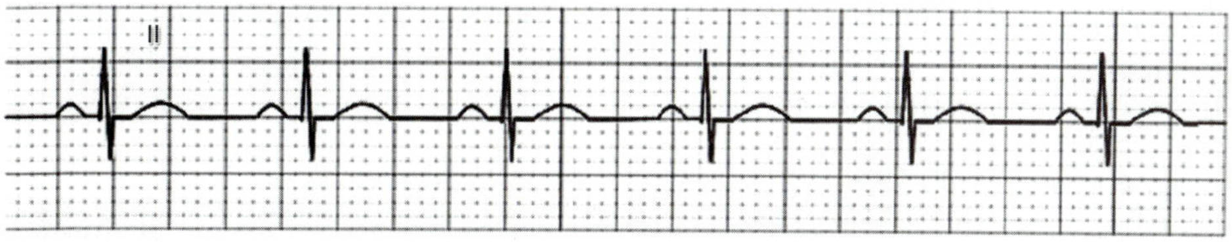

Fig. 40.7: *ECG showing sinus rhythm: each narrow complex is preceded by a normal P wave in lead II*

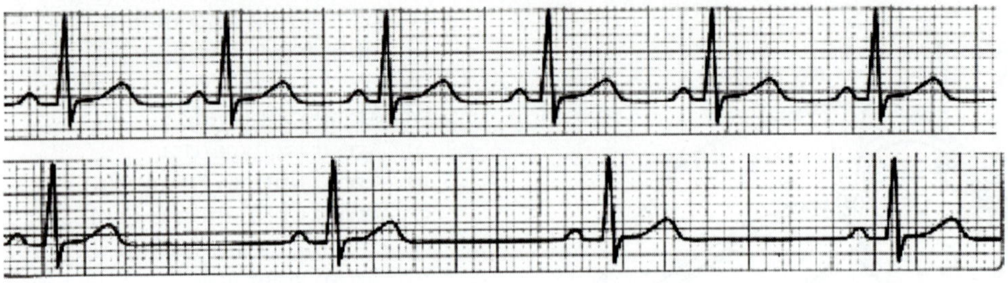

Fig. 40.8: *The EKG on the top shows normal sinus rhythm. The EKG at the bottom shows sinus bradycardia*

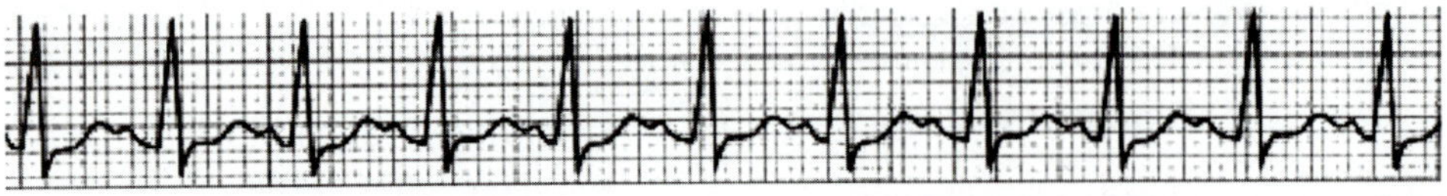

Fig. 40.9: *The EKG at the bottom shows sinus tachycardia*

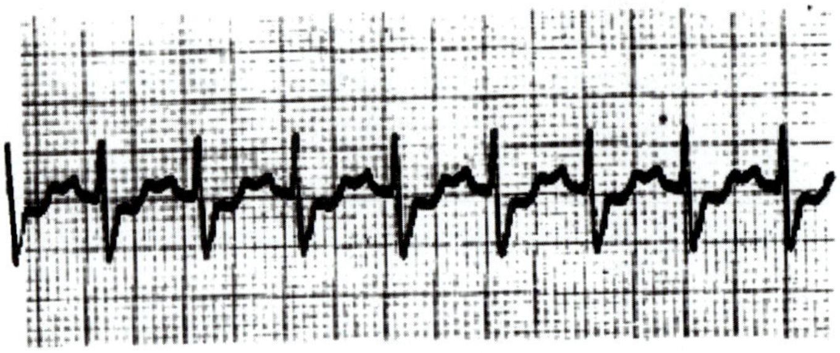

Fig. 40.10: *ECG showing paroxysmal sinus tachycardia*

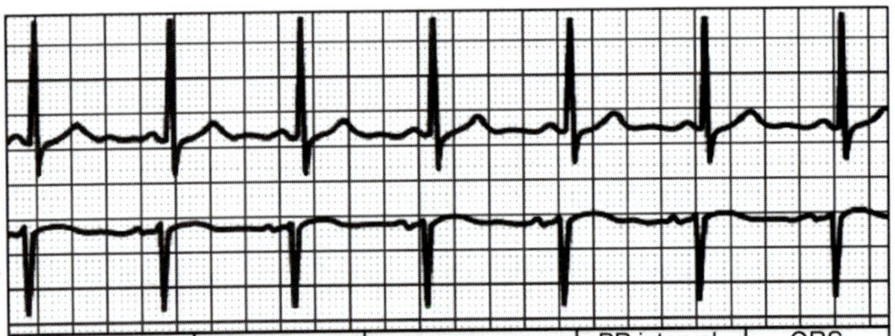

Heart rate	Rhythm	P wave	PR interval (in seconds)	QRS (in seconds)
60-100 bpm	Regular	Before each QRS, identical	.12 to .20	<.12

Fig. 40.11: *ECG showing normal rhythm strip in lead II and V1*

The arrhythmias, which originate in the sinus (or sinoatrial SA) node, are classified as sinus tachycardia, sinus bradycardia, sinus arrhythmia, SA block, SA nodal reentry, sick sinus syndrome, and sinus arrest. In all these conditions, the sinus node is the pacemaker of the heart, though its rate may be too fast, too slow, irregular, or inconsistent.

Sinus Tachycardia (Figs 40.10 and 40.13)

In a patient with sinus tachycardia, there is regular sinus rhythm of more than 100 beats/min. It can be considered as one of the first signs of congestive heart failure, cardiogenic shock, pulmonary embolism, or infarct extension.

ECG Characteristics

1. Rate : 100 beats/min
2. Rhythm : Regular
3. PR interval : Normal, although the PR may be too long or too short because of other conditions. All the P waves have the same shape and are upright in leads I, II, aVF, and V_4 to V_6
4. QRS complex : Normal but may be prolonged due to other associated conditions.

Causes

1. **Drug**
   (i) atropine, (ii) isoproterenol (isuprel), (iii) quinidine, (iv) epinephrine (adrenalin)
2. Exercise, emotions, fever or pain
3. Hyperthyroidism
4. Conditions involving increased sympathetic stimulation.

Sinus tachycardias vary only if they are part of a bradycardia-tachycardia syndrome or because of associated conditions, such as AV block, bundle-branch block, PVCs, or PACs.

The diagnosis of sinus tachycardia is always made by identifying uniform P wave with regular rhythm.

Treatment

The basic treatment is of the underlying cause. Beta-blockers will slow down the rate. Sinus tachycardia caused by thyrotoxicosis will respond to beta-blockers; on the other hand. Sinus tachycardia resulting from left ventricular dysfunction, usually, should not be treated with beta-blockers as these drugs may precipitate heart failure.

Sinus Bradycardia

Sinus bradycardia can be diagnosed both clinically and electrocardiographically when the peripheral pulse is of regular rhythm with heart rate less than 60 beats/min, and has regular sinus rhythm character.

ECG Characteristics

1. Rate : 60 beats/min
2. Rhythm : Regular
3. PR interval : Normal, although the PR may be too long or too short because of other conditions. All the P waves have the same shape and are upright in leads I, II, aVF, and V_4 to V_6
4. QRS complex : Normal, although the QRS may be prolonged as a result of other associated conditions.

Causes:

1. During fast sleep
2. Cardiac response in atheletes
3. Increased vagal tone
4. Therapy with bata-adrenergic drugs

Sinus bradycardias vary only if they are part of a bradycardia-tachycardia or because of associated conditions, such as AV block, bundle-branch block, PVCs or PACs. The diagnosis of sinus bradycardia is always established by looking at the underlying rhythm.

Treatment

It is treated only if the patient is symptomatic or if the condition is associated with haemodynamic deterioration and marked decrease in cardiac output. Acute treatment

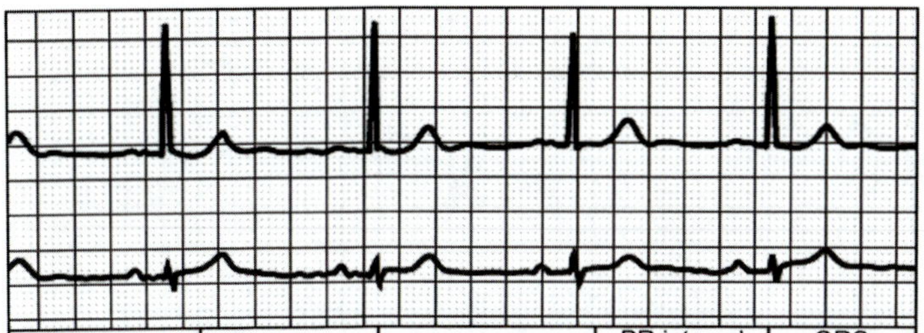

Heart rate	Rhythm	P wave	PR interval (in seconds)	QRS (in seconds)
< 60 bpm	Regular	Before each QRS, identical	.12 to .20	<.12

Fig. 40.12: *ECG showing sinus bradycardia*

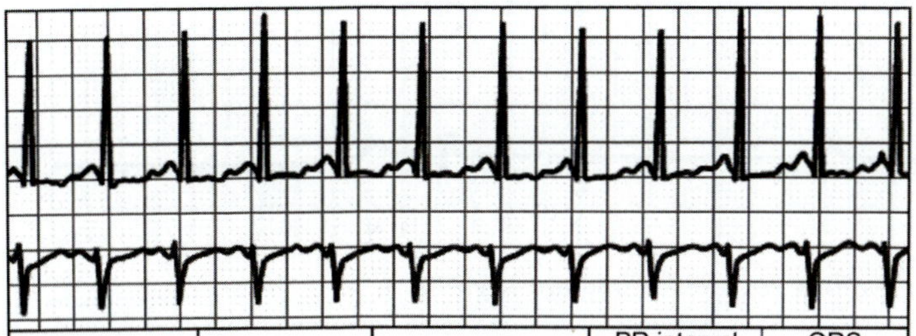

Heart rate	Rhythm	P wave	PR interval (in seconds)	QRS (in seconds)
> 100 bpm	Regular	Before each QRS, identical	.12 to .20	<.12

Fig. 40.13: *ECG showing sinus tachycardia*

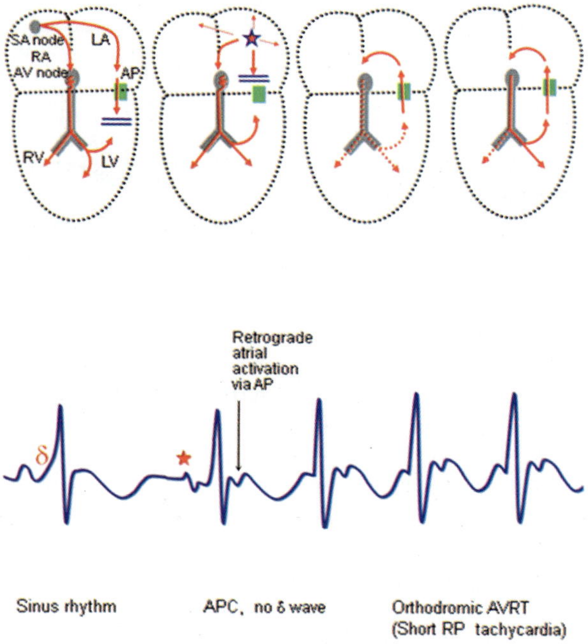

Fig. 40.14: *Orthodromic AV reciprocating tachycardia in a patient with left-sided AP*

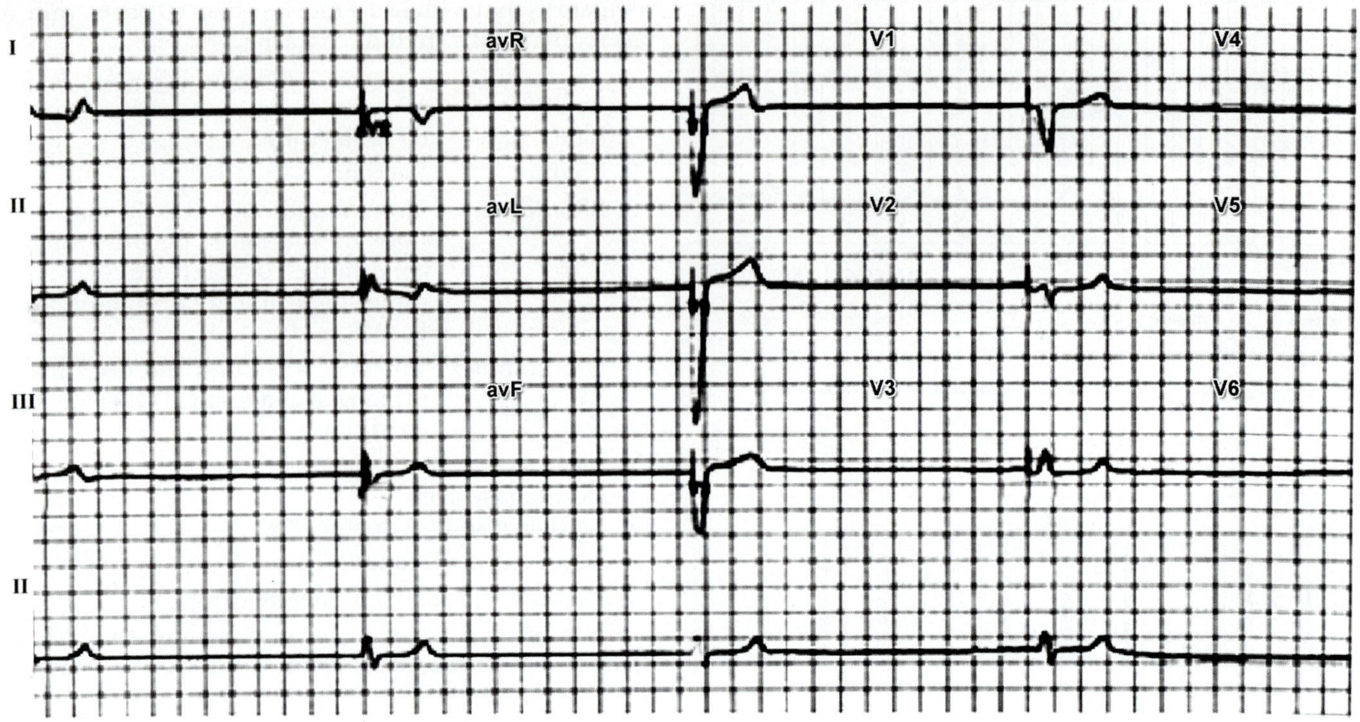

Fig. 40.15: *ECG showing sinus arrest with a ventricular escape rhythm*

in the sick sinus syndrome includes 0.5 mg of atropine sulfate I/v, administered every 5 minutes until the desired response is achieved or a 2 mg total does has been employed. If this is unsuccessful, isoproterenol may be administered in infusion form, which is monitored according to heart and response. These patients do need permanent pacemaker implantation in case where stokes-adams attacks are manifested frequently.

Sinus Arrhythmia

Sinus arrhythmia can be diagnosed by an irregular sinus rhythm in which the cycles lengths vary so that the difference between the shortest PP interval and the longest PP interval is 0.12 sec.

ECG Characteristics

1. Rate : It varies with respiration: Faster with inspiration-slower with expiration
2. Rhythm : Irregular
3. PR interval : Normal, although the PR may be too long or too short because of other conditions. All the P waves have the same shape and are upright in leads. I,II, aVF, and $V_4$to V_6
4. QRS complex : Normal, although the QRS may be prolonged as a result of other conditions.

It can be isolated from other conditions by the presence of varying rate, cyclical, irregular rhythm, and uniform shape of the P waves.

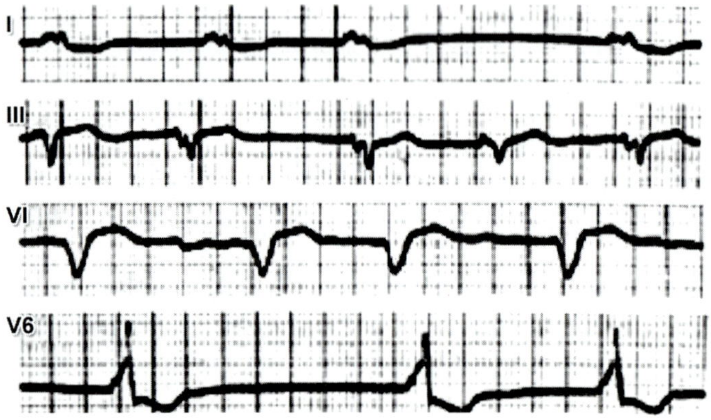

Fig. 40.16: *ECG trace shows sick sinus syndrome with A-V nodal rhythm with retrograde conduction at rate 31 beats/min*

Causes

Normal respiratory pattern

Sinus arrhythmia can be differentiated from SA nodal re-entry due to the presence of transition with abrupt faster rate which is, usually, not related to respiration although P waves may remain of similar morphology in both the conditions.

SA Block

SA block is characterized by the absence of P waves, intermittently, due to incomplete conduction of sinus P waves as they emerge from the sinus pacemaker.

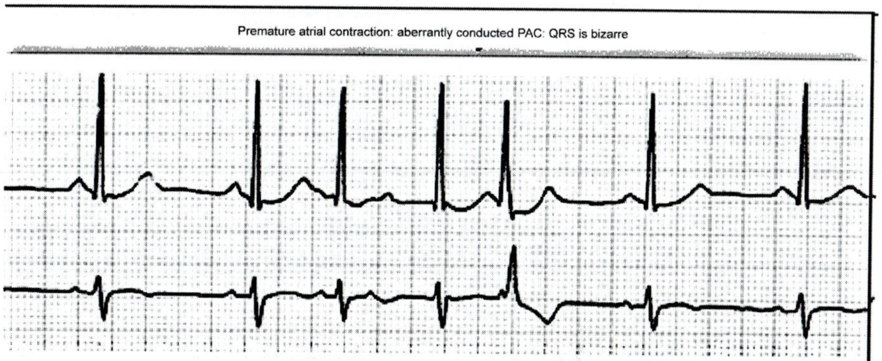

Heart rate	Rhythm	P wave	PR interval (in seconds)	QRS (in seconds)
N/A	Irregular	Premature and abnormal or hidden	<.20	<.12 abnormal shape

Fig. 40.17: *ECG showing PAC with RBBB aberrant conduction*

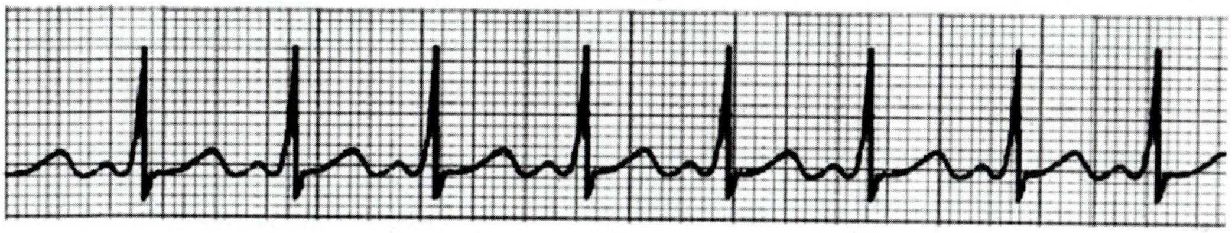

Fig. 40.18: *The EKG shows delta wave in ascending limb of QRS in Wolff-Parkinson-White syndrome*

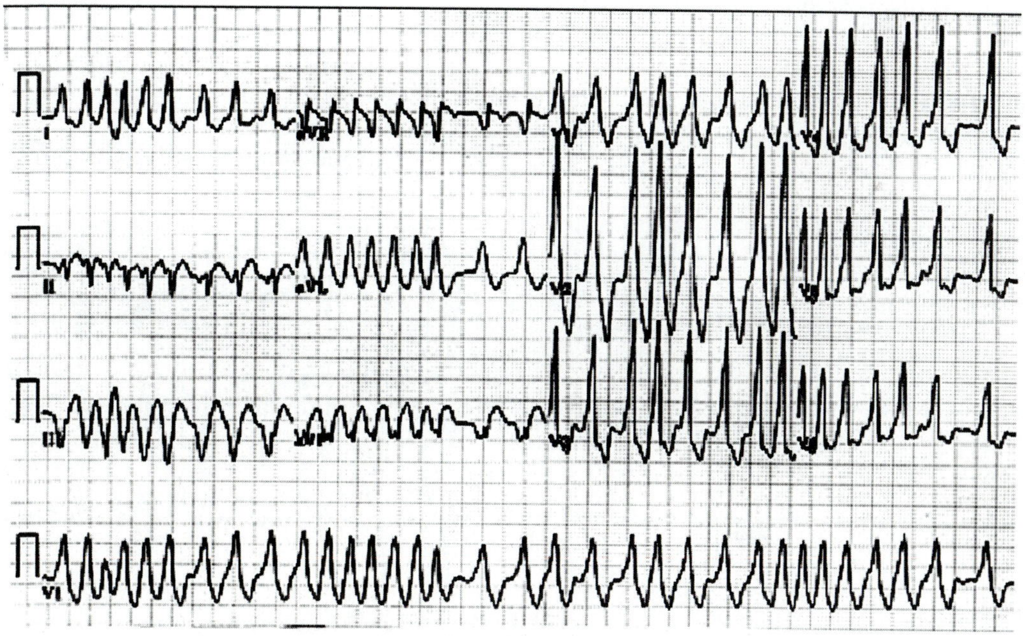

Fig. 40.19: *ECG shows aberrant conduction through AV pathways*

ECG Characteristics

1. Rate : Normal, but varies because of pauses.
2. Rhythm : Irregular
3. PR interval : Normal, although the PR may too long or too short because of other conditions. All the P waves have the same shape

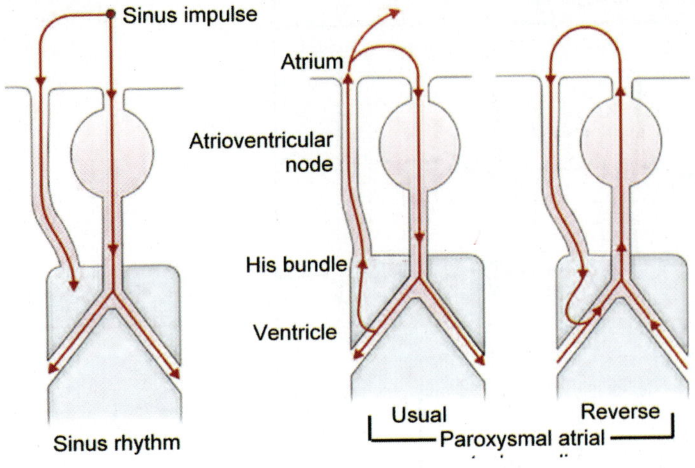

Fig. 40.20: *Normal conduction system and the accessary atrioventricular connection showing the conduction sequence during sinus rhythm in the left hand panel and during tachycardia in the middle and right hand panels*

and upright in leads I,II, aVF, and V_4 to V_6

4. QRS complex : Normal, although the QRS may be prolonged as a result of other conditions.

Causes

1. Acute infection
2. Digitalis, quinidine, or salicylates
3. Carotid sinus sensitivity and increased vagal tone.
4. Coronary artery disease.

Distinguishing Features

Type-I (Wenchebach) SA block: PP intervals shorten until a P wave is dropped; pauses are less than twice the shortest cycle.

Type-II SA block: PP intervals are an exact multiple of the sinus cycle and are regular before and after the dropped P wave.

Differential Diagnosis

Nonconducted PACs are far more common and should be suspected first, Usually, the P wave can be seen distorting the T wave before the pause. The diagnosis of sinus arrest can be made after ruling out nonconducted PACs and SA block.

Sinus Arrest

Sinus arrest may be defined as that condition in which the sinus impulses are not generated with the result that one may find occasional absent P waves. In case this type of rhythm persists, it may lead to atrial standstill.

ECG Characteristics

1. Rate : Normal, but varies because of pauses.
2. Rhythm : Irregular
3. PR interval : Normal, althought the PR may be too long or too short as a result of other conditions. All the P waves have the same shape and are upright in leads I, II, aVF, and V_4 to V_6
4. QRS complex : Normal, although the QRS may be prolonged. Because of other conditions.
5. Distinguishing features : Abrupt interruption of the sinus rhythm. PP interval of the pause is not a multiple of the sinus cycle.

Causes

1. Digitalis, quinidine or salicylates
2. Coronary artery disease
3. Acute infection
4. Carotid sinus sensitivity and increased vagal tone.

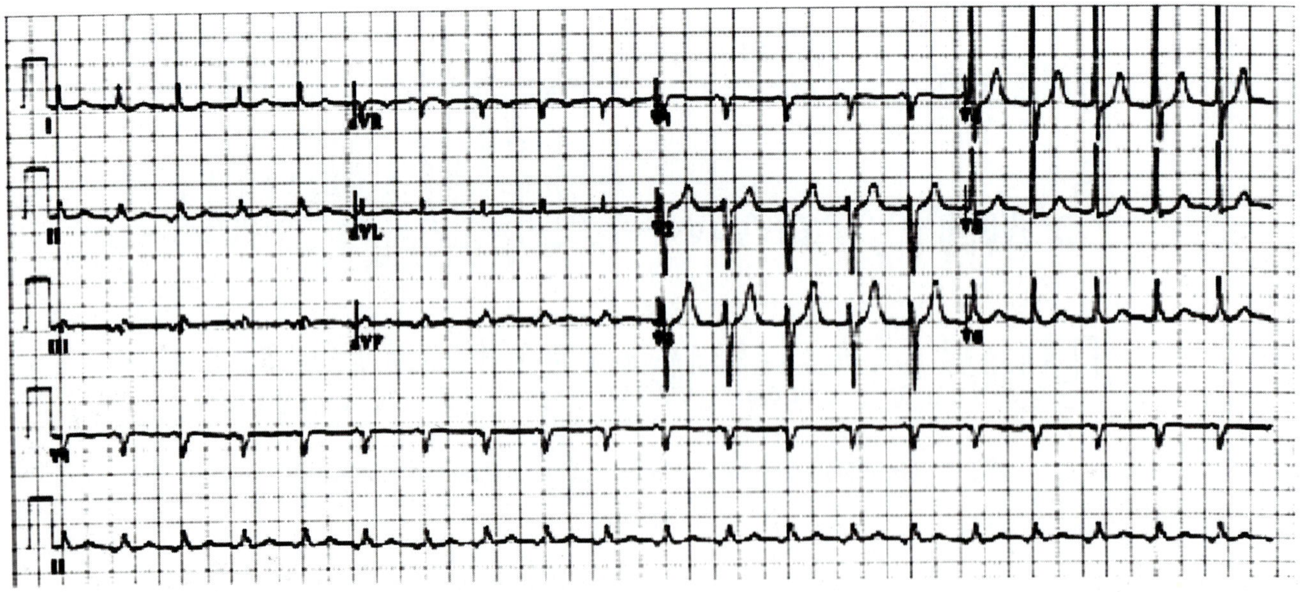

Fig. 40.21: *ECG trace showing ectopic atrial tachycardia: there is a narrow complex tachycardia at 120 bpm. Each QRS complex is preceded by an abnormal P wave-upright in V1, inverted in the inferior leads II, III and aVF*

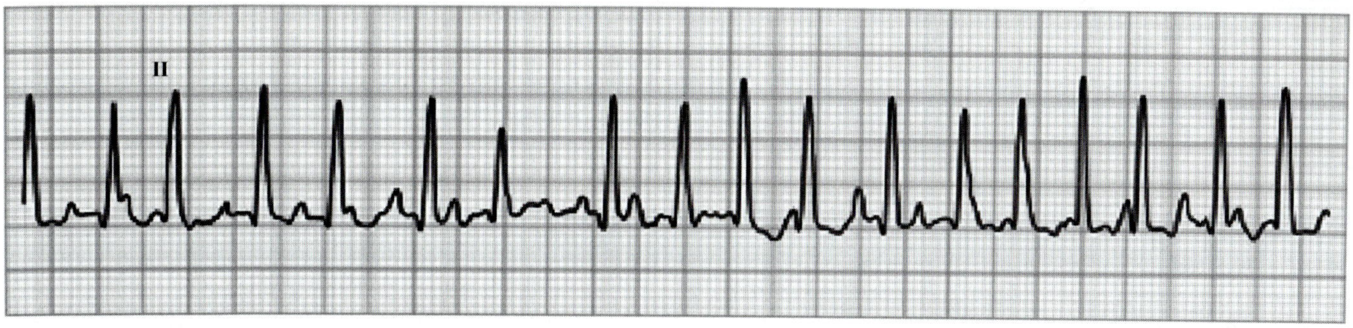

Fig. 40.22: *ECG showing multifocal atrial tachycardia in lead II*

Differential Diagnosis

Nonconducted PACs are far common and are always suspected first. Usually, the P wave can be seen distorting the T wave before the pause. The diagnosis of sinus arrest can be made after ruling out nonconducted PACs and SA block.

Sick Sinus Syndrome

Sick sinus syndrome may be defined clinically by the presence of near syncope, syncope, convulsions, fatigue, angina pectoris and other symptoms of hypoperfusion of the brain and electrocardiographic manifestations of bradycardia and tachycardia along with other features of cardiac arrhythmia due to sinus node dysfunction and failure of an adequate escape pacemaker.

ECG Characteristics

1. Rate : Too fast or too slow
2. Rhythm : Irregular
3. PR interval : May be abnormal
4. QRS complex : Normal, although the QRS may be prolonged because of other conditions.

Distinguishing features: Any of the following arrhythmias may be present and associated with syncope:

a. Severe sinus bradycardia
b. Sinu arrest
c. Atrial stand still
d. SA block
e. Sinus bradycardia with recurring atrial fibrillation
f. Bradycardia-tachycardia
g. Temporary asystole following tachycardia or following electrical cardioversion of atrial tachyarrhythmia
h. Paroxysmal atrial fibrillation
i. Failure of the sinus node to accelerate in response to fever or exercise.

Causes

1. Ischaemic disease due to obstructive blood supply to the sinus node
2. Inflammatory disease of sinus node
3. Amyloidosis: Infilteration of the sinus node with amlyoid material
4. Collagen disease
5. Metastatic disease
6. Surgical injury
7. Idiopathic.

Variations

There are many variations among which are:

a. SSS with type II second-degree SA block
b. SSS in the form of a bradycardia-tachycardia syndrome
c. SSS with inappropriate overdrive suppression following an early PAC (in the T wave before the pause).

Treatment

Before a pacemaker is inserted, ensure that no drugs have been given at all for several days. The arrhythmia may be drug related.

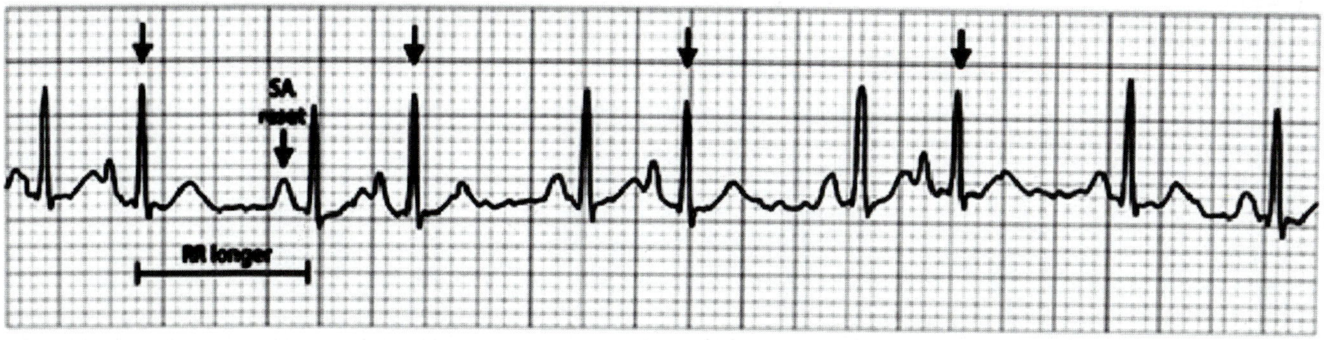

Fig. 40.23: *This rhythm strip displays the typical pattern of frequent PACs (arrows) separated by post-extrasystolic pauses*

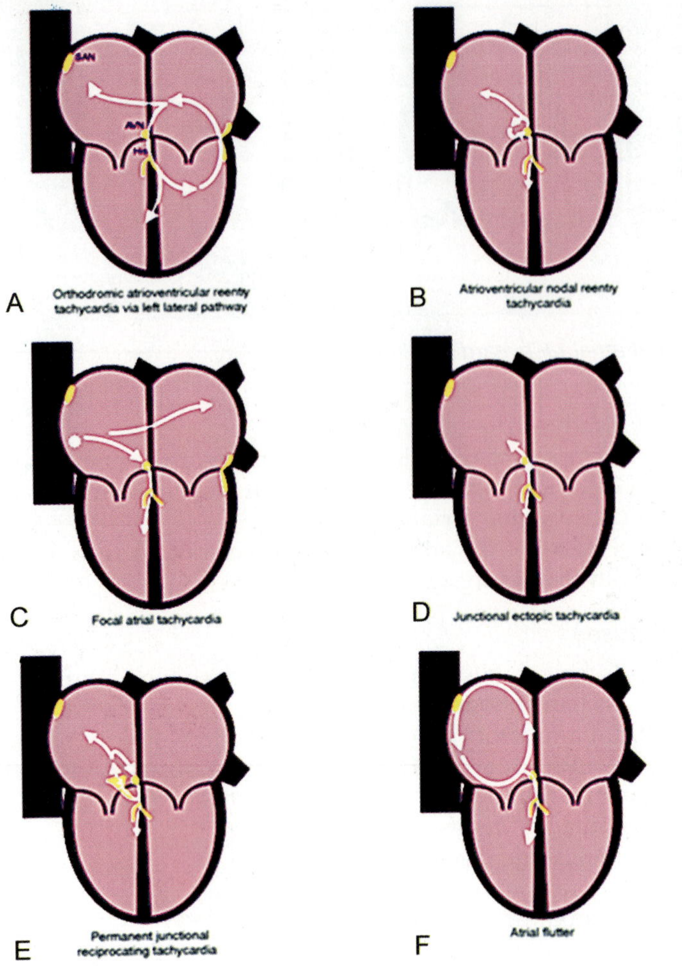

Fig. 40.24: *Different sites, origin and spread of abnormal impulse along the aberrant pathways of conduction in the genesis of different kinds of cardiac arrhythmia*

Paroxysmal Sinus Tachycardia Resulting from Nodal Reentry

Paroxysmal sinus tachycardia is the sudden onset of the sinus tachycardia.

ECG Characteristics

1. Rate : Too fast
2. Rhythm : Irregular
3. PR interval : Normal although the PR may be too long or too short because of other conditions. All the P waves have the same shape and are upright in leads I, II, aVF, and V_4 to V_6
4. QRS complex : Normal, although the QRS may be prolonged as a result of other conditions.
5. Distinguishing features:
   a. Heart rate suddenly accelerates; tachycardia ends abruptly
   b. Rhythm of the tachycardia, usually, regular
   c. Normal sinus P waves.

Causes

a. Ischaemia
b. Cardiomyopathy.

Differential Diagnosis

Sinus arrhythmia.

Treatment

Short paroxysms may require no treatment.

1. Termination may often be achieved by vagal manoeuvres, but carotra artery message should not be advised in patients with or at risk for carotid artery disease
2. Intravenous verapamil is considered by some to be treatment of choice, but should be used cautiously in those patients who had poor left ventricular functions.

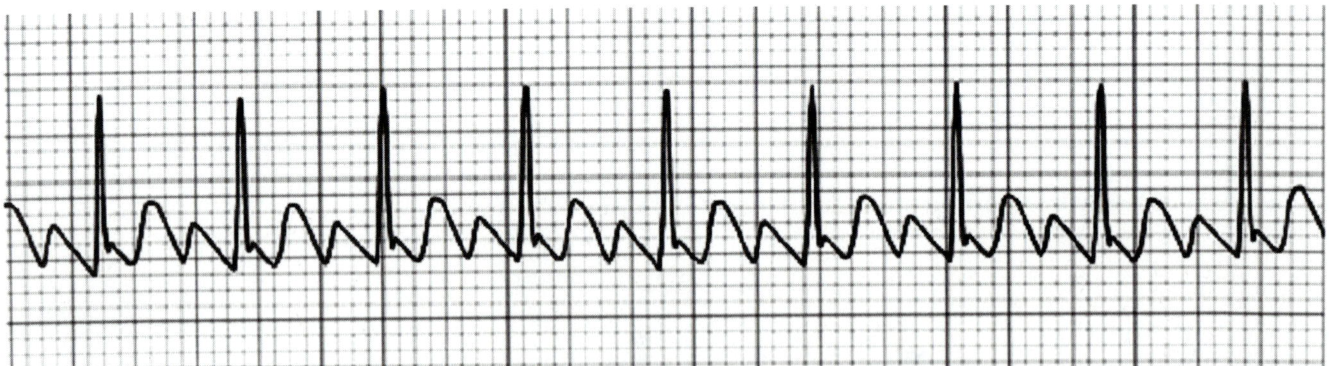

Fig. 40.25: *ECG trace showing atrial flutter: narrow QRS complexes are associated with regular flutter waves*

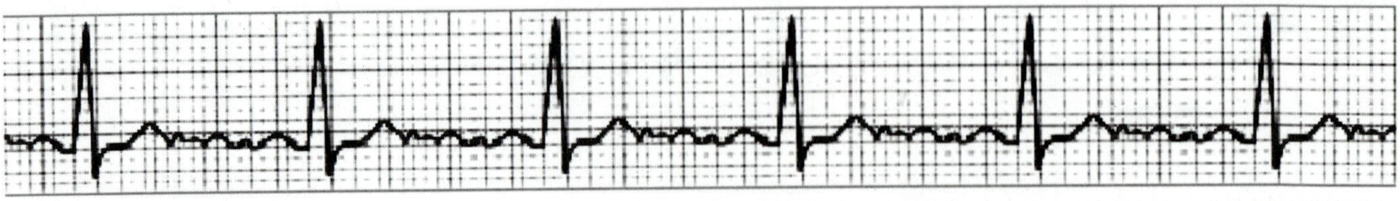

Fig. 40.26: *Atrial fibrillation. The ECG trace shows irregularily irregular heart rate in atrial fibrillation with 1 fibrillatory waves*

3. Digitalis and beta-blockers, which prolong AV nodal conduction and refractoriness in both alpha and beta pathways are usually, effective.
4. Type IA antiarrhythmic agents may be useful.
5. Oral diltizaem, 90 mg three times a day, may be effective in preventing recurrence.

In situations where one can find severe haemodynamic disturbances, direct synchronous cardioversion, using 40/ w/s, is, often, quite contributory.

Supraventricular Arrhythmia

1. Premature atrial contraction (PAC)
2. Atrial flutter
3. Atrial fibrillation
4. Atrial tachycardia
5. Atrial fusion
6. Atrial parasystole
7. Paraxysmal supraventricular tachycardia (PSVT)
8. Wandering pacemaker
9. Premature junctional contraction (PJC)
10. Accelerated junctional rhythm
11. Junctional tachycardia.

Mechanism

Cardiac arrhythmia, which usually, has it origin outside the sinus node and above the branching portion of the bundle of His, can be called as supraventricular arrhythmia, manifesting, initially, as ectopic(s). They may be either abnormal premature mechanisms or normal escape mechanisms, occurring in response to an abnormality in the sinus node. The two most common mechanisms involved are enhanced automaticity in the atria or AV junction (bundle of His) and AV nodal reentry or reentry, using an accessory pathway (WPW syndrome).

Enhanced automaticity may be secondary to digitalis, electrolyte imbalance, hypoxia, myocardial stretch, or acute myocardial infarction, and may result in single PACs or PJCs, ectopic atrial tachycardia, accelerated junctional rhythm, or junctional tachycardia.

An AV nodal reentry mechanism may be initiated by a single premature atrial, junctional, or ventricular complex, resulting in paroxysmal supraventricular tachycardia (PSVT).

Premature Atrial Ectopics (PAC)

PACs are premature atrial beats that originate outside the sinus node. The resulting ECG deflection is called a P' (P prime) wave.

Pathophysiology and Mechanism

PACs are a result of enhanced automaticity or after depolarizations. The mechanisms of AV conduction and compensatory pauses, following PACs are described here.

AV conduction: The PAC may be so premature that it is not conducted at all, because both bundle branches are refractory: or, it may be conducted down only one bundle branch and be blocked in the other (aberrant ventricular conduction).

Less than full compensatory pause: The PAC resets the SA node, causing the next expected sinus P wave to be on time if measured from the PAC, but earlier than it would have if the sinus node had not been disturbed.

Full or more than full compensatory pause: The PAC may suppress the SA node (overdrive suppression) and cause the next few sinus cycles to lengthen.

ECG Characteristics

1.	Rate	: That of the underlying rhythm
2.	Rhythm	: Irregular, resulting from PACs (underlying rhythm may be regular)
3.	PR interval	: Normal, although the PR interval may be too long or too short because of other conditions. All the P waves have the same shape and upright in leads I, II, aVF, and V_4 to V_6

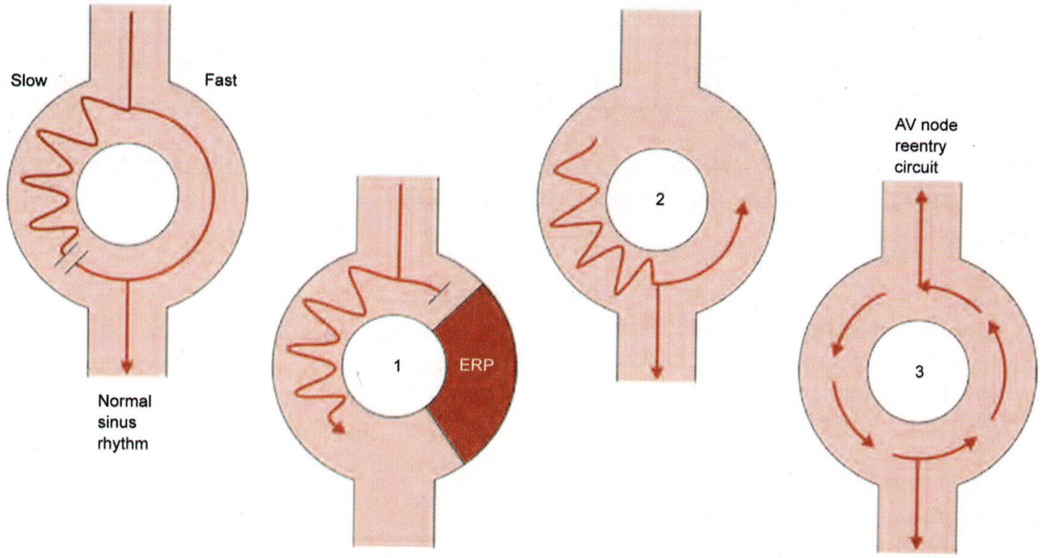

Fig. 40.27: *Diagram depicting mechanism of reentry in "slow-fast" AVNRT (ERP, effective refractory period)*

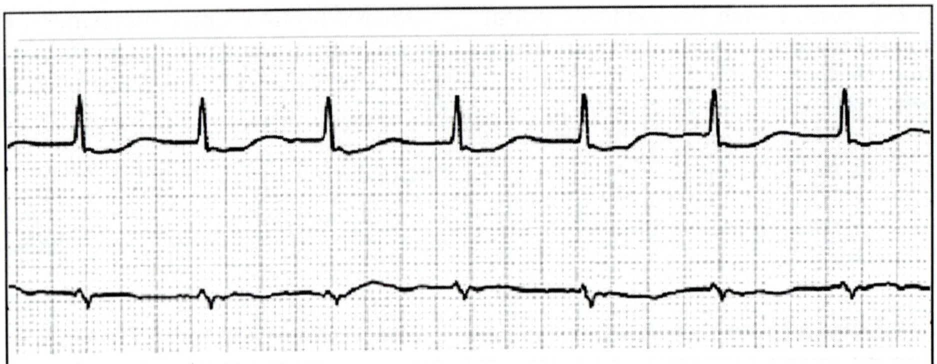

Heart rate	Rhythm	P wave	PR interval (in seconds)	QRS (in seconds)
60-100 bpm	Regular	Inverted, absent or after QRS	<.12	<.12

Fig. 40.28: *ECG showing accelerated junctional rhythm: This is an active junctional pacemaker rhythm caused by events that perturb pacemaker cells (e.g. ischemia, drugs and electrolyte abnormalities). The rate is 60–100 bpm).*

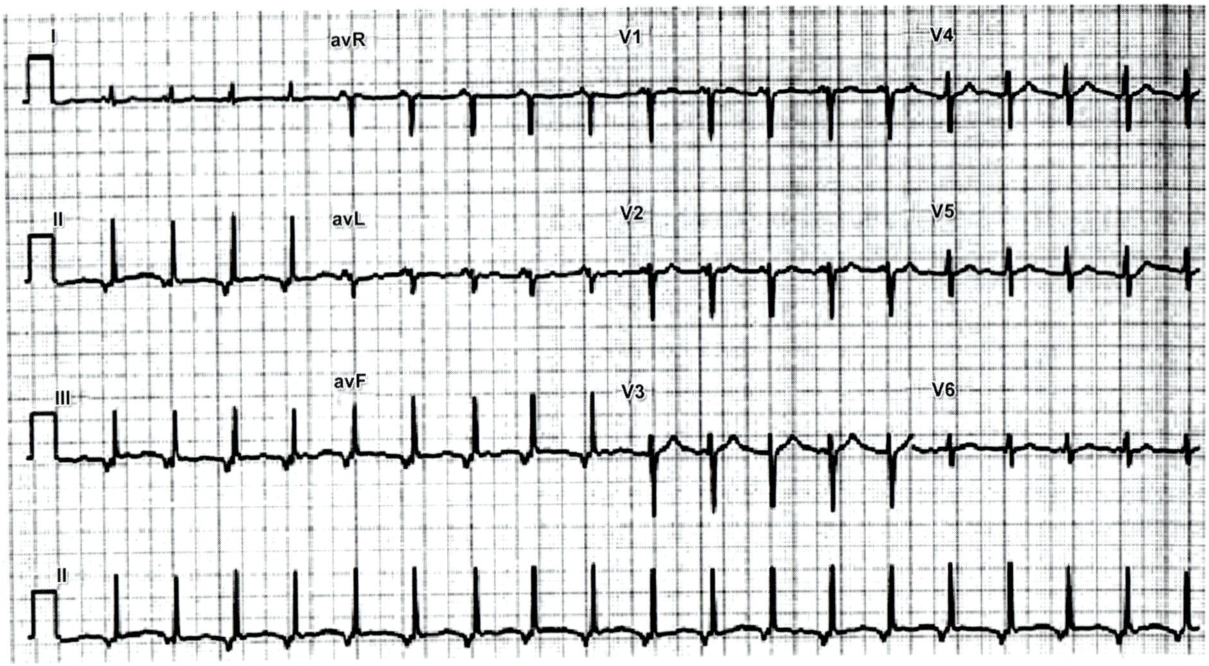

Fig. 40.29: *ECG trace showing accelerated junctional rhythm: narrow complex tachycardia at 115 bpm. Retrograde P waves-inverted in II, III and aVF; upright in V1 and aVR. Short PR interval (< 120 ms) indicates a junctional rather than atrial focus*

(The PR interval may be the same, longer, or shorter than the PR interval, or the P wave may not be conducted to the ventricles (a blocked PAC).

4. QRS complex : Normal, although the QRS may be prolonged as a result of aberrancy or other conditions
5. Distinguishing features: Normal QRS and a P wave that is premature and different in shape from the sinus P wave.

Etiological Factors

1. Various stimuli—emotion, tobacco, or coffee
2. Congestive heart failure (in the setting of myocardial infarction).
3. Atrial dilation or hypertrophy, resulting from mitral stenosis or atrial septal defect
4. Electrolyte imbalance
5. Hypoxia
6. Digitalis toxicity

Variations

i. PACs hidden in T waves
ii. Bigeminal PACs
iii. Nonconducted PACs
iv. Bigeminal nonconducted PACs.

Differential Diagnosis

Sinus arrest or SA block: Nonconducted PACs are statistically far more common and can, usually, be stotted distorting the T wave.

Treatment

PACs are not treated, but in association with acute myocardial infarction, their cause is identified and treated.

Atrial Tachycardia

Atrial tachycardia is an ectopic atrial rhythm with a rate of 140–250 beats/min.

ECG Features

1. Rate : 140–250 beats/min (atrial). The ventricular rate depends on the AV conduction ratio
2. Rhythm : Regular
3. PR interval : Not applicable; PR interval may be normal or prolonged. The P waves are ectopic.
4. QRS complex : Normal, although the QRS may be prolonged because of other conditions.

Distinguishing features: Rate and AV conduction ratio, which is, usually, 2:1. In digitalis toxicity, the P wave axis is, often, superior-inferior (positive in inferior leads), and often, in 2:1 block. The PP interval, across the QRS, is shorter than the one without a QRS (ventriculo-phasic PP interval).

Causes

1. Digitalis toxicity
2. Heart disease.

Variations

Atrial tachycardia with 4:1 AV conduction (other conduction ratios are also possible).

Chaotic Atrial Tachycardia (CAT)

Chaotic atrial tachycardia is a multifocal atrial tachycardia.

ECG Features

1. Rate : 100 to 250 beats/min.
2. Rhythm : Irregular
3. PR interval : May or may not be normal. PR intervals may vary.
4. QRS complex : Normal
5. Distinguishing features : P waves of several different shapes and an irregular rhythm.

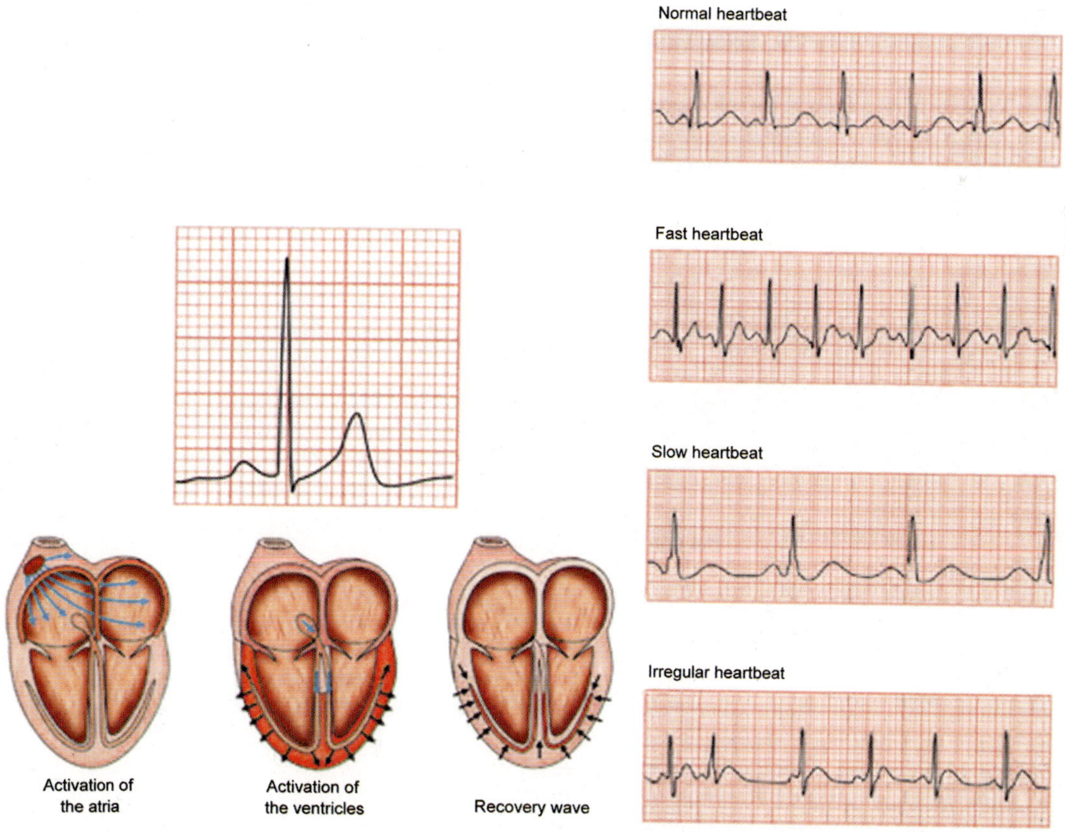

Fig. 40.30: *Activation of conducting tissues of both atria and ventricles (left) and variations in rate and rhythm of the heart (right)*

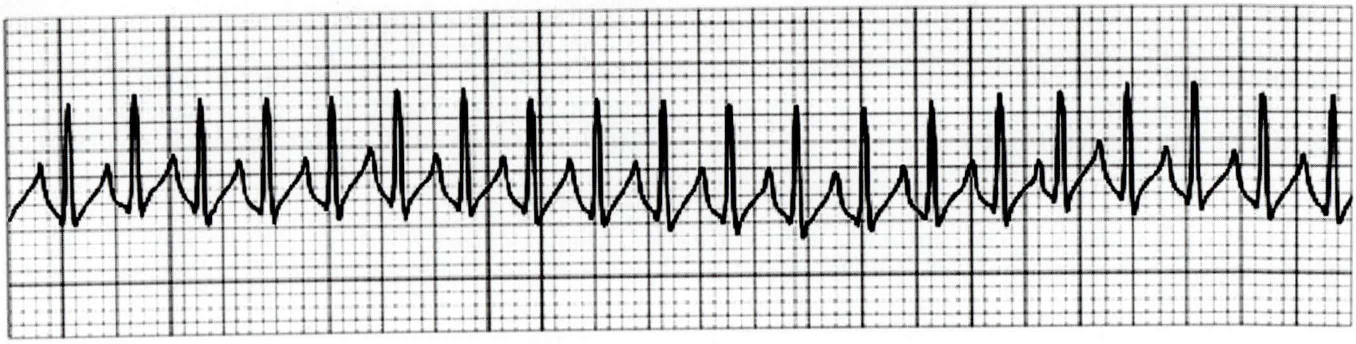

Fig. 40.31: *ECG trace shows junctional tachycardia: narrow QRS complexes with no visible P waves*

Etiological Factors

1. Chronic pulmonary disease
2. Hypoxia
3. Electrolyte imbalance.

Differential Diagnosis

Atrial fibrillation.

Treatment

Verapamil is found to be effective but basic underlying causes, leading to such abnormality, is important to manage first.

Atrial Flutter

Atrial flutter is a rapid atrial tachycardia of two types.

ECG Characteristics

1. Rate : Type-I (classical): The atrial rate ranges from 230–250 beats/min.
   Type-II: The range is 340–430 beats/min.
2. Rhythm : Atrial rhythm is regular, ventricular rhythm depends on the AV conduction pattern.
3. PR interval : 0.26–0.46 sec
4. QRS complex : Normal
5. Distinguishing features
   Regular sawtooth pattern in II, III, aVF sharp positive P waves in V_1. Normal QRS complexes AV conduction in 2:1 to 8:1 ratios T wave may distort the flutter pattern.

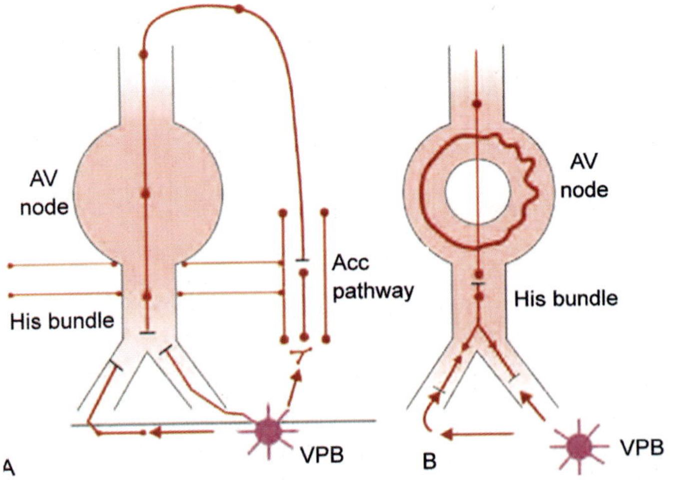

Fig. 40.32: *Different ways for ventricular premature beat (VPB) to gain access to the tachycardia circuit and to terminate tachycardia in AV nodal tachycardia and in circus movement tachycardia using an accessary pathway for ventriculoatrial conduction*

Causes

1. Any form of heart disease: Such as rheumatic heart disease, coronary artery disease, preexcitation syndrome, etc.
2. Acute illness.

Variations

1. Varying degrees of AV conduction ratios
2. Atrial flutter with AV dissociation (an accelerated idioventricular rhythm).

Differential Diagnosis

When the conduction ratio is 2:1, atrial flutter is, often, mistaken for sinus tachycardia of 140–175 beats/min. The ventricular rate makes one suspicious of a hidden flutter wave, and usually, the onset of the R wave is distorted by the flutter wave.

Treatment

1. The haemodynamic compromise is present due to a fast ventricular rate, direct synchronous cardioversion with 40–50 w/s should be administered.
2. Fast ventricular response rate can be controlled with digitalis. Propranolol or verapamil can also be used but are less effective. Normal rhythm can be achieved, usually, by the administration of these drugs.

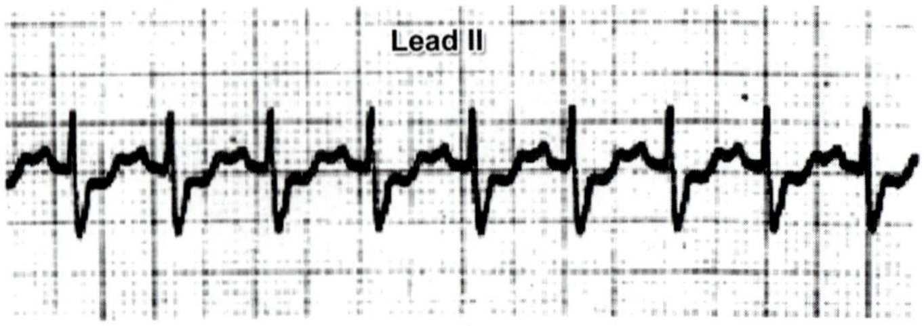

Fig. 40.33: *ECG showing atrial tachycardia in lead II*

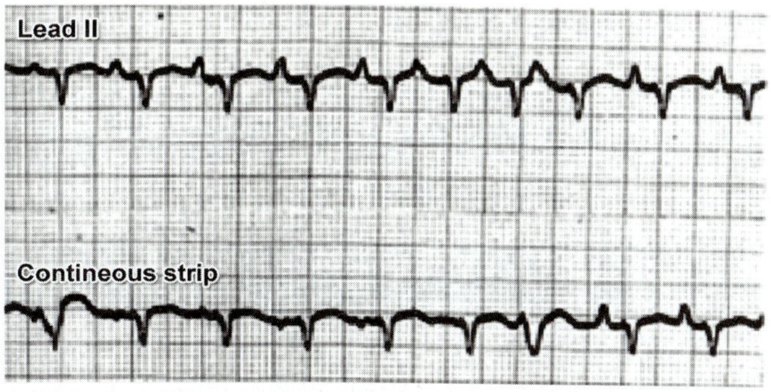

Fig. 40.34: *ECG trace showing chaotic atrial tachycardia (Cat)*

3. Digoxin and verapamil should not be prescribed to patients with flutter associated with Wolff-Parkinson-White syndrome.
4. Reversion to sinus rhythm may also be, often, achieved with the use of a type IA antiarrhythmic agents.
5. A patient should not be administered quinidine until digitalization is achieved since quinidine may facilitate AV conduction. Procainamide may rarely increase the ventricular response to atrial flutter by slowing the flutter rate; the AV node may conduct every second atrial depolarization instead of every third, producing an increased ventricular rate.
6. Atrial flutter can be converted to sinus rhythm with temporary overdrive pacing. It is done by pacing 115–125% of the spontaneous atrial rate at a critical duration. Overdrive pacing can also be successful, utilizing a special esophageal electrode.
7. If an artial thrombus has been diagnosed by echocardiography, the patient should be given warfarin with the prothrombin time, 1.2 to 1.5 times of control, for 3 weeks. If there is an abnormal slow atrial flutter rate or a high degree of AV block when the patient is receiving no antiarrythmic agernts, disease of the AV node should be suspected, and backup temporary pacing should be done till the rhythm is converted to normal rate response.

Atrial Fibrillation

Atrial fibrillation is an ectopic atrial arrhythmia characterized by erratic depolarization of the atrial.

Newer Classification of AF

Some of the workers have classified atrial fibrillation into three different types on electrophysiological studies. They observed that all patients had uniform conduction in the free wall of the right atrium, during sinus rhythm, rapid atrial pacing procedure.

Type I: Seen in 40% of patients in whom there are uniform, single broad wave fronts that propagate through the atrial wall without significant conduction delay. There may be short areas of conduction block, small areas of slow conduction, that do not interfere with the main course of propagation. The cycle length is somewhat slow (median 174 ms), there is almost no reentry, and no source of activation waves is visible, despite the persistence of atrial fibrillation.

Type II, found in 32% of patients in which there is intermediate pattern, which describes either a single wave associated with major areas of conduction block and /or slow conduction or two wavelets, separated by a line of functional conduction block.

Type III which manifests with a highly fragmented and complex pattern, seen in 28% of cases, and characterized by three or more wavelets, associated with lines of functional conduction block under the mapping electrode. This type of fibrillation is associated with a shorter cycle length (median interval, 136 ms) than type I and with a wide 100 ms variation in cycle length spanning very short and very long cycles.

It may also be kept in mind that the three types of atrial fibrillation do not constitute three separate entities, but rather a continuous spectrum of increasing complexity.

ECG Characteristics

1. Rate	: Uncontrolled, 110–180 beats/min. controlled, 70–80 beats
2. Rhythm	: Irregular
3. PR interval	: Absent P waves
4. QRS complex	: Normal
5. Distinguishing features	: Absent P waves and irregular ventricular response.

Causes

i. Mitral valve disease
ii. Ischaemic disease, particularly acute myocardial infarction.
iii. Hypertension
iv. Thyrotoxicosis
v. Increasing left-atrial size in elderly patients
vi. Idiopathic (lone) type of atrial fibrillations.

Variations

A. Coarse atrial fibrillation with signs of digitalis toxicity (regularization of the ventricular response)
B. Fine atrial fibrillation with uncontrolled ventricular response.
C. Atrial fibrillation with complete AV block
D. Atrial fibrillation with conduction over an accessory pathway.

Treatment

1. Therapy with digoxin still remains the basic method of treatment of atrial fibrillation in controlling the ventricular response. Depending upon the clinical urgency and the ventricular rate, it may be given orally or intravenously. Digoxin is strongly contraindicated in atrial fibrillation with antegrade preexcitation by an accessory pathway. Verapamil is also contraindicated in this situation.
2. If severe haemodynamic compromise is present due to atrial fibrillation with a rapid ventricular response, synchronous cardioversion is considered. After

Table 40.5: *Drugs commonly used to control ventricular rate in patients with atrial fibrillation*

Drug	*Initial dosing*	*Maintenance dosing*	*Comments*
Calcium channel blockers			
Diltiazem (cardizem)	15–20 mg IV over 2 minutes; may repeat in 15 minutes	5–15 mg per hour by continuous IV infusion	Convenient; easy to titrate to heart rate goal
Verapamil (calan, isoptin)	5–10 mg IV over 2 minutes; may repeat in 30 minutes	Not standardized	More myocardial depression and hypotension than with diltiazem
Beta blockers			
Esmolol (brevibloc)	Bolus of 500 mcg per kg IV over 1 minute; may repeat in 5 minutes	50–300 mcg per kg per minute by continuous IV infusion	Very short-acting; easy to titrate to heart rate goal
Propranolol	1 mg IV over 2 minutes; (inderal) 5 minutes to maximum of 5 mg	1–3 mg IV every 4 hours may repeat every	Short duration of action; hence, need for repeat dosing
Digoxin (lanoxin)	0.25–0.5 mg IV; then 0.25 mg IV every 4–6 hours to maximum of 1 mg	0.125–0.25 mg per day IV or orally	Adjunctive therapy; less effective for rate control than beta-blockers or calcium channel blockers

IV = intravenous.

Adapted with permission from Li H, Easley A, Barrington W, Windle J. Evaluation and management of atrial fibrillation in the emergency department. Emerg Med Clin North Am 1998;16:389–403.

cardioversion, it may be helpful to administer digitalis and/or to start procainamide or quinidine to help maintain the patient in sinus rhythm.

3. In a stable patient, one should determine if the rhythm is acute or chronic and whether electrical cardioversion is required. The patient should be anticoagulated with warfrain for 3 weeks if the rhythm has been present for more than 2 days or if the duration is uncertain, prior to cardioversion. The prothrombin time should be 1.2 to 1.5 times of the control. While the patient is being anticoagulated, the ventricular response should be controlled with digitalis, at times, adding either beta-blockers or verapamil. The digoxin may be initated intravenously, and, when the ventricular rate is brought under check, it should be switched over to the oral medication. Acute short-term heparinization does not exclude the possibility of embolic episode, following cardioversion, and should not be employed. Quinidine or procainamide is, usually, started 24–48 hours to elective cardioversion. Occasionally, this will produce cardioversion, and usually, the medication should be continued after successful electrical cardioversion to prevent recurrence.
4. Long-term administration of anticoagulation be considered in patients with chronic atrial fibrillation.
5. If atrial fibrillation is as short as 2–3 days' duration, medical cardioversion may be considered by administering 1–2 mg of digoxin over 24 hours. If the patient fails to achieve normal rhythm, procainamide or quinidine is added. A patient should be fully digitalized prior to starting quinidine which may increase the ventricular response.
6. Electrical cardioversion is usually, successful, but atrial fibrillation may return if the underlying cause is not removed. Quinidine or procainamide should be given, after cardioversion, to check further reoccurance of atrial fibrillation.
7. Electrical or medical cardioversion should be avoided in sick sinus syndrome, if the ventricular rate is less than 80 beats per minute, or if digitalis toxicity is suspected. If necessary, such patients may be electively cardioverted, after a temporary pacing catheter is inserted, to avoid a bout of asystole.
8. Beta-blockers and diltiazem may show some therapeutic response on rare occasions when added to the therapeutic does of digioxin to control the ventricular rate in chronic atrial fibrillation.

Wandering Pacemaker

It may be defined as that of atrial arrhythmia in which there is shifting of impulse formation from focus to focus within the atrial tissue virtually with every beat. Sinus beats may be interspersed throughout. P waves are of many forms, and the cadence tends to be somewhat irregular. Ventricular complexes are without alteration.

ECG Characteristics

1. Rate : Normal or 50 beats/min
2. Rhythm : Slightly irregular
3. PR interval : Normal
4. QRS complex : Normal
5. Distinguishing features : A sinus rhythm that gives way to an ectopic atrial or junctional rhythm,

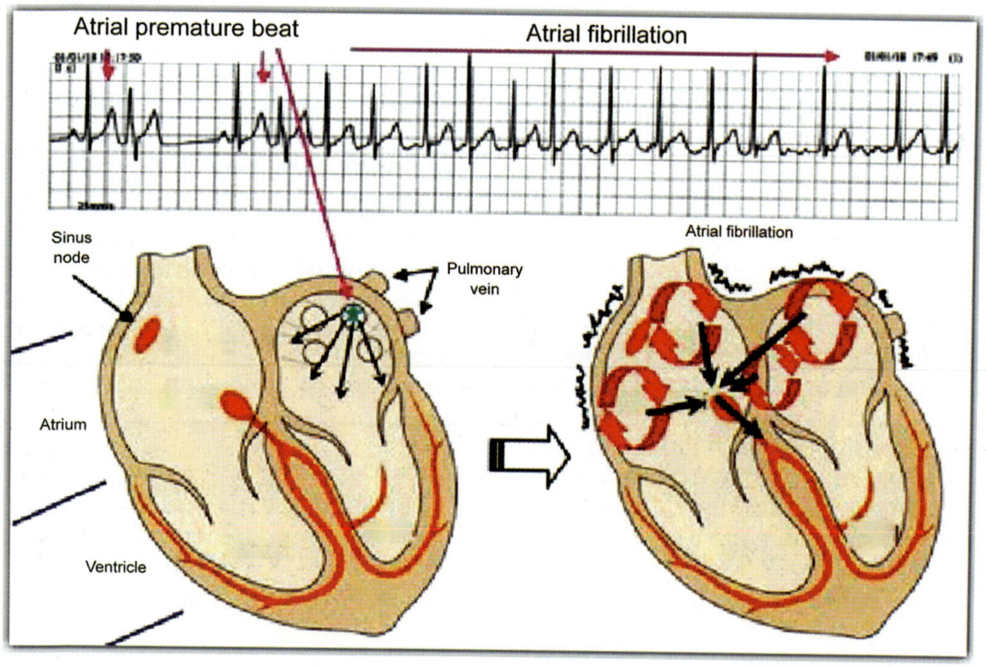

Fig. 40.35: *Mechanism of onset of atrial fibrillation*

often, with atrial beats at the transitions; there is retrograde conduction to the atria from junctional focus.

Causes

1. It is associated with ischaemic heart disease, involving the sinus node.
2. Acute rheumatic fever
3. Digilatis toxicity enhancing vagal tone
4. Normal heart due to vagotonia.

Variations

Normal sinus rhythm with an accelerated junctional or atrial rhythm.

Treatment

If there is a normal escape mechanism, no treatment is indicated unless there is haemodynamic deterioration, and then, IV atropine may be appropriate, ask the patient to cough; coughing decreases vagal tone and promotes the reappearance of the sinus rhythm. If the ectopic rhythm is enhanced, then the cause should be sought and treated.

Junctional ectopic mechanisms: premature and escape junctional beats (PJCs)

A junctional beat takes its origin from the bundle of His and may be either premature or escape, and it may or may not follow retrograde conduction to the atria.

ECG Characteristics

1. Rate : It is of the underlying rhythm
2. Rhythm : Irregular as a result of the PJCs (underlying rhythm may be regular)
3. PR interval : Normal in the underlying sinus rhythm. The P wave associated with the junctional beat may be absent if there is no retrograde conduction to the atria, if present, it is negative in II, III and aVF, and may appear before, during or after the QRS complex.
4. QRS complex : It is normal although it may be prolonged due to other conditions.
5. Distinguishing features : Normal QRS complex and a P wave that is not seen, buried in the QRS complex, or negative in II, III and aVF. If the P wave precedes the QRS, it does so by no more than 0.12 sec.

Etiological Factors

1. Digitalis
2. Acute inferior-wall myocardial infarction
3. Tricuspid prosthesis
4. Rheumatic fever

Escape junctional beats are caused by excessively long pauses in the cardiac cycle.

Variations

Premature junctional contraction (PJC) with the preceding the QRs complex

- PJC with the P hidden in the QRS complex
- PJC with the P following the QRS complex.

Treatment

Normally, PJC are not treated, but if their cause is identified, these should be appropriately treated.

Accelerated Idiojunctional Rhythm

it may be defined as that ectopic rhythm which originates from the bundle of His and monitors the ventricles at a rate of 60–100 beats/min. When the rate exceeds 100 beats/min, it is called junctional tachycardia.

ECG Features

1. Rate : 60–100 beats/min
2. Rhythm : Regular
3. PR interval : Normal in the underlying sinus rhythm. When the junctional focus begins to take over. The PR interval may appear to shorten. However. When this happens, there is no relationship between the P wave and the QRS complex (AV dissociation).
4. QRS complex : Normal, although the QRS complex may be prolonged as a result of other conditions.
5. Distinguish features : A junctional rhythm reveals itself when its rate is about the same as that of the sinus node. Resulting in AV dissociation. P waves get closer and closer to the QRS complex as the rate of the junctional focus exceeds that of the sinus node.

Etiological Factors

1. Myocardial infarction
2. Digitalis toxicity.

Treatment

No treatment is advisable unless it is associated with haemodynamic disturbances when 0.5–1.0 mg atropine I/V may be required for the treatment.

Junctional Tachycardia (Figs 40.39–40.46)

This kind of ectopic rhythm is produced as a result of focus, with enhanced automaticity, lying in the bundle of His, and controlling the ventricles at a rate of 100–130 beats/min. if the rate is less than 100 beats/min, it is termed accelerated junctional or idiojunctional rhythm.

ECG Features

1. Rate : 100 to beats/min
2. Rhythm : Regular
3. PR interval : When the junctional focus begins to take over. The PR interval may appear to shorten: however, when this happens, there is no relationship between the P and the QRS complex (AV dissociation). The P wave will be absent if there is no retrograde conduction to the atria; if present, it is negative in II, III, and aVF and may be before during, or after the QRS complex depending on the relative speed of anterograde and retrograde conduction and the location of the ectopic focus in the bundle of His.

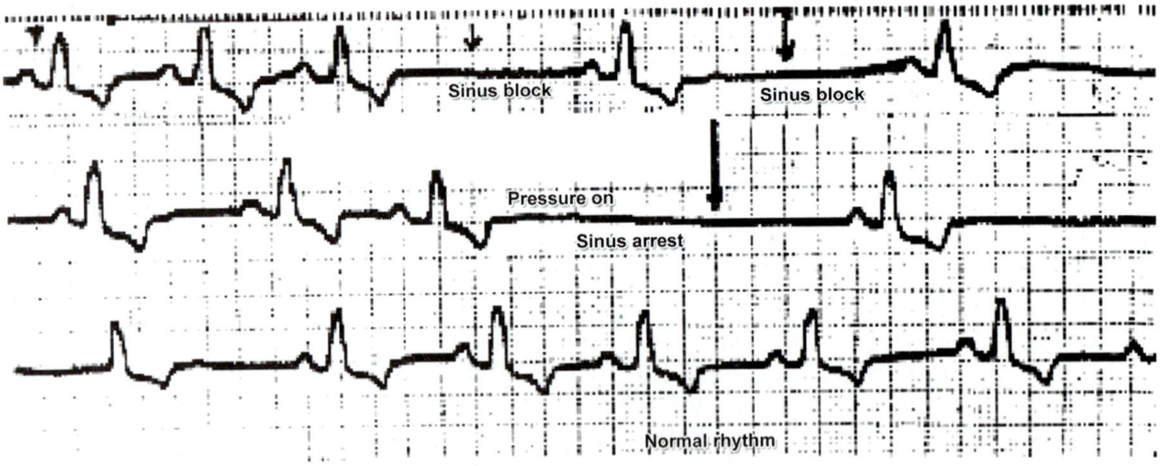

Fig. 40.36: *Graph explaining as to how pressure on carotid sinus produces sinus arrest or sinus block*

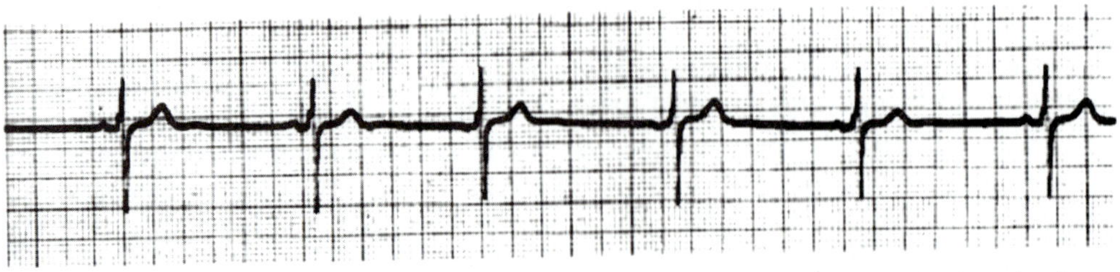

Fig. 40.37: *Graph showing changing P wave morphology between sinus node and atrioventricular junction in wandering pacemaker rhythm in limb lead II*

Table 40.6: *Showing classwise antirrhythmic drugs*

Class	*Known as*	*Examples*	*Mechanism*	*Clinical uses in cardiology*
Ia	Fast-channel blockers-affect QRS complex	• Quinidine • Procainamide • Disopyramide	Na^+ channel block (intermediate association/dissociation)	• Ventricular arrhythmias • Prevention of paroxysmal recurrent atrial fibrillation (triggered by vagal overactivity) • Procainamide in Wolff-Parkinson-White syndrome
Ib-do not affect QRS complex		• Lidocaine • Phenytoin • Mexiletine • Tocainide	Na^+ channel block (fast association/dissociation)	• Treatment and prevention during and immediately after myocardial infarction, though this practice is now discouraged given the increased risk of asystole • Ventricular tachycardia • Atrial fibrillation
Ic	—	• Flecainide • Propafenone • Moricizine	Na^+ channel block (slow association/dissociation)	• Prevents paroxysmal atrial fibrillation • Treats recurrent tachyarrhythmias of abnormal conduction system. • Contraindicated immediately post-myocardial infarction
II	Beta-blockers	• Propranolol • Esmolol • Timolol • Metoprolol • Atenolol • Bisoprolol	Beta blocking Propranolol also shows some class I action	• Decrease myocardial infarction mortality • Prevent recurrence of tachyarrhythmias
III		• Amiodarone • Sotalol • Ibutilide • Dofetilide • Dronedarone • E-4031	K^+ channel blocker Sotalol is also a beta-blocker Amiodarone has class I, II, III and IV activity	• In Wolff-Parkinson-White syndrome • Sotalol: Ventricular tachycardias and atrial fibrillation • Ibutilide: atrial flutter and atrial fibrillation
IV	Slow-channel blockers	• Verapamil • Diltiazem	Ca^{2+} channel blocker	• Prevent recurrence of paroxysmal supraventricular tachycardia • Reduce ventricular rate in patients with atrial fibrillation
V		• Adenosine • Digoxin • Magnesium sulfate	Work by other or unknown mechanisms (direct nodal inhibition).	Used in supraventricular arrhythmias, especially in heart failure with atrial fibrillation, contraindicated in ventricular arrhythmias. Or in the case of magnesium sulfate, used in torsades de pointes.

Table 40.7: There is a popular **mnemonic** to remember the class I agents:

Class Ia	*Disopyramide, quinidine, procainamide*	*Double quarter pounder* *Police department questions* (procainamide, disopyramide, quinidine)
Class Ib	*Lidocaine, mexiletine, tocainide*	*Lettuce, mayo, tomato* *The little man* (tocainide, lidocaine, mexiletine)
Class Ic	*Moricizine, flecainide, propafenone*	*More fries please.* (note there are two "M"s in the mnemonic, but *moricizine* and *more* can clarify which is which) *For pushing ecstasy* (*molly* or *ecstasy* may be used to denote moricizine or encainide)

4. QRS compex : Normal, although the QRS complex may be prolonged as a result of other conditions.
5. Distinguishing features : A junctional rhythm of more than 100 beats/min. The QRS complex will be narrow if there is no associated intraventricular conduction problem.

Differential diagnosis: There is hardly any other condition which closely resembles the junctional tachycardia

Table 40.8: *Recommendations for antithrombotic therapy in cardioversion for atrial fibrillation*

Timing of cardioversion	*Anticoagulation*
Early cardioversion in patients with atrial fibrillation for less than 48 hours	Heparin during cardioversion period to achieve PTT of 1.5–2.5 times the baseline value
Early cardioversion in patients with atrial fibrillation for more than 48 hours or an unknown duration, but without documented atrial thrombi	Heparin during cardioversion period to achieve PTT of 1.5–2.5 times the baseline value Warfarin (coumadin) for 4 weeks after cardioversion to achieve target INR of 2.5 (range: 2.0–3.0)
Elective cardioversion in patients with atrial fibrillation for more than 48 hours or an unknown duration	Warfarin for 3 weeks before and 4 weeks after cardioversion to achieve target INR of 2.5 (range: 2.0–3.0)

Table 40.9: *Recommendations for antithrombotic therapy in chronic atrial fibrillation*

Stroke risk	*Anticoagulation*
High risk	Warfin (coumadin) to achieve target INR of 2.5 (range: 2.0–3.0)
Previous stroke, transient ischemic attack, or systemic icembolus	
History of hypertension	
Poor left ventricular systolic function	
Patient age >75 years	
Rheumatic mitral valve disease	
Prosthetic heart valve	

unless its rate exceeds 130 beats/min, and then, there may difficulty in differentiating it from an AV node reentry mechanism (PSVT). A vagal manaeuvre, usually, interrupts the PSVT and has no effect on junctional tachycardia.

Treatment

Identify and treat the cause.

Paroxysmal Supraventricular Tachycardia (PSVT) Resulting from AV Nodal Reentry

It has it supraventricular origin and, usually, comes in recurrent episodes, and, hence, termed as paroxysmal supraventricular tachycardia. It is characterized by spontaneous and abrupt termination. It may be, further, supported by either an AV nodal reentry or by an AV reentry circuit and achieves rates of 170–250 beats/min.

ECG Characteristics

1. Rate : 170–250 beats/min
2. Rhythm : Regular
3. PR interval : It may be normal in the sinus rhythm. The PR interval at the onset of the tachycardia is, abnormally, long
4. QRS complex : Identical features of the sinus conducted QRS complex. It may be aberrantly, conducted at times.
5. Distinguishing features : Anarrow QRS tachycardia that, usually, exceeds 170 beats/min and begins, abruptly, with a prolonged PR interval. This is necessary to accommodate the refractoriness, and establish the reentry circuit. The rest of the P waves will either not be seen or they will distort the end of the QRS (P waves just barely showing). There is no alternans of the QRS after the first 5–6 seconds: may be interrupted by a vagal manoeuvre.

Etiological Factors

1. One early PAC
2. Rarely, a PJC.

Variations

A. AV nodal reentry, using a slow anterograde intranodal pathway and a fast retrograde pathway, causing simultaneous atrial and ventricular activation (P buried within or peeking out at the end of the QRS).
B. AV nodal reentry, using a fast anterograde intranodal pathway and a slow retrograde pathway, causing atrial activation to follow ventricular activation with a long PR interval.

Treatment

Short paroxysms may require no treatment

1. Termination may, often, be achieved by vagal manoeuvres, but carotid artery massage should not be advised in patients having or likely to have carotid artery disease.
2. Intravenous verapamil is considered by some to the treatment of choice, but should be used cautiously in those patients who had poor left ventricular functions.

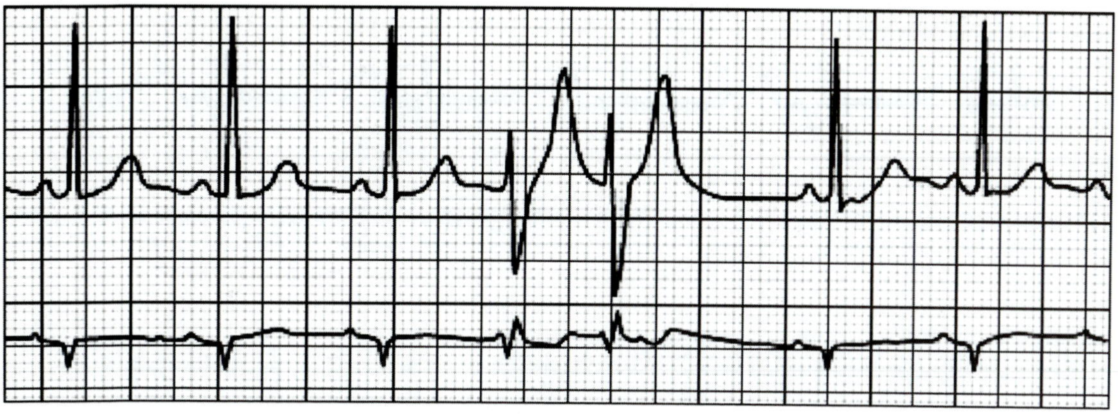

Fig. 40.38: *ECG showing coupled PVCs; occurs in pairs*

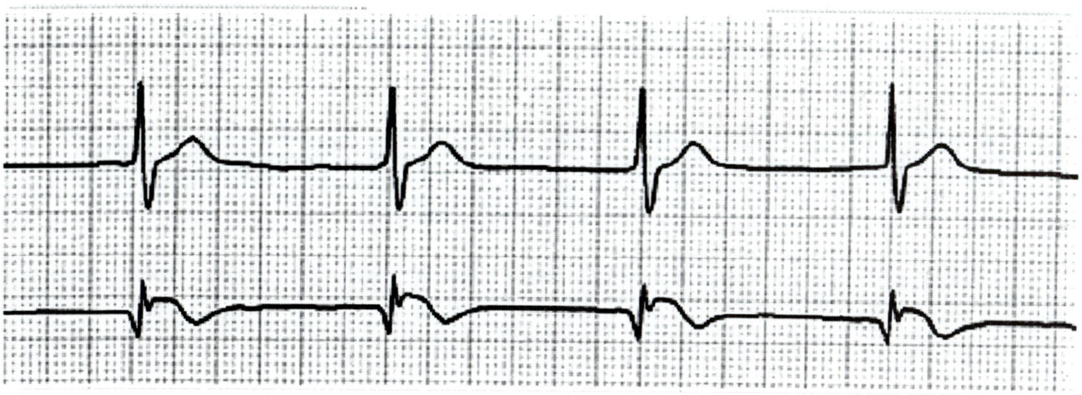

Heart rate	Rhythm	P wave	PR interval (in seconds)	QRS (in seconds)
40-60 bpm	Regular	Inverted, absent or after QRS	<.12	<.12

Fig. 40.39: *ECG showing junctional escape rhythm: This is a sequence of 3 or more junctional escapes occurring by default at a rate of 40–60 bpm. There may be AV dissociation or the atria may be captured retrogradely by the junctional pacemaker. In the ECG example below the retrograde P waves are not seen and must be hidden in the QRS's; the significant "Q" wave with ST elevation in the bottom strip suggests an acute MI*

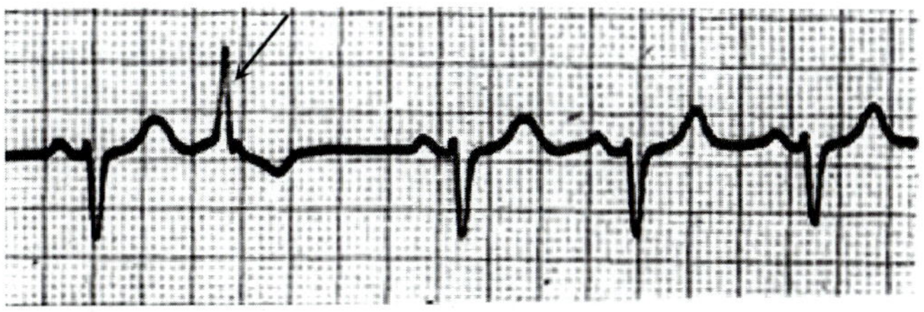

Fig. 40.40: *ECG trace showing junctional ectopic*

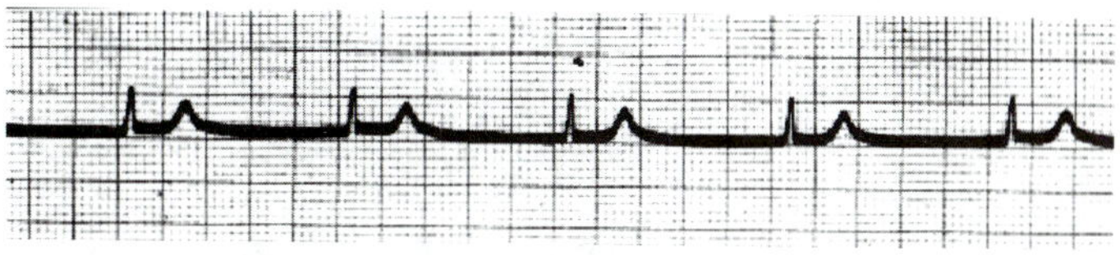

Fig. 40.41: *ECG trace showing atrioventricular junctional rhythm with P waves buried in QRST complex*

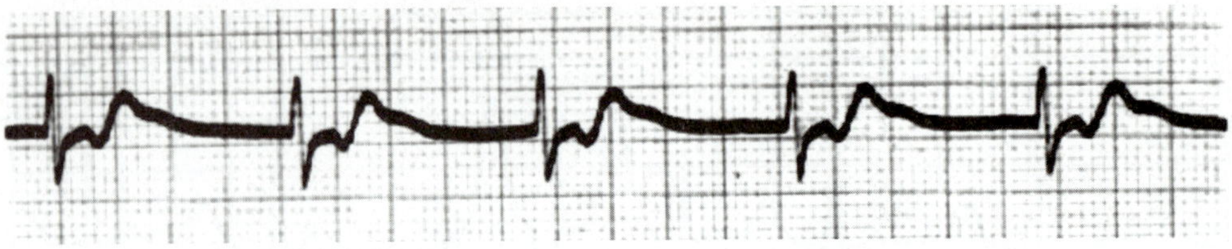

Fig. 40.42: *ECG trace showing atrioventricular junctional rhythm with P waves follow the QRS complexes and distorts ST segment*

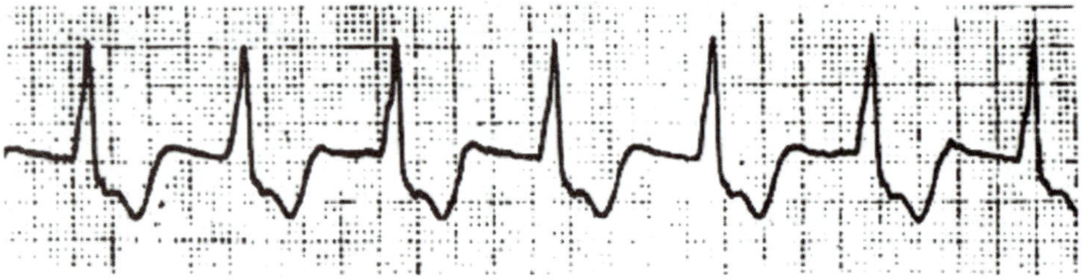

Fig. 40.43: *ECG trace showing accelerated idiojunctional rhythm*

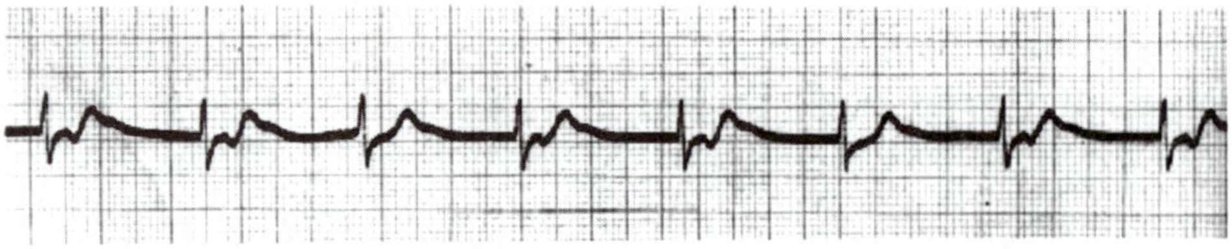

Fig. 40.44: *ECG trace showing atrioventricular junctional rhythm with 2.1 retrograde block*

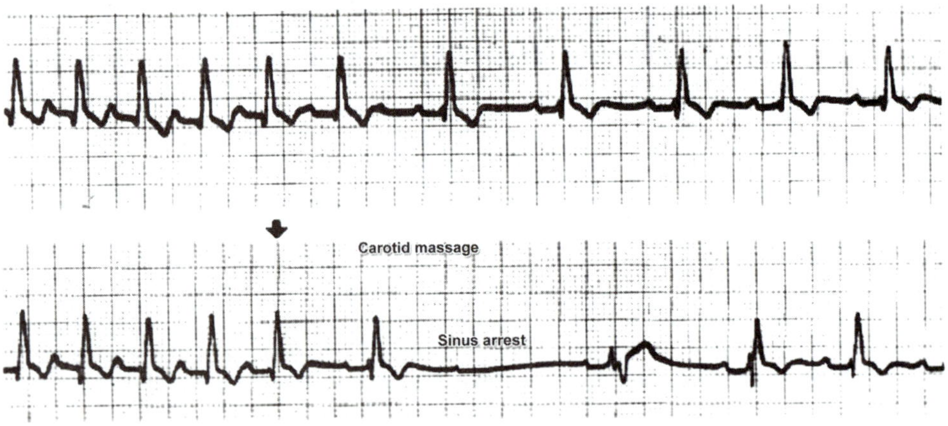

Fig. 40.45: *ECG trace showing paroxysmal supraventricular tachycardia and effect of carotid sinus massage*

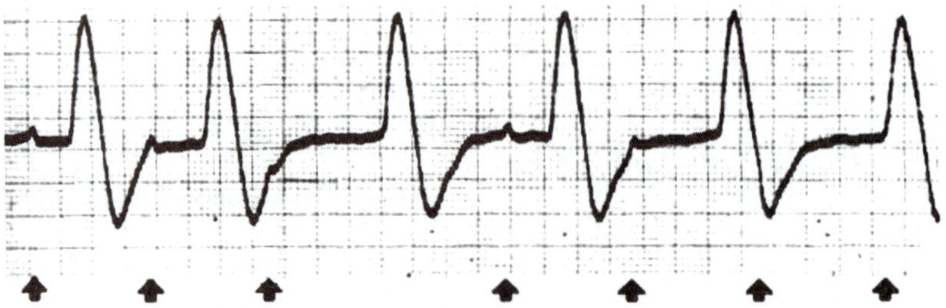

Fig. 40.46: *ECG trace showing accelerated idioventricular rhythm*

3. Digitalis and beta-blockers, which prolong AV nodal conduction and refractoriness in both alpha and beta pathways, are usually, effective.
4. Type IA antiarrhythmic agents may be useful.
5. Oral diltiazem, 90 mg, three times a day, may be effective in preventing recurrence.

In situations, where one can find severe haemodynamic disturbances, direct synchronous cardioversion, using 40 w/s, is often, quite contributory.

Vagotonic Manoeuvres for PSV

1. Carotid Sinus Stimulation (Figs 40.36, 40.45, 40.48)

Out of vagotonic manoeuvres, carotid sinus stimulation is, commonly, practised by physicians and quite reliable test when done by an experienced health worker. The main purpose of this test is to create an elevation of blood pressure in the carotid sinus so that there will be reflex slowing of AV conduction. This is achieved by pressing the carotid sinus against the lateral processes of the vertebra. It will cause pain for a seconds for which the individual should be educated before performing this manoeuvre.

Technical aspects: To start with, grip the patient's chin, with your right palm, and swing your right thumb around; you will find that it, automatically, falls at the angle of the jaw, the location of the carotid bifurcation. This area, then, is pressed with tolerable force with the thumb for not more than 3 seconds as a longer duration of pressure, with greater force, may lead to dangerous complications. Prior to the performance of this manoeuvre, one should always record the history of transient ischaemic attacks and listen to the carotid bruit. One should never perform sinus stimulation test without ECG monitoring so that the results can be observed and acted upon, if required. This manoeuvre is relatively safe and effective.

2. Gagging

This is a good vegotonic manoeuvre. If the episodes of PSVT occur, instruct the patient to try to vomit.

3. Trendelenburg Position

The patient can be instructed to perform this at home.

4. Valsalva Manoeuvre

Blowing against a closed glottis is an effective vegotonic manoeuvre.

5. Squatting

Squatting with hands, gripped across the belly and pulling in, is a fairly easy thing to do and is very effective. This is obvious not for the older patient who cannot squat. It is, usually, prescribed for a younger patient. It is not only ineffective, but it is also dangerous as it may lead to retinal detachment in a few elderly patients.

Atrial Fusion Complexes

The collision of two atrial impulses, within atria, leads to the formation of a new complex, which is termed as atrial fusion complex.

ECG Characteristics

1. Rate : That of the underlying rhythm
2. Rhythm : Regular
3. PR interval : The PR interval of the fusion beat is the same as that of the sinus rhythm. The P wave of the fusion beat is, sometimes, isoelectric or intermediate between the P waves of the fusing impulses.
4. QRS complex : It is same as that of the underlying rhythm.
5. Distinguishing features : There are other atrial ectopic beats in the tracing, and there is reason to believe that one beat was due at the same time as the sinus P wave.

Causative Factors

These are the same as those of the atrial ectopics or atrial rhythm.

Variations

1. Atrial parasystole
2. Wandering pacemaker.

Atrial Parasystole

Atrial parasystole is an independent and undisturbable ectopic rhythm whose pacemaker cannot be discharged by impulses of the dominant (usually, sinus) rhythm. It is far less common than the ventricular parasystole.

ECG Characteristics

1. Rate : That of the underlying rhythm.
2. Rhythm : Irregular, because of atrial premature beats
3. PR interval : Normal
4. QRS Complex : Normal
5. Distinguishing features : Atrial ectopic with no fixed coupling interectopic intervals that are multiples of a common denominator.

Fusion Beats

Causes

Myocardial infarction.

Differential Diagnosis

PACs.

Ventricular Arrhythmia

1. Premature ventricular contractions (PVC)
2. Ventricular tachycardia
3. Ventricular fibrillation
4. Torsades de pointes
5. Accelerated idioventricular rhythm
6. Ventricular parasystole
7. Ventricular fusion
8. Ventricular flutter.

Ventricular Escape

Ventricular ectopics are produced as a result of enhanced automaticity reentry, or altered depolarizations. These manifest as premature beats, ventricular tachycardia, ventricular fibrillation, accelerated idioventricular rhythm, or parasystole. Premature ventricular complexes (PVCs) may be right or left ventricular, unifocal, multifocal, bigeminal, interpolated, R-on-T, end- diastolic, or fusion

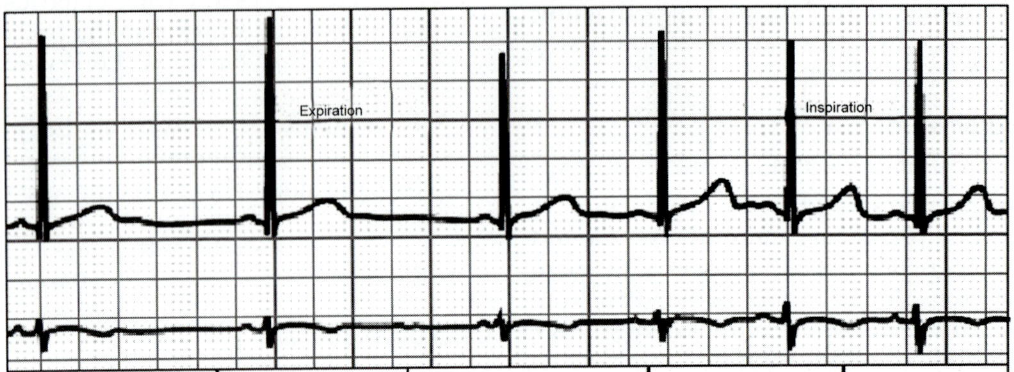

Heart rate	Rhythm	P wave	PR interval (in seconds)	QRS (in seconds)
Usually 60-100 bpm	Irregular	Before each QRS, identical	.12 to .20	<.12

Fig. 40.47: *ECG lead II showing normal sinus rhythm with sinus arrhythmia in a healthy person. Note the marked variation in the P-P intervals induced by respiration*

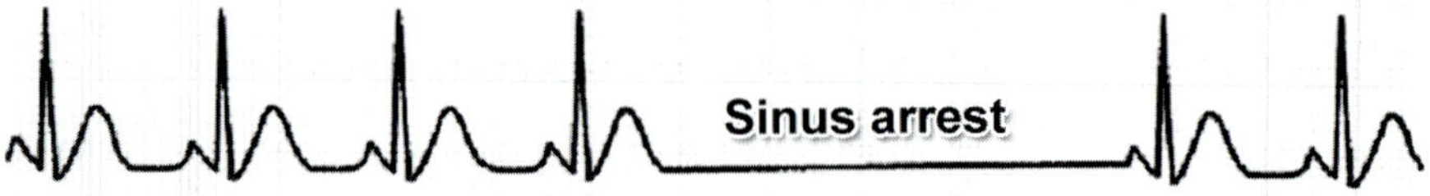

Fig. 40.48: *ECG trace showing sinus arrest. The basic rhythm is regular. The length of the pause is not a multiple of the sinus interval*

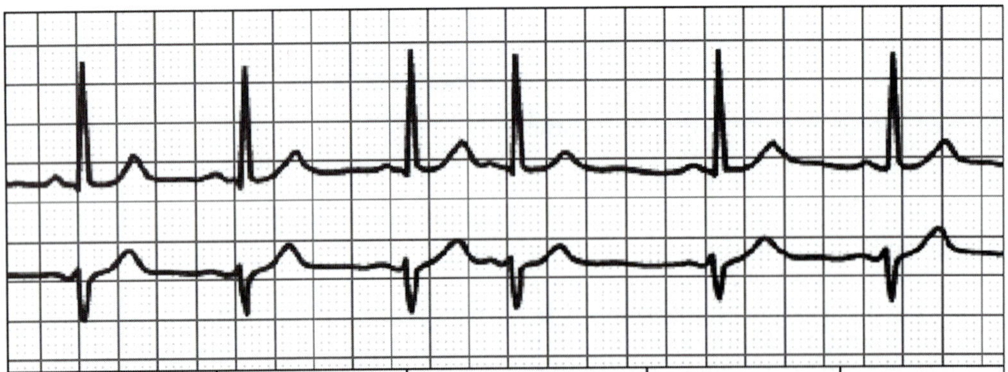

Heart rate	Rhythm	P wave	PR interval (in seconds)	QRS (in seconds)
N/A	Irregular	Before each QRS, identical	.12 to .20	<.12

Fig. 40.49: *ECG showing premature atrial contraction with pause*

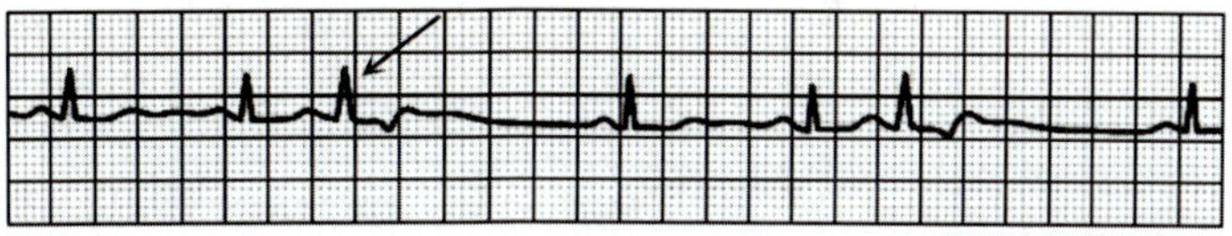

Fig. 40.50: *ECG trace showing junctional ectopic with pause*

beats; in the setting of acute myocardial infarction, they produce dangerous consequences and are treated on emergency basis.

Premature Ventricular Complexes (PVCS) (Figs 40.83–40.85)

PVCs are premature ectopics, which are generated in the ventricles below the branching of the bundle of His.

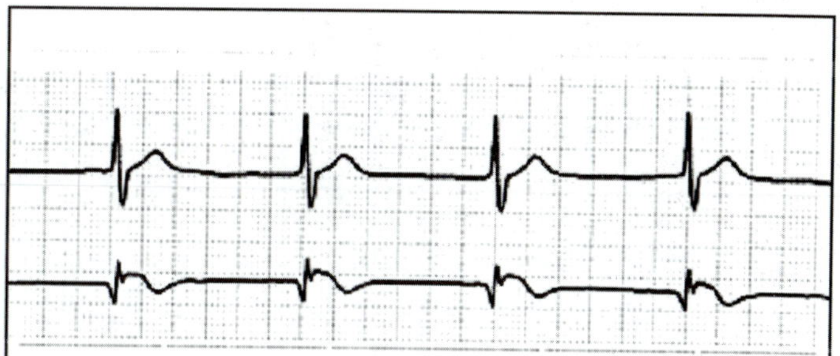

Heart rate	Rhythm	P wave	PR interval (in seconds)	QRS (in seconds)
40-60 bpm	Regular	Inverted, absent or after QRS	<.12	<.12

Fig. 40.51: *ECG showing junctional rhythm without pause*

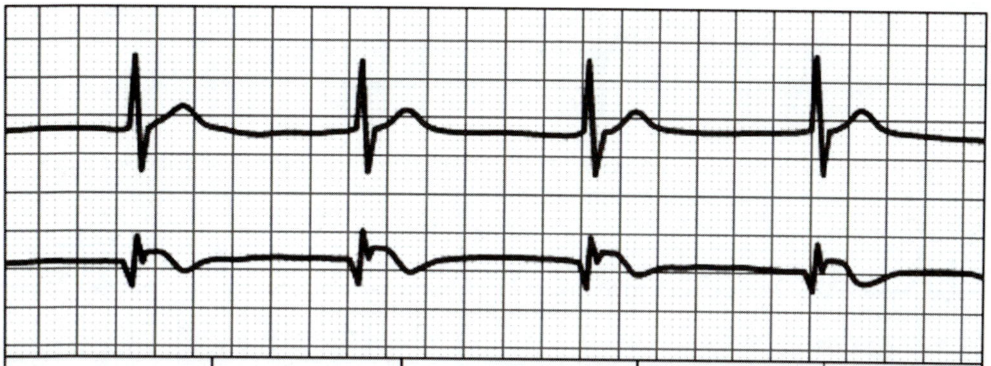

Heart rate	Rhythm	P wave	PR interval (in seconds)	QRS (in seconds)
40-60 bpm	Regular	Inverted, absent or after QRS	<.12	<.12

Fig. 40.52: *ECG showing junctional bradycardia*

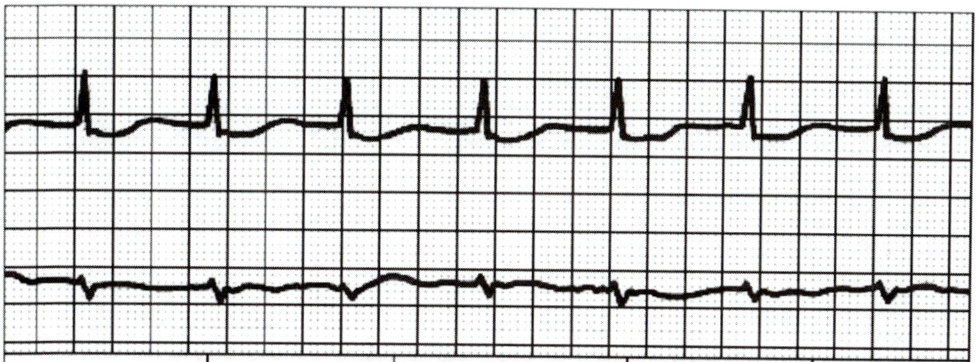

Heart rate	Rhythm	P wave	PR interval (in seconds)	QRS (in seconds)
60-100 bpm	Regular	Inverted, absent or after QRS	<.12	<.12

Fig. 40.53: *ECG showing accelerated junctional rhythm*

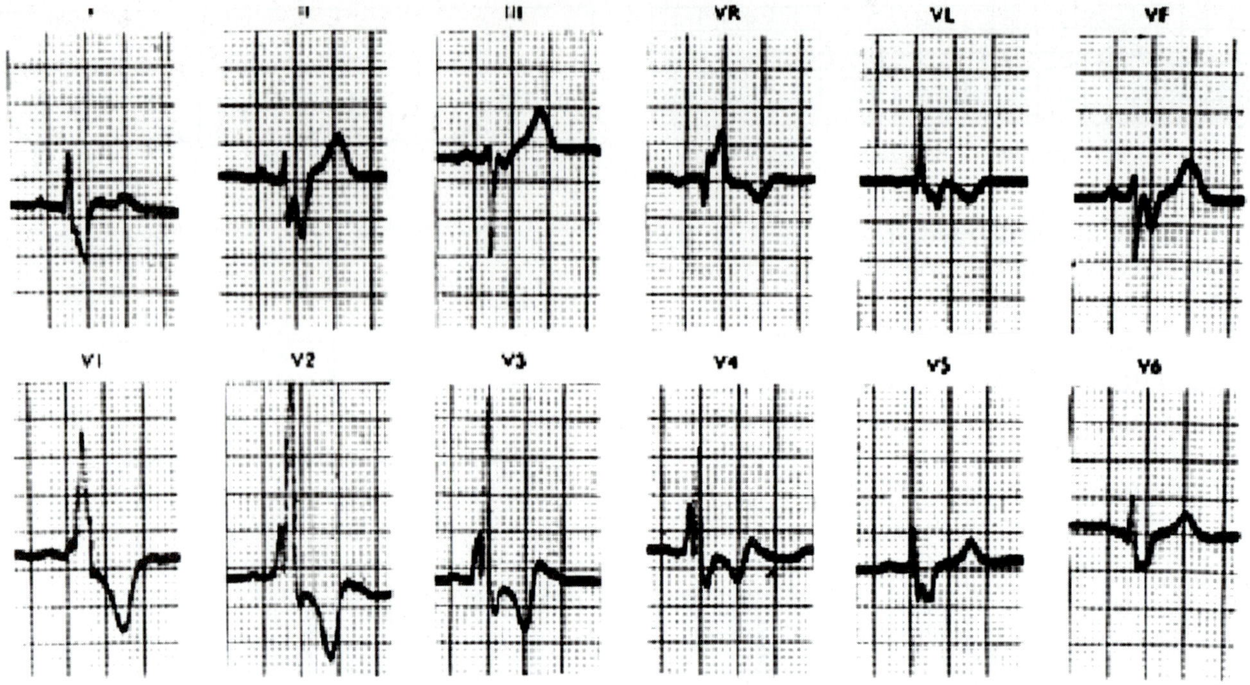

Fig. 40.54: *12 leads ECG showing left axis deviation and RBBB in bifascicular block*

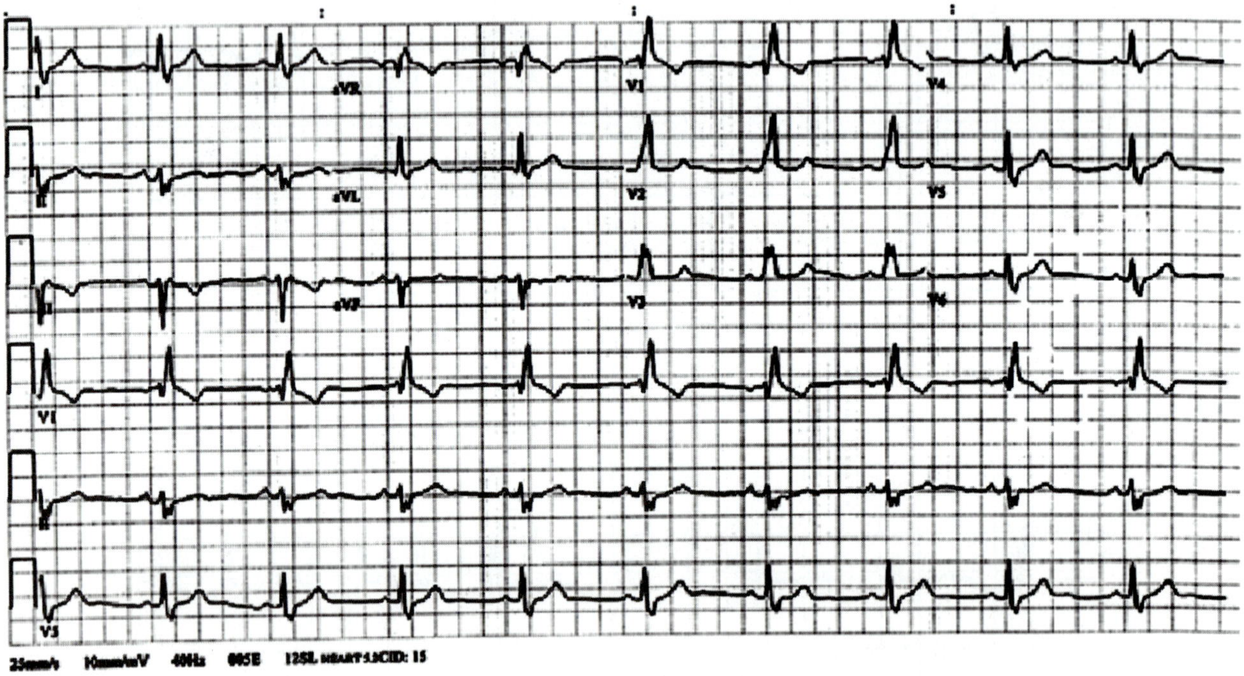

Fig. 40.55: *12 leads ECG showing bifascicular blocks RBBB + LAFB, i.e. RBBB + LAD*

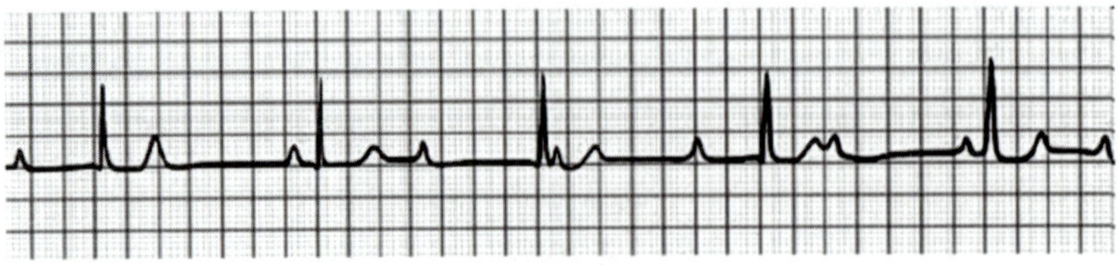

Fig. 40.56: *ECG trace showing complete heart block, there is complete absence of AV conduction—none of the supraventricular impulses are conducted to the ventricles*

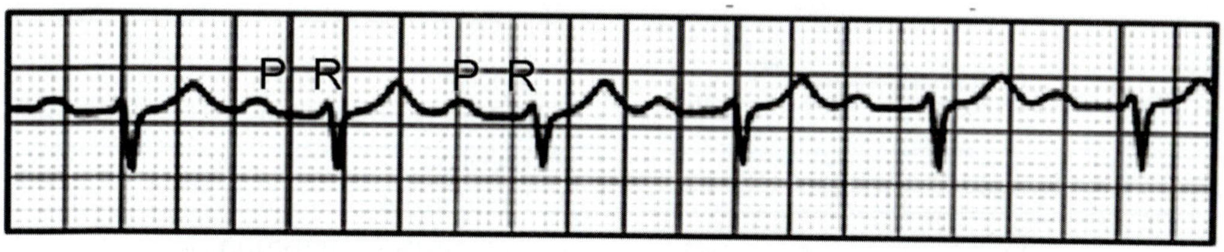

Fig. 40.57: *ECG trace showing 1st degree AV block (PR = 280 ms)*

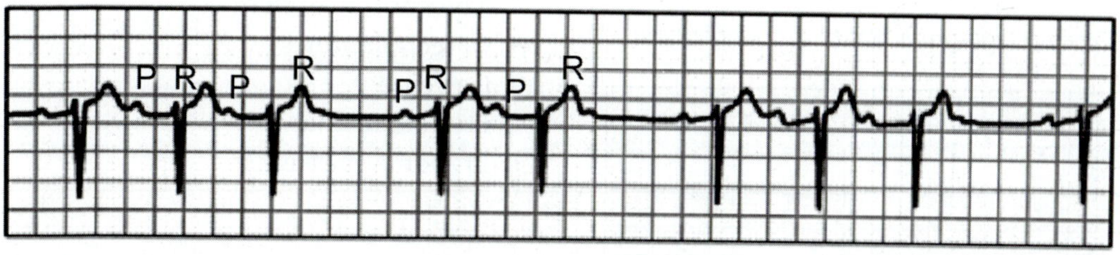

Fig. 40.58: *ECG trace showing type 1 AV block (classic Wenckebach phenomenon) with varying in PR interval till nonconducted P wave appears*

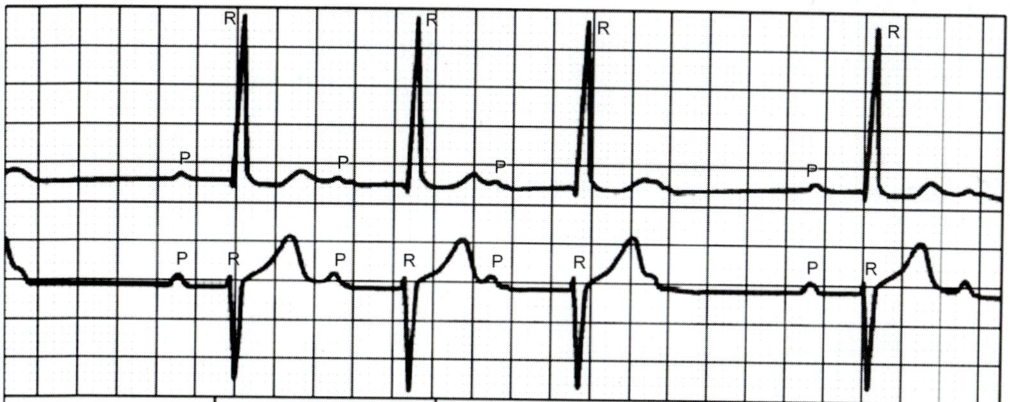

Heart rate	PR interval (in seconds)	QRS (in seconds)	Characteristics
Conduction intermittant	Increasingly prolonged	Before each QRS, identical	QRS dropped in a repeating pattern

Fig. 40.59: *Second degree AV block (Mobitz type 11). The PR interval are constant untill a nonconducted P wave appears*

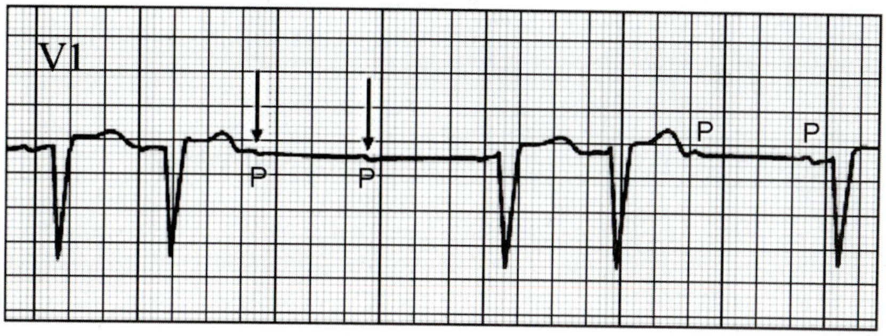

Fig. 40.60: *Second degree AV block (Mobitz type 11). The PR interval are constant untill a nonconducted P waves appears*

ECG Characteristics

1. Rate : It is of the underlying rhythm.
2. Rhythm : It is irregular due to PVC
3. PR interval : It is of the underlying rhythm. There is no P wave associated with the PVC.
4. QRS complex : It is wider due to PVC and may be normal with the basic underlying rhythm
5. Distinguishing features : No related P wave: premature, broad QRS complex; T wave of opposite polarity

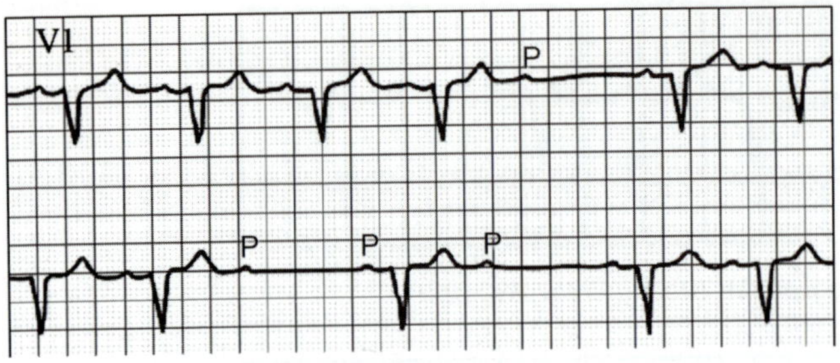

Fig. 40.61: *ECG showing high grade AV block (Mobiz type 11)*

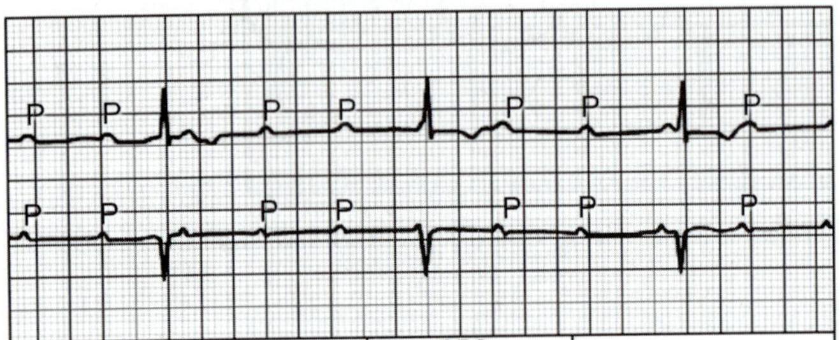

P wave	PR interval (in seconds)	QRS (in seconds)	Characteristics
Normal but not related to QRS	None	N/A	No relationship between P&RS

Fig. 40.62: *ECG showing third degree (complete) AV block with dissociation between P waves and QRS complexes variable PR interval and fixed RR interval*

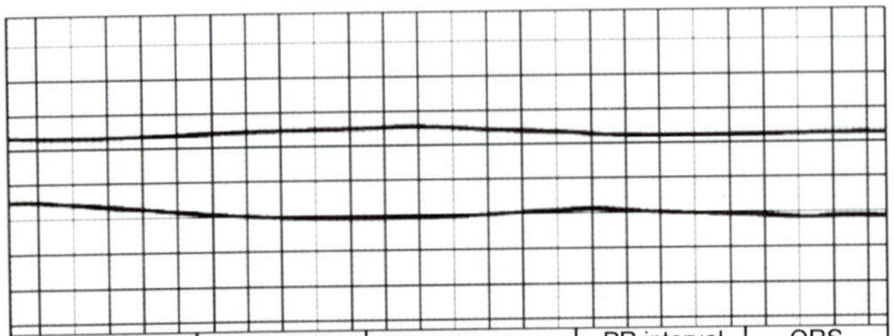

Heart rate	Rhythm	P wave	PR interval (in seconds)	QRS (in seconds)
Absent	Absent	Absent or present	N/A	Absent

Fig. 40.63: *ECG showing ventricular asystole (standstill)*

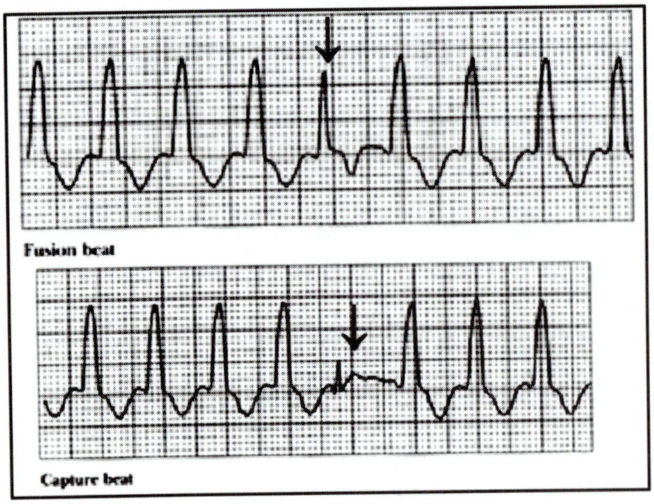

Fig. 40.64: *ECG showing formation and propagation of fusion beat (top arrow) and capture beat (bottom arrow)*

Etiological Factors

1. Digitalis
2. Drugs (epinephrine, isoproterenol, or aminophylline)
3. Hypoxia
4. Ischaemia
5. Myocardial infarction
6. Significant anaemia
7. Myocardial stretch
8. Catecholamines
9. Caffeine
10. Hypokalaemia
11. Hypomagnesaemia.

Variations

1. Unifocal PVCs and ventricular bigeminy
2. Ventricular trigeminy (one normal and two PVCs)
3. Paired PVCs
4. R-on-T PVCs
5. End-diastolic PVC
6. Interpolated PVC
7. PVC with retrograde conduction to the atria
8. Right ventricular PVC
9. Left ventricular PVC

Differential Diagnosis

Premature atrial contraction with aberrant ventricular unless a P wave comes in front of the broad beat or there is morphological proof of ventricular aberrancy. One should always make the diagnosis of ventricular ectopy unless proved otherwise.

Treatment

In the diseased, ischaemic, or infracted heart,anti- arrhythmics (lidocaine or procainamide) are given.

Ventricular Tachycardia (Figs 40.67–40.81)

When ventricular ectopics takes the shape of a rhythm with a rate of 100–170 beats/min, it is called as ventricular tachycardia.

ECG Characteristics

1. Rate : 100–170 beats/min
2. Rhythm : Regular 75% of the time
3. PR interval : Not applicable
4. QRS complex : 0.12 sec and most often 0.14 sec
5. Distinguishing features : Broad QRS complex with a regular rhythm and a rate between 100 and 170 beats/min left-axis deviation, and, in VI,a monophasic R, QR, qR, RS, or a "rabbit ear" configuration (that is, two peaks, the first being the tallest). In slower rates, AV dissociation may be seen; however, in 40% cases, there is retrograde conduction to the atria.

Key points: *Supraventricular tachycardias*

- The following groups of patients may benefit from referral to a cardiac electrophysiologists
  1. All patients with regular SVT on antiarrhythmic drugs
  2. All patients with recurrent regular SVT
  3. Patients with established AF in whom control of the ventricular response is suboptimal
  4. Patients with lone paroxysmal AF in whom maintenance of sinus rhythm cannot be achieved with class Ic antiarrhythmics
- It is likely that an effective curative catheter ablation procedure for established AF will be established within the next 10 years

Etiological Factors

1. Drugs (digitalis, isoproterenol)
2. Coronary artery disease
3. Acute myocardial infarction
4. Significant underlying cardiac disease
5. May occur in the absence of structural heart disease.

Variations

A. Ventricular tachycardia with retrograde conduction to the atria
B. Bidirectional ventricular tachycardia
C. Torsades de pointes
D. Ventricular flutter.

Treatment

If there is haemodynamic deterioration, cardioversion is indicated; otherwise, lidocaine or procainamide may be given. Cardioversion attempts with 10 watt-seconds should be started and increments increased until results are obtained.

Ventricular Fibrillation

It may be defined as disorganized electrical activity in the ventricles, resulting into inadequate contraction of the ventrical, incapable of maintaining sufficient cardiac output.

Differential Diagnosis

Ventricular fibrillation should always be distinguished from that of an erratic fibrillatory line within QRS complex.

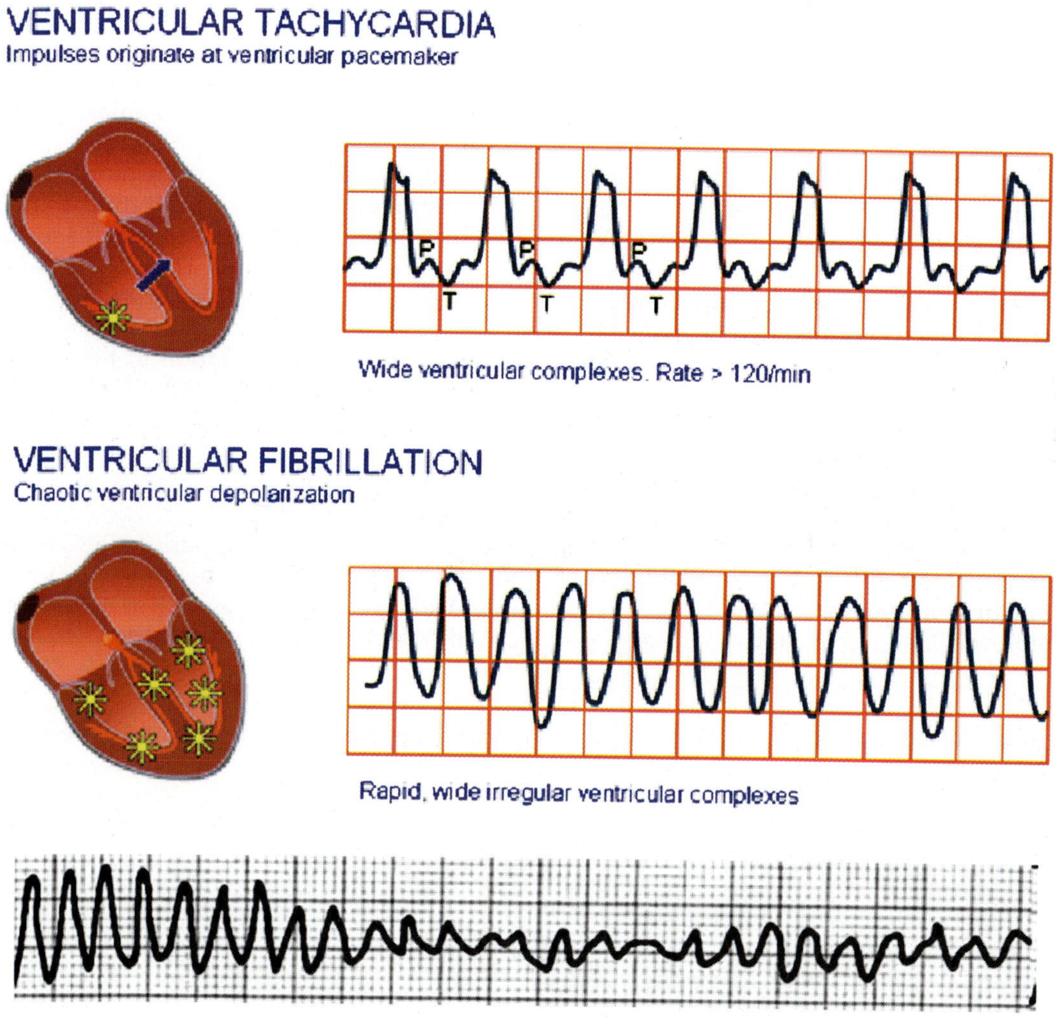

Fig. 40.65: *Ventricular tachy cardia and fibrillation*

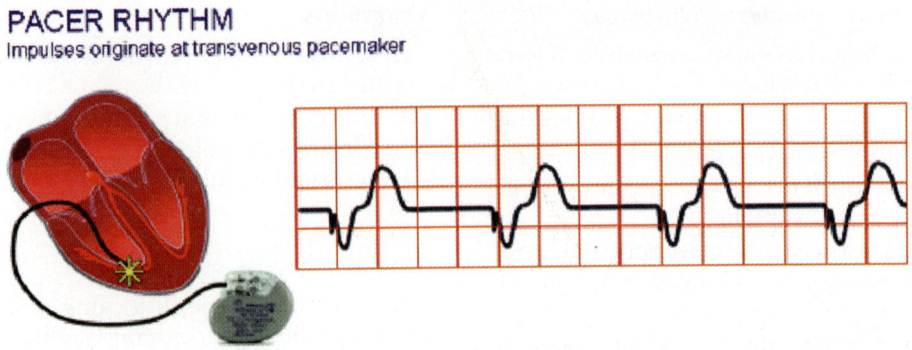

Fig. 40.66: *Wide ventricular complexes preceded by pacemaker spike. Rate is the pacer rhythm*

Etiological Factors

1. Myocardial infarction
2. Myocardial ischaemia
3. R-on-T, frequent, paired, or multifocal PVCs in the setting of acute myocardial infarction.

Variations

A. Coarse ventricular fibrillation
B. Fine ventricular fibrillation.

Treatment of ventricular fibrillation (VF)

1. Cough, CPR, if patient awake and able to cough
2. Defibrillate with 200 joules; repeat once if necessary
3. If successful, administer lidocaine, a bolus and an infusion per protocol.
4. If VF persists initiate chest compression and positive pressure ventilation. Start IV line.
5. Epinephrine 1:10,000, 5–10 mL (0.5 to 1 mg) IV or intratracheal.
6. After 30–60 sec of ventilation and chest compression, defibrillate with 300–400 joules; may repeat once.
7. Bretylium 5 mg/kg IV bolus.
8. Sodium bicarbonate 1 mEq.Kg IV push, especially if metabolic acidosis is documented by arterial blood gases.
9. If VF persists, attempt improvement of ventilation and oxygenation, continuous CPR, obtain arterial blood gases. Further sodium bicarbonate administration guided by arterial blood gas results, if available, if not, repeat one-half dose in 10 min.
10. Repeat epinephrine 0.5–1 mg IV stat.
11. Repeat defibrillation 300–400 joules
12. Repeat defibrillation 300–400 joules
13. Consider other drugs-magnesium, nitroglycerine, or additional bretylium.
14. Consider methods of "new CPR".

Torsades De Pointes

Torsades de pointes (twists of pointes) is a polymorphous ventricular tachycardia, associated with a prolonged Q-T interval.

ECG Characteristics

1.	Rate	: 150–250 beats/min
2.	Rhythm	: May be regular or irregular
3.	PR interval	: Not applicable
4.	QRS complex	: 0.12 sec; usually, 0.14 sec
5.	Distinguishing features	: In sinus rhythm, the QT interval is too long (0.46–0.50 sec or 33% of base-line). This measurement is absolute as opposed to the corrected. A ventricular tachycardia with phasic variation in the electrical polarity of the QRS complex. The tachycardia may be paroxysmal, repetitive, the patient remaining fully conscious.

Etiological Factors

Any of the factors, which leads to the lengthening of the Q-T interval, as mentioned below, can lead to this disorder:

1. Antiarrhythmic drugs such as quinidine, procainamide, disopyramide or amiodarone.

Table 40.10: *Modified lown classification for ventricular ectopy and common synonyms used for description of ventricular arrhythmias on long-term monitoring*

0	No ectopy		
1	Occasional VPBs (30/hours)	"Isolated"	
2	Frequent VPBs (>30/hours)		Low grade
3	Multiform VPBs		Moderate grade
4a	Couplets		
4b	VT or VF	"Repetitive"	High grade
5	Early VPB (R on T)		

VPB, ventricular premature beta; VT, ventricular tachycardia (≥ 3 consecutive beats): and VF, ventricular fibrillation

2. Hypokalaemia
3. Hypomagnesaemia
4. Psychotropic drugs
5. Unilateral alteration of sympathetic tone
6. Profound bradycardia
7. Intracerebral pathology.

Differential Diagnosis

Coarse ventricular fibrillation without preceding QT lengthening; ventricular flutter.

Treatment

It consists of removing any predisposing cause and suppressing the rapid ventricular rhythm. The anti arrhythmic drugs such as quinidine, procainamide, disopyramide, and most others that may prolong the QT interval should be avoided. Magnesium may be effective, especially when the rhythm is related to an antiarrhythmic drug. For acute management, isoproterenol infusion may be useful, particularly if there is underlying bradycardia. Atrial or ventricular overdrive pacing is also frequently very effective in acutely suppressing the rhythm. It should, usually, be continued for 24 hours. Prolonged episodes may require electrical defibrillation. If the rhythm recurs after all possible predisposing causes have been excluded, the patient should be treated with a beta-adrenergic blocking agent, which, usually, is successful. Occasionally refractory patient needs operation in which a left stellate ganglion sympathectomy or implantation of an automatic, defibrillation device is considered.

Temporary overdrive ventricular or atrial pacing IV magnesium sulfate (IV push: 2 g over 1–2 min: IV infusion: 1–2 g/hr for 4–6 hr).

Accelerated Idioventricular Rhythm

The accelerated idioventricular rhythm (AIVR) is an ectopic ventricular rhythm with a rate of 40–100 beats/min.

ECG Characteristics

1. Rate : 40–100 beats/min
2. Rhythm : Regular
3. PR interval : Not applicable, but that of the underlying rhythm may be normal.
4. QRS complex : 0.12 sec; usually, 0.14 sec
5. Distinguishing features : A ventricular ectopic rhythm that, often, begins and ends with fusion beats and misifests itself when its rate is approximately that of the sinus node.

Cause

Acute myocardial infarction.

Variations

Accelerated idioventricular rhythm with atrial flutter.

Ventricular Fusion Complexes

It may be defined as the type of resultant complex when two impulses collide with each other in the ventricles, like the one, seen in atrial fusion beats in atria.

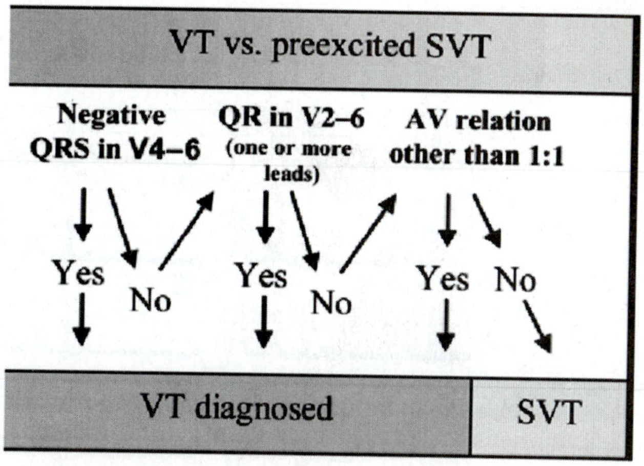

Fig. 40.67: *VTs and SVTs were in the comparison*

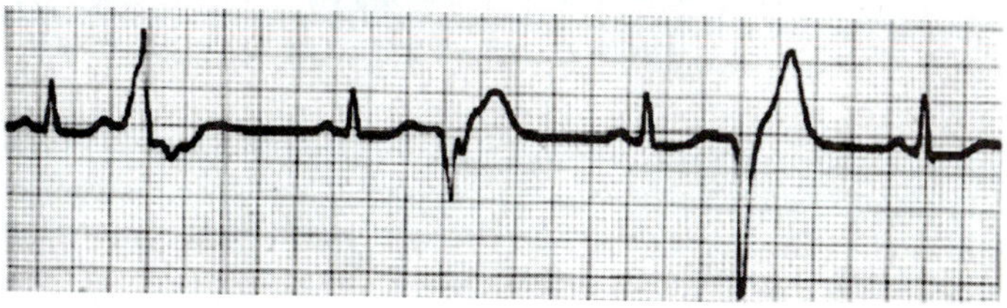

Fig. 40.68: *ECG trace showing multifocal ventricular ectopics*

ECG Characteristics

1. Rate : That of the underlying rhythm
2. Rhythm : Regular
3. PR interval : PR interval of the fusion beat may be the same as or shorter than that of the sinus rhythm, but is never more than 0.06 sec shorter than the dominant PR interval.
4. QRS complex : Normal in the underlying rhythm, but may be variable in the fusion beats.
5. Distinguishing features : It should be differentiated from other ventricular ectopic beats by critically analyzing the basic rhythm.

QRS of the fusion beat has a contour intermediate between that of the fusing impulses.

Causes

That of the ventricular ectopic beat or rhythm.

Variations

1. Ventricular parasystole
2. Accelerated idioventricular rhythm
3. Electronic pacemaker fusion beat
4. End-diastolic PVCs
5. Bigeminal end-diastolic PVCs.

Differential Diagnosis

Electrical alternans vs bigeminal end-diastolic PVCs.

Ventricular Parasystole

These are usually unifocal premature ventricular contractions which have varying coupling intervals at regular

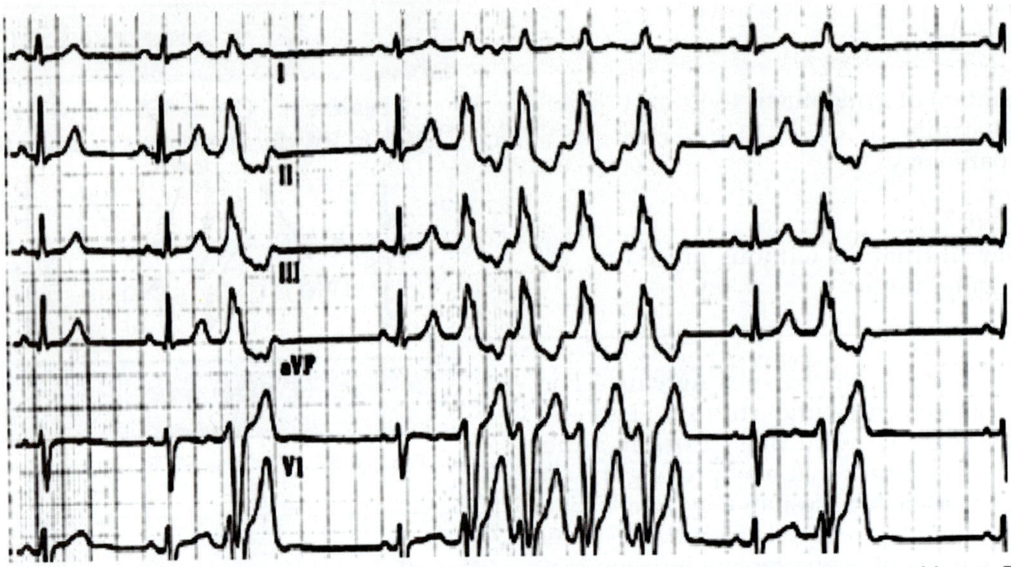

Fig. 40.69: *ECG showing repetitive monomorphic ventricular tachycardia (VT) with a structurally normal heart. This ECG pattern is typical for idiopathic VT arising from the right ventricular outflow tract. This rhythm is often exertional and, unlike ischemic VT, suppressed by beta-blockade or verapamil. The prognosis is good with the following exceptions: (1) sudden death may be seen if right ventricular dysplasia or exceptionally rapid VT is encountered, and (2) occasionally, patients with incessant VT develop congestive heart failure due to tachycardia-induced cardiomyopathy or frequent ectopy. The cardiomyopathy resolves when the tachycardia is treated*

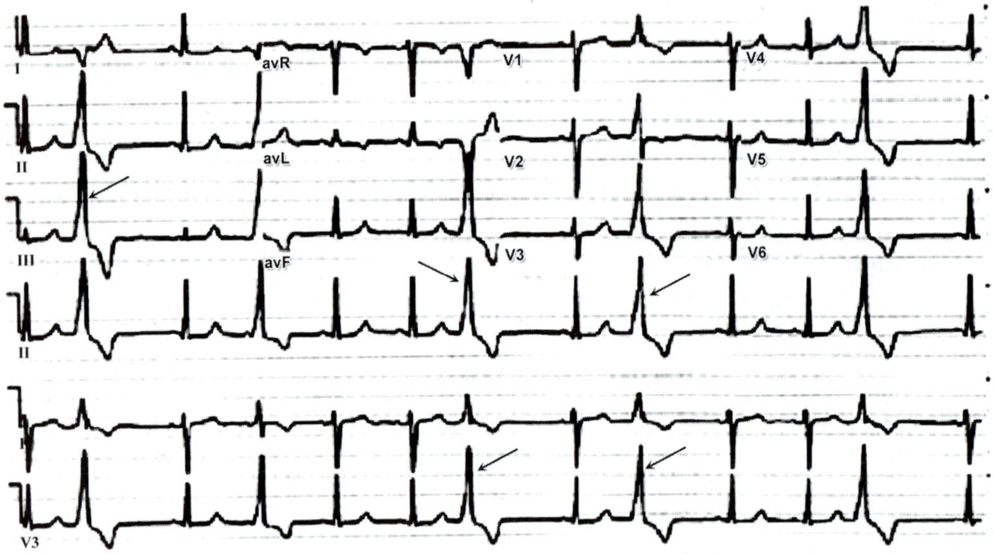

Fig. 40.70: *Holter ECG A 18-year-young person complaining of recurrent palpitation was advised Holter monitoring. On Holter study, he had bigeminy pattern of cardiac arrhythmia*

cadence. Such a constantly recurring ectopic beat is termed as parasystole. Parasystole is diagnosed by observing on active focus of automaticity, usually, in the region of ventricle, which operates independently of the dominant pacemaker. The rhythmic discharges are, somewhat, not affected by the propagation of the primary impulse. In this condition, both the dominant and the parasystolic rhythms have separate and independent cadences.

In classical ventricular parasystole, the rate of impulses from the ectopic focus is considerably slower than that of the sinus node, because the sinus node and the ventricular ectopic focus are firing independently of one another and at different rates. Premature ventricular contractions produced by this mechanism, usually, will show marked variation in coupling (R-V) intervals. Electrocardiographic analysis will reveal that the intervals, between successive premature ventricular contractions, are all multiples of a manifest or calculated minimum V-V interval. Clinically, it seems to be benign condition. The parasystolic arrhythmia is, frequently, resistant to antiarrhythmic drug therapy.

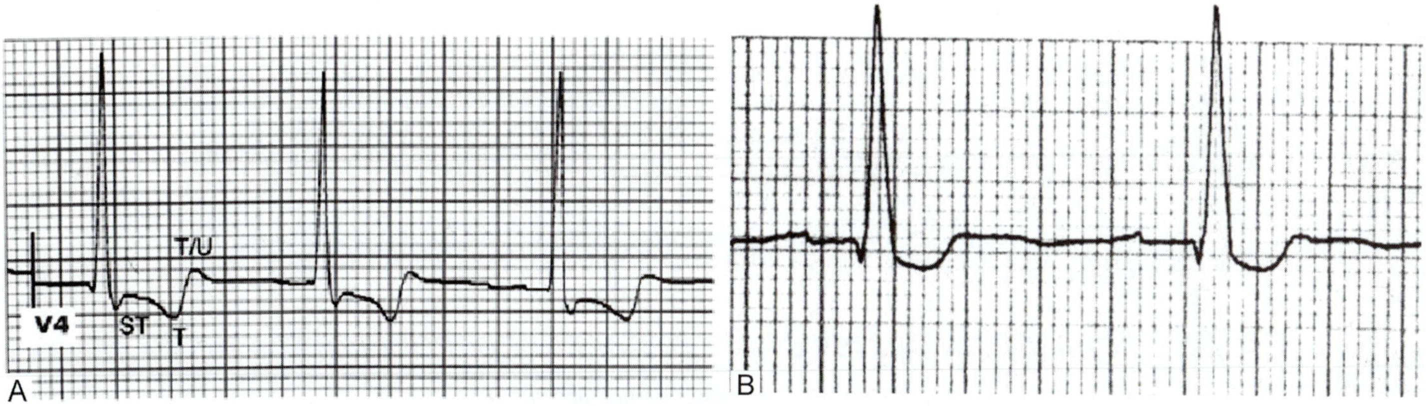

Fig. 40.71: *(A) The ECG features of digoxin effect are seen with therapeutic doses of digoxin and are due to: Shortening of the atrial and ventricular refractory periods—producing a short QT interval with secondary repolarisation abnormalities affecting the ST segments, T waves and U waves. Increased vagal effects at the AV node—causing a prolonged PR interval. (B) Overdose changes are reflected on the ECG by a decrease in ventricular response rate PR-interval prolongation, QT-interval shortening, and ST-segment and T-wave forces opposite the direction of the major QRS forces (scooped ST segment). This results in the characteristic digitalis effect*

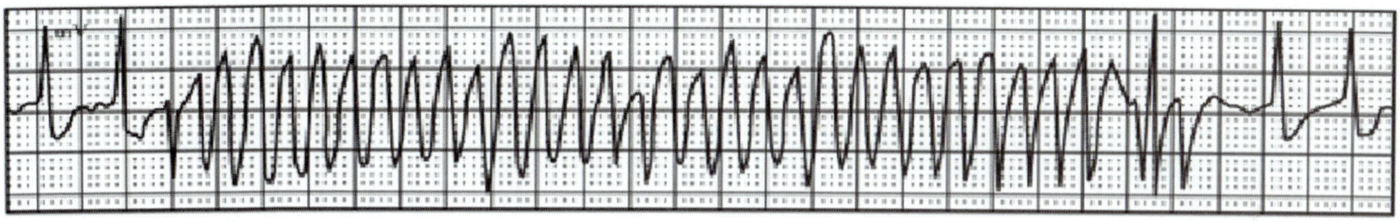

Fig. 40.72: *ECG trace showing torsades de pointes, or "twisting around a point" is the description of an arrhythmia similar to ventricular fibrillation. This arrhythmia, shown in the next figure, results in ineffective cardiac output and cardiac arrest if it is not converted to a more effective rhythm. Torsades de pointes can convert back to a normal rhythm spontaneously or after defibrillation*

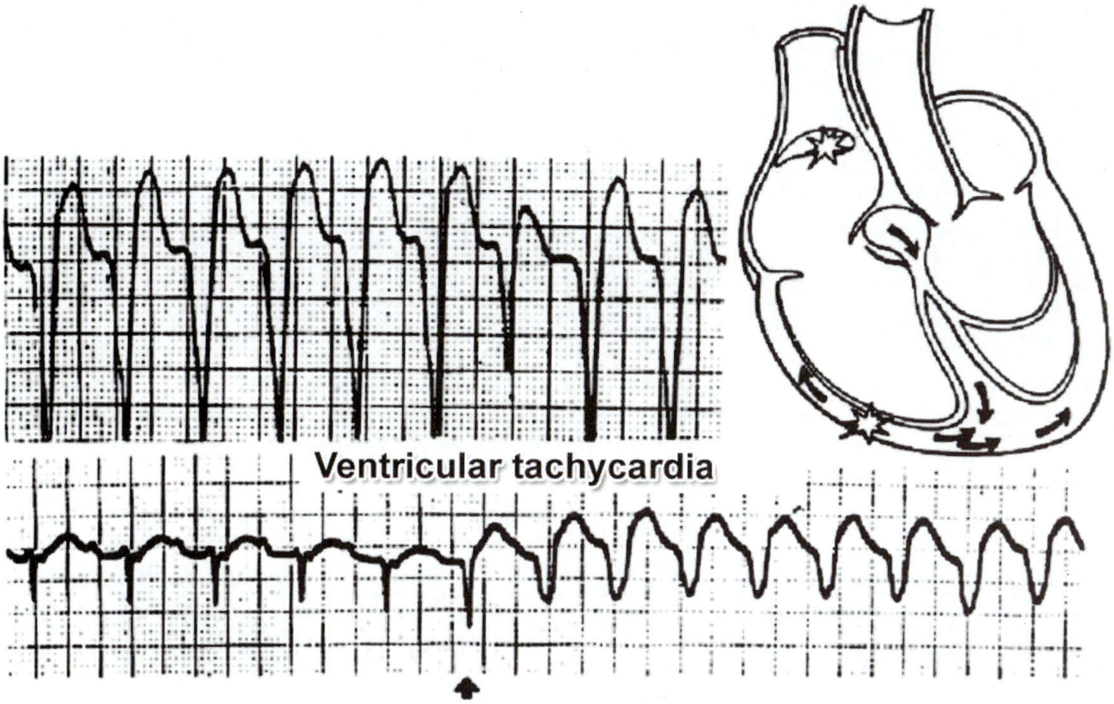

Fig. 40.73: *ECG showing ventricular tachycardia (upper panel) and fusion beat as indicated (lower panel) and diagram showing the genesis of fusion beats (upper right panel)*

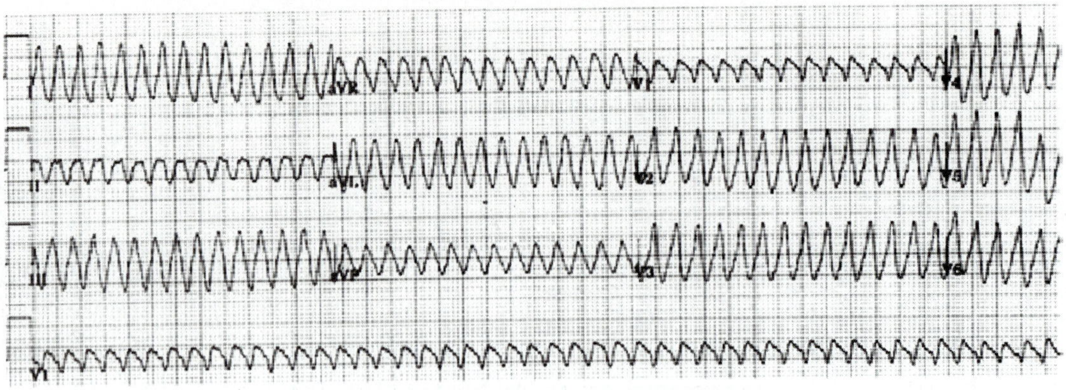

Fig. 40.74: *ECG showing ventricular flutter*

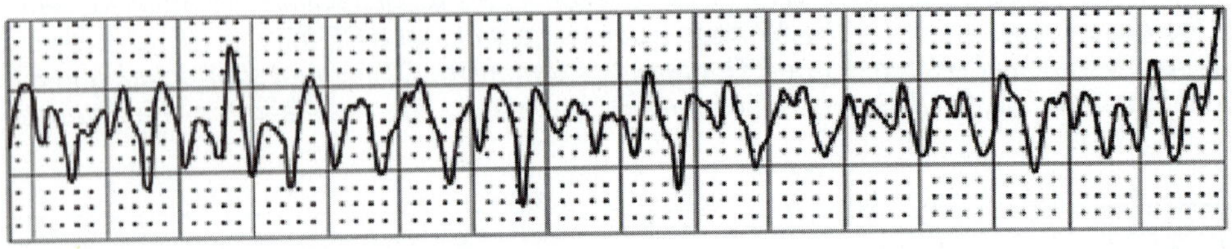

Fig. 40.75: *ECG showing ventricular fibrillation is an arrhythmia resulting from rapid and uncoordinated electrical discharges from the ventricle. It results in a lack of cardiac output and a cardiac arrest. The only treatment for ventricular fibrillation is defibrillation*

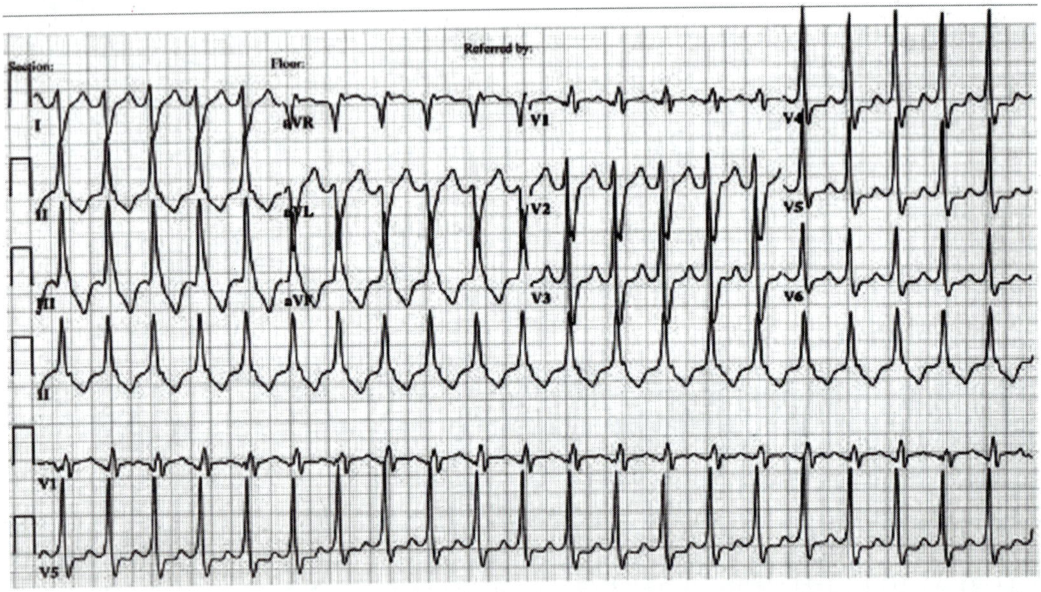

Fig. 40.76: *Electrocardiogram illustrating left ventricular outflow tract ventricular tachycardia (LVOT VT). The S wave in L1 and R-wave transition in V1 suggest LVOT VT. In addition, an R:S amplitude ratio of 30% and an R:QRS duration ratio of 50% are seen. Presence of an S wave in leads V5 and V6 suggests an infravalvular origin of the tachycardia*

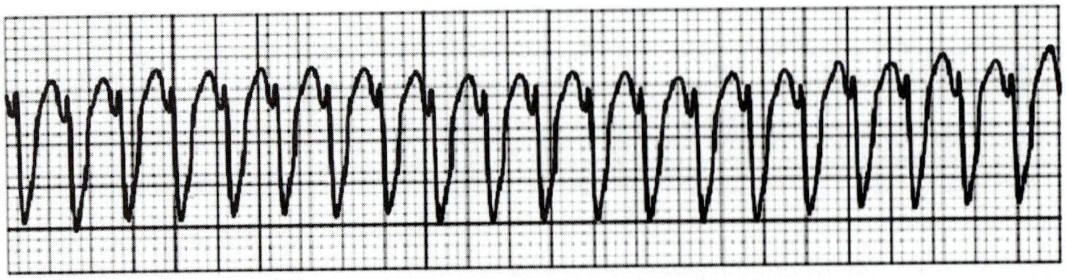

Fig. 40.77: *ECG trace showing ventricular tachycardia: broad QRS complexes with no visible P waves*

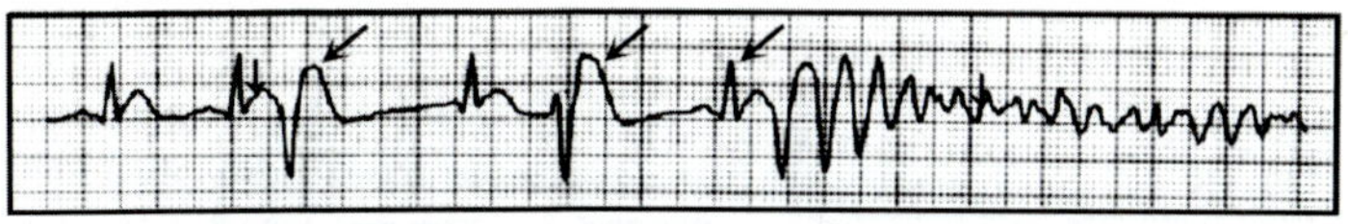

Fig. 40.78: *ECG trace showing R on T phenomenon (arrow) giving rise to ventricular fibrillation (arrow)*

ECG Characteristics

1. Rate : That of the underlying rhythm
2. Rhythm : Irregular, as a result of extrasytoles
3. PR interval : Normal is the underlying rhythm
4. QRS complex : Normal in the underlying rhythm; broad in the parasystolic beats
5. Distinguishing features : a. No fixed coupling
   b. Interectopic intervals that have a common denominator
   c. Fusion beats

Variations

Fixed coupling in parasystole if the rates of the two pacemaker happen to be mathematically related. No fixed coupling, but interectopic intervals are not exact multiples, because the ectopic focus is influenced, but not reset, by the sinus impulses.

Differential Diagnosis

Accelerated idioventricular rhythm.

Ventricular Flutter and Fibrillation

The electrocardiographic diagraphic of ventricular flutter is made the ventricular tachyarrhythmias is greater than 200 beats/min, and large sinusoidal or zig-zag waves are observed. The rate, is, frequently, between 240 beats/min and 280 beats/min. In ventricular flutter, QRS complex cannot be clearly distinguished from ST-T waves. The diagnosis of ventricular flutter may be applied when the rate is less than 200 beats/ min if the ECG morphology is absolutely typical.

Ventricular fibrillation is recognized on ECG tracing by the absence of QRS complex and T waves and the presence of low-amplitude baseline undulations which are quite variable, both in amplitude and periodicity.

Clinically, ventricular flutter is, rarely, recorded, perhaps, due to its highly unstable rhythm that tends to convert to sinus-rhythm or, more often, to ventricular fibrillation. Ventricular flutter, nearly always, leads to severe and symptomatic haemodynamic impairment.

Ventricular fibrillation on the other hand is the most catastrophic cardiac arrhythmia. It is usually, observed in myocardial infarction, hypokalamia marked hypothermia, electrocution and drug toxicity, i.e. with digitalis, quinidine, procainamide or tricyclic antidepressants. Ventricular fibrillation can lead to death, within a short period due to cardiogenic collapse if such a rhythm is not converted to haemodynamically effective rhythm.

ECG Characteristics

1. Rate : 150–300 beats/min
2. Rhythm : Regular or irregular
3. PR interval : Not applicable
4. QRS complex : Broad and poorly defined
5. Distinguishing features : A zig-zag, almost a sine wave configuration, instead of clearly defined QRS complex.

Etiological Factors

1. Myocardial infarction
2. Myocardial ischaemia
3. R-on-T frequent, paired, or multifocal PVCs in the setting of acute myocardial infarction.
4. An interim arrhythmia between ventricular tachycardia and fibrillation.
5. Drugs (digitalis, procainamide, quinidine and tricyclic antidepressants).
6. Electrolyte imbalance, i.e. hypokalaemia.

Differential Diagnosis

Torsades de pointes.

Ventricular Escape

It is ectopic beat which takes its origin in the ventricle and is followed by a long pause. It, usually, has it rate the same as that of the underlying rhythm. It is caused by the failure of the sinus node or AV conduction along with failure of the junctional escape mechanism. Electrocardiographically, it usually, has irregular rhythm with broad QRS complex. followed by along pause. It should always be differentiated from late junctional escape with phase 4 aberration.

Treatment

That of the underlying cause.

Long QT Syndrome (Fig. 40.87)

Patients with a prolonged QT interval are more prone to the risk of recurrent syncope and sudden death due to ventricular tachycardia or ventricular fibrillation. The idiopathic long QT syndrome ventricular fibrillation. The idiopathic long QT syndrome may be either autosomal recessive or autosomal dominant.

Prolongation of the QT interval may be

a. Acquired by patients having electrolyte-imbalance,
b. Taking antiarrhythmic drugs
c. Taking psychotropic drugs
d. Having myocarditis
e. Myocardial ischemia
f. Sinus node disease or
g. Central nervous system disease
h. Consuming liquid protein diets.

It is associated with a specific type of ventricular arrhythmia, torsade de pointes, which is characterized by the cycles of alternating electrical polarity of the QRS complex peaks that oscillate or twist around the isoelectric line. The alternating cycles may be interrupted by periods of rapid tachycardia and polarity. The rhythm rate varies from 160 to 280 beats per minute and most often is between

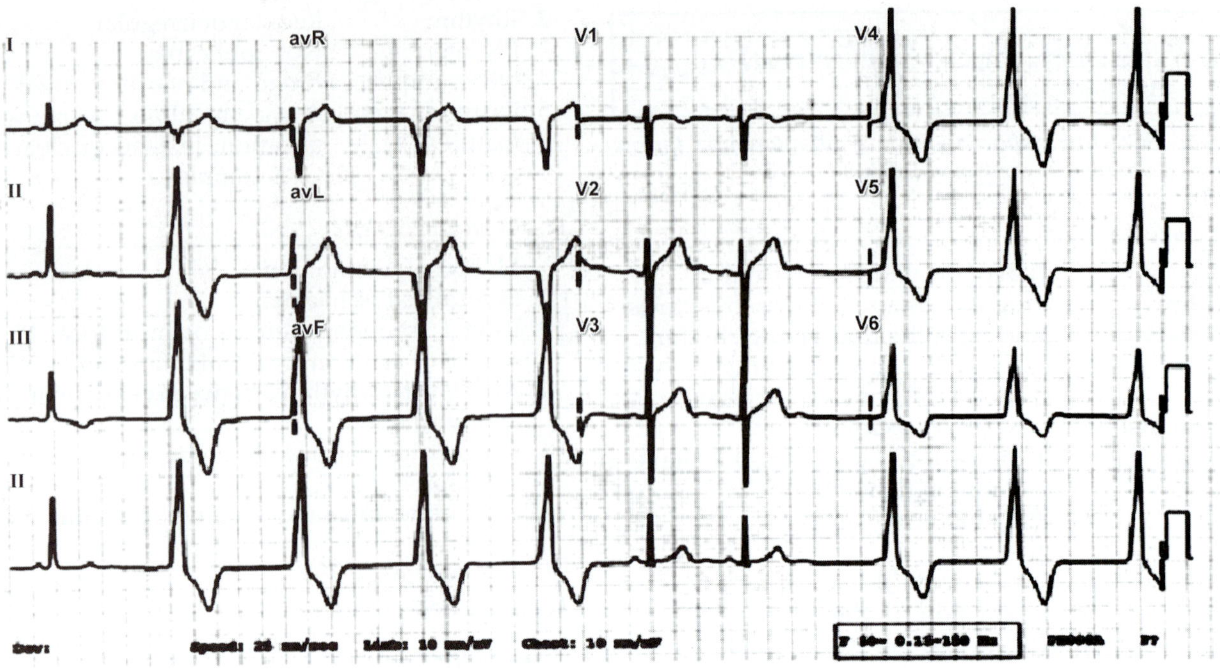

Fig. 40.79: *ECG showing accelerated idioventricular rhythm (AIVR), sinus capture beats, isorhythmic AV dissociation, sinus arrhythmia*

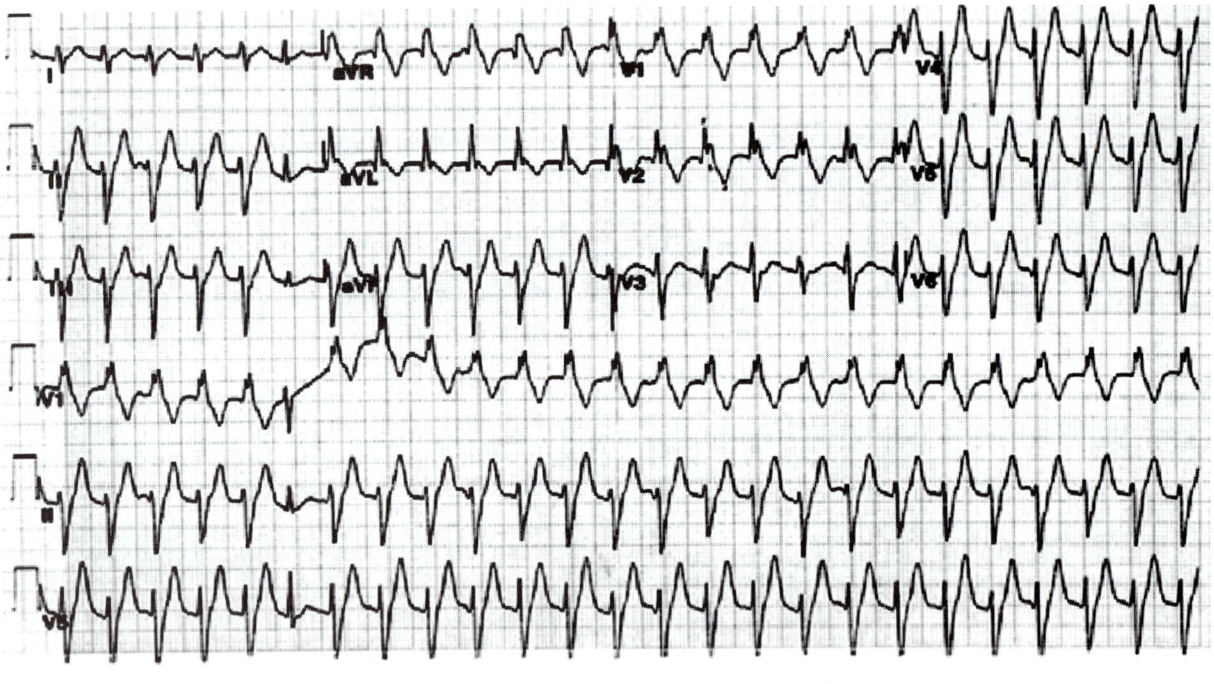

Fig. 40.80: *12 leads ECG showing idiopathic fascicular VT*

200 and 250 beats per minute. Assessment and treatment of ventricular tachyarrhythmias present extraordinary challenges to the clinician. Moreover, the prognosis for patients is quite variable with these characteristically sudden-onset, unpredictable, and transitory arrhythmias. In some patients, ventricular ectopic activity may be benign and without sequelae, but in other patients, comparable ectopy is a harbinger of ventricular fibrillation and sudden cardiac death.

Short QT Syndrome (Fig. 40.88)

Short QT syndrome is a genetic disease of the electrical system of the heart. It consists of a constellation of signs and symptoms, consisting of a short QT interval interval on EKG (300 ms) that doesn't significantly change with heart rate, tall and peaked T waves, and a structurally normal heart. Short QT syndrome appears to be inherited in an autosomal dominant pattern, and a few affected

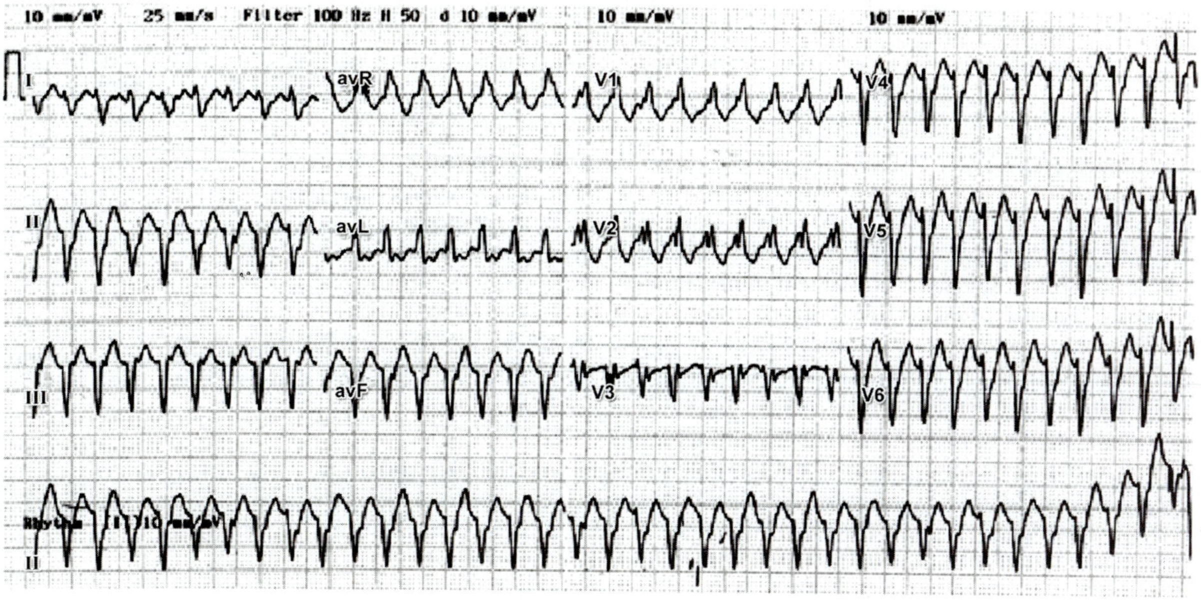

Fig. 40.81: *ECG showing features of monomorphic VT*

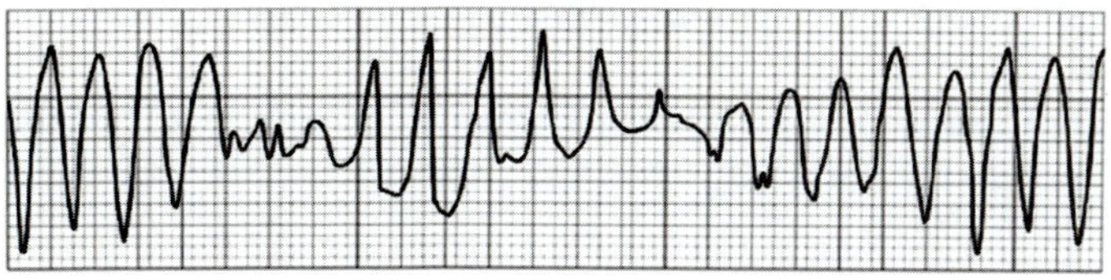

Fig. 40.82: *ECG trace showing torsades de pointes*

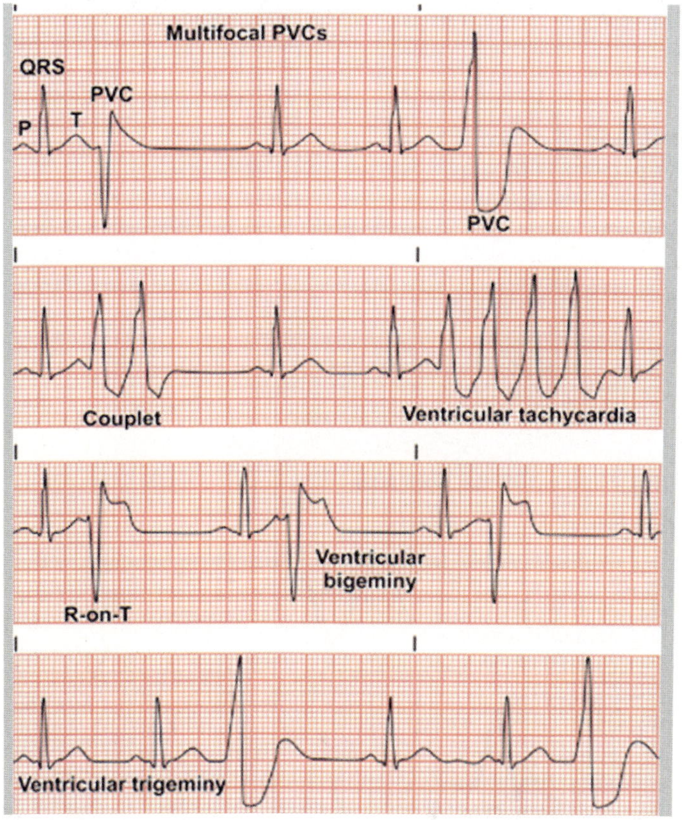

Fig. 40.83: *Illustration shows various forms of premature contractions (PVCS) in lead 11*

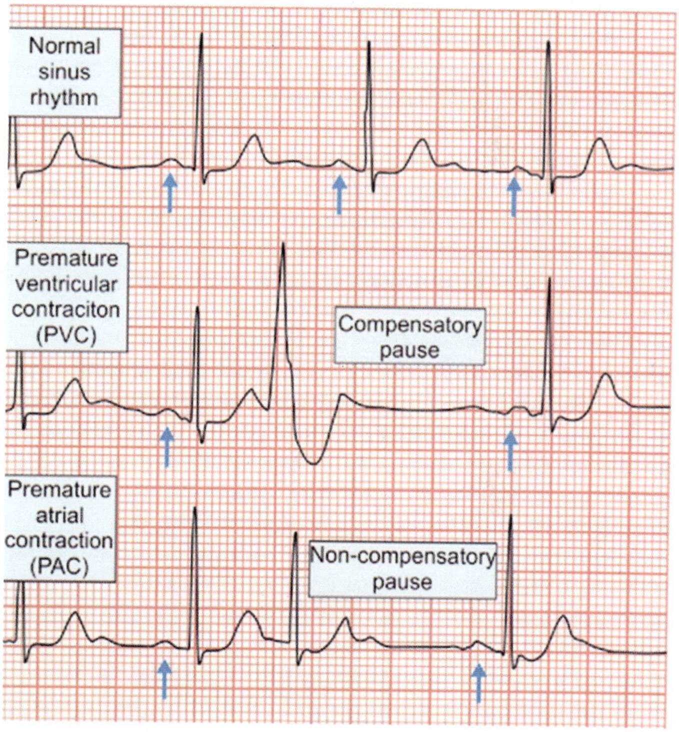

Fig. 40.84: *ECG showing compensatory and noncompensatory pause in relation to PVC and PAC*

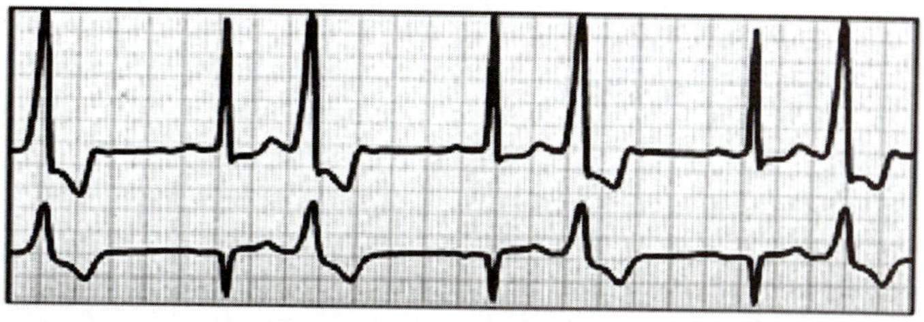

Fig. 40.85: *ECG shows bigeminal PVCS, every other beat is a PVC*

Table 40.11: *Summarizes drugs used in the emergency management of life-threatening ventricular arrhythmias*

Medication	*VF pulseless VT*	*Stable monomorphic VT*	*Stable wide complex tachycardia etiology uncertain*	*Unstable monomorphic VT*	*Torsades de pointes*
Amiodarone	Initial:300 mg Recurrent/ persistent: 150 mg diluted in 100 mL D5W over 10 min	150 mg diluted in 100 mL D5W over 10 min. Follow with continuous infusion 1 mg/min for 6 hr, then 0.5 mg/min for 18 hr	150 mg diluted in 100 mL D5W over with continuous infusion 1 mg/min for 6 hr, then 0.5 mg/min for 18 hr	Not first treatment of choice	Not treatment of choice
Lidocaine	Recurrent/ persistent: 1–1.5 mg/kg IV push. May follow with repeat bolus every 5–10 mins. Maximum total dose: 3 mg/kg	1.5 mg/kg IV push. May follow with repeat bolus of 0.5–0.75 mg/kg every 5 to 10 mins to max total dose of 3 mg/kg or maintenance infusion of 2–4 mg/min (30–50 mcg/ kg/min)	Not treatment of choice	Not first treatment of choice	Not treatment of choice
Magnesium sulfate	Only indicated if hypomagnesemia is suspected or known	Only indicated if hypo-magnesemia is suspected or known	Only indicated if hypomagnesemia is suspected	Only indicated if hypomagesemia is suspected	For cardiac arrest: 1–2 grams over a maximum of 15 mins given IV push
Procainamide	Persistent/ recurrent Loading dose: 20–50 mg/min (or 100 mg every 5 mins) IV infusion	Loading dose: 20–50 mg/ min (or 100 mg every 5 mins) IV infusion Maintenance infusion: 1–4 mg/min Maximum dose: 17 mg/kg Not drug of choice for persons with reduced ventricular function	Loading dose: 20–50 mg/min (or 100 mg every 5 mins) IV infusion Maintenance infusion: 1–4 mg/min Not drug of choice for persons with reduced ventricular function	Not first treatment of choice	Not treatment of choice

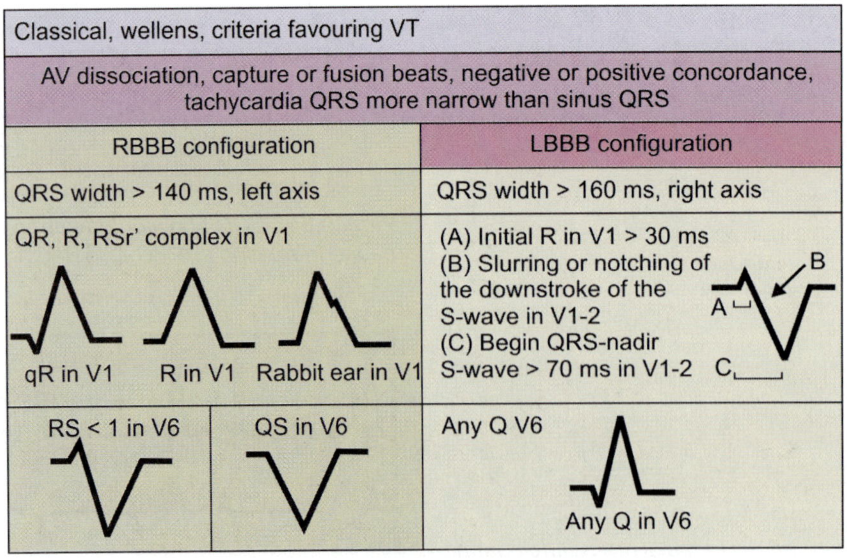

Fig. 40.86: *Classical "Wellens" criteria favouring VT*

families have been identified. Short QT syndrome is inherited in an autosmal dominant patterns. Individuals with short QT syndrome frequently complain of palpitations and may have syncope (loss of consciousness) that is unexplained. Mutations in the $KCNH_2$, $KCNJ_2$, and KCNQ1 genes cause short QT syndrome. These genes provide instructions for making proteins that act as channels across the cell membrane. These channels transport positively charged atoms (ions) of potassium into and out of cells. In cardiac muscle, these ion channels play critical roles in maintaining the heart's normal rhythm. Mutations in the $KCNH_2$, $KCNJ_2$, or KCNQ1 gene increase the activity of the channels, which changes the flow of potassium ions between cells. This disruption in ion transport alters the way the heart beats, leading to the abnormal heart rhythm characteristic of short QT syndrome. Short QT syndrome appears to have an autosomal dominant pattern of inheritance. Due to the autosomal dominant inheritance pattern, most individuals will have family members with a history of unexplained or sudden death at a young age (even in infancy), palpitations, or atrial fibrillation. Short QT syndrome is associated with an increased risk of sudden cardiac death, most likely due to ventricular fibrillation.

Diagnosis: The diagnosis of short QT syndrome consists of characteristic history and findings on EKG and electrophysiologic testing. There are currently no set guidelines for the diagnosis of short QT syndrome.

Electrocardiogram: The characteristic findings of short QT syndrome on EKG are a short QT interval, typically 300 ms, that doesn't significantly change with the heart rate. Tall, peaked T waves may also be noted. Individuals may also have an underlying atrial rhythm of atrial fibrillation.

Brugada Syndrome (Fig. 40.89)

In 1992, Brugada and colleagues described a clinical syndrome consisting of apparently healthy adults presenting with syncope or sudden death. Their ECGs showed coved ST segment elevation and negative T waves in leads VI and V2 (V3) in the absence of RBBB pattern This ECG pattern has become to be known as the "Brugada-ECG". These patients were thought to have no evidence of structural heart disease, and were at high risk for recurrent syncope or sudden death. In 15% to 20% of patients a genetic defect in the cardiac sodium channel was found. It has been proposed that there is a premature termination of the epicardial action potential with loss of the phase-2 dome pattern. The ECG changes are believed to be due to regional epicardial, endocardial voltage gradient during the plateau phase of the action potential. This voltage gradient may give rise to VT due to phase-2 reentry caused by inhomogeneity of the voltage in adjacent areas of the myocardium. In patients with the Brugada syndrome, syncope and sudden death are due to polymorphic VT. Since the original descripion, it has been observed that the "Brugada-ECG" type ST segment elevation in V1 in the right precordial leads can be:

1. Cove shaped
2. Saddle shaped
3. Transient
4. Be present in a multitude of clinical-conditions.

There has been a recent attempt to standardize this diagnostic ECG feature as follows:

Type I: Coved-shaped right precordial ST elevation, in more than one right precordial lead (VI-V3), of > 2 mm followed by a negative T wave:

Type II: Saddle-shaped ST elevation

Type III: ST elevation of < 2 mm.

Only type I is said to be diagnostic of Brugada syndrome. These ST elevations are sensitive to heart rate and the effects of autonomic stimulation. Furthermore, sodium channel-blocking antiarrhythmic drugs such as procainamide or lecainide have been shown to "provoke" these ECG changes in patients with otherwise normal baseline ECG, and have been proposed as a screening tool in patients suspected to have the Brugada syndrome. However, the sensitive, specificity and reproducibility of this drug provocation are not well established. Of interest, certain gene mutations are sensitive to temperature with regard

Table 40.12: *Ventricular arrhythmias: who to refer and who not to refer to an electrophysiologist*

Do not refer:	*Do refer*
• Patients with mildly symptomatic or asymptomatic ventricular ectopic activity	• Patients with highly symptomatic ventricular ectopic activity
• Asymptomatic patients with "benign" ventricular tachycardia on or off antiarrhythmic drug treatment	• Symptomatic patients with "benign" ventricular tachycardia or controlled only with unacceptable side effects from antiarrhythmic drugs
• Patients who are candiates for prophylactic ICD implantation but without symptomatic arrhythmia	• Patients who are candidates for prophylactic ICD implantation but with symptomatic arrhythmia
	• Any patient with symptomatic ventricular tachycardia with or without prophylactic ICD indication
	• Any patient suspected of having a "sudden cardiac death syndrome"
	• Any patient in whom arrhythmia mechanism is uncertain

ICD, implantable cardioverter-defibrillator.

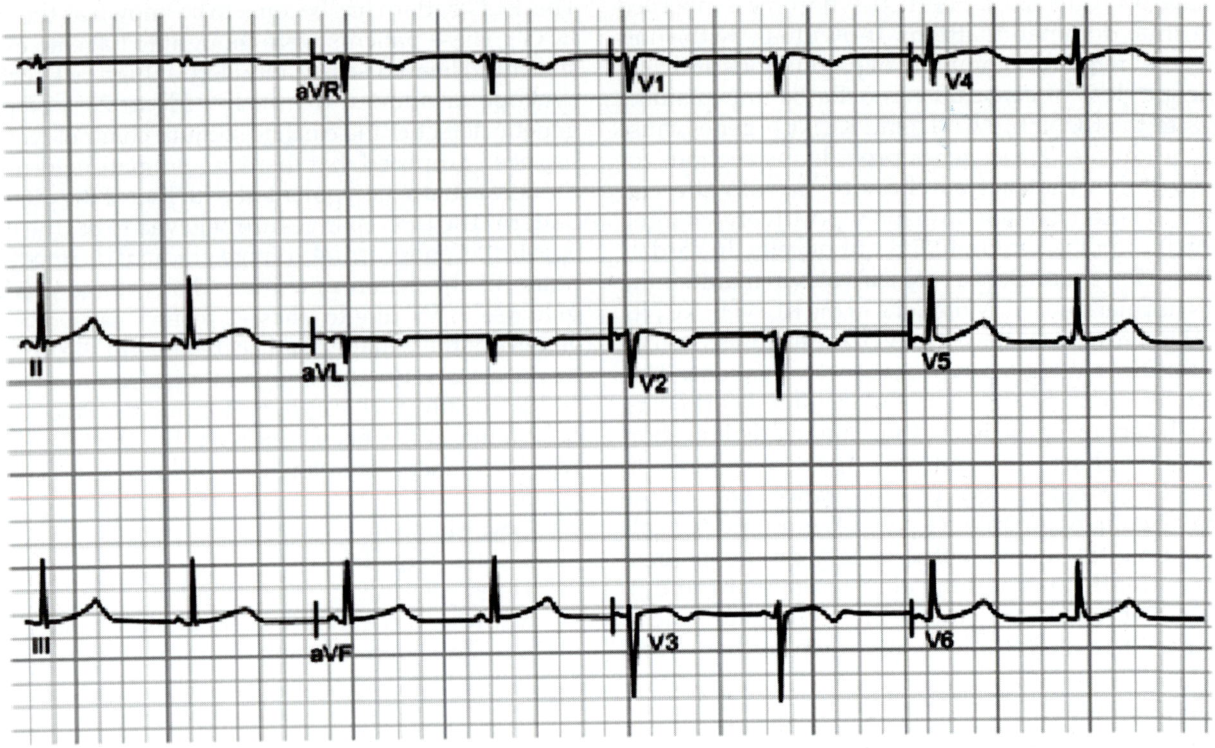

Fig. 40.87: *12 leads ECG showing long QTc (620 ms) due to severe hypothermia*

to their phenotypic expression. Indeed, Brugada-type ECG changes have been seen in patients only during febrile illness. Some speculate that seizures during febrile illness may be related to self-terminating ventricular arrhythmias due to a temperature sensitive mutation in the sodium channel, giving rise to the "Brugada syndrome".

Patients with resuscitated sudden death or syncope or with a family history of premature sudden death and typical type I Brudaga ECG changes are at increased risk of recurrent events, and should be considered for ICD" therapy. Asymptomatic patients who have an unprovoked typical Brudaga ECG (type I) are also at increased risk for arrhythmic events, but the magnitude of the risk is unclear. In one study the event rate over a mean of 24 months follow-up was 8% in these patients. Those presenting with typical Brugada ECG (type I) only after drug exposure or those presenting with nondiagnostic right precordial ECG abnormalities (type II, type III) are believed to be at low risk. The role of electrophysiologic study and prognostic value of inducible VF remain controversial.

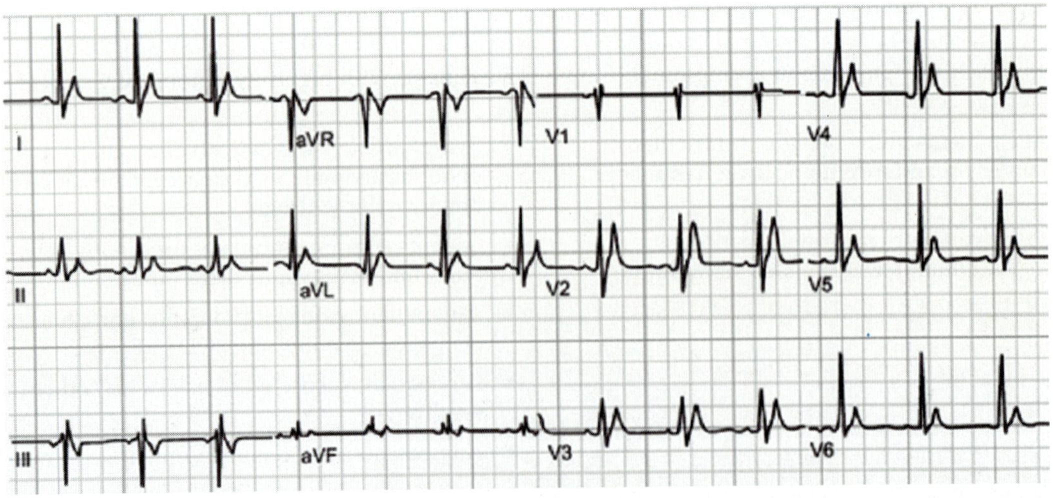

Fig. 40.88: *12 leads ECG showing very short QTc (280 ms) with tall, peaked T waves due to congenital short QT syndrome*

How is an Arrhythmia Diagnosed?

If you have symptoms of an arrhythmia, you should make an appointment with a cardiologist. You may want to see an electrophysiologist—a cardiologist who has additional specialized training in the diagnosis and treatment of heart rhythm disorders.

After evaluating your symptoms and performing a physical examination, the cardiologist may perform a variety of diagnostic tests to help confirm the presence of an arrhythmia and indicate its causes.

Some tests that may be done to confirm the presence of an irregular heart rhythm include:

- **Electrocardiogram (ECG or EKG):** A picture of the electrical impulses traveling through the heart muscle. An ECG is recorded on graph paper, through the use of electrodes (small, sticky patches) that are attached to your skin on the chest, arms and legs.
- **Ambulatory monitors**, such as:
  - **Holter monitor:** A small portable recorder that is attached to electrodes on your chest. It continuously records your heart's rhythm for 24 hours.
  - **Transtelephonic monitor:** A small monitor is attached to electrode leads, usually on your finger or wrist. With the help of this device, your heart's rhythm is transmitted over the phone line to your doctor's office.
  - **Transtelephonic monitor with a memory loop:** A small, portable recorder that is worn continuously for an extended period of time to record and save information about your heart's rhythm around the time you experience an arrhythmia. The recording is triggered by pushing a button (event button). The rhythm is recorded, saved and transmitted over the phone line.
- **Stress test:** A test used to record arrhythmias that start or are worsened with exercise. This test also may be helpful in determining if there is underlying heart disease or coronary artery disease associated with an arrhythmia.
- **Echocardiogram:** A type of ultrasound used to provide a view of the heart to determine if there is heart muscle or valve disease that may be causing an arrhythmia. This test may be performed at rest or with activity.
- **Cardiac catheterization:** Using a local anesthetic, a catheter (small, hollow, flexible tube) is inserted into a blood vessel and guided to the heart with the help of an X-ray machine. A contrast dye is injected through the catheter so X-ray movies of your coronary arteries, heart chambers and valves may be taken. This test helps your doctor determine if the cause of an arrhythmia is coronary artery disease. This test also provides information about how well your heart muscle and valves are working.
- **Electrophysiology study (EPS):** A special heart catheterization that evaluates your heart's electrical system. Catheters are inserted into your heart to record the electrical activity. The EPS is used to find the cause of the abnormal rhythm and determine the best treatment for you. During the test, the arrhythmia can be safely reproduced and terminated (Figs 40.90–40.93, 40.94).
- **Tilt table test (also called a passive head-up tilt test or head upright tilt test):** Records your blood pressure and heart rate on a minute-by-minute basis while the table is tilted in a head-up position at different levels. The test results may be used to evaluate heart rhythm, blood pressure and sometimes other measurements as you change position.

Cardiac Arrhythmia Treatment

There are many kinds of arrhythmia treatments a doctor may recommend:

- Rate control medication
- Rhythm control medication.

Nonpharmacological Options (Figs 40.94–40.97)

You will want to discuss with your doctor(s) the various treatment options in detail, so you understand the potential benefits and risks, as well as costs and other important factors.

Arrhythmia treatments may include one or more of the following:

- Lifestyle changes
- Medicine to prevent and control arrhythmias and to treat related conditions such as high blood pressure, coronary artery disease and heart failure
- Anticoagulant medication to reduce the risk of blood clots and stroke
- A pacemaker that uses batteries to help your heart beat more regularly
- Cardiac defibrillation and implanted cardioverter defibrillators (ICDs)
- Cardiac ablation
- Surgery.

There are many factors your doctor(s) may wish to consider in your treatment plan:

- The nature or cause of the arrhythmia (where it starts in the heart)
- The severity of the arrhythmia
- The severity of your symptoms
- If you have other health problems/medications you take
- Your age, overall health, and personal and family medical history.

Cardiac ablation—a safe and effective arrhythmia treatment option

Cardiac ablation offers new advances in medicine with the potential to reduce or eliminate the arrhythmia and the symptoms.

Medications a doctor may prescribe to treat cardiac arrhythmias including atrial fibrillation

Heart medications have different effects on the body. Some medications act to slow the rate of the heart. These are called "rate control" medicines. Other medications act to help maintain a normal heart rhythm. These are called "rhythm control" medications or antiarrhythmic drugs.

Antiarrhythmic drugs are being used less, with more care and often in conjunction with implantable cardioverter defibrillators (ICDs) or cardiac ablation (anchor link to cardiac ablation para below), explained further on in this section. Many of the prescription medications reviewed here are also used to treat other kinds of heart-related conditions, including heart failure, high blood pressure, and angina (chest pain). The choice of medication used is based on the needs of the individual patient. In the following information you will learn about some of the medications used to treat arrhythmias and the differences between "rate" and "rhythm" control medicines.

1. Rate and Rhythm Medications

Rate and rhythm medications are often a first course of action in managing atrial fibrillation. Rate control medications are used to slow the heart rate to less than 100 beats per minute. If rate control doesn't work, then a rhythm control medication may be used to try to restore your heart's normal sinus rhythm. Rhythm control medication is also called "drug cardioversion". If rate control medications are unsuccessful, then rhythm control medications are often used to restore the heart's normal sinus rhythm.

2. Rate Control Heart Medications

Beta-Blockers

Beta-blockers slow heart rate, relax the blood vessels and make it easier for the heart to pump blood.

Examples of Beta-blockers

Acebutolol (sectral), atenolol (tenormin), carvedilol (coreg), metoprolol (toprol-XL, lopressor), sotalol (betapace)

Calcium Channel Blockers

Calcium channel blockers are also called "calcium antagonists". These medicines work by interrupting the movement of calcium into heart and blood vessel tissue to slow heart rate.

Examples of calcium channel blockers[3]

Diltiazem (cardizem®, tiazac) and verapamil (calan covera-HS isoptin)

Rhythm control heart medications:

- Sodium channel blockers: Sodium channel blockers slow the electrical conductivity of the heart to improve rhythm problems.

Examples of sodium channel blockers

Flecainide (Tambocor™), Propafenone (Rythmol®) and Quinidine (Cardioquin, Quinaglute Dura-Tabs, Quinidex).

Anticoagulants

Anticoagulant medications help to prevent new clots from forming in the blood or existing clots from getting larger. They are often prescribed for patients with atrial fibrillation to help reduce stroke risk. Aspirin also is often recommended for these patients in addition to or instead of prescription anticoagulants.

Talk to your doctor about possible medication side effects and risks

All medications have potential side effects and risks. Antiarrhythmic drugs must be taken daily and indefinitely. There are also side effects that can be hard to manage. These

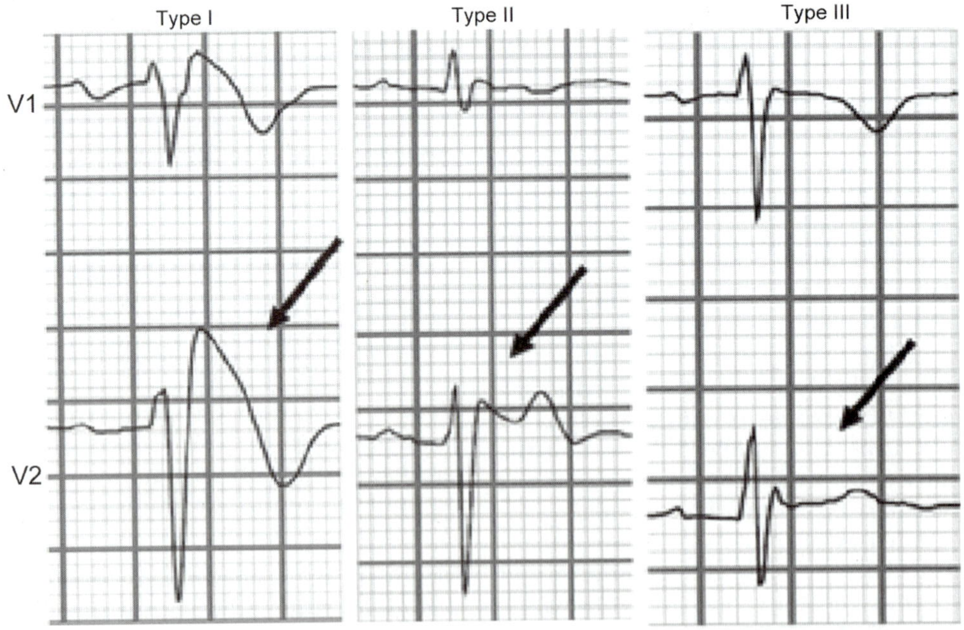

Fig. 40.89: *ECG abnormality diagnostic or suspected of Brugada syndrome. Type 1: ECG (coved-type ST-segment elevation) is the only diagnostic ECG in Brugada syndrome and is defined as a J-wave amplitude or an ST-segment elevation of >2 mm or 0.2 mV at its peak (followed by a negative T wave with little or no isoelectric separation). Type 2: ECG (saddle-back-type ST-segment elevation), defined as a J-wave amplitude of >2 mm, gives rise to a gradually descending ST-segment elevation (remaining >1 mm above the baseline) followed by a positive or biphasic T wave that results in a saddle-back configuration. Type 3: ECG is a right precordial ST-segment elevation (saddle-back type, coved type, or both) without meeting the aforementioned criteria*

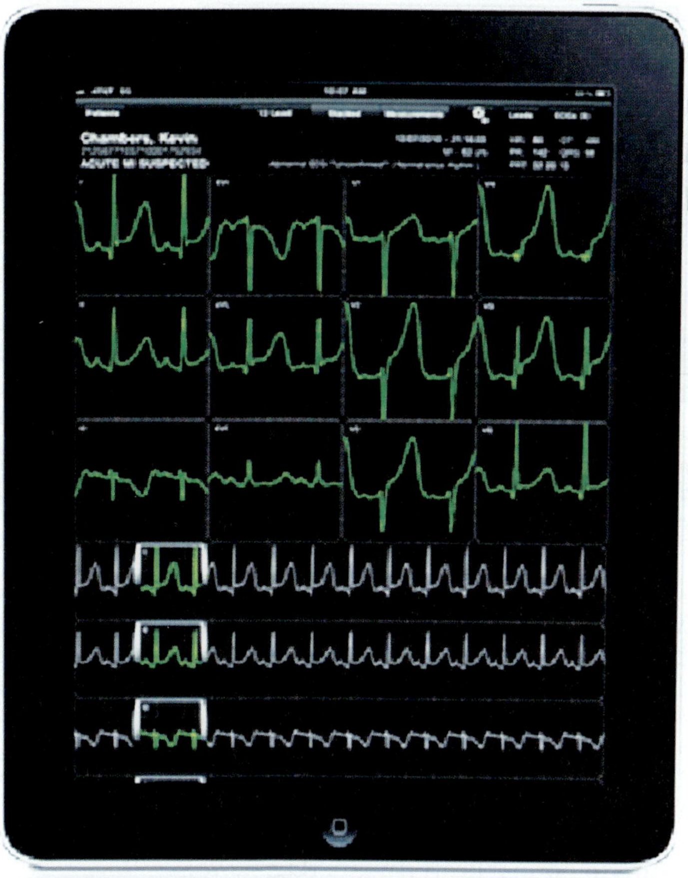

Fig. 40.90: *ECG measurements are challenging because changes as small as 0.5 millimeters can indicate the presence of a serious or emergency heart condition. AirStrip Cardiology's high resolution can detect such small differences through completely interactive iPad or iPhone views. Unlike traditional remote diagnostics, zooming in on waveforms does not affect visual clarity. With AirStrip Cardiology, clinical information is available from 12- and 15-lead ECGs, supporting high precision levels. Clinicians can view current data and historical tests conducted up to 1 year ago, in 10-second increments. Regardless of where remote cardiologists are when a critical decision is needed, they can leverage AirStrip Cardiology to quickly determine the best treatment paths for their patients. This may reduce the need to return to the hospital or access a computer connected to the hospital network. A remote cardiologist can now use AirStrip Cardiology to precisely measure ECG waveforms, helping on-site ED clinicians determine, for example, if a patient requires cath lab intervention*

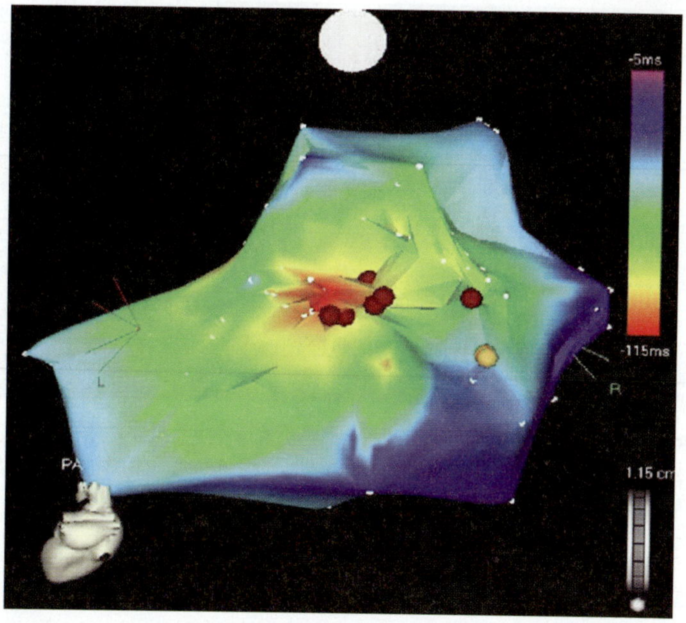

Fig. 40.91: *Shows a posteroanterior view of a right ventricular endocardial activation map during ventricular tachycardia in a patient with a prior septal myocardial infarction. Earliest activation is recorded in red; late activation shows as blue to magenta. Fragmented low amplitude diastolic local electrograms were recorded adjacent to the earliest (red) breakout area, and local ablation in this scarred zone (red dots) resulted in termination and noninducibility of this previously incessant arrhythmia*

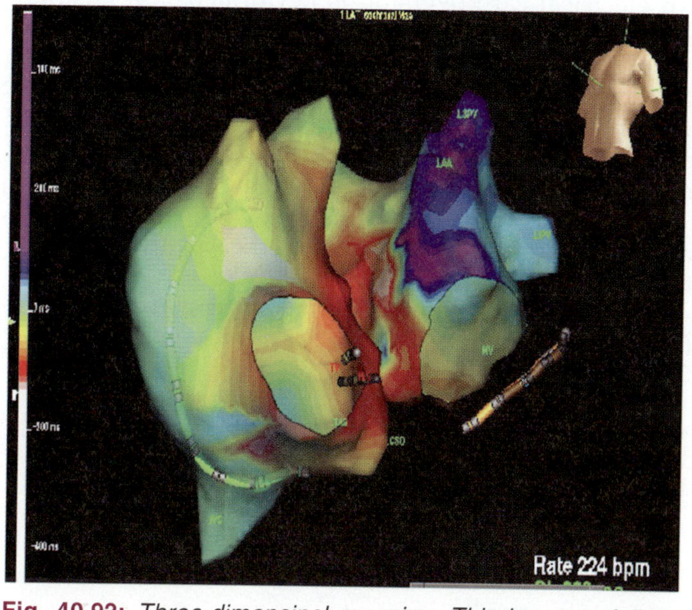

Fig. 40.92: *Three-dimensinal mapping. This is a specialized mapping technique which utilizes a computer to delineate the source of complex arrhythmias. It works by projecting a virtual three-demensional image of the heart in the computer to help the cardiac electrophysiologist navigate his catheters, in ways very similar to what GPS does for driving a car or flying an airplane. For many types of ablation, such as those for atrial fibrillation, 3D mapping is essential to ensure optimal success rates and safety for the patients*

side effects may include proarrhythmia. Proarrhythmia means that the drug has caused your arrhythmia to actually get worse or you develop a new arrhythmia as bad or worse than the original problem.

When medication proves unsuccessfull, the American College of Cardiology and the American Heart Association suggest catheter (cardiac) ablation or surgical ablation be considered a safe and effective treatment option.

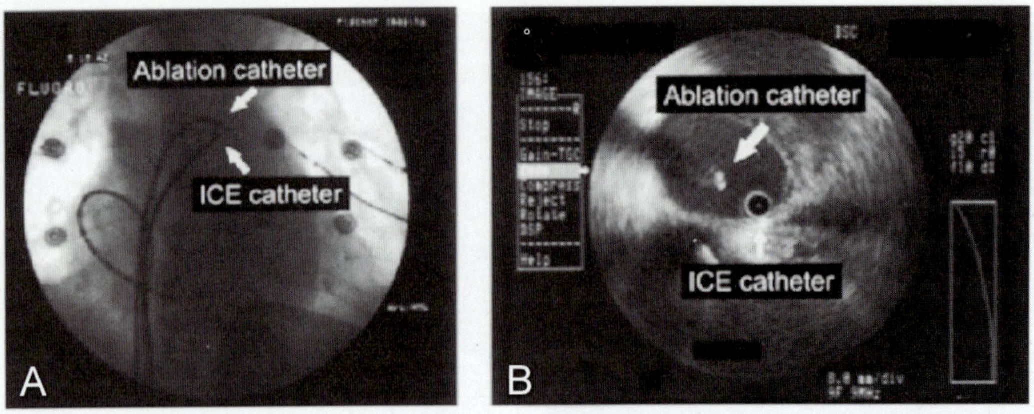

Fig. 40.93: *Intracardiac echocardiography (ICE) placed in left superior pulmonary vein (LSPV). An ablation catheter and ICE catheter are placed within the LSPV to guide radiofrequency ablation. (A) Fluoroscopic image of intracardiac catheters: duodecapolar catheter in right atrium with ICE and ablation catheter in LSPV. (B) Concomitant image from ICE visualizing the ablation catheter within the LSPV lumen (arrow)*

3. Nonpharmacological Options

Devices: Implantable cardioverter defibrillator (ICD): This device is inserted into the patient's chest like a pacemaker. When an episode of fast, irregular heartbeat begins, the device delivers a shock to end the tachycardia, preventing the heart from going into ventricular fibrillation, which is frequently fatal (Figs 40.95–40.97).

Cardioversion: This treatment can be chemical (implemented through fast-acting drugs) or electric (implemented through a direct current using paddles over the chest) and is used to restore the heart's normal rhythm. An electrical cardioversion is performed in a hospital setting such as an emergency room, intensive care unit, recovery room, special procedure room, or electrophysiology laboratory. This split-second interruption of the abnormal beat allows the heart's electrical system to regain control and restore a normal heartbeat. This method does not provide a permanent solution to the problem.

Cardiac ablation: A nonsurgical technique that neutralizes parts of the abnormal electrical pathway (tissue) that is causing the arrhythmia. The technique utilizes a variety of imaging and monitoring systems that navigate flexible wires (catheters) to the heart through an artery or vein, locate the precise location of abnormal electric activity (where ablation is needed), and evaluate their progress. Once in the heart, one or more catheters are used to pinpoint the source of the abnormal electrical signals. When the source of the arrhythmia is located, the catheter delivers bursts of high-energy waves that eliminates the abnormal areas. Most patients who receive this treatment experience a long-term reduction in the number of episodes of arrhythmia and the severity of symptoms, or a permanent return to normal heart rhythm (Fig. 40.94).

Cardiac surgery: Cardiac surgery is an invasive procedure where surgeons will remove abnormal sites (tissue) in the heart that are causing the arrhythmia. In comparison, cardiac ablation is the most effective treatment option for a range of common cardiac arrhythmias.

Newer Antirrhythmic Drugs

Dronedarone

Amiodarone is generally accepted to be a valuable antiarrhythmic drug, but it accumulates in tissues during long-term therapy, which may result in significant toxicity in several organ systems. Several compounds that were designed to be similar in structure and electrophysiological

Box 40.2: *Indications for implantable cardioverter-defibrillator*

Primary prevention
- Dilated or ischemic cardiomyopathy: EF d"35%, based on MADIT-II, SCD-HeFT, definite criteria

Secondary prevention
- Survivors of sudden cardiac death or documented hemodynamically unstable or sustained VT or VF

Biventricular ICD
- Dilated or ischemic cardiomyopathy, EF <35%, QRS interval >120 msec, functional class III
- Investigational: Biventricular ICD in normal QRS and echocardiographic evidence of biventricular dyssynchrony (Rethinq trial) or biventricular ICD in heart failure, conduction disturbance in functional class I or II (MADIT-CRT)

Other rare indications for ICD
- Brugada syndrome
- Hypertrophic cardiomyopathy
- Long QT syndrome

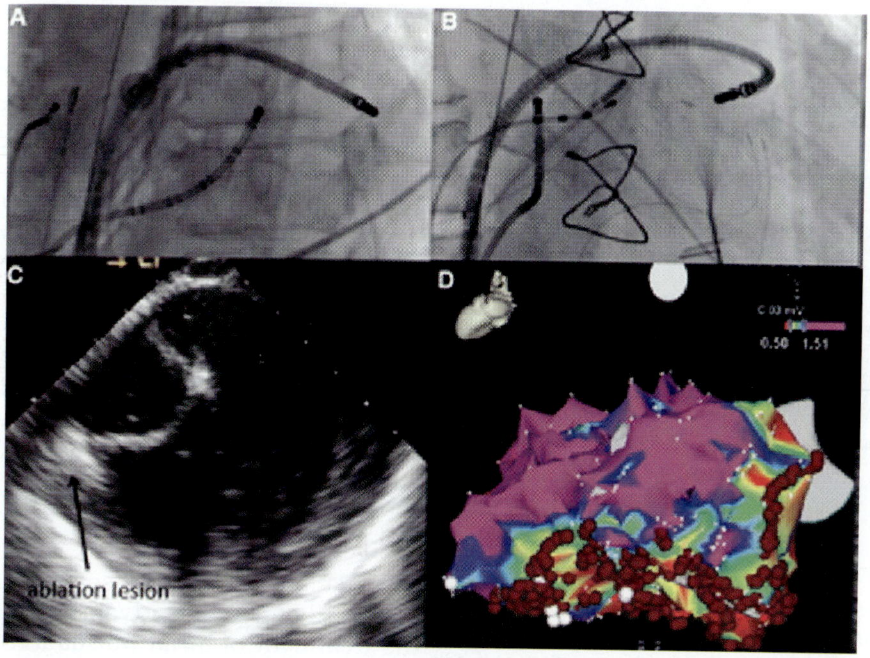

Fig. 40.94: *Mapping and ablation of a basal lateral scar. (A and B) Robotic catheter position in left and right anterior oblique fluoroscopic views, respectively. The mid-lateral wall is being mapped. (C) Intracardiac echocardiographic image showing catheter contact and lesion formation in the left ventricular lateral wall. (D) Three-dimensional map of the lateral scar and the ablation lesions created*

effects to amiodarone have completed or are now in clinical trials.

Dronedarone is, like amiodarone, a benzofuranyl compound with iodine removed and a methane sulfonyl group added. Removing iodine from the molecule was intended to eliminate or reduce iodine-related organ toxicity. The side chain modification decreased lipophilicity, resulting in a shorter elimination half-life with less potential for tissue accumulation. The basic and clinical pharmacology of dronedarone has been recently reviewed.

Dronedarone retains many of amiodarone's electrophysiological effects. It is a multichannel blocker with effects on the rapid and slow components of the delayed rectifier current (IKr and IKs), L-type calcium currents, (ICa-L), the inward sodium current (INa), and the inward rectifier potassium current (IK1). Dronedarone also inhibits the acetylcholine receptor-dependent K^+ current (IKAch) and the pacemaker current (If) and is a noncompetitive a- and β-adrenergic antagonist. Dronedarone reduces sinus rate and prolongs AV nodal conduction and refractoriness. Effects on the QT and QTc intervals have been variable when studied in different species. In several animal models of ischemia or reperfusion-induced arrhythmias, dronedarone effectively prevents spontaneous and induced ventricular fibrillation.

Budiodarone

Unlike dronedarone, **budiodarone** (AT1-2042), another compound that structurally resembles amiodarone, retains iodine atoms in its molecular structure. A sec-butyl acetate side chain has been added at position 2 of the benzofuranyl ring. This ester modification changes the compound's metabolic pathways such that budiodarone undergoes rapid degradation by plasma and tissue esterases, not by CYP3A-mediated oxidation, to an inactive compound. During in vitro studies, budiodarone has shown electrophysiological properties similar to amiodarone.

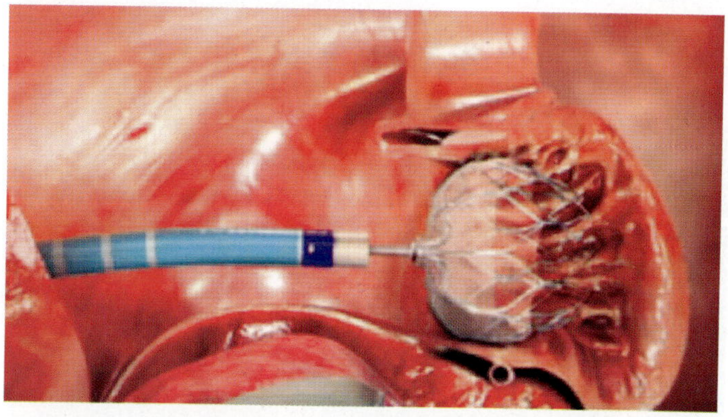

Fig. 40.95: *Left atrial appendage closure device. Patients with atrial fibrillation (AF) are at an increased risk of stroke that can originate in the left atrial appendage (LAA) WATCHMAN device from Boston Scientific was developed to fill the space of the LAA and capture any clots that form within. Now the company received expanded indication approval in Europe to offer this treatment to AF patients that have a contraindication to the currently available anticoagulants*

Only limited clinical data on budiodarone are available. One study assessed twice-daily placebo or doses of 200, 400, 600, and 800 mg during sequential 2-week periods in a very small group of patients with paroxysmal atrial fibrillation and implanted pacemakers. Atrial fibrillation burden (defined as percent time in atrial fibrillation) was

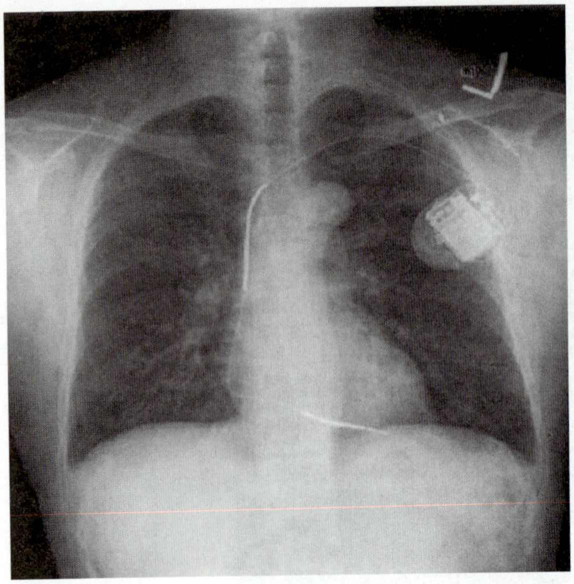

Fig. 40.96: *Chest X-ray showing an implantable cardioverter-defibrillator (ICD), with its battery fixed at left subclavicular region and is connected with a wire placed in the trabecular part of the right ventricular apex*

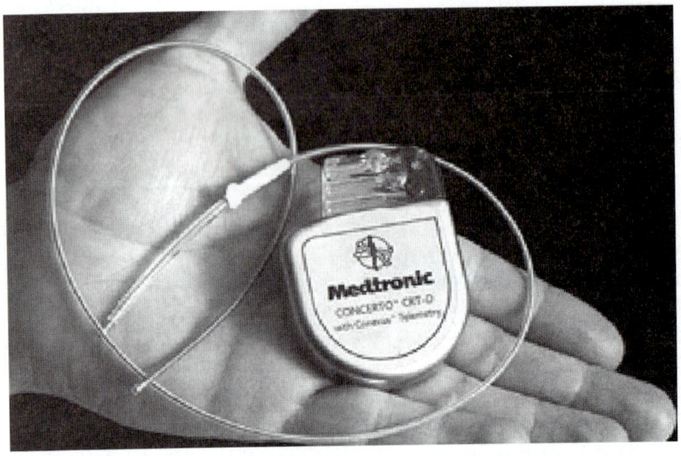

Fig. 40.97: *Closeup view of an ICD*

calculated during each period. Budiodarone reduced total atrial fibrillation burden by reducing the duration but not the number of atrial fibrillation episodes. Preliminary data from a similar but a larger phase 2 trial compared placebo and budiodarone (200, 400, and 600 mg twice daily) in 72 patients with pacemakers and paroxysmal atrial fibrillation. There were 54.4% and 75% reductions in AF burden in the 400 mg and 600 mg groups. Some patients manifested a rise in thyroid-stimulating hormone, but clinical symptoms of thyroid disease did not appear.

Celivarone

Celivarone (SSR149744C) is another noniodinated benzofuran derivative with electrophysiological effects similar to amiodarone. Few clinical data have been published in manuscript form, but a phase 2 trial tested celivarone's efficacy at 300- or 600 mg daily doses for conversion of atrial fibrillation and flutter (CORYFEE, NCT00232310) and a dose ranging study compared celivarone at 50, 100, 200, or 300 mg once daily with amiodarone for maintenance of sinus rhythm (MAIA, NCT00233441) have been completed but not yet published. A preliminary report from the dose-ranging study showed the lowest rate of atrial fibrillation recurrence at the 50 mg dose with no enhanced efficacy at the higher doses. In another study in patients with ICDs, 2 doses of celivarone (100 and 300 mg daily) were compared with placebo over 6 months of therapy. A 46% reduction in the number of sustained ventricular arrhythmia episodes requiring ICD therapy was noted in the 300 mg daily group, but this reduction did not achieve statistical significance (P = 0.172). Additional trials in patients with ventricular arrhythmias and ICDs are planned.

Vernakalant

Vernakalant is an atrial-selective, multiple ion channel blocker that is in the advanced stages of investigation for the treatment of atrial fibrillation. Both intravenous and oral forms of vernakalant have undergone clinical trials. The intravenous form has been recommended for approval by the cardiorenal advisory committee of the food and drug administration, but a formal letter of approval has not been issued. Vernakalant is an atrial repolarization-delaying agent with its major target IKur. Vernakalant also blocks Ito and INa, although there is little effect on IKr or IKs. As IKur is present in higher density in the atria, vernakalant is relatively atrial selective. The INa inhibition is rate- and voltage-dependent. Vernakalant has, therefore, a much greater effect in fibrillating atria than in the ventricle and is less likely to be proarrhythmic.

Vernakalant is hepatically metabolized by CYP2D6. It is not clear what effect abnormal liver function has on the metabolism of the drug. In a study of intravenous vernakalant, coadministration of CYP2D6 inhibitors did not appear to decrease clearance, and little difference was seen in maximum plasma concentrations between CYP2D6 poor and extensive metabolizers. Differences in renal function, age, sex, race, blood pressure, and heart failure status have not been shown to affect the pharmacokinetics of vernakalant. Vernakalant demonstrates two-compartment elimination pharmacokinetics, and its half-life after intravenous administration is 2–5 hours. The oral bioavailability of vernakalant is approximately 20%. During oral therapy in the dose range of 300–600 mg twice daily, steady-state concentrations are achieved in 4 days. It remains to be seen whether CYP2D6 poor and extensive metabolizers will require different doses during chronic oral therapy.

Phase 3 trials have not been completed for oral vernakalant, although phase 2 trials have been promising for the long-term maintenance of sinus rhythm. The phase 2a trial was double-blinded, randomized, and compared a 300-mg dosage, a 600-mg dosage, and placebo for 25 days after cardioversion. Electrical cardioversion was permitted for patients who did not convert within 3 days after initiation of the medication. Significantly more patients

Table 40.13: *Types of cardiac arrhythmia associated with congenital cardiac anomalies*

Arrhythmias	*Associated defects*
	VSD indicates ventricular septal defect
Tachycardias	
Accessory pathways	Ebstein's anomaly, L-TGA
Twin AV nodes	Heterotaxy syndrome
Intra-atrial reentrant tachycardia (atrial flutter)	Postoperative mustard, postoperative senning, postoperative fontan, others
Atrial fibrillation	Mitral valve disease, aortic stenosis, unrepaired single ventricle
Ventricular tachycardia	Tetralogy of fallot, congenital aortic stenosis, others
Bradycardias	
Congenital sinus node dysfunction	Heterotaxy syndrome
Acquired sinus node dysfunction	Postoperative mustard, postoperative senning, postoperative fontan, posterative glenn, others
Congenital AV block	Endocardial cushion defects, L-TGA
Acquired AV block	VSD closure, subaortic stenosis relief, AV valve replacement

remained in sinus rhythm at the end of the trial period in the 300-mg dosing group and in the combined 300- and 600-mg groups, when compared with placebo. The phase 2b trial compared 150-, 300-, and 500-mg dosages with placebo, and the trial duration was 90 days. The 500-mg dosage group showed durable maintenance of sinus rhythm at 90 days compared with placebo, with low incidence of side effects. There were no reported cases of torsades de pointes.

In summary, intravenous vernakalant for cardioversion of recent onset AF is moderately effective for rapid termination of atrial fibrillation with durable maintenance of sinus rhythm up to 24 hours. The side effect profile shows relatively modest potential for toxicity. Age, sex, ethnicity, and concomitant illnesses do not appear to alter efficacy. Of course, drugs used only for the acute conversion of atrial fibrillation must also be compared with electrical cardioversion as well as other agents. Oral vernakalant may prove useful for maintenance of sinus rhythm, but phase 3 trials have yet to be completed. If these trials show efficacy, vernakalant probably will be more widely used in conversion attempts as a step to long-term therapy. There are no clinical data on the effects of vernakalant in ventricular arrhythmias, and its mechanisms of action suggest it would not be useful.

Ranolazine

Ranolazine is currently approved for the treatment of chronic angina pectoris. Ranolazine reduces myocardial ischemia by its effects on the late inward Na^+ current (INaL). During myocardial ischemia and heart failure, INaL is augmented. This results in increased sodium entry and, via sodium-calcium exchange, increased cytosolic calcium concentrations. These changes produce action potential prolongation and increased susceptibility to early after depolarizations. Ranolazine is an inactivated sodium channel blocker. At concentrations near its therapeutic range for angina (2–6 μmol/L, IC50 60 μmol/L), ranolazine inhibits INaL. In the same concentration range, ranolazine inhibits peak INa in the atrium but not the ventricle. This effect results in reduced atrial excitability and a rate-dependent increase in postrepolarization atrial refractoriness. In experiments using an isolated canine ventricular wedge preparation, ranolazine results in either no change or a decrease in transmural ventricular dispersion of refractoriness and does not produce early afterdepolarizations, triggered activity, or polymorphic ventricular tachycardia. In other experiments, ranolazine has been shown to suppress excitability and triggered activity in an isolated canine pulmonary vein sleeve preparation, terminate acetylcholine- and isoproterenol-induced atrial fibrillation, and prevent its reinitiation.

Ranolazine has variable systemic availability after oral administration due to its extensive first-pass metabolism in the gut and liver. Metabolism is mainly via CYP3A4 and, to a lesser extent, CYP2D6. The terminal elimination half-life is 7 hours. The recommended dosage in patients with angina is 500–1,000 mg twice daily. Ranolazine should not be used as concurrent therapy with strong CYP3A4 inhibitors (e.g. ketoconazole), and dose reduction is recommended with moderate CYP3A4 inhibitors (e.g. diltiazem) or P-glycoprotein inhibitors. Ranolazine is a weak inhibitor of CYP3A4 and a moderate inhibitor of CYP2D6 and P-glycoprotein.

Ranolazine's effects on ECG intervals underwent extensive study during its development for its current indication of chronic angina. Ranolazine results in a 2- to 6 ms mean increase in the QTc interval, but drug-induced polymorphic ventricular tachycardia has not been observed. The MERLIN-TIMI trial enrolled 6,560 patients with a non-ST-elevation acute coronary syndrome who were randomly assigned to either ranolazine (intravenous initiation, then 1,000 mg twice daily) or matched placebo, in addition to standard medical therapy. No significant improvement was shown in the primary end-point of death and recurrent ischemic events with ranolazine in MERLIN-TIMI, but data from continuous ambulatory ECG recordings during the first 7 days of therapy were recently reported. Significant decreases in the frequency of nonsustained ventricular and supraventricular tachycardia were noted. A trend toward less frequent new-onset atrial fibrillation was also seen. A single case report on the successful use of ranolazine to suppress high-density ventricular tachycardia has been reported. An uncontrolled case series has also described control of recurrent atrial fibrillation in 4 of 7 patients with drug-resistant arrhythmia. Controlled trials with ranolazine as an antiarrhythmic drug in patients with atrial fibrillation are in the planning stages.

One form of the long-QT syndrome (LQT3) is caused by mutations in the SCN5A sodium channel that lead to enhanced and sustained activity of late INa. Moss et al administered intravenous ranolazine to 5 patients with LQT3. During the infusion, ranolazine shortened QTcf by 26 ± 3 ms. Diastolic function on echocardiography was also improved. Ranolazine may also prove useful in another form of the long-QT syndrome. The Timothy syndrome (LQT8) is a multisystem disorder characterized by facial dysmorphism, syndactyly, QT prolongation, and premature sudden death. The syndrome is caused by a missense mutation in Cav1.2, the gene that encodes the a-subunit of the L-type calcium channel, resulting in a gain in function of the L-type calcium current. In an animal model of the Timothy syndrome, ranolazine suppressed polymorphic ventricular tachycardia induced by the calcium channel agonist BayK8644. Clinical data on the chronic treatment of arrhythmias in LQT3 and Timothy syndrome patients are not available.

At present, the only approved indication for ranolazine is the treatment of angina. It remains to be proven whether it will also be useful as an antiarrhythmic agent.

Ivabradine

Ivabradine selectively inhibits the spontaneous pacemaker activity of the sinus node by blocking the 1h current. This reduces the heart rate without altering myocardial contractility or other hemodynamics. Ivabradine has been approved for use as an antianginal in Europe. It has also been used off-label in Europe as a treatment for inappropriate sinus tachycardia. It has not yet been approved for any use in the United States. The blockage of the 1h current is dose-dependent and heart rate-dependent. There is a greater efficiency in blocking 1h at faster heart rates, limiting the risks of symptomatic bradycardia. Electrophysiological studies of ivabradine in humans have shown little effect on the conduction system or on atrial and ventricular refractoriness. Some remodeling of the sinus node appears to occur in response to ivabradine, but no rebound tachycardia has been seen after discontinuing the drug.

Ivabradine is 80% hepatically metabolized by the CYP3A4 enzyme and cannot be used concomitantly with drugs that inhibit this enzyme, such as azoles and macrolide antibiotics. There does not appear to be a difference in heart rate response between patients who are CYP3A4 rapid metabolizers and those who are slow metabolizers. It is 20% renally cleared. The oral bioavailability is approximately 40% and it takes 60–90 minutes to reach maximal plasma concentrations. The half-life is approximately 2 hours.

The major trial that evaluated ivabradine is the BEAUTIFUL study. This randomized, double-blind, placebo-controlled trial enrolled 10,917 patients with ischemic cardiomyopathy to receive ivabradine versus placebo. There was no difference in the primary end-point of cardiovascular death or admissions for acute infarction or heart failure. In patients with baseline heart rates >70 bpm, however, the secondary end-points of admission for fatal and nonfatal infarction and the need for revascularization were significantly reduced. The heart rate reduction due to ivabradine was 6 ± 2 bpm. A previous study compared ivabradine with atenolol for treatment of patients with stable angina and found that ivabradine was as effective as atenolol. It is on this basis that it was approved for use in Europe.

Composite data from phase 2 and phase 3 trials suggest that most side effects are dose-related. Ion channels in the retina that generate the Ih current are also affected by ivabradine. This is the mechanism for ivabradine's major side effect, visual luminous phenomena, also known as phosphenes (14.5%). Phosphenes usually resolve with continued treatment and are a rare cause of drug discontinuation. Severe bradycardia is seen in 3.3% of patients. Other less common side effects include palpitations, nausea, headaches, vertigo, muscle cramps, hypereosinophilia, and hyperuricemia.

Little trial data exists regarding the treatment of atrial tachyarrhythmias with ivabradine. The mechanism of action suggests that ivabradine may benefit patients with inappropriate sinus tachycardia. In Europe, where the drug is being marketed, it is used off-label in the treatment of inappropriate sinus tachycardia. Further data will be needed as to its effectiveness in treating this condition.

Adenosine A1 Receptor Agonists

Adenosine is frequently used for termination of supraventricular tachycardias (SVT). Adenosine terminates SVT in patient with AV nodal or AV reentry by stimulating the A1 adenosine receptor to produce transient AV block. However, adenosine induces atrial fibrillation in up to 15% of patients by decreasing the refractory period of the atrium.

In addition, adenosine also stimulates the A2A, A2B, and A3 adenosine receptor subtypes, which contribute to its adverse effect profile. Stimulation of these receptors leads to a variety of systemic side effects including flushing (18%), dyspnea (12%), and chest pain (7%). Efforts have been made to identify A1 receptor-selective agonists for both the termination of SVT and rate control for atrial fibrillation. Several are under investigation currently including tecadenoson, selodenoson, and PJ-875. Tecadenoson is the furthest along in the development process. A phase 3 trial has been completed evaluating tecadenoson for the termination of SVT, and preclinical data are promising for rate control of atrial fibrillation. Selodenoson and PJ-875 are both in the early stages of evaluation for treatment of atrial fibrillation.

Preclinical trials indicate that tecadenoson is a potent and selective agonist of the A1 receptor. Studies in animal models showed that it caused significant prolongation of AV nodal conduction and refractoriness without causing hypotension or negative inotropic effects. In addition, those effects were dose-dependent and persistent with chronic administration of the drug. A phase 1 dose-escalation trial in 32 patients showed a dose-dependent prolongation of the AH interval. There was no effect on the HV interval. The peak effect on AH interval was at 1 minute, and resolution occurred at 20 minutes. Four patients had significant heart block and three patients had atrial fibrillation (2 after atrial pacing). Two patients had neurological effects. There is incomplete published information regarding the pharmacokinetics tecadenoson. It appears to follow a 2-compartment model and has a longer half-life than adenosine (20–30 minutes).

The most significant trial to evaluate tecadenoson to date is the phase 3 TEMPEST trial. This study was a multicenter, double-blinded, placebo-controlled trial that randomly assigned 181 patients to receive placebo versus 1 of several dose-escalating regimens of tecadenoson for termination of SVT. Overall, the conversion rates were 73.5% in the tecadenoson-treated patients and 6.7% in the placebo group. The rates of conversion did improve with dose escalation. Side effects were relatively mild and increased with dose escalation. Twelve patients had second-degree heart block. Two patients had complete heart block, and both of those patients were in the highest dose treatment group. Five patients in the two highest dose treatment groups developed transient atrial fibrillation or atrial flutter. The rates of flushing, dyspnea, and chest pain were 4%, 2.6%, and 3%, respectively. No patients in this study had alterations in blood pressure.

An animal study of tecadenoson for rate control of atrial fibrillation has shown promising results. In combination with metoprolol, rate control was improved with tecadenoson compared with either agent alone. Improved rate control was seen with exercise and with rest. A phase 2 clinical trial to evaluate the safety of tecadenoson to treat atrial fibrillation has been completed. Results have not yet been released.

In summary, the available data regarding adenosine A1 receptor agonists, particularly tecadenoson, is promising for the conversion of SVT and for short-term rate-control of atrial fibrillation. The rate of conversion for SVT is similar to that of adenosine, but the systemic side effects are milder. In addition, although adenosine A1 receptor stimulation is the presumed mechanism for the induction of atrial fibrillation, tecadenoson appears less likely to cause atrial fibrillation, perhaps because the maximal action potential shortening seen with a bolus of adenosine is not observed with longer-acting agents.

It is now recognized that atrial fibrillation originates from atrial tissue that has altered structure or function. Fibrosis within the atrium is one of the major mechanisms of atrial remodeling, which provides the substrate for atrial fibrillation generation and maintenance. Efforts have been made to develop "upstream" therapies for atrial fibrillation. The renin-angiotensin-aldosterone system has been implicated in the fibrotic process. Therapies that alter renin-angiotensin-aldosterone system, as well as antiinflammatory and antioxidative drugs, are being investigated both alone and in combination with traditional antiarrhythmic drugs. For some newer drugs, data have only been generated in animal models. Further studies will be needed to delineate the full potential benefits of these and other therapies.

BIBLIOGRAPHY

1. Blomstöm-Lundqvist C, Scheinman MM, Aliot EM, et al: ACC/AHA/ESC Guidelines for the management of patients with supraventricular arrhythmias—executive.
2. Summary: a report of the American College of Cardiology/American Heart Association Task Force on Practice Guidelines and the European Society of Cardiology Committee for Practice Guidelines (Writing Committee to Develop Guidelines for the Management of Patients with Supraventricular Arrhythmias). Circulation 108:1871, 2003.
3. Mehta D, Wafa S, Ward DE, et al: Relative efficacy of various physical manoeuvres in the termination of junctional tachycardia. Lancet 1:1181, 1988.
4. Kay GN, Pressley JC, Packer DL, et al: Value of the 12-lead electrocardiogram in discriminating atrioventricular nodal reciprocating tachycardia from circus movement atrioventricular tachycardia utilizing a retrograde accessory pathway. Am J Cardiol 59:296, 1987.
5. Brugada P, Brugada J, Mont L, et al: A new approach to the differential diagnosis of a regular tachycardia with a wide QRS complex. Circulation 83:1649, 1991.
6. Wellens HJ, Bar FW, Lie KI: The value of the electrocardiogram in the differential diagnosis of a tachycardia with a widened QRS complex. Am J Med 64:27, 1978.
7. Akhtar M, Jazayeri MR, Sra J, et al: Atrioventricular nodal reentry: clinical, electrophysiological, and therapeutic considerations. Circulation 88:282, 1993
8. Sung RJ, Waxman HL, Saksena S, et al: Sequence of retrograde atrial activation in patients with dual atrioventricular nodal pathways. Circulation 64:1059, 1981.
9. Amsterdam EA, Kulcyski J, Ridgeway MG: Efficacy of cardioselective beta-adrenergic blockade with intravenously administered metoprolol in the treatment of supraventricular tachyarrhythmias. J Clin Pharmacol 31:714, 1991.
10. Lee KL, Chun HM, Liem LB, et al: Effect of adenosine and verapamil in catecholamine-induced accelerated atrioventricular junctional rhythm: insights into the underlying mechanism. Pacing Clin Electrophysiol 22:866, 1999.
11. Overholt ED, Rheuban KS, Gutgesell HP, et al: Usefulness of adenosine for arrhythmias in infants and children. Am J Cardiol 61:336, 1988.

12. Mauritson DR, Winniford MD, Walker WS, et al: Oral verapamil for paroxysmal supraventricular tachycardia: a long-term, double-blind randomized trial. Ann Intern Med 96:409, 1982.
13. Winniford MD, Fulton KL, Hillis LD: Long-term therapy of paroxysmal supraventricular tachycardia: arandomized, double-blind comparison of digoxin, propranolol and verapamil. Am J Cardiol 54:1138, 1984.
14. Flecainide acetate prevents recurrence of symptomatic paroxysmal supraventricular tachycardia. The Flecainide Supraventricular Tachycardia Study Group: Circulation 83:119, 1991 Long-term safety and efficacy of flecainide in the treatment of supraventricular tachyarrhythmias: the United States experience. The Flecainide Supraventricular Tachy arrhythmia Investigators: Am J Cardiol 70:11A, 1992.
15. A randomized, placebo-controlled trial of propafenone in the prophylaxis of paroxysmal supraventricular tachycardia and paroxysmal atrial fibrillation. UK Propafenone PSVT Study Group: Circulation 92:2550, 1995.
16. Yeh SJ, Lin FC, Chou YY, et al: Termination of paroxysmal supraventricular tachycardia with a single oral dose of diltiazem and propranolol. Circulation 71:1041985.
17. Clague JR, Dagres N, Kottkamp H, et al: Targeting the slow pathway for atrioventricular nodal reentrant tachycardia: initial results and long-term follow-up in 379 consecutive patients. Eur Heart J 22:82, 2001.
18. Scheinman MM, Huang S: The 1998 NASPE prospectiveScheinman MM, Huang S: The 1998 NASPE prospective catheter ablation registry. Pacing Clin Electrophysiol 23:1020, 2000.
19. Ross DL, Uther JB: Diagnosis of concealed accessory pathways in supraventricular tachycardia. Pacing Clin Electrophysiol 7:1069, 1984.
20. Dreifus LS, Haiat R, Watanabe Y, et al: Ventricular fibrillation: a possible mechanism of sudden death in patients and Wolff-Parkinson-White syndrome. Circulation 43:520, 1971.
21. Klein GJ, Bashore TM, Sellers TD, et al: Ventricular fibrillation in the Wolff-Parkinson-White syndrome. N Engl J Med 301:1080, 1979.
22. Timmermans C, Smeets JL, Rodriguez LM, et al: Aborted sudden death in the Wolff-Parkinson-White syndrome. Am J Cardiol 76:492, 1995.
23. Campbell RW, Smith RA, Gallagher JJ, et al: Atrial fibrillation in the preexcitation syndrome. Am J Cardiol 40:514, 1977.
24. Kottkamp H, Hügl B, Krauss B, et al. Electromagnetic versus fluoroscopic mapping of the inferior isthmus for ablation of typical atrial flutter: A prospective randomized study. Circulation. 2000;102(17):2082–2086.
25. Willems S, Weiss C, Ventura R, et al. Catheter ablation of atrial flutter guided by electroanatomic mapping (CARTO): a randomized comparison to the conventional approach. J Cardiovasc Electrophysiol. 2000;11(11): 1223–1230.
26. Tsai CF, Tai CT, Yu WC, et al. Is 8-mm more effective than 4-mm tip electrode catheter for ablation of typical atrial flutter? Circulation. 1999;100(7):768–771.
27. Paydak H, Kall JG, Burke MC, et al. Atrial fibrillation after radiofrequency ablation of type I atrial flutter: time to onset, determinants, and clinical course. Circulation 1998;98(4):315–322.
28. Pérez FJ, Schubert CM, Parvez B, Pathak V, Ellenbogen KA, Wood MA. Long-term outcomes after catheter ablation of cavotricuspid isthmus dependent atrial flutter: a meta-analysis. Circ Arrhythmia Electrophysiol 2009;2(4):393–401.
29. Savelieva I, Camm AJ. Anti-arrhythmic drug therapy for atrial fibrillation: current anti-arrhythmic drugs, investigational agents, and innovative approaches. Europace 2008;10:647–665.
30. Ehrlich JR, Biliczki P, Hohnloser SH, Nattel S. Atrial-selective approaches for the treatment of atrial fibrillation. J Am Coll Cardiol 2008;51:787–792.
31. Dale KM, White CM. Dronedarone: an amiodarone analog for the treatment of atrial fibrillation and atrial flutter. Ann Pharmacother 2007;41:599–605.
32. Tafreshi MJ, Rowles J. A review of the investigational antiarrhythmic agent dronedarone. J Cardiovasc Phamacol Ther 2007;12:15–26.
33. Clinical Investigator's Brochure: SR33589B Dronedarone. Bridgewater, NJ, Sanofi-Syntholabe Recherche. Edition: E07, 2006.
34. Tschuppert Y, Buclin T, Rothuizen LE, Decosterd LA, Galleyrand J, Gaud C, Bioffaz J. Effect of dronedarone on renal function in healthy subjects. Br J Clin Pharmacol 2007;64:785–791.
35. Touboul P, Brugada J, Cappucci A, Crijns HJGM, Edvardsso N, Hohnloser SH. Dronedarone for prevention of atrial fibrillation: a dose-ranging study. Eur Heart J. 2003;24:1481–1487.
36. Singh BN, Connolly SJ, Crijns HJGM, Roy D, Kowey PR, Cappucci A, Radzik D, Aliot EM, Hohnloser SH, for the EURIDIS and ADONIS Investigators. Dronedarone for maintenance of sinus rhythm in atrial fibrillation or flutter. N Engl J Med 2007;357:23–35.

41 Artificial Pacemaker Therapy in Children and Adolescents

Pacemaker therapy in children involves unique issues regarding patient size, growth, development, and possible presence of congenital heart disease; accordingly, this topic reviews unique aspects of pediatric pacemaker implantation and follow-up, with particular attention to the difficulties encountered with smaller children and patients with coexistent congenital heart defects.

Transvenous pacemaker implantation in young patients previously was limited by generator size and lead diameter in comparison to vascular dimensions and capacitance. Historically, epicardial pacing was more common in children. As technology has improved, generators and leads have become smaller and more advanced, allowing transvenous pacing systems in children; pacemaker therapy is even technically feasible in infants and neonates.

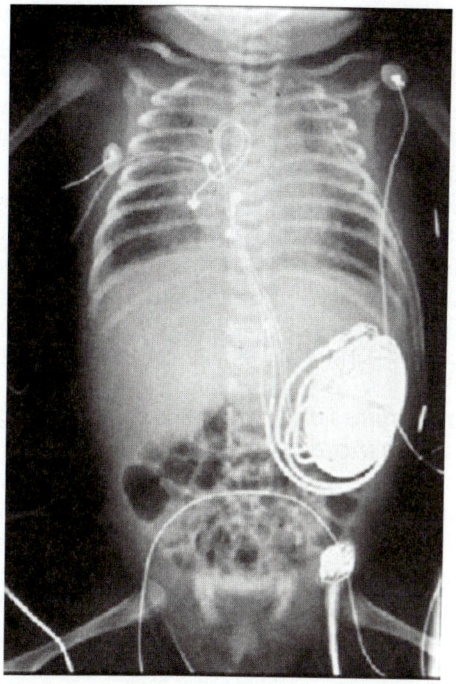

Fig. 41.1: *Skiagram chest and abdomen showing dual chamber pacemaker with epicardial electrodes implanted through a median sternotomy and pulse generator seen in abdominal region in a newborn with complete heart block*

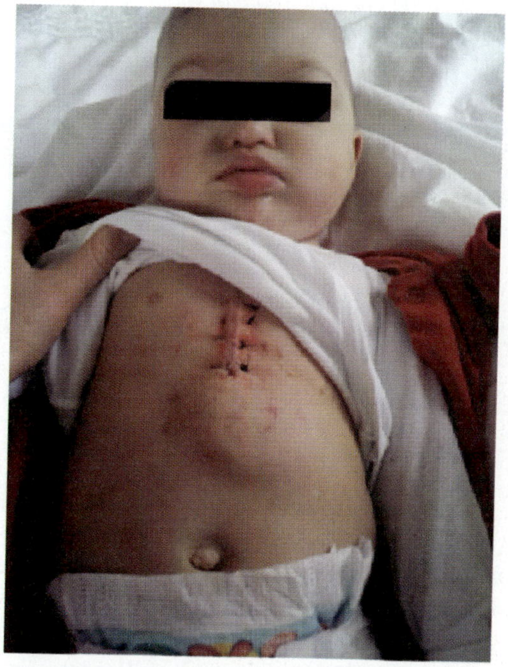

Fig. 41.2: *Dual chamber pacemaker implanted through a median sternotomy (see scarover the chest) in a newborn with complete heart block*

Pediatric pacemaker implantation is performed primarily to treat abnormalities of sinoatrial (SA) node (i.e. sinus node) or atrioventricular (AV) node function that lead to an insufficient heart rate. In addition, pacemakers are used (though less commonly) for other disorders, such as congenital long QT syndrome and cardiomyopathy. A specialized type of pacemaker therapy known as cardiac resynchronization therapy (CRT) has been used adjunctively in pediatric patients with heart failure.

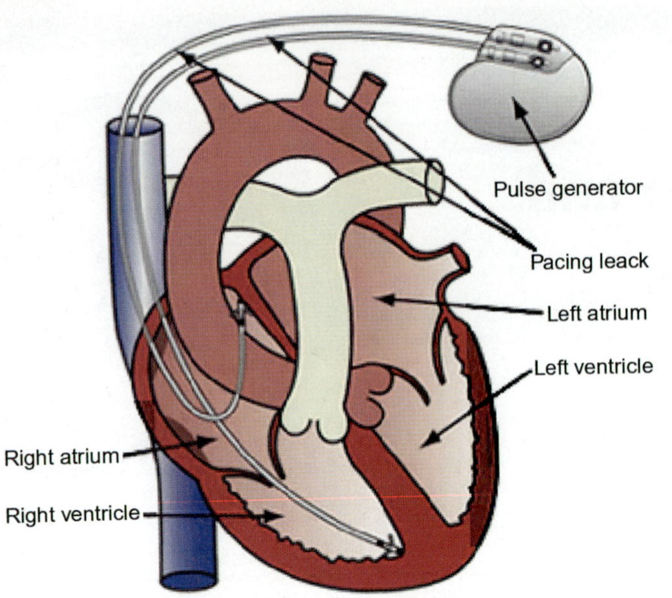

Fig. 41.3: *Drawing showing route of wires and fixation of battery in a commonly used transvenous ventricular pacemaker in a young child*

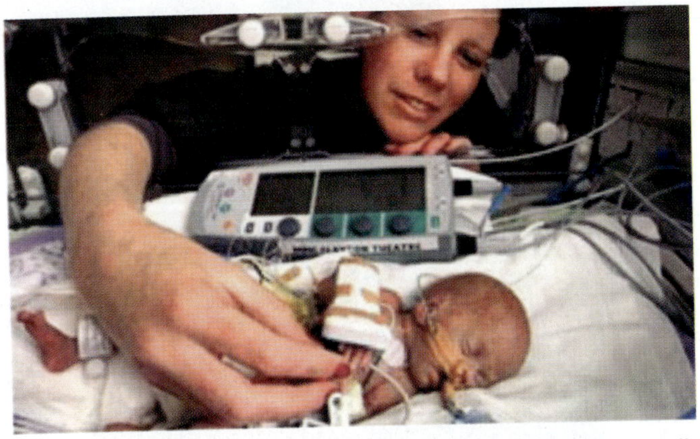

Fig. 41.4: *World's youngest girl who was tilted with cardiac pacemaker for her critical cardiac defect. Doctors decided to fit DDIP pacemaker in this baby*

AV blocks occur in 3° of severity as follows:
- *First degree:* The impulse is conducted through the AV node, albeit delayed
- *Second degree:* Not all impulses are conducted through the AV node
- *Third degree:* AV block is complete, and none of the impulses are conducted across the AV node

Causes of SA or AV node dysfunction can be divided into two distinct categories: congenital and acquired. Congenital causes include congenital AV block and congenital SA node dysfunction, which is notably less common. Congenital heart block is often due to autoantibody production from maternal systemic lupus erythematosus (SLE). Also, congenital heart block may be associated with congenital heart disease.

Acquired forms of heart block or SA node dysfunction are caused by infection or injury. Infections include viral myocarditis and lyme disease. Surgical repair of congenital heart disease is the predominant cause of nodal or conduction tissue injury.

Permanent pacing in children is a successful procedure that results in physiologic heart rates. Pacing also allows the patient to return to normal activity and lifestyle. The prognosis is excellent, because modern generation pacing systems allow physiologic atrial-synchronous, rate-responsive pacing in the vast majority of patients, even small infants and children with congenital heart disease.

Indications and Contraindications of Pacemaker Implantation (Table 41.1)

Although indications for pacing in children differ from those in adults, both include abnormalities in SA node and AV node function. The American Heart Association (AHA) and the American College of Cardiology (ACC) have published updated guidelines for implanting pacing systems in children. The AHA's scientific statements on pacing in children and adolescents divide the recommendations for pacemaker implantation in children into several classes reflecting the strength (or the absence) of the indication (Table 41.3).

Class I signifies that pacing is indicated and includes the following:
- Advanced second- or third-degree AV block with symptomatic bradycardia, ventricular dysfunction, or low cardiac output
- SA node dysfunction with symptoms during age-inappropriate bradycardia (the definition varies with the patient's age and expected heart rate)
- Postoperative advanced second- or third-degree AV block that is not expected to resolve or that persists at least 7 days
- Congenital third-degree AV block with a wide QRS escape rhythm, complex ventricular ectopy, or ventricular dysfunction
- Congenital third-degree AV block in an infant with a heart rate lower than 50–55 beats/min or with congenital heart disease and a heart rate lower than 70 beats/min.
- Sustained pause-dependent ventricular tachycardia with or without prolonged QT, with thoroughly documented pacing efficacy (Figs 41.39–41.43, 41.47–41.49).

Class IIa signifies that there is general agreement that pacing is indicated and includes the following:
- Bradycardia-tachycardia syndrome with need for long-term antiarrhythmic treatment (Figs 41.51–41.53, 41.58)
- Congenital third-degree AV block beyond the first year of life, with an average heart rate lower than 50 beats/min, abrupt pauses in ventricular rate that are 2–3 times the basic cycle length, or symptoms due to chronotropic incompetence
- Long QT syndrome with 2:1 AV or third-degree AV block
- Asymptomatic sinus bradycardia in a child with complex heart disease, with a heart rate lower than 40 beats/min or pauses exceeding 3 seconds

- Patients with congenital heart disease and impaired hemodynamics due to sinus bradycardia or loss of AV synchrony.

Class IIb signifies that although there is no consensus, implantation may reasonably be considered for the following:

- Transient postoperative third-degree AV block that reverts to sinus rhythm with residual bifascicular block
- Congenital third-degree AV block in an asymptomatic infant, child, or young adult with acceptable rate and function and narrow QRS
- Asymptomatic sinus bradycardia in congenital heart disease with a heart rate lower than 40 beats/min or pauses exceeding 3 seconds
- Neuromuscular disease with any degree of AV block (including first degree) with or without symptoms as there may be unpredictable progression of AV block

Class III signifies that pacing is not indicated and includes the following:

- Transient postoperative AV block with return of normal AV conduction
- Asymptomatic postoperative bifascicular block with or without first-degree AV block
- Asymptomatic type I second-degree AV block
- Asymptomatic sinus bradycardia in adolescents with longest R-R shorter than 3 seconds and a minimum heart rate higher than 40 beats/min.

In addition, expected survival of less than 6 months is a relative contraindication to permanent pacing therapy for patients who are terminally ill. Patients who fully regain normal conduction after transient postoperative heart block typically do not need to receive a permanent pacemaker.

Techniques in Implantation of Pacemakers in Infants and Children (Figs 41.5A and 41.5B)

Congenital (or acquired) structural heart disease presents additional issues for pacemaker implantation in children. These patients may have a more critical reliance on adequate hemodynamic status. Optimal hemodynamic performance is achieved with atrial synchronous pacing. Maintaining AV synchrony in this population is often more important than in children who have structurally normal hearts. For example, in a newborn with congenital complete

Table 41.1: *Indications for permanent pacing in children and adolescents*

Class I
1. Advanced second- or third-degree AV block associated with symptomatic bradycardia, congestive heart failure, or low cardiac output. *(Level of evidence: C)*
2. Sinus node dysfunction with correlation of symptoms during age-inappropriate bradycardia. The definition of bradycardia varies with the patient's age and expected heart rate. *(Level of evidence: B)*
3. Postoperative advanced second- or third-degree AV block that is not expected to resolve or persists at least 7 days after cardiac surgery. *(Level of evidence: B, C)*
4. Congenital third-degree AV block with a wide QRS escape rhythm or ventricular dysfunction. *(Level of evidence: B)*
5. Congenital third-degree AV block in the infant with a ventricular rate <50 to 55 bpm or with congenital heart disease and a ventricular rate <70 bpm. *(Level of evidence: B, C)*
6. Sustained pause-dependent VT, with or without prolonged QT, in which the efficacy of pacing is thoroughly documented. *(Level of evidence: B)*
Class IIa
1. Bradycardia-tachycardia syndrome with the need for long-term antiarrhythmic treatment other than digitalis. *(Level of evidence: C)*
2. Congenital third-degree AV block beyond the first year of life with an average heart rate <50 bpm or abrupt pauses in ventricular rate that are two or three times the basic cycle length. *(Level of evidence: B)*
3. Long QT syndrome with 2:1 AV or third-degree AV block. *(Level of evidence: B)*
4. Asymptomatic sinus bradycardia in the child with complex congenital heart disease with resting heart rate <35 bpm or pauses in ventricular rate >3 seconds. *(Level of evidence: C)*
Class IIb
1. Transient postoperative third-degree AV block that reverts to sinus rhythm with residual bifascicular block. *(Level of evidence: C)*
2. Congenital third-degree AV block in the asymptomatic neonate, child, or adolescent with an acceptable rate, narrow QRS complex, and normal ventricular function. *(Level of evidence: B)*
3. Asymptomatic sinus bradycardia in the adolescent with congenital heart disease with resting heart rate <35 bpm or pauses in ventricular rate >3 seconds. *(Level of evidence: C)*
Class III
1. Transient postoperative AV block with return of normal AV conduction within 7 days. *(Level of evidence: B)*
2. Asymptomatic postoperative bifascicular block with or without first-degree AV block. *(Level of evidence: C)*
3. Asymptomatic type I second-degree AV block. *(Level of evidence: C)*
4. Asymptomatic sinus bradycardia in the adolescent when the longest RR interval is <3 seconds and the minimum heart rate is >40 bpm. *(Level of evidence: C)*

heart block but a structurally normal heart, an epicardial ventricular pacing system initially suffices to meet hemodynamic needs. In contrast, a newborn with significant structural heart disease and congestive heart block may benefit more from a dual-chamber system to obtain AV synchrony and meet hemodynamic needs.

In general, the transvenous route is a reasonable approach for children weighing at least 10 kg although other authors have reported successful transvenous pacing in neonates without complications. Physical considerations include absence of intracardiac shunting, low-flow states, and anatomic barriers (e.g. mechanical valves that block pacing leads).

Transvenous lead placement in congenital heart patients often requires nonstandard positioning because of variations in venous and intracardiac anatomy. The atrial appendage is often concurrently amputated with cannulation for cardiac bypass, and atrial anatomy is often different from usual in pacemaker patients. The use of active-fixation leads allows easier sampling of nonstandard pacing sites and easier removal. In specific operations for congenital heart disease, such as the Fontan procedure, the right medial wall often is viable; in postoperative Mustard and Senning procedures, superior aspects of the systemic venous atrium are optimal. High-output pacing is imperative testing for diaphragmatic or phrenic nerve stimulation, particularly in lateral pacing sites. The active pacing lead tip may be used for mapping of optimal tissue implant sites.

Although anticoagulation is not universally recommended, it may help patients who have leads implanted in low-flow chambers. It is also important to consider the possibility of future rhythm complications in children who have undergone palliative repairs. For example, a child who develops heart block after a Fontan procedure needs ventricular pacing. These children are also at risk for SA node dysfunction; thus, placing an atrial pacing lead concurrent with placing a ventricular lead may prove beneficial.

Table 41.2: *Result of intraoperative measurements*

Parameter	*Desirable*	*Acceptable*	*Unacceptable*
Pacing threshold V	≤ 0.5 V	≤ 1.0 V	> 1.0 V
R wave	> 8.0 mV	> 4.0 mV	≤ 4.0 mV
Pacing threshold A	≤ 1.0 V	≤ 1.5 V	> 1.5 V
P wave	> 4.0 mV	> 2.0 mV	≤ 2.0 mV

Table 41.3: *Matching pacemaker type to medical indication*

Clinical indication	*AAI*	*AAIR*	*VVI*	*VVIR*	*VDD*	*DDD*	*DDDR*
Sinus node dysfunction with symptomatic bradycardia; AV node function normal	Yes	Yes	Yes	Yes	No	Yes	Yes
Sinus node dysfunction with symptomatic bradycardia; AV node function normal; AV synchrony needed	Yes	Yes	No	No	No	Yes	Yes
Sinus node dysfunction with symptomatic bradycardia; AV node function normal; AV synchrony needed; chronotropic incompetence present	No	Yes	No	Yes	No	Yes	Yes
Sinus node dysfunction with symptomatic bradycardia; AV node function abnormal; AV synchrony needed	No	No	No	No	No	Yes	Yes
Sinus node dysfunction with symptomatic bradycardia; AV node function abnormal; AV synchrony needed; chronotropic incompetence present	No	No	No	No	No	No	Yes
Symptomatic sinus node chronotropic incompetence; AV node function normal	No	Yes	No	Yes	No	No	Yes
Symptomatic sinus node chronotripic incompetence; AV node function abnormal	No	Yes	No	Yes	No	No	Yes
Third-degree AV block with symptomatic bradycardia; intact sinus node	No	No	Yes	Yes	Yes	Yes	Yes
Third-degree AV block induced by AV node ablation; underlying atrial flutter present	No	No	Yes	Yes	No	No	No
Third-degree AV block induced by AV node ablation; absence of underlying atrial fibrillation or atrial flutter	No	No	Yes	Yes	Yes	Yes	Yes
Second-degree type II AV block with symptomatic bradycardia; intact sinus node function	No	No	Yes	Yes	Yes	Yes	Yes
Chronic atrial fibrillation/atrial flutter with slow ventricular response	No	No	Yes	Yes	No	No	No
Hypersensitive carotid sinus syndrome (mixed etiology) with intact sinus node function; AV synchrony required	No	No	No	No	Yes	Yes	Yes
Hypersensitive carotid sinus syndrome (mixed etiology) with chronic atrial fibrillation	No	No	Yes	Yes	No	No	No

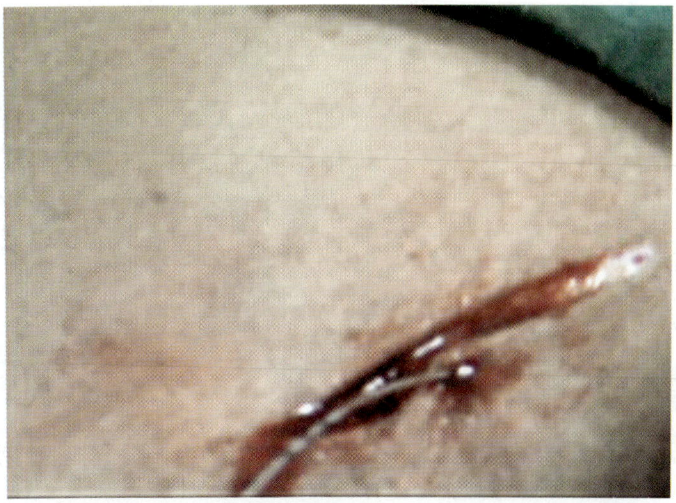

Step 1. *To make skin incision under left collar bone*

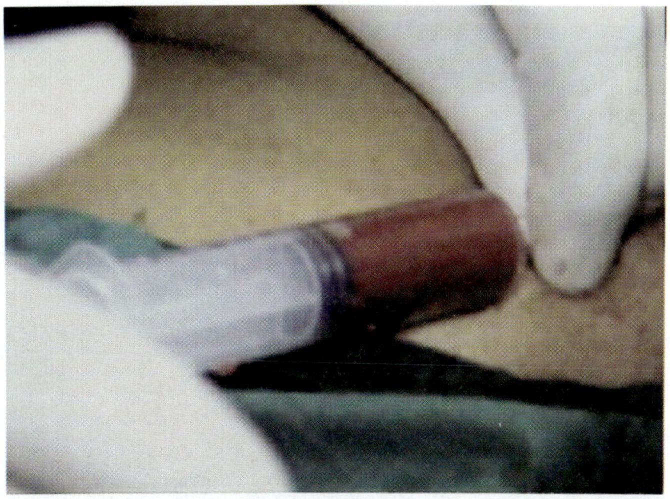

Step 2: *Stepwise minimal surgical intervention in the implantation of intracardiac pacemaker*

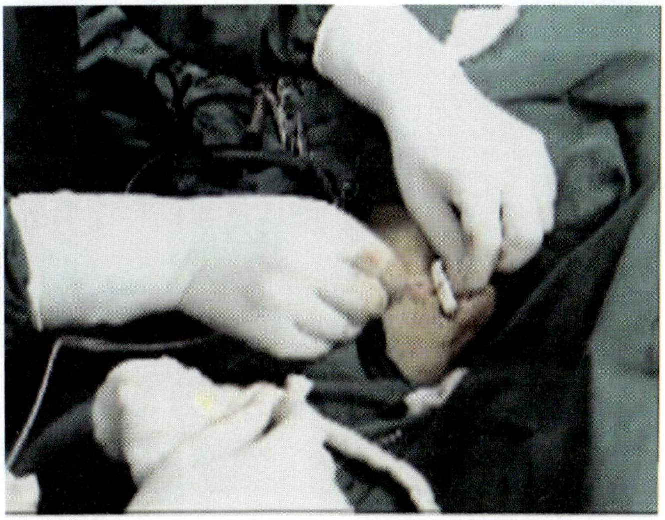

Step 3: *Guidewire being inserted*

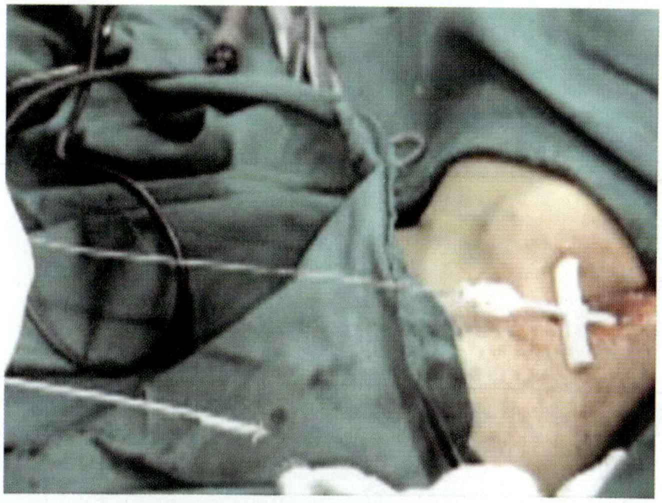

Step 4: *Left subclavian vein catheterized*

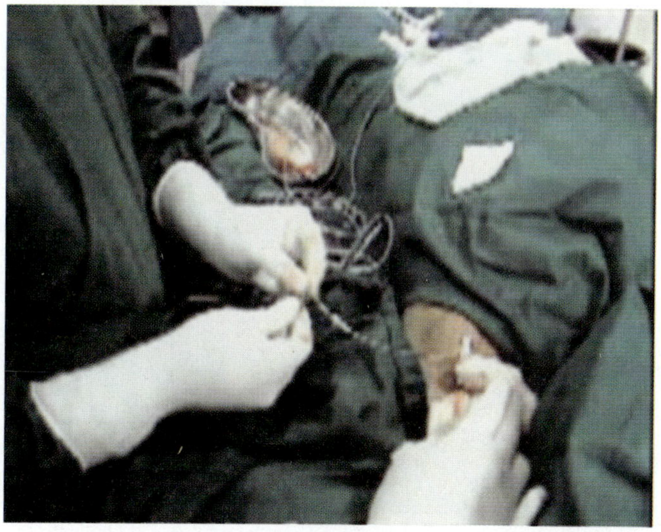

Step 5: *External pacing done to check the lead's*

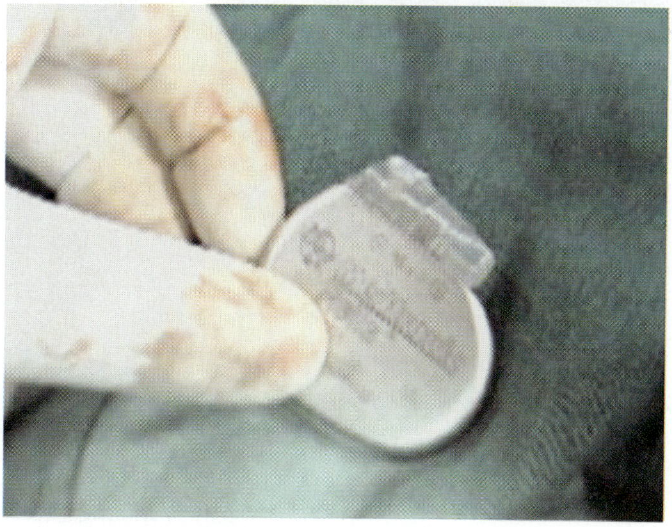

Step 6: *Depiction of smaller size pacemaker (recent)*

Fig. 41.5A: ***(Steps 1 to 6)*** *Stepwise minimal surgical intervention in the implantation of intracardiac pacemaker*

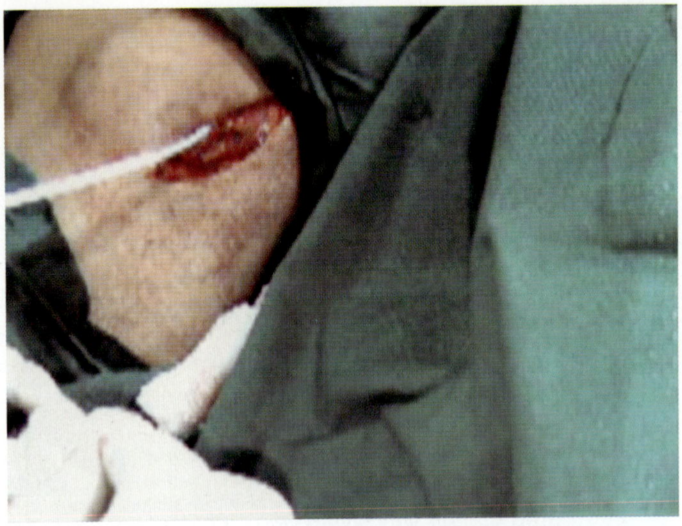

Step 7: *Pocket prepared under the left collar bone*

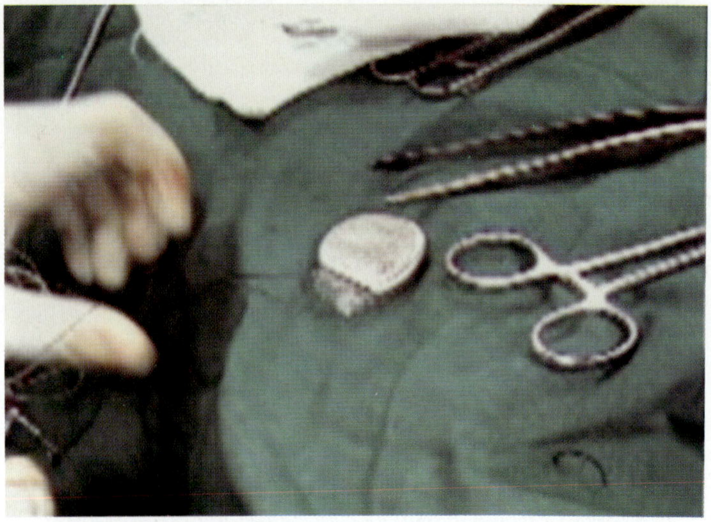

Step 10: *Pacemaker connected with leads*

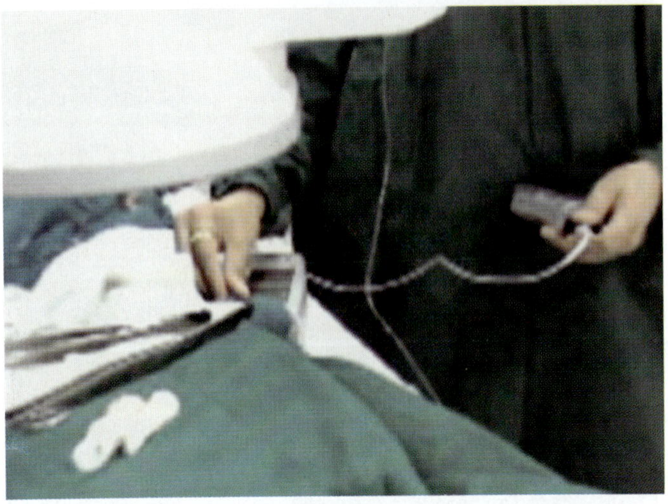

Step 8: *Pacemaker pulse rate being set*

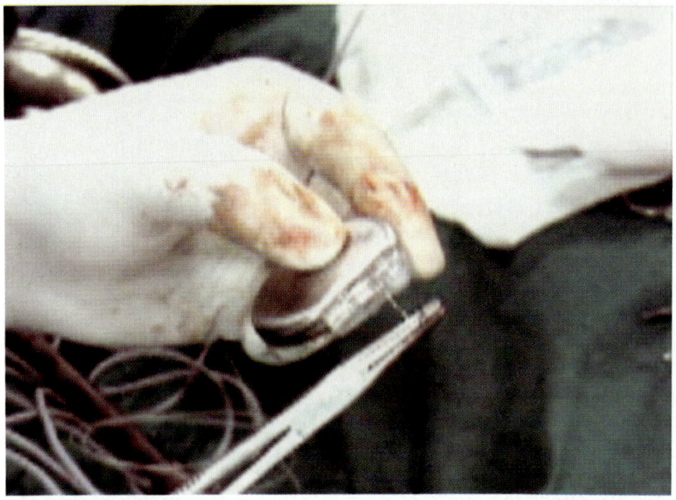

Step 11: *An anchoring suture is applied to the pacemaker*

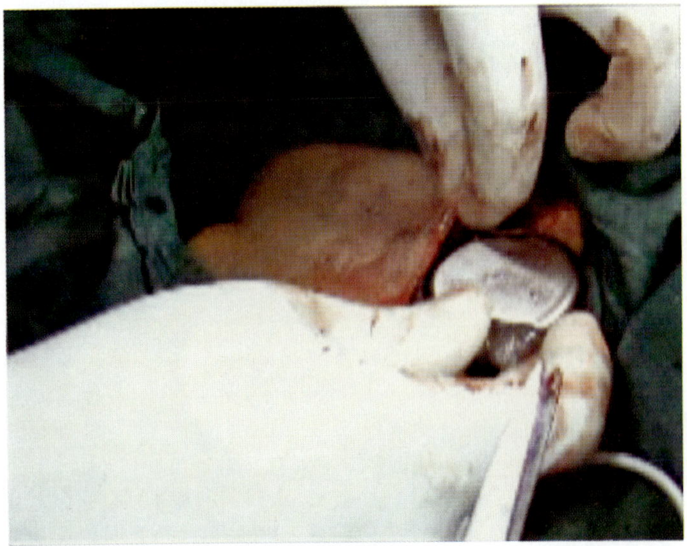

Step 9: *Pacemaker being inserted in the skin pocket*

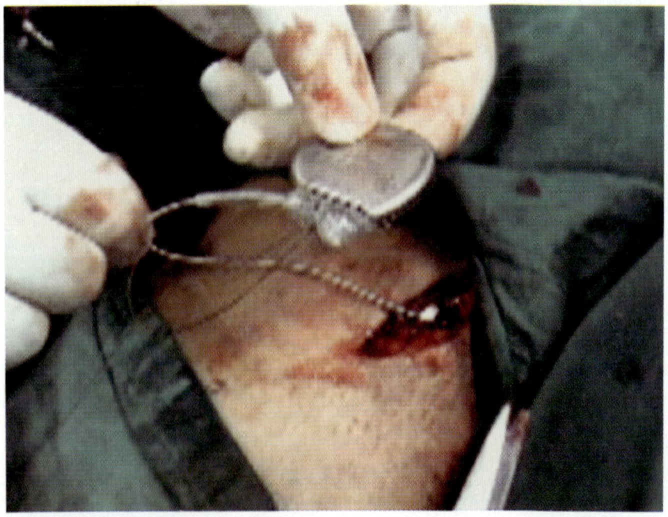

Step 12: *Pacemaker ready to be kept in pocket already prepared under subclavicular region*

Fig. 41.5B: ***(Steps 7 to 12)*** *Stepwise minimal surgical intervention in the implantation of intracardiac pacemaker*

Table 41.4: The revised NASPE/BPEG generic code for antibradycardia pacing

I	*II*	*III*	*IV*	*V*
Chamber(s) paced	Chamber(s) sensed	Response to sensing	Rate modulation	Multisite pacing
O = None	O = None	O = None	O = None	O = None
A = Atrium	A = Atrium	T = Triggered	R = Rate modulation	A = Atrium
V = Ventricle	V = Ventricle	I = Inhibited		V = Ventricle
D = Dual (A+V)	D = Dual (A+V)	D = Dual (T+I)		D = Dual (A+V)

Table 41.5: Clinical problems faced by the physician after PPI

Abnormality	*Time of appearance after pacemaker implant*	*Possible fault*	*Management*
1. Dizziness and missed beats; recurrence of initial symptoms	Hours to days	Lead displacement or penetration resulting in the loss of capture	Reposition lead; occassionally
2. Frequent, irregular beats	Hours to days	Lead displacement resulting in the loss of sensing	Reprogramming is possible
3. Painful pacer site with or without pyrexia	Usually days or weeks	Infected pacer pocket	Removal of pacing system and resetting
4. Dizziness and syncope	Often months or	Myoinhibition years	Programme to R wave triggered or change to bipolar system
5. Dizziness and heavy palpitations	Variable	Retrograde conduction pacemaker syndrome	Change to dual chamber system if symptoms severe
6. Recurrence of initial symptoms	Years	Lead fracture or pacemaker failure	Replace faulty part
7. Tachycardia with dual chamber	Variable	Pacemaker mediated tachycardia	Reprogramme pacemaker

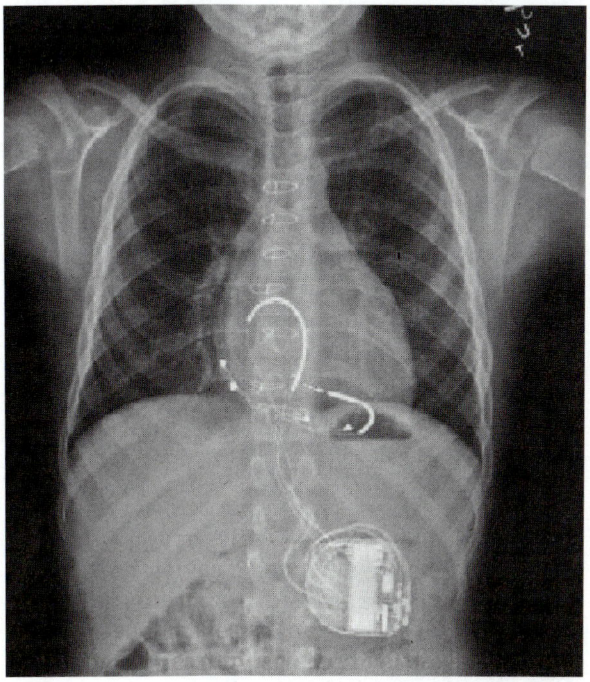

Fig. 41.6: Skiagram of cheast PA view showing on pacing and implantable cardioverter defibrillators in a young child

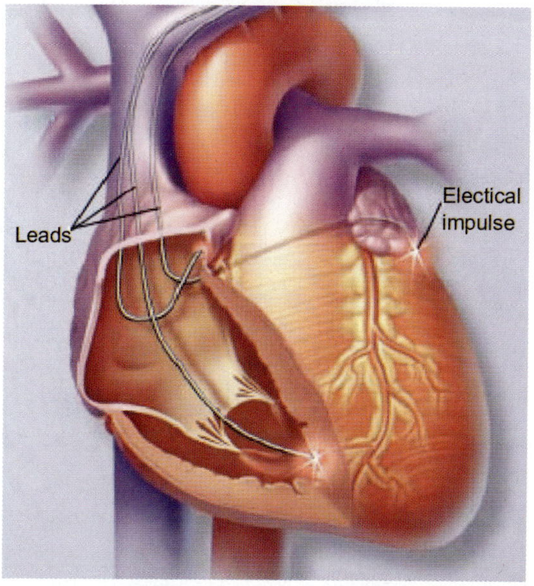

Fig. 41.7: Diagram showing endocardial and epicardial leads in biventricular pacing along with their respective areas of connection for CRT

Certain populations are at greater risk for the development of atrial tachycardia; therefore, pacemaker type is important. A patient with SA node dysfunction who is at risk for atrial tachycardia should probably have a generator placed that also allows antitachycardia pacing, either manual or automatic. There are now automatic atrial antitachycardia pacemakers that have been shown to be effective in pediatric congenital heart disease patients.

Implantable Cardioverter Defibrillator (ICD)

Additional concerns include patients who require a pacemaker but who also are at risk for ventricular arrhythmias (e.g. an older patient with previous repaired tetralogy of Fallot). If these patients require a pacemaker, avoidance of placement in the left subclavian vein and pectoral pocket may be prudent, thus reserving this area for future potential placement of an implantable cardioverter defibrillator (ICD) (Fig. 41.6).

Cardiac Resynchronization Therapy (CRT) (Fig. 41.7)

For those patients with heart failure, CRT may be used in conjunction with medical therapy to improve cardiac function and quality of life. Although indications for CRT in pediatrics remain controversial, important anatomic considerations are noted. CRT requires two strategically placed leads in the ventricles (typically 1 in the right ventricle and 1 in the left) that pace 2 ventricular areas to synchronize ventricular contraction.

A transvenous approach requires a patent coronary venous system that is accessed via the coronary sinus.

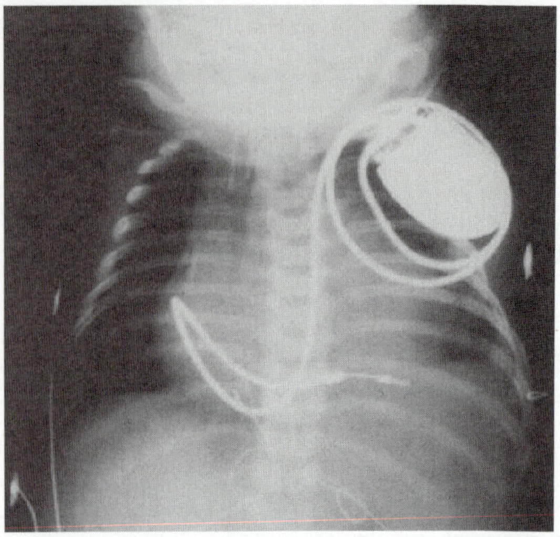

Fig. 41.8: *Transvenous pacing system in a newborn via left superior vena cava to right ventricle (bipolar steroid eluting Medtronic screw in 4068-52cm) with the pulse generator (Medtronic MicroMinix 8360) in a subcutaneous left pectoral pouch*

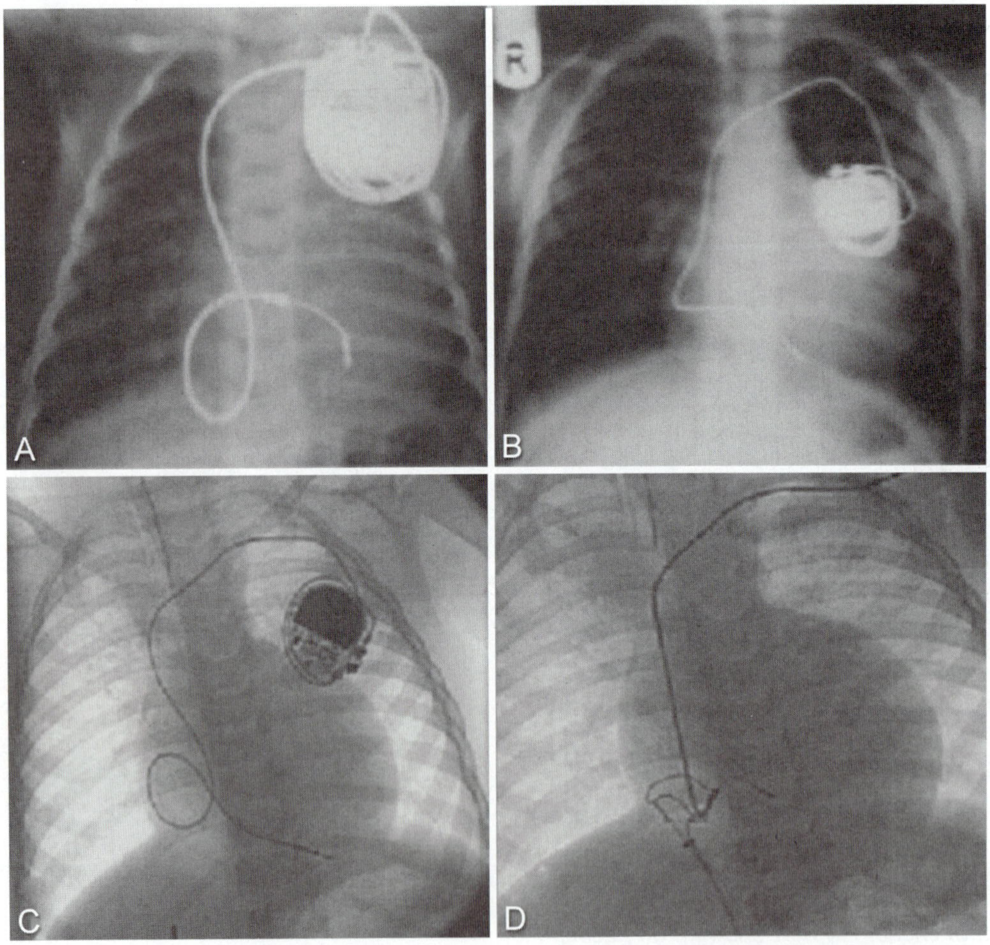

Fig. 41.9: *An infant with congenitally corrected transposition (cTGA) developed heart failure with the onset of complete heart block and was paced at 6 weeks of age (A). At 4 years the generator reached its end of life with some remaining lead slack (B). During the generator change, the lead was inadvertently damaged and had to be replaced. Angiography revealed an occluded subclavian vein (C). To avoid the use of large countertraction sheaths from the subclavian approach, a coronary guidewire was passed into the lead stylet channel and was drawn out the femoral sheath with the lead after snaring the lead with the help of a tip deflector wire (D). Over the subclavian-femoral guidewire circuit, a new sheath was placed to implant a new ventricular lead*

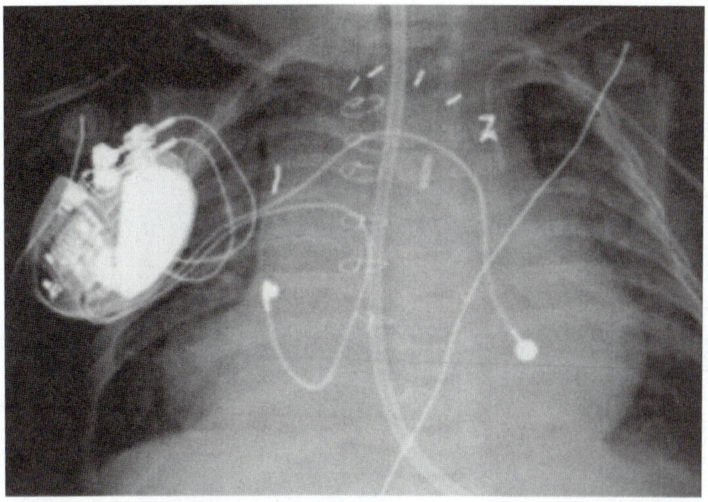

Fig. 41.10: *Epicardial dual-chamber pacemaker lead configuration in a newborn with complex congenital heart disease (heterotaxy). The pacemaker is implanted in the right pectoral region, and the leads are tunneled through the chest wall to the atrium and ventricle. This unusual approach was required because the infant had an associated abdominal wall defect*

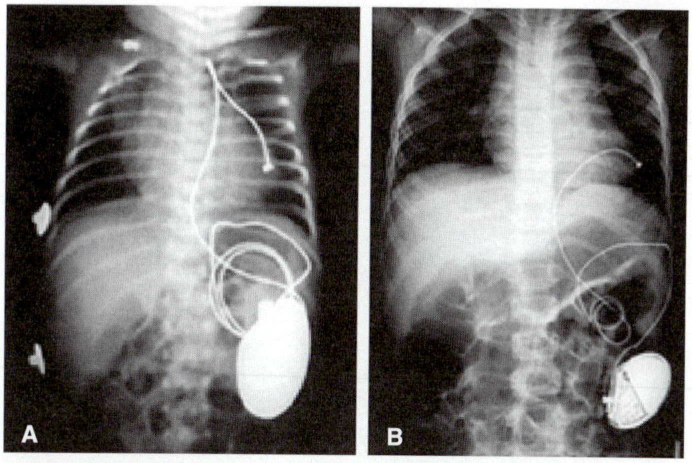

Fig. 41.11: *(A) Anteroposterior roentgenogram taken after primary pacemaker implantation at 1 month of life shows the large generator in the peritoneal cavity. The lead is looped in the pericardial cavity and the subcutaneous layer of the left side of the abdomen. (B) Anteroposterior roentgenogram taken after generator exchange at 4 years 6 months of life. The generator is placed into the layer between the internal and external oblique muscles. The lead has shortened in the pericardium with growth of the patient*

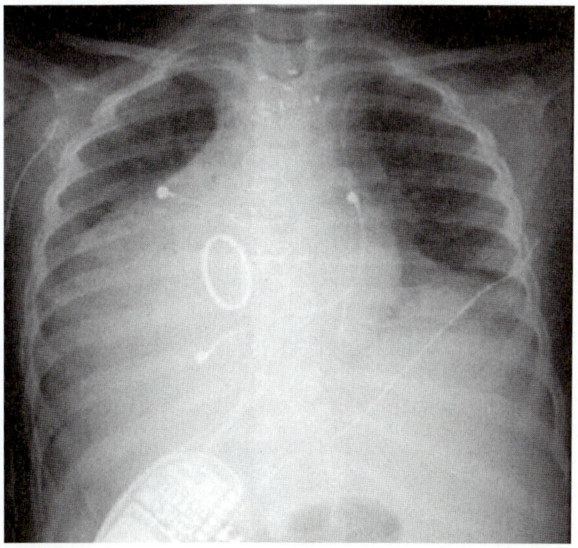

Fig. 41.12: *Epicardial lead placement for cardiac resynchronization therapy (CRT) in a 2-year-old child with dextrocardia, complex congenital heart disease, and ventricular dysfunction associated with severe mitral insufficiency. The atrial lead is at the high left atrial border. There are two ventricular leads, one at the anterior apex of the ventricles overlying the ventricular septum and the other at the posterobasal aspect of the systemic ventricle. CRT resulted in shortening the QRS duration from 120 ms to 80 ms and gradual improvement in ejection fraction from 20% to 35%, which allowed the patient to undergo successful mitral valve replacement.*

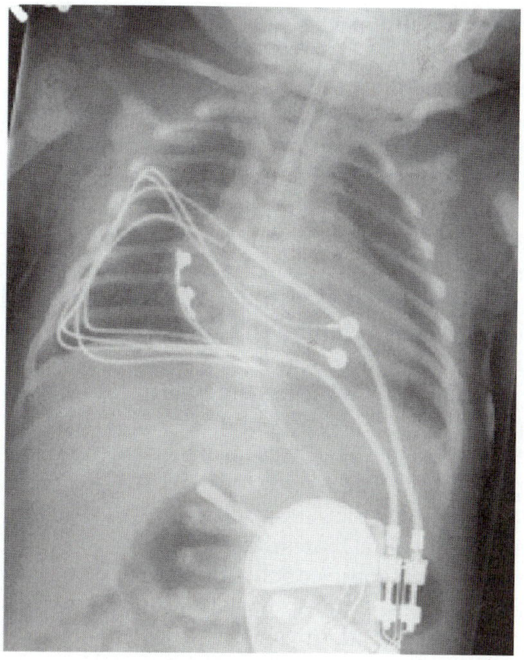

Fig. 41.13: *X-ray chest PA and frontal abdominal views showing epicardial pacemaker leads attached proximally with heart and is supported with external battery fitted in the abdomen distally in a 4-yrs-old boy*

Typically, the left ventricular lead is placed through the coronary sinus and then carefully maneuvered into one of the tributary cardiac veins of the left ventricle. Patients with congenital heart disease often have distorted coronary venous anatomy; in these patients, CRT may require an epicardial approach.

Selection of Pacemaker in Children

Single-chamber Versus Dual-chamber Pacing

Whether dual-chamber synchronous pacing is superior to single-chamber ventricular pacing remains subject to debate atrial-based pacing, which includes AAI(R), DDD,

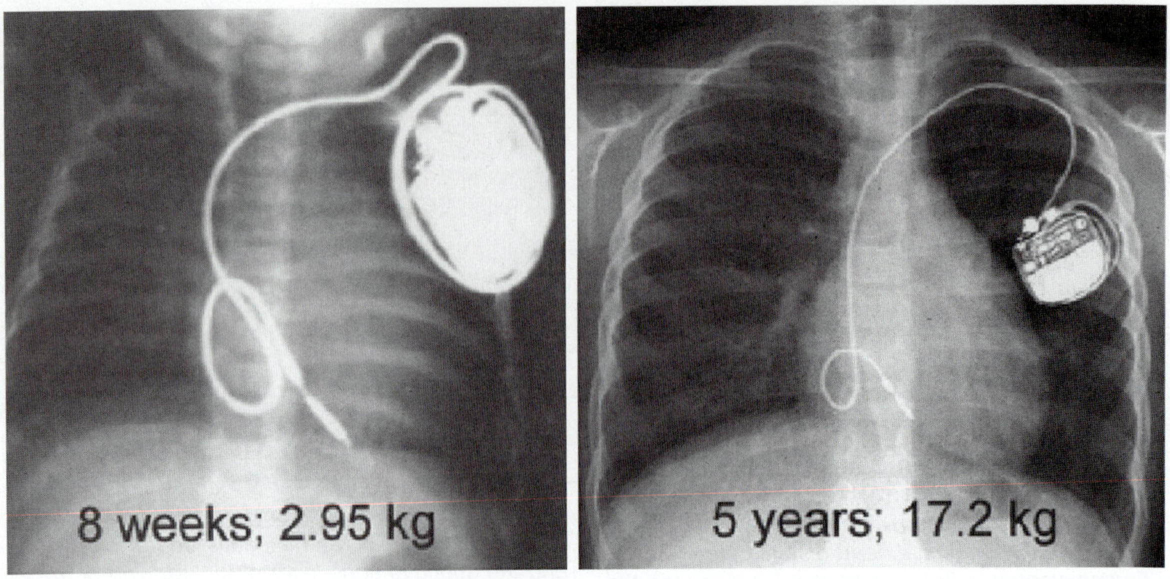

Fig. 41.14: *Left panel shows lead position in a baby with congenital complete heart block who was born prematurely with hydrops. A transvenous endocardial pacemaker was implanted at the age of 8 weeks when she weighed 2.95 kg. At 5 years of age (weight 17.2 kg), she still has the initial lead and generator (right panel). The redundant loop of lead formed in the right atrium has not yet been taken up and will allow generator replacement without the need for lead advancemenrt*

and VDD(R) pacing modes, has been shown to be superior to ventricular-based (VVIR) pacing in studies of adults, although controversy regarding DDD versus VVI pacing continues. Several large-scale prospective studies are under way to help illuminate these issues.

In adult studies, dual-chamber pacing may have lower morbidity and mortality compared with ventricular pacing in patients with congestive heart failure, valvular heart diseases, and hypertensive heart disease. Studies indicate higher incidences of death, stroke, atrial fibrillation, pacemaker syndrome, and heart failure during VVI pacing than during DDD pacing.

An apparently convincing argument advocates atrial-based pacing [either single-chamber AAI (R)] or dual-chamber modes) over ventricular-based pacing modalities, although whether DDD is better than AAI(R) for patients with intact atrioventricular conduction is less clear.

Experimental data that address pacing in children are more limited, and some conclusions are extrapolated from adult patient series. Common pacing indications in children are similar to those in adults (e.g. SA or AV node dysfunction) though concomitant cardiac, medical, psychological, and size-related issues often differ markedly. Rate-responsive ventricular pacing often has been used in children with complete AV block. Rate-responsive ventricular pacing also responds adequately to the physiologic requirements of healthy active children.

Many pediatric patients, however, have underlying structural heart disease, tachyarrhythmia, and hemodynamic derangements that compromise ventricular performance. In addition, pediatric patients frequently have structural anatomic barriers to implantation and limited access to cardiac chambers.

Many patients who have previously undergone atrial surgical procedures (e.g. Fontan, Mustard, or Senning procedures) have both bradyarrhythmia and tachyarrhythmia. Some studies have demonstrated higher atrial-pacing failure rates in these patients, presumably as a consequence of higher atrial pressures, scarring, and ischemia.

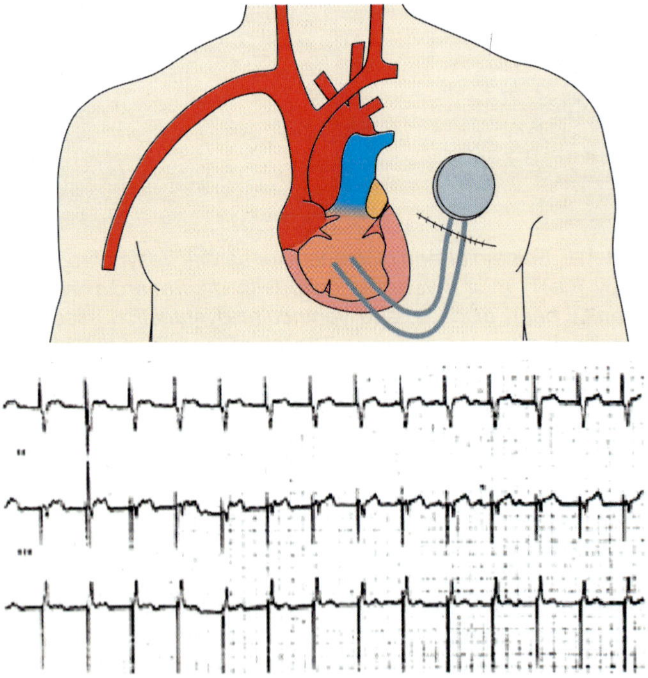

Fig. 41.15: *(Upper) Diagram shows implantation of epicardial pacemaker in children. (Bottom) shows ECG features of normally functioning epicardial pacemaker*

A large retrospective series from Boston Children's Hospital revealed no significant differences between many patients who had undergone Fontan or atrial switch procedures. Investigators compared these patients with others who underwent Fontan surgery and received no permanent pacemaker, an atrial single-chamber pacemaker, a ventricular-based pacing system, or a dual-chamber pacing system. No clear choice of pacing modality emerged for pediatric single-ventricle patients.

Epicardial Versus Endocardial Pacing Sites

The main difference in lead implantation is route of placement. Although the vast majority of adult pacemaker patients have transvenous lead placement, children have an almost even distribution of transvenous and epicardial lead implantation (Figs 41.10–41.13, 41.15 and 41.16).

For sometime, epimyocardial pacing was the most common pediatric pacing application. At present, epicardial pacing is primarily used when transvenous pacing is contraindicated or for patients undergoing concomitant heart surgery. Contraindications to transvenous pacing include prosthetic tricuspid valves, right-to-left intracardiac shunts, congenital heart disease, surgery precluding transvenous access to cardiac chambers, recurrent transvenous lead dislodgment, and, probably, minimum patient size (Fig. 14.29).

Advantages of epicardial implantation include the absence of a need to provide vascular continuity with cardiac chambers and the avoidance of concerns about venous thrombosis. Disadvantages include more frequent reports of sensing and capture failure, higher rates of insulation

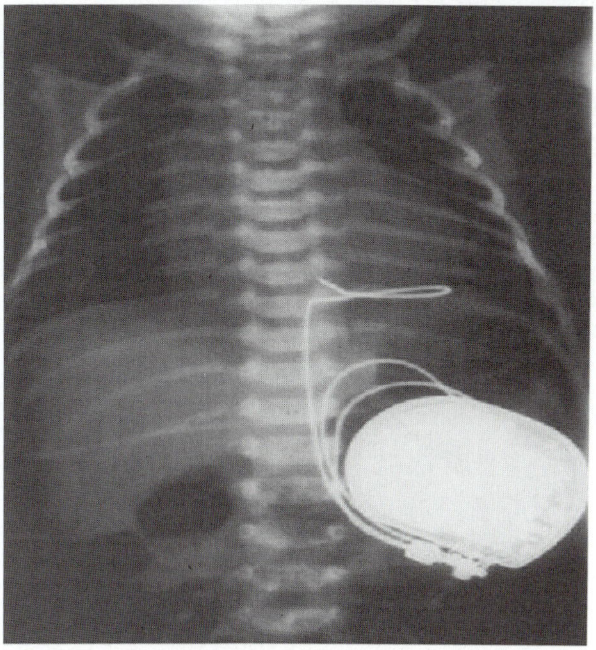

Fig. 41.16: *A baby girl was born prematurely at 34 weeks, weighing 1.5 Kg .The baby was diagnosed with a complete heart block in the 28th week of mothers pregnancy. The baby had a permanent pacemaker during 20th minute of her life. This is considered as the Worlds smallest baby to receive a permanent cardiac pacemaker on 5th march 2015 in mumbai*

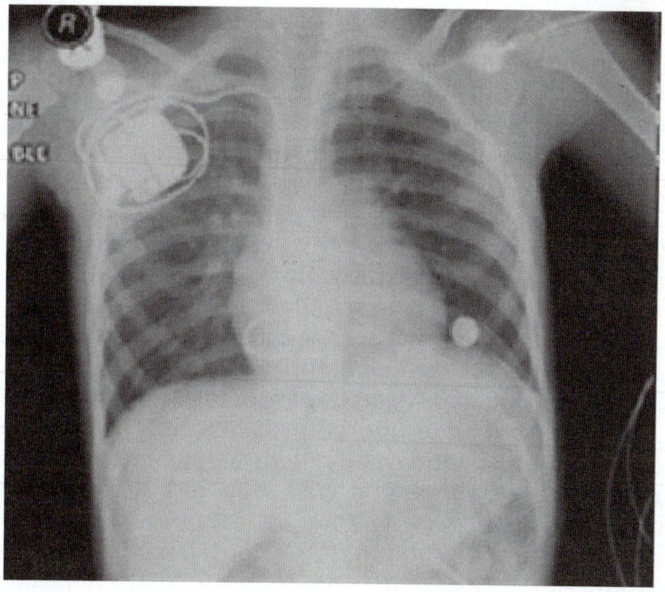

Fig. 41.17: *X-ray depicting the endocardial pacemaker inserted through the right subclavian vein*

and conductor fractures, and the need for an open chest approach (e.g. via a thoracotomy, a sternotomy, or a subxiphoid or subcostal incision).

Transvenous pacing is certainly feasible in infants and small children. Smaller pacemaker generators and thinner lead diameters now simplify placement of permanent transvenous pacing systems. However, the easier placement of transvenous leads in small patients does not imply that this approach is necessarily superior to others. Current practice suggests that transvenous pacing leads routinely can be placed in children who weigh more than 10 kg. As pacing technology continues to reduce lead body diameter, it is likely that children with even smaller body weights can be considered for transvenous placement. However, because of continued growth and vigorous activity, pediatric patients have lead fracture and failure rates distinctly higher than adults.

Actual survival comparisons have been performed for transvenous pacing leads in children. These comparisons show progressive lead failure over time from fracture, insulation discontinuities, adapter or header failures, or pacing exit block.

Advantages of the transvenous route include avoidance of thoracotomy, lower pacing thresholds (and thus longer battery life), and lower incidences of exit block and lead fractures. Disadvantages include a slightly higher dislodgment rate (e.g. with passive fixation devices), potential venous occlusion, possible embolic events (e.g. from an intracardiac shunt), a slight risk of endocarditis, and subclavian crush syndrome.

Twiddler syndrome can also occur in children with potential lead dislodgment, generator migration, or pacing failure due to twisting of leads or generator in the pocket. Significant vascular access challenges can also relate to congenital heart diseases and surgical corrections.

Preoperative Evaluation in Pacemaker Implantation

For patients with congenital or idiopathic atrioventricular (AV) block, test for **maternal lupus antibodies (anti-Ro, anti-La), and measure Lyme titers**. AV block due to Lyme carditis is typically reversible with appropriate antibiotic treatment.

Echocardiography is used to determine the underlying anatomy, particularly the presence of L-looping of the ventricles (i.e. physiologically corrected transposition of the great arteries), which has a high association with the development of AV block. Echocardiographic data are also useful to assess ventricular function and to determine presence of congenital heart disease or intracardiac shunts.

Phlebography may be helpful before transvenous pacemaker implantation, particularly for patients who have undergone prior surgery or central venous line placement. Arm phlebography can outline the course of the venous system and confirm continuity with the heart. Variants (e.g. left superior vena cava to coronary sinus connections and other vascular anomalies) can be easily identified.

Performing chest radiography before pacemaker implantation to identify heart chamber sizes and potential vascular abnormalities (e.g. right aortic arch) is reasonable. In addition, imaging should be performed in patients with existing pacing systems to visualize the lead positions.

Electrocardiography (ECG) is essential for documenting the rhythm before the pacemaker is implanted.

Equipment Required in Pacemaker Implantation

Pacemaker Size and Type (Figs 41.18–41.21 and 41.25)

Size is an important factor in pacemaker selection, particularly for infants and smaller children. Modern generators have markedly reduced mass, width, and circumference, and single-chamber and dual-chamber devices are now similarly sized.

No pacemaker is specifically designed for pediatric use. Each generator has special features and options, which vary among different manufacturers and specific models. Some features may be particularly appropriate or inappropriate

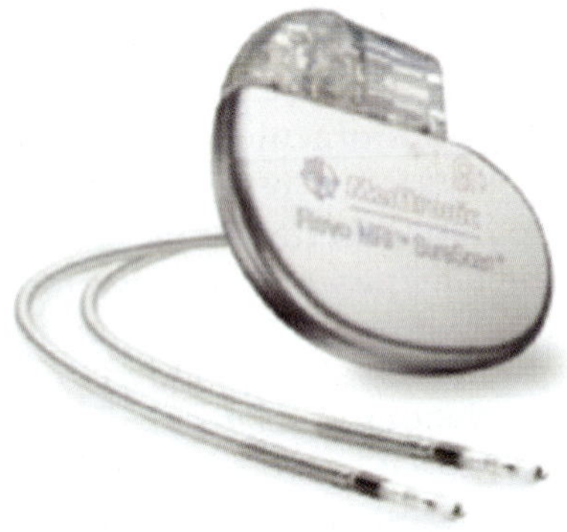

Fig. 41.18: *Revo MRITM SureScan pacing system, the first MR-conditional pacing system designed, tested and FDA approved for use in the magnetic resonance imaging (MRI) environment*

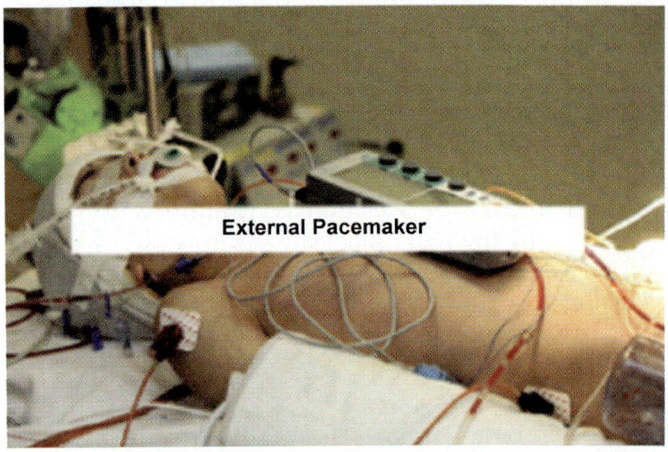

Fig. 41.20: *External pacemaker during child heart surgery*

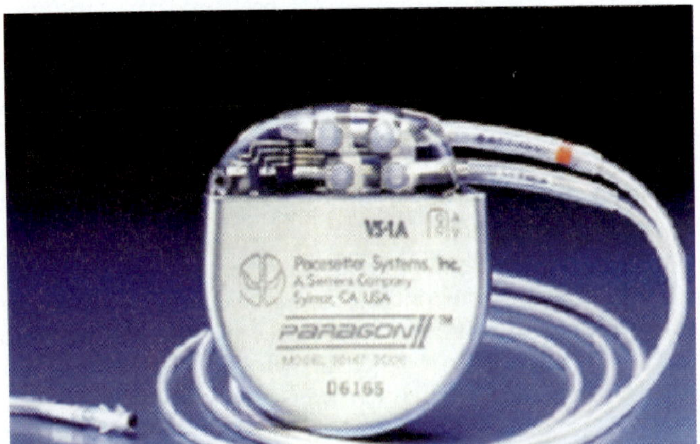

Fig. 41.19: *Showing DDDC type of pacemaker model*

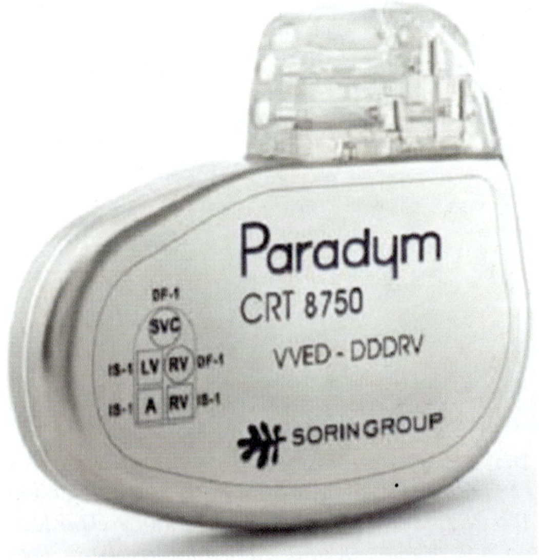

Fig. 41.21: *Showing world's most powerful cardiac resynchronization therapy defibrillator sorin group (Milan, Italy)*

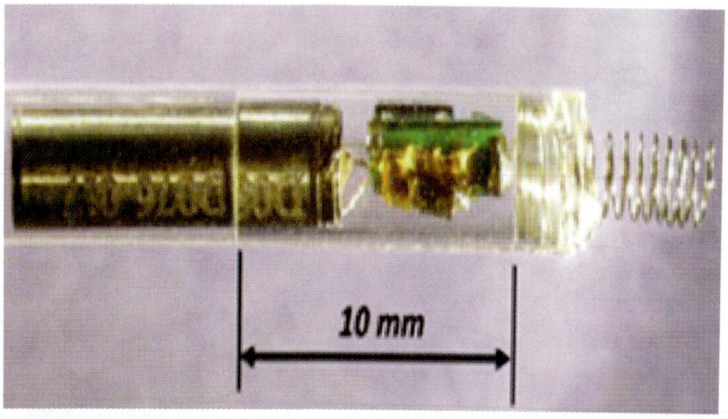

Fig. 41.22: *Original mechanical concept for the fetal pacemaker and its deployment. University of Southern California's fetal pacemaker measures just 20 millimeters and is implanted directly onto the baby's heart using a cannula during noninvasive surgery. If successful, researchers hope that this type of pacemaker could someday be used to treat adults as well*

for children. For example, because pacemakers are designed primarily for adults, the resting heart rate is expected to be lower than 100 beats/min. Most pacemakers released before 1996 had a maximum rate limit of 120–130 beats/min, which may be inadequate for a neonate or critically ill postoperative infant.

A programmable lower and upper rate limit may require a higher setting in children to compensate for increased demands on myocardial oxygen consumption, cardiac output response to exercise, and increased predicted maximum heart rates with exertion. Unfortunately, battery longevity is sacrificed in favor of optimizing hemodynamic performance. Because cardiac output is more critically dependent on heart rate in children, the requirement for faster pacing rates increases battery expenditure.

Pacemaker Leads (Figs 41.22–41.24)

Fixation mechanisms in transvenous leads are divided into active-fixation tips and passive-fixation leads. In general, active-fixation leads are now more commonly used in children because they can be more easily removed if necessary.

Active-fixation leads have a screw on the end that penetrates the endocardium. These mechanisms either are covered in a dissolvable material (e.g. gelatin, sugar cap) to protect the delicate veins during insertion or have an intricate screw extension-retraction mechanism that allows the operator to enter the vein and cardiac chambers without an exposed screw.

Active-fixation leads can be fixated almost anywhere in the endocardium; they may be especially valuable for patients with left ventricular lead placements (e.g. corrected transposition of great arteries) or those without a right atrial appendage (e.g. most postoperative patients with congenital heart disease). Active-fixation leads are more easily removed, even after being implanted for many years. This feature is a distinct advantage for young patients, who may need multiple pacemaker system replacements over a lifetime.

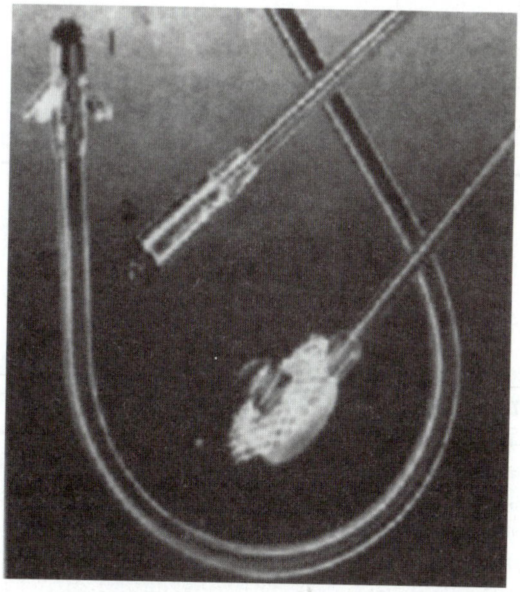

Fig. 41.23: *Photograph showing different types of tips of pacing electrode in current use (1. steroid impregnated porous transvenous lead. 2. and 3. screw type of tip for epicardial paclng)*

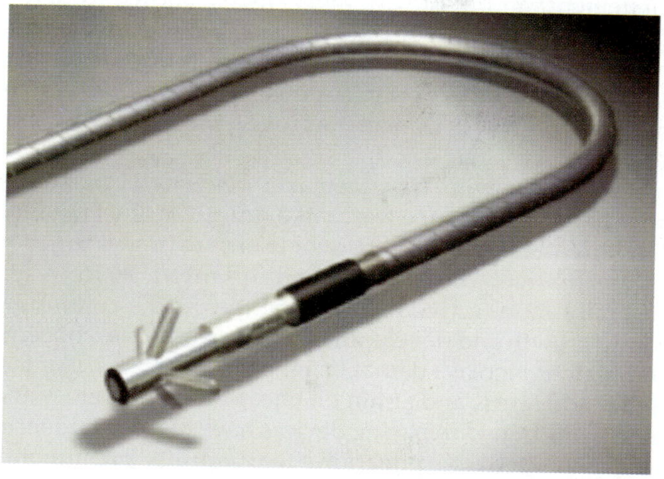

Fig. 41.24: *Showing Medtronic's MR-conditional CapSure Sense MRI SureScan pacing lead. The CapSure Sense MRI SureScan(R) leads address an unmet clinical need for thoroughly tested MRI conditional passive fixation leads*

Passive-fixation mechanisms use small tines or fins near the distal tip, which become entrapped in the right ventricular trabeculations and lodge within scar over time. These leads do not require a screw-in device but are facilitated by placement in a trabeculated region, which may not be routinely available in patients with congenital heart disease. Passive-fixation leads are more difficult to extract when implanted for long periods and may be less appropriate for pediatric patients because multiple revisions are anticipated.

The tips of the leads may have special coatings to improve pacing characteristics or to decrease surrounding tissue inflammation. The most common is a steroid-eluting tip, which continually disperses a tiny amount of dexamethasone (or another corticosteroid) into the local tip-tissue interface. These steroid-eluting leads, available in both passive-fixation and active-fixation tips, prevent subacute threshold rise, which is seen several weeks after lead implantation. This benefit can be critically important in children, who typically have a greater inflammatory response to tissue injury and a larger threshold rise.

Titanium nitride and other metallic compounds also have been used to increase the surface area at the tip-tissue interface; this increased surface area should improve pacing and sensing performance.

Monitoring and follow-up care of implanted pacemaker during immediate and on longterm basis

(Figs 41.25 and 41.26)

Follow-up is routine and simplified. During the initial few months after surgery, evaluate the patient to assess for a possible rise in capture thresholds secondary to inflammation and exit block. Program a safety margin to avoid possible loss of capture because of a subacute threshold rise, which may be seen in the first several weeks, particularly with epimyocardial implants or nonsteroid-eluting leads (Tables 41.2, 41.4 and 41.5).

Transtelephonic pacing system evaluation is simple, convenient, and relatively inexpensive, allowing follow-up with fewer cardiology office visits. These systems have become more sophisticated and more automated over the past few years, permitting extensive pacemaker system information to be transmitted over the telephone and internet (Figs 41.26, 41.59).

For patients who are pacemaker-dependent, dizziness, presyncope, or syncope warrants a full device interrogation of both leads and pulse generator to ensure proper function of the device. Children with implanted devices are generally more active than adults; the child's continuing bodily growth and development create additional concerns and further increase demands on pacing systems. Contact sports add stress and strain on pacemaker generators and leads. Children with pacing devices have higher incidences of lead-related complications than adults, presumably secondary to growth and vigorous exertion. Younger patients are more apt to participate in contact sports and to continue to engage in vigorous activities.

Resumption of normal activities, as feasible, and promotion of healthy development without incurring significant additional risks are important goals of pediatric health care. Physicians must identify potential concerns and obstacles that patients and families may encounter and must offer strategies to guide them through their adjustment.

Approach Considerations (Figs 41.27 and 41.28)

Provide a thorough and adequate explanation of pacemaker implantation procedures to the patient. Document indications for permanent pacing and outline the plan for route of access. Make relevant surgical decisions after comprehensive consideration of the following factors:

- **Transvenous versus epicardial approach**
- **Single-chamber pacing versus dual-chamber pacing versus cardiac resynchronization therapy (CRT)**

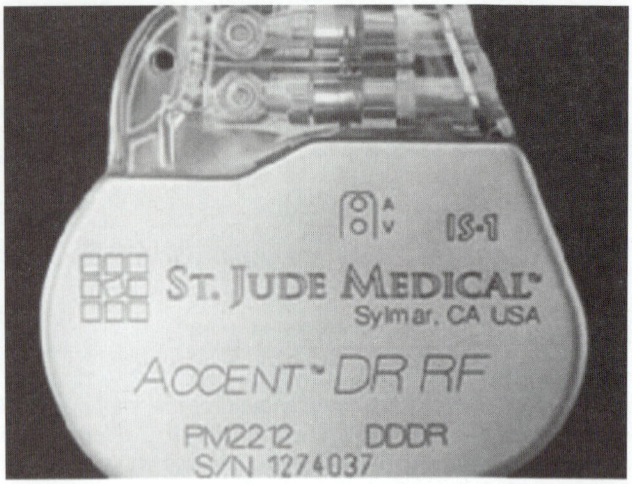

Fig. 41.25: *The accent RF pacemaker is the first to simplify patient management from implant through follow-up with wireless monitoring. With the intelligence to sense and automatically adjust device parameters, the accent RF device, a wireless monitoring pacemaker, is designed to maintain effective therapy and enhance patient safety. The accent RF pacemaker provides intelligent sensing and adjustment of selected device parameters and remote monitoring to help streamline follow-ups, simplify therapy optimization and enhance clinic efficiency*

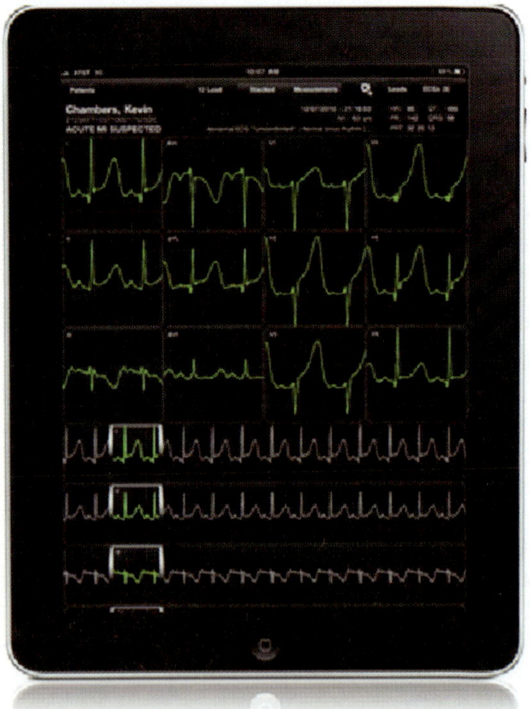

Fig. 41.26: *Showing live patient ECG's from GE's MUSE Cardiology on Your iOS Device. Regardless of where remote cardiologists are when a critical decision is needed, they can leverage AirStrip cardiology to quickly determine the best treatment paths for their patients. This may reduce the need to return to the hospital or access a computer connected to the hospital network. A remote cardiologist can now use AirStrip cardiology to precisely measure ECG waveforms, helping on-site ED clinicians determine, for example, if a patient requires cath lab intervention*

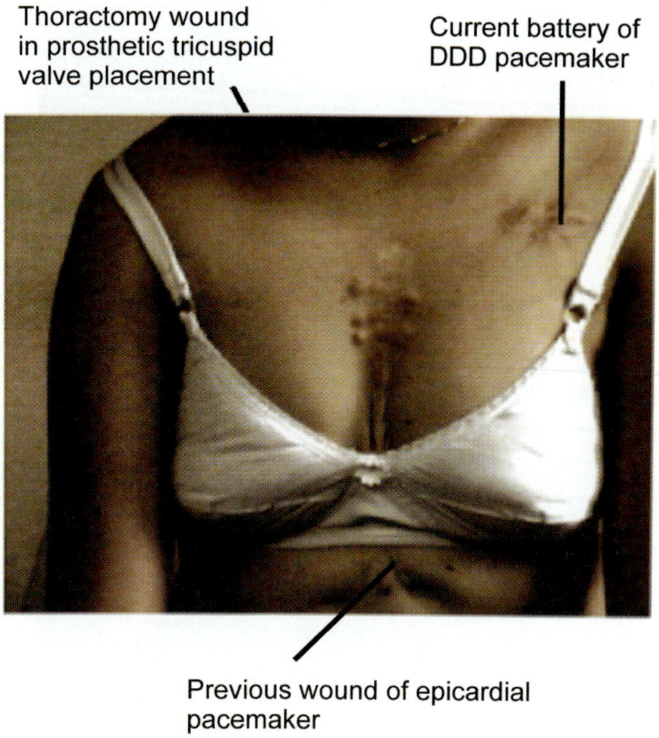

Fig. 41.27: *Patient at the age of 20 yrs, her epicardial pacemaker and prosthetic tricuspid valve completely failed to work satisfactorily after 16 yrs. She was managed with implantation of DDD pacemaker for cardiac arrhythmia and prosthetic tricuspid valve was also replaced with synthetic tissue valve for severe type of primary tricuspid regurgitation (See Fig. 41.28)*

- Vascular access and continuity
- Prepectoral versus submuscular pocket (Fig. 41.17)
- Handedness of the patient and left-side versus right-side implantation
- Presence of structural heart disease, intracardiac shunts, and obstruction to the right heart chambers
- Relevant medical, surgical, and anesthesia history
- Allergies
- Risks of the procedure including pacemaker-specific risks
- Finite battery longevity, lead failure, and likely potential for reoperation
- Implantation of pacemaker in children (Figs 41.5A and 41.5B)
- A sterile environment is absolutely essential for implantation. Proper facilities include an operating room, a cardiac catheterization laboratory, or an electrophysiology laboratory. The implantation procedure may be performed with either general or local anesthesia, depending on the patient's age and the planned route of implantation.
- For the transvenous approach, one can perform either a cephalic vein cutdown or percutaneous subclavian (or axillary) vein puncture to access the venous system. Position a wire in the right heart with pacing leads positioned in the right atrium or ventricle. Testing is performed using cables to a pacing system analyzer, which can ascertain adequate sensing of intrinsic waves, capture thresholds, and lead impedances.
- The generator is then connected to the leads, and a pacemaker pocket is fashioned either prepectorally or subpectorally, usually with blunt dissection, cauterization, or both. The generator is placed in the pocket, and the incision is closed in multiple layers.
- Leaving a generous amount of slack in the lead to allow uncurling may reduce the risk of lead fracture or dislodgment with linear growth (see the image below). Studies have been performed to estimate the amount of

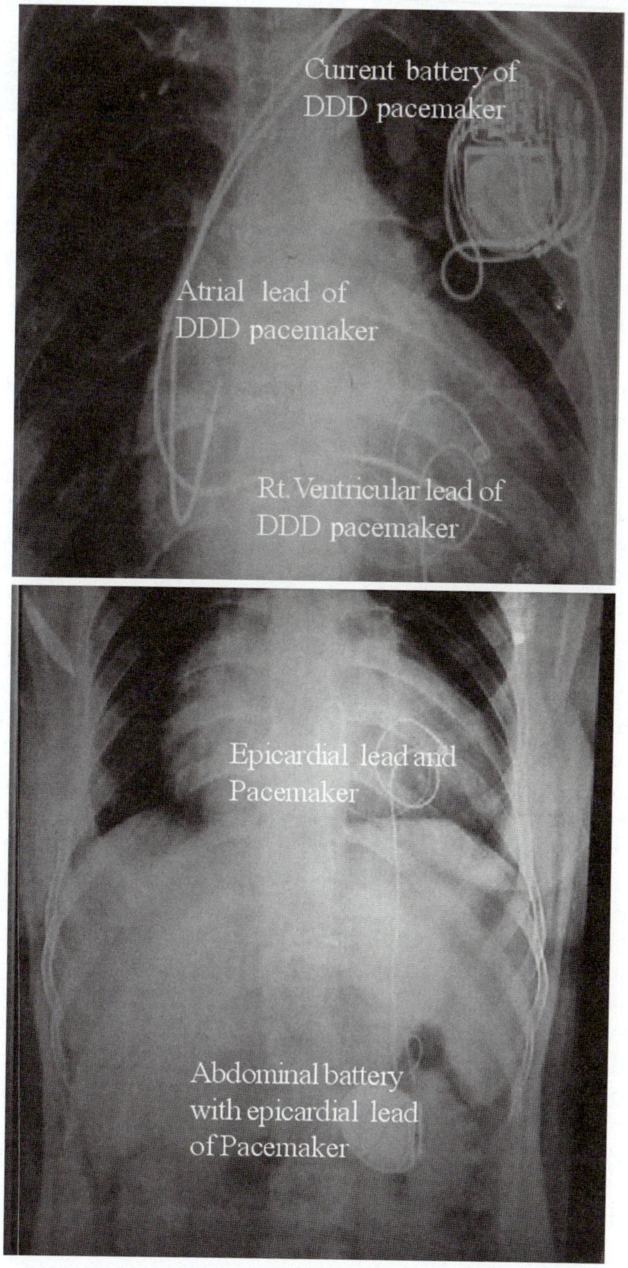

Fig. 41.28: *Redosurgery at the age of 20 yrs (Upper) X-ray chest shows implantation of DDD pacemaker with battery on the left subclavicular region. (Bottom) X-ray chest shows epicardial pacemaker with battery placed in the abdominal region while she was at very young age of only 6 years*

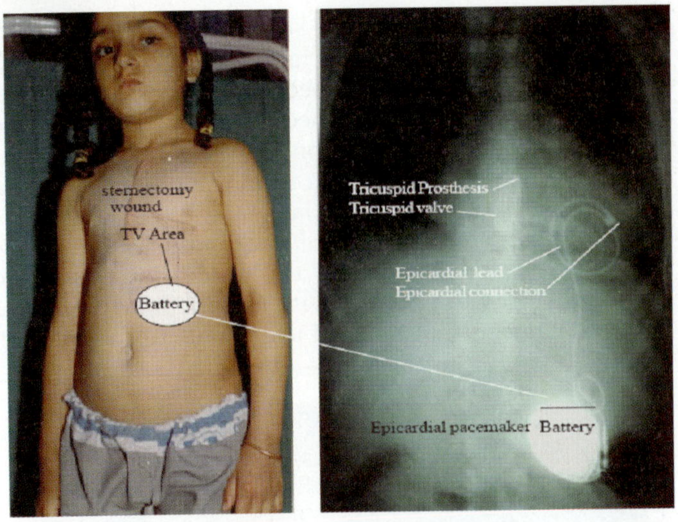

Fig. 41.29: *Epicardial pacemaker was inserted in the heart in a 6-years old child with primary tricuspid regurgitation when during fixing the prosthetic tricuspid valve she developed complete heart block and life was saved by selectively implanting the pacer. (left) Right panel shows the X-ray of chest visualising tricupid prosthesis and abdomen where epicardial lead has been shown connected with the battery placed into the abdominal region*

intracardiac lead redundancy necessary to allow for anticipated growth.

- **The epicardial approach** is typically performed via a subcostal or subxiphoid incision, a thoracotomy, or a sternotomy. The pacing leads are attached to epicardial surfaces and then tested for capture, sensing, and lead impedances. As with the transvenous approach, a pocket is created, typically in the subrectus region of the abdomen (or in the pectoral region), with subcutaneous tunneling of the leads from epicardial sites to the pocket.
- As a rule, most patients remain hospitalized for 12–48 hours after the operation, depending on age, complexity, and route of access.
- Aside from several weeks' restriction from heavy lifting, extreme stretching of the accessed shoulder (for transvenous implants), and vigorous activities, patients may resume normal activities of daily living after the procedure. These restrictions are particularly important after passive lead implantation to avoid dislodgment. The incision must be kept clean and dry and typically heals within 7–10 days.
- Antibiotic prophylaxis after the first 24 hours has not been demonstrated to reduce the risk of pacemaker system or pocket infection. Patients are instructed to immediately report any symptoms of possible infection.
- For patients with newly implanted CRT devices, clinicians may choose to optimize the system (specifically the pacemaker timings) with the help of echocardiography.
- **Complications of pacemaker implantation**
- Complications involve immune response to artificial materials and response of the body to the pacemaker system.
- **Pacemaker generators** are typically very reliable and have a low failure rate. The lithium iodide battery has a

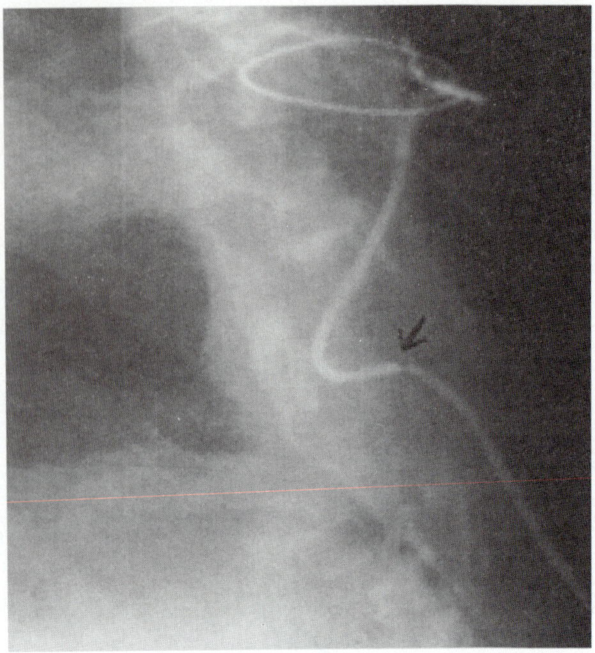

Fig. 41.30: *Fracture of epicardial lead (arrow)*

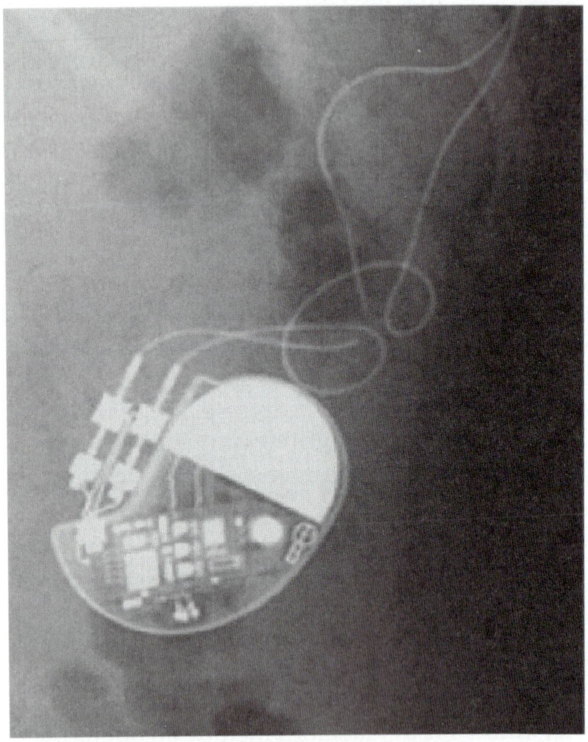

Fig. 41.31: *Abdominal flat plate film of a patient with an atrial lead fracture several years after the Fontan procedure. This lead fracture is at the most common site, immediately below the left costal margin, which is a site of repetitive flexion. The patient was relatively asymptomatic, as pacing in the VVI mode occurred by default in the absence of atrial sensing*

limited longevity of 5–15 years. Battery depletion is not a complication but a normal occurrence.

- **Pacing leads are more prone to failure,** particularly in children. Leads may fail at the conductor wires or in the

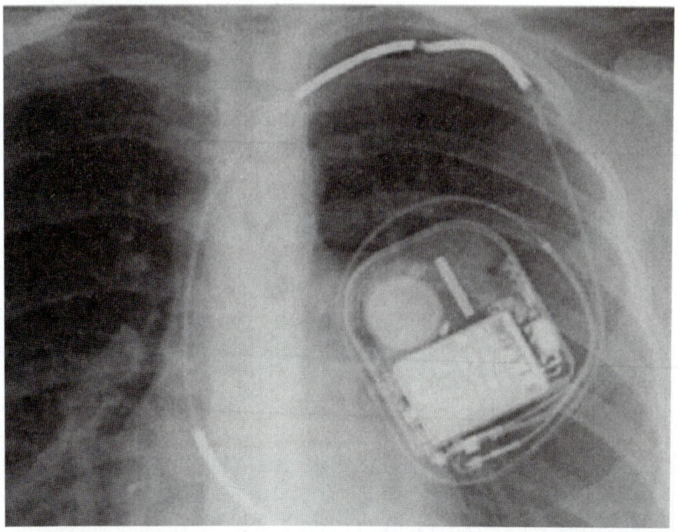

Fig. 41.32: *Implantable cardioverter-defibrillator (ICD) lead fracture in a 12-year-old child with long QT syndrome. The ICD lead initially had been implanted with a redundant loop in the right atrium and the proximal coil at the superior vena cava—innominate vein junction. However, 6 months later, the loop had uncoiled, and the proximal coil had migrated from the superior vena cava to the entry point of the left subclavian vein. Of note, lead testing of threshold and impedance (at the distal electrodes) did not identify a defect in either conductance or insulation. This lead was removed and replaced with a single coil lead at the right ventricular apex. This finding emphasizes the need for periodic radiographic examination of all pacemaker and ICD lead systems in growing children*

insulation material (polyurethane or silicone). Lead failure typically results in inappropriate sensing or capture (i.e. underpacing or overpacing) (Figs 41.30 and 41.31).

- **Infection** of the pacemaker system is a serious complication and almost always necessitates complete system removal, intravenous antibiotics, and system replacement at a remote site. However, in selected cases, pacemaker system infection can occasionally be effectively treated with a prolonged course of antibiotics, without system removal.
- **Twiddler syndrome** is an interesting finding caused by repetitive and often unintentional twisting of the generator in the pacemaker pocket, causing lead dislodgment or fracture and pacemaker failure. It is most commonly observed in patients with behavioral issues.
- **Significant vascular access** challenges can also relate to congenital heart diseases and surgical corrections.
- Finally, chronic right ventricular pacing over long periods (e.g. decades) has been shown in a small group of patients to lead to decreased cardiac function.

A pacemaker is an electronic device, approximately the size of a pocket watch, that senses intrinsic heart rhythms and provides electrical stimulation when indicated. Cardiac pacing can be either temporary or permanent.

Permanent pacing is most commonly accomplished through transvenous placement of leads to the endocardium (i.e. right atrium or ventricle) or epicardium (i.e. to the left

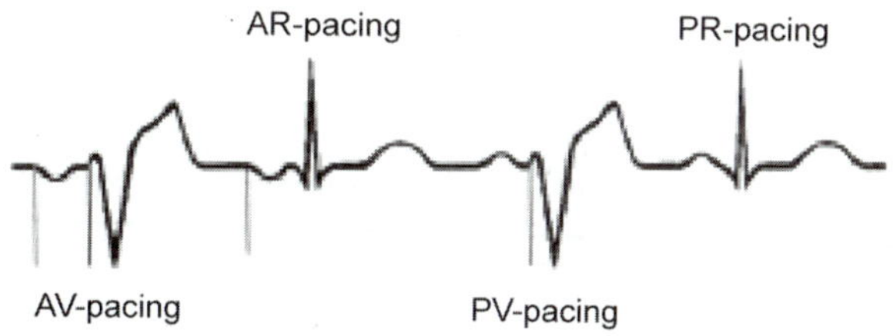

Fig. 41.33: *ECG morphology in different modes of pacing*

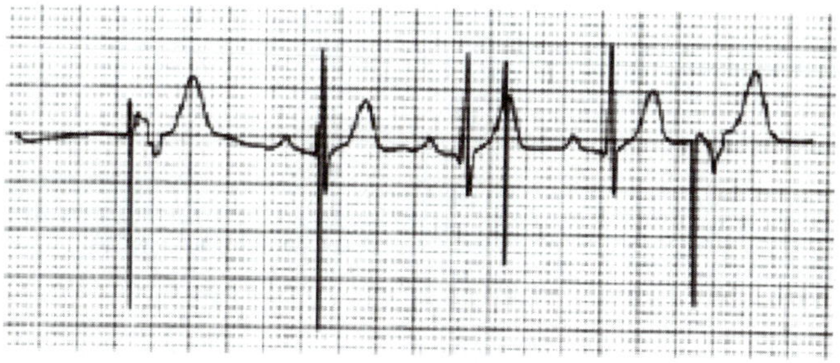

Fig. 41.34: *Loss of ventricular sensing. The first and the fifth complexes are ventricular paced beats. The second to fourth complexes are the patient's intrinsic rhythm, which have not been sensed, hence the inappropriately timed pacing spike*

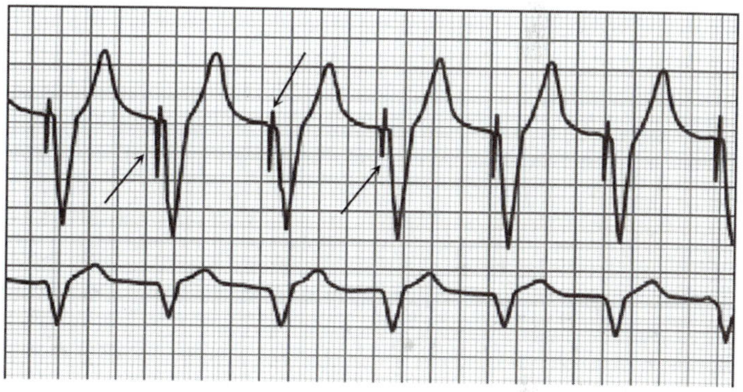

Fig. 41.35: *Artificially induces electronic stimulus that paces the patient's rhythm causing a blip or spike on the ECG waveform*

ventricular surface via the coronary sinus), which are subsequently connected to a pacing generator placed subcutaneously in the infraclavicular region.

Pacemaker Malfunction Detection by Routine EKG

With a demand pacemaker there may be a loss of either sensing or capturing.

Sensing Malfunction

Undersensing (Fig. 41.44)

When it has lost its ability to sense it functions as a fixed-rate asynchronous pacemaker.

Sometimes exercise will increase the native heart rate and expose a failure to sense.

May not always be due to pulse generator malfunction. It may be due to scar tissue, inadequate myocardial or

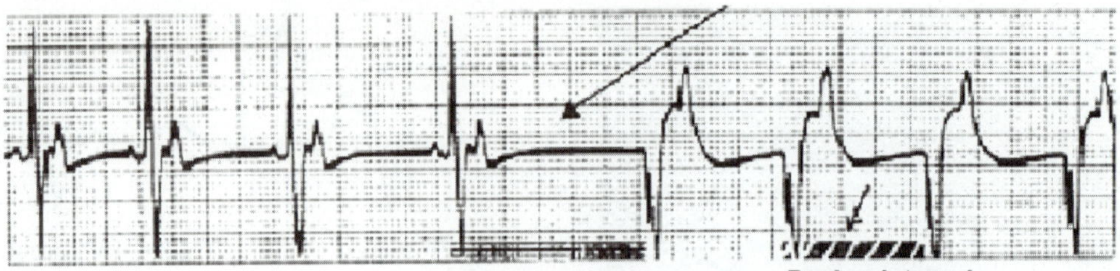

Fig. 41.36: *Graph showing method of calculation of hysteresis and pacing intervals in hysteresis programming In the evaluation of pacemaker function (arrows)*

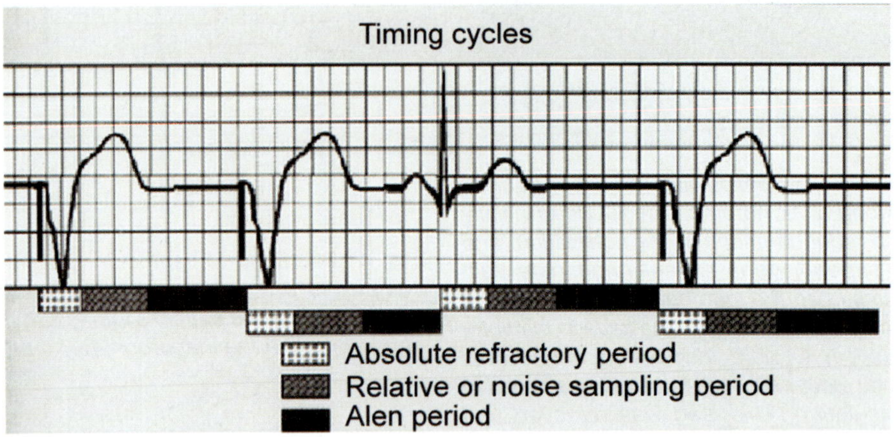

Fig. 41.37: *Showing timing cycles in relation to absolute refractory, relative and alert periods*

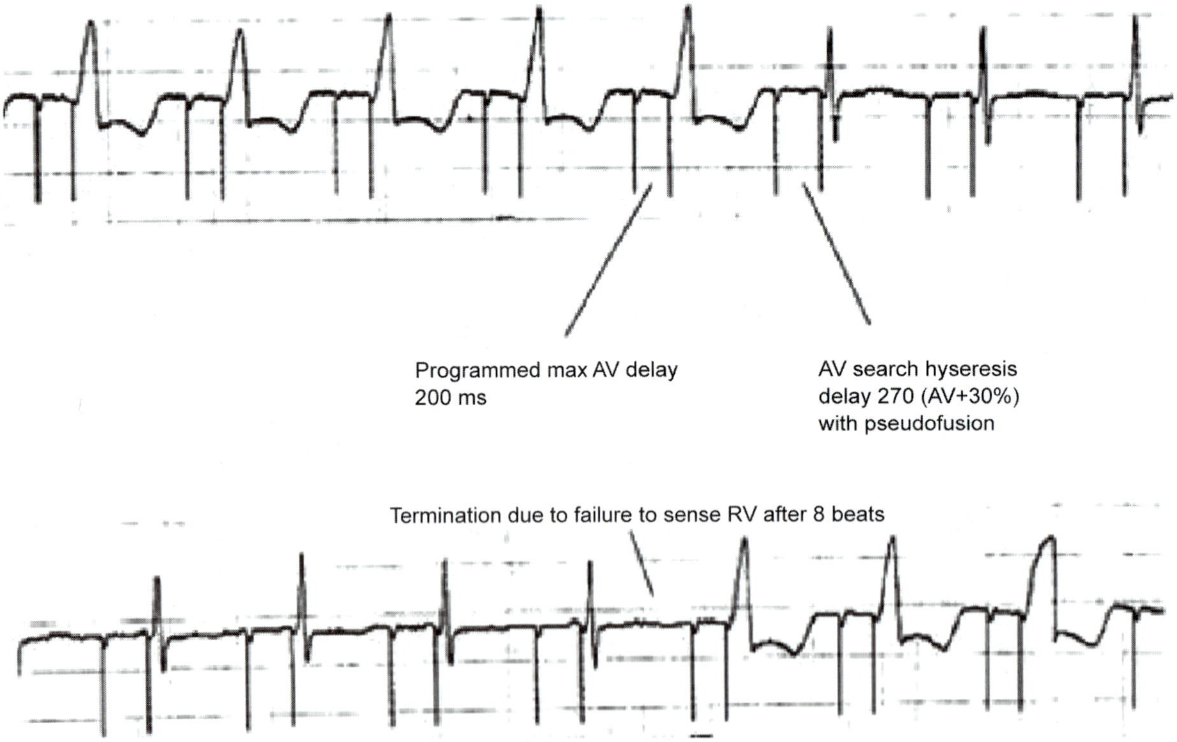

Fig. 41.38: *An example of AV search hysteresis on telemetry is shown. The dual chamber pacemaker (Guidant Insignia I Plus; DDDR 70-130; base-rate AV delay 200 ms) is pacing at the lower rate limit at the longest of the dynamic AV delay. The AV delay increases to almost 270 ms, 30% longer than the programmed AV delay for 8 cycles. In this case, the algorithm failed to sense the intrinsic narrow QRS as it fell just beyond the extended AV delay, resulting in pseudofusion. Due to the lack of sensing during the 8 cycles, the AV delay then shortens to the programmed delay of 200 ms and reattempts the algorithm in 32 cycles*

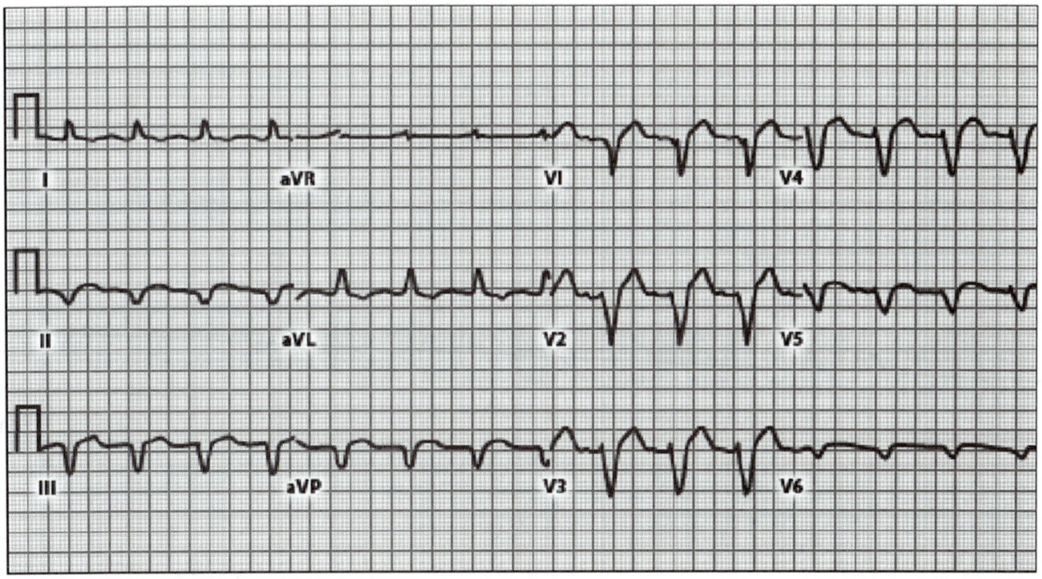

Fig. 41.39: *ECG showing small pacemaker spikes before the QRS complexes in many of the leads. In addition, the QRS complex in V1 exhibits ventricular ectopic morphology. There is a slur or notch at the beginning of the S wave*

Atrial pacemaker (single chamber)

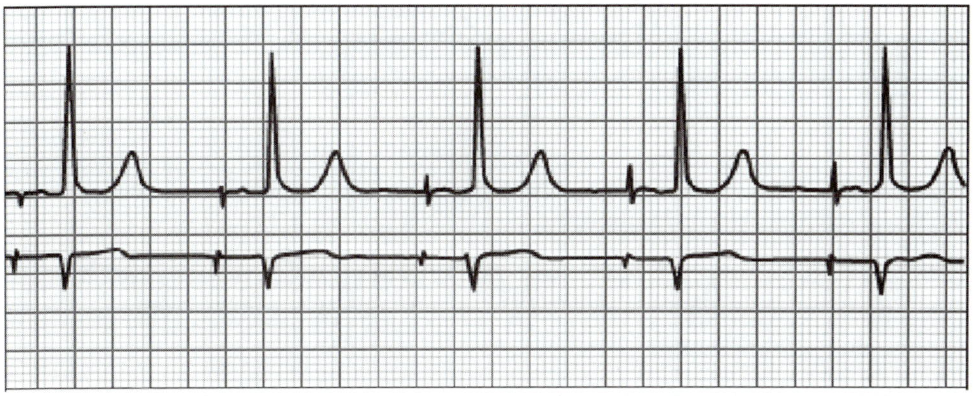

Fig. 41.40: *ECG showing one spike producing an abnormal P wave (atrial capture) followed by a normal QRS*

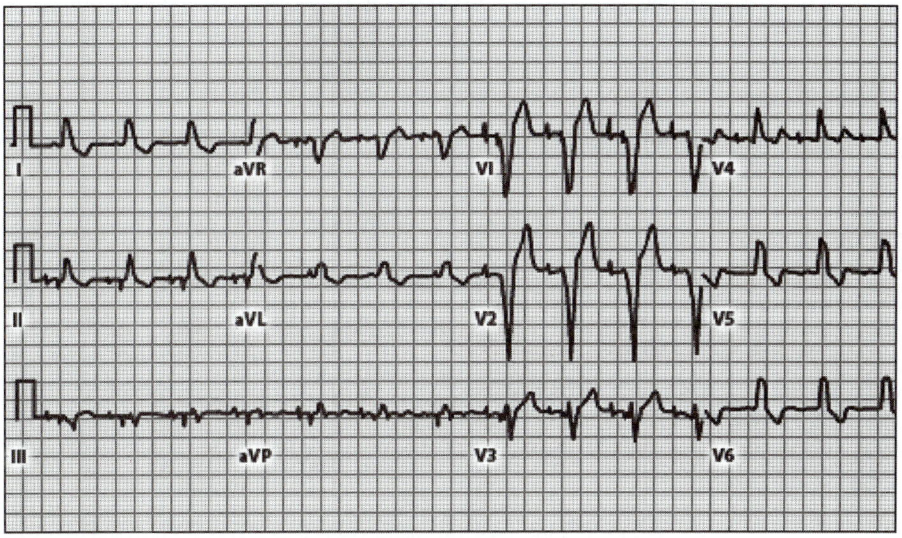

Fig. 41.41: *AV sequential pacing. In this ECG, both atria and ventricles are being paced. Two pacemaker spikes are seen before each QRS, one for the atria and one for the ventricles (best seen in lead V1)*

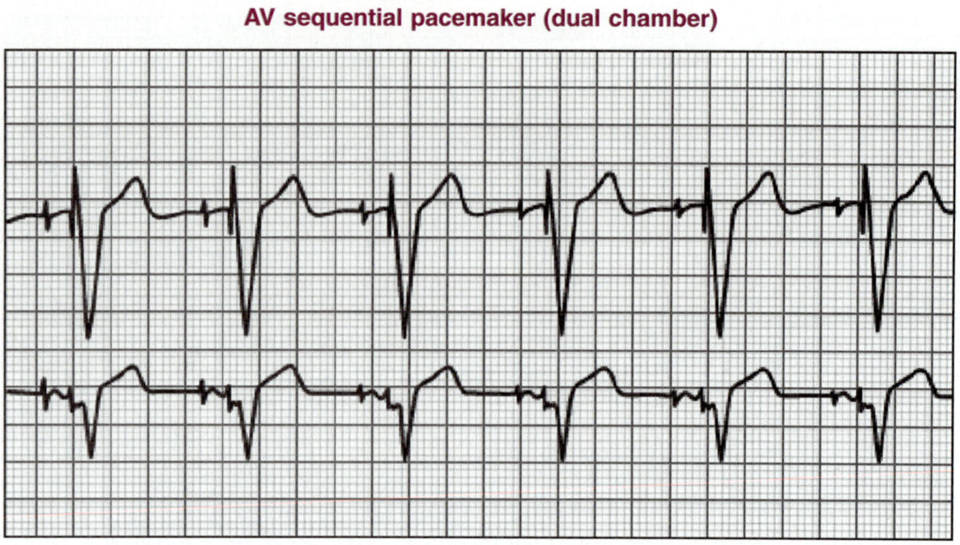

Fig. 41.42: *ECG showing one spike followed by an abnormal P (atrial capture) followed by a second spike productng a wide QRS (ventricle capture)*

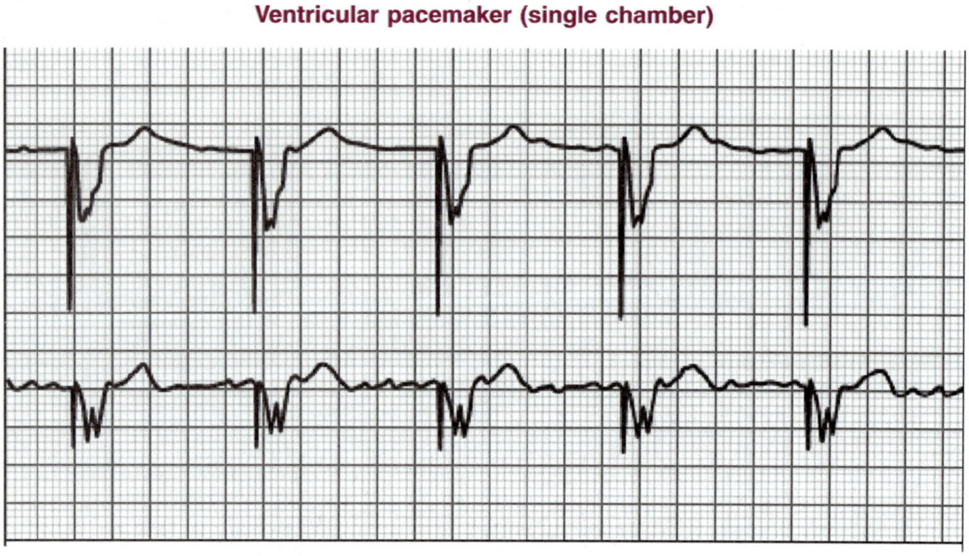

Fig. 41.43: *ECG showing one spike producing a wide QRS (ventricular capture)*

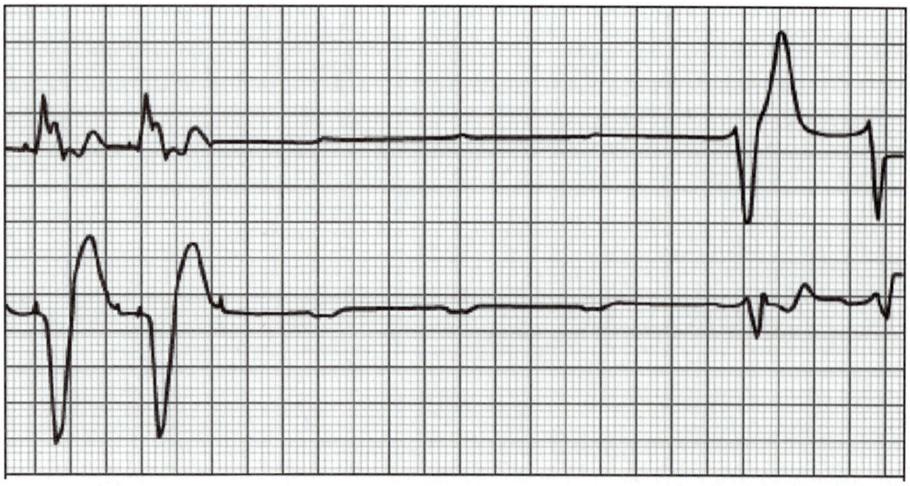

Fig. 41.44: *ECG showing the pacemaker does not recognize normal beats and generates an unnecessary pacemaker spike*

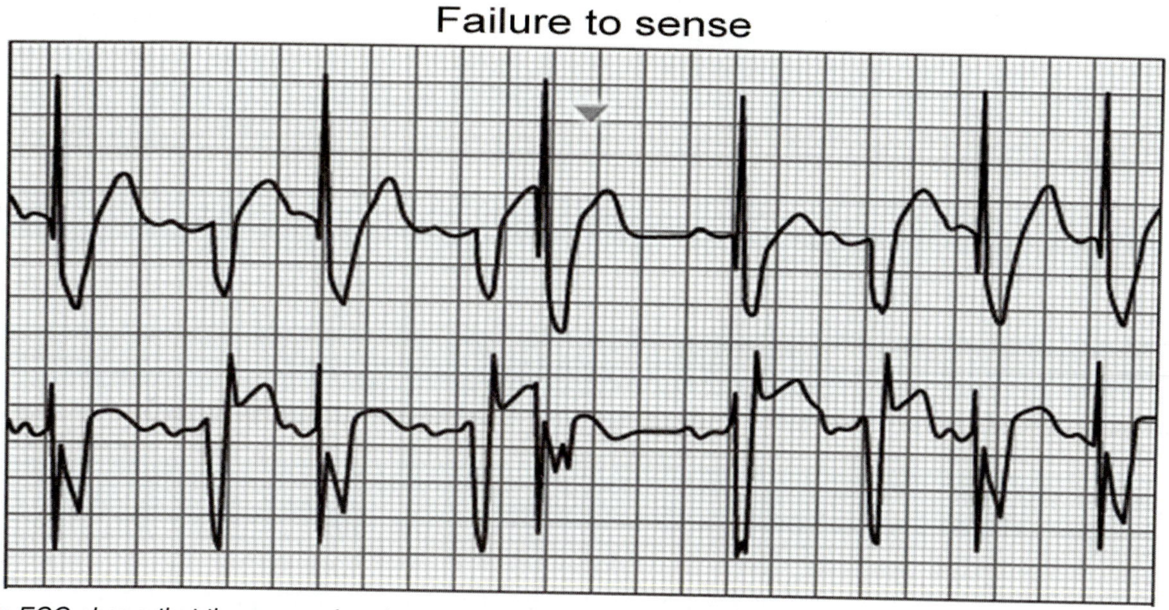

Fig. 41.45: *ECG shows that the pacemaker does not recognize normal beats and generates an unnecessary pacemaker spike*

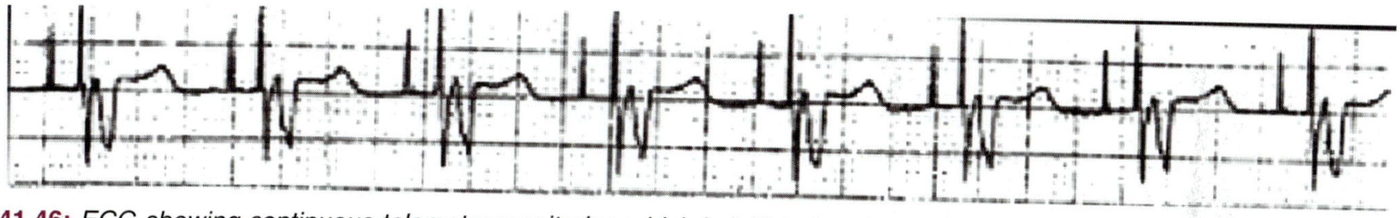

Fig. 41.46: *ECG showing continuous telemetry monitoring which is initiated and strip is obtained. It does not show any evidence of pacing problems; each beat is initiated by a P wave, and each beat is followed by a paced QRS complex. Every QRS is paced, and the rate falls within the rate setting programmed for the pacemaker*

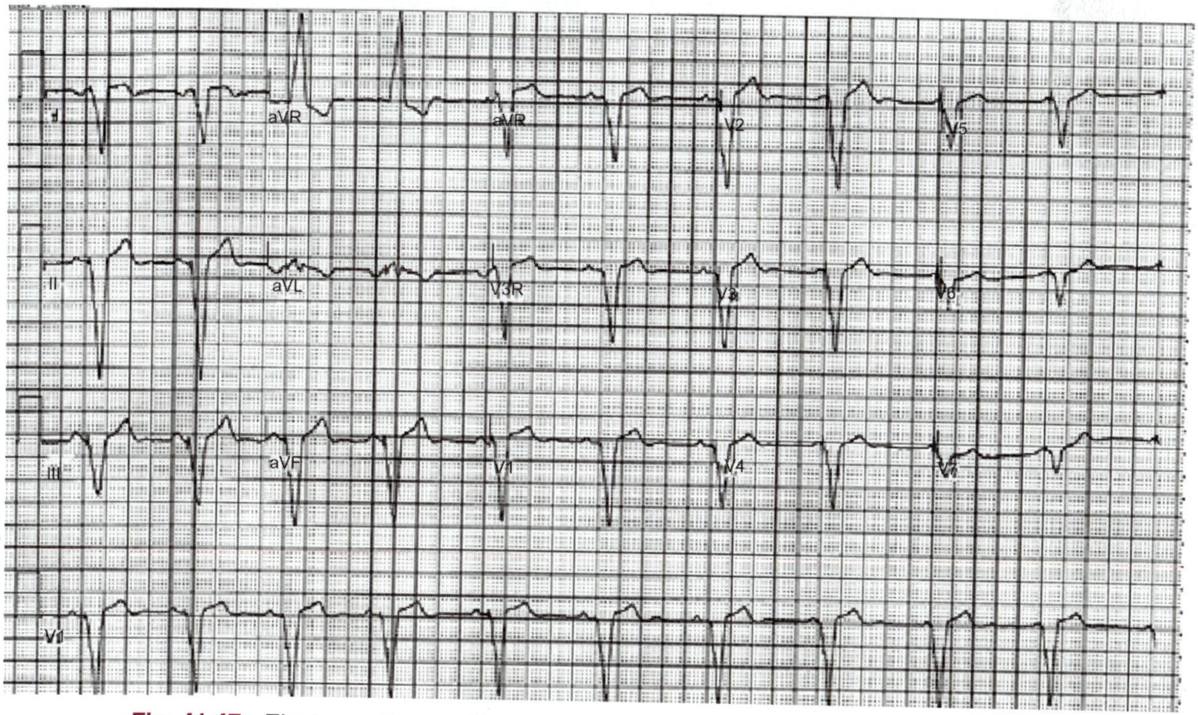

Fig. 41.47: *Electrocardiogram illustrates atrial-synchronous, ventricular paced rhythm*

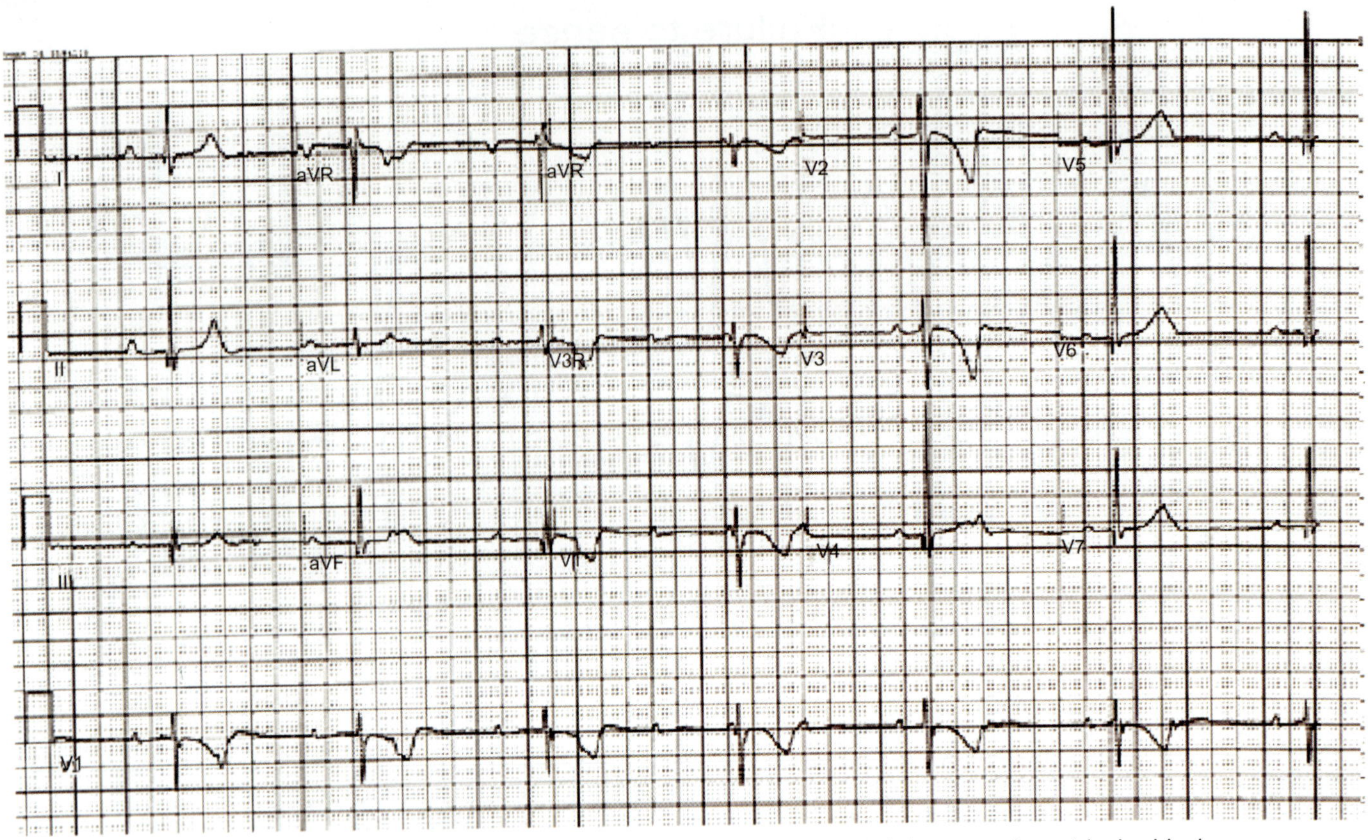

Fig. 41.48: *Electrocardiogram illustrates 2-year-old child with third-degree atrioventricular block*

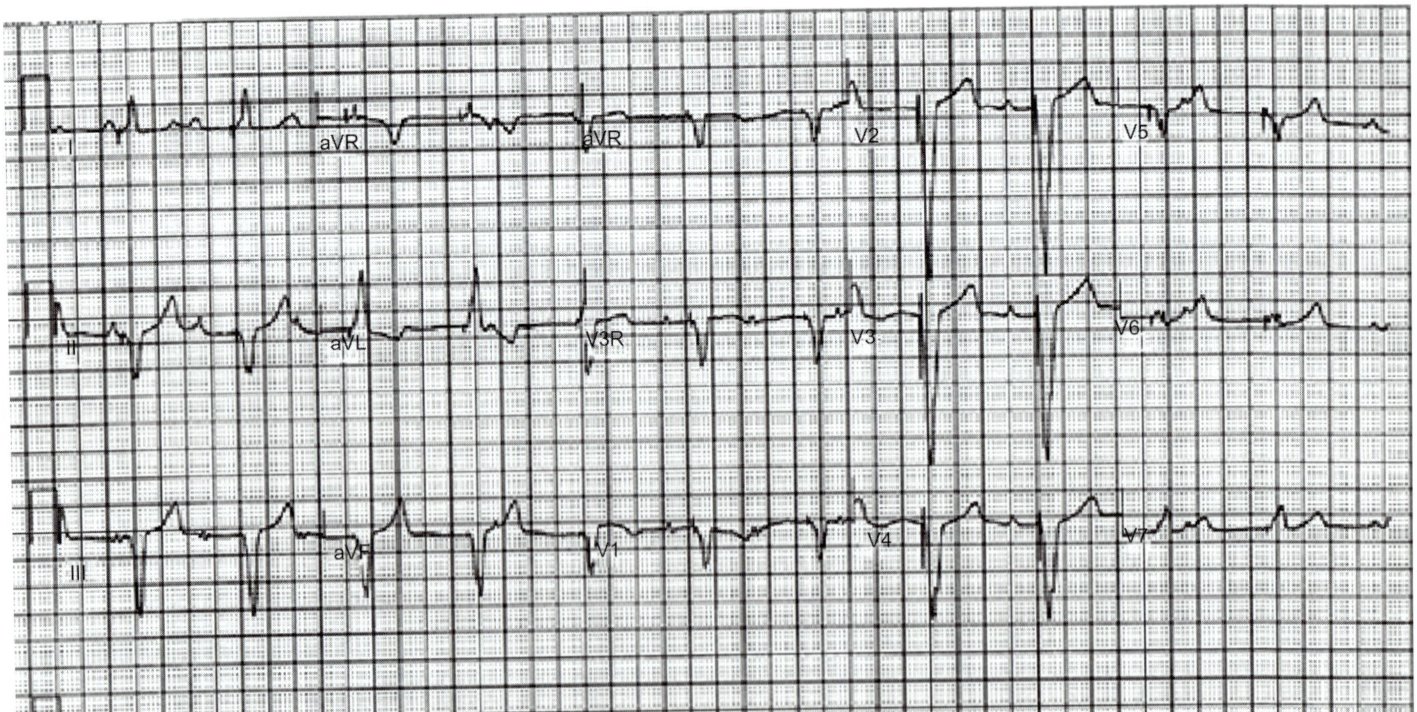

Fig. 41.49: *Electrocardiogram reveals sinus atrial mechanism with complete atrioventricular block and ventricular paced rhythm*

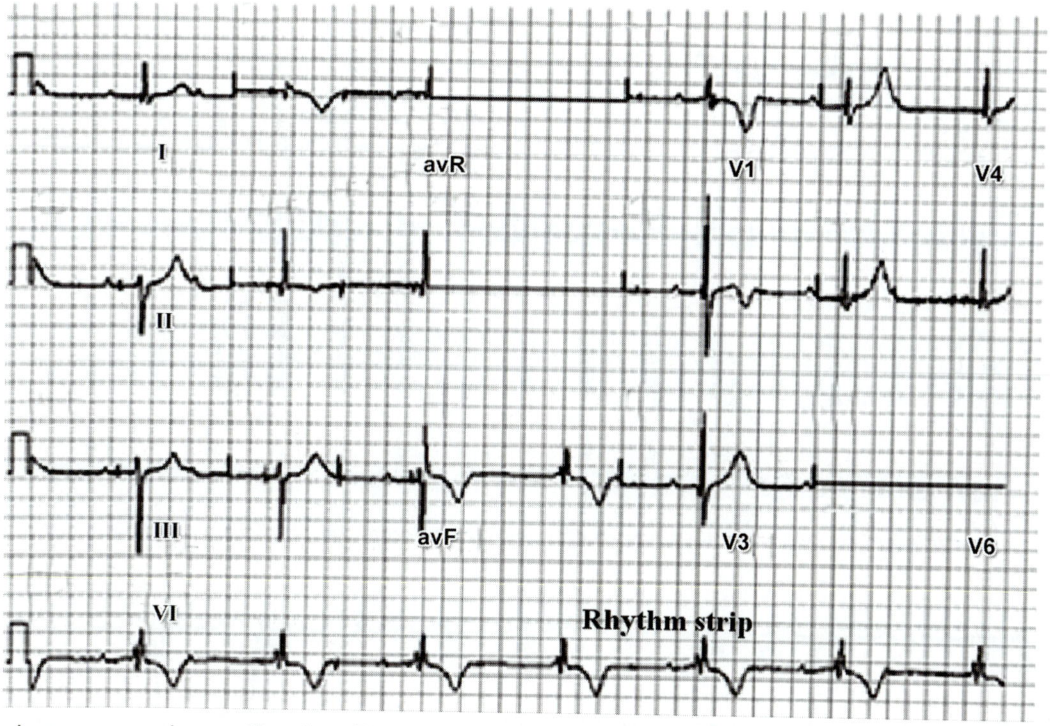

Fig. 41.50: *ECG shows pacemaker malfunction. Electrocardiogram obtained in an 8-year-old child with congenital complete heart block treated with an epicardial ventricular pacemaker at 2 months of age. The tracing shows failure to capture the pacemaker spikes. The ventricular escape rate is 41. The patient was subsequently documented to have a break in the pacemaker wire*

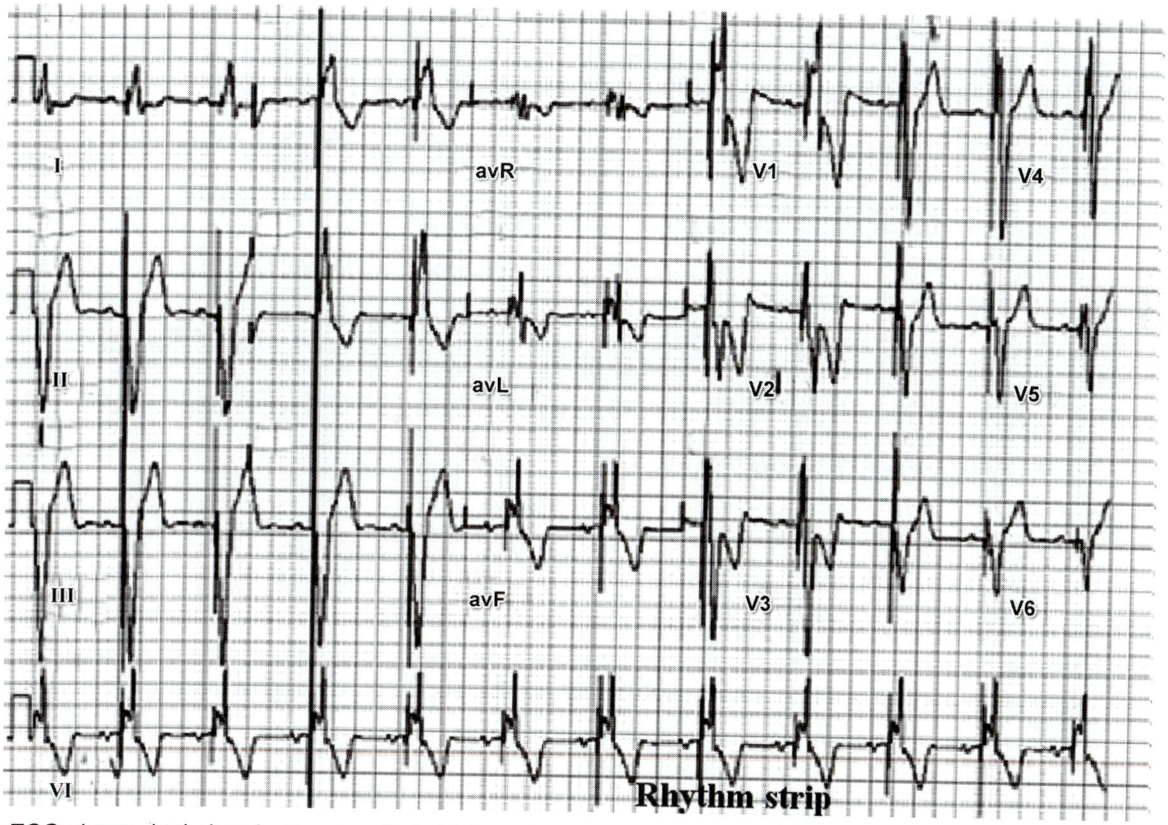

Fig. 41.51: *ECG shows dual chamber pacemaker-atrial sense, ventricular pace. Electrocardiogram obtained in a 10-year-old child with Shone's syndrome, s/p multiple surgical procedures including ventricular septal defect closure complicated by the development of complete heart block. The patient has a transvenous DDD dual chamber pacemaker system. The tracing shows atrial sensing and ventricular pacing (spike before the QRS complex). There is no spike before the P wave*

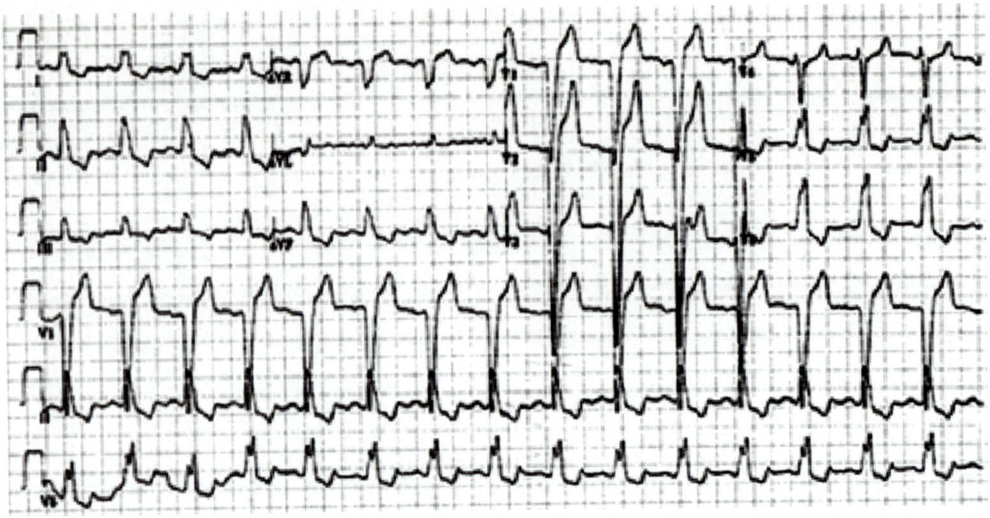

Fig. 41.52A: *Electrocardiogram showing normal sinus rhythm with left bundle-branch block. Note that QRS duration is 152 ms*

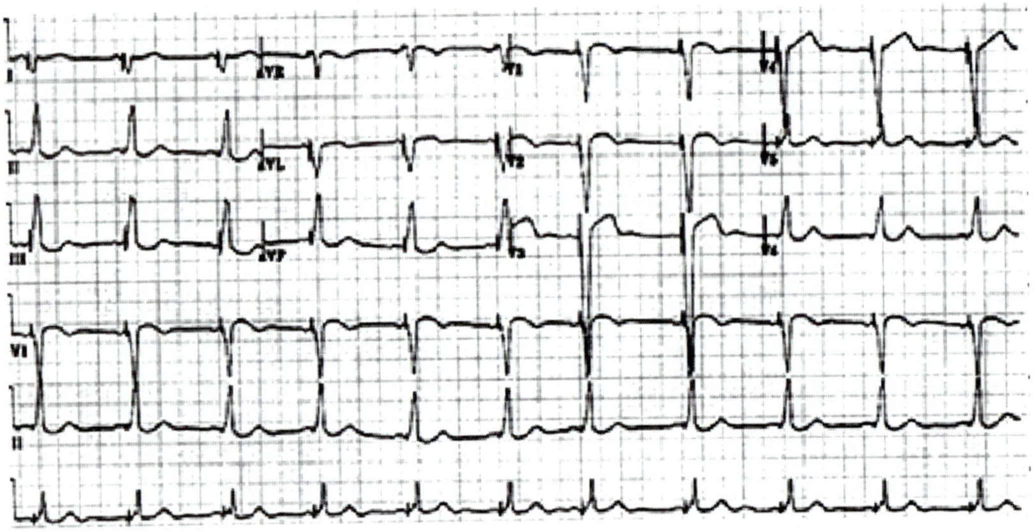

Fig. 41.52B: *Electrocardiogram (ECG) after cardiac resynchronization therapy with defibrillator implantation. Note that QRS duration (130 ms) is narrowed compare with previous ECG*

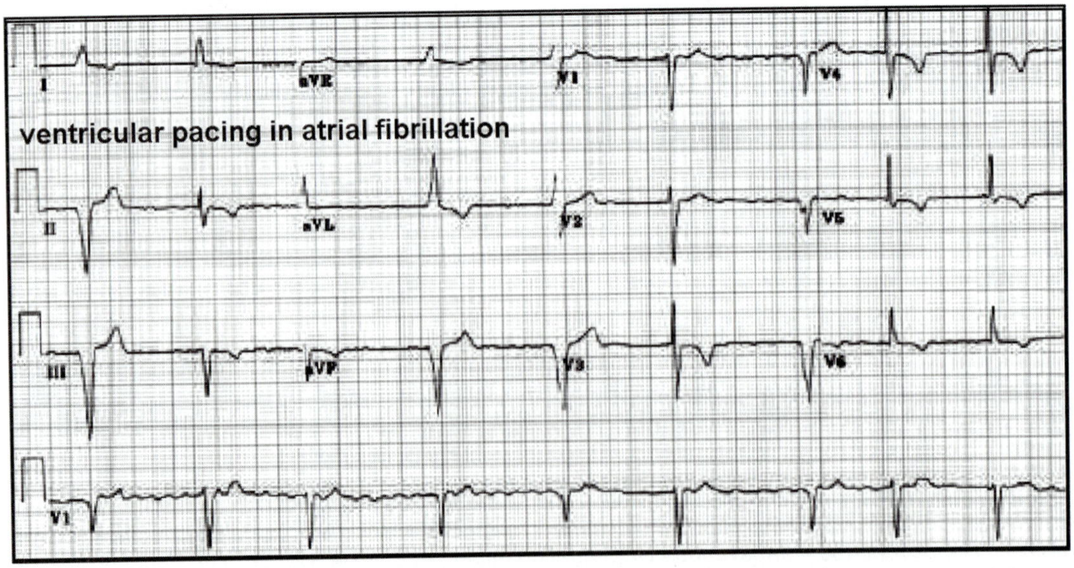

Fig. 41.53: *ECG showing DDD pacemaker which is programmed to the VVI mode with no atrial sensing*

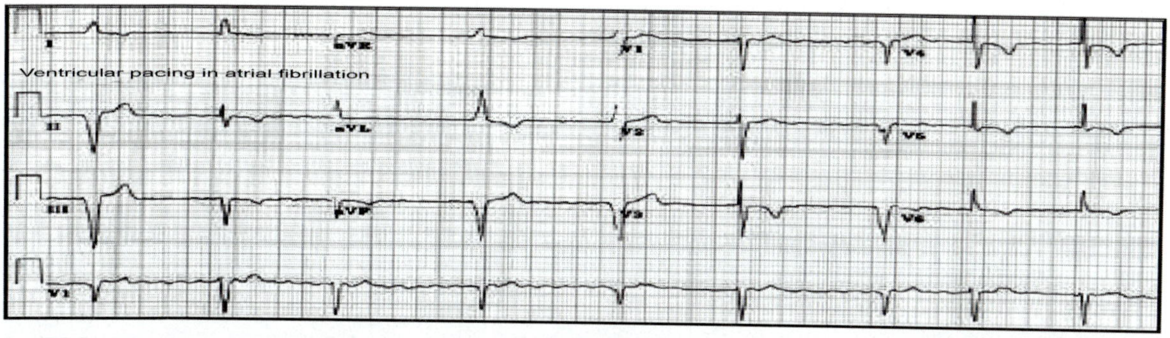

Fig. 41.54: *ECG showing loss of atrial pacing because of oversensing preceding T wave. Ventricular pacing set at a low rate*

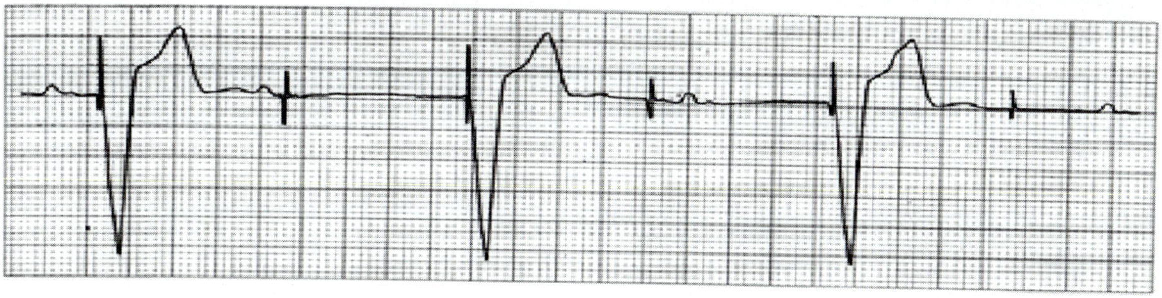

Fig. 41.55: *ECG showing VVI pacemaker with intermittent failure to capture. Every second pacemaker beat captures. The rest of the time, pacemaker spikes are seen but not associated with capture*

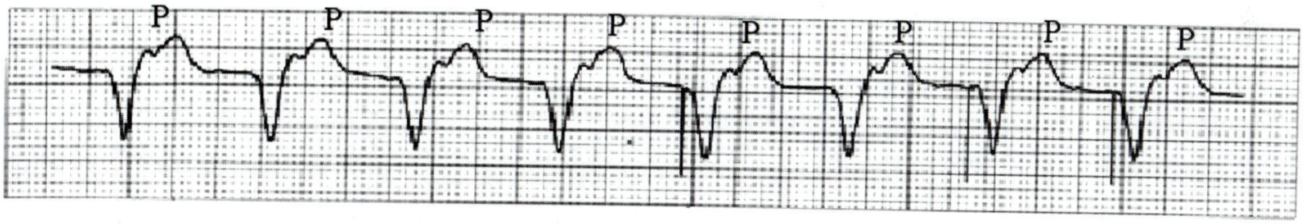

Fig. 41.56: *ECG shows pacemaker syndrome: retrograde P waves are evident*

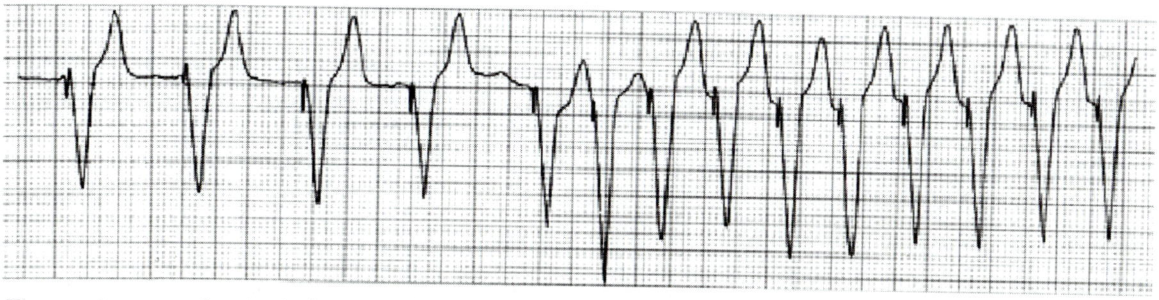

Fig. 41.57: *The most commonly reported pacemaker mediated tachycardia which is "endless loop tachycardia" and occurs in patients with dual chamber pacemakers*

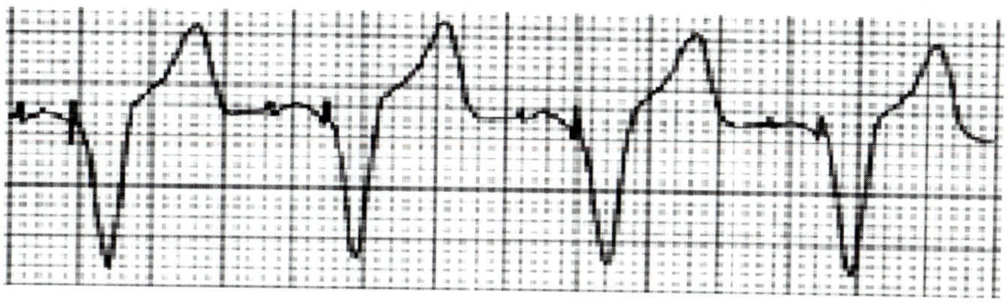

Fig. 41.58: *Typical ECG tracing produced by DDD pacer*

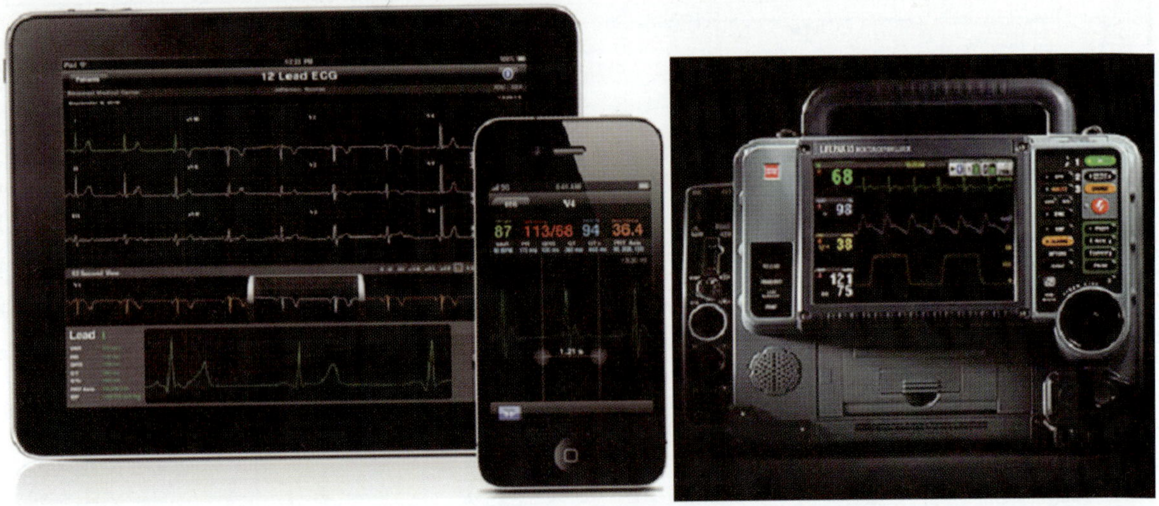

Fig. 41.59: *Showing defibrillator/monitors to transmit cardiac data to physician allowing doctors to provide immediate assistance to EMS crews handling complicated patients.The integrated solution empowers clinicians to communicate immediately with the EMS crew to provide the clinical assistance needed to properly care for the patient while en route, direct them to the appropriate care facility and prepare for the arrival of the patient accordingly. With the integrated solution, these capabilities are available to clinicians anytime, anywhere on their smartphone or tablet device*

endocardial contact, poor orientation of a bipolar electrode, or inappropriate programming of amplifier sensitivity in a newly placed pacemaker (Fig. 41.34).

Late sensing loss may be due to acute MI, growth of insulating tissue around the electrode, or myocardial perforation with the electrode migrating to a poor signal area. Broken leads or wire insulation are now uncommon causes as the quality of the wires has improved.

Oversensing (Fig. 41.54)

Uncommon to oversense physiologic intracardiac voltage. Occasionally very tall P waves or t waves may be mistaken for QRS complexes.

Myopectoral inhibition may occur when the pectoralis muscle inhibits the pacer.

Radar, TV, radiotransmitters and electrocautery may inhibit the pacemaker.

Microwave and weapon detector equipment no longer cause a problem in modern equipment.

DC countershock and XRT may damage pulse generators.

Pacing Malfunction (Figs 41.45, 41,50, 41.55, 41.57, 41.60)

It can only be recognized of the patient's rate is slow enough to permit pacer spikes.

If the patient's rate is too rapid, then a magnet can be applied to convert the pacer to a fixed-rate mode.

A change in the spike to spike interval of more than 10 m/sec may indicate early battery depletion. Such a change in the rate is difficult to determine from the routine EKG, and a change of 1 to 2 beats per minute may be due to a change in the paper speed.

Generally, a slowing of more than 4 beats per minute is an indication of battery depletion.

Some pacemakers now allow the detection of a reduction in the pulse width or pulse amplitude of the spike.

Myocardial perforation may be responsible for pacing failure.

RV endocardial leads may perforate either the interventricular septum or more commonly the free wall of the RV, ECG would then change from a LBBB to a RBBB.

DDD (Atrioventricular Universal Pacemakers)

The most common dual chamber device implanted today. Senses both the atrium and the ventricle.

It may be inhibited or triggered to pace the atrium or ventricle or both according to the programmed rate limits and AV interval.

The rate is often programmed to be 60 beats/min, the upper rate is 150 beats/min and the AV interval is 200 msec. If the rate is faster than 60 beats/min (if a P wave appears is less than 800 msec from the preceding QRS) and the AV conduction time is less than 200 msec (the programmed intervals) then no pacing stimulus is seen.

There are built in features to prevent pacemaker-induced arrhythmias so that no ventricular stimulus is delivered in less than 400 msec from the preceding QRS interval. This is the same as an upper rate limit of 150 beats/min.

If a PVC is sensed less than 800 msec after the preceding QRS, both atrial and ventricular pacing is inhibited. The atrial and the ventricular response is reset by the PVC. Application of a magnet results in DOO pacing (asynchronous pacing in both the atria and the ventricles).

DDD Pacemaker Related Tachycardias (Fig. 41.57)

Wenckebach pacemaker response

It occurs when the atrial rate is faster than the programmed DDD pacemaker upper rate limit. In this situation, the atrial pacemaker is inhibited. The ventricle does not necessarily fire at the preset AV interval, it will wait until the upper rate limit (the upper VV interval) is reached.

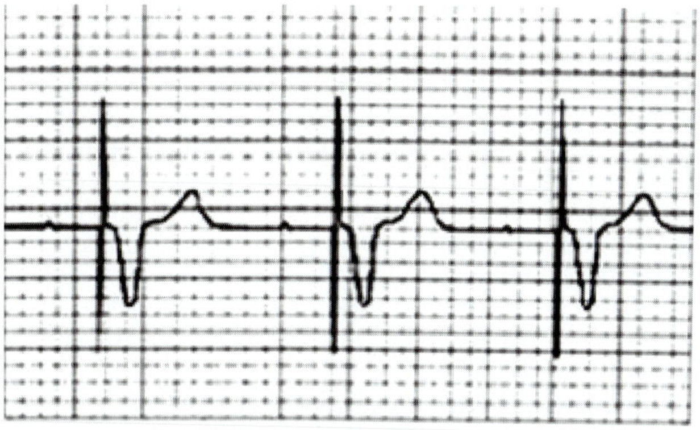

Fig. 41.60: *Graph showing retrograde P wave in a patient with pacemaker syndrome in whom permnent pacemake was implanted a few years back*

Therefore there is prolongation of the P to V interval, the degree to which is proportional to the preceding VP interval.

Pacemaker circus movement tachycardia

Also called endless loop tachycardia. The cause is retrograde P waves. Such a retrograde P wave is sensed by the atrial component of the pacemaker, which in turn triggers the delivery of a ventricular stimulus, resulting in a paced QRS complex with retrograde atrial capture.

The rate is limited by the upper rate of the pacemaker.

Lengthening the atrial refractory period of the pacemaker may decrease the incidence of, but does not eliminate this potential complication.

Hysteresis, Fallback Response, Cross Talk

With regard to atrial hysteresis, there are two AV intervals. The AV interval of a sensed atrial event is shorter than that which follows an atrial stimulus. The reason for this is to make the AV intervals the same in actuality to maintain the hemodynamic benefit of the atrial contraction.

The reason that the interval following a sensed atrial beat is that there is a time delay between when the pacemaker senses the atrial activity. When atrial activity is sensed, atrial contraction is likely to have begun.

Rate hysteresis is present when the pacemaker escape interval is longer than the pacing interval. This allows the patient's own sinus rhythm, which is more physiological, to be maintained at a lower rate than the pacing rate (Figs 41.36–41.38).

In patients who cannot tolerate a sustained upper rate, the fallback response mechanism returns the ventricular response rate to more tolerable levels. AV synchrony may not be maintained during the fallback synchrony may not be maintained during the fallback response.

Cross talk refers to the phenomenon whereby the ventricular channel senses the atrial impulse and is thereby inhibited. To overcome this, the ventricular sensing circuit is turned off shortly after the atrial stimulus.

Pacemaker Syndrome (Figs 41.56, 14.60)

Refers to dizziness, near syncope, and fatigue even though there is no pacemaker malfunction. This syndrome is the

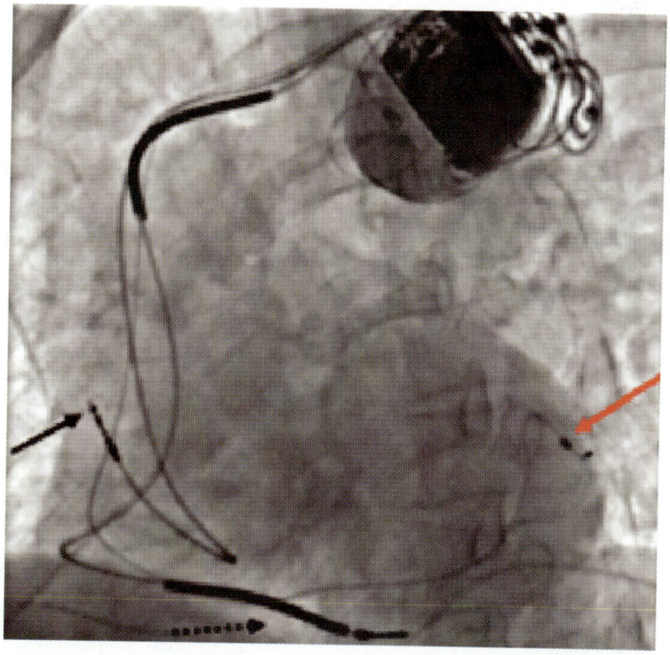

Fig. 41.61: *Three leads can be seen in this example of a cardiac resynchronization device: a right atrial lead (solid black arrow), a right ventricular lead (dashed black arrow), and a coronary sinus lead (red arrow). The coronary sinus lead wraps around the outside of the left ventricle, enabling pacing of the left ventricle. Note that the right ventricular lead in this case has 2 thickened aspects that represent conduction coils and that the generator is larger than typical pacemaker generators, demonstrating that this device is both a pacemaker and a cardioverter-defibrillator, capable of delivering electrical shocks for dangerously fast abnormal ventricular rhythms*

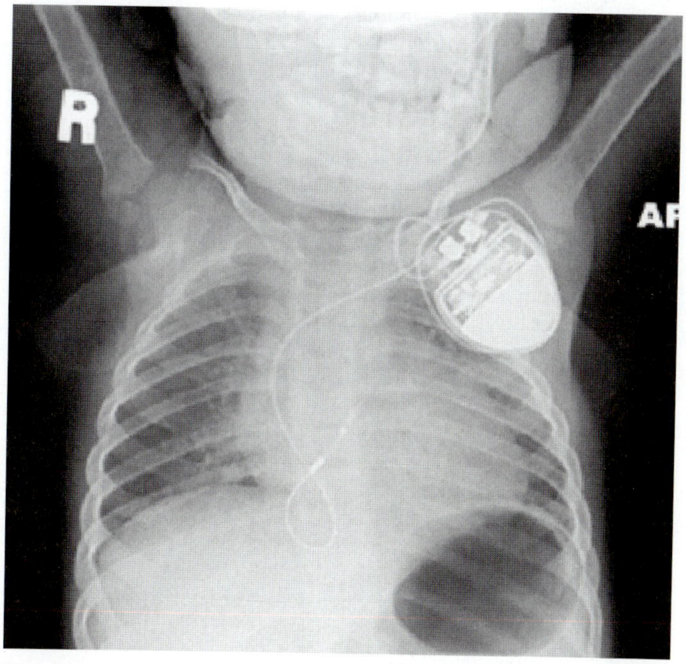

Fig. 41.62: *Epicardial dual chamber implantable cardioverter defibrillator in neonate with congenital complete atrioventricular block. Two bipolar suture-on leads (1 on atrium and 1 on ventricle) are attached to DDDR pacemaker*

result of unfavorable hemodynamic consequences of AV asynchrony.

The incidence is higher in patients with VA conduction.

Implantable Pacemakers

Permanent pacemakers are implantable devices that sense intrinsic cardiac electric potentials and, if these are too infrequent or absent, transmit electrical impulses to the heart to stimulate myocardial contraction. A specialized type of pacemaker therapy, cardiac resynchronization therapy (CRT) with biventricular pacing, with or without an implantable cardioverter-defibrillator (ICD), has been used as adjunctive therapy for patients with heart failure.

Implantable Defibrillators (Figs 41.32, 41.59, 41.61, 41.62)

The implantable cardioverter-defibrillator (ICD) is first-line treatment and prophylaxis for patients at risk for ventricular tachycardia (VT) or ventricular fibrillation (VF). Current devices offer tiered therapy with programmable antitachycardia pacing schemes, as well as low-energy and high-energy shocks in multiple tachycardia zones.

Dual-chamber, rate-responsive bradycardia pacing is now available in all ICDs, and sophisticated discrimination algorithms minimize shocks for atrial fibrillation, sinus tachycardia, and other nonlife-threatening supraventricular tachyarrhythmias. Diagnostic functions including stored electrograms, allow for verification of shock appropriateness.

BIBLIOGRAPHY

1. Bink-Boelkens MTHE: Cardiac pacing in infants and children. Neth J Cardiol 1992;5:199–202.
2. Smyth CN: Medical Electronics. London 1960. (Elmquist R, Senning A: An implantable pacemaker for the heart. Second International Conference, Paris 1959).
3. Bevilacqua L, Hordof A: Cardiac pacing in children. Curr Opin Cardiol 1998;13:48–55.
4. Mann C, Antretter H, Hammerer I: Pacemaker therapy in a pediatric patient with hypertrophic obstructive cardiomyopathy and rapid intrinsic atrioventricular conduction. Pediatr Cardiol 1999; 20: 229–231.
5. Rishi F, Hulse E, Auld DO, et al.: Effects of dual-chamber pacing for pediatric patients with hypertrophic obstructive cardiomyopathy. JACC 1997;29:734–740.
6. Dorostkar PC, Eldar M, Belhassen B, et al: Long-term-follow-up of patients with Long-QT syndrom treated with b-blockers and continuous pacing. Circulation 1999;100:2431–2436.
7. Dreifus LS, Fisch C, Griffin JC, et al. Giudelines for implantation of cardiac pacemakers and antiarrhythmia devices. A report of the American College of Cardiology/American Heart Association Task Force on Assessment of Diagnostic and Therapeutic Cardiovascular Procedures. J Am Coll Cardiol 1991;18:1–13.
8. Friedman RA, Collins E, Fenrich AL: Pacing in Children: Indications and techniques. Progress Ped Cardiol 1995;4:21–29.
9. Antretter H, Fritz M, Bonatti J, et al. : Left superior vena cava pacemaker implantation in a neonate. Eur J C P E 1995;5: 324.
10. Rao V, Williams WG, Hamilton RH, et al.: Trends in pediatric cardiac pacing. Can J Cardiol 1995;11:993–999.
11. Molina JE, Dunnigan AC, Crosson JE: Implantation of transvenous pacemakers in infants and small children. Ann Thorac Surg 1995;59:689–694.
12. Campbell RM, Raviele AA, Hulse EJ, et al: Experience with a low profile bipolar, active fixation pacing lead in pediatric patients. PACE 1999;22:1152–1157.
13. Rosenthal E, Bostock J: Use of an atrial loop to extend the duration of endocardial pacing in a neonate. PACE 1997;20: 2489–2491.
14. Gheissari A, Hordof AJ, Spotnitz HM: Transvenous pacemaker in children: relation of lead length to anticipated growth. Ann Thorac Surg 1991;52:118–121.
15. Gasparini M, Mantica M, Galimbert P, et al.: Inferior vena cava loop of the implantable cardioverter defibrillator endocardial lead: A possible solution to the growth problem in pediatric implantation. PACE 2000;23:2108–2112.
16. Antretter H, Hangler H, Colvin J, et al.: Inferior vena caval loop of an endocardial pacing lead did not solve the growth problem in a child. PACE 2001;24:1706–1708.
17. Alexander ME, Cecchin F, Walsh EP, Triedman JK, Bevilacqua LM, Berul CI. Implications of implantable cardioverter defibrillator therapy in congenital heart disease and pediatrics. J Cardiovasc Electrophysiol. Jan 2004; 15(1):72–6.
18. O'Sullivan JJ, Jameson S, Gold RG, Wren C: Endocardial pacemaker in children: lead length and allowance for growth. PACE 1993;16:267–271.
19. Rao G: Letter to the editor. PACE 1998;21:1496.
20. Friedmann RA, Moak JP, Garson A Jr: Active fixation of endocardial pacing leads: the preferred method of pediatric pacing. PACE 1991;14:1213–1216.
21. Antretter H, Klaus A, Hintringer F, et al.: Ist die Schrittmacher-elektroden-Extraktion ein riskanter Eingriff. Retrospektive Analyse von 37 Patienten. Herzschrittmacher 1999;19:168–175.
22. Ceviz N, Celiker A, Kucukosmanoglu O, et al: Comparison of mid-term clinical experience with steroid-eluting active and passive fixation ventricular electrodes in children. PACE 2000;23:1245–1249.
23. Siwik ES, Van Hare GF: Severe cyanosis in a newborn after transvenous pacing wire placement. Pediatr Cardiol 1998; 19:168–170.
24. Chandra Bose Reddy S, Saxena A, Iyer KS: In advertent but asymptomatic right atrial perforation with epicardial pacing in a neonate: a rare complication of temporary transvenous cardiac pacing. PACE 1997;20:368–369.
25. Ing FF, Mullins CE, Grifka RG, et al.: Stent dilation of superior vena cava and innominate vein obstructions permits transvenous pacing lead implantation. PACE 1998;21:1517–1530.
26. Antretter H: Schrittmacher - Implantationstechniken: Standardzugange und Alternativen. Herzschrittmacher 1999; 19:231–240.
27. Gilette PC, Shannon C, Blair H: Transvenous pacing in pediatric patients. Am Heart J 1983;105:843–847.
28. Esperer HD, Singer H, Riede FT, et al.: Permanent epicardial and transvenous single- and dual-chamber cardiac pacing in children. Thorac Cardiovasc Surg 1993;41:21–27.
29. Goldman Cutler N, Karpawich PP, Cavitt D, et al.: Steroid eluting epicardial pacing electrodes: six year experience of pacing thresholds in a growing pediatric population. PACE 1997;20:2943–2948.
30. Beafort-Krol GC, Mulder H, Nagelkerke D, et al.: Comparison of longevity, pacing and sensing characteristics of steroid eluting epicardial versus conventional endocardial

pacing leads in children. J Thorac Cardiovasc Surg 1999;117:523–528.
31. Bauersfeld U, Nowak B, Molinari L, et al.: Low-energy epicardial pacing in children: the benefit of autocapture. Ann Thorac Surg: 1999;68:1380–1383.
32. Sachweh JS, Vazquez-Jimenez JF, Schondube FA, et al.: Twenty years experience with pediatric pacing: epicardial and transvenous stimulation. Eur J Cardio Thorac Surg 2000; 17:455–461.
33. Byrd CL, Schwartz SJ. Transatrial implantation of transvenous pacing leads as an alternative to implantation of epicardial leads. PACE 1990:13:1856–1859.
34. Hoyer MH, Beermann LB, Ettedgui JA, et al.: Transatrial lead placement for endocardial pacing in children. Ann Thorac Surg 1994;58:97–101.
35. Antretter H, Klaus A: Letter to the editor. PACE 1999;22: 1274.
36. Gillette PC, Edgerton J, Kratz J, Zeigler V: The subpectoral pocket: the preferred implant site for pediatric pacemakers. PACE 1991;14:1089–1092.
37. Andersen C, Horder K, Kristensen L, Mickley H: Psychosocial aspects and mental health in children after permanent pacemaker implantation. Acta Cardiol 1994;49:405–418.
38. Abrams S, Peart I: Twiddler's syndrome in children: an unusual cause of pacemaker failure. Br Heart J 1995;73:190–192.
39. Rosenheck S, Elami A, Amikam S, et al.: Single pass lead VDD pacing in children and adolescents. PACE 1997;20:1961–1966.
40. Rosenthal E, Bostock J, Qureshi SH, et al.: Single pass VDD pacing in children and adolsecents. PACE 1997;20:1975–1982.
41. Rosenthal E, Bostock J: VDD pacing in children with congenital complete heart block: advantages of a single pass lead. PACE 1997;20:2102–2106.
42. Harcombe AA, Newell SA, Ludman PF, et al.: Late complications following permanent pacemaker implantation or elective unit replacement. Heart 1998;80:240–244.
43. Parsonnet V, Bernstein AD, Neglia D: Nonthoracotomy ICD implantation: lessons to be learned from permanent pacemaker implantation. PACE 1995;18:1597–1600.
44. Tantengco MVT, Thomas RL, Karpawich PP: Left ventricular dysfunction after long-term right ventricular apical pacing in the young. JACC 2001;37:2093–2100.
45. Karpawich PP, Rabah R, Haas JE: Altered cardiac histology following apical right ventricular pacing in patients with congenital atrioventricular block. PACE 1999;22:1372–1377.
46. DeMaso DR, Lauretti A, Spieth L, et al. Psychosocial factors and quality of life in children and adolescents with implantable cardioverter–defibrillators. 2004;93:582–7.
47. Silka MJ, Bar-Cohen Y. Pacemakers and implantable cardioverter-defibrillators in pediatric patients. Heart Rhythm. Nov 2006;3(11):1360–6.
48. Smerup M, Hjertholm T, Johnsen SP, et al. Pacemaker implantation after congenital heart surgery: risk and prognosis in a population-based follow-up study. Eur J Cardiothorac Surg. Jul 2005;28(1):61–8.
49. Chintala K, Forbes TJ, Karpawich PP. Effectiveness of transvenous pacemaker leads placed through intravascular stents in patients with congenital heart disease. Am J Cardiol. Feb 1 2005;95(3):424–7.
50. Cecchin F, Frangini PA, Brown DW, et al. Cardiac Resynchronization Therapy (and Multisite Pacing) in Pediatrics and Congenital Heart Disease: Five Years Experience in a Single Institution. J Cardiovasc Electrophysiol. Sep 3 2008.
51. Dubin AM, Janousek J, Rhee E, et al. Resynchronization therapy in pediatric and congenital heart disease patients: an international multicenter study. J Am Coll Cardiol. Dec 20 2005;46(12):2277–83.
52. Epstein AE, DiMarco JP, Ellenbogen KA, et al. ACC/AHA/HRS 2008 Guidelines for Device-Based Therapy of Cardiac Rhythm Abnormalities: a report of the American College of Cardiology/American Heart Association Task Force on Practice Guidelines (Writing Committee to Revise the ACC/AHA/NASPE 2002 Guideline Update for Implantation of Cardiac Pacemakers and Antiarrhythmia Devices) developed in collaboration with the American Association for Thoracic Surgery and Society of Thoracic Surgeons. J Am Coll Cardiol. May 27 2008;51(21):e1–62.
53. Gregoratos G, Abrams J, Epstein AE, et al. ACC/AHA/NASPE 2002 guideline update for implantation of cardiac pacemakersand antiarrhythmia devices: summary article: a report of the American College of Cardiology/American Heart Association Task Force on Practice Guidelines (ACC/AHA/NASPE Committee t. Circulation. Oct 15 2002;106(16):2145–61.
54. Gregoratos G, Cheitlin MD, Conill A. ACC/AHA guidelines for implantation of cardiac pacemakers and antiarrhythmia devices: a report of the American College of Cardiology/American Heart Association Task Force on Practice Guidelines (Committee on Pacemaker Implantation). J Am Coll Cardiol. Apr 1998;31(5):1175–209.
55. Horenstein MS, Karpawich PP. Pacemaker syndrome in the young: do children need dual chamber as the initial pacing mode?. Pacing Clin Electrophysiol. May 2004;27(5):600–5.
56. Mathony U, Schmidt H, Groger C, et al. Optimal maximum tracking rate of dual-chamber pacemakers required by children and young adults for a maximal cardiorespiratory performance. Pacing Clin Electrophysiol. May 2005;28(5): 378–83.
57. Ovsyshcher IE, Hayes DL, Furman S. Dual-chamber pacing is superior to ventricular pacing: fact or controversy? [comment]. Circulation. Jun 16 1998;97(23):2368–70.
58. Silvetti MS, Drago F. Upgrade of single chamber pacemakers with transvenous leads to dual chamber pacemakers in pediatric and young adult patients. Pacing Clin Electrophysiol. Aug 2004;27(8):1094–8.
59. Fishberger SB, Wernovsky G, Gentles TL, et al. Long-term outcome in patients with pacemakers following the Fontan operation. Am J Cardiol. Apr 15 1996;77(10):887–9.
60. Noiseux N, Khairy P, Fournier A, Vobecky SJ. Thirty years of experience with epicardial pacing in children. Cardiol Young. Oct 2004;14(5):512–9.
61. Stojanov P, Vranes M, Velimirovic D, et al. Prevalence of venous obstruction in permanent endovenous pacing in newborns and infants: follow-up study. Pacing Clin Electrophysiol. May 2005;28(5):361–5.
62. Fortescue EB, Berul CI, Cecchin F, Walsh EP, Triedman JK, Alexander ME. Comparison of modern steroid-eluting epicardial and thin transvenous pacemaker leads in pediatric and congenital heart disease patients. J Interv Card Electrophysiol. Oct 2005;14(1):27–36.
63. Fortescue EB, Berul CI, Cecchin F, Walsh EP, Triedman JK, Alexander ME. Patient, procedural, and hardware factors associated with pacemaker lead failures in pediatrics and congenital heart disease. Heart Rhythm. Jul 2004;1(2):150–9.
64. Berul CI, Hill SL, Estes NA 3rd. A teenager with pacemaker twiddler syndrome. J Pediatr. Sep 1997;131(3):496–7.
65. Molina JE, Dunnigan AC, Crosson JE. Implantation of transvenous pacemakers in infants and small children. Ann Thorac Surg. Mar 1995;59(3):689–94.

42 Sudden Infant Death Syndrome (SIDS)

Sudden infant death syndrome (SIDS) is a medical term that describes the sudden death of an infant which remains unexplained after all known and possible causes have been carefully ruled out through autopsy, death scene investigation, and review of the medical history. SIDS is responsible for more deaths than any other cause in childhood for babies 1 month to 1 year of age, claiming 150,000 victims in the United States in this generation alone –7,000 babies each year *-nearly* 1 baby every hour of every day. It strikes families of all races, ethnic and socioeconomic origins without warning; neither parent nor physician can predict that something is going wrong. In fact, most SIDS victims appear healthy prior to death (Fig. 42.1).

Sudden infant death syndrome (SIDS) is a syndrome marked by the symptoms of sudden and unexplained death of an apparently healthy infant aged 1 month to 1 year. The term cot death is often used in the United Kingdom, Australia and New Zealand, while crib death is sometimes used in North America. Typically the infant is found dead after having been put to bed, and exhibits no signs of having suffered.

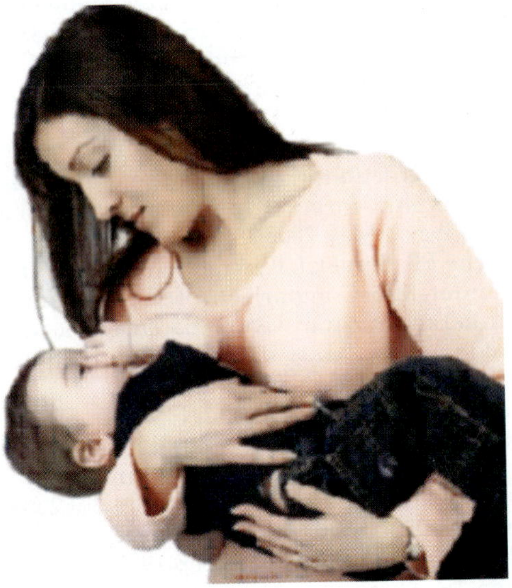

Fig. 42.1: In SIDS history infant apparently looking healthy in mother's arms

SIDS is a diagnosis of exclusion. It can only be applied to an infant whose death is sudden and unexpected, and remains unexplained after the performance of an adequate postmortem investigation (Fig. 42.2).

Etiological Factors

The cause (or causes) of SIDS is still unknown. Despite the dramatic decrease in the incidence of SIDS in the United States in recent years, SIDS remains one of the leading causes of death during infancy beyond the first 30 days after birth. It is generally accepted that SIDS may be a reflection of multiple interacting factors.

- **Infant development:** A leading hypothesis is that SIDS may reflect a delay in the development of nerve cells within the brain that are critical to normal heart and lung function. Research examinations of the brain stems of

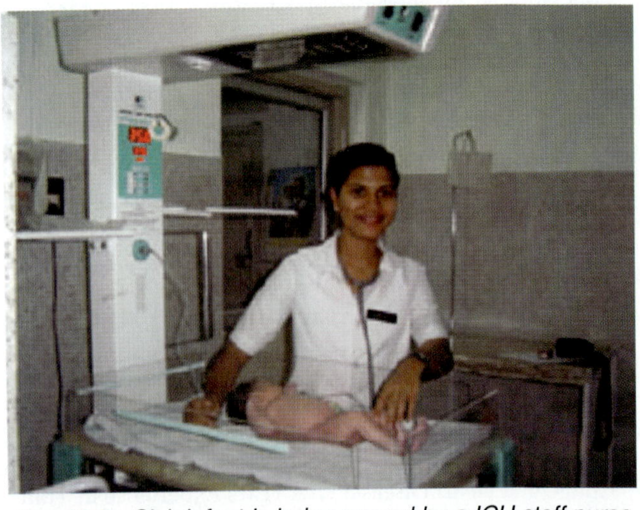

Fig. 42.2: Sick infant is being nursed by a ICU staff nurse

infants who died with a diagnosis of SIDS have revealed a developmental delay in formation and function of several serotonin-binding nerve pathways within the brain (serotonin is an example of a brain chemical known as a neurotransmitter that is important for brain function). These pathways are thought to be crucial to regulating breathing, heart rate, and blood pressure responses.

- The hypothesis is that certain infants, for reasons yet to be determined, may experience abnormal or delayed development of specific, critical areas of their brain. This could negatively affect the function and connectivity to regions regulating arousal.
- Arousal, in this context, refers to an infant's ability to awaken and/or respond to a variety of physiological stimuli. For example, a child sleeping facedown may move his or her face into such a position so that the nose and mouth are completely obstructed. This may alter the levels of oxygen or carbon dioxide in the infant's blood.
- Trigger arousal responses, prompting the infant to move his or her head to the side to alleviate this obstruction.
- In addition, other normally protective responses to stressful stimuli may be defective in infants who are vulnerable to SIDS. One such reflex is the laryngeal chemoreflex. This reflex results in changes in breathing, heart rate, and blood pressure when portions of the airway are stimulated by fluids like saliva or regurgitated stomach contents. Having saliva in the airway may activate this reflex, and swallowing may be important to keep the airway clear. When an infant is in the facedown position, the rate of swallowing is decreased. Protective arousal responses to these laryngeal reflexes are also diminished in active sleep in the facedown position.
- *Rebreathing asphyxia:* When a baby is facedown, air movement around the mouth may be impaired. This can cause the baby to re-breathe carbon dioxide that the baby has just exhaled. Soft bedding and gas-trapping objects, such as blankets, comforters, water beds, and soft mattresses, are other types of sleep surfaces that may impair normal air movement around the baby's mouth and nose when positioned facedown.

Table 42.1: *Factors contributing to SIDS*

- Baby sleeping on tummy or on his/her side
- Family history of sudden infant death syndrome
- Low family income, which makes a baby receive less care
- Lack of proper nutrition
- The age of the mother being less than 20, at the time of pregnancy
- The mother receiving little or no prenatal care
- Smoking by the mother during pregnancy
- Consumption of drugs by the mother during pregnancy
- Premature birth of the baby
- Low weight of the baby at the time of the birth
- Baby being exposed to second hand smoking (when someone smokes while they are around the baby)

Hyperthermia (increased temperature): Overdressing, using excessive coverings, or increasing the air temperature may lead to an increased metabolic rate in these infants and eventual loss of breathing control. However, it is unclear whether the increased temperature is an independent factor or if it is just a reflection of the use of more clothing or blankets that may act as objects obstructing the airway.

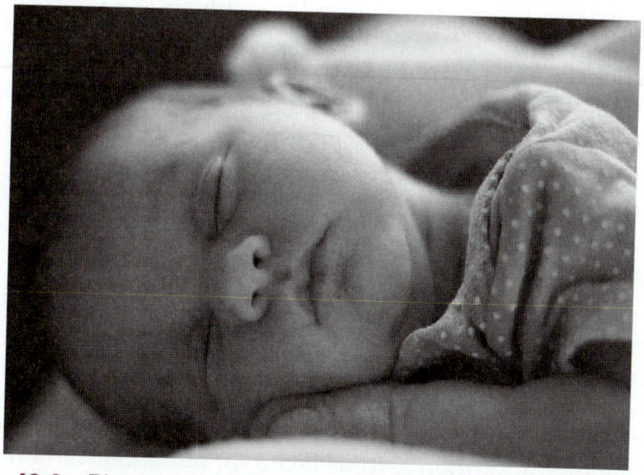

Fig. 42.3: *Photograph showing dead infant under SIDS category*

Clinical Features of SIDS

Sudden infant death syndrome remains an unpredictable, unpreventable, and largely inexplicable tragedy. The baby is seemingly healthy without any sign of distress or significant illness prior to the incident.

- Death occurs rapidly while the infant is sleeping. Typically, it is a silent event. The baby does not cry. The infant usually appears to be well developed, well nourished, and is generally felt to be in good health prior to death. Minor upper respiratory or gastrointestinal symptoms are not uncommon in the last 2 weeks preceding SIDS (Fig. 42.3).

Examination and laboratory tests: SIDS is a diagnosis of exclusion, meaning that other causes of death must be ruled out. The cause of an infant's death can be determined only through a process of collecting information and conducting sometimes-complex forensic tests and procedures. All other recognizable causes of death are investigated prior to making the diagnosis of SIDS. Four major avenues of investigation aid in the determination of a SIDS death.

1. Postmortem laboratory tests
2. Autopsy
3. Death-scene investigation
4. Review of victim and family case history.

Postmortem laboratory tests are done to rule out other causes of death (for example, electrolytes are checked to rule out-dehydration and electrolyte imbalance; cultures are obtained to evaluate whether an infection was present). In SIDS, these laboratory tests are generally not revealing. An autopsy provides clues as to the cause of death. In 15–25% of sudden, unexpected infant deaths, specific abnormalities of the brain or central nervous system, the heart or lungs, or infection may be identified as the cause of death. The autopsy findings in SIDS victims are typically subtle and yield only supportive, rather than conclusive, findings to explain SIDS.

- A thorough investigation of the death scene consists of interviewing the parents, other caregivers, and family members, collecting items from the death scene, and evaluating that information. A detailed scene investigation may reveal a recognizable and possibly preventable cause of death.
- A parent or caregiver may be asked these questions:
- Where was the baby discovered?
- What position was the baby in?
- When was the baby last checked?

Last fed?

- How was the baby sleeping?
- Where there any recent signs of illness?
- Was the infant taking any medication, either prescription or over the counter?

You should let your doctor know about any family or infant medical history. It is important to note that family history would include any previous history of unexplained infant death, sudden cardiac death, or metabolic or genetic disorders, for example. SIDS is responsible for roughly 1 death per 2,000 births in the US. It is responsible for far fewer deaths than congenital disorders and disorders related to short gestation though it is the leading cause of death in healthy babies after 1 month of age.

Undiagnosed conditions: Some conditions that may be undiagnosed and thus result in a diagnosis of SIDS include

1. Medium chain acyl CoA dehydrogenase
2. Deficiency MCAD
3. Infant botulism
4. Long QT syndrome
5. Shaken baby syndrome
6. Infections with the bacteria called *Helicobacter pylori*.

Risk factors: Very little is certain about the possible causes of SIDS, and there is no proven method for prevention. Although studies have identified risk factors for SIDS, such as putting infants to bed on their stomachs, there has been little understanding of the syndrome's biological cause or causes. The frequency of SIDS appears to be a strong function of infant sex and the age, ethnicity, and the education and socioeconomic status of the parents.

According to a study published in October 2007 in the Journal of the American Medical Association, babies who die of SIDS have abnormalities in the part of the brain called the medulla which helps control functions like breathing, blood pressure and arousal. Researchers examined the brains of 31 babies who had died of SIDS and 10 who had died from other causes. It was discovered that the medulla had neurons that released a chemical called serotonin. The number of these neurons was greater than normal in 55% of the brains of the babies who had died of SIDS. They also found that babies had fewer receptors for serotonin and that abnormalities in the brain stem appear to affect the ability to use and recycle serotonin, which is responsible for regulating mood as well as vital body functions. According to the National Institutes of Health, which funded the study, the new finding is the strongest evidence to date suggesting that innate differences in a specific part of the brain may place some at increased risk of dying from SIDS. In a British study released May 29, 2008 researchers discovered that the common bacterial infections *Staphylococcus aureus* (staph) and *Escherichia coli* (E. coli) appear to be the cause of some cases of Sudden Infant Death Syndrome. Both the "staph" and E. coli bacteria had a greater presence in the unexplained deaths of infants. SIDS cases peak between the ages of 8–10 weeks of age, which is also the time frame in which the antibodies that were passed along from mother to child are starting to disappear and babies have not yet made their own antibodies.

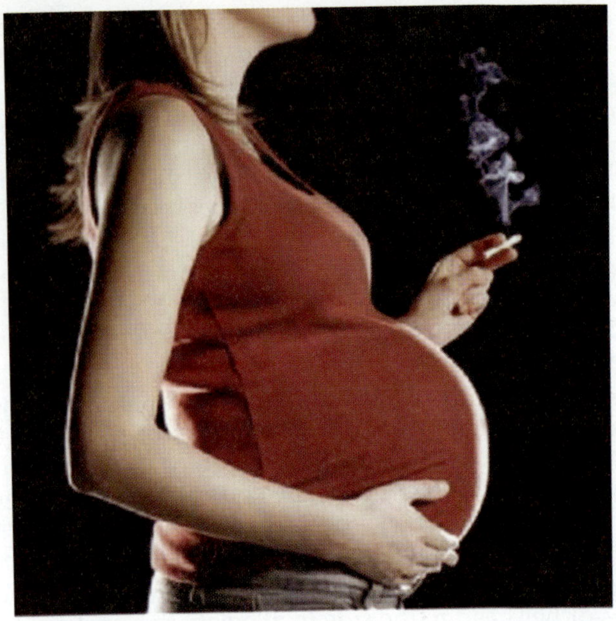

Fig. 42.4: *Photograph of a smoking cigarette by a pregnant mother is one of the risk factors to SIDS*

Listed below are several factors associated with increased probability of the syndrome based on information available prior to this recent study (Table 42.1).

Prenatal Risks

Maternal nicotine use e.g. tobacco or nicotine patch inadequate prenatal care inadequate prenatal nutrition use of heroin subsequent births less than 1 year apart alcohol abuse.

Obesity

Teen pregnancy (the more babies a teen mother) has the greater the risk.

Postnatal risks

- Low birth weight [especially less than 1.5 kg (<.3lb)]
- Exposure to tobacco smoke
- Laying an infant to sleep on their stomach
- Not breastfeeding
- Excess clothing and overheating

- Excess bedding, soft sleep surface and stuffed animals
- Infant's sex (61% of SIDS cases) occur in males
- Iinfant's age (incidence rises from zero at birth) is highest from 2–4 months, and declines towards zero at 1 year
- Premature birth (increase risk of SIDS) death by 50 times.

Risk reduction for SIDS: Though SIDS cannot be prevented, parents of infants are encouraged to take several precautions in order to reduce the likelihood of SIDS.

Sleep positioning: Sleeping on the back has been recommended by (among others) the American Academy of Pediatrics (starting in 1992) to avoid SIDS with the catchphrase "Back to Bed" and "Back to Sleep". The incidence of SIDS has fallen sharply in a number of countries in which the back to bed recommendation has been widely adopted, such as the US and New Zealand. However, the absolute incidence of SIDS prior to the back to sleep campaign was already low in the US among the theories supporting the back to sleep recommendation is the idea that small infants with little or no control of their heads may, while face down, inhale their exhaled breath (high in carbon dioxide) or smother themselves on their bedding—the brainstem anomaly research (above) suggests that babies with that particular genetic makeup do not react "normally" by moving away from the pooled CO_2 and thus smother. Another theory is that babies sleep more soundly when placed on their stomachs, and are unable to rouse themselves when they have an incidence of sleep apnea, which is thought to be common in infants. Arguments against infant back-sleeping include concerns that an infant could choke on fluids it brings up. Hospital staff commonly place newborns on their side although they advise parents to place their infants on their backs after going home from the hospital (Fig. 42.9).

Other concerns raised about the back to sleep campaign have included the possible increase the risk of positional facial and head deformities (see positional plagiocephaly), possible interference with development of good sleep habits (which in turn may have other bad effects) and possible interference with motor skills development (as infants delay attempts to lift their heads, crawl, etc.).

Breastfeeding: A 2003 study published in pediatrics, which investigated racial disparities in infant mortality in Chicago, found that previously or currently breastfeeding infants in the study had 1/5 the rate of SIDS as non-breastfed infants, but that "it became nonsignificant in the multivariate model that included the other environmental factors. These results are consistent with most published reports and suggest that other factors associated with breastfeeding, rather than breastfeeding itself, are protective".

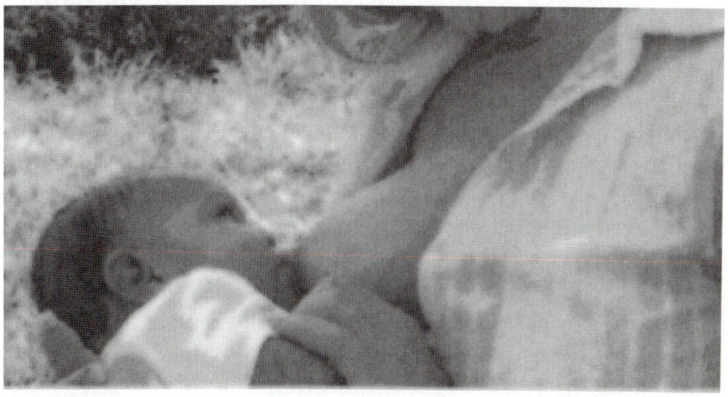

Fig. 42.5: *Breastfeeding is useful in the prevention of SIDS*

Co-sleeping: A controversial approach to lowering SIDS rates is limiting co-sleeping. A 2005 policy statement by the American Academy of Pediatrics on sleep environment and the risk of SIDS condemned all co-sleeping and bedsharing as unsafe. However, some data has suggested that almost all SIDS deaths in adult beds occur when other prevention methods, such as placing infants on their backs, are not used.

Secondhand smoke reduction: According to the US surgeon general's report, secondhand smoke is connected to SIDS. Infants who die from SIDS tend to have higher concentrations of nicotine and cotinine (a biological marker for secondhand smoke exposure) in their lungs than those who die from other causes. Infants exposed to secondhand smoke after birth are also at a greater risk of SIDS. Parents who smoke can significantly reduce their children's risk of SIDS by either quitting or smoking only outside and leaving their house completely smoke-free (Figs 42.4 and 42.10).

Bedding

To prevent SIDS, many families use firm mattresses with tight-fitting sheets in cribs or bassinets. The families do not allow pillows, stuffed animals, or fluffy bedding in the cribs. In cold weather, the families dress the infants warmly in well-fitted clothing. The infants blankets should also not be placed over their heads. It has been recommended that the infants are only covered up to their chest with their arms exposed. This will help to eliminate the chances of the infant moving the blanket over their heads (Fig. 42.6).

Sleep sacks: In colder environments where bedding is required to maintain a baby's body temperature, the use of a sleep sack is becoming more popular. A study published in the European Journal of Pediatrics in August 1998 has shown the protective effects of a sleep sack as reducing the incidence of turning from back to front during sleep, reinforcing putting a baby to sleep on their back for placement into the sleep sack and preventing bedding from coming up over the face which leads to increased temperature and carbon dioxide rebreathing. They conclude in their study "The use of a sleeping-sack should be particularly promoted for infants with a low birth weight".

Pacifiers: A 2005 study indicated that use of a pacifier is associated with a 90% reduction in the risk of SIDS. It has been speculated that the raised surface of the pacifier holds the infant's face away from the mattress, reducing the risk of suffocation. Although suffocation is an actual cause, while SIDS refers to an unexplained infant death, in the absence of sufficient postmortem investigation, a SIDS diagnosis may result (Figs 42.7 and 42.8).

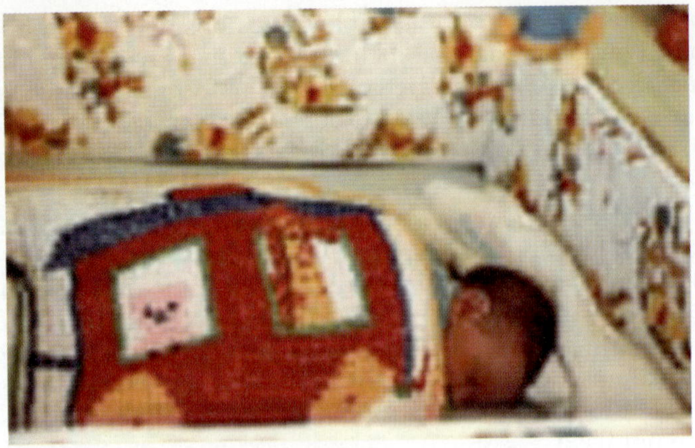

Fig. 42.6: *Infant's proper bedding and sleeping position may be helpful in the prevention of SIDS*

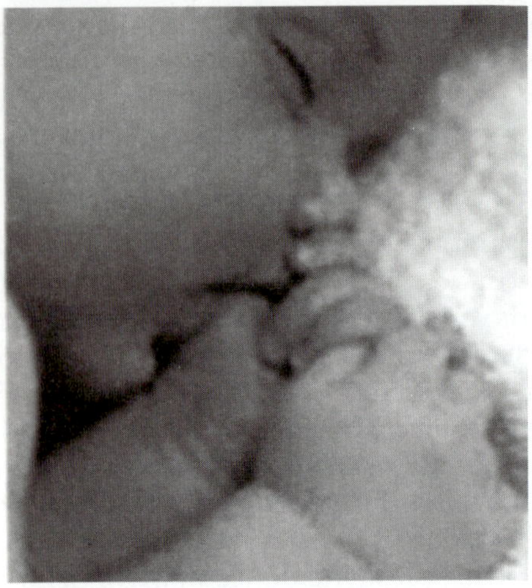

Fig. 42.8: *Dead infant lying on side with thumb in his mouth*

Bumper Pads

Bumper pads may be a contributing factor in SIDS deaths and should be removed. Health Canada, the Canadian Government's Health Department, issued an advisory recommending against the use of bumper pads, with the warning that they may decrease the amount of oxygen rich air available to the baby: The presence of bumper pads in a crib may also be a contributing factor for Sudden Infant Death Syndrome (SIDS). These products may reduce the flow of oxygen rich air to the infant in the crib. Furthermore, proposed theories indicate that the rebreathing of carbon dioxide plays a role in the occurrence of SIDS. Speculated associations: a number of theoretical causes have been proposed as a trigger for SIDS, but many of them are unproven or have not been thoroughly studied and peer-reviewed.

Mattress bugs: A 2002 study hypothesized that bugs feeding on baby vomit and dust could be fatal for small children, creating "supertoxins" which spur the baby's body into overreacting, leading to anaphylactic shock.

Brain disorder: A recently published research article in the journal of the American Medical Association showed evidence that cells in the brainstem fail to develop receptors for serotonin in the womb. This abnormality continues until after birth, supposedly until the end of their first year. This would account for there being few to no SIDS deaths after the first year of infancy and the reason the risk is more for premature infants. The SIDS Alliance/First Candle has posted a message about this along with a link to the abstract on their website (www.firstcandle.com), which can be accessed from the front page.

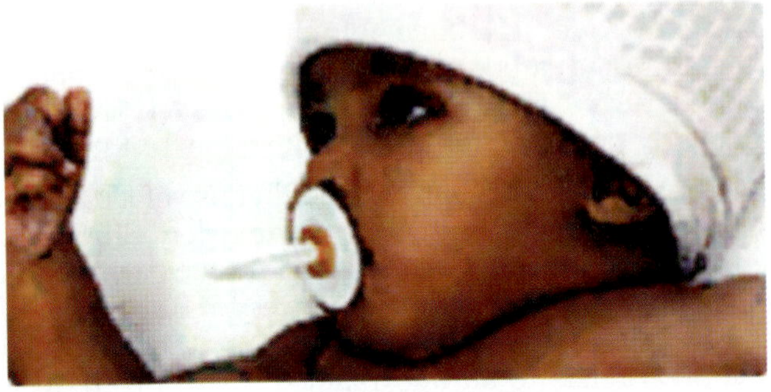

Fig. 42.7: *Infant's different types of pacifiers under use may be useful in the prevention of SIDS*

Vitamin C: According to a 1993 article in journal of Orthomolecular Medicine, Australian medical doctor Archie Kalokerinos performed research showing that high doses of vitamin C eliminates SIDS. As SIDS was shown to be caused solely by vitamin deficiency, the article stated that it was no longer a syndrome, and that the proper disease name is now SID. As of January 2007, the Journal of Orthomolecular Medicine was not included among journals selected by the US National Library of Medicine for inclusion in their medline database.

Toxic Gases

In 1989, a controversial piece of research by UK Scientist Barry Richardson claimed that all cot deaths were the result of toxic nerve gases being produced through the action of fungus in mattresses on compounds of phosphorus, arsenic and antimony. These chemicals are frequently used to make mattresses fire-retardant. A major plank in this explanation is the widely-observed phenomenon that the risk of cot death rises from one sibling to the next. Richardson claims that the cause is that parents are more likely to buy new bedding for their first child, and to reuse that bedding for later children. The more frequently used the bedding is, the more chance there will be that fungus has become resident in the material; thus, a higher chance of cot death. In 1994, the New Zealand Government, under the advice of Dr Jim Sprott, issued advice recommending new parents to either buy bedding free of the toxic compounds or to wrap the mattresses in a barrier film to prevent the escape of the gases. Dr Sprott claims that no case of cot death has ever been traced back to a properly manufactured or wrapped mattress.

However, a final report of The Expert group to investigate Cot Death Theories: Toxic Gas Hypothesis, published in May 1998, concluded that "there was no evidence to substantiate the toxic gas hypothesis that antimony- and phosphorus-containing compounds used as fire retardants in PVC and other cot mattress materials are a cause of SIDS. Neither was there any evidence to believe that these chemicals could pose any other health risk to infants". The report also states that "in normal cot-like conditions it is not possible to generate toxic gas from antimony in mattresses" and "babies have also been found to die on wrapped mattresses". Dr Sprott's website, however, claims that the study does not actually refute his theory: contrary to media publicity, the 1998 UK Limerick Report did not disprove the toxic gas theory as a highly qualified environmental scientist has stated in the New Zealand Medical Journal. In fact, the Limerick Committee's experiments proved the fungal generation of toxic gases (forms of stibine and arsine) from cot mattress materials. According to Dr Sprott, as of 2006, the New Zealand Government has not reported any SIDS deaths when babies have slept on mattresses wrapped according to his method. While the Limerick report claims that babies have been found to die on wrapped mattresses, Dr Sprott argues that a chemical analysis of the bedding should be performed. He additionally claims that this part of the report was flawed: In February 2000, Dr Peter Fleming (a co-author of the Limerick Report and principal author of the UK CESDI Report) conceded that the claim that three babies in the United Kingdom had died of cot death on polythene-covered mattresses could not be substantiated.

Central Respiratory Pattern Deficiency

There is ongoing research in the pediatric/neonatal community that has begun to associate apnea-like breathing cessations in animal models with unusual neural architecture or signal transduction in central pattern generator circuits including the pre-Bötzinger complex. It is possible that irregularities in neurotransmitter release (such as GABA, adenosine, and NMDA) or deficiencies in their associated receptors (including both $GABA_A$, $GABA_B$ subtypes and NMDA-glutamate receptors) are linked to incomplete prenatal development as is evident in preterm infants. Genetic factors are also being studied with several rat and mouse knockouts.

Upper cervical spinal cord injury as a result of birth trauma: During birth if the infant's head is traumatically turned side to side, upper cervical spinal injury can result. Difficulty breathing is a classic sign of upper spinal cord and brainstem injury. When infants with undiagnosed upper cervical spinal cord injury are continually placed on their stomach for sleep, they are forced to turn their head to the side to breathe. This is hypothesized to aggravate and prolong the spinal cord injury sustained during birth, preventing proper healing and ultimately leading to fatal breathing difficulty.

Sex distribution: There is a consistent 50% male excess in SIDS per 1,000 live births of each sex. Given a 5% male excess birth rate (105 male to 100 female live births) there appear to be 3.15 male SIDS per 2 female SIDS for a male fraction of 0.61. The X-linkage hypotheses for SIDS and the male excess in infant mortality have shown that the 50% male excess could be caused by a dominant X-linked allele that occurs with a frequency of S! that is protective of transient cerebral anoxia. An unprotected XY male would occur with a frequency of T! and an unprotected XX female would occur with a frequency of $^4D_9$. The ratio of T! to $^4D_9$ is 1.5 to 1 which matches the observed male 50% excess rate of SIDS. Although many authors have found autosomal and mitochondrial genetic risk factors for SIDS they cannot explain the male excess because such gene loci have the same frequencies for males and females. Supporting evidence is found by examination of other causes of infant respiratory death, such as inhalation of food and other foreign objects. Although food is prepared identically for male and female infants, there is a 50% male excess of death from such causes indicating that males are more susceptible to the cerebral anoxia created by such incidents in exactly the same proportion as found in SIDS. The study which indicated that there was a relationship between fewer serotonin binding sites and SIDS noted that the boys "had significantly fewer serotonin binding sites than girls".

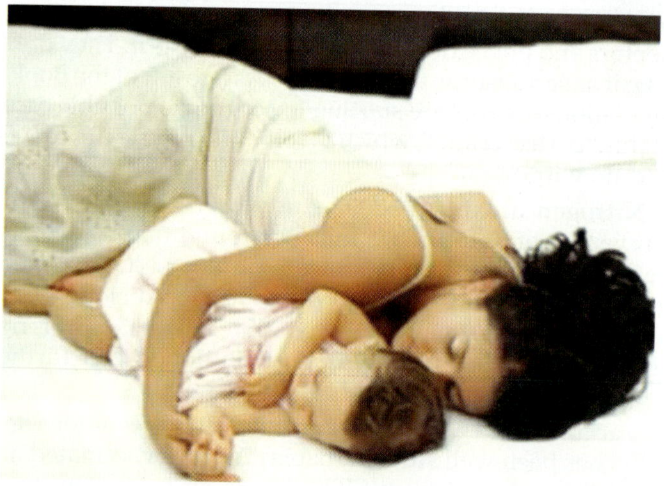

Fig. 42.9: *Co-sleeping of mother and child. Latest British study claims that sharing a bed with a baby becomes dangerous only if other factors are also prominent which include parents drinking alcohol, parents smoking or taking drugs, or excessively tired parents, use of heavy bedding, adult pillows and soft mattresses*

SIDS and child abuse: British former pediatrician Roy Meadow believes that many cases diagnosed as SIDS are really the result of child abuse on the part of a parent displaying Munchausen Syndrome by Proxy (a condition which he was first to describe, in 1977). During the 1990s and early 2000s, a number of mothers of multiple apparent SIDS victims were convicted of murder, to varying degrees on the basis of Meadow's opinion. In 2003, a number of high-profile acquittals brought Sir Meadow's theories into disrepute, and many now doubt their credibility. Several hundred murder convictions were reviewed, leading to several high-profile cases being reopened and convictions overturned. The Royal Statistical Society issued a media release refuting the expert testimony in one UK case in which the conviction was subsequently overturned. Stating The misdiagnosis of infanticide as SIDS "happens all over"

Ms Talan, a medical reporter at News day, said. "A lot of doctors and police don't know how to handle it. They don't take it as seriously as they should". As a result of the book's revelations, people are starting to scrutinize possible cases of this "perfect crime", which involves no physical evidence and no witnesses.

Nitrogen dioxide: A 2005 study by researchers at the University of California, San Diego found that "SIDS may be related to high levels of acute outdoor NO_2 exposure during the last day of life". While nitrogen dioxide (NO_2) exposure may be one of many possible risk factors, it is not considered causal, and the report cautioned that further studies were needed to replicate the result.

Vaccination: The relationship between vaccinations and SIDS has been well studied. Babies that are vaccinated are possibly protected from SIDS according to one study in the British Medical Journal. Other studies indicate that there is no significant difference in risk.

Inner ear samage: Records of hearing tests administered to certain infants show that those who later died of SIDS had a unique pattern of partial hearing loss, according to the journal early human development. One suggestion for the cause of SIDS is that the deaths are caused by disturbances in respiratory control (from other than suffocation). The vestibular apparatus of the inner ear has been shown to play an important role in respiratory control during sleep. It is speculated that this inner ear damage could be linked to SIDS. It is speculated that the damage occurs during delivery, particularly when prolonged contractions create greater blood pressure in the placenta. The right ear is directly in the "line of fire" for blood entering the fetus from the placenta, and thus could be most susceptible to damage. If the findings are relevant, it may be possible to take corrective measures. Researchers are beginning animal studies to explore the connection.

Unfavourable effects of SIDS risk reduction recommendations: Dr Rafael Pelayo from Stanford University and a number of other pediatric sleep researchers in the US have stated that they believe that the American Academy of Pediatrics recommendations regarding cosleeping and pacifier use may have unintended consequences. They have stated that the SIDS prevention strategy of the American Academy of Pediatrics which keeps infants at a low arousal threshold and reduces the time in quiet sleep may be unhealthy for children. They state that slow wave sleep is the most restorative form of sleep and limiting this sleep in the first 12 months of life may have unintended consequences to both the sleep and the infant. According to 1998 study by British researchers that compared back sleeping infants to stomach sleeping infants, there were developmental differences at 6 months of age between the two groups. At 6 months of age the stomach sleeping infants had higher gross motor scores, social skills scores, and total development skills scores than the back sleeping infants. The differences were apparent at the 5% statistical significant level. But, at 18 months the differences were no longer apparent. The researchers deemed the lower development scores of back sleeping infants at 6 months of age to be transient and stated that they do not believe the back sleeping recommendations should be changed. Other scientists have stated that the conclusion that the negative effects of back sleep at 18 months of age is transient is based upon very little evidence and that no long-term randomized trials have been completed.

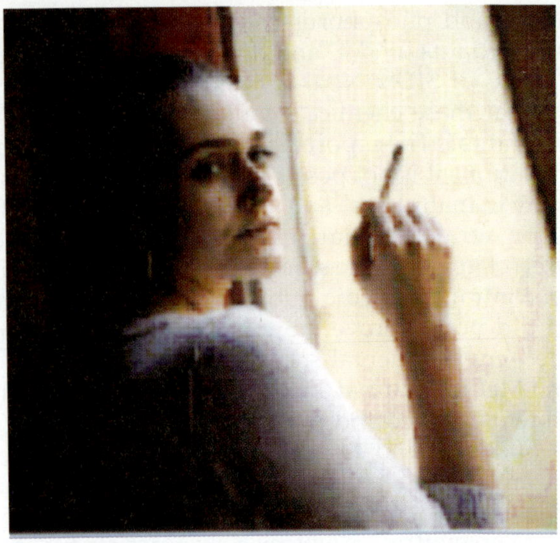

Fig. 42.10: *Exposure to cigarette smoke induces abnormalities in babies' brains, putting them at increased risk of sudden infant death syndrome*

Other side effects of the back sleeping position include: Increased rates of shoulder retraction, positional plagiocephaly, and positional torticollis. Some scientists dispute that plagiocephaly is a negative side effect. Dr Peter Fleming, who is co-author of the study that deemed delays at 6 months of age to be transient, has stated that he does not think plagiocephaly is a negative side effect of back sleep. In an interview with the Guardian Dr Fleming stated "I do not think it is a medical problem, it is more of a cosmetic one. Mothers may feel it is a syndrome and a problem when it really is nonsense. A research study on children with plagiocephaly found that 26% had mild to severe psychomotor delay. This study also showed that 10% of infants with plagiocephaly had mild to severe mental development delay. Because of the delays caused by back sleep some medical professionals have suggested that the "normal" ages at which children had previously attained developmental milestones should be pushed back. This would enable medical professionals to consider "normal" children who previously were considered developmentally delayed.

Prevention of sudden infant death syndrome (SIDS): By definition, the cause of SIDS is unknown. In fact, it is likely that SIDS is the end result of many different processes. That makes prevention of all SIDS a difficult task. New evidence suggests that a subtle form of suffocation may be the true culprit in one-quarter to one-half of all suspected SIDS cases. There is strong evidence that the prone position in which babies sleep (face down) is associated with SIDS. Several studies, particularly those from Australia and New Zealand, have linked the prone position to elevated SIDS risk. Based on the careful evaluation of numerous studies, health officials now want to change the way. American babies sleep in the hope of preventing SIDS. The campaign to educate parents about the importance of sleep position for babies is called "Back to Sleep" and is supported and endorsed by the surgeon general's office, the US consumer product safety commission and the American Academy of Pediatrics. The specific advice is to let the baby fuss on his or her back (for no more than a few minutes) during the first few months of life before calming him down and trying again. If you try for 20–30 minutes three nights in a row and the baby still will not go to sleep on his back, let him fall asleep on the stomach and then turn him onto his back or wait a few days and try positioning him again. Parents can buy special wedges that help to maintain the baby's position on the back or side. Furthermore, babies should not be placed asleep on any blankets or with any pillows or stuffed animals. The goal is to not have any objects that can block the baby's face and hinder breathing.

The underlying mechanism for these cases of SIDS appears to be an abnormal response to stressors such as changes in blood levels of oxygen or carbon dioxide. This may explain the high frequency in the first half year of life that subsequently declines with increasing developmental maturity.

Another cause that has been postulated is a specific heart dysrhythmia called prolonged QT syndrome. Although this can be screened for, it is unclear what the exact risk is and if treatment would be successful. Still another cause is metabolic defects.

Unfortunately, some cases of SIDS are due to infanticide. This possibility makes a thorough examination of each case all the more important.

Home monitoring has long been utilized as preventative measure in higher risk children and those who have already experienced an ALTE. However, there is almost no evidence to suggest that home monitoring is effective for this purpose.

Precautions to Reduce the Chance of SIDS

- Have good medical care and adequate nutrition during pregnancy.
- Keep baby in smoke-free surroundings (smoking by either parent as well as secondhand smoke are clearly linked with SIDS).
- Put baby to sleep on a firm mattress.
- Breastfeed if possible (Fig. 42.5).
- If "blue spells" are noticed in the infant, get prompt medical advice.
- Try not to let the baby get too hot (don't over-swaddle).
- Never have the infant's face covered by bedclothes.
- Avoid thick blankets, pillows or bumpers in the crib.
- Try not to let the infant sleep on his/her stomach.
- Put the baby to sleep on his/her side or back. (A rolled-up towel along his/her back will help to keep the baby on his/her side.)

Babies seem to be at above-SIDS risk where the following conditions are present:

- In winter time
- If their mothers smoke cigarettes during and/or after pregnancy
- If their mothers are drug addicts
- If their mothers received insufficient health care while pregnant (poor uterine environment)
- If parts of the baby's brain that regulate breathing remain immature (delayed development)—perhaps due to short bouts of oxygen shortage
- If infants are overheated (faulty body temperature control)—Over-swaddling or heavy bedding may make the body work too hard to keep down body temperature.
- If babies are overweight at birth, slow to gain weight or premature—especially with lung disorders
- If they have had serious apnea (temporary breathing stoppage). Several "blue spells" may signal a flaw in breathing control.
- If bottlefed rather than breastfed.

How can I reduce the SIDS risk?

Health care providers don't know what exactly causes SIDS, but they do know certain things can help to reduce the risk of SIDS.

- **Always place babies on their backs to sleep:** Babies who sleep on their backs are less likely to die of SIDS than babies who sleep on their stomachs or sides. Placing your baby on his or her back to sleep is the number one way to reduce the risk of SIDS.
- **Use the back sleep position every time:** Babies who usually sleep on their backs but who are then placed on their stomachs, like for a nap, are at very high risk for SIDS. So, it is important for babies to sleep on their backs every time for naps and at night.
- **Place your baby on a firm sleep surface, such as a safety-approved crib mattress covered with a fitted sheet:** Never place a baby to sleep on a pillow, quilt, sheepskin, or other soft surface.
- **Keep soft objects, toys, and loose bedding out of your baby's sleep area:** Don't use pillows, blankets, quilts, sheepskins, or pillow-like bumpers in your baby's sleep area. Keep all items away from the baby's face.
- **Avoid letting your baby overheat during sleep:** Dress your baby in light sleep clothing and keep the room at a temperature that is comfortable for an adult.
- **Think about using a clean, dry pacifier when placing your baby down to sleep**, but don't force the baby to take it. (If you're breastfeeding, wait until your child is 1 month old, or is used to breastfeeding before using a pacifier.)

BIBLIOGRAPHY

1. Adgent MA. Environmental tobacco smoke and sudden infant death syndrome: a review. (review). Birth Defects Research. Part B. Developmental and Reproductive Toxicology 77(1): 69–85, 2006.
2. Alm B; Lagercrantz H; Wennergren G. Stop SIDS: Sleeping solitary supine, sucking soother, stopping smoking substitutes. Acta Paediatrica 95(3): 260–262, 2006.

3. Bajanowski T; Brinkmann B; Mitchell EA; Vennemann MM; Leukel HW; Larsch KP, et al. Nicotine and cotinine in infants dying from sudden infant death syndrome. International Journal of Legal Medicine 122(1): 23–28, 2008.
4. Burd L; Klug MG; Martsolf JT. Increased sibling mortality in children with fetal alcohol syndrome. Addiction Biology 9(2): 179–186, 2004.
5. Chan-Yeung M; Dimich-Ward H. Respiratory health effects of exposure to environmental tobacco smoke. Respirology 8(2): 131–139, 2003.
6. Chong DSY; Yip PSF; Karlberg J. Maternal smoking: An increasing unique risk factor for sudden infant death syndrome in Sweden. Acta Paediatrica 93(4): 471–478, 2004.
7. Fleming P; Blair PS. Sudden Infant Death Syndrome and parental smoking. Early Human Development 83(11): 721–725, 2007.
8. Friend KB; Goodwin MS; Lipsitt LP. Alcohol use and sudden infant death syndrome. Developmental Review 24(3): 235–251, 2004.
9. Hafstrom A; Milerad J; Sandberg KL; Sundell HW. Cardiorespiratory effects of nicotine exposure during development. Respiratory Physiology and Neurobiology 149(1–3): 325–341, 2005.
10. Gingras JL; Mitchell EA; Grattan KJ; Stewart AW. Effects of maternal cigarette smoking and cocaine use in pregnancy on fetal response to vibroacoustic stimulation and habituation. Acta Paediatrica 93(11): 1479 –1485, 2004.
11. Horne RSC; Franco P; Adamson TM; Groswasser J; Kahn A. Influences of maternal cigarette smoking on infant arousability. Early Human Development 79(1): 49–58, 2004.
12. Hunt CE; Hauck FR. Sudden infant death syndrome. (review). Canadian Medical Association Journal 174(13): 1861–1869, 2006.
13. Howard LM; Hannam S. Sudden infant death syndrome and psychiatric disorders. British Journal of Psychiatry 182(5): 379–380, 2003.
14. James C; Klenka H; Manning D. Sudden infant death syndrome: bed sharing with mothers who smoke. Archives of Disease in Childhood 88(2): 112–113, 2003.
15. Rushton L; Courage C; Green E. Estimation of the impact on children's health of environmental tobacco smoke in England and Wales. Journal of the Royal Society for the Promotion of Health 123(3): 175–180, 2003.
16. Sawnani H; Jackson T; Murphy T; Beckerman R; Simakajornborn N. The effect of maternal smoking on respiratory and arousal patterns in preterm infants during sleep. American Journal of Respiratory and Critical Care Medicine 169(6): 733–738, 2004.
17. Sundell HW. SIDS prevention: Good progress, but now we need to focus on avoiding nicotine. (editorial). Acta Paediatrica 93(4): 450–452, 2004.

43 Sudden Cardiac Death in Children and Adolescents

Sudden cardiac death (SCD) is an unexpected death due to cardiac causes occurring in a short time period (generally within 1 h of symptom onset) in a person with known or unknown cardiac disease in whom no previously diagnosed fatal condition is apparent. Most cases of SCD are related to cardiac arrhythmias. Approximately half of all cardiac deaths can be classified as SCDs. SCD occurs as the first expression of cardiac disease in many individuals presenting as out-of-hospital patients with cardiac arrest. Sudden death in childhood is rare. About 10% of paediatric deaths after the first year of life are sudden and population based studies put the individual age related risk at around 1:20 000 to 1:50 000 per year. About half of these deaths are related to a previously known abnormality, the most common being epilepsy, asthma, and cardiovascular abnormalities. Another third are attributed to an abnormality discovered at necropsy, usually either an infection or a cardiovascular abnormality. At least one sudden death in six remains unexplained, but this is almost certainly an underestimate as some deaths attributed by the coroner's pathologist to epilepsy or respiratory infection are probably more accurately described as being unexplained by findings at necropsy (Figs 43.1 and 43.2).

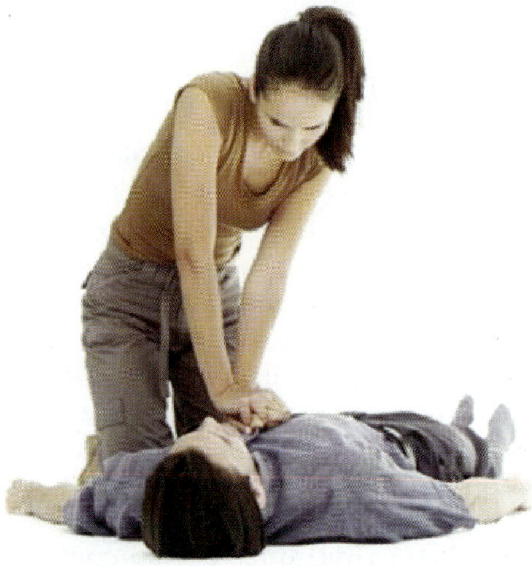

Fig. 43.1: *A modified form of CPR involving chest compression only, is being conducted on teenager who suddenly collapsed on the road side*

Pathophysiology

One report of terminal electrical activity in paediatric patients dying in hospital documented bradycardic arrest in 88% of neonates, 67% of infants, and 64% of children. Ventricular tachycardia or fibrillation was more likely in those with heart disease and in older children. The term "sudden death" should not be confused with nonfatal cardiac arrest.

The most common electrophysiologic mechanisms leading to SCD are tachyarrhythmias such as VF or VT. Interruption of tachyarrhythmias, using either an automatic external defibrillator (AED) or an implantable cardioverter defibrillator (ICD), has been shown to reduce mortality and morbidity from SCD. Patients with tachyarrhythmias, especially VT, carry the best overall prognosis of SCD patients because of the success of defibrillation. In patients

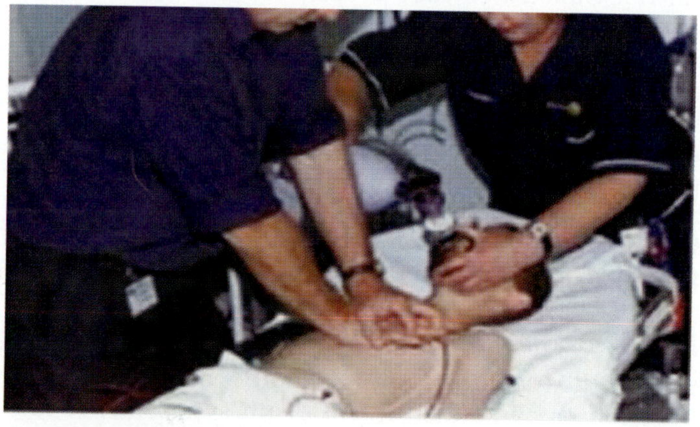

Fig. 43.2: *Cardiopulmonary resuscitation is being carried out in a young patient with SCD*

with ischemic heart disease, the most common form of VT is monomorphic, which arises from a reentrant circuit.

Approximately 20–30% of patients from all documented sudden death events have bradyarrhythmia or asystole at the time of initial contact. Oftentimes, it is difficult to determine with certainty the initiating event in a patient presenting with a bradyarrhythmia because asystole and pulseless electrical activity (PEA) may result from a sustained VT. Conversely, an initial bradyarrhythmia producing myocardial ischemia may then provoke VT or VF. Most cases of SCD occur in patients with structural abnormalities of the heart, related to either a prior myocardial infarction (MI) or a congenital abnormality. Acute thrombosis in an atherosclerotic coronary artery may present as unstable angina, acute myocardial infarction (MI), or SCD. Although more than 80% of SCD events occur in individuals with coronary artery disease (CAD), evidence of acute MI is far less common. Hypertrophic cardiomyopathy (HCM) and dilated cardiomyopathy (DCM) both are associated with increased risk of SCD. Heart failure and various valvular diseases such as aortic stenosis are associated with increased risk of SCD. The strongest predictor of SCD is left ventricular dysfunction of any cause. Acute illnesses, such as myocarditis, may provide both an initial and sustained risk of SCD due to inflammation and fibrosis of the myocardium. Less commonly, SCD happens in patients who may not have apparent structural heart disease. These conditions usually are inherited arrhythmia syndromes.

At the molecular level, VT and VF can be caused by altered Ca hemodynamics, neurohormonal changes, altered K hemodynamics especially in ischemia, or mutations resulting in dysfunction of a sodium channel (Na channelopathy) resulting in enhanced automaticity or reentry with unidirectional block. In patients who survive a myocardial infarction (MI), it has been demonstrated that the presence of premature ventricular contractions (PVCs), particularly complex forms, such as multiform PVCs, short coupling intervals (R-on-T phenomenon), or VT (salvos of 3 or more ectopic beats), reflect an increased risk of sudden death.

Even though many patients have anatomic and functional cardiac substrates that predispose them to develop ventricular arrhythmias, only a small percentage develop SCD. The interplay between the regional ischemia, LV dysfunction, and transient inciting events (e.g. worsened ischemia, acidosis, hypoxemia, wall tension, drugs, metabolic disturbances) has been proposed as being the precipitator of sudden death of 0.1–0.2% per year in the adult population. SCD commonly is the first expression of CAD and is responsible for approximately 50% of deaths from CAD.

Deaths Occuring During Infancy

Sudden death in infancy is usually caused either by infection or by sudden infant death syndrome. A few neonatal or infant deaths are caused by unrecognized congenital cardiovascular malformations, particularly duct dependent abnormalities or obstructive left heart malformations. Primary arrhythmias are rare causes of death in infancy but fatal ventricular arrhythmias are described. Complete atrioventricular block is usually recognized in utero or soon after birth but may cause death if unrecognized or untreated.

Complications in postoperative period in children with congenital heart disease (Fig. 43.3)

In the 1960s and 1970s, sudden cardiac death most often occurred in children with irreversible pulmonary vascular disease associated with unoperated congenital heart disease or in children with unoperated aortic valve stenosis. In recent years, surgical repair has been performed earlier and more effectively so that those most at risk of sudden death now are children with repaired heart disease. In a population based study of late postoperative sudden death, Silk a and colleagues identified an average risk of 0.9 per 1,000 patient-years follow-up for the most common surgically repaired malformations. Those patients with a risk above the average had aortic valve stenosis, transposition of the great arteries, tetralogy of Fallot or coarctation of the aorta. Death was attributed to "arrhythmia" in the majority, based on the history, but in only a few was an arrhythmia identified in life.

Deaths among adults with congenital heart diseases

Among patients in an adult congenital heart follow-up clinic in Toronto, not all of whom had undergone surgery, the reported sudden death rate was 5.3 per 1,000 patient-years. The most common abnormalities in those who died suddenly were Eisenmenger's syndrome, tetralogy of Fallot, and transposition of the great arteries, but the risk for individual diagnoses could not be assessed for lack of a denominator. In a more recent report from the same unit, 8% of adult patients died during follow-up—65% of deaths were cardiovascular and 26% were sudden. Although numbers for individual diagnoses were small, the highest proportion of deaths were sudden in patients with coarctation of the aorta, Ebstein's anomaly, and congenitally corrected transposition of the great arteries. The highest number of sudden deaths in the clinic population occurred in patients who had undergone repair of tetralogy of Fallot.

Complications after repair of tetralogy of Fallot

Of the various problems encountered late after surgical repair of tetralogy of Fallot, sudden death is the most difficult to predict. It usually occurs many years after operation and thus affects young adults more than children, with an average risk of 1.4 per 1,000 patient years, or about 1 in 700 per year. Many risk factors for sudden death have been identified retrospectively, but prospectively, even in combination, they are not useful in predicting risk. Although ventricular tachycardia or fibrillation is thought to be the most common mechanism of sudden death, more minor ventricular arrhythmias are so common as to be unhelpful in predicting risk. An important recent "pseudo-prospective" multicentre study involving six centres in the UK, USA, Canada and Japan retrospectively identified 793

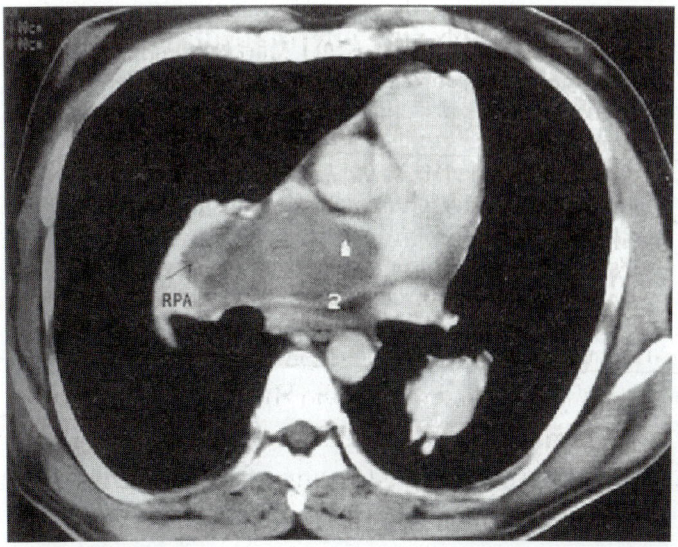

Fig. 43.3: *CT scan of the thorax with contrast injection showing the large MPA and a thrombus in the RPA (arrow) in Eisenmenger syndrome*

patients alive in 1985 and "followed" their progress for the next 10 years, yielding more than 7,500 patient-years follow-up. Thirty three patients developed sustained monomorphic ventricular tachycardia, 29 developed atrial flutter or fibrillation, 16 died suddenly, and 715 remained free from arrhythmia. There were no deaths in those who presented with ventricular tachycardia and there was only one death among patients presenting with atrial arrhythmia. The risk profile for ventricular tachycardia and sudden death was similar, with most of the patients having pulmonary regurgitation and right ventricular dysfunction. The authors suggest that surgical preservation or restoration of pulmonary valve function may reduce the risk of sudden death, but this remains unproven.

After atrial repair among patients with transposition of the great arteries

Most major published reports of experience of the Senning and Mustard operations for atrial repair of transposition of the great arteries give a risk of 5–6 per 1,000 patient-years or of about 1 in 180 per year. The relation between late sudden death and arrhythmia is not clear. There is a progressive loss of sinus rhythm so that fewer than half of patients have normal rhythm after 10 years. Junctional rhythm is common but asymptomatic bradycardia does not require treatment. Bradycardia seems not to be a risk factor for sudden death and pacemaker implantation offers no protection against it. One widely accepted theory is that the sudden onset of atrial flutter with 1:1 atrioventricular conduction may lead to sudden death, particularly if it is associated with impaired right ventricular function or atrial baffle obstruction, but as yet there is only circumstantial evidence for this. There is a complicated interrelation between arrhythmia, impaired ventricular function, and sudden death, which has yet to be explored fully. Other possible causes for late death after atrial repair of transposition include ventricular arrhythmias or acute heart failure.

Sudden death after repair of other malformations

Late sudden death after surgical repair of other common cardiovascular malformations is rare, with an incidence of around 0.1 per 1,000 patient-years. Surgical repair of some less common cardiac malformations may be associated with a higher risk of late sudden death. In a report of experience with the Rastelli operation for repair of complex transposition of the great arteries from Boston, there were five late sudden deaths in a group of 94 survivors of surgery who were followed for a median of 8.5 years (6.3 deaths per 1,000 patient years). Deaths were thought to be caused by the development of ventricular arrhythmias or atrioventricular block. The late postoperative sudden death rate in patients with heart defects characterized by double outlet right ventricle may be even higher. Among 89 patients the sudden death rate was 26 per 1,000 patient years, with 50% of deaths within 1 year of surgery. Risk factors for late death included perioperative ventricular tachycardia and atrioventricular block. The risk in rare conditions is harder to define but in some, such as pulmonary atresia, it may be significant.

Sudden death in children with unoperated heart disease (Table 43.1)

One would hope that most significant cardiovascular malformations would be detected early in life, preferably at an asymptomatic stage. However, despite health screening some significant problems go unrecognized, and may cause sudden death. Deaths from obstructive left heart malformations are unusual but they do occur. Postoperative deaths in such patients were ascribed to "arrhythmia" in the study by Silka and colleagues, but syncope in aortic valve stenosis is probably not primarily arrhythmic in origin. Congenital abnormalities of the coronary arteries are rarely diagnosed in life and prodromal syncope is uncommon. The most frequently recognized abnormalities after sudden death are anomalous origin of the left or right coronary arteries from the contralateral aortic sinus, with a proximal course between the aorta and the main pulmonary artery. Although the prevalence of such anomalies is hard to define precisely, the risk of sudden death is probably high enough to warrant surgical treatment. Sudden death in other specific conditions, such as Williams syndrome, is also reported and may be caused, in some cases at least, by coronary artery stenosis or malformation.

Cardiomyopathies

Hypertrophic Obstructive Cardiomyopathy (Figs 43.4 and 43.5)

The risk of sudden death in childhood from hypertrophic cardiomyopathy diagnosed in life is impossible to establish for lack of a denominator. Hypertrophic cardiomyopathy is said to affect as many as 1 in 500 of the adult population, but it is much less common in childhood. The impression given by published reports from specialized referral units is that the risk of sudden death is high whereas evidence from the few population based studies does not support this. "Risk stratification" is encouraged and may identify a few

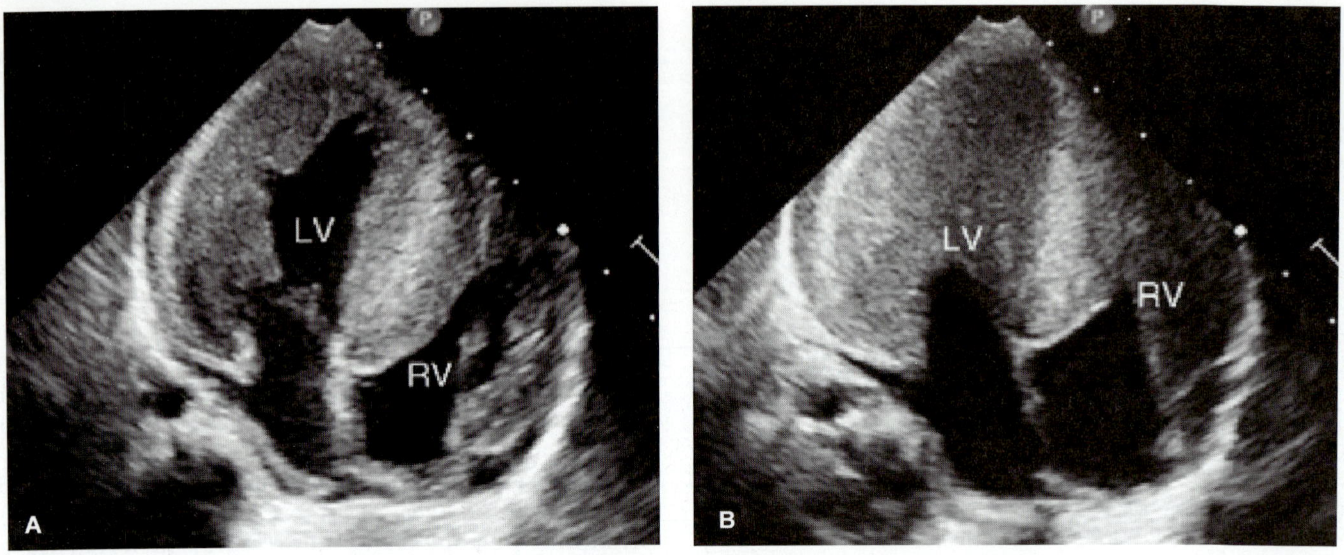

Fig. 43.4: *Echocardiograms showing a hypertrophic cardiomyopathy in diastole (a) and sistole (b) of the heart, respectively. The measurements indicate gross thickening of the left ventricular myocardium*

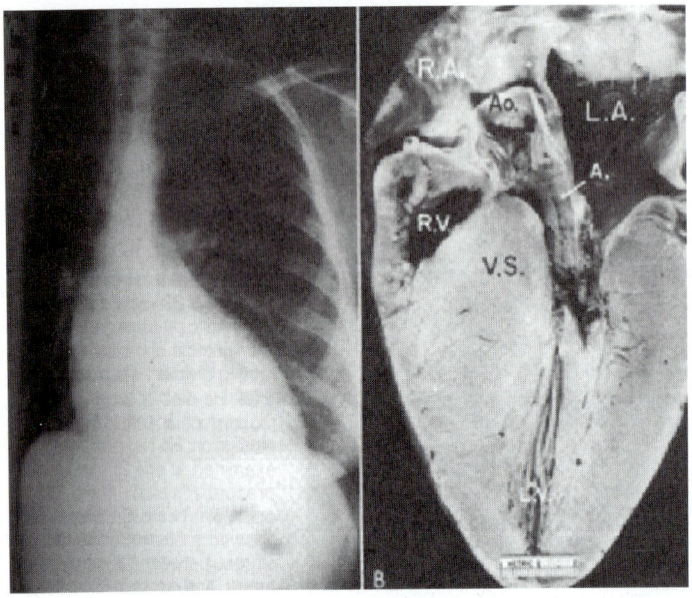

Fig. 43.5: *Photograph of X-ray chest (left) and cadaver model of heart (right) showing marked hypertrophy of both IVS and posterior left ventricular wall reducing LV cavity to a slit in patient with hypertrophic cardiomyopathy*

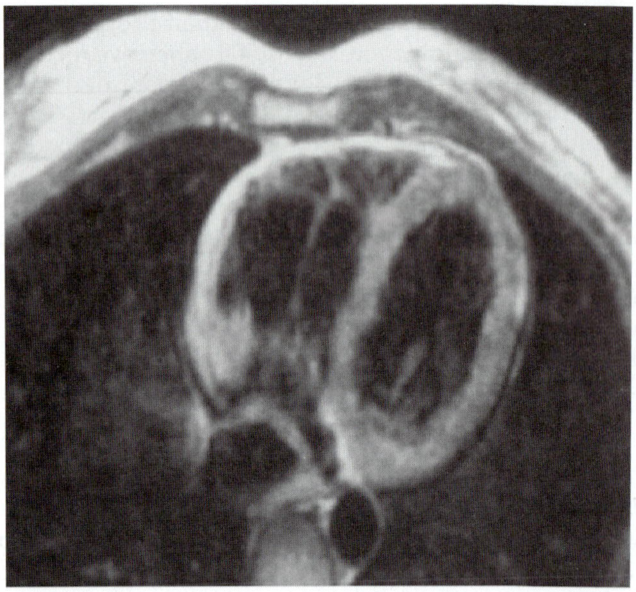

Fig. 43.6: *MRI findings in a 22 year adolescent with a history of dizziness and sustained ventricular tachycardia with an LBBB pattern. Short-axis view showing a dilated right ventricle with a brighter signal from a thin anterior free wall. Spin-echo nuclear magnetic resonance for tissue characterisation in arrhythmogenic right ventricular cardiomyopathy*

individuals at increased risk. "Risk factors" have been identified but are absent in most children. Risk factors for an increased risk of sudden death in adults include a family history of sudden death from hypertrophic cardiomyopathy, recurrent syncope, nonsustained ventricular tachycardia on an ambulatory ECG, and extreme left ventricular hypertrophy, but their presence does not reliably identify individuals at risk. A recent study of the use of implantable cardioverter-defibrillators (ICDs) in primary and secondary prevention has shown benefit. Appropriate discharges were triggered by ventricular tachycardia or fibrillation, providing insight into the mechanism of sudden death and an incentive for better risk stratification. However, only eight of 128 patients receiving an ICD were children. In a study of 99 children with hypertrophic cardiomyopathy in Toronto, the reported annual combined risk of sudden death and cardiac arrest was 2.7% between the ages of 8 and 18 years. In this study, syncope did not predict sudden death whereas cardiac arrest did and ventricular tachycardia on ambulatory ECG was a significant risk factor. The risk of sudden death is low for the majority of children, especially in the absence of symptoms. There is no evidence that treatment of asymptomatic patients has any effect on outcome. Because some sudden deaths occur

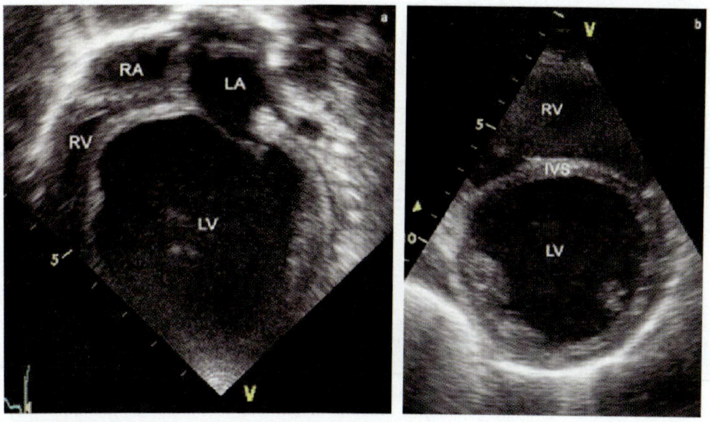

Fig. 43.7: *Dilated cardiomyopathy. (A) A four chamber echocardiogram showing a hugely dilated left ventricle that is squashing the right ventricle. (B) is a short-axis view. The myocardium is thinned*

during or after exercise it is often recommended that affected children should avoid sports or intense physical exertion. While such advice may seem sensible, there is no evidence that this leads to any reduction in risk.

Sudden death from *previously unsuspected* hypertrophic cardiomyopathy is rare—with an age specific risk in apparently normal children or adolescents of less than 1 in 1,000,000 per year. Because hypertrophic cardiomyopathy typically has dominant inheritance, diagnosis at necropsy should lead to screening of other family members. Often no further cases are identified, either because of variable penetrance or because the index case represents a new mutation. Clinical exclusion of the diagnosis is often very difficult as detectable cardiovascular abnormalities may only develop during adolescence. Gene testing is not generally available at present. A nonhypertrophic variant of hypertrophic cardiomyopathy has also been described recently. Troponin T mutations produce characteristic histological myocardial disarray and seem to have a particularly poor prognosis in the few families described but their prevalence is unknown.

Table 43.1: *Main causes of sudden cardiac death in children*

Cardiovascular malformations

Atrial repair of transposition of the great arteries (Mustard and Senning operations)

- Repaired tetralogy of Fallot
- Aortic valve stenosis
- Coarctation of the aorta
- Pulmonary atresia
- Pulmonary vascular disease (Eisenmenger syndrome)
- Coronary artery malformations

Other structural heart abnormalities

Hypertrophic cardiomyopathy

- Myocarditis
- Dilated cardiomyopathy
- Kawasaki disease
- Arrhythmogenic right ventricular cardiomyopathy (Fig. 43.6)

Primary arrhythmias

- Long QT syndrome
- Wolff-Parkinson-White syndrome
- Atrioventricular block
- Other ventricular arrhythmia (for example, catecholaminergic ventricular tachycardia, Brugada syndrome, etc)
- Nonhypertrophic varieties of hypertrophic cardiomyopathy (troponin T mutation)

Dilated Cardiomyopathy (Fig. 43.7)

Sudden death in dilated cardiomyopathy is uncommon. A study of 63 children from Houston documented 16% mortality over 10 years, but only 1 of 5 deaths was sudden.

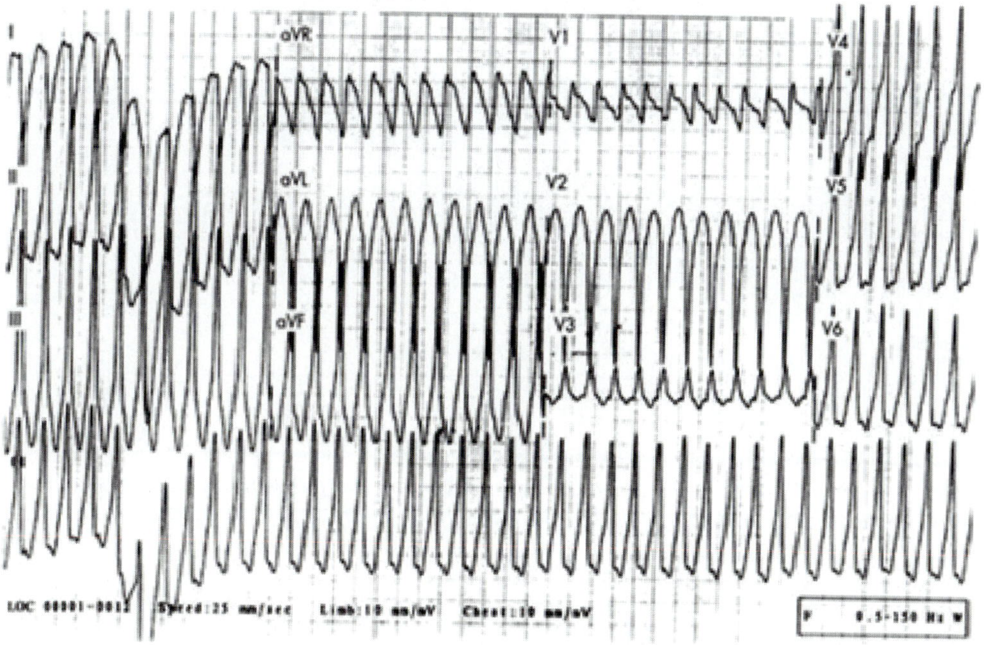

Fig. 43.8: *Postoperative ventricular tachycardia in a 14-year-old boy with a Rastelli repair of complex transposition who presented with syncope. The left bundle branch-block pattern and inferior frontal plane vector indicate an origin from the right ventricular side*

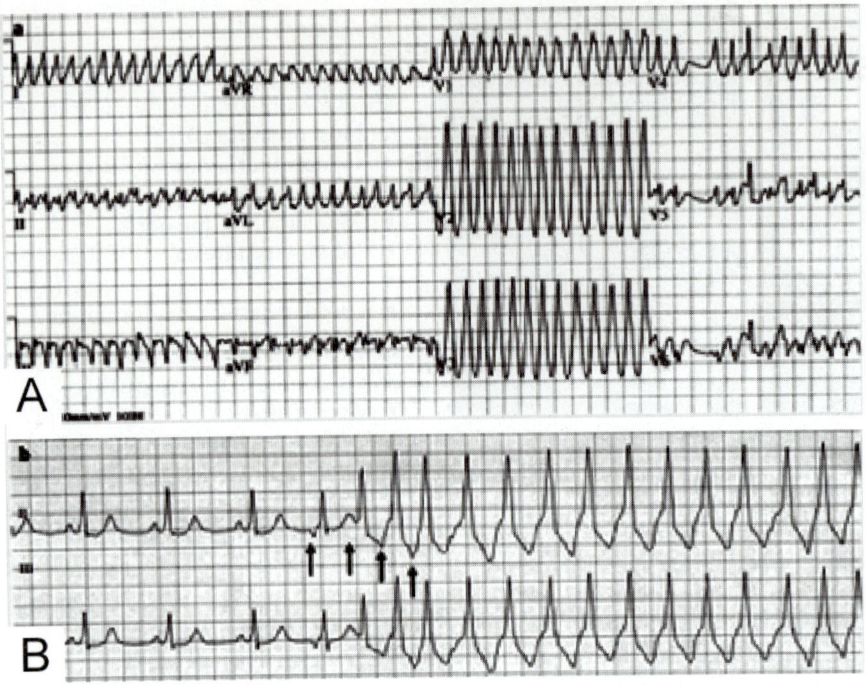

Fig. 43.9: *Wolff-Parkinson-White syndrome. (A) Preexcited atrial fibrillation. The teenager presented in cardiovascular shock requiring DC cardioversion. The rhythm resembles polymorphic VT, although the upward slope at the start resembles a delta wave in several leads and it is more organized than polymorphic VT, but less regular than monomorphic VT. The diagnosis was confirmed when a delta wave was seen on the resting 12-lead ECG after cardioversion. (B) A rhythm strip here shows initially sinus rhythm, with a delta wave demonstrating some ventricular preexcitation. At the first arrow, an atrial tachycardia starts up - the p wave is clearly different and the rate quicker, the subsequent three arrows indicate inverted p waves. After this the delta wave is more obvious, as the AV node no longer conducts, and conduction to the ventricle is preferentially via the accessory pathway*

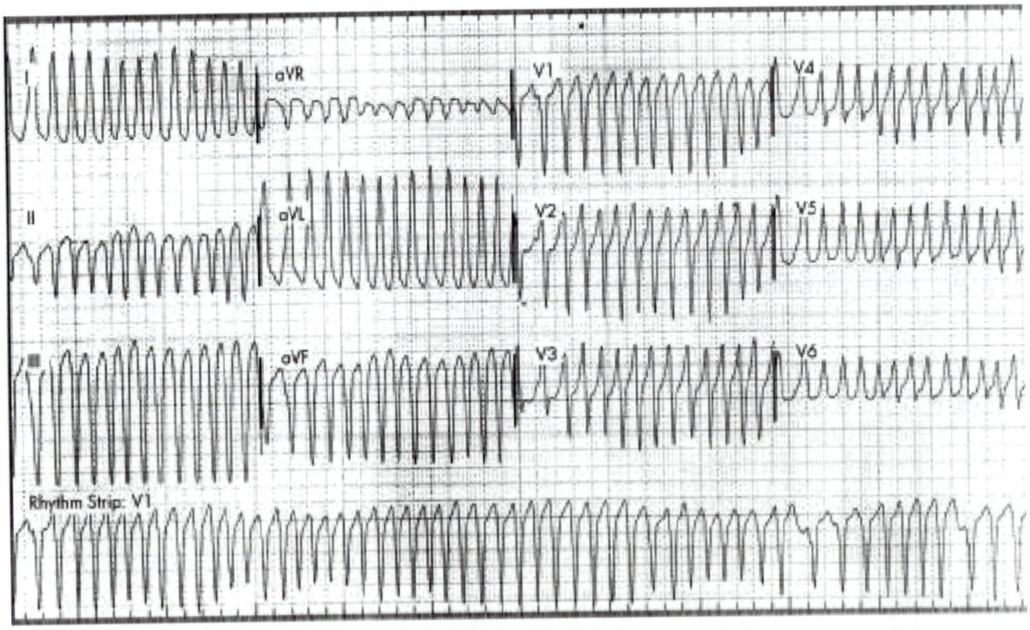

Fig. 43.10: *Atrial fibrillation in Wolff-Parkinson-White syndrome in a 10-year-old girl with a history of recurrent syncope. There is a rapid, irregular, wide QRS tachycardia with a morphology which matched the preexcitation seen in sinus rhythm*

In a report from Heidelberg 4 of 28 children died suddenly during a mean follow-up of 4.1 years. In both studies, arrhythmias of various types were present in at least half of the children, but they were unhelpful in risk prediction.

Restrictive Cardiomyopathy

Restrictive cardiomyopathy is a rare diagnosis at any age. There is a high mortality in childhood with a 2 year survival of only 50%. Most deaths are sudden. The main predictors

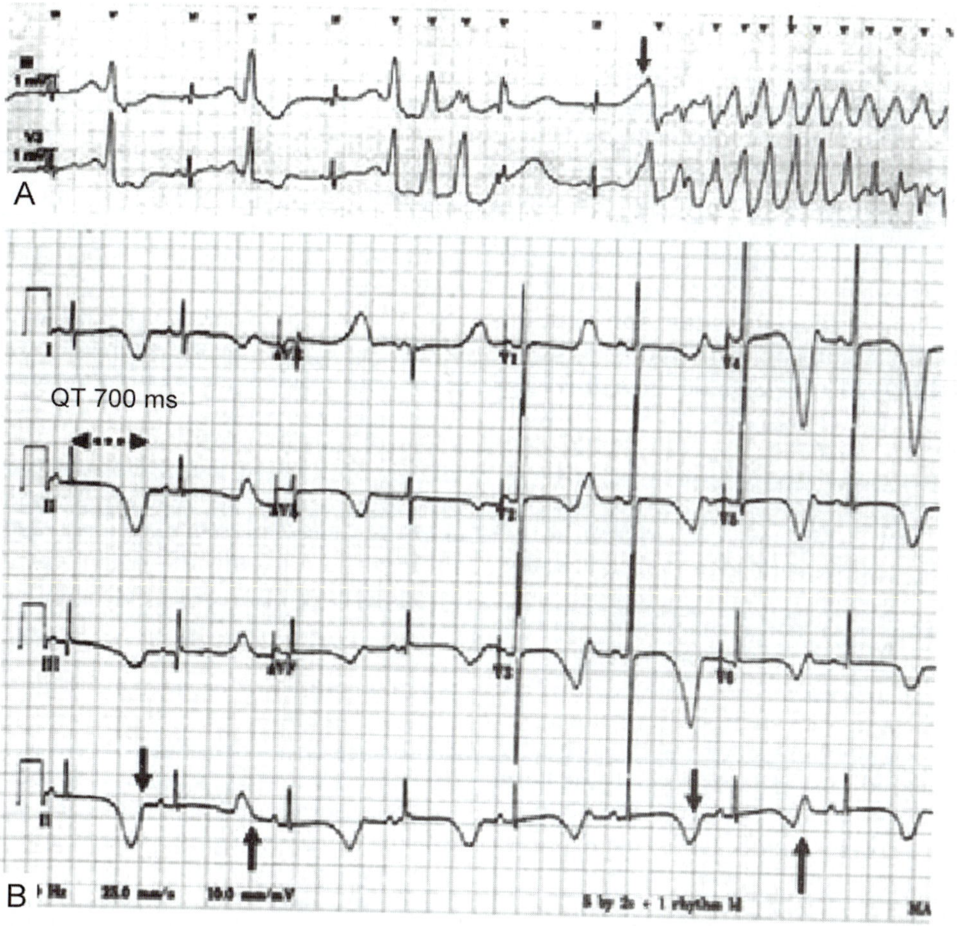

Fig. 43.11: *ECGs from an 8-year-old boy with catecholaminaergic-polymorphic VT .(A) This event was recorded on an implanted digital loop recorder. In fact, the asystole was detected by the device; the preceding rapid polymorphic VT had not been detected (it had been mistaken for electrical noise). Shortly afterwards he returns to sinus rhythm. (B) An exercise test in the same boy indicates normal QT interval, but there are multiple ventricular ectopics of bidirectional type (shown by the asterix), and a run of VT at the end of the screen (arrow)*

of mortality are syncope, chest pain, ischaemic changes on the ECG and female sex. Cardiac transplantation is the only treatment to offer an improvement in outcome. Arrhythmogenic right ventricular cardiomyopathy is a familial disease which usually affects young adult men. True diagnoses in childhood are exceptional. The disease may present with syncope, or with ventricular tachycardia with left bundle-branch block morphology (that is, right ventricular origin). It may cause death in young athletes and seems to be particularly common in Italy. Risk assessment and therapeutic strategies are not well developed.

The incidence of sudden death in apparently normal children beyond the first year of life is probably around 1–1.5 per 100,000 per year. In addition to the various types of cardiomyopathy and coronary artery abnormalities discussed above, diagnoses first established after death include myocarditis. Exact mode of death in myocarditis is uncertain but it is probably caused by an arrhythmia. In other children, death may remain unexplained after necropsy, but the circumstances may lead to a retrospective presumed diagnosis of a primary cardiac arrhythmia.

Cardiac Arrhythmia (Figs 43.8–43.14, 43.16–43.21 and 43.30)

Primary Cardiac Arrhythmia

Most sudden cardiac deaths that remain unexplained after necropsy are probably caused by primary cardiac arrhythmias. Arrhythmias which are known to be potentially fatal, and which would leave no trace after death include polymorphic ventricular tachycardia in congenital long QT syndrome, other primary ventricular arrhythmias such as those described by Brugada and Coumel, atrial fibrillation in Wolff-Parkinson-White syndrome, and congenital complete atrioventricular block. Retrospective confirmation of an arrhythmia is not possible unless a familial condition (such as long QT syndrome) is subsequently recognised in a family member. This group of arrhythmias also comprises the majority of diagnoses made after resuscitation from out of hospital cardiac arrest.

Congenital Long QT Syndrome

Congenital long QT syndrome is characterised by QT prolongation on the ECG in association with polymorphic ventricular tachycardia, and may affect as many as one child in 7,000. It is usually amenable to treatment with a blocker, but some patients require pacemaker or defibrillator implantation. It is difficult to establish the overall mortality risk as death may be the first symptom, but 8% of 287 patients reported by the Pediatric Electrophysiology Society died suddenly during a mean follow-up of 5 years. The main predictors of sudden death in that report were extreme QTc prolongation (> 600 ms) and poor compliance with blocker medication. Congenital long QT syndrome has dominant inheritance. Despite this, in the Pediatric Electrophysiology Society report only 39% of children with a clinical diagnosis had a positive family history of long QT syndrome, probably explained either by variable penetrance or because they represent new mutations. Diagnosis in a child should lead to screening of first degree relatives. However, long QT syndrome can be difficult to diagnose or to exclude because of the overlap of QT intervals in gene carriers and in the normal population. Although several gene defects causing long QT syndrome have been identified, genetic analysis is costly and time consuming and the diagnosis remains clinical in most cases. Because a normal phenotype in the presence of an abnormal genotype is associated with a risk of syncope or death, there may be an indication for genetic investigation of family members with apparently normal or borderline ECGs. Acquired long QT syndrome is the term sometimes used to describe QT prolongation seen in metabolic disturbances or with use of pharmacological agents. It may also be familial and may cause arrhythmias and sudden death (Fig. 43.17).

Serious ventricular arrhythmias leading to sudden death

Catecholaminergic ventricular tachycardia, as described by Coumel, has some similarities with long QT syndrome. However, the QT interval is normal and polymorphic ventricular tachycardia is preceded by increasingly complex ventricular arrhythmias including a characteristic bidirectional ventricular tachycardia. The exercise test and ambulatory ECG are often positive and are helpful in making the diagnosis. Treatment with a blocker is usually effective but poor compliance with medication is associated with a high risk of death. Brugada syndrome describes the association of polymorphic ventricular tachycardia or ventricular fibrillation with ST segment elevation in right precordial leads on the ECG. It is a familial condition, usually not causing symptoms until early adult life, and is probably very rare in children. Diagnosis is difficult as the characteristic ECG changes are intermittent and can be very subtle. The only means of preventing sudden death in affected individuals is an implantable defibrillator.

Wolff-Parkinson-White Syndrome (Figs 43.9, 49.10, 49.21)

Wolff-Parkinson-White syndrome is one of the most common causes of arrhythmias in childhood, but sudden deaths are rare. The overall mortality risk is very difficult to quantify but may be around 1.5 per 1,000 patient-years. Sudden death is probably caused by ventricular fibrillation which, in turn, is precipitated by atrial fibrillation in patients with a very short anterograde accessory pathway refractory period. Cardiac arrest and sudden death mainly occur in adolescents and young adults and are very rare in younger children. Resuscitation from cardiac arrest is (perhaps not surprisingly) a strong predictor of risk, but

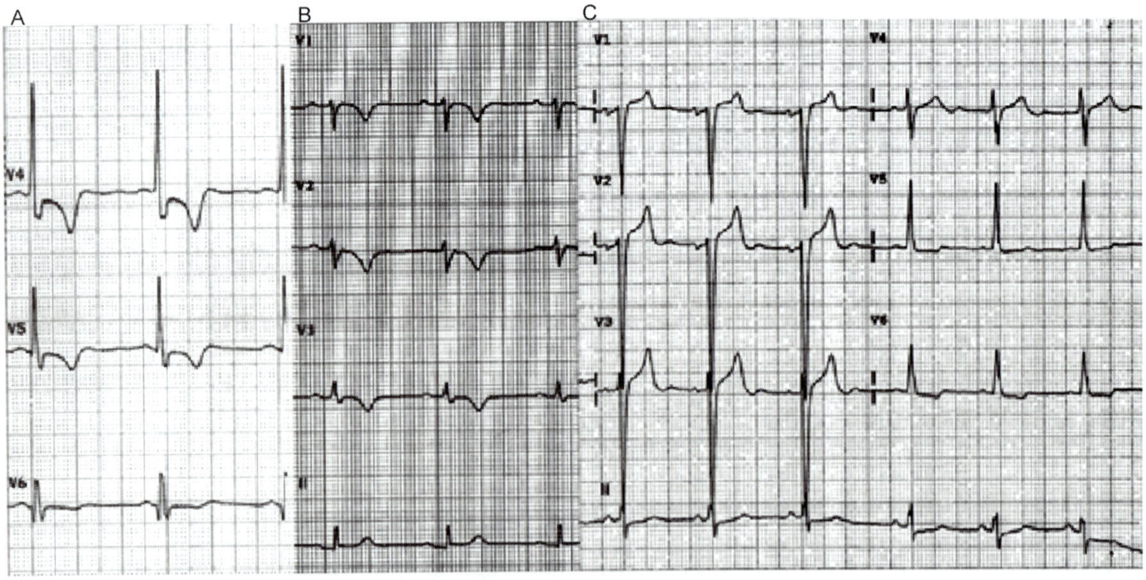

Fig. 43.12: *Patients with inherited cardiomyopathy. (A) Lateral precordial leads of a patient with hypertrophic cardiomyopathy showing Q wave (V6), ST depression, and T wave inversion associated with large voltage QRS complexes. (B) Right precordial leads of a patient with arrhythmogenic right ventricular cardiomyopathy showing epsilon wave (V2), QT prolongation, and T wave inversion. (C) Precordial leads of a patient with dilated cardiomyopathy showing incomplete left bundle-branch block and electrocardiographic left atrial enlargement. These children are at higher risk for sudden cardiac death*

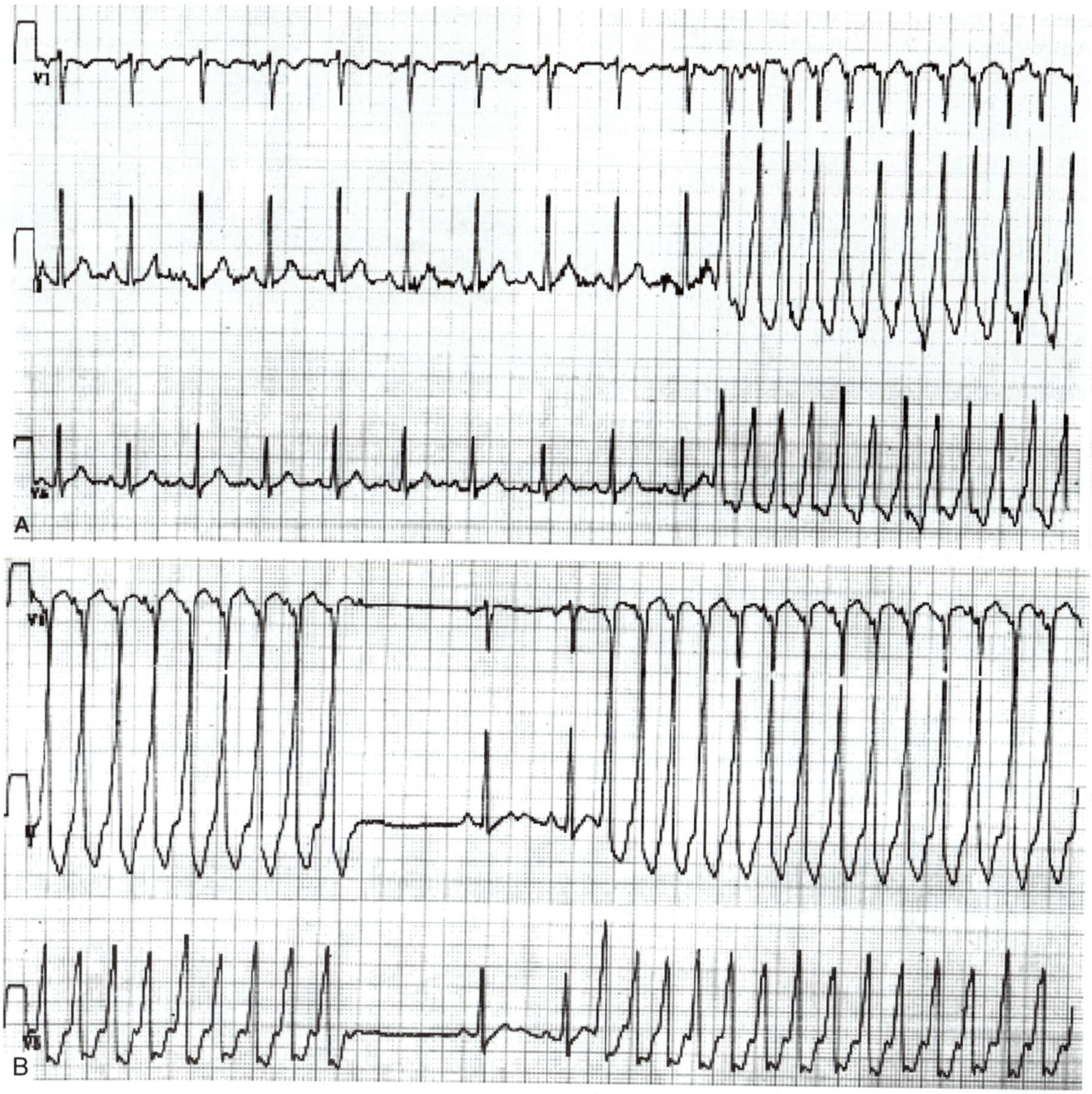

Figs 43.13A and B: *Exercise induced ventricular tachycardia during TMT in an athlete*

syncope and atrial fibrillation have poor predictive value, although they would be indications for catheter ablation in any case. Although a short anterograde refractory period of the accessory pathway is thought to be the best electrophysiological indicator of risk, the predictive value of such a finding is poor. Patients with significant symptoms require treatment, irrespective of any associated small risk, but the role of risk stratification by invasive electrophysiology study in children with few or no symptoms remains unclear.

Sudden Death in Congenital Atrioventricular Block

Congenital complete atrioventricular block affects around one baby in every 20,000. Not all are recognised at birth, or even in infancy. The risk of sudden death is probably mainly related to the ventricular rate. The development of symptoms is an indication for pacemaker implantation, but absence of symptoms in childhood or adult life does not imply absence of risk of sudden death. Risk stratification in asymptomatic patients is imperfect but pacemaker implantation is usually advisable in infants with a resting ventricular rate below 55 per minute, or in children below 50 per minute, especially if there are other arrhythmias or other findings on ambulatory monitoring.

- Long QT syndrome
- Idiopathic long QT syndrome, in which patients have a prolonged QT with a propensity to develop malignant ventricular arrhythmias, is a rare familial disorder.
- Two forms of congenital long QT syndrome have been described.

The Jervell-Lange-Nielsen syndrome, associated with congenital deafness, has an autosomal-recessive pattern of inheritance. **The Romano-Ward syndrome** is not associated with deafness and has an autosomal dominant pattern of inheritance with variable penetration. This syndrome accounts for 90% of long QT syndrome cases. More than 200 mutations in the 7 genes related to long QT syndrome have been found. Among the most common are mutations of *SCN5A* on chromosome 3, the *HERG* gene on chromosome 7, and the *KVLTQT1* gene on chromosome 11. Alteration in the function of a myocellular channel protein that regulates the potassium flux during electrical repolarization is thought to be causative, though in some subsets of long QT syndrome, such as those with mutations in *SCN5A* (long QT3), Na channels are primarily impaired. A relationship with sympathetic nervous system imbalance also appears to exist. The prolongation that occurs makes these patients susceptible to develop a specific form of VT called torsade de pointes.

- The clinical course of patients with long QT syndrome is quite variable, with some patients remaining asymptomatic while others develop torsade de pointes with syncope and sudden death. Symptoms and SCD are more common among homozygous individuals (those with two copies of the mutant allele), compared with heterozygous individuals (who have a single mutant allele). The risk of SCD is impacted by environmental factors such as hypokalemia, medications and the presence of sinus pauses. SCD in these patients also has been associated with emotional extremes, auditory auras or stimulation, and vigorous physical activity. Symptoms usually begin in childhood or adolescence.
- The probability of having congenital long QT syndrome is divided to low, intermediate, and high.

Acquired Long QT Syndrome

- A number of antiarrhythmics (especially class Ia and class III) and other medications, electrolyte abnormalities, cerebrovascular diseases, and altered nutritional states are known to cause QT prolongation and put patients at risk for torsade de pointes. This usually occurs when QT prolongation is associated with a slow heart rate and hypokalemia.

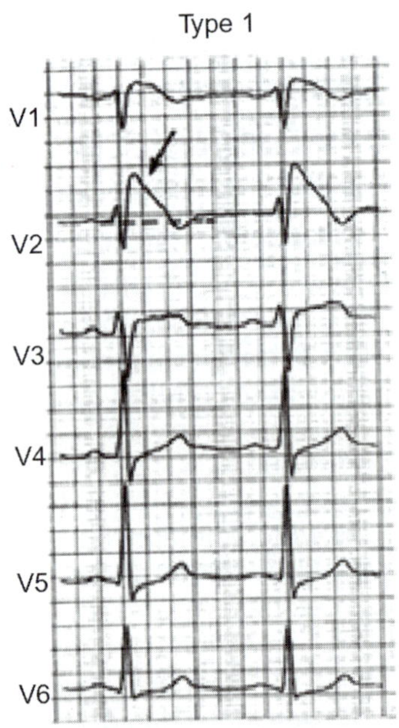

Fig. 43.14: *Precordial ECG leads (25 mm/s; 10 mm/mV) of different ECG patterns in Brugada syndrome. Type I: coved ST segment elevation > in leads VI and V2 (and V3) followed by a negative T wave. Type II: saddleback-type ST segment elevation < 1 mm. Type III: saddleback-type ST segment elevation < 1 mm*

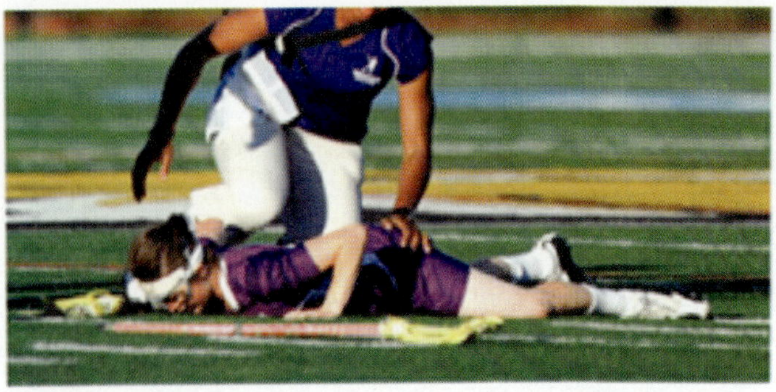

Fig. 43.15: *Athletes trainer saves the life of a teenager in the playing ground*

- The QT interval is prolonged in as many as 32% of patients with intracranial hemorrhage (especially in subarachnoid hemorrhages). Lesions in the hypothalamus are thought to lead to this phenomenon.
  Reports of sudden death due to ventricular arrhythmia in patients with hypocalcemia, hypothyroidism, nutritional deficiencies associated with modified starvation diets, and in patients who are obese and on severe weight-loss programs have been reported.
- Class Ia antiarrhythmic drugs that cause acquired long QT syndrome include quinidine, disopyramide, and procainamide. Class III antiarrhythmic drugs that cause acquired long QT syndrome include sotalol, *N*-acetyl procainamide, bretylium, amiodarone and ibutilide.
- Other drugs that cause acquired long QT syndrome include bepridil, probucol, tricyclic and tetracyclic antidepressants, phenothiazines, haldol, antihistamines (e.g. terfenadine, astemizole), antibiotics (e.g. erythromycin, sulfamethoxazole/trimethoprim), chemotherapeutics (e.g. pentamidine, anthracycline), serotonin antagonists (e.g. ketanserin, zimeldine) and organophosphorus insecticides.

Electrolyte abnormalities that cause acquired long QT syndrome include hypokalemia, hypomagnesemia and hypocalcemia.

Altered nutritional states and cerebrovascular disease that cause acquired long QT syndrome include intracranial and subarachnoid hemorrhages, stroke and intracranial trauma.

- Hypothyroidism and altered autonomic status (e.g. diabetic neuropathy) can cause acquired long QT syndrome.

Short QT syndrome: The short QT syndrome is a newly recognized syndrome, first time described in 2000, which can lead to lethal arrhythmias and SCD. Three mutations in potassium channels have been described that lead to gain of function in potassium channels and shortening of action potential and decreased QT interval (Fig. 43.16).

- To diagnose short QT syndrome, the QTc should be less than 330 msec and tall and peaked T waves should be

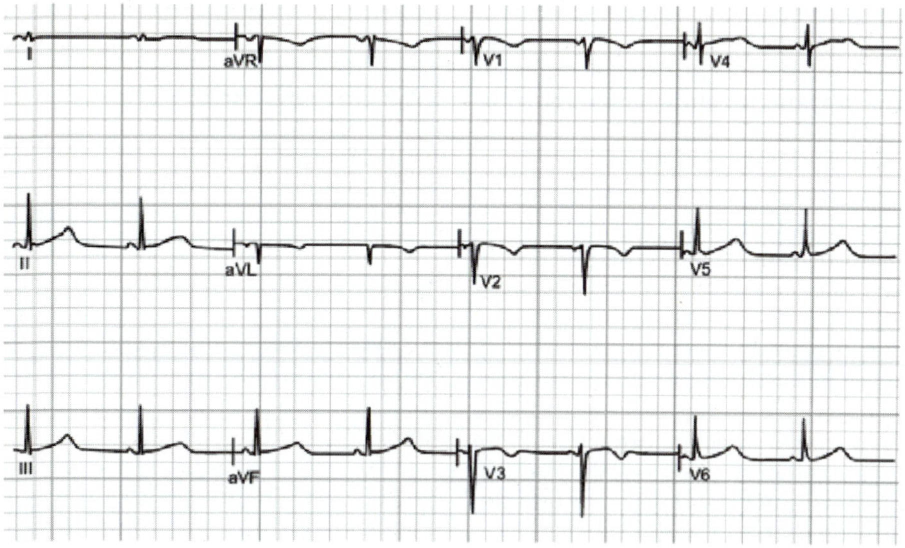

Fig. 43.16: *ECG showing very short QTc (280 ms) with tall, peaked T waves due to congenital short QT syndrome*

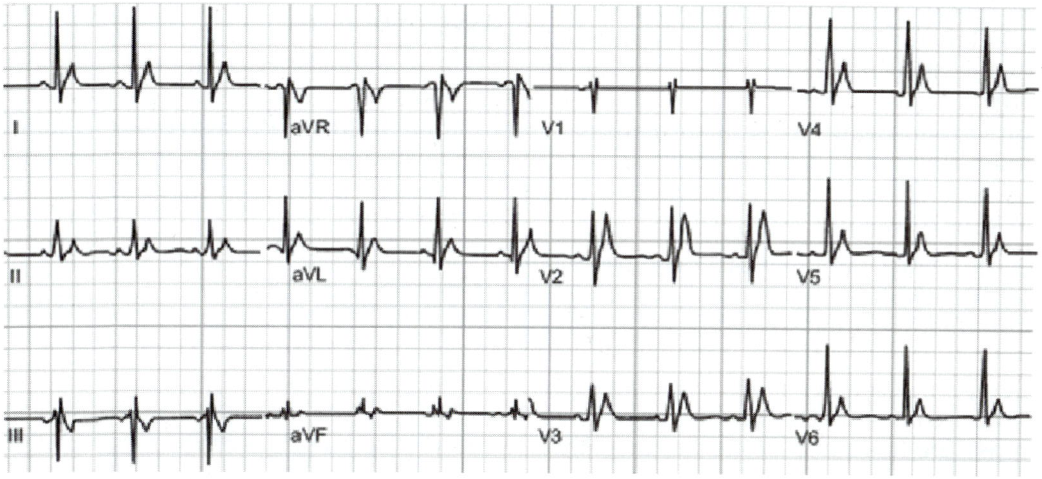

Fig. 43.17: *ECG showing QTc 550ms due to congenital long QT syndrome*

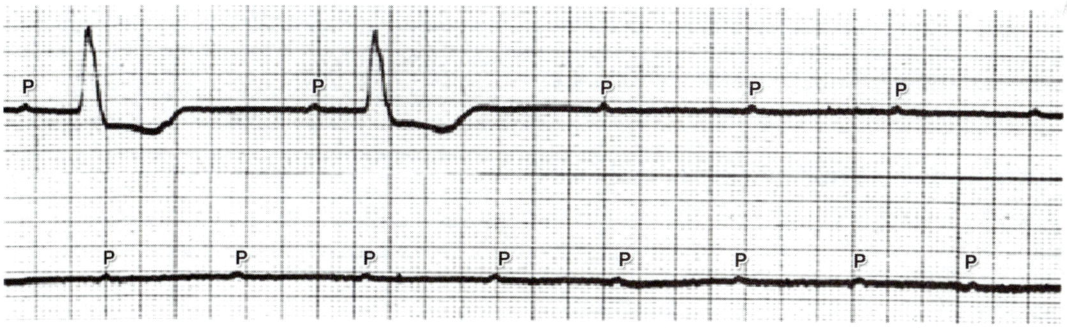

Fig. 43.18: *ECG showing complete A-V dissociation in patient with Stokes-Adam attack*

present. Clinical manifestations are variable from no symptoms, to palpitation due to atrial fibrillation, syncope due to VT, and SCD. VF is easily inducible at electrophysiology study in these patients, and SCD can happen at any age.

- Although antiarrhythmic medications, such as sotalol, ibutilide, and procainamide, have been proposed as a therapy (to prolong the QT), data to support this approach are insufficient at present. ICD placement may be considered to prevent VT and SCD, although T-wave oversensing, resulting in inappropriate ICD discharges, has been problematic.
- **Right ventricular outflow tract ventricular tachycardia:** Right ventricular outflow tract (RVOT) tachycardia is the

most common form of idiopathic VT, comprising 70–80% of all idiopathic VTs. RVOT tachycardia is a rare cause of SCD. It also has been referred to as exercise-induced VT, adenosine-sensitive VT, and repetitive monomorphic VT.

- RVOT tachycardia occurs in patients without structural heart disease and arises from the RV outflow region. Current data suggest that triggered activity is the underlying mechanism of RVOT tachycardia. RVOT tachycardia is believed to be receptor-mediated because exogenous and endogenous adenosine can terminate this process. Maneuvers that increase endogenous acetylcholine also have been demonstrated to antagonize this process.
- Symptoms typical of RVOT tachycardia include palpitations and presyncope or syncope often occurring during or after exercise or emotional stress. VT also can occur at rest. The ECG during VT displays a left bundle-branch block/inferior axis morphology.
- Treatment is based on frequency and severity of symptoms. The first line of therapy is a beta-blocker or calcium channel blocker. Patients with symptoms not relieved by medical therapy are best treated with radiofrequency catheter ablation. Successful ablation is reported in 83–100% of cases.
- Other causes of sudden death: Two major causes of sudden cardiopulmonary death deserve mention.

Sudden Death in Young Athletes (Fig. 43.14)

Deaths during sports attract publicity but they are rare events. Estimates from the USA suggest that 5 per 100,000 young athletes (including children, teenagers, and young adults) have a predisposing condition and that about 10–25 such deaths per year occur in the US population of 260,000,000. The most common structural abnormalities identified at necropsy are hypertrophic cardiomyopathy, coronary artery abnormalities, right ventricular cardiomyopathy and aortic valve stenosis._"Unexplained" cases may be caused by ventricular arrhythmia or atrial fibrillation in Wolff-Parkinson-White syndrome (as discussed above). Health screening programmes are in place for some young athletes but their efficacy has not been prospectively evaluated.

Syncope in Healthy Looking Children (Table 43.2)

Syncope is a frequent problem in childhood. The common causes are benign whereas some rare causes are potentially dangerous. A "simple faint", or vasovagal syncope, is said to occur in up to 15% of the normal population at some time during childhood. Other "vascular" but benign causes of syncope include neurocardiogenic syncope in older children and "pallid syncope" or "reflex asystolic syncope" in younger children. The mechanisms of these may be similar with inappropriate reflex bradycardia and hypotension. In the former syncope is often postural and in the latter a frequent trigger is surprise, minor hurt or frustration. Children or adults with repaired or unoperated congenital heart disease and children with other known heart disease should already be under review in a specialist follow-up clinic. Syncope in such patients may be an indication for urgent reassessment or investigation.

Table 43.2: *Possible ECG abnormalities in children with syncope*

- QT prolongation
- Ventricular preexcitation
- Atrioventricular block
- Left ventricular hypertrophy or ST/T abnormalities in hypertrophic cardiomyopathy
- ST elevation in V1–V3 in Brugada syndrome

Studies that examine children presenting with syncope rarely identify any diagnoses with a significant risk of death because such problems are rare. However, the spectrum of underlying abnormalities in children resuscitated from cardiac arrest is, not surprisingly, very different and more malignant. Diagnoses include various types of cardiomyopathy and substrates for primary arrhythmias including QT prolongation and ventricular preexcitation, all discussed above.

Valvular Disease

- **Aortic stenosis:** Prior to the advent of surgical therapy for valvular heart disease, SCD was fairly common in patients with progressive aortic stenosis. Most aortic stenosis deaths were sudden. In a study by Chizner et al

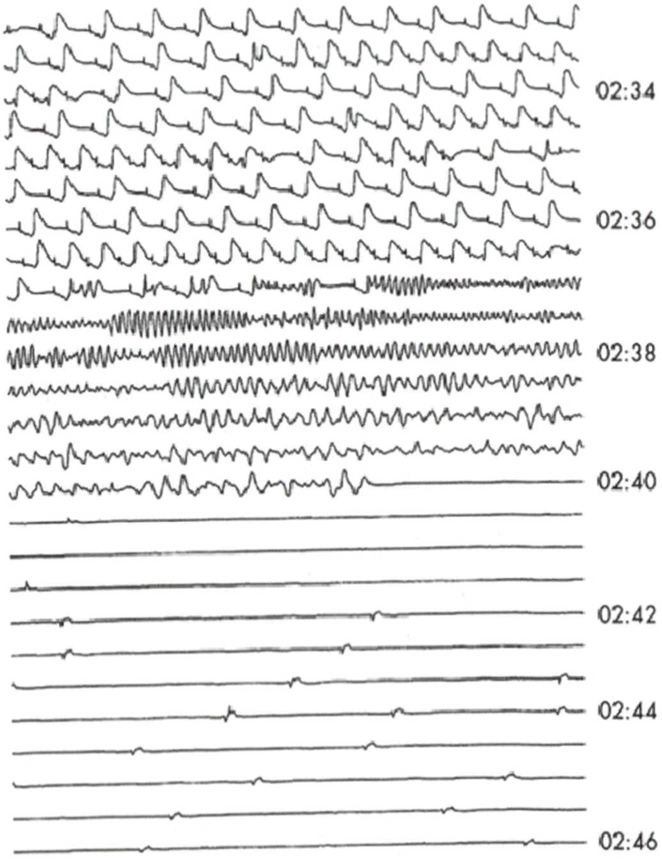

Fig. 43.19: *Sudden death in acquired QT prolongation. The ambulatory recording shows development of polymorphic ventricular tachycardia which degenerates into ventricular fibrillation and then asystole*

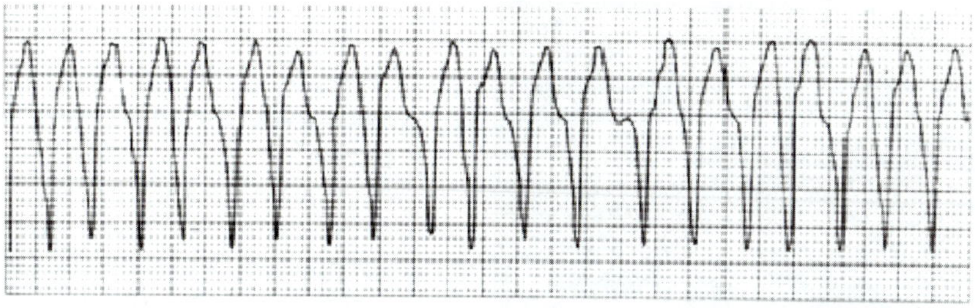

Fig. 43.20: *ECG showing polymorphic ventricular tachycardia*

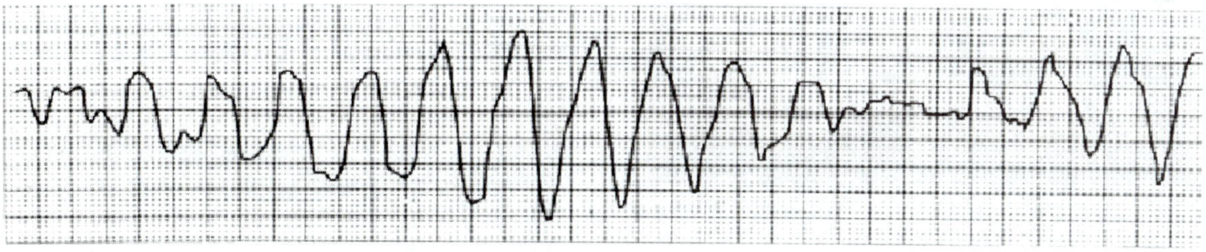

Fig. 43.21: *ECG showing atrial fibrillation in W-P-W syndrome with irregular QRS complexes*

of 42 patients who had isolated aortic stenosis and did not undergo valve replacement, as many as 56% of deaths were sudden at 5 years of follow-up. Of these 42 patients, 32 were symptomatic and 10 were asymptomatic. The mechanism of sudden death is unclear, and both malignant ventricular arrhythmia and bradyarrhythmia have been documented (Fig. 43.22).

The incidence of SCD has decreased significantly with advent of aortic valve replacement. However, it still accounts for the second most common cause of death postoperatively in this population and especially in those with prosthetic and heterograft aortic valve replacement. The incidence of SCD after aortic valve surgery is highest

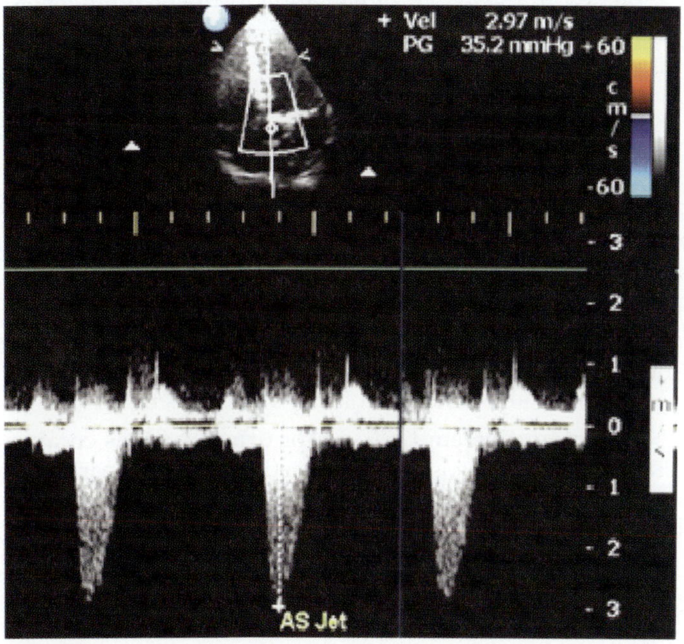

Fig. 43.22: *Color flow-guided evaluation of aortic stenosis jet from apical five chamber view with continuous wave Doppler interrogation*

in the first 3 weeks after the procedure and then plateaus at 6 months of follow-up.

- **Other valvular lesions:** The risk of SCD is much lower in other valvular diseases compared with aortic stenosis. Aortic insufficiency usually presents with signs of heart failure and progressive LV dilatation. As part of this process reentrant or automatic ventricular foci may develop and ultimately lead to a symptomatic ventricular arrhythmia.

After valve replacement, LV wall tension can be expected to reduce and the risk of arrhythmia can be expected to decrease.

- **Mitral stenosis** is becoming increasingly uncommon in the United States because of widespread use of antibiotics in primary streptococcal infections. SCD due to mitral stenosis is very rare (Fig. 43.23).
- The incidence of SCD is low in patients with mitral valve prolapse (MVP). MVP has a 5–7% incidence in the general population. In clinically significant MVP, the risk of SCD seems to rise along with total mortality. Kligfield et al estimated that the incidence of sudden death varies with the presence of symptoms and the severity of mitral regurgitation. Ventricular tachyarrhythmias are the most frequent arrhythmia in patients with SCD. Risk factors for SCD to consider in these patients include a family history of SCD, echocardiographic evidence of a redundant mitral valve, repolarization abnormalities, and lengthening of the corrected QT interval (>420 ms in women and >450 ms in men).
- **Congenital heart disease:** In the pediatric and adolescent age groups, SCD occurs with an incidence of 1.3–8.5 cases per 100,000 patients annually, accounting for approximately 5% of all deaths in this group. The causes of SCD are much more diverse in children than adults. In reviewing 13 studies involving 61 children and adolescents with SCD, Driscoll found 50% of cases were due to HCM; 25% were due to anomalous origin of the left coronary

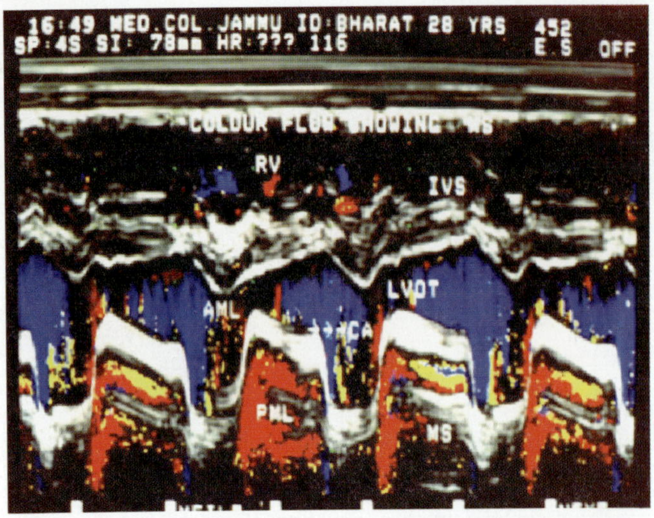

Fig. 43.23: *Color flow M-mode showing markedly thickened anterior and posterior mitral leaflets with paradoxical movement of posterior leaflet in patient with rheumatic mitral native valvular stenosis along with dilated and hypertrophied RV*

artery; and the remaining patients had aortic stenosis, cystic medial necrosis, and sinus node artery obstruction. The following is a classification of SCD in the pediatric population:

In patients with known, previously recognized (including repaired) heart disease, congenital causes of SCD include the following:

Tetralogy of Fallot

Transposition of the great arteries

- Fontan operation
- Aortic stenosis ·

Marfan syndrome

- Mitral valve prolapse
- Hypoplastic left heart syndrome

Eisenmenger syndrome

Congenital heart block

- Ebstein anomaly
- In patients with known, previously recognized (including repaired) heart disease.

Acquired causes of SCD include the following:

- Kawasaki syndrome
  DCM or myocarditis
  In patients with previously unrecognized heart disease who have structural heart disease.
- HCM
- Congenital coronary artery abnormalities
- Arrhythmogenic RV dysplasia
- In patients with previously unrecognized heart disease who do not have structural heart disease.
- Long QT syndrome
- WPW syndrome
- Primary VT and VF
- Primary pulmonary hypertension.

Commotio cordis: Traumatic blow to the chest wall (e.g. from a hockey puck or baseball) causing VT/VF and SCD in the absence of significant identifiable trauma.

- The predominant mechanism is ventricular arrhythmias. In tetralogy of Fallot after postoperative correction of the anomaly, as many as 10% of these patients have VT and the incidence of sudden death is 2–3%. In the Fontan procedure, i.e. to correct a physiologic single ventricle, even atrial arrhythmias can cause severe hemodynamic compromise and arrhythmic death. Patients who develop secondary pulmonary hypertension (Eisenmenger syndrome), despite attempted correction of the anatomic defects, have a very poor prognosis. The terminal event may be bradycardia or VT progressing to VF.
- ***Primary electrophysiologic abnormalities:*** This generally represents a group of abnormalities in which patients have no apparent structural heart disease but have a primary electrophysiologic abnormality that predisposes them to VT or VF. Some imaging techniques have detected abnormal sympathetic neural function in these patients. An ECG study can provide clues to the diagnosis; consider a familial component to these conditions.
- **Pulmonary embolism** is a frequent cause of sudden death in people at risk. Risk factors include previous personal or family history of deep venous thromboembolism, malignancy, hypercoagulable states, and recent mechanical trauma such as hip or knee surgery.
- **Aortic dissection or aneurysmal rupture** is the other major cause of out-of-hospital nonarrhythmic cardiovascular death. Predisposing factors for aortic dissection include genetic deficiencies of collagen such as Marfan syndrome, Ehlers-Danlos syndrome, and aortic cystic medial necrosis (Figs 43.24 and 43.25).

Laboratory Studies

Cardiac enzymes (creatine kinase, myoglobin, troponin): Elevations in these enzyme levels may indicate ischemia and MI. The extent of myocardial damage usually can be correlated to the extent of elevation in the enzyme levels. Patients are at increased risk for arrhythmia in the peri-infarct period.

Electrolytes, calcium, and magnesium: Severe metabolic acidosis, hypokalemia, hyperkalemia, hypocalcemia and hypomagnesemia are some of the conditions that can increase the risk for arrhythmia and sudden death.

Quantitative drug levels (quinidine, procainamide, tricyclic antidepressants, digoxin): Drug levels higher than the levels indicated in the therapeutic index may have a proarrhythmic effect. Subtherapeutic levels of these drugs in patients being treated for specific cardiac conditions also can lead to an increased risk for arrhythmia. Most of the antiarrhythmia medications also have a proarrhythmic effect.

Toxicology screen: Looking for drugs, such as cocaine, that can lead to vasospasm-induced ischemia is warranted if suspicion exists. Obtaining levels of drugs (antiarrhythmics) also may be warranted.

Thyroid-stimulating hormone: Hyperthyroidism can lead to tachycardia and tachyarrhythmias. Over a period of time, it also can lead to heart failure.

- **Brain natriuretic peptide (BNP):** BNP has predictive value especially in post-MI patients and in patients with

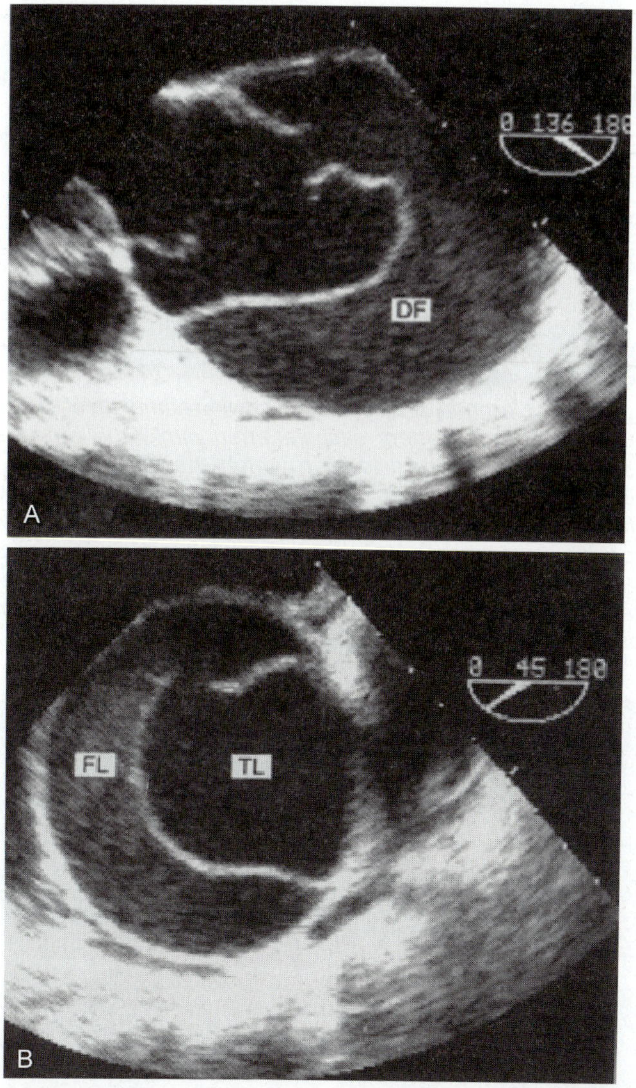

Fig. 43.24: *(A) Transesophageal echocardiography of dissection flap (DF). (B) In cross-section the true lumen (TL) and false lumen (FL) can be seen*

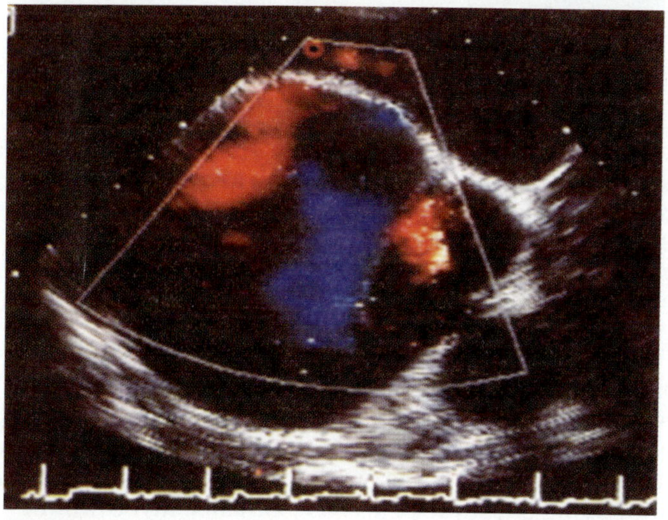

Fig. 43.25: *TEE scan showing dissection of ascending aorta in patient with hypertension admitted in emergency department with acute chest pain*

HF. Although preliminary and not conclusive, emerging data support the notion that an elevated BNP level may provide prognostic information on the risk of SCD, independent of clinical information and LVEF.

Imaging Studies in Sudden Cardiac Death

- **Chest X-ray:** This may reveal whether someone is in congestive heart failure. It also can show signs of LV hypertrophy or RV hypertrophy. Signs of pulmonary hypertension also may be evident on the chest X-ray.
- **Echocardiography:** Two dimensional echocardiography with Doppler is essential in the evaluation of SCD. A number of studies have demonstrated that the use of two dimensional echocardiogram to evaluate left wall motion abnormalities after an acute MI (using the LV wall-motion score index) is useful in predicting the risk for major cardiac events, including sudden death. A decrease in the ejection fraction and worsening wall motion abnormalities upon exercise echocardiography in patients who have had an MI has been suggested to confer increased risk of cardiac death.

Nuclear imaging techniques: Resting thallium or technetium-99m scintigraphy is helpful in assessing myocardial damage after MI. A larger defect has been associated with greater risk for future cardiac events. Exercise nuclear scintigraphy is very sensitive when detecting the presence, extent, and location of myocardial ischemia. Gibson et al found that pharmacologic-stress nuclear (dipyridamole or adenosine) scintigraphy was better than submaximal exercise ECG and coronary

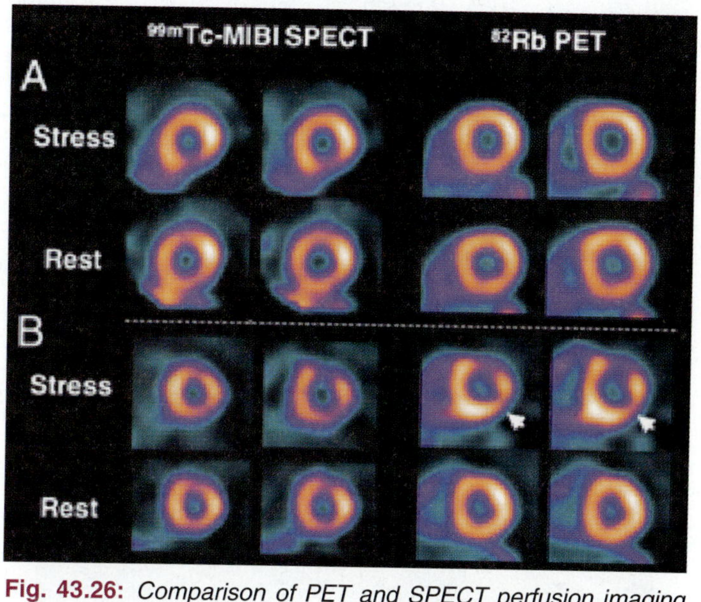

Fig. 43.26: *Comparison of PET and SPECT perfusion imaging shown are matched, representative short-axis slices for single-photon emission computed tomography (SPECT) (left) and positron emission tomography (PET) (right) in 2 subjects with suspected coronary artery disease. Panel A illustrates improved specificity with PET. A fixed defect in the inferior wall on SPECT is absent on PET, suggesting the presence of a SPECT attenuation artefact. Panel B illustrates improved sensitivity with PET. Stress-induced perfusion defects in the anterior and inferolateral walls (arrows) are more clearly shown with PET versus SPECT*

angiography in predicting cardiac death and other cardiac events. These tests can be very helpful in patients with low functional capacity such as chronic obstructive pulmonary disease, peripheral vascular disease, or orthopedic problems. The Multi-Center Post-Infarction Research Group provided evidence that resting ejection fraction was the most important noninvasive predictor of SCD and other cardiac events in patients with MI (Fig. 43.26).

Other Tests

Electrocardiogram: This study is indicated in all patients. Evidence of MI, prolonged QT interval, short QT interval, epsilon wave, Brugada sign, short PR, a WPW pattern, or other conditions should be sought (Fig. 43.27).

- Signal-averaged ECG (SAECG) has been variably reported to be useful in analysis of patients with SCD. What appears to be more useful is analysis of T wave alternans in patients with VT, VF, and/or SCD. Small changes in T amplitude are not detected in 12-lead ECG. Microvolt T wave alternans (MTWA) amplifies the alternans and may be used in the workup to predict the risk of SCD.
- **Genetic testing:** The value of genetic testing in conditions such as congenital long QT and HCM is still being evaluated. Some studies have recommended the testing of siblings and close relatives of people with SCD due to these conditions.

Procedures (Figs 43.28 and 43.29): *Coronary angiography:* Perform cardiac catheterization in patients who survive SCD to assess the state of ventricular function and the severity and extent of CAD. The number of vessels with severe obstruction and the degree of LV dysfunction are important variables in predicting cardiac events. Ejection fraction is the best predictor of significant cardiac events and survival (Figs 43.28 and 43.29).

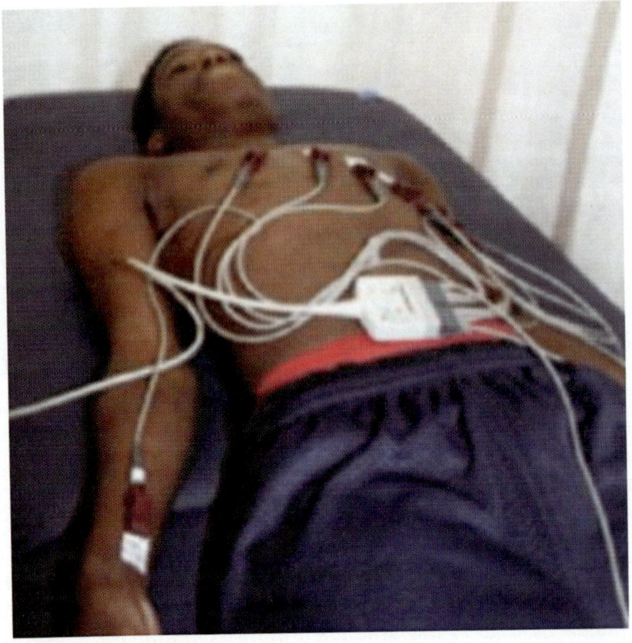

Fig. 43.27: *ECG test is underway for screening of athlete for SCD*

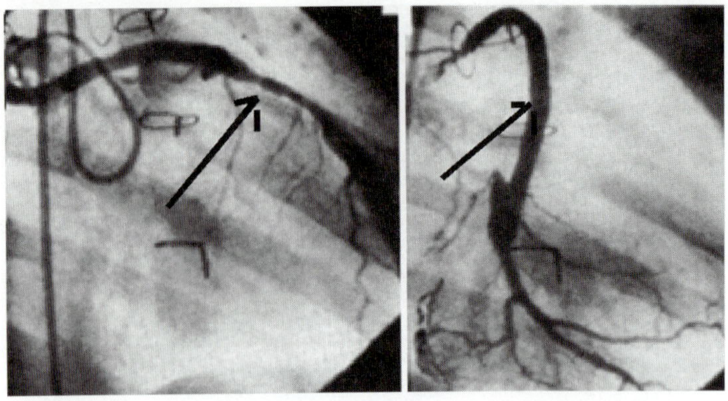

Fig. 43.28: *Coronary arteriograms showing complete obstruction of the right coronary artery, saccular aneurysm of the left anterior descending coronary artery, in which the distal site of the aneurysm is narrowed, and narrowing of the most proximal portion of the left circumflex coronary artery; a left ventriculogram showed hypokinesis of the inferior aspect of the left ventricular wall and an ejection fraction of 60% (left), ACBG was perfonned 5 years after the onset of the illness, and postoperatively, the bypass graft was arteriographically patent (right)*

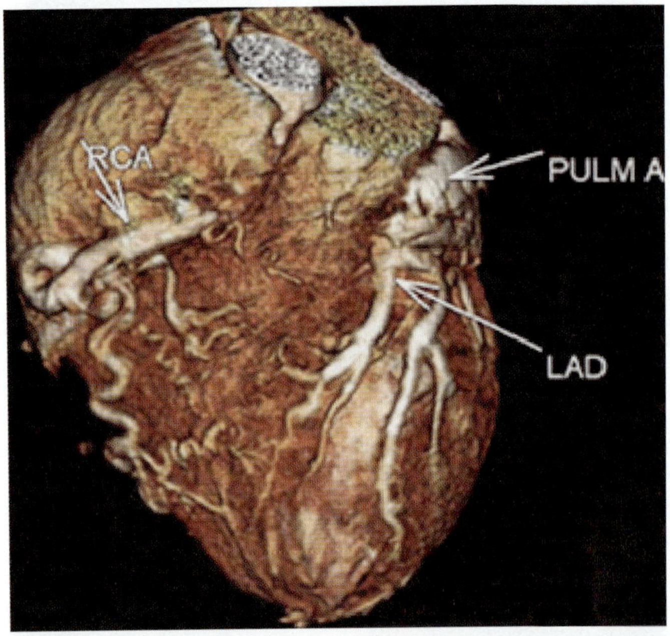

Fig. 43.29: *CT angiography volume rendered image. Right coronary artery is dilated and tortious with a large number of collaterals feeding the left coronary system. Left coronary artery is emerging from pulmonary artery trunk. The left anterior descending artery and their diagonal branches are also dilated and tortuous*

Coronary angiography also can help to identify coronary anomalies and other forms of congenital heart disease. Angiography is performed with the aim of identifying patients who may benefit from revascularization. Revascularization is the single greatest treatment for the underlying substrate of VT/VF, ischemic myocardium.

- **Electrophysiology studies:** In targeted patients, EPS play diagnostic, prognostic, and therapeutic roles. EPS usually are performed after ischemic and structural heart disease has been diagnosed and addressed. These studies have been used to identify patients who have inducible versus noninducible sustained monomorphic VT. The presence of inducible sustained VT, at baseline or when the patient is on antiarrhythmic medications, confers a higher risk for sudden death. Significantly, lower ventricular function also has been observed in patients with inducible sustained VT. Inducible bundle-branch reentrant VT can be seen in patients with DCM and in the postoperative period after valvular replacement. As many as 20% of patients with HCM have inducible sustained monomorphic VT. The identification of accessory pathways also is possible with these studies. EPS are performed with an eye toward the following:

- Ablation of VT foci, e.g. bundle branch VT, RVOT VT, and some cases of idiopathic LV tachycardia.
- **ICD implantation,** which generally is the case in survivors of SCD (Figs 43.30 and 43.31).

Medical Care

- Advanced cardiac life support (ACLS): In the event of cardiac arrest, the immediate implementation of ACLS guidelines is indicated. Widespread interest in improving rates of public ACLS training with a special emphasis on use of early defibrillation by public service personnel (e.g. police, fire, airline attendants) exists. Through these measures, the greatest public health benefits can be achieved in the fight against sudden death.

Medical stabilization: Careful postresuscitative care is essential to survival because studies have shown a 50% repeat in-hospital arrest rate for people admitted after an SCD event. Treatment of myocardial ischemia, heart failure, and electrolyte disturbances are all justified by the results of multiple acute MI and CHF randomized trials. Empiric beta-blockers are reasonable in many circumstances because of favorable properties Empiric antiarrhythmics including amiodarone, should not supersede ICD implantation unless control of recurrent VT is needed while the patient is in the hospital.

Surgical Care

- **Radiofrequency ablation:** Radiofrequency ablation, now routinely available, may be indicated for patients with atrioventricular bypass tracts, bundle-branch block VT, RVOT VT, idiopathic LV tachycardia, and more rare forms of automatic foci VT. Unfortunately, most cases of SCD are not amenable to radiofrequency ablation and require ICD implantation. Radiofrequency ablation may be useful in the treatment of patients with SCD who experience frequent recurrent VT/VF after ICD placement, especially those who require frequent defibrillation.
- Several multicenter trials examining the prophylactic use of cardioverter defibrillator therapy in patients at high risk for SCD have been performed.
- The annual SCD rate in patients with these devices has been reduced from 25% to 1–2%. Studies have shown that in patients at high risk in whom electrophysiologic-

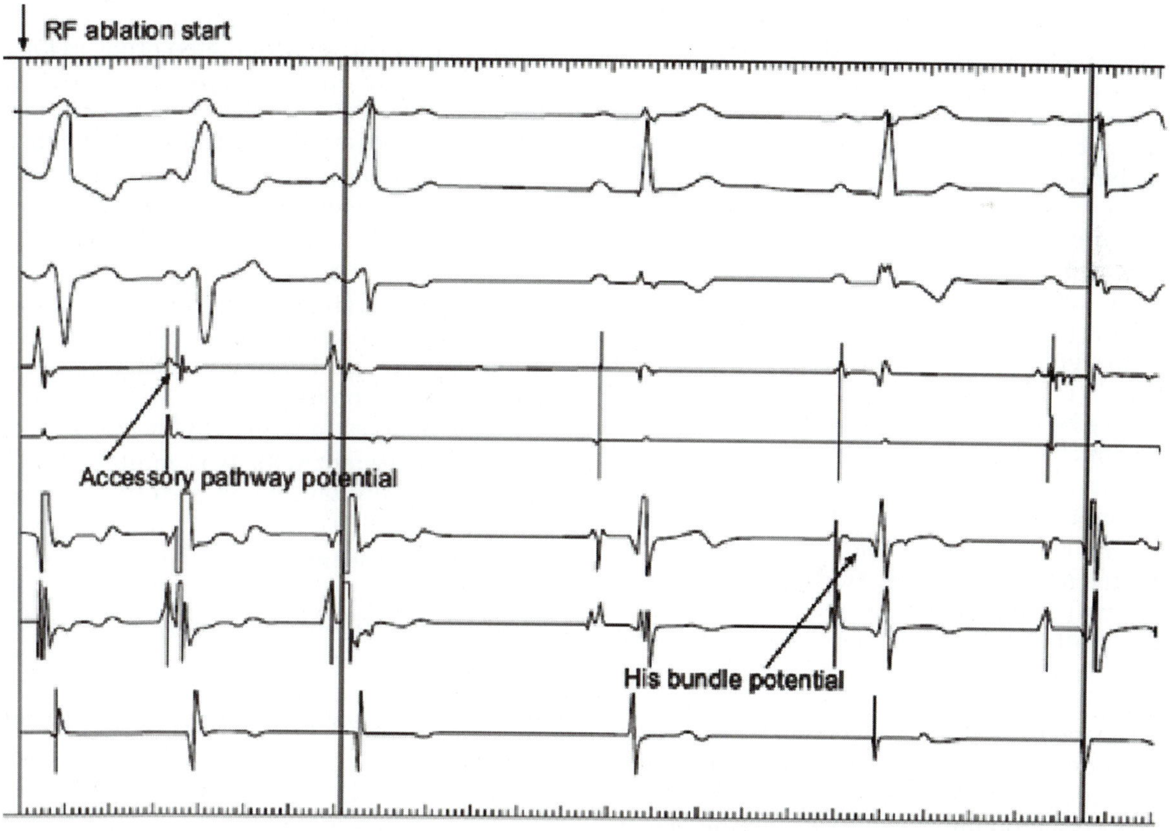

Fig. 43.30: *EPS shows accessory pathway potential and local AV fusion at successful RF ablation site with loss of preexcitation and return of normal HV interval*

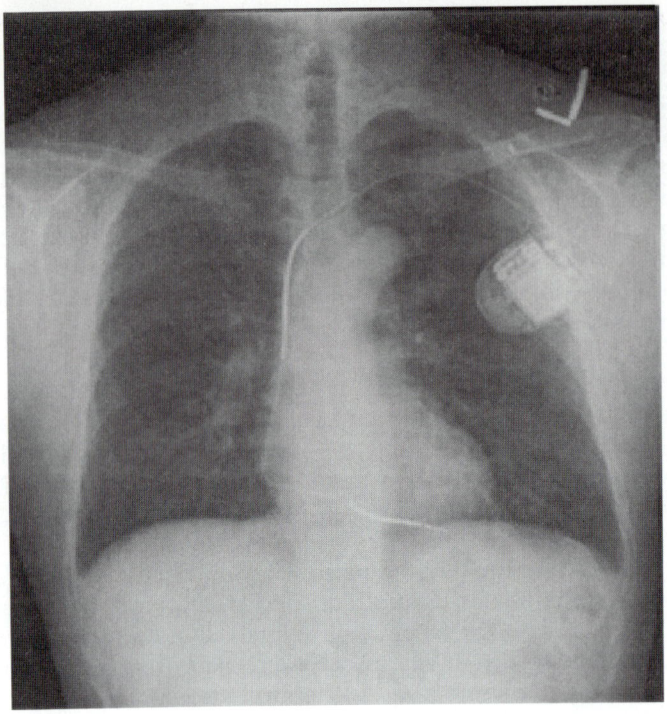

Fig. 43.31: *Photograph of X-ray chest (PA) view showing implanted ICD in a patient with drug resistant ventricular tachycardia*

guided therapy with antiarrhythmics has failed. ICD placement is beneficial. In several studies comparing ICD placement to antiarrhythmic therapy in patients with VT and/or prior cardiac arrest, ICD placement has been shown to be associated with decreased mortality.

- The use of ICDs as primary prevention for SCD is now standard care for anyone with LVEF less than 35%. Newer ICDs have pacing capabilities and have addressed bradyarrhythmias either causing or complicating VT or VF.
- Cardiac surgery can be a primary treatment for SCD via a variety of strategies.
- Surgical treatment in patients with ventricular arrhythmias and ischemic heart disease includes coronary artery bypass grafting (CABG). The CASS study illustrated that patients with significant CAD and operable vessels who underwent CABG had a decrease in the incidence of sudden death when compared to patients on conventional medical treatment. The reduction was most evident in patients who had three-vessel disease and CHF.

Surgical treatment of ventricular arrhythmias in patients with nonischemic heart disease includes excision of VT foci after endocardial mapping and excision of LV aneurysms. This is performed with decreasing frequency because of perioperative mortality and the alternative, transvenous ICD implantation.

- Aortic valve replacement is associated with improved outcome in patients with hemodynamically significant valvular stenosis and well-preserved ventricular function. In patients with MVP associated with significant valvular regurgitation and LV dysfunction, malignant tachyarrhythmias and SCD have been reported. These patients are candidates for mitral valve replacement.
- Orthotopic heart transplantation is indicated in cases of SCD and refractory heart failure in which significant improvement in actuarial survival is expected. Given a limited donor service, this form of treatment is expected to be beneficial for very few people who survive SCD.
- Patients with long QT syndrome who do not respond to beta-blockers are candidates for ICD implantation or high thoracic left sympathectomy.

Diet

- Patients with CAD are advised to follow a diet low in fat and cholesterol. Patients with severe heart failure should monitor their fluid and sodium intake. Medications are prescribed on an individual basis, depending on the underlying cause of SCD.

Transfer

- Patients should be at centers where intensive cardiac monitoring and appropriate invasive and noninvasive studies can be performed. In general, a cardiovascular service including interventional cardiology, electrophysiology, and cardiac surgery, is needed.

Prognosis

- Prognosis of morbidity and mortality for people who have had SCD can be made using the cardiac arrest score developed by McCullough and Thompson. The detection of the underlying cause of SCD and available treatment options play an important role in the natural history and prognosis of SCD.
- SCD is a frequently encountered problem for emergency physicians, internists and cardiologists. Ischemic cardiomyopathy in all adult cases and HCM in pediatric and adolescent cases are at the top of the differential diagnosis.
- **The clinical course**, once the patient is resuscitated, largely is predicted by the ED presentation of hemodynamic stability, early neurologic recovery, and the duration of the resuscitation.
- Patients who survive the initial phases require a systematic evaluation of LV performance, myocardial perfusion, and electrophysiologic instability. Survivors of SCD have a recurrence rate on the order of 20–25% per year, making ICD implantation important in the majority of patients.
- **Modern treatment with ICD implantation** has saved lives and likely will be an area of continued clinical growth (Fig. 43.31).
- **Preventive measures,** at their roots, are measures of CAD prevention. Efforts to inform and train the public about external defibrillator use likely will have the greatest public health impact on improving survival rates of SCD.

Population Screening for Unsuspected Heart Disease

The infrequency of prodromal symptoms and the absence of physical signs in children who die suddenly and are found at necropsy to have a cardiac problem may seem to be an indication for screening of the general population. However, there is no evidence that population screening

Box 1: Sudden death in children and adolescents: key points

- Sudden death accounts for about 10% of all deaths in children
- Structural cardiac abnormalities that may cause sudden death in apparently normal children include hypertrophic cardiomyopathy, other cardiomyopathies, and coronary artery malformations
- The operations with the most significant risk of late sudden death are the Senning or Mustard operations for transposition of the great arteries and repair of tetralogy of Fallot
- At least one sudden death in six remains unexplained—an age specific incidence of around 1 in 200,000 per year
- Deaths which remain unexplained after necropsy are probably caused by primary cardiac arrhythmias, such as those in long QT syndrome, other primary ventricular arrhythmias, Wolff-Parkinson-White syndrome, and congenital atrioventricular block

of children for abnormalities such as hypertrophic cardiomyopathy is either feasible or appropriate, and no evidence that either early detection or treatment in the absence of symptoms has any effect on outcome. The only prospective population wide screening programme of normal children has been undertaken in Tokyo. The reported prevalence of hypertrophic cardiomyopathy is around 1 in 15,000 and those children identified seemed to be at particularly low risk. The programme does also detect children with long QT syndrome, atrioventricular block, and Wolff-Parkinson-White syndrome by routine ECG but these problems are rare. So far, it has not been possible to show that screening prevents sudden death.

Conclusion

Many children who suffer sudden cardiac death are already known to have a heart problem. Many of these have had surgery for congenital heart disease and the risk of sudden death in such patients probably increases with time. The risks for such patients are probably decreasing with better and earlier surgical repair, but prospective identification of individuals at significant risk remains an elusive goal. In some children who die suddenly, the necropsy reveals the cause of death. In others, who are apparently normal, the likely cause is a primary cardiac arrhythmia. Only a minority of children who die suddenly have previously experienced syncope.

Most children who experience syncope are not at risk of sudden death. Worrying features which would be an indication for investigation include syncope during or immediately after exercise, collapse in a swimming pool, a family history of premature sudden death or of potentially life-threatening cardiac problems, and abnormalities on clinical examination or ECG.

Several potentially fatal conditions are genetic in origin but unfortunately, at present, many of them are easier to confirm than to exclude. For instance, an echocardiogram during childhood cannot rule out the possibility of later manifestation of hypertrophic cardiomyopathy; some gene carriers of long QT syndrome have normal ECGs and yet 2.5% of normal children have a QT interval above the "upper limit of normal"; and the characteristic ECG appearances of Brugada syndrome are intermittent. For the moment, identification of these conditions remains a clinical problem but in the future they will probably be simple genetic diagnoses. Some of the clinical management dilemmas, however, will probably remain.

BIBLIOGRAPHY

1. Molander N. Sudden natural death in later childhood and adolescence. Arch Dis Child 1982;57:572–6.
2. Driscoll DJ, Edwards WD. Sudden unexpected death in children and adolescents. J Am Coll Cardiol1985;5:118B–21B.
3. Neuspiel DR, Kuller LH. Sudden and unexpected natural death in childhood and adolescence. JAMA1985;254:1321–5.
4. Wren C, O'Sullivan JJ, Wright C. Sudden death in children and adolescents. Heart 2000;83:410–3.
5. Walsh CK, Krongrad E. Terminal cardiac electrical activity in pediatric patients. Am J Cardiol1983;51:557–61.
6. Berul CI. Neonatal long QT syndrome and sudden cardiac death. Prog Pediatr Cardiol 2001;11:47–54.
7. Silka MJ, Hardy BG, Menashe VD, et al. A population-based prospective evaluation of risk of sudden cardiac death after operation for common congenital heart defects. J Am Coll Cardiol 1998;32:245–51.
8. Harrison DA, Connelly M, Harris L, et al. Sudden cardiac death in the adult with congenital heart disease. Can J Cardiol 1996;12:1161–3.
9. Wren C. Late postoperative arrhythmias. In: Wren C, Campbell RWF, eds. Paediatric cardiac arrhythmias. Oxford: Oxford University Press, 1996:238–59.
10. Saul JP, Alexander ME. Preventing sudden death after repair of tetralogy of Fallot: complex therapy for complex patients. J Cardiovasc Electrophysiol 1999;10:1271–87.
11. Gatzoulis MA, Balaji S, Webber SA, et al. Risk factors for arrhythmia and sudden cardiac death late after repair of tetralogy of Fallot: a multicentre study. Lancet 2000;356:975–81.
12. Watkins H. Sudden death in hypertrophic cardiomyopathy. N Engl J Med 2000;342:422–4.
13. McKenna WJ, Behr ER. Hypertrophic cardiomyopathy: management, risk stratification, and prevention of sudden death. Heart 2002;87:169–76.
14. Vincent GM. Role of DNA testing for diagnosis, management, and genetic screening in long QT syndrome, hypertrophic cardiomyopathy, and Marfan syndrome. Heart 2001;86:12–4.
15. Corrado D, Basso C, Thiene G. Arrhythmogenic right ventricular cardiomyopathy: diagnosis, prognosis and treatment. Heart 2000;83:588–95.
16. Maron BJ, Shirani J, Poliac LC, et al. Sudden death in young competitive athletes. JAMA1996;276:199andndash;204.
17. Garson A Jr, Dick M, Fournier A, et al. The long QT syndrome children. An international study of 287 patients. Circulation 1993;87:1866–72.
18. Liberthson RR. Sudden death from cardiac causes in children and young adults. N Engl J Med1996;334:1039–44.
19. McLeod KA. Dizziness and syncope in adolescence. Heart 2001;86:350andndash;4.
20. Ino T, Yabuta K, Yamauchi K. Heart disease screening in Japanese children. BMJ 1993;306:1128.

21 Altemose GT, Buxton AE: Idiopathic ventricular tachycardia. Annu Rev Med 1999; 50: 159–77.
22 Anderson KP, Freedman RA, Mason JW: Sudden death in idiopathic dilated cardiomyopathy. Ann Intern Med 1987 Jul; 107(1): 104–6.
23. Antiarrhythmics Versus Implantable Defibrillators Investigators: A comparison of antiarrhythmic-drug therapy with implantable defibrillators in patients resuscitated from near-fatal ventricular arrhythmias. N Engl J Med 1997 Nov 27; 337(22): 1576–83.
24. Bayes de Luna A, Coumel P, Leclercq JF: Ambulatory sudden cardiac death: mechanisms of production of fatal arrhythmia on the basis of data from 157 cases. Am Heart J 1989 Jan; 117(1): 151–9.
25. Belhassen B, Viskin S: Idiopathic ventricular tachycardia and fibrillation. J Cardiovasc Electrophysiol 1993 Jun; 4(3): 356–68.
26. Benditt DG, Pritchett LC, Smith WM, et al: Characteristics of atrioventricular conduction and the spectrum of arrhythmias in Lown-Ganong-Levine syndrome. Circulation 1978 Mar; 57(3): 454–65.
27. Berger S, Dhala A, Friedberg DZ: Sudden cardiac death in infants, children, and adolescents. Pediatr Clin North Am 1999 Apr; 46(2): 221–34.
28. Beta-blocker Heart Attack Research Group: A randomized trial of propranolol in patients with acute myocardial infarction. I. Mortality results. JAMA 1982 Mar 26; 247(12): 1707–14.
29. Bigger JT, Fleiss JL, Kleiger R: The relationships among ventricular arrhythmias, left ventricular dysfunction, and mortality in the 2 years after myocardial infarction. Circulation 1984 Feb; 69(2): 250–8.
30. Bigger JT: Prophylactic use of implanted cardiac defibrillators in patients at high risk for ventricular arrhythmias after coronary-artery bypass graft surgery. Coronary Artery Bypass Graft (CABG) Patch Trial Investigators. N Engl J Med 1997 Nov 27; 337(22): 1569–75.
31. Blackstone EH, Kirklin JW: Death and other time-related events after valve replacement. Circulation 1985 Oct; 72(4): 753–67.
32. Bromberg BI, Lindsay BD, Cain ME: Impact of clinical history and electrophysiologic characterization of accessory pathways on management strategies to reduce sudden death among children with Wolff-Parkinson-White syndrome. J Am Coll Cardiol 1996 Mar 1; 27(3): 690–5.
33. Brugada J, Brugada R, Brugada P: Right bundle-branch block and ST-segment elevation in leads V1 through V3: a marker for sudden death in patients without demonstrable structural heart disease. Circulation 1998 Feb 10; 97(5): 457–60.
34. Brugada P, Brugada J: A distinct clinical and echocardiographic syndrome: right bundle branch block, persistent ST segment elevation with normal QT interval and sudden cardiac death. PACE 1991; 14: 746–51.
35. Brugada R, Hong K, Cordeiro JM: Short QT syndrome. CMAJ 2005; 173(11): 1349–54.
36. Burkart F, Pfisterer M, Kiowski W: Effect of antiarrhythmic therapy on mortality in survivors of myocardial infarction with asymptomatic complex ventricular arrhythmias: Basel Antiarrhythmic Study of Infarct Survival (BASIS). J Am Coll Cardiol 1990 Dec; 16(7): 1711–8.
37. Burke AP, Farb A, Malcom GT: Coronary risk factors and plaque morphology in men with coronary disease who died suddenly. N Engl J Med 1997 May 1; 336(18): 1276–82.
38. Cairns JA, Connolly SJ, Roberts R: Randomised trial of outcome after myocardial infarction in patients with frequent or repetitive ventricular premature depolarisations: CAMIAT. Canadian Amiodarone Myocardial Infarction Arrhythmia Trial Investigators. Lancet 1997 Mar 8; 349(9053): 675–82.
39. Cardiac Arrhythmia Suppression Trial Investigators: Preliminary report: effect of encainide and flecainide on mortality in a randomized trial of arrhythmia suppression after myocardial infarction. N Engl J Med 1989 Aug 10; 321(6): 406–12.
40. Chang D, Goldstein S: Sudden cardiac death in ischemic heart disease. Compr Ther 1997 Feb; 23(2): 95–103.
41. Chizner MA, Pearle DL, deLeon AC: The natural history of aortic stenosis in adults. Am Heart J 1980 Apr; 99(4): 419–24.
42. Corrado D, Basso C, Thiene G: Spectrum of clinicopathologic manifestations of arrhythmogenic right ventricular cardiomyopathy/dysplasia: a multicenter study. J Am Coll Cardiol 1997 Nov 15; 30(6): 1512–20.
43. Davies MJ, Thomas A: Thrombosis and acute coronary-artery lesions in sudden cardiac ischemic death. N Engl J Med 1984 May 3; 310(18): 1137–40.
44. Davies MJ: The investigation of sudden cardiac death. Histopathology 1999 Feb; 34(2): 93–8.
45. de Vreede-Swagemakers JJ, Gorgels AP, Dubois-Arbouw WI: Out-of-hospital cardiac arrest in the 1990's: a population-based study in the Maastricht area on incidence, characteristics and survival. J Am Coll Cardiol 1997 Nov 15; 30(6): 1500–5.
46. DeRose JJ, Banas JS, Winters SL: Current perspectives on sudden cardiac death in hypertrophic cardiomyopathy. Prog Cardiovasc Dis 1994 May-Jun; 36(6): 475–84.
47. Domanski MJ, Zipes DP, Schron E: Treatment of sudden cardiac death. Current understandings from randomized trials and future research directions. Circulation 1997 Jun 17; 95(12): 2694–9.
48. Doval HC, Nul DR, Grancelli HO: Nonsustained ventricular tachycardia in severe heart failure. Independent marker of increased mortality due to sudden death. GESICA- GEMA Investigators. Circulation 1996 Dec 15; 94(12): 3198–203.
49. Doyle JT, Kannel WB, McNamara PM: Factors related to suddenness of death from coronary disease: combined Albany-Framingham studies. Am J Cardiol 1976 Jun; 37(7): 1073–8.
50. Driscoll DJ, Edwards WD: Sudden unexpected death in children and adolescents. J Am Coll Cardiol 1985 Jun; 5(6 Suppl): 118B–121B.
51. Echt DS, Liebson PR, Mitchell LB: Mortality and morbidity in patients receiving encainide, flecainide, or placebo. The Cardiac Arrhythmia Suppression Trial. N Engl J Med 1991 Mar 21; 324(12): 781–8.
52. Ehtisham J, Watkins H: Is Wolff-Parkinson-White syndrome a genetic disease? J Cardiovasc Electrophysiol 2005; 16(11): 1258–62.
53. Garson A, McNamara DG: Sudden death in a pediatric cardiology population, 1958 to 1983: relation to prior arrhythmias. J Am Coll Cardiol 1985 Jun; 5(6 Suppl): 134B–137B.
54. Gillum RF: Sudden coronary death in the United States: 1980–1985. Circulation 1989 Apr; 79(4): 756–65.
55. Gillum RF: Coronary heart disease in black populations. I. Mortality and morbidity. Am Heart J 1982 Oct; 104(4 Pt 1): 839–51.

56. Gilman JK, Jalal S, Naccarelli GV: Predicting and preventing sudden death from cardiac causes. Circulation 1994 Aug; 90(2): 1083–92.
57. Goldberger JJ: Treatment and prevention of sudden cardiac death: effect of recent clinical trials. Arch Intern Med 1999 Jun 28; 159(12): 1281–7.
58. Goldstein S, Landis JR, Leighton R: Characteristics of the resuscitated out-of-hospital cardiac arrest victim with coronary heart disease. Circulation 1981 Nov; 64(5): 977–84.
59. Goldstein S: The necessity of a uniform definition of sudden coronary death: witnessed death within 1 hour of the onset of acute symptoms. Am Heart J 1982 Jan; 103(1): 156–9.
60. Gottlieb SS: The use of antiarrhythmic agents in heart failure: implications of CAST. Am Heart J 1989 Nov; 118(5 Pt 1): 1074–7.
61. Holmes DR, Davis KB, Mock MB: The effect of medical and surgical treatment on subsequent sudden cardiac death in patients with coronary artery disease: a report from the Coronary Artery Surgery Study. Circulation 1986 Jun; 73(6): 1254–63.
62. Iseri LT, Humphrey SB, Siner EJ: Prehospital brady-asystolic cardiac arrest. Ann Intern Med 1978 Jun; 88(6): 741–5.
63. Itoh H, Horie M, Ito M: Arrhythmogenesis in the short-QT syndrome associated with combined HERG channel gating defects: a simulation study. Circ J 2006; 70(4): 502–8.
64. Jaoude SA, Leclercq JF, Coumel P: Progressive ECG changes in arrhythmogenic right ventricular disease. Evidence for an evolving disease. Eur Heart J 1996 Nov; 17(11): 1717–22.
65. Kannel WB, Cupples LA, D'Agostino RB: Sudden death risk in overt coronary heart disease: the Framingham Study. Am Heart J 1987 Mar; 113(3): 799–804.
66. Kuller LH: Sudden death—definition and epidemiologic considerations. Prog Cardiovasc Dis 1980 Jul-Aug; 23(1): 1–12.
67. Kunavarapu C, Bloomfield DM: Role of noninvasive studies in risk stratification for sudden cardiac death. Clin Cardiol 2004; 27(4): 192–7.
68. Ladich E, Virmani R, Burke A: Sudden cardiac death not related to coronary atherosclerosis. Toxicol Pathol 2006; 34(1): 52–7.
69. Latini R, Maggioni AP, Flather M: ACE inhibitor use in patients with myocardial infarction. Summary of evidence from clinical trials. Circulation 1995 Nov 15; 92(10): 3132–7.
70. Lerman BB, Stein KM, Markowitz SM: Idiopathic right ventricular outflow tract tachycardia: a clinical approach. Pacing Clin Electrophysiol 1996 Dec; 19(12 Pt 1): 2120–37.
71. Lombardi G, Gallagher J, Gennis P: Outcome of out-of-hospital cardiac arrest in New York City. The Pre- Hospital Arrest Survival Evaluation (PHASE) Study. JAMA 1994 Mar 2; 271(9): 678–83.
72. Makikallio TH, Barthel P, Schneider R: Frequency of sudden cardiac death among acute myocardial infarction survivors with optimized medical and revascularization therapy. Am J Cardiol 2006; 15;97(4): 480–4.
73. Marcus FI, Fontaine GH, Guiraudon G: Right ventricular dysplasia: a report of 24 adult cases. Circulation 1982 Feb; 65(2): 384–98.
74. Maron BJ, Bonow RO, Cannon RO: Hypertrophic cardiomyopathy. Interrelations of clinical manifestations, pathophysiology, and therapy (2). N Engl J Med 1987 Apr 2; 316(14): 844–52.
75. Maron BJ, Shirani J, Poliac LC: Sudden death in young competitive athletes. Clinical, demographic, and pathological profiles. JAMA 1996 Jul 17; 276(3): 199–204.
76. Maron BJ, Epstein SE, Roberts WC: Causes of sudden death in competitive athletes. J Am Coll Cardiol 1986 Jan; 7(1): 204–14.
77. Maseri A, Severi S, Marzullo P: Role of coronary arterial spasm in sudden coronary ischemic death. Ann N Y Acad Sci 1982; 382: 204–17.
78. McCullough PA, Thompson RJ, Tobin KJ: Validation of a decision support tool for the evaluation of.
79. McCullough PA, Thompson RJ, Tobin KJ: Validation of a decision support tool for the evaluation of cardiac arrest victims. Clin Cardiol 1998 Mar; 21(3): 195–200.
80. Metoprolol in Acute Myocardial Infarction Trial Research Group: Metoprolol in acute myocardial infarction (MIAMI). A randomised placebo-controlled international trial. Eur Heart J 1985 Mar; 6(3): 199–226.
81. Moss AJ, Hall WJ, Cannom DS: Improved survival with an implanted defibrillator in patients with coronary disease at high risk for ventricular arrhythmia. Multicenter Automatic Defibrillator Implantation Trial Investigators. N Engl J Med 1996 Dec 26; 335(26): 1933–40.
82. Moss AJ: Prognosis after myocardial infarction. Am J Cardiol 1983 Oct 1; 52(7): 667–9.
83. Moss AJ, Schwartz PJ, Crampton RS: The long QT syndrome. Prospective longitudinal study of 328 families. Circulation 1991 Sep; 84(3): 1136–44.
84. Moss AJ, Hall WJ, Cannom DS: Improved survival with an implanted defibrillator in patients with coronary disease at high risk for ventricular arrhythmia. Multicenter Automatic Defibrillator Implantation Trial Investigators. N Engl J Med 1996 Dec 26; 335(26): 1933–40.
85. Myerburg RJ, Castellanos A: Cardiac arrest and sudden cardiac death. In: Brunwald E, ed. Heart Disease: A Textbook of Cardiovascular Medicine. 4th ed. Philadelphia, Pa: WB Saunders; 1992: 756–89.
86. Myerburg RJ, Kessler KM, Castellanos A: Sudden cardiac death. Structure, function, and time-dependence of risk. Circulation 1992 Jan; 85(1 Suppl): 12–10.
87. Myerburg RJ, Estes D, Zaman L: Outcome of resuscitation from bradyarrhythmic or asystolic prehospital cardiac arrest. J Am Coll Cardiol 1984 Dec; 4(6): 1118–22.
88. Nademanee K, Singh BN, Stevenson WG: Amiodarone and post-MI patients. Circulation 1993 Aug; 88(2): 764–74.
89. Napolitano C, Bloise R, Priori SG: Long QT syndrome and short QT syndrome: how to make correct diagnosis and what about eligibility for sports activity. J Cardiovasc Med (Hagerstown) 2006; 7(4): 250–6.
90. Narasimhan C, Jazayeri MR, Sra J: Ventricular tachycardia in valvular heart disease: facilitation of sustained bundle-branch reentry by valve surgery. Circulation 1997 Dec 16; 96(12): 4307–13·
91. Neuspiel DR, Kuller LH: Sudden and unexpected natural death in childhood and adolescence. JAMA 1985 Sep 13; 254(10): 1321–5.
92. Prystowsky EN: Prevention of sudden cardiac death. Clin Cardiol 2005; 28(11 Suppl 1): I12–8.
93. Rosen MR, Jause MJ, Myerburg RJ: Arrhythmias induced by coronary artery occlusion: what are the electrophysiologic mechanisms? In: Hearse DJ, Mannings AS, Janse M, eds. Life-Threatening Arrhythmias During Ischemia and Infarction. New York.

44 Cardiovascular Disorders in Young Athletes

The majority of sudden deaths in young athletes occur in the context of underlying inherited or genetic cardiac disorders. The evaluation of every athlete regarding underlying cardiac disease is impractical and therefore needs to be targeted at those who are at a higher risk. A practical approach would be to channel efforts towards athletes with cardiac symptoms, those with a family history of inherited cardiac disease, and those with a family history of premature sudden death. There are potential pitfalls in the evaluation of young athletes using noninvasive tests when making the distinction between physiological adaptations to exercise and cardiac pathology. Physicians

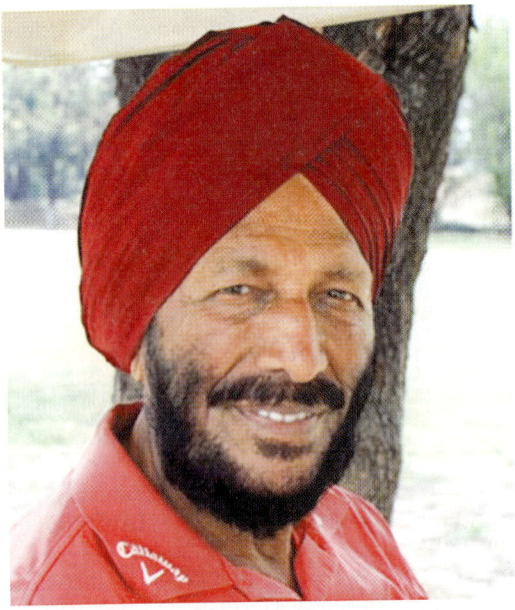

Fig. 44.1: *Milkha Singh, India's athletics icon. Milkha Singh who is encouraging many Indian young athletes to take part in different games. Playing games tones up your cardiovascular system and prolonges your life and one may remain drug and disease free even more than 80 years like Milkha Singh of India*

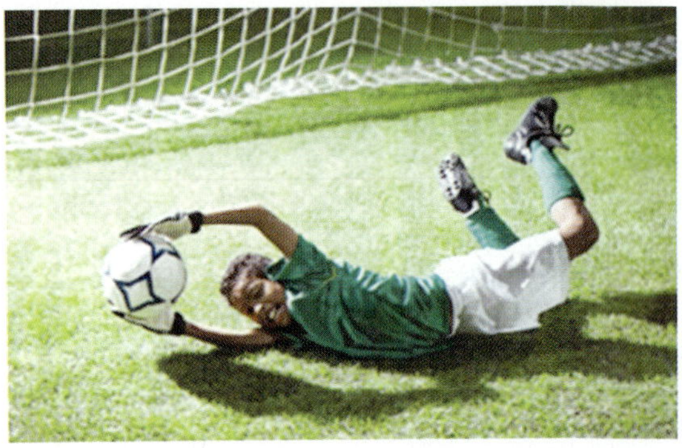

Fig. 44.2: *Young athlete is busy in playing football game*

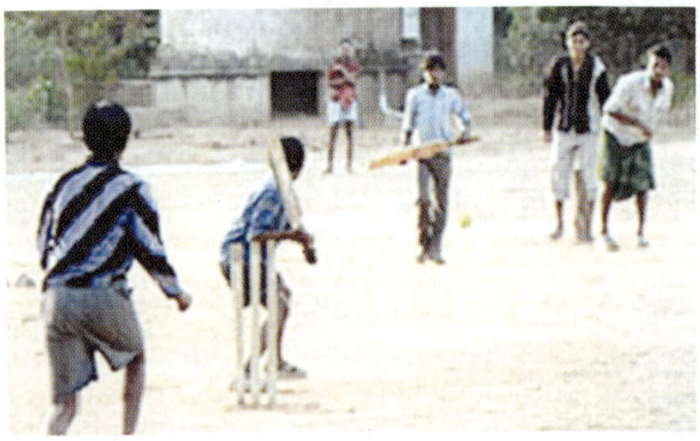

Fig. 44.3: *Young children are busy in playing the popular game of cricket*

evaluating young athletes need to be aware of the spectrum of physiological adaptations and to be familiar with conditions responsible for sudden death in this population.

Athlete's heart is a constellation of structural and functional changes that occur in the heart of people who train for > 1 h most days. The changes are asymptomatic; signs include bradycardia, a systolic murmur, and extra heart sounds. ECG abnormalities are common. Diagnosis is clinical or by echocardiography. No treatment is necessary. Athlete's heart is significant because it must be

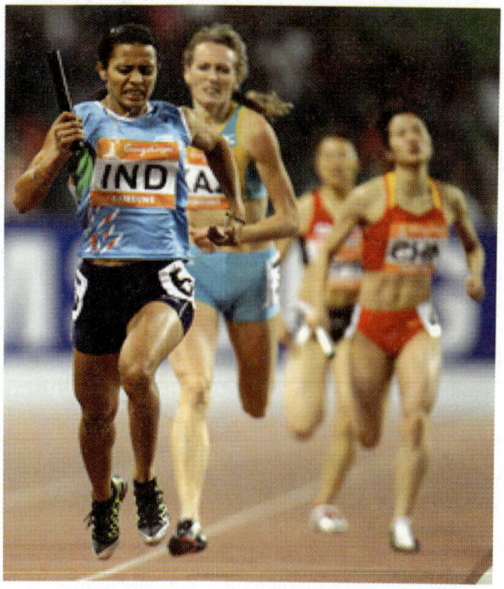

Fig. 44.4: *Young international athletes including Indian taking part in running competition*

distinguished from serious cardiac disorders. Intensive, prolonged endurance and strength training produces many physiologic adaptations. Volume and pressure loads in the left ventricle (LV) increase, which, over time, increase LV muscle mass, wall thickness and chamber size. Maximal stroke volume and cardiac output increase, contributing to a lower resting heart rate and longer diastolic filling time.

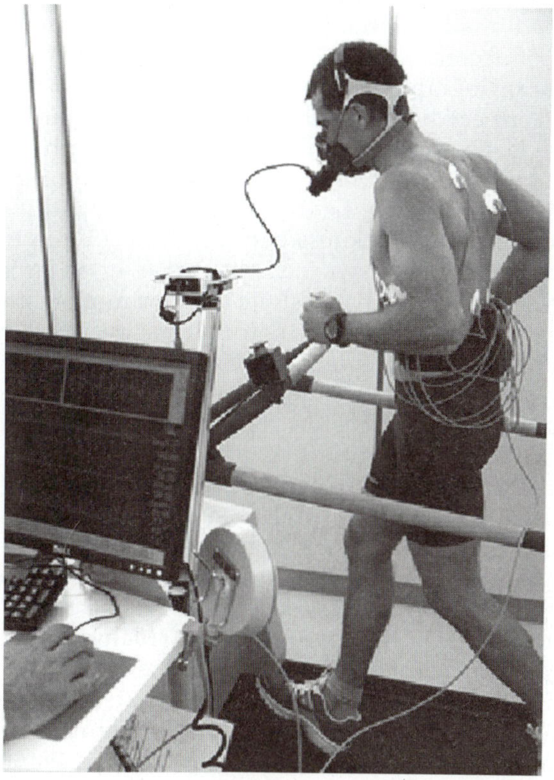

Fig. 44.5: *Exercise stress testing is being conducted for participation in atheletic events*

Lower heart rate results primarily from increased vagal tone, but decreased sympathetic activation and other nonautonomic factors that decrease intrinsic sinus node activity may play a role. Bradycardia decreases myocardial O_2 demand; at the same time, increases in total Hb and blood volume enhance O_2 transport. Despite these changes, systolic function and diastolic function remain normal. Structural changes in women are typically less than those in men of the same age, body size, and training. While the entity of athlete's heart has been recognized for over 100 years, only in the past two decades has the application of echocardiography and other noninvasive imaging techniques permitted definition with some precision of the alterations in cardiac dimensions associated with athletic conditioning. Echocardiography has demonstrated that long-term athletic training leads to an increase in left ventricular mass due to increases in left ventricular diastolic cavity dimension, wall thickness, or both. These changes in cardiac morphology are relatively mild in absolute terms, and the differences between athlete and nonathlete populations are statistically significant but generally small. Furthermore, cardiac alterations associated with training differ somewhat depending on the particular sport in which the individual athlete participates. In particular, the changes in left ventricular wall thickness, cavity dimension, or both associated with long-term athletic training may be more striking in certain sports such as distance running, swimming, cycling, and rowing/canoeing. The differential diagnosis with cardiac disease is more likely to be raised in athletes training in such sports (Figs 44.1–44.3).

Symptoms and Signs

There are no symptoms. Signs vary but may include bradycardia; an LV impulse that is laterally displaced, enlarged, and increased in amplitude; a systolic ejection (flow) murmur at the left lower sternal border; a 3rd heart sound (S3) due to early, rapid diastolic ventricular filling; a 4th heart sound (S4), heard best during resting bradycardia because diastolic filling time is increased; and hyperdynamic carotid pulses. These signs reflect structural cardiac changes that are adaptive for intense exercise.

Diagnosis

Clinical Evaluation (Table 44.1)

Findings are typically detected during routine screening or during evaluation of unrelated symptoms. Most athletes do not require extensive testing although ECG is often

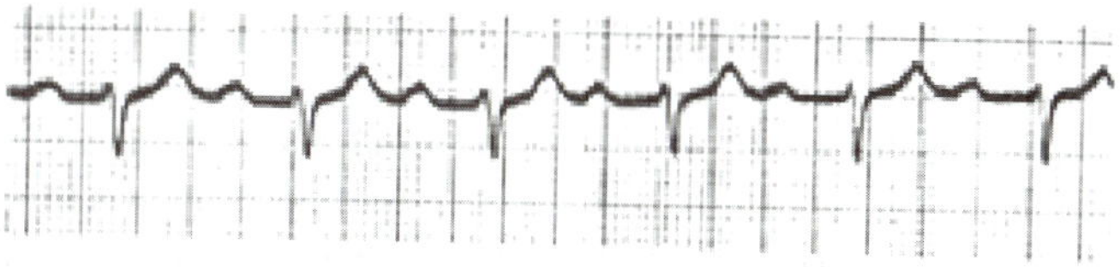

Fig. 44.6: *The normal PR interval is 0.12–0.20 sec, or 120–200 ms. First degree AV block is defined by PR intervals greater than 200 ms. This may be caused by drugs, such as digoxin; excessive vagal tone; ischemia; or intrinsic disease in the AV junction or bundle-branch system*

Table 44.1: *Specific athlete characteristics needed for cardiovascular testing according to American Heart Association recommendations*

Type of examination	*Characteristics*
Personal history	• Exertional chest pain or discomfort • Unexplained syncope or near-syncope, assumed not vasovagal • History of hypertension • Excessive exertional and unexplained dyspnea/fatigue • History of previously recognized heart murmur
Family history	• Sudden and unexpected premature death in at least one relative before age 50 years • Disability from heart disease in a close relative < 50 years old • Previously diagnosed inheritable heart disease in family members including, but not limited to, hypertrophic cardiomyopathy, dilated cardiomyopathy, congenital long QT syndrome or other ion channelopathies, Marfan syndrome, or clinically important arrhythmias
Physical examination	• Heart murmur • Abnormal femoral pulses, suggestive of aortic coarctation • Physical stigmata of Marfan syndrome • Abnormal brachial artery blood pressure for age (taken in both arms in a sitting position)

Table 44.2: *Common ECG findings in athletes. Training-related ECG alterations are common, physiological adaptations to regular exercise and are considered normal variants in athletes*

Normal ECG finding
Sinus bradycardia
Sinus arrhythmia
First-degree AV block
Incomplete RBBB
Early repolarisation
Isolated QRS voltage criteria for LVH

- Isolated increases in QRS amplitude are common in trained athletes. However, QRS voltage criteria for LVH+ any non-voltage criteria for LVH (such as atrial enlargement, left axis deviation, a strain pattern of repolarisation, ST-segment depression, T-wave inversion or pathological Q waves) are abnormal and require further evaluation
- AV, atrioventricular; LVH, left ventricular hypertrophy, RBBB, right bundle-branch block

warranted. If symptoms suggest a cardiac disorder (e.g. palpitations, chest pain), ECG, echocardiography, and exercise stress testing are done. Athlete's heart is a diagnosis of exclusion; it must be distinguished from disorders that cause similar findings but are life-threatening (e.g. hypertrophic or dilated cardiomyopathies, ischemic heart disease, arrhythmogenic right ventricular dysplasia).

Electrocardiography: Numerous changes in rhythm and ECG morphology can occur; they correlate poorly with level of training and cardiovascular performance. The most common ECG finding is **sinus bradycardia.**

Rarely, heart rate is <40 beats/min. Sinus arrhythmia often accompanies the slow heart rate. Resting bradycardia may also predispose to (Tables 44.2, 44.4–44.6).

- Atrial or ventricular ectopy (including couplets and bursts of nonsustained ventricular tachycardia); pauses after ectopic beats do not exceed 4 sec.
- Wandering supraventricular pacemaker (Fig. 44.16)
- Atrial fibrillation (Figs 44.13 and 44.23)

Other ECG findings that may occur include:

- First-degree atrioventricular (AV) block (in up to one third of athletes) (Fig. 44.6)
- **Second degree AV block (mainly type I):** This finding occurs during rest and disappears with exercise (Fig. 44.14)
- **High voltage QRS with inferolateral T-wave changes (reflecting LV hypertrophy)** (Figs 44.8, 44.9 and 44.26)

Deep anterolateral T-wave inversion incomplete right bundle-branch block. However, third-degree AV block is abnormal and should be investigated thoroughly. These ECG and rhythm changes have not been associated with adverse clinical events, suggesting that various arrhythmias are not abnormal in athletes. The arrhythmias are usually abolished or substantially reduced after a relatively brief period of deconditioning.

Echocardiography: It can usually distinguish athlete's heart from cardiomyopathies but the distinction is not always clear because there is a continuum from physiologic to pathologic cardiac enlargement. The zone of overlap between the athlete's heart and cardiomyopathy is left ventricular septal thickness between 13 to 15 mm in men and 11 to 13 mm in women. In this overlap area, the presence of mitral valve systolic anterior motion strongly suggests hypertrophic cardiomyopathy. In general, echocardiographic changes correlate poorly with level of training and cardiovascular performance. Trace mitral regurgitation and tricuspid regurgitation are commonly detected (Fig. 44.7A and B).

Stress testing: During exercise stress testing, heart rate remains lower than normal at submaximal stress and increases appropriately and comparably to nonathletes at maximal stress; it rapidly recovers after exercise. BP response is normal: systolic BP increases, diastolic BP falls, and mean BP stays relatively constant. Many resting ECG changes decrease or disappear during exercise; this finding is unique to athlete's heart, distinguishing it from pathologic conditions. However, pseudonormalization of T-wave inversions could reflect myocardial ischemia and thus warrants further investigation in older athletes (Figs 44.5, 44.21 and 44.24).

Table 44.3: *Abnormal ECG criteria in athletes. Any abnormal findings is considered training-unrelated and suggests the possibility of underlying pathological disease, required further diagnostic investigation*

Abnormal ECG finding	*Definition*
T-wave inversion	>1 mm in depth from baseline in two or more adjacent leads not including aVR or V1
ST-segment depression	≥ 1 mm in depth in two or more adjacent leads
Pathological Q waves	> 3 mm in depth or >0.04 s in duration in two or more leads
Complete left bundle-branch block	QRS > 0.12s, predominantly negative QRS complex in lead V_1 (QS or rS and upright monophasic R wave in leads I and V_6
Complete right bundle	QRS >0.12 s, terminal R wave in lead V_1 (rsR′) and wide terminal S wave in leads I and V_6.
Intraventricular conduction delay	Nonspecific, QRS > 0.12 s
Left atrial enlargement	Prolonged P wave duration of >0.12 s in lead I or II with negative portion of the P wave ≥1 mm in depth and ≥ 0.04 s in duration in lead V_1
Left axis deviation	–30° to 90°
Right atrial enlargement	High/pointed P wave ≥ 2.5 mm in lead II and III or V_1
Right ventricular hypertrophy	Right axis deviation ≥ 120°, tall R wave in V1 + persistent precordial S wave ($R - V_1 + S - V_5 >$ 10.5 mm)
Mobitz type II 2° AV block	Intermittently nonconducted P wave not preceded by PR prolongation and not followed by PR shortening
3° AV block	Complete heart block
Ventricular preexcitation	PR interval < 0.12 s with a S wave (slurred upstroke in the QRS complex)
Long QT interval	QTc ≥ 0.47 s (99% men) QTc ≥ 0.18 s (99% women) QTc ≥ 0.50 s (unequivocal LQTS)
Short QT interval	QTc ≤ 0.34 s
Brugada-like ECG pattern	High take-off and downsloping ST-segment elevation in V_1–V_3
Epsilon wave	Small negative deflection just beyond the QRS in V_1 or V_2
Profound sinus bradycardia	< 30 BPM or sinus pauses ≥ 3 s
Atrial tachyarrhythmias	Supraventricular tachycardia, atrioventricular nodal reentrant tachycardia, atrial fibrillation, atrial flutter
Premature ventricular contractions	≥ 2 per tracing
Ventricular arrhythmias	Couplets, triplets, nonsustained ventricular tachycardia

- AV, atrioventricular; BPM, beats per minute; LQTS, long QT syndrome.

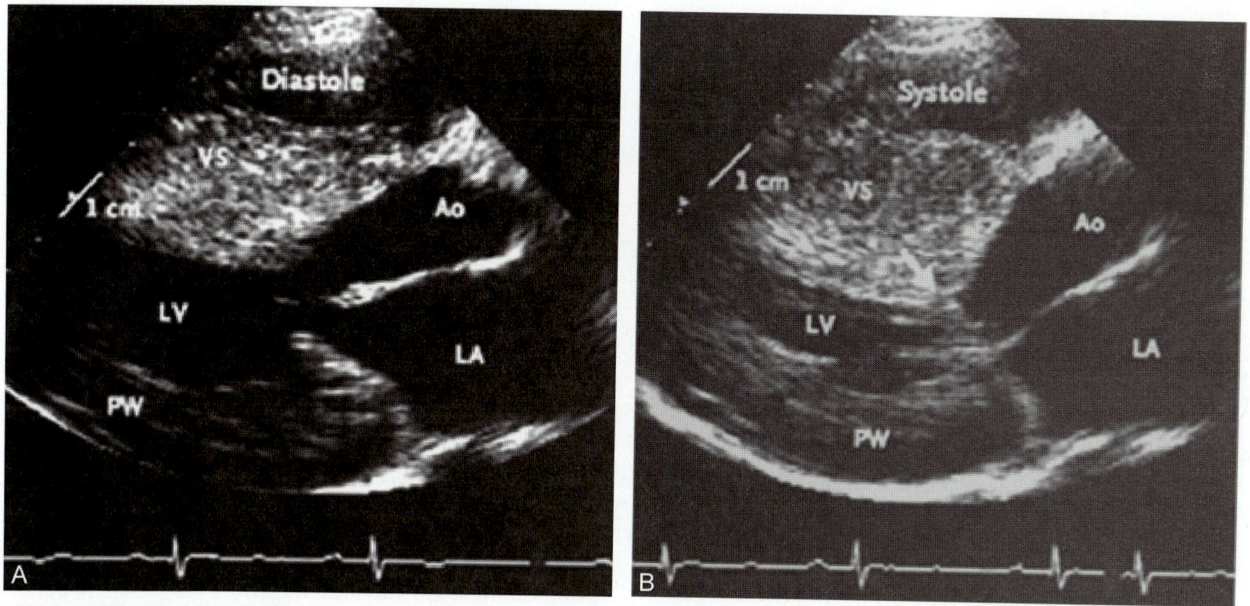

Fig. 44.7(A and B): *Two dimensional echocardiogram in a patient with severe hypertrophic obstructive cardiomyopathy. Marked asymmetrical hypertrophy can be seen in the ventricular septum (VS). Diastole is shown (A). During systole (B), the outflow tract from the left ventricle (LV) becomes obstructed. Abbreviations: Ao, aorta; LA, left atrium; PW, posterior wall*

Table 44.4: *Criteria for positive 12-lead ECG in athletes*

P wave

Left atrial enlargement: negative portion of the P wave in lead V1 = 0.1 mV in depth and 0.04 s in duration

Right atrial enlargement: peaked P wave in leads II and III or V1 = 0.25 mV in amplitude

QRS complex

Frontal plane axis deviation: right = +120° or left –30° to –90°

increased voltage amplitude of R or S wave in a standard lead = 2 mV, S wave in lead V1 or V2 = 3 mV, or R wave in lead V5 or V6 = 3 mV; abnormal Q waves = 0.04 s in duration or = 25% of the height of the ensuring R wave or QS pattern in two or more leads; right or left bundle-branch block with QRS duration = 0.12 s; R or R′ wave in lead V1 = 0.5 mV in amplitude and R/S ratio = 1.

ST-segment, T-waves and QT interval

ST-segment depression or T-wave flattening or inversion in two or more leads

prolongation of heart rate corrected QT interval > 0.44 s in males and > 0.46 s in females

Rhythm and conduction abnormalities

Premature ventricular beats or more severe ventricular arrhythmias

Supraventricular tachycardias, atrial flutter, or atrial fibrillation; short PR interval (< 0.12 s) with or without delta wave; sinus bradycardia with resting heart rate = 40 beats/min first (PR = 0.21 s)[a], second or third degree atrioventricular block.

[a]Not shortening with hyperventillation or limited exercise test. Modified from corrado et al.

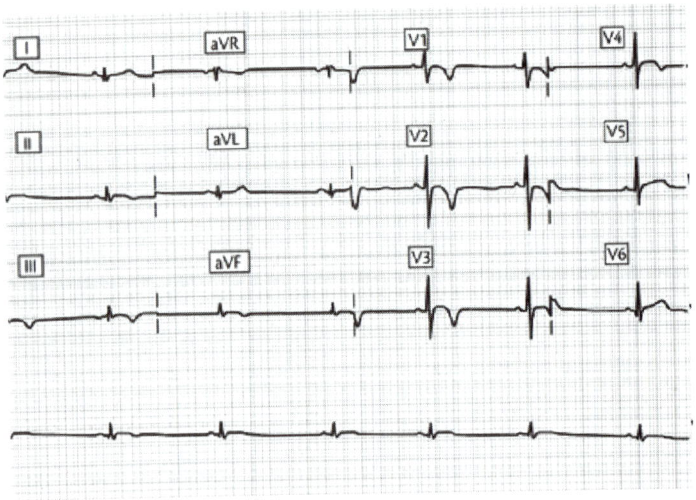

Fig. 44.8: *Twelve-lead ECG in an asymptomatic athlete with ARVC. The athlete was referred for further echocardiographic examination and cardiac magnetic resonance because of ECG abnormalities found at preparticipation evaluation which consisted of inverted T-waves in the inferior and anteroseptal leads and low QRS voltages in the peripheral leads*

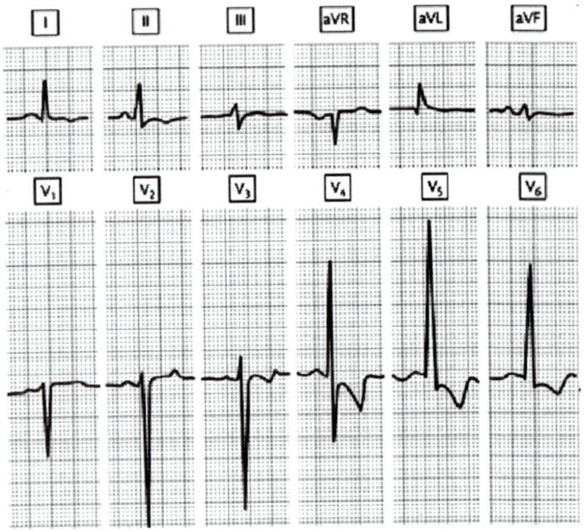

Fig. 44.9: *Twelve-lead ECG of an asymptomatic athlete with HCM. The disease was suspected at preparticipation evaluation thanks to ECG abnormalities consisting of increased QRS voltages and inverted T-waves in lateral leads. HCM was diagnosed by echocardiography afterwards*

Table 44.5: *Classification of abnormalities of the athlete's electrocardiogram*

Group 1: Common and training-related ECG changes	*Group 2: Uncommon and training-unrelated ECG changes*
Sinus bradycardia	T-wave inversion
First-degree AV block	ST-segement depression
Incomplete RBBB	Pathological Q-waves
Early repolarization	Left atrial enlargement
Isolated QRS voltage criteria for left ventricualr hypertrophy	Left-axis deviation/left anterior hemiblock
	Right-axis deviation/left posterior hemiblock
	Right ventricular hypertrophy
	Ventricular preexcitation
	Complete LBBB or RBBB
	Long or short-QT interval
	Brugada-like early repolarization

RBBB, right bundle-branch block; LBBB, left bundle-branch block.

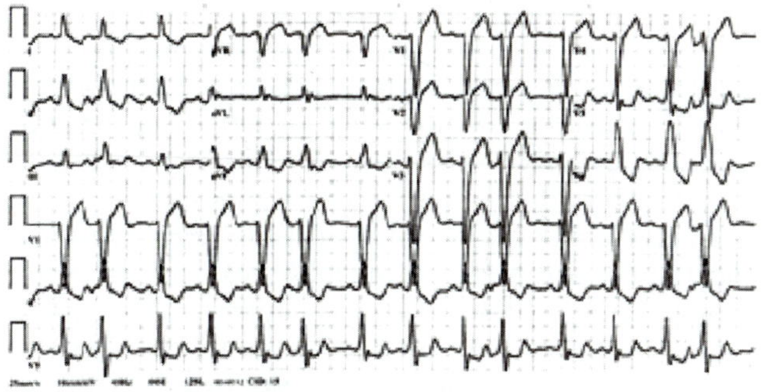

Fig. 44.10: *Electrocardiogram showing left bundle-branch block and irregular rhythm due to supraventricular extrasystoles*

Cardiovascular Causes of Sudden Death

A variety of cardiovascular diseases have been identified as potential causes of sudden death in young competitive athletes (<35 years old). The vast majority of these deaths occur on the athletic field during severe exertion in the context of training or competition. Each of the responsible diseases is also known to cause sudden death in nonathletes. The most common cause of sudden death in young athletes appears to be HCM. Less common causes are a variety of congenital coronary artery anomalies, myocarditis, dilated cardiomyopathy, Marfan's syndrome, and right ventricular dysplasia (in one series). Uncommon but reported causes of these athletic field catastrophies include sarcoid, mitral valve prolapse, aortic valve stenosis, atherosclerotic coronary artery disease, and QT-interval prolongation syndromes (Table 44.8 and Fig. 44.11).

Differential Diagnosis between Athlete's Heart and Cardiovascular Disease

Dilated cardiomyopathy: In an important minority of athletes, the increase in left ventricular diastolic cavity dimension that occurs with training overlaps with that characteristic of certain known pathological entities. For example, while left ventricular end-diastolic cavity dimension in athletes is usually in the range of 53– 58 mm, in some individuals it may extend into what may be regarded as the pathological range of >58 mm and thereby resemble dilated cardiomyopathy. However, the absence of left ventricular systolic dysfunction is usually sufficient to distinguish this physiological ventricular enlargement induced by training from that due to dilated cardiomyopathy.

Table 44.6: *Prevalence of ECG abnormalities in an unselected population of 32,652 young individuals undergoing the preparticipation cardiovascular screening*

ECG abnormalities	*Athletes, n (%)*
Negative T-waves in precordial/standard leads	751 (2.3)
RBBB	351 (1.0)
Increased R/S wave voltage (suggestive of LVH)	247 (0.8)
Left anterior fascicular block	162 (0.5)
Preexcitation pattern	42 (0.1)
LBBB	19 (0.1)
Prolonged corrected QT interval	1 (0.003)
Other (incomplete RBBB, prolonged PR interval, early repolarization pattern)	2280 (7.0)
Total	3853 (11.8)

RBBB, right bundle-branch block; LVH, left ventricular hypertrophy, LBBB, left bundle-branch block

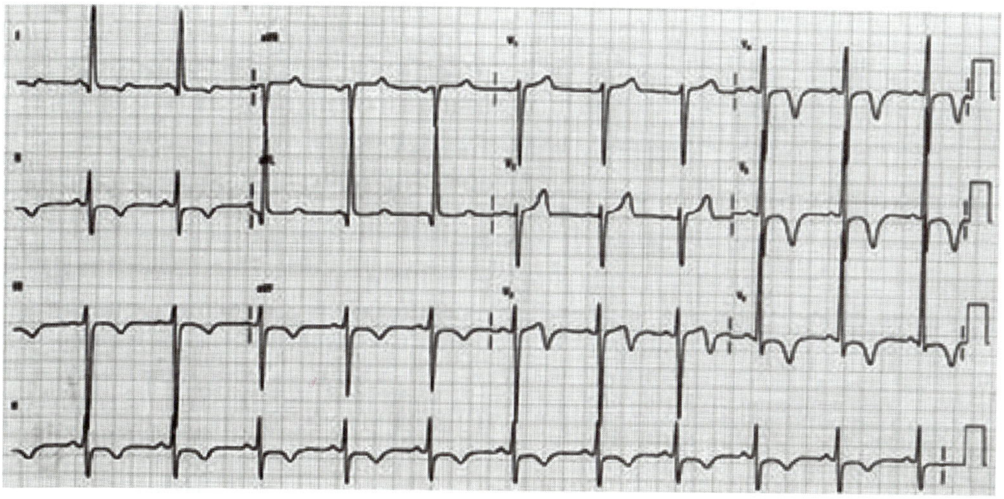

Fig. 44.11: *12-lead ECG of a young male with hypertrophic cardiomyopathy demonstrating voltage criteria for LV hypertrophy and repolarisation changes*

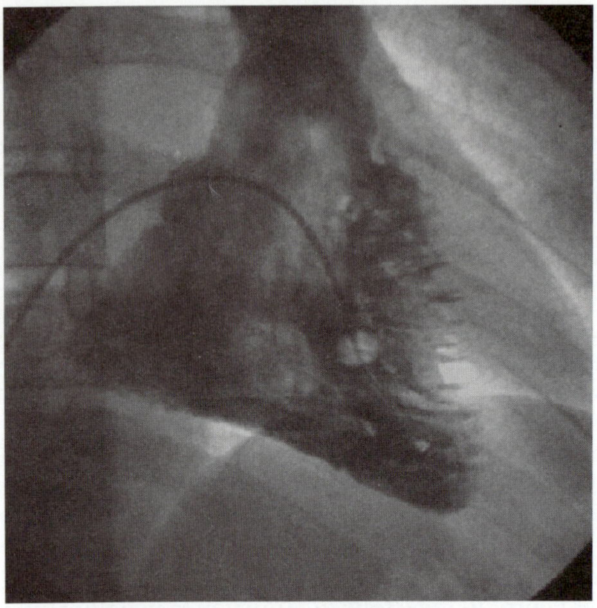

Fig. 44.12: *Right ventriculogram showing akinetic/dyskinetic areas with diastolic septal bulge ("stack of coins") compatible with arrhythmogenic right ventricular dysplasia*

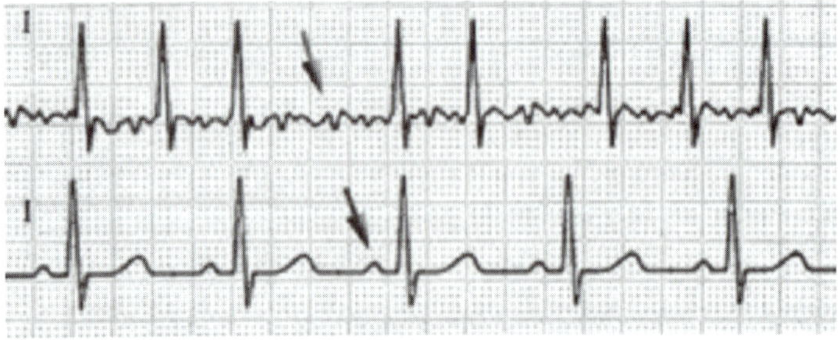

Fig. 44.13: *ECG of atrial fibrillation (top) and normal sinus rhythm (bottom). The purple arrow indicates a P wave which is lost in atrial fibrillation*

Myocarditis: Myocarditis, a disorder associated with a heterogeneous clinical profile, has recently been incriminated as the possible cause of some highly publicized deaths in athletes. While myocarditis usually has an infectious origin, it can also be a consequence of drug abuse Sudden cardiac death may occur in its active or healed phases as a consequence of complex arrhythmias that develop in the setting of an unstable myocardial electrical substrate. In an athlete with myocarditis, left ventricular cavity enlargement may be due to the disease, to athletic training, or to a combination of these, but the differential diagnosis with athlete's heart is usually resolved by the presence of clinically relevant and overt arrhythmias, cardiac symptoms such as syncope, presyncope and palpitations, or heart failure with systolic dysfunction. In some instances, the diagnosis may also be clarified by histological examination of myocardium obtained by endomyocardial biopsy.

Right ventricular dysplasia: Arrhythmogenic right ventricular dysplasia (or cardiomyopathy) is a heart muscle disorder of unknown cause that is characterized pathologically by fibrofatty replacement of the right ventricular myocardium. The clinical and phenotypic profile is variable but includes structural and functional abnormalities of the right ventricle, ventricular and supraventricular arrhythmias, familial occurrence, and the risk for sudden cardiac death. Indeed, it has been suggested that right ventricular dysplasia is an important cause of sudden death in the young including competitive athletes, largely on the basis of reports from the northeastern (Veneto) region of Italy (Figs 44.8, 44.12, 44.18 and 44.21).

Because highly trained athletes may demonstrate right ventricular enlargement and a variety of depolarization, repolarization, and conduction abnormalities on the ECG, the differential diagnosis between athlete's heart and right ventricular dysplasia may arise. Noninvasive identification

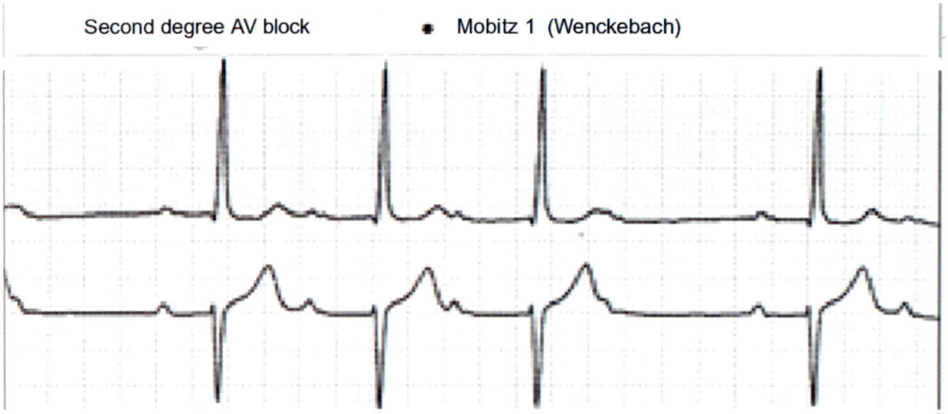

P wave	PR interval (in seconds)	QRS (in seconds)	Characleristics
Conduction intermittant	Increasingly prolonged	<.12	QRS dropped in a repeating pattern

Fig. 44.14: *Second degree AV block, type I (Wenckebach)*

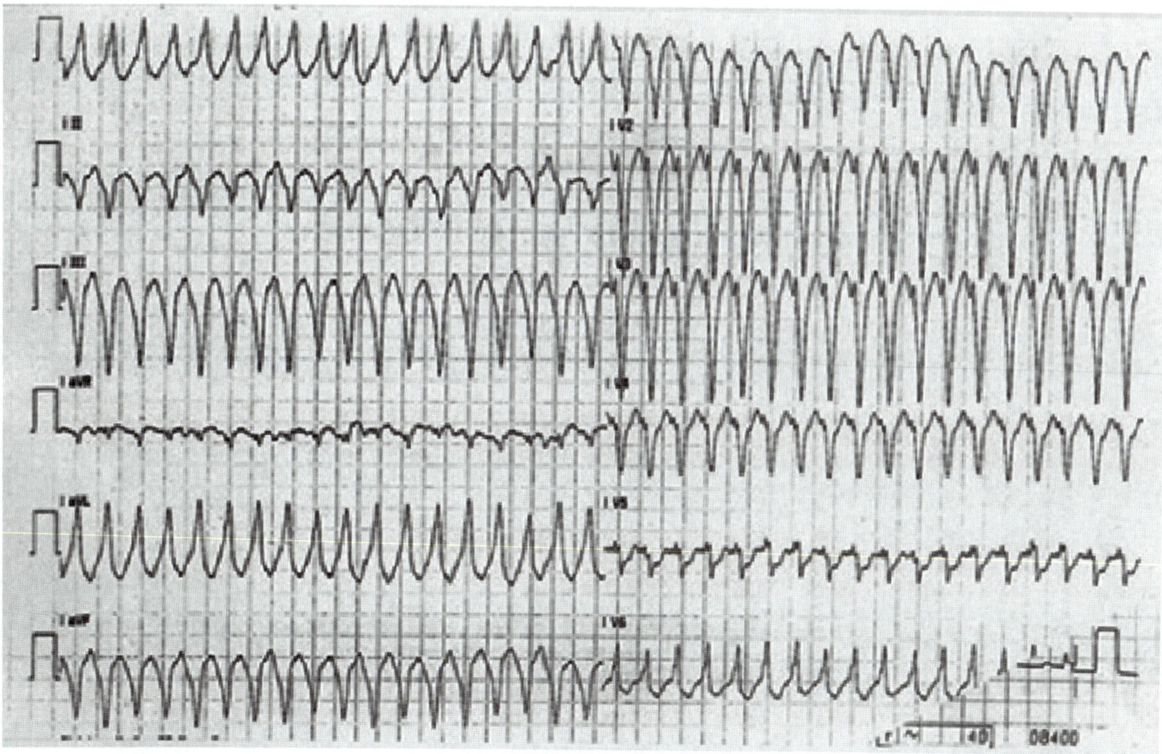

Fig. 44.15: *12 lead ECG recording of VT with left bundle-branch block (LBBB) morphology*

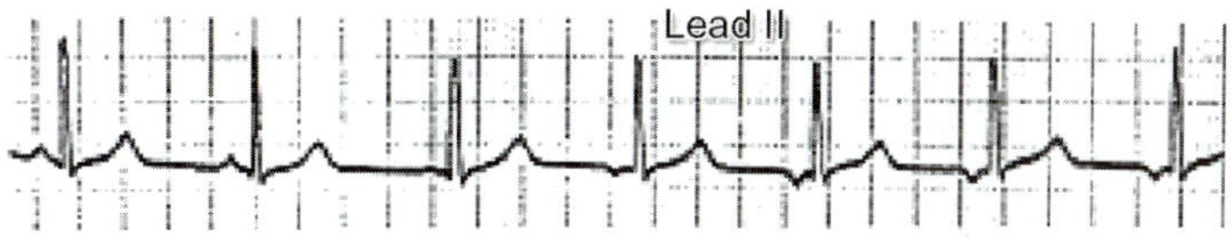

Fig. 44.16: *Wandering atrial pacemaker is a benign rhythm change where the pacemaker site shifts from the sinus node into the atrial tissues. P-wave morphology varies with the pacemaker site*

of right ventricular dysplasia by echocardiography may be difficult because of technical limitations in imaging right ventricular structure and assessing function in these patients and because the spectrum of the disease is broad and includes mild morphological forms with subtle manifestations. Magnetic resonance imaging, however, promises enhanced noninvasive diagnosis of this condition. The demonstration of right ventricular segmental or global dysfunction or substantial right ventricular cavity enlargement would support the diagnosis of right ventricular dysplasia; alternatively, thickening or enlargement of the left ventricle would be most consistent with athlete's heart.

Hypertrophic cardiomyopathy: The greatest difficulty in distinguishing clinically between athlete's heart and structural heart disease most frequently arises with respect to HCM, since many of the other cardiac disorders that cause sudden death in a young athletic population can be identified independently of any changes in cardiac morphology typically associated with training. The basic definition of HCM used here is that of a patient (or athlete) with evidence of a hypertrophied and nondilated left ventricle in the absence of another cardiac or systemic disease that could itself cause hypertrophy of the magnitude present in that individual (Figs 44.9, 44.11 and 44.32).

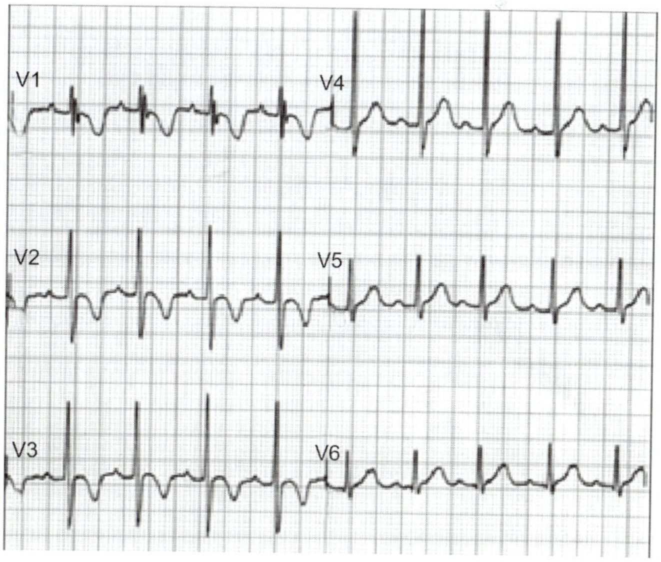

Fig. 44.17: *Incomplete RBBB in a child (RSR' in V1, QRS < 120 ms)*

Wall thickness: In the vast majority of competitive athletes, absolute left ventricular wall thickness is normal or only mildly increased (12 mm). In some athletes, however, the increase in left ventricular wall thickness may be more substantial, up to 16 mm, unavoidably raising the possibility of HCM. In patients with HCM, the increase in left ventricular wall thickness is usually marked; the

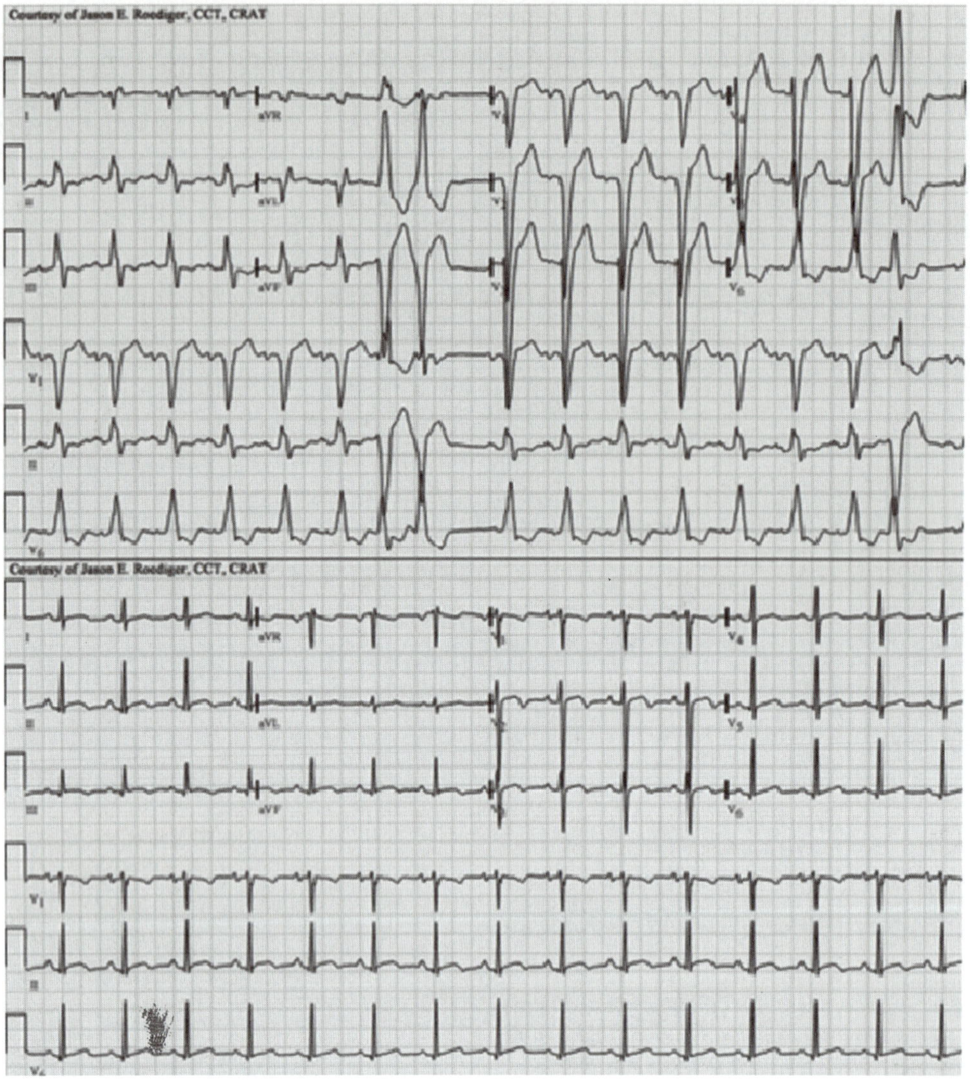

Fig. 44.18: *12-lead ECGs from a 19-year-old black adolescent with arrythmogenic cardiomyopathy. (Top): Sinus tachycardia (rate about 101/min) with LBBB accompanied by RAD (here about 108°). Frequent multifocal PVCs (both singly and in pairs) and left atrial enlargement. (Bottom): Same patient about 5 months later was fitted with orthotopic heart transplant*

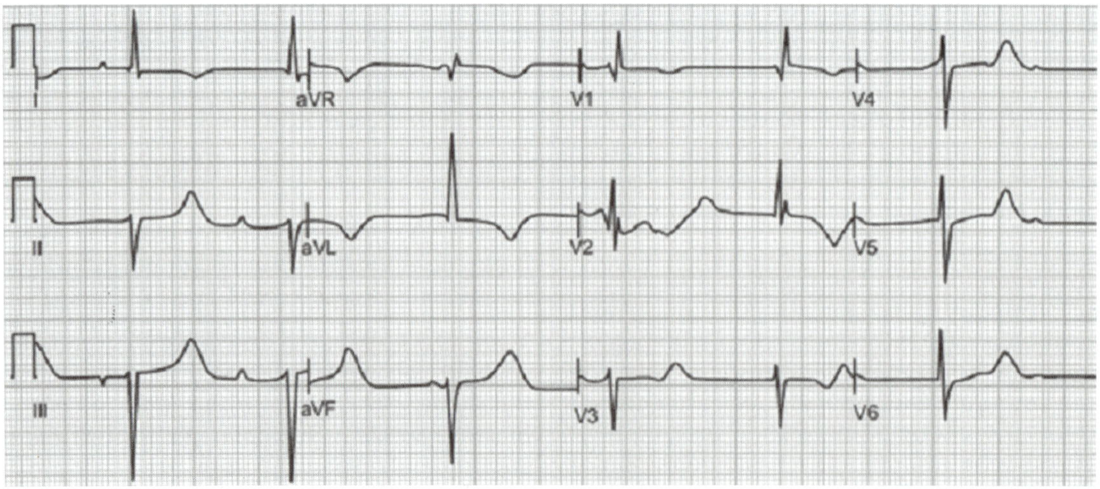

Fig. 44.19: *ECG showing long QTc (620 ms) due to severe hypothermia*

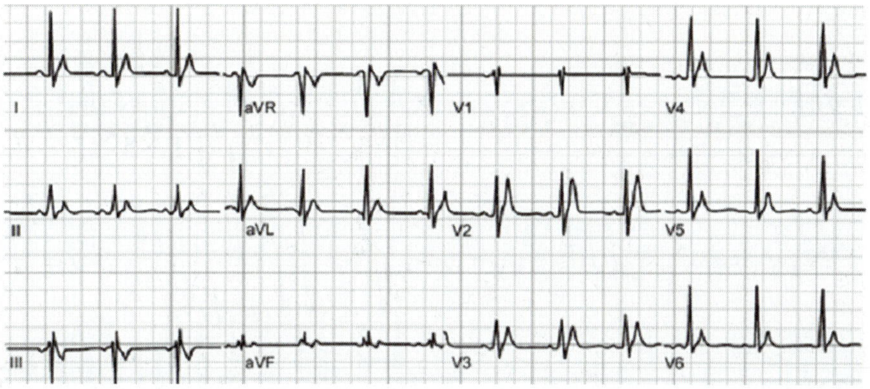

Fig. 44.20: *ECG showing very short QTc (280 ms) with tall, packed T waves due to congenital short QT syndrome*

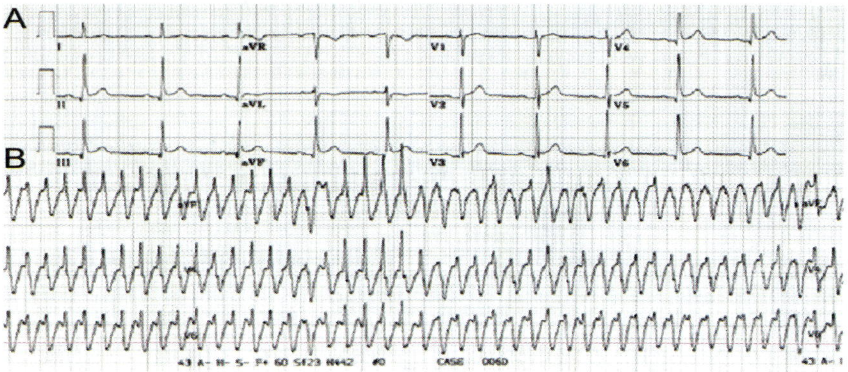

Fig. 44.21: *ECG showing, the features of ERPV in the baseline ECG (A) recorded immediately before an exercise stress test (B) that resulted in Torsade de Pointes ventricular tachycardia*

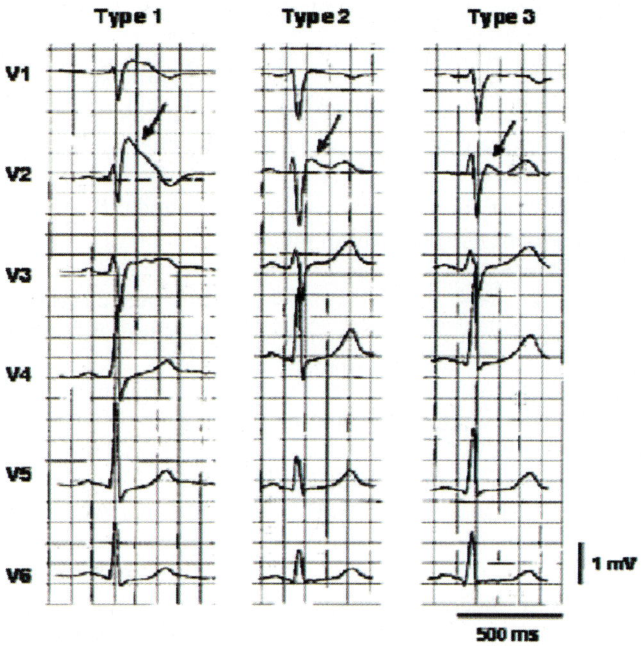

Fig. 44.22: *Three types of ST-segment elevation in Brugada syndrome as shown in the precordial leads on ECG in the same patient at different times. Left panel shows a type 1 ECG pattern with pronounced elevation of the J point (arrow), a coved-type ST segment, and an inverted T wave in V1 and V2. The middle panel illustrates a type 2 pattern with a saddleback ST-segment elevated by >1 mm. The right panel shows a type 3 pattern in which the ST segment is elevated < 1 mm. According to a consensus report (Antzelevitch, 2005), the type 1 ECG pattern is diagnostic of Brugada syndrome. (Modified from Wilde, 2002)*

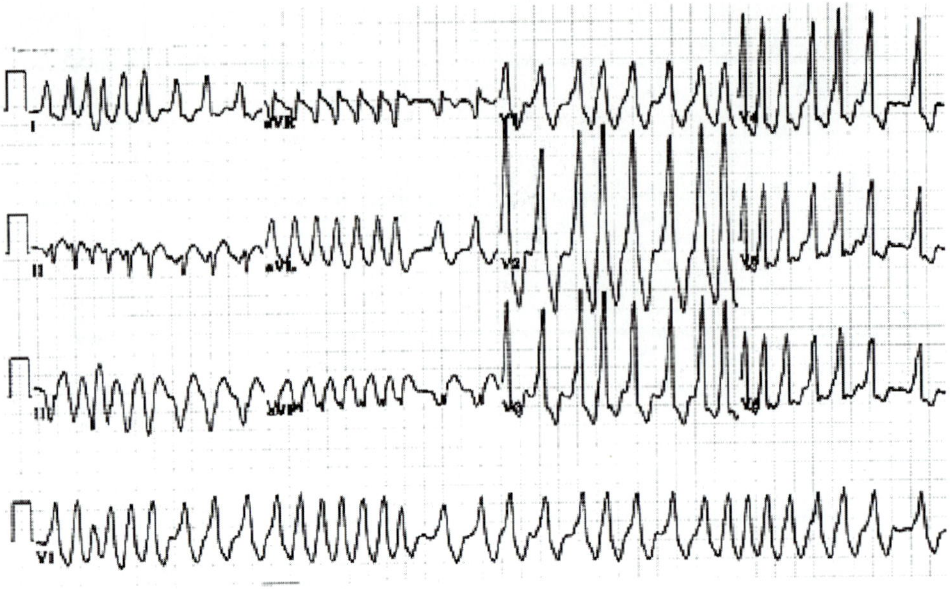

Fig. 44.23: *ECG showing bizzare wide QRS tachycardia is "irregularly irregular", indicative of atrial fibrillation with a fast ventricular response. The bizzare QRS morphology is due to ventricular activation being initiated from the AV bypass track (bundle of Kent) which conducts faster than the AV node*

average wall thickness reported in most echocardiographic studies of this disease is 20 mm, ranging to >50 mm. However, an important minority of patients with HCM show relatively mild left ventricular hypertrophy with wall thickness values in the range of 13–15 mm, and many of these patients are asymptomatic. Therefore, a diagnostic dilemma arises in those athletes who fall into this morphological "gray zone" between physiological hypertrophy and HCM. While this distinction cannot be resolved with certainty in some of these athletes, careful analysis of several echocardiographic and clinical features permits this diagnostic differentiation in most (Table 44.7).

Table 44.7: *Major and minor criteria for diagnosis of ARVC. A patient needs either 2 major criteria, 1 major and 2 minor criteria, or 4 minor criteria from different categories*

Category	*Major criteria*	*Minor criteria*
RV dysfunction	• Severe dilation with reduction of RV EF with little or no LV impairment • Localized RV aneurysms • Severe segmental RV dilation	• Mild global RV dilation and/or EF reduction with normal LV • Mild segmental RV dilation • Regional RV hypokinesis
Tissue characterization of wall	• Fibro-fatty replacement of myocardium on endomyocardial biopsy	
Repolarization abnormalities		• Inverted T waves in right precordial leads (V_2 and V_3) (applies for patients aged > 12 years old, in absence of RBBB)
Depolarization or conduction abnormalities	• Epsilon waves in V_1–V_3 • Localized prolongation of QRS complex > 110 ms in leads V_1–V_3	• Late potentials in a signal-averaged ECG
Arrhythmias	• Any of the arrhythmias in minor criteria listed at right plus inverted T waves in V_2 and V_3	• LBBB-type VT (either sustained or nonsustained) found on ECG, Holter, or exercise testing • Frequent ventricular extrasystoles (> 1,000/24 hours) found on Holter monitoring
Family history	• Familial disease confirmed at necropsy or surgery	• Family history of premature sudden cardiac death (< 35 years old) with ARVC as suspected cause • Family history of ARVC (with diagnosis based on these criteria)

Abbreviations: ARVC, arrhythmogenic right ventricular cardiomyopathy; EF, ejection fraction; LBBB, left bundle-branch block; LV, left ventricle; RBBB, right bundle-branch block; RV, right ventricle; VT, ventricular tachycardia.

Table 44.8: *Differences between atheletic heart syndrome and cardiomyopathy*

Feature	*Athletic heart syndrome*	*Cardiomyopathy*
Left ventricular hypertrophy	< 13 mm	> 15 mm
Left ventricular end-diastolic diameter	< 60 mm	> 70 mm
Diastolic function	Normal (E:A ratio > 1)	Abnormal (E:A ratio < 1)
Septal hypertrophy	Symmetric	Asymmetric (in hypertrophic cardiomyopathy)
Family history	None	May be present
BP response to exercise	Normal	Normal or reduced systolic BP response
Deconditioning	Left ventricular hypertrophy regression	No left ventricular hypertrophy regression

Cardiac Arrhythmia in Young Athletes

(Figs 44.7–44.10, 44.12, 44.14–44.22)

Treatment of atrial fibrillation in young athletes is similar to other young patient populations. There is little evidence that calcium channel blockers and β-blockers reduce episodes of atrial fibrillation, but rather make them less symptomatic when they occur. Antiarrhythmic drugs are typically quite effective in individuals without heart disease. Type 1C agents such as flecainide or propafenone are generally preferred as initial agents because of the safety profile and efficacy of these drugs. Rapid atrial flutter can be especially troubling with flecainide and for this reason a rate controlling agent such as a β-blocker or calcium channel blocker is generally recommended. The use of amiodarone is not advised because of the young age of the athletes and the long-term toxicity of amiodarone. Whether dronedarone will play a role in the management of atrial fibrillation in young athletes is not yet clear. Ablation of atrial fibrillation is a particularly attractive option for athletes as they generally are young, have normal hearts and face a lifetime of atrial fibrillation risk. Pulmonary vein isolation would be a reasonable first step in the ablation of atrial fibrillation in athletes with more aggressive ablation options reserved for those who fail pulmonary vein isolation (Figs 44.10 and 44.13).

Atrial flutter is unusual in the individual without heart disease; when present, a stress test and echocardiogram are necessary to rule out the presence of structural heart disease. Radiofrequency ablation is preferable to antiarrhythmic agents in individuals with atrial flutter because of the high likelihood of cure and the low risk of the procedure.

Anticoagulation in atrial fibrillation and atrial flutter is no different than in nonathletes. The CHADS2 (congestive heart failure, hypertension, age >75, diabetes, history of stroke or transient ischemic attach) score can be utilized to ascertain individual risk of thromboembolism; most athletes would have a CHADS2 score of zero, therefore, by the current guidelines anticoagulation with aspirin alone would be sufficient.

Wolf-Parkinson-White (WPW) is not more common in the athlete, but athletes with WPW may be at higher risk for sudden death due to the high sympathetic drive seen with competition and with training. For this reason most authorities recommended risk stratification of individuals with WPW. Risk stratification may be performed by rapid atrial pacing, by induction of atrial fibrillation in the electrophysiological laboratory and sometimes by stress testing. The 36th Bethesda guidelines recommend ablation for multiple bypass tracts or if the bypass tract can conduct rapidly enough to sustain a tachycardia of greater than 240 bpm. ESC Guidelines are more aggressive and recommend ablation for all asymptomatic WPW athletes age 12 years because of the relative ease of ablation and the life-long risk of SCD. In individuals who refuse ablation, competitive sports are allowed provided that short preexcited cycle lengths of <240 ms at rest and <220 on isoproterenol or exercise during atrial fibrillation are not present. Both European and Bethesda Guidelines recommend radiofrequency ablation for the symptomatic athlete with WPW (Fig. 44.23).

Other supraventricular tachycardias such as AV nodal reentrant tachycardia, AV reciprocating tachycardia, and atrial tachycardia are not more common in athletes. Similar to nonathletes, when these arrhythmias occur initial treatment may be with β-blockers and calcium channel blockers. However, in both the 36th Bethesda Guidelines and the European Guidelines, definitive treatment such as ablation is generally preferred because of the young age and lifetime risk of these arrhythmias. Atrial premature contractions are common in many individuals and may be symptomatic or asymptomatic. If symptomatic, atrial premature beats can be treated with β-blockers; however, reassurance is usually reasonable enough treatment.

Idiopathic Ventricular Tachycardia

(Figs 44.15, 44.21 and 44.30)

The two most common cardiac regions for idiopathic ventricular tachycardias are the right ventricular outflow tract and the left posterior fascicle. Both of these ventricular tachycardias can be triggered by exercise and both these ventricular tachycardias are readily curable with ablation. They are also adenosine and verapamil sensitive. In individuals with these idiopathic ventricular tachycardias strong consideration should be given to ablation as the ablation is curative and of relatively low risk.

Deep vein thrombosis (DVT) or pulmonary embolism (PE) in athletes, The diagnosis of deep vein thrombosis (DVT) or pulmonary embolism (PE) in athletes, who exhibit classic symptoms (Table 44.1), may be delayed or even missed because such medical problems are often not considered by healthcare providers or by the affected

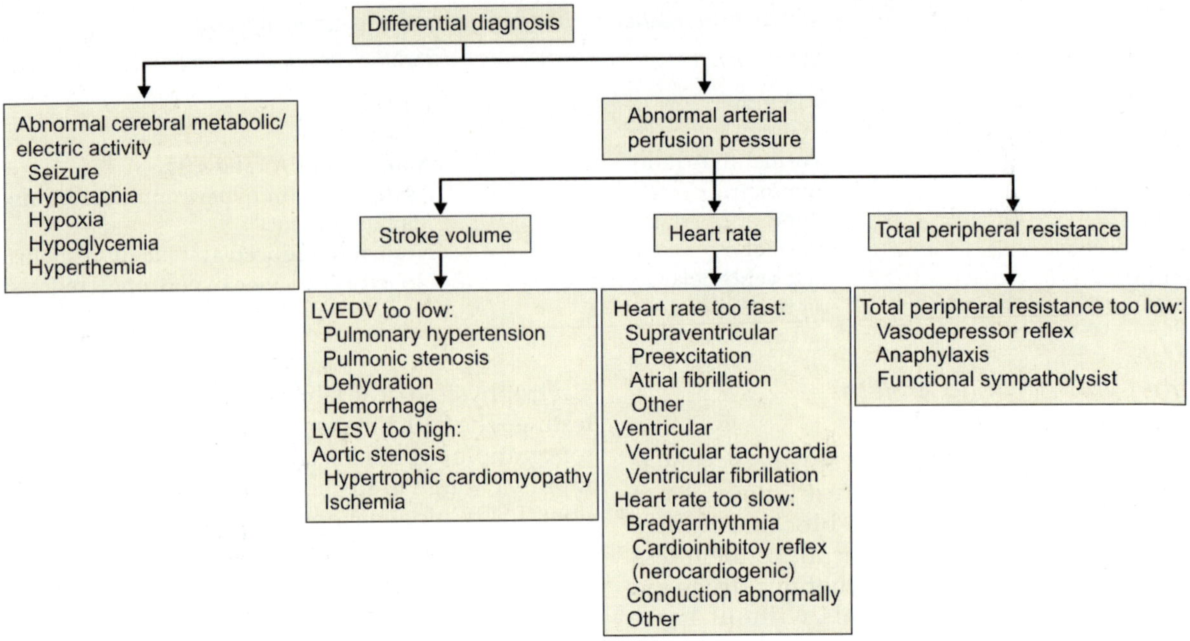

Fig. 44.24: *Differential diagnosis of exercise-related syncope in young athletes. Arterial perfusion pressure is a function of the "triple product" of heart rate 3 stroke volume 3 total peripheral resistance. LVEDV, left ventricular end diastolic volume; LVESV, left ventricular end systolic volume (Information from Levine BD, Buckey JC, Fritsch JM, Yancy CW Jr, Watenpaugh DE, Snell PG. Physical fitness and cardiovascular regulation: mechanisms of orthostatic intolerance. J Appl Physiol 1991;70:112-22)*

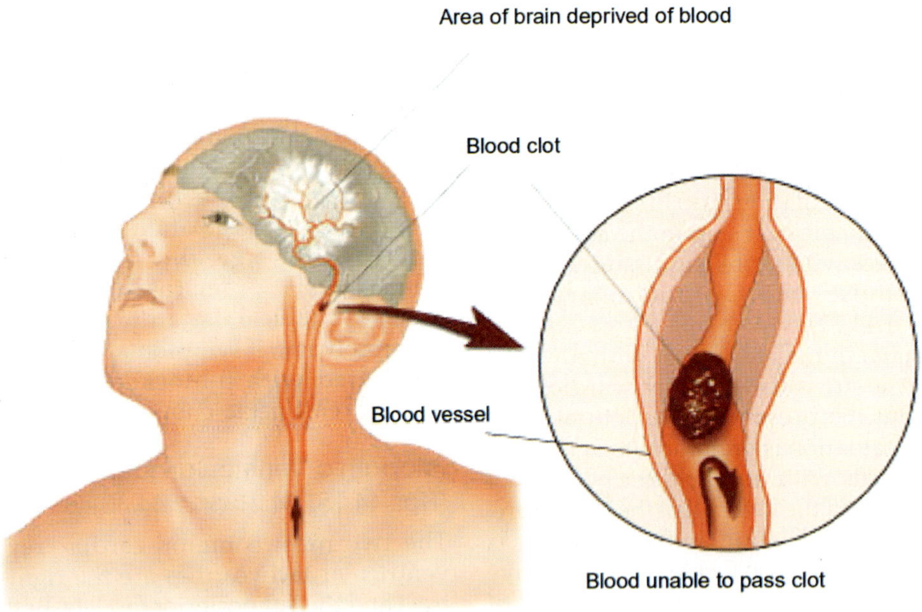

Fig. 44.25: *University of Colorado School of Medicine has explored the link between lack of oxygen, called hypoxia, and the inflammation that can injure or kill some athletes who undergo surgery. Lack of oxygen during a surgery can injure kidneys, lungs or heart muscles and this can lead to inflammation. However, athletes deliberately train at high altitude so as to adapt their bodies to the reduced oxygen*

athlete. No studies have been done to determine whether athletes are at a higher, the same, or lower risk for developing blood clots than nonathletes. Blood clots are uncommon in young, healthy individuals—and most athletes are young and healthy. So, for that reason, DVT, PE, and arterial clots in athletes are not the norm.

To understand the problematic issues facing an athlete and the attending caregiver it is important to first understand the condition terminology. Our body is composed of an endless tunnel of arteries and veins through which blood flows throughout the body. Arteries are the blood vessels through which the blood flows from the heart into the periphery: the brain, the internal organs, the legs, and the arms. A clot in an artery leads to stroke, heart attack, or limb-threatening peripheral arterial clot causing a painful, cold, and pale extremity (Fig. 44.32).

Many people think of blood clots as a problem occurring in elderly people, but not in young and apparently healthy individuals. Symptoms may, therefore, be misinterpreted as something less serious. The leg symptoms from DVT are often interpreted as "muscle tear", a "Charlie horse", a "twisted ankle", or shin splints, while the chest symptoms from PE are attributed to a pulled muscle, costochondritis (inflammation of the joint between ribs and breast bone), bronchitis, or a "touch of pneumonia".

Veins are the vessels through which blood is carried back to the heart. A clot in the deep veins of legs, arms, pelvis, abdomen, or around the brain is called a deep vein thrombosis (DVT). If a piece of clot breaks off from a leg or arm DVT. It can travel into the lung causing a life- threatening condition known as a pulmonary embolism (PE).

Athlete-Specific Risk Factors for Clots

Being apparently healthy and being an athlete does not prevent a person from developing blood clots. Several circumstances put the athlete, as well as the nonathlete, at increased risk for DVT and PE (Table 44.1). Athletes, coaches and trainers should be particularly aware of these risk factors.

Blood Clots can Occur When (Fig. 44.25)

- There is a disparity between the two systems that balance the clotting process in our blood; either (A) too much activity of the proteins and blood platelets that form clots (the procoagulant system), or (B) too little activity of the system that dissolves blood clots as they form (the fibrinolytic system) (Fig. 44.25).
- There is trauma to the blood vessel wall, as may occur after a bone fracture or in thoracic outlet obstruction (see discussion below).
- Blood return from the extremities to the heart is impaired, such as when sitting with bent legs in cramped positions for a prolonged period of time.
- The blood is "thicker" than usual, as occurs when an athlete is dehydrated, using the drug erythropoietin (EPO), or has received excessive blood transfusions (blood doping).

Unfortunately, there are few studies investigating the influence that physical training has on blood clot formation and dissolution. So, the exact net effect of training on this equilibrium is unknown. It is known, for example, that blood levels of the clotting protein "factor VIII" increase with exercise and that the elevation persists during recovery. Theoretically, this could lead to an increased risk of blood clots in athletes. However, data also indicate that the fibrinolytic system that dissolves blood clots is overactive in people who exercise. With this over activity present, the athlete would be protected from having a blood clot. Yet, the net effect of these changes in the athlete is not known.

A detailed scientific discussion of the coagulation issues relevant to exercise and training can be found in a recently published review. However, the conclusions are sparse and

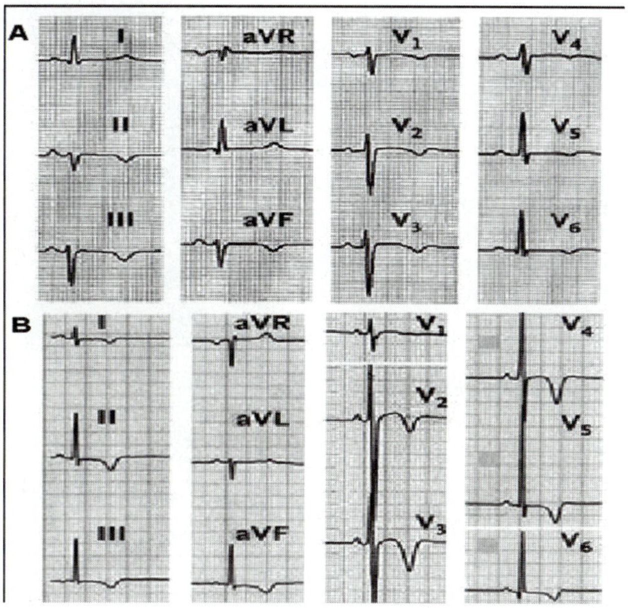

Fig. 44.26: *Three 12-lead electrocardiograms (ECGs), obtained in trained athletes at initial evaluation, showing evidence of marked repolarization abnormalities. The ECG from a young person shows diffuse T-wave inversion (Panel A). The athlete died suddenly during exercise 12 months after evaluation, of undetected arrhythmogenic right ventricular cardiomyopathy. (Panel B) shows the ECG from a 26-year-old regional-level soccer player without left ventricular hypertrophy on echocardiography at the initial evaluation. The ECG shows markedly increased R- and S-wave voltage in the precordial leads (V2-V6) in association with deep T-wave inversion in standard (I, II, III, aVF) and precordial(V_2 to V_6) leads. The athlete showed phenotypic evidence of nonobstructive hypertrophic cardiomyopathy 7 years later*

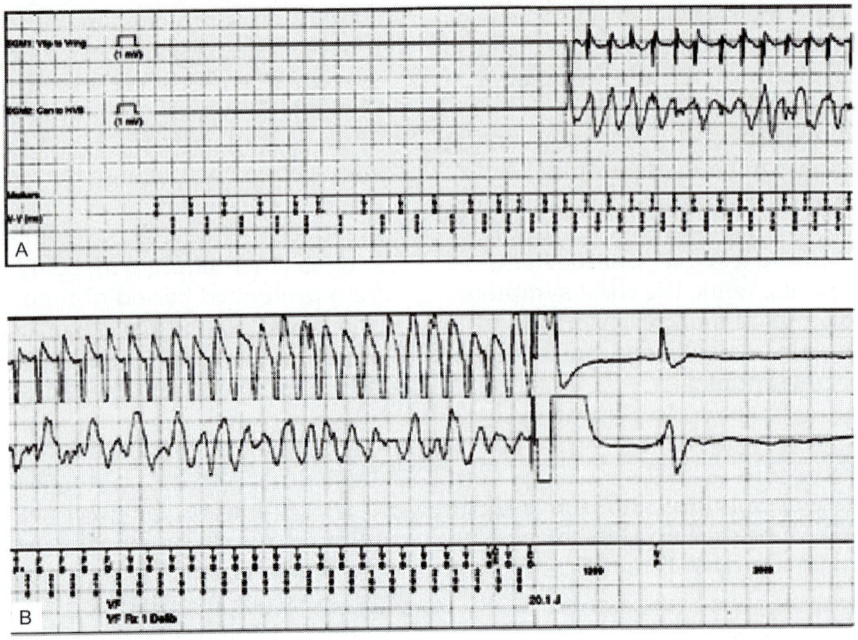

Fig. 44.27: *Initiation (A) and termination (B) of ventricular fibrillation in a 9-year-old boy with hypertrophic cardiomyopathy and an ICD. He presented 3 months earlier with syncope during a school gym class and was found to have hypertrophic cardiomyopathy. Because of the syncope and hypertrophic cardiomyopathy, an ICD was recommended and placed. This current episode also caused syncope and the ICD promptly defibrillated him*

vague, because of a lack of data and conflicting results from different studies.

Risk Factors for DVT and PE in Athletes

The most common clots occurring in athletes are DVT of the leg and PE. Factors that increase the risk for an athlete, as well as the nonathlete, are listed in Table 44.2. A few unique risk factors predisposing the young and the athlete to DVT and PE are:

Thoracic outlet obstruction

In some individuals an extra (cervical) rib or excess muscle or tendon tissue compress the big vein in the upper chest (subclavian vein) that drains the blood from the arm. This compression typically gets worse when the arm is lifted up. This obstruction, often combined with repeated trauma to the vein (due to throwing activities or gymnastics maneuvers), may cause a DVT to form in this area, extending into the arm veins. This is termed "effort thrombosis" or "thoracic outlet obstruction/syndrome". If the DVT resolves, such as after clot buster treatment, resection of the extra rib or the excess tissue may be indicated to increase space in the thoracic outlet.

Table 44.9: *Cardiovascular causes of sudden death in young competitive athletes*

Most common
Hypertrophic cardiomyopathy
Congenital coronary artery anomaly
Less common
Myocarditis
Aortic rupture (Marfan syndrome)
Mitral valve prolapse
Uncommon
Arrhythmogenic RV cardiomyopathy
Atherosclerotic coronary artery disease
Conduction system abnormalities
Aortic valve stenosis

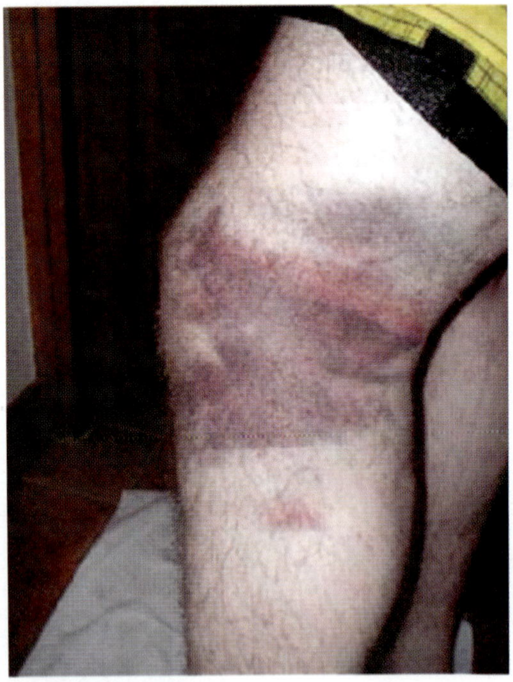

Fig. 44.28: *Bruise can cause a serious blood clot in athletes*

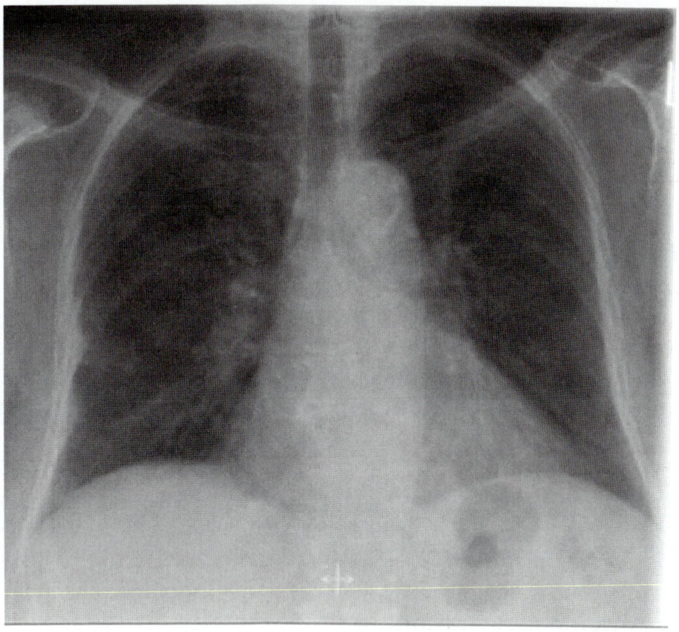

Fig. 44.29: *Pulmonary embolism with lung infarction. Notice the peripheral wedge of airspace opacity lateral in the middle lobe, the "Hampton's hump"*

May-Thurner syndrome

This is a common congenital anatomic variation that predisposes to DVT in the left leg because the main left pelvic vein is compressed by the overlying main right pelvic artery. This increases the risk of clot formation at the site of this narrowing in the left pelvis with extension of clot down into the left leg. If the DVT resolves, such as after clot buster (thrombolytic) treatment, the narrowing can be opened up by a radiologist with a balloon angioplasty and then kept open by placing a stent (Fig. 44.28).

Congenital Absence or Malformation of the Vena Cava

Congenital abnormalities of the anatomy of the big vein in the abdomen (vena cava) or pelvic veins can be a cause of DVT in young people. The abnormal anatomy probably leads to disturbed blood flow and an increased risk of clotting. Treatment decisions for people affected with blood clots must be individualized. This is particularly true for young, apparently healthy individuals, such as athletes. In the case of unexplained DVT, testing for an inherited or acquired clotting disorder may be appropriate. When first diagnosed with the DVT, clot buster medication (fibrinolytic or thrombolytic therapy) should be considered to quickly dissolve the clot. However, clot buster treatment has not been systematically studied to determine whether it really decreases the risk for long-term damage to the veins of the leg and arm, i.e. the postthrombotic syndrome.

Athlete-Specific Challenges and Questions

Most often, an active individual—be it an athlete or one who remains physically fit through routine training and exercise—is suddenly stymied by the affects of his/her clotting incident. Questions, lots of questions, are poised to the caregiver. Of paramount importance for the athlete are particularly the two following issues:

(a) Can I continue my sport while on warfarin?

A solid medical assessment should be made whether the person who has had a blood clot can come off warfarin or should remain on it. Being on warfarin increases the risk for bleeding. Therefore, contact sports and sports

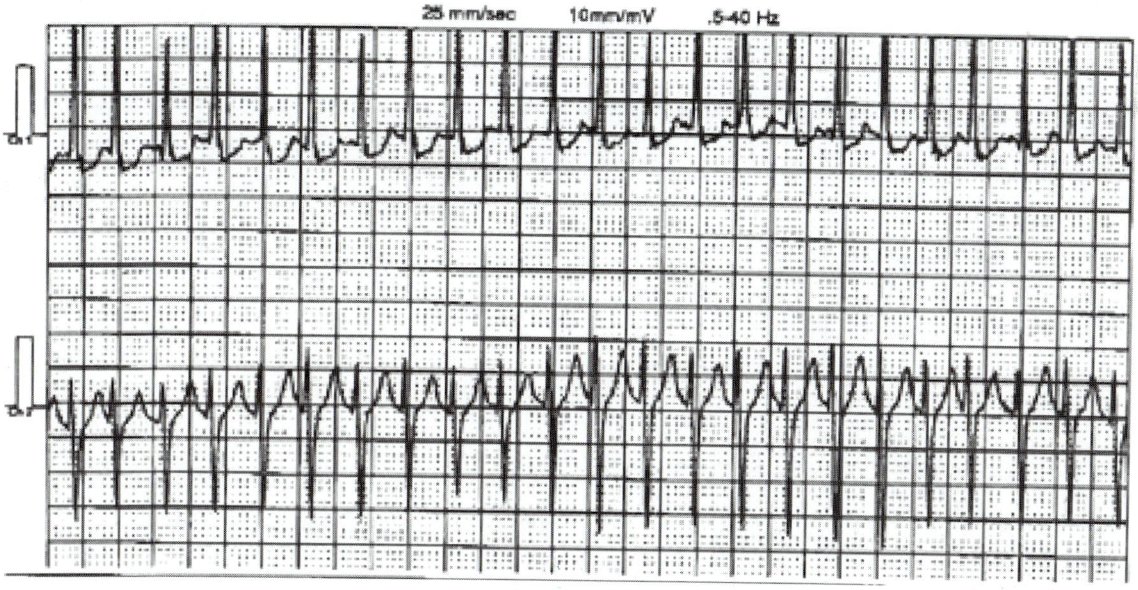

Fig. 44.30: *Loop monitor recording of a 20-year-old female who, during basketball games, had sudden onset of palpitations, lightheadedness, and fatigue, limiting but not eliminating her ability to play ball. Her coaches thought that she wasn't trying hard enough until this loop monitor documented a narrow complex tachycardia that was the cause of her symptoms. At an invasive electrophysiologic evaluation she was found to have AV nodal reentrant tachycardia which was successfully ablated*

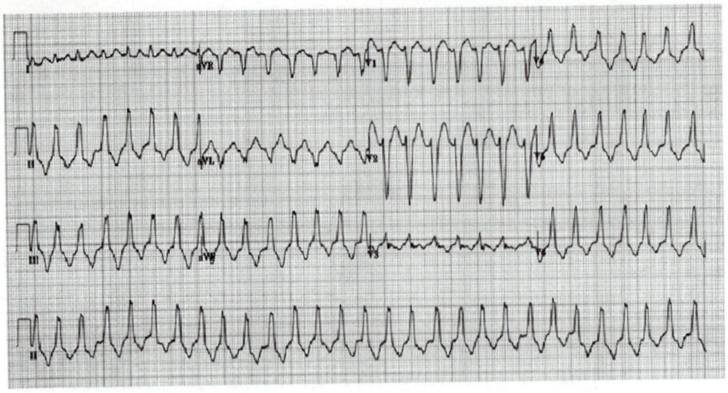

Fig. 44.31: *The ECG from a patient with ARVC, had paroxysmal episodes of ventricular tachycardia with a LBBB morphology (i.e. RV, VT)*

with a risk for serious injury, such as football, hockey, basketball, soccer, gymnastics, alpine skiing, or boxing should not be pursued by a person on warfarin. However, athletes such as runners, bicyclists or triathletes may be able to continue their sport, but they should adapt their activities to avoid trauma that might put them at risk for bleeding (avoid situations leading to bicycle crashes, etc.). Individual blood thinning treatment plans can also be designed, such as (a) a decrease in warfarin dosage a few days prior to athletic events that would otherwise put the person at increased risk for bleeding, (b) switching the athlete who should be on long-term blood thinners to low molecular weight heparin shots during the athletic season and interrupting the shots for competitions that pose a risk for bleeding, (c) stopping blood thinners during the season and accepting a higher risk for blood clots during that time, but restarting warfarin during the off season. Finally, an athlete may decide to switch from a high risk bleeding competitive sport to one with a lower risk. Obviously, these are all very individual treatment decisions that should be thoroughly discussed between the patient's personal physician, the patient, and the team physician (if the patient is participating in a team sport).

(b) How soon after a DVT or PE can I go back to training? (Fig. 44.32)

Patients with a DVT may have significant extremity swelling and pain which may improve only slowly over weeks and months. Some residual symptoms may persist long-term, this is termed "postthrombotic syndrome". It appears that being highly active 1 month after a DVT is not detrimental; it may, actually be beneficial and lead to less symptoms of postthrombotic syndrome. This can be used as an argument to encourage individuals to return to physical activity relatively soon after a DVT. Also, wearing individually fitted compression stockings decreases the long-term risk for postthrombotic syndrome.

No official guidelines exist as to when and how quickly an athlete might return to exercising. Each patient will need an individualized exercise plan. It seems appropriate to refrain from any athletic activities for the first 10–14 days after an acute DVT or PE until the clot is more adherent to the blood vessel wall and the risk of having the clot break loose (causing a PE) has decreased. To lessen deconditioning during this period of relative inactivity, the athlete may do some strength training—arm and trunk exercises in the case of a leg DVT, leg and trunk exercises in the case of an arm DVT. The athlete may then increase activity between week 2 and 4 and return to preclot activity levels by week 4.

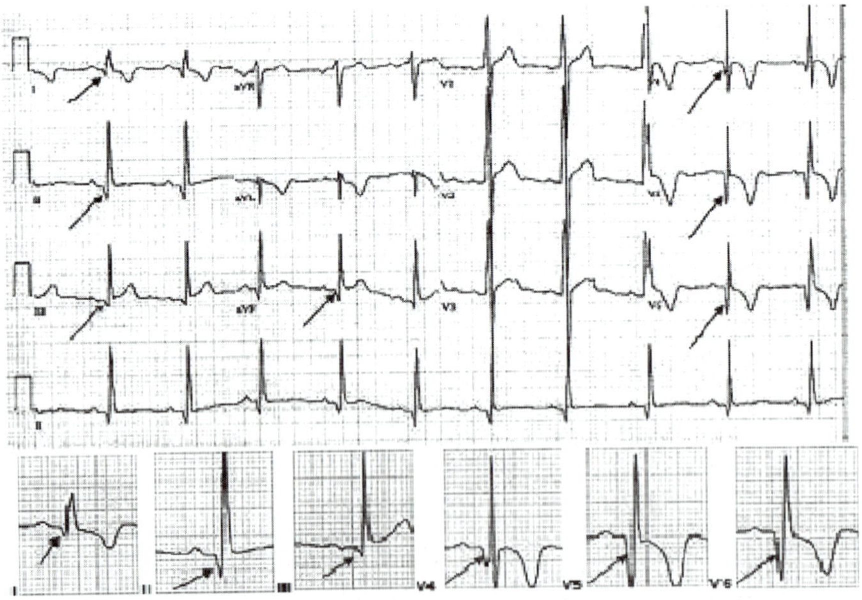

Fig. 44.32: *ECG in HOCM. Producing pseudo Q wave in HOCM (hypertrophic obstructive cardiomyopathy) usually has LVH pattern. Left ventricular hypertrophy results in increased precordial voltages and nonspecific ST segment and T-wave abnormalities. Asymmetrical septal hypertrophy produces deep, narrow ("dagger-like") Q waves in the lateral (V5-6, I, aVL) and inferior (II, III, aVF) leads. These may mimic prior myocardial infarction, although the Q-wave morphology is different: infarction Q waves are typically > 40 ms duration while septal Q waves in HCM are < 40 ms. Lateral Q waves are more common than inferior Q waves in HCM*

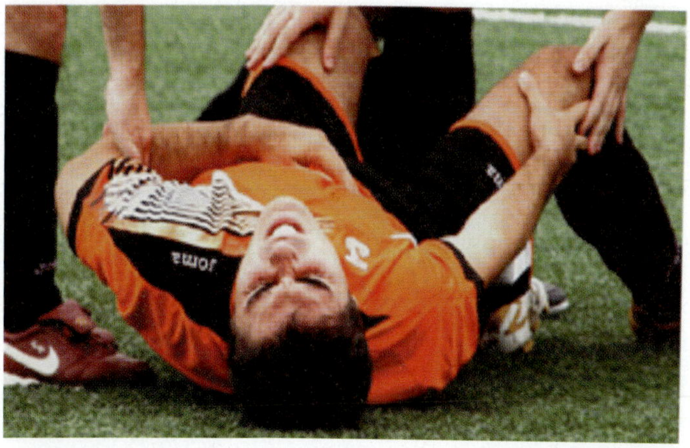

Fig. 44.33: *A young athlete is found collapsing from cardiac arrest in playing ground*

Psychosocial Implications

Athletes need to appreciate that significant deconditioning can occur after a DVT or PE. Depression can also set in after such a life-changing event. This is not surprising, given that athletes often view themselves as healthy and, from a health point of view, invincible, and now suddenly realize that they are vulnerable, sick, and sometimes even disabled. Patient support groups may be helpful in this situation, as may antidepressants.

How to Minimize the Risk for Clots

Measures that the athlete and, for that matter, the non-athlete should take to minimize the risk for DVT or PE are listed in Table 44.3. For the athlete, the most important ones are probably to (a) avoid dehydration, and (b) take breaks when traveling long distances.

Prognosis: Although gross structural changes resemble those in some cardiac disorders, no adverse effects are apparent. In most cases, structural changes and bradycardia regress with detraining although up to 20% of elite athletes have residual chamber enlargement, raising questions, in the absence of long-term data, about whether athlete's heart is truly benign.

Treatment: No treatment is required, although 3 months of deconditioning may be needed to monitor LV regression as a way of distinguishing this syndrome from cardiomyopathy. Such deconditioning can greatly interfere with an athlete's life and may meet with resistance.

Hypercoagulability in Athletes

Risk factors for thromboembolism are well known, and athletes are placed under conditions that can result in exposure to several of these risk factors, which include travel, trauma, immobilization, hemoconcentration, and polycythemia. Presence of a genetic hypercoagulable disorder adds additional risk. Overall management is no different than in nonathletes. Thrombolysis is strongly recommended for upper extremity deep venous thrombosis (DVT) coupled with surgical decompression of obstructive structures if indicated. Thrombolytic therapy does not appear to be necessary for treatment of lower extremity DVT. Prevention of DVT with travel can be achieved through general techniques such as leg exercises, hydration, and loose fitting clothes. Aspirin before travel shows some benefits of protection, but individuals at higher risk may need low molecular weight heparin. Athletes should be screened during preparticipation physicals for thromboembolic risk. Individuals on anticoagulation therapy should not participate in collision or contact sports. Return to play with gradual increase in intensity is recommended with careful monitoring for recurrent venous thromboembolism and management of postthrombotic symptoms.

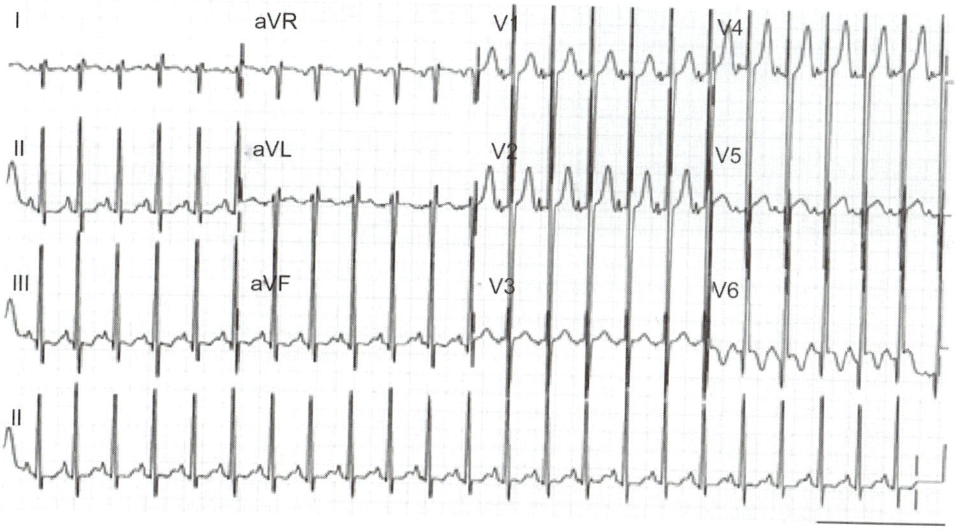

Fig. 44.34: *ECG presentation in patient with ALCAPA. Typical prominent Q waves are present in lead V6. Conversely, typical abrupt loss of R waves in midprecordial leads and prominent Q waves in leads I and aVL associated with ALCAPA are not present*

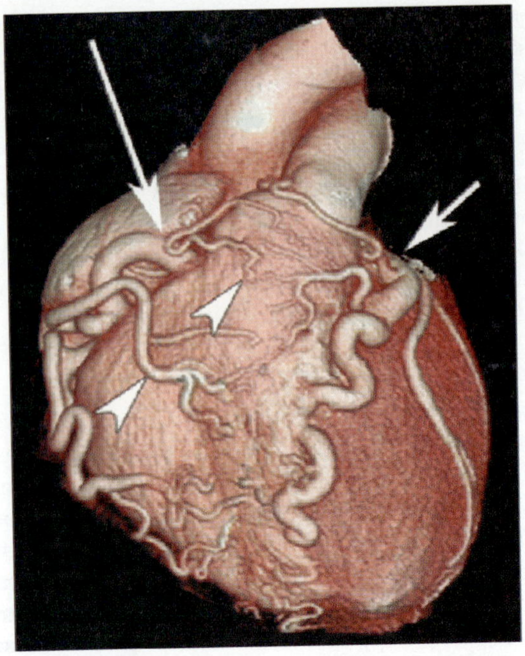

Fig. 44.35: *Three dimensional volume-rendered multidetector CT angiogram shows dilated intercoronary collateral arteries (arrowheads), which connect the tortuous RCA (long arrow) to the LCA (short arrow)*

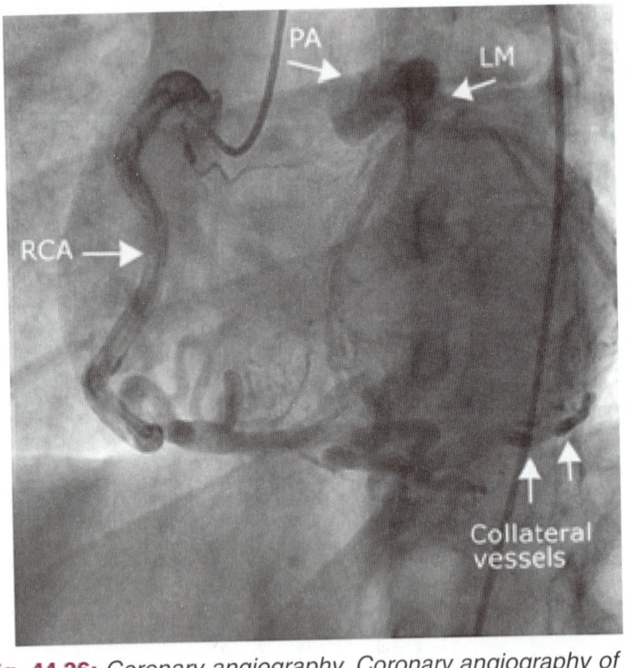

Fig. 44.36: *Coronary angiography. Coronary angiography of the right coronary artery with collateral filling of the left coronary vascular territory, which connects directly to the pulmonary trunk*

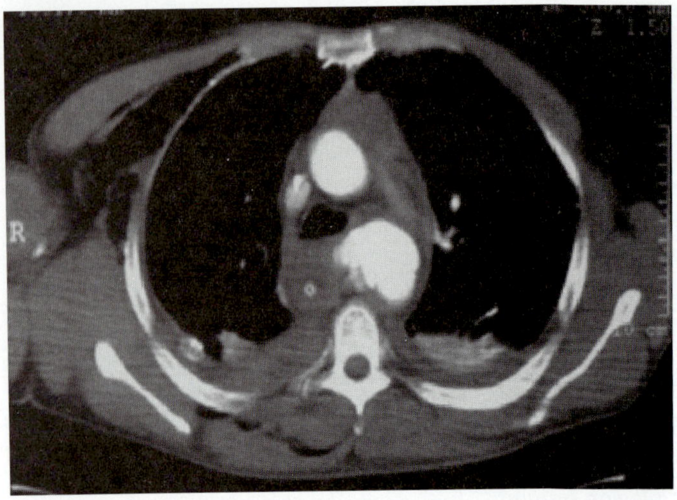

Fig. 44.37: *Axial source image of CT angiography traumatic aortic dissection*

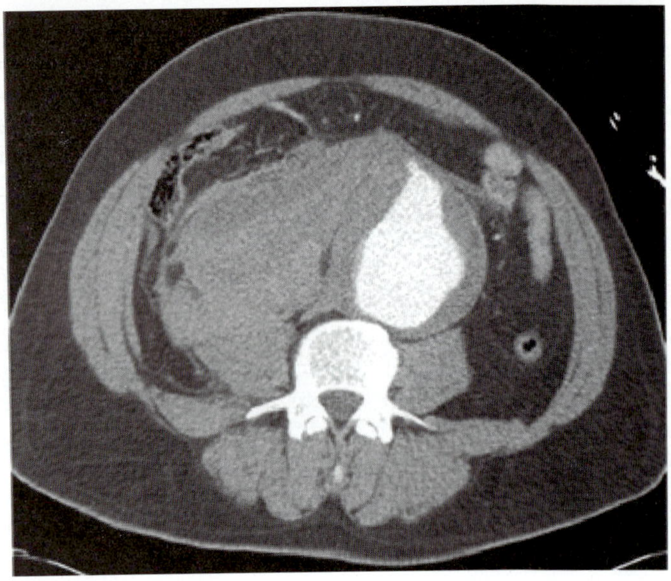

Fig. 44.38: *Axial source image of CT angiography showing ruptured ascending aorta*

Sudden Cardiac Arrest in Young Athletes (Figs 44.3, 44.34–44.36)

Each year between 10–12 million kids in the US participate in sports. The tragedy of a sudden death in an otherwise "presumably healthy" child causes not only sadness, but concern as to how the death might have been prevented. Doctors are often asked, "isn't there a test or something to prevent this?" (Tables 44.9).

Depending on the studies I have read, the sudden cardiac death of a child or adolescent accounts for about 100 deaths a year in the US. The prevalence rate for sudden cardiac death is 1:100,000–200,000 and is higher among males than females. Statistics show that 90% of these sudden deaths occur immediately posttraining or competition with football and basketball having the highest incidence.

In 2007, the American Heart Association came out with guidelines to evaluate athletes who may be at risk for sudden cardiac death. The most important screening mechanism has been found to be the "gold standard" in medicine, a thorough history and physical examination. The history that should be taken on any athlete who is being screened for sports participation should include a history of any unexplained or sudden death in a family member.

Are there any family members with unexplained fainting episodes or seizures? Are there family members who had unexplained deaths (drowning or single car accidents)? Are there any family members with a known genetic disorder that predisposes to sudden cardiac death? The history should also ask about any fainting (syncope) in the athlete. After a good history is taken (which should be updated yearly), the child/adolescent needs a complete and thorough physical examination. This examination should include blood pressure measurements, and a careful cardiac examination looking for new murmurs. Symptoms such as palpitations during exercise, visual changes, fainting while exercising or immediately after exercise, and chest pain should all warrant further evaluation. Studies show that about half of pediatric patients who succumb to sudden cardiac death had experienced a warning sign.

There are about 20 causes for SCD, with the most common causes being hypertrophic cardiomyopathy, anomalous coronary artery, and myocarditis. While some may advocate routine EKG screening and echocardiograms on athletes (this is done in Italy), many studies have been done which show that it would take the screening of 200,000 student athletes to prevent 1 death. At the same time, you will certainly identify some children with clear risk factors for SCD, but for every positive finding there may be 10–20 athletes who have "borderline" or questionable findings that would require even more expensive follow-up. These pediatric patients might also be told they cannot participate in sports during the evaluation time and some might be told that they cannot participate even if they were not found to have disease, but were excluded just due to liability concerns.

There does not seem to be one right answer to this issue. If your child is going to begin competitive sports make sure to see your pediatrician for a complete physical examination including a good family history. Also advocate that your school have automatic external defibrillators viable at all times and personnel that know how to use them. That's your daily dose for today. We'll chat again tomorrow.

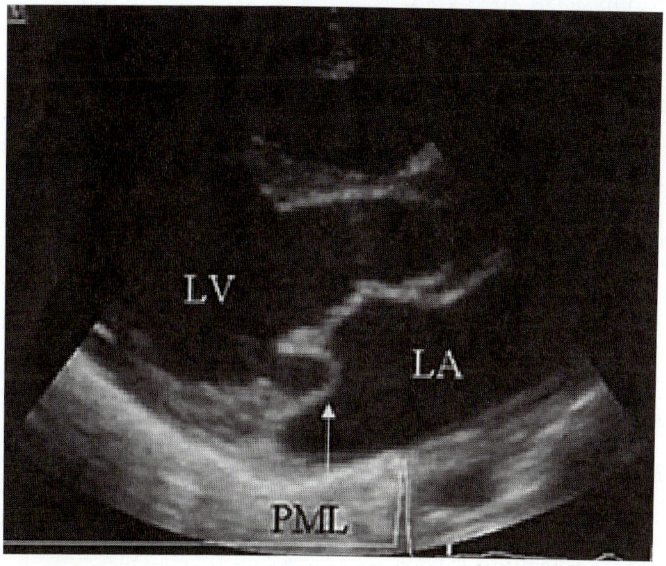

Fig. 44.39: *2D echocardiography in LAX view showing mitral valve prolapse in young athlete with cardiac arrhythmia*

Cardiovascular Causes of Sudden Death in Young Individuals Including Athletes

From 1978 to 1993 in the Veneto region, we collected 200 cases of sudden death in the young (<35 years). Sudden death was cerebral in 15 cases (7.5%), respiratory in 10 (5%), and cardiovascular in 163 (81.5%), whereas it remained unexplained in 12 cases (6%). Among cardiovascular sudden death, obstructive coronary atherosclerosis accounted for 23% of cases, arrhythmogenic right ventricular cardiomyopathy for 12.5%, mitral valve prolapse for 10%, conduction system abnormalities for 10%, congenital coronary artery anomalies for 8.5%, myocarditis for 7.5%, hypertrophic cardiomyopathy for 5.5%, aortic rupture for 5.5%, dilated cardiomyopathy for 5%, nonatherosclerotic-acquired coronary artery disease for 3.5%, postoperative congenital heart disease for 3%, aortic stenosis for 2%, pulmonary embolism for 2%, and other causes for 2%. Cardiac arrest remained unexplained in 6% of the cases. Specific pathology and pathogenetic mechanisms of each disease were investigated and correlated with clinical signs and symptoms in detail. A large spectrum of cardiovascular disorders, both congenital and acquired, may represent the organic substrate of sudden death in the young. The underlying abnormality is frequently concealed and discovered only at postmortem examination. Most of the diseases, although asymptomatic, are potentially detectable during life with proper imaging tests (Figs 44.34–44.36).

Risk of Sudden Death During Sports Performance

Little is known about the risk of sudden death associated with exercise in young competitive athletes, and whether the benefits of sports activity outweigh the hazards of exercise-related fatal events is a clinical dilemma. For the purpose of this consensus document, we consider young competitive athletic individuals who are aged 35 years or less and are engaged in a regular fashion in exercise training as well as participating in official athletic competitions. Competition is intended as an organized team or individual sport event, placing high premium on athletic excellence and achievement. Characteristics of competitive athletes are their strong inclination to extend themselves physically to their limits and to improve performance.

Recently, Corrado et al assessed the incidence of sudden death in the athletic and nonathletic young population (12–35 years old) of the Veneto Region of Italy and showed that competitive sports activity enhances by 2.5-fold the risk of sudden death in adolescents and young adults. In this study, young competitive athletes who died suddenly were affected by silent cardiovascular diseases, predominantly consisting of cardiomyopathies, premature coronary artery disease, and congenital coronary anomalies. Therefore, sports activity was not per se a cause of the increased mortality; rather, it acted as a trigger of cardiac arrest upon those underlying cardiovascular

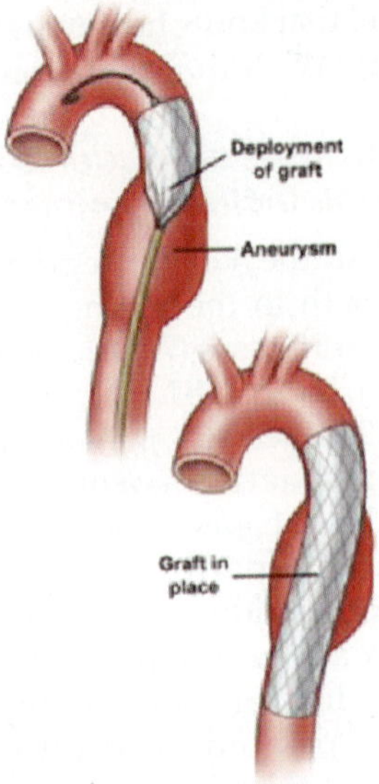

Fig. 44.40: *Surgical repair in a athlete with Marfan syndrome*

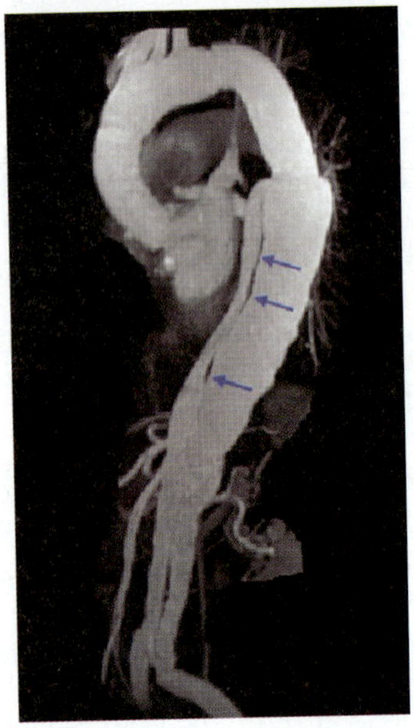

Fig. 44.41: *MRI of type B aortic dissection (blue arrows) in a athlete with Marfan syndrome*

diseases predisposing to life-threatening ventricular arrhythmias. Thus, it seems ethically and clinically justifiable that every effort should be made to recognize in good time such diseases that the athlete is at risk, with the perspective that disqualification of affected individuals makes the prevention of athletic field death possible.

Acute Aortic Dissection

(Figs 44.37, 44.38 and 44.40 and 44.41)

Acute aortic dissection can occur at the time of intense physical exertion in strength-trained athletes like weightlifters, bodybuilders, throwers and wrestlers.

Rapid rise in blood pressure and history of hypertension are the most common causes of aortic dissection in athletes. It is a very tragic event because of its high mortality rate of about 32% in young patients.

Mitral valve prolapse: definition and implications in athletes

Mitral valve prolapse is probably the most common cardiac valve disorder, affecting approximately 5% of the population. Although it is genetically determined, its clinical manifestations do not usually become evident before adulthood. In the setting of a cardiology referral center, a mitral valve prolapse syndrome, consisting of nonspecific symptoms, repolarization changes on the electrocardiogram and arrhythmias, has been identified. However, doubt has recently been expressed about the existence of such a syndrome. The prognosis of mitral valve prolapse is generally favorable but infrequent complications do occur and include transient ischemic attacks, progression of mitral regurgitation with or without ruptured chordae tendineae, infective endocarditis and sudden death. The symptoms and the complications are not usually related to physical activity. A permissive attitude toward participation of patients with mitral valve prolapse in competitive athletics is probably warranted; however, it would appear reasonable to disqualify athletes with mitral valve prolapse in the following circumstances: history of syncope; disabling chest pain; complex ventricular arrhythmias, particularly if induced or worsened by exercise; significant mitral regurgitation; prolonged QT interval; Marfan's syndrome; and family history of sudden death (Figs 44.19–44.22).

BIBLIOGRAPHY

1. Lohr, John Thoman. (1999). Athletic Heart Syndrome. Gale Encyclopedia of Medicine.
2. Alexander RW, Schlant RC, Fuster V (editors). The Heart. 9th ed. New York: McGraw-Hill, 1998.
3. Drezner, Jonathan A. Sudden cardiac death in young athletes. Postgraduate Medicine, October 2000.
4. O'Conner, Francis G, et al. Sudden death in young athletes: screening for the needle in a haystack. American Family Physician, June 1998.
5. Maron BJ, Mitchell JH. Revised eligibility recommendations for competitive athletes with cardiovascular abnormalities: the introduction to Bethesda Conference #26. J Am Coll Cardiol. 1994; 24:846–848.
6. Maron BJ. Structural features of the athlete heart as defined by echocardiography. J Am Coll Cardiol. 1986;7:190–203.
7. Rost R. The athlete's heart. Eur Heart J. 1982;3(suppl A):193–198.
8. Hutson TP, Puffer JC, MacMillan W. The athlete heart syndrome. N Engl J Med. 1985;313:24–32.
9. Maron BJ, Roberts WC, McAllister HA, Rosing DR, Epstein SE. Sudden death in young athletes. Circulation. 1980;62:218–229.
10. Maron BJ, Epstein SE, Roberts WC. Causes of sudden death in the competitive athlete. J Am Coll Cardiol. 1986;7:204–214.
11. Maron BJ, Shirani J, Mueller FO, Cantu RC, Roberts WC. Cardiovascular causes of "athletic field" deaths: analysis of sudden death in 84 competitive athletes. Circulation. 1993;88(suppl I):I–50.
12. Lewis JF, Maron BJ, Diggs JA, Spencer JE, Mehrotra PP, Curry CL. Preparticipation echocardiographic screening for

cardiovascular disease in a large predominantly black population of collegiate athletes. Am J Cardiol. 1989;64:1029–1033.
13. Maron BJ, Bodison S, Wesley Y, Tucker E, Green KJ. Results of screening a large population of intercollegiate athletes for cardiovascular disease. J Am Coll Cardiol. 1987;10:1214–1222.
14. Maron BJ. Sudden death in young athletes: lessons from the Hank Gathers affair. N Engl J Med. 1993;329:55–57.
15. Kassirer JP. Diagnosis in the public domain. N Engl J Med. 1993;329:50–51.
16. The death of Reggie Lewis: a search for answers. Boston Globe, September 12, 1993:69–76.
17. Maron BJ, Mitchell JH. 26th Bethesda Conference: recommendations for determining eligibility for competition in athletes with cardiovascular abnormalities. J Am Coll Cardiol. 1994;24:845–899.
18. Ehsani AA, Hagberg JM, Hickson RC. Rapid changes in left ventricular dimensions and mass in response to physical conditioning and deconditioning. Am J Cardiol. 1978;42:52–56.
19. Fagard R, Aubert A, Lysens R, Staessen J, Vanhees L, Amery A. Noninvasive assessment of seasonal variations in cardiac structure and function in cyclists. Circulation. 1983;67:896–901.
20. Shapiro LM. Physiological left ventricular hypertrophy. Br Heart J. 1984;52:130–135.
21. Shapiro LM, Kleinebenne A, McKenna WJ. The distribution of left ventricular hypertrophy in hypertrophic cardiomyopathy: comparison of athletes and hypertensives. Eur Heart J. 1985;6:967–974.
22. Milliken MC, Stray–Gundersen J, Peshock RM, Katz J, Mitchell JH. Left ventricular mass as determined by magnetic resonance imaging in male endurance athletes. Am J Cardiol. 1988;62:301–305.
23. Douglas PS, O'Toole ML, Hiller DB, Reichek N. Left ventricular structure and function by echocardiography in ultraendurance athletes. Am J Cardiol. 1986;58:805–809.
24. Pelliccia A, Maron BJ, Spataro A, Caselli G. Absence of left ventricular hypertrophy in athletes engaged in intense power training. Am J Cardiol. 1993;72:1048–1054.
25. Pelliccia A, Maron BJ, Spataro A, Proschan MA, Spirito P. The upper limit of physiologic cardiac hypertrophy in highly trained elite athletes. N Engl J Med. 1991;324:295–301.
26. Nishimura T, Yamada Y, Kawai C. Echocardiographic evaluation of long-term effects of exercise on left ventricular hypertrophy and function in professional bicyclists. Circulation. 1980;61:832–840.
27. Morganroth J, Maron BJ, Henry WL, Epstein SE. Comparative left ventricular dimensions in trained athletes. Ann Intern Med. 1975;82:521–524.
28. Gilbert CA, Nutter DO, Felner JM, Perkins JV, Heymsfield SB, Schlant RC. Echocardiographic study of cardiac dimensions and functions in the endurance-trained athlete. Am J Cardiol. 1977;40:528–533.
29. Keul J, Dickhuth H-H, Simon G, Lehmann M. Effect of static and dynamic exercise on heart volume, contractility, and left ventricular dimensions. Circ Res. 1981;48(suppl I):I-162-I-170.
30. Ikaheimo MJ, Palatsi IJ, Takkunen JT. Noninvasive evaluation of the athletic heart: sprinters versus endurance runners. Am J Cardiol. 1979;44:24–30.
31. Longhurst JC, Kelly AR, Gonyea WJ, Mitchell JH. Chronic training with static and dynamic exercise: cardiovascular adaptation and response to exercise. Circ Res. 1981;48(suppl I):I–171-I-178.
32. El-Sayed MS, et al: Exercise and training effects on blood haemostasis in health and disease: an update. Sports Med 2004;34(3):181–200.
33. Shrier I, Kahn SR: Effect of physical activity after recent deep venous thrombosis: a cohort study. Medicine and Science in Sports and Exercise 2005;37: 630–634.
34. Roberts WO, Christie DM: Return to training and competition after deep venous calf thrombosis. Medicine and Science in Sports and Exercise 1992;24:2.

45 Hypothermia in Children and Adolescents

Hypothermia in children presents several challenges. It is common enough that clinicians will need to recognize and treat it, but uncommon enough that the details of care are hard to recall. The diagnosis is surprisingly easy to overlook, and its treatment alters some standard practices. Although generally harmful, severe hypothermia may also provide cerebral protection against anoxia, allowing cases of remarkable survival after cardiac arrest (Figs 45.1 and 45.2).

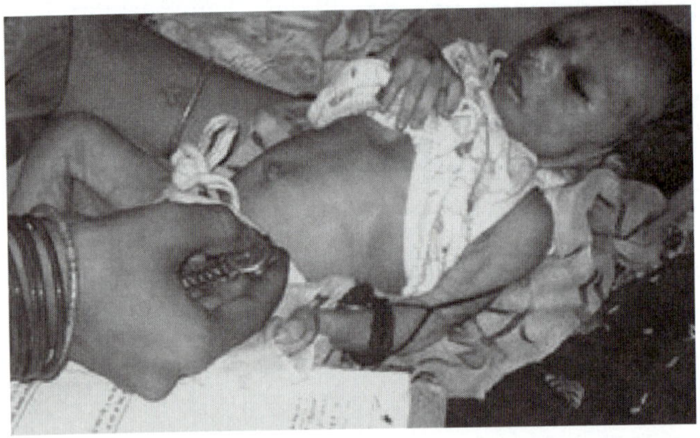

Fig. 45.1: *Infant with septecemia who was very weak with high respiratory rate and hypothermia*

Hypothermia (from Greek, is a condition in which core temperature drops below the required temperature for normal metabolism and body functions which is defined as 35.0°C (95.0°F). Body temperature is usually maintained near a constant level of 36.5–37.5°C (98–100°F) through biologic homeostasis or thermoregulation. If exposed to cold and the internal mechanisms are unable to replenish the heat that is being lost, a drop in core temperature occurs. As body temperature decreases, characteristic symptoms occur such as shivering and mental confusion.

Hypothermia is the opposite of hyperthermia which is present in heat exhaustion and heat stroke. The lowest documented body temperature from which anyone has recovered was 13.0°C (55.4°F), in a drowning incident involving a 7-year-old girl in Sweden in December 2010.

Classification

Normal human body temperature in adults is 34.4–37.8°C (94–100°F). Sometimes a narrower range is stated, such as 36.5–37.5°C (98–100°F). Hypothermia is defined as any body temperature below 35.0°C (95.0°F). It is subdivided into four different degrees:

1. Mild, 32–35°C (90–95°F)
2. Moderate, 28–32°C (82–90°F)
3. Severe, 20–28°C (68–82°F)
4. **Profound** at less than 20°C (68°F). This is in contrast to hyperthermia and fever which are defined as a temperature of greater than 37.5°C (99.5°F)–38.3°C (100.9°F).

Pathophysiology

The body's core temperature is tightly regulated in the "thermoneutral zone" between 36.5°C and 37.5°C, outside

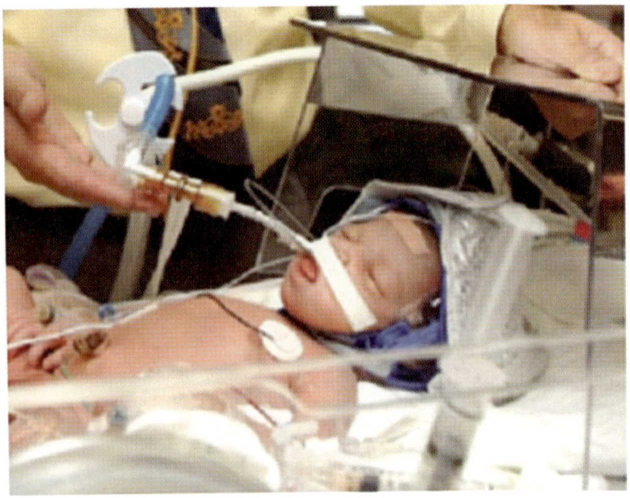

Fig. 45.2: *Neonatal hypothermia treatment with cooling cap*

of which thermoregulatory responses are usually activated. The body maintains a stable core temperature through balancing heat production and heat loss. At rest, humans produce 40–60 kilocalories (kcal) of heat per square meter of body surface area through generation by cellular metabolism, most prominently in the liver and the heart. Heat production increases with striated muscle contraction; shivering increases the rate of heat production 2–5 times. Heat loss occurs via several mechanisms, the most significant of which, under dry conditions, is radiation (55–65% of heat loss). Conduction and convection account for about 15% of additional heat loss, and respiration and evaporation account for the remainder. Conductive and convective heat loss, or direct transfer of heat to another object or circulating air, respectively, are the most common causes of accidental hypothermia. Conduction is a particularly significant mechanism of heat loss in drowning/immersion accidents as thermal conductivity of water is up to 30 times that of air (Fig. 45.3).

The hypothalamus controls thermoregulation via increased heat conservation (peripheral vasoconstriction and behavior responses) and heat production (shivering and increasing levels of thyroxine and epinephrine). Alterations of the CNS may impair these mechanisms. The threshold for shivering is 1° lower than that of vasoconstriction and is considered a last resort mechanism by the body to maintain temperature. The mechanisms for heat preservation may be overwhelmed in the face of cold stress and core temperature can drop secondary to fatigue or glycogen depletion.

Hypothermia affects virtually all organ systems. Perhaps the most significant effects are seen in the cardiovascular system and the CNS. Hypothermia results in decreased depolarization of cardiac pacemaker cells, causing bradycardia. Since this bradycardia is not vagally mediated, it can be refractory to standard therapies such as atropine. Mean arterial pressure and cardiac output decrease, and an electrocardiogram (ECG) may show characteristic J or Osborne J waves (*see* the image below). While generally associated with hypothermia, the J wave may be a normal variant and is seen occasionally in sepsis and myocardial ischemia.

Osborne (J) waves (V3) in a patient with a rectal core temperature of 26.7°C (80.1°F). ECG courtesy of Heather Murphy-Lavoie of Charity Hospital, New Orleans.

Atrial and ventricular arrhythmias can result from hypothermia; asystole and ventricular fibrillation have been noted to begin spontaneously at core temperatures below 25–28°C.

Hypothermia progressively depresses the CNS, decreasing CNS metabolism in a linear fashion as the core temperature drops. At core temperatures less than 33°C, brain electrical activity becomes abnormal; between 19°C and 20°C, an electroencephalogram (EEG) may appear consistent with brain death. Tissues have decreased oxygen consumption at lower temperatures; it is not clear whether this is due to decreases in metabolic rate at lower temperatures or a greater hemoglobin affinity for oxygen coupled with impaired oxygen extraction of hypothermic tissues.

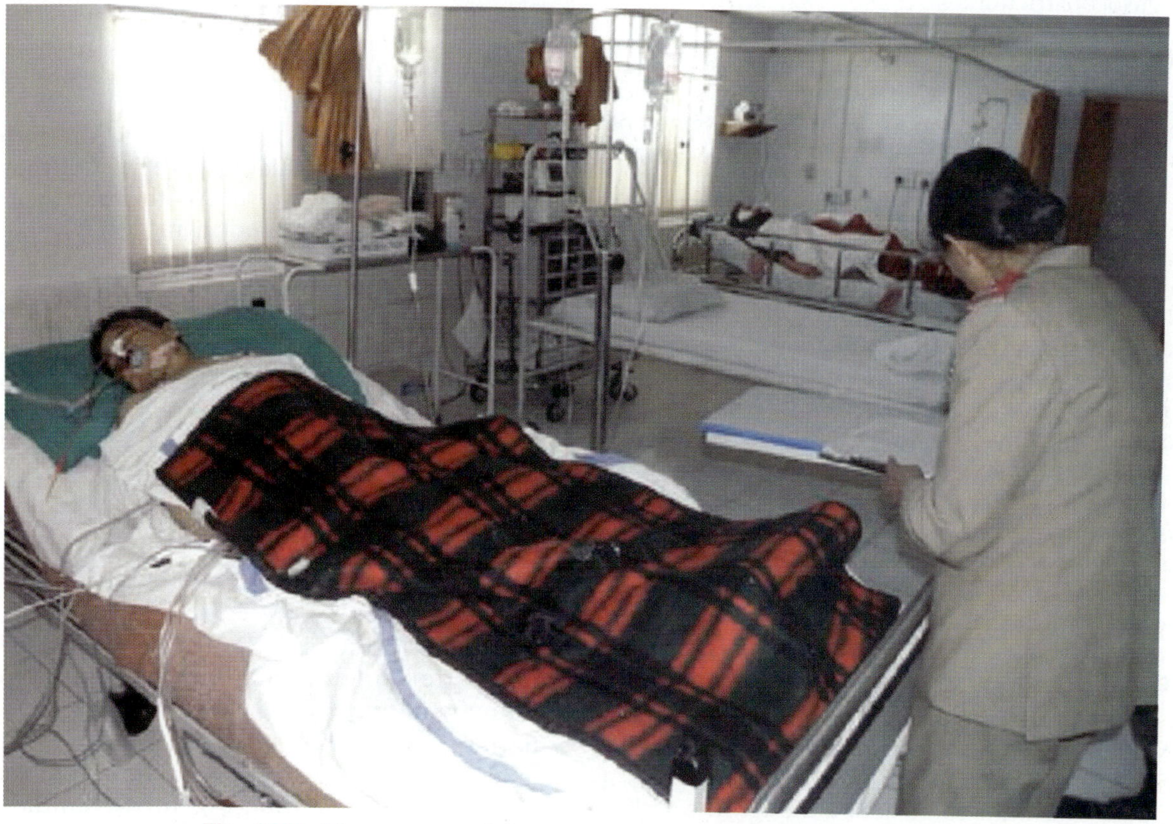

Fig. 45.3: *Management of the patient in the hospital with hypothermia*

The term "core temperature after drop" refers to a further decrease in core temperature and associated clinical deterioration of a patient after rewarming has been initiated. The current theory of this documented phenomenon is that as peripheral tissues are warmed, vasodilation allows cooler blood in the extremities to circulate back into the body core. Other mechanisms may be in operation as well. Some believe that after drop is most likely to occur in patients with frostbite or long-standing hypothermia.

Heat Loss Occurs through: Radiation, Conduction, Convection, Evaporation

- Hypothermia results in multiple organ failure.
- Shivering increases metabolic rate (2–5 times) but only while glycogen stores last and above 30°C.
- Vasoconstriction fails at temperatures below 24°C
- Tachycardia is followed by bradycardia, hypotension and fall in cardiac output.
- Arrhythmias are common, may be refractory to treatment. Asystole and VF may occur spontaneously < 25°C.
- Cerebrovascular autoregulation is lost at 24°C. Cerebral metabolism falls and EEG becomes flat at 20°C when the patient appears dead.
- Respiration rate stimulation is followed by depression as metabolism slows.
- In severe hypothermia CO_2 retention respiratory acidosis indicate disturbance of normal respiratory responses.
- Renal blood flow falls. There may be a large diuresis due to initial vasoconstriction.

Signs and Symptoms (Table 45.1)

The signs and symptoms vary depending on the degree of hypothermia and may be divided by the three stages of severity.

Mild

Symptoms of mild hypothermia may be vague with sympathetic nervous system excitation (shivering, hypertension, tachycardia, tachypnea and vasoconstriction). These are all physiological responses to preserve heat. Cold diuresis, mental confusion, as well as hepatic dysfunction may also be present. Hyperglycemia may be present, as glucose consumption by cells and insulin secretion both decrease, and tissue sensitivity to insulin may be blunted. Sympathetic activation also releases glucose from the liver. In many cases, however, especially in alcoholic patients, hypoglycemia appears to be a more common presentation. Hypoglycemia is also found in many hypothermic patients because hypothermia often is a result of hypoglycemia.

Moderate

Low body temperature results in shivering becoming more violent. Muscle miscoordination becomes apparent. Movements are slow and labored, accompanied by a stumbling pace and mild confusion, although the victim may appear alert. Surface blood vessels contract further as the body focuses its remaining resources on keeping the vital organs warm. The victim becomes pale. Lips, ears, fingers and toes may become blue.

Profound

Difficulty in speaking, sluggish thinking, and amnesia start to appear; inability to use hands and stumbling is also usually present. Cellular metabolic processes shut down. Below 30°C (86°F), the exposed skin becomes blue and puffy, muscle coordination becomes very poor, walking becomes almost impossible, and the victim exhibits incoherent/irrational behavior including terminal burrowing or even a stupor. Pulse and respiration rates decrease significantly, but fast heart rates (ventricular tachycardia, atrial fibrillation) can occur. Major organs fail. Clinical death occurs. Because of decreased cellular activity in stage 3 hypothermia, the body will actually take longer to undergo brain death.

As the temperature decreases further physiological systems falter and heart rate, respiratory rate, and blood pressure all decreases. This results in an expected HR in the 30s with a temperature of 28°C (82°F).

Paradoxical Undressing

Twenty to fifty percent of hypothermia deaths are associated with paradoxical undressing. This typically occurs during moderate to severe hypothermia, as the person becomes disoriented, confused, and combative. They may begin discarding their clothing, which, in turn, increases the rate of heat loss.

Rescuers who are trained in mountain survival techniques are taught to expect this; however, some may assume incorrectly that urban victims of hypothermia have been subjected to a sexual assault.

One explanation for the effect is a cold-induced malfunction of the hypothalamus, the part of the brain that regulates body temperature. Another explanation is that the muscles contracting peripheral blood vessels become exhausted (known as a loss of vasomotor tone) and relax, leading to a sudden surge of blood (and heat) to the extremities, fooling the person into feeling overheated.

Terminal Burrowing

In the final stages of hypothermia, the brain stem produces a burrowing-like behavior. Similar to hibernation behavior in animals, individuals with severe hypothermia are often found in small, enclosed spaces, such as under the bed or behind wardrobes.

Imaging Studies

- A chest radiograph is indicated in patients with hypoxia. Aspiration pneumonia and pulmonary edema are common findings.
- Patients with trauma or altered mental status of indeterminate cause may need a noncontrast head CT scan and further imaging for a standard trauma evaluation.

Table 45.1: *Causes of hypothermia*

General
Young and old
Systemic illness
Sepsis
Malnutrition
Environmental
Cold, wet, windy conditions
Cold water immersion
Exhaustion
Marathon runners
Trauma
Multiple trauma
Minor trauma, immobility
Major burns
Drugs
Ethanol
Sedatives (e.g. bdz, TCAs, opioids OD)
Phenothiazines (impaired shivering)
Neurological
CVA
Paraplegia
Parkinson's disease
Endocrine
Hypoglycaemia and diabetes
Hypothyroidism
Hypoadrenalism

Laboratory Investigations

U and E

- Hypo- or hyperkalaemia - rhabdomyolysis may occur.
- Raised urea and creatinine.

Glucose

- Hypo- or hyperglycaemia
- Hyperamylasaemia
- Pancreatitis is common.

CK

- May be elevated.

FBC

- Increased haematocrit due to intravascular volume depletion
- Thrombocytopaenia.

Clotting

- Coagulopathy including DIC is common.

ABG

- Hypothermia is protective against hypoxia by shifting O_2 - Hb curve to the left
- Initial respiratory alkalosis followed by a respiratory and metabolic acidosis
- Use measured values not "corrected" for temperature.

ECG

- Bradycardia and AF (physiological arrhythmias of hypothermia)
- Systole prolonged > diastole.

Increased conduction time > relative refractory period predisposes to re-entrant arrhythmias.

Prolonged PQ, QRS and QT intervals Osborne wave J wave)—most common in II and V3–V6 image

Management

Prehospital Care

Prehospital management focuses on preventing further heat loss, rewarming the body core temperature, and avoiding precipitating ventricular fibrillation or another malignant cardiac rhythm. This should be the preeminent concern. Conscious patients can develop ventricular fibrillation suddenly; prehospital workers, particularly those operating in remote search-and-rescue operations, should avoid inadvertent jerky movement of severely hypothermic patients. Patients who develop hypothermia-induced dysrhythmia in the field may be beyond resuscitation. How the hypothermic heart deteriorates into the rhythm of ventricular fibrillation remains under debate. Patients developing hypothermia from cold-water immersion appear to be at high risk of fibrillation; rescuers probably are justified in instructing such patients to minimize motion and to await careful extrication.

Anecdotal reports of sudden cardiac death associated with tracheal intubation appear to be exaggerated, particularly if a patient is adequately preoxygenated.

Both cardiac pacing and atropine are generally ineffective for bradyarrhythmia.

Lidocaine is ineffective in preventing hypothermia-induced ventricular dysrhythmias.

Many authors have advocated prophylactic bretylium in cases of severe hypothermia when spontaneous conversion to ventricular fibrillation is possible. This recommendation is due to the success of such therapy both in controlled animal studies and in anecdotal human reports.

- Cardiac dysrhythmias begin to develop at a core temperature of 30°C.
- Ventricular fibrillation susceptibility is greatest below the core temperature of 22°C.
- Bretylium (5 mg/kg initially) is recommended for any hypothermic patient manifesting significant new ventricular ectopy or frank dysrhythmia. However, bretylium has been discontinued by all manufacturers resulting in a worldwide shortage and has been unavailable to many centers since 1999.
- Although the optimal dosage and ideal infusion rate for bretylium are unknown, consider prophylactic bretylium for patients with core temperatures below 30°C.
- To prevent cardiac dysrhythmia with continued hypothermia, rescuers or paramedics should attempt rewarming in the field. (A notable exception would be isolated frostbite injury in which limb rewarming would preclude self-rescue because of pain.)
- Gently place patients in an environment most favorable to reducing further heat loss from evaporation, radiation, conduction or convection.

- Remove wet clothing, and replace it with dry blankets or sleeping bags.
- Initiate active external rewarming with heat packs (e.g. hot water bottles, chemical packs) placed in the axillae, on the groin, and on the abdomen.
- Be aware of the risk of causing body surface burns from exuberant active external rewarming.
- In dire circumstances, when heat packs are unavailable, rescuers can provide skin-to-skin contact with patients.

Ventricular fibrillation in a cold patient is a desperate event. Generally, defibrillation is ineffective at hypothermic core temperatures and when equipment for heroic attempts at resuscitation is unavailable. In such circumstances, attempt a round of chemical conversion with intravenous bretylium (if available), followed by extended cardiopulmonary resuscitation (CPR) until rescuers can begin active rewarming and perform successful defibrillation.

Emergency Department Care

Patients with respiratory failure should be endotracheally intubated and placed on a mechanical ventilator. Intubation and insertion of vascular catheters should not be delayed but performed gently while closely monitoring cardiac rhythm for ventricular fibrillation.

Measure core temperatures using a low-reading esophageal, rectal, or bladder thermometer. Tympanic thermometers are unreliable in a setting of profound hypothermia and should not be used. If using a rectal probe, be careful not to insert it into stool.

Determine whether a cold patient is profoundly or mildly hypothermic. Profoundly hypothermic patients present with stupor or cardiac dysrhythmia (regardless of the recorded temperature) and a core temperature of 30°C or lower. Mildly hypothermic patients may be rewarmed in any available manner (e.g. warm blankets, removal of cold, wet clothing) since their risk for cardiac dysrhythmia is low. Surface rewarming is adequate in these cases, but it is ineffective in very low body temperatures and carries an additional risk of temperature after drops and shock secondary to peripheral vasodilation.

Remove any Wet Clothing, and Replace it with Warm, Dry Materials

Profound hypothermia is a true emergency, warranting the same resource-intensive resuscitation as myocardial infarction. Direct treatment at maintaining or restoring cardiac perfusion; maximizing oxygenation is indicated for a prolonged period of time until the core temperature is at least 32°C.

Do not attempt resuscitation on the patient with a frozen chest where compressions are not possible.

Gingerly handle patients identified with profound hypothermia, and take immediate measures to prevent degeneration of cardiac activity into malignant dysrhythmia.

Profoundly hypothermic patients who demonstrate cardiac ectopy may be ideal candidates for bretylium if available. Administer an initial dose of 5 mg/kg IV (repeated at 10 mg/kg, as needed) to prevent ventricular fibrillation. Lidocaine is ineffective for treatment of hypothermia-induced dysrhythmias. While no randomized human trials have been reported, at least four animal trials and two human case reports support using bretylium for any patient with profound hypothermia. Based on such evidence, the US Wilderness Emergency Medical Services Institute recommends using empiric bretylium for profound hypothermia.

Initiate warmed, humidified oxygen; provide heated intravenous saline; and place warmed blankets or heat lamps around a hypothermic patient.

Although many texts suggest that intravenous fluids be heated to 45°C, this temperature choice is based on convenience of previous study designs rather than any hard evidence. A trial using fluids heated to 65°C demonstrated more efficacy in treating severe hypothermia. Emergency departments that routinely treat hypothermia can keep blankets and intravenous fluid bags in a shared heater. In urgent situations, intravenous fluids that contain no dextrose or blood can be heated in a microwave oven. Once these simple measures have been applied, consider more difficult rewarming therapies.

Optimal rewarming techniques depend upon a patient's condition. Treatment is often limited by hospital availability and physician inexperience with rewarming approaches. If core body temperature does not respond to warming efforts, underlying infection or endocrine derangements must be considered.

A patient who is not becoming progressively colder, is conscious, and has a perfusing cardiac rhythm may not require intensive intervention beyond the methods already discussed.

Debate centers on interventions for patients who are worsening, are comatose, have nonperfusing rhythms, or appear dead. Most texts advocate aggressive therapy for severely hypothermic patients, basing the recommendation on anecdotal reports of success.

Researchers recently confirmed justification for aggressive treatment in a 16-year longitudinal review of profound hypothermia. In this series of 32, Swiss patients presenting with hypothermia and cardiac arrest, 15 patients were resuscitated with aggressive techniques, and all 15 patients showed full neurologic recovery.

In an older review, rewarming at rates faster than 2°C/h was noted to reduce mortality when compared with slower rates.

An optimal warming strategy is elusive. Some have postulated that rapidly warming a patient to 33°C and maintaining him or her at that temperature, using hypothermia therapeutically as though he or she was a cardiac arrest patient might be beneficial.

For simplicity, aggressive rewarming methods can be categorized as slow, moderate, or rapid. Slow rewarming provides heat from 17–30 kcal/h, corresponding to increasing temperature by 0.3–1.2°C/h. (Comparisons are somewhat difficult since different study groups used different measurements of heat gain.) Slow rewarming methods include IV solutions heated to 45°C (17 kcal/h); heated, humidified oxygen by mask (30 kcal/h or 0.7°C/

h); warmed blankets (0.9°C/h); and heated, humidified oxygen via endotracheal tube (1.2°C/h). If intact, a patient's endogenous physiologic mechanisms (other than shivering) provide similar rates of rewarming (30 kcal/h).

Moderate rewarming methods provide heat at approximately 3°C/h. Methods include warmed gastric lavage (2.8°C/h), intravenous solutions heated to 65°C (2.9°C/h), and peritoneal lavage with 45°C fluid at 4 L/h (70 kcal/h or 3°C/h).

Rapid rewarming methods provide heat at levels higher than 100 kcal/h. Methods include thoracic lavage at 500 mL/min (6.1°C/h), cardiopulmonary bypass (400 kcal/h or 18°C/h), thoracic lavage at 2 L/min (19.7°C/h), ECMO, and AV dialysis [1–4° per hour, and warm-water immersion (1500 kcal/h)].

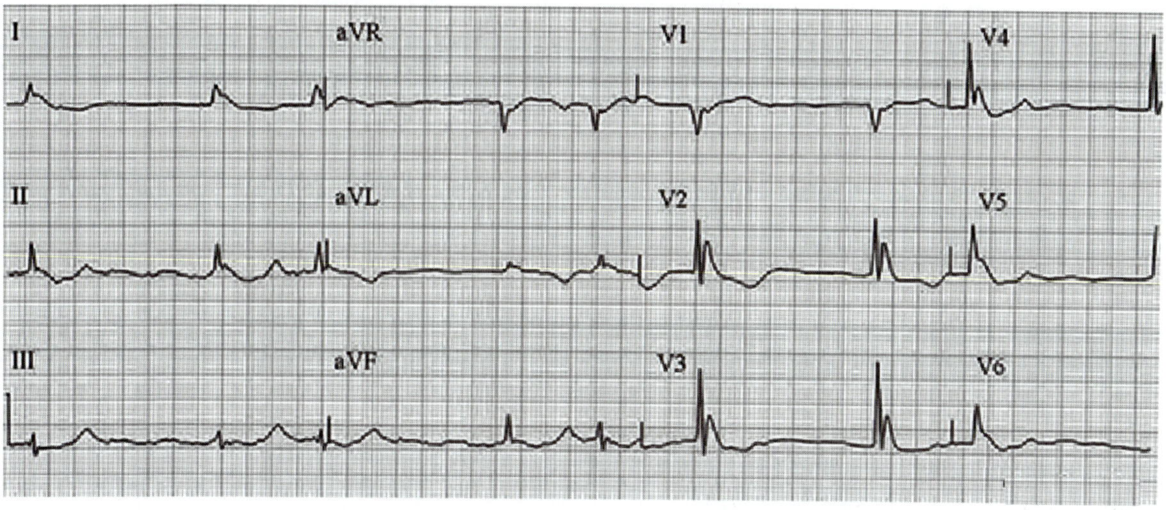

Fig. 45.4: *Atrial fibrillation and Osborne J waves in a person with hypothermia*

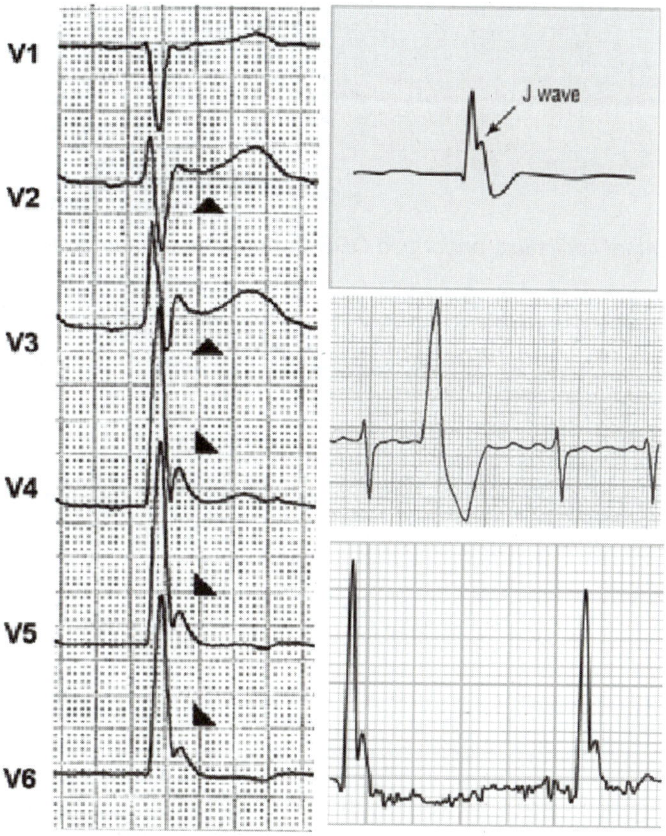

Fig. 45.5: *(Left panel) Detail of the admission ECG shows the Osborne waves and the Brugada-like ECG pattern with saddleback-type ST-segment elevation in V1 and V2. Right Panel (upper) showing J wave as Osborne wave (middle) showing ventricular ectopic and (bottom) shows J waves along with shivering pattern in different severity of hypothermia*

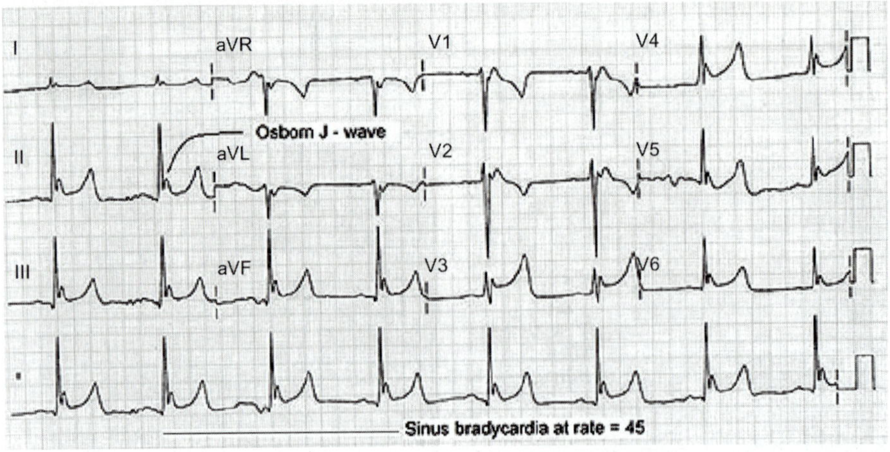

Fig. 45.6: *ECG showing classical Osborn-J-wave and sinus brady cardia in patient with hypothermia*

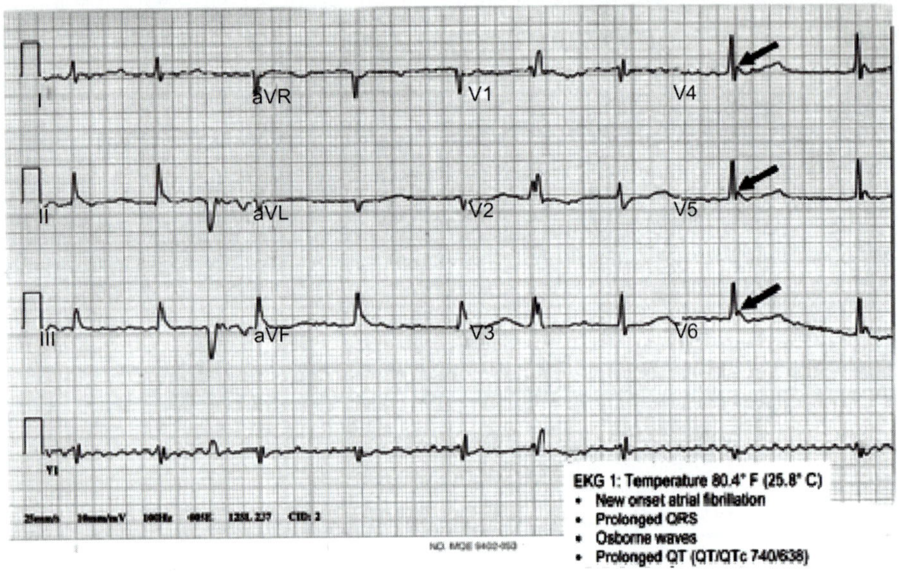

Fig. 45.7: *ECG showing new onset atrial fibrillation, prolonged QRS, Osborn-J-wave and prolonged QT_c interval in patient with body temperature of 80.4°C*

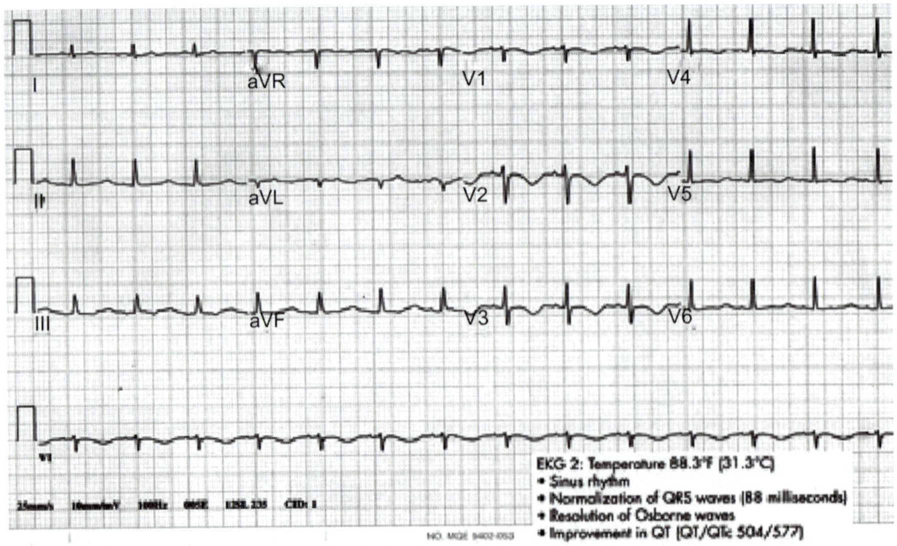

Fig. 45.8: *ECG showing sinus rhythm, normalization of QRS waves (88 miliseconds), resolution of Osborn-J-waves and improvement in QT_c interval in patient with body temperature of 88.3F (31.3°C)*

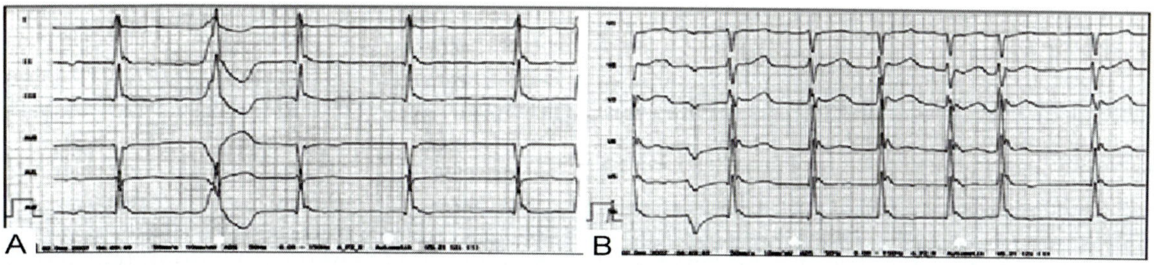

Figs 45.9A and B: *A 12-channel surface ECG obtained at the patient's admission shows sinus bradycardia, QT-interval prolongation, atrial and ventricular ectopy, prominent Osborne waves in all leads, a right bundle-branch block pattern, and a saddleback-type ST-segment elevation in V_1 and V_2*

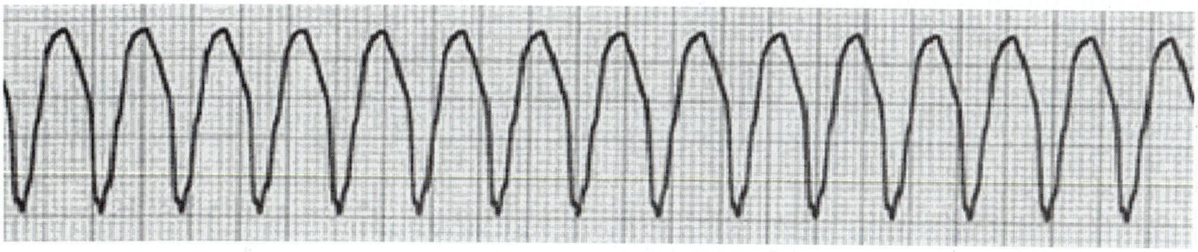

Fig. 45.10: *ECG showing monomorphic ventricular tachycardia in severe hypothermia*

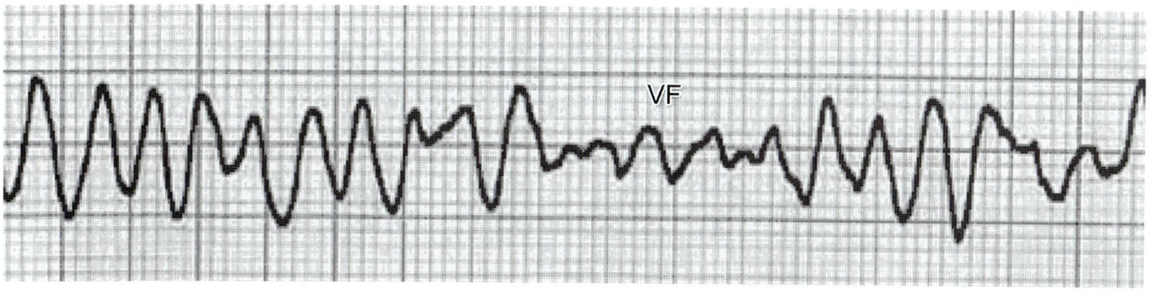

Fig. 45.11: *ECG rhythm, rate, P wave, PR interval, T wave, can not be determined, the duration of the QRS can not be determined. VF appears as fibrillatory waves with no recognisable pattern*

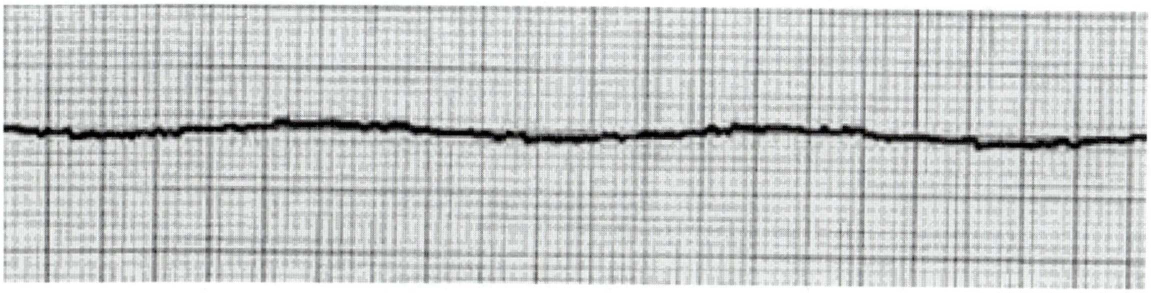

Fig. 45.12: *ECG showing asystole as ventricular standstill. Patient unresponsive with no electrical activity in the heart and no CO_2. This is an arrest situation*

In comparison, endogenous shivering provides rewarming at a rate of 300 kcal/h. No noninvasive technique rewarms as rapidly as full-body immersion in warm water. Known as the Hubbard tank technique, immersion has successfully rewarmed humans with severe hypothermia. Unfortunately, patients who require rapid rewarming in the emergency department also need cardiac monitoring and intravenous therapy, both of which are difficult to manage under water.

Defibrillation also is difficult; however, defibrillation is likely futile once a patient's core temperature falls below 30°C.

Initiate CPR for hypothermic patients who deteriorate into ventricular fibrillation. These patients also warrant immediate weight-based defibrillation (2 J/kg), along with prompt administration of high-dose bretylium (10 mg/kg). Consider initiating cardiopulmonary bypass for any case of ventricular fibrillation or profound hypothermia with deterioration. Patients with this degree of hypothermia have optimized outcomes with procedures such as cardiopulmonary bypass and pleural lavage. However, these methods are invasive, often unavailable, and infrequently used and as such are subject to user-inexperience.

Ventricular fibrillation should be treated immediately with defibrillation, despite the fact that most other dysrhythmias will correct with warming alone. If initial attempts at defibrillation are unsuccessful, further attempts at defibrillation and antiarrhythmic intravenous medications should be held until the patient is warmed to above 30°C. During this interval, basic life support is continued. If ventricular fibrillation persists despite rewarming, current AHA guidelines recommend administration of amiodarone.

Although studies in emergency medicine are lacking, cardiothoracic surgeons who induce hypothermia to perform open-heart procedures rewarm patients on a daily basis using open cardiac massage with warmed saline solution. Therefore, a desperate case of severe hypothermia may warrant consideration of direct cardiac rewarming via open emergency department thoracotomy with open cardiac massage.

Cardiothoracic bypass has been successful for treating cases of accidental hypothermia with prolonged cardiac arrest. To be successful, bypass must be performed rapidly. If a delay is expected, the physician can expedite bypass during an interim period by placing cordis catheters in the patient's femoral vein and artery. Groin cutdowns may be necessary to facilitate such placement; if cutdowns are needed, perform them without hesitation. If bypass is unavailable or delayed, two previously described methods of internal rewarming are available: heated thoracic lavage and arteriovenous (AV) heated countercurrent exchange.

The literature describes two methods of thoracic lavage; the simplest method uses available equipment and provides rewarming rates equivalent to cardiopulmonary bypass.

The technique involves placing two left-sided, 38 French chest tubes (third intercostal space midclavicular line and sixth intercostal space midaxillary line). Isotonic saline, in 3-liter bags heated to at least 41°C, is infused through the anterior tube at 2 L/min, then drained by gravity via the posterior tube. When warmed saline was not available, physicians successfully infused warmed tap water.

The AV heating method, developed at the University of Washington, uses a modified bypass technique for rapid blood rewarming using a level one fluid warmer that is familiar to physicians experienced in trauma resuscitation. The treatment is preferred for patients with profound hypothermia and markedly depressed hemodynamic status or cardiac arrest. AV heating requires a spontaneous pulse, since the patient's intrinsic blood pressure drives flow through the countercurrent module. (In true cardiothoracic bypass, an external pump is built into the machine.) Catheters are placed into the femoral artery and venous cordis.

Once catheters are placed, the arterial output is connected to the inflow port of a level one countercurrent warmer, where intravenous fluids are connected. The outflow port is connected to the femoral venous catheter. Water is circulated, at a temperature preset on the level one device, around the blood-containing tubing; the blood warms as it flows through the countercurrent module. The AV method has rewarmed profoundly hypothermic patients 5 times more rapidly (39 min vs 199 min) than standard methods and was demonstrated to decrease the mortality rate.

In an alternative endovascular warming technique, a catheter is advanced into the inferior vena cava and circulates warmed fluids. The catheter acts as indwelling radiator as it is connected to an esophageal temperature probe and uses a feedback loop to attain and maintain programmed patient temperature. By this method, the core body temperature may be elevated at a rate of 3 degrees an hour. Additionally, it is an invasive technique to raise core temperature that utilizes skills that emergency physicians are already well trained and comfortable with.

Vasodilation increases the vascular space; consequently, patients that have been hypothermic for more than 45–60 minutes often require fluid administration. Hypotension should be addressed with volume resuscitation; inotropic agents, such as dopamine, should be avoided unless the hypotension is refractory to intravenous fluids due to the possible cardiac stimulation/ectopy that pressors may induce.

Probes for pulse oximetry placed on the ears or the forehead appear to be less influenced by the peripheral vasoconstriction of the digits associated with decreased body temperature.

Assessment should include a total body survey to exclude local cold-induced injuries.

Further Inpatient Care

Medical complications from hypothermia often result and necessitate admission to the hospital in moderate and severe hypothermia. Severely hypothermic patients should be admitted to an intensive care unit where their respiratory and cardiac function and temperature may be closely monitored.

Acute pulmonary edema should be treated with oxygen, empirical antibiotics for aspiration pneumonia, and diuretics as necessary.

Frostbite and other localized cold injuries result in deep tissue damage. Surgical exploration and debridement may be necessary. Affected body parts may have to be amputated if gangrene develops. Such a procedure is usually performed at some delayed time interval once a line of demarkation has declared itself days to weeks later. The development of rhabdomyolysis should be monitored.

Deterrence/Prevention

- Preparation is key to avoiding accidental hypothermia.
- Appropriate cold weather clothing and survival bags are a necessity if walking or climbing in a cold climate.
- Persons should avoid alcohol if anticipating exposure to cold because alcohol can disrupt temperature homeostasis by causing vasodilation.

- Individuals should remain alert to early symptoms and initiate preventive measures (e.g. drinking warm fluids).
- Adequate heat in the home should be maintained.
- Patients should be referred to a social service agency for help with adequate housing, heat, and/or clothing.

General Measures

- ABC
- Intubation as required, as gently as possible
- Warmed, humidified oxygen at 40–46°C
- Remove wet clothing and insulate to prevent further heat loss
- Gentle handling at all times—may precipitate dysrhythmias
- Consider coexistent pathology
- IV, urinary and gastric catheters if necessary
- Temperature and cardiac monitoring
- Warmed fluid resuscitation (dehydration is frequently present)
- Dextrose containing fluids will also provide energy substrate
- Avoid Ringer's lactate
- Avoid central lines and Swan Ganz catheters.

Endogenous Rewarming

- Ideal for mild hypothermia
- A part of all rewarming protocols
- Requires some endogenous thermogenesis
- Warm environment, warm clothing and insulation.

External Exogenous Warming

- External application of heat
- Required at temperatures <32°C
- Purported link with peripheral vasodilatation, hypotension and core temperature after-drop
- Immersion is not recommended
- Forced air warming blanket (Bair Hugger)
- Should achieve warming rate of 2° per hour.

Core Exogenous Rewarming

- Application of heat to the core
- Warmed humidified inhaled oxygen
- Warmed IV fluids provide little heat but prevent ongoing loss
- Insulate IV lines
- Blood warmer for blood and IV fluids
- Cardiopulmonary bypass or left pleural lavage is life-saving measure in arrested hypothermics
- Most other methods are less effective

Frostbite and other injuries may require treatment.

Arrhythmias (Figs 45.4–45.12)

- VF may occur spontaneously or be precipitated by rough handling with temperatures <29°C
- Sinus bradycardia and AF with slow ventricular response are common and should be regarded as physiological arrhythmias of hypothermia
- AF usually reverts spontaneously during rewarming (Other atrial arrhythmias should be regarded as innocent)
- Transient ventricular arrhythmias should be ignored
- Magnesium may be effective (lignocaine appears to be less effective, procainamide should be avoided).

CPR in Hypothermia

- Misdiagnosis of cardiac arrest is a hazard in the prehospital setting
- Chest wall elasticity and myocardial compliance are reduced and may make chest compression difficult
- CPR rate as for normothermic victims
- Drug metabolism is reduced and accumulation
- Epinephrine and other drugs are often withheld until core body temperature is >30°C
- Above 30°C intervals between doses should be doubled and the lowest doses recommended used
- Ventricular fibrillation may not respond to defibrillation if the core temperature is less than 30°C
- If no response to 3 initial shocks, subsequent shocks should be delayed until the core temperature >30°C
- Initiate CPR in accidental hypothermia unless guidelines of the Wilderness Medical Society, USA
- Not for resuscitation status is documented and verified
- Obvious lethal injuries are present
- Chest wall decompression is impossible
- Any signs of life are present
- Rescuers are endangered by evacuation delays or altered triage conditions
- Bypass is better that external rewarming in hypothermic cardiac arrest.

Prognostic Factors in Hypothermia

No strong indicators to predict death or permanent neurological dysfunction in patients with significant hypothermia.

No definitive indicators to suggest which patients can or cannot be resuscitated successfully.

Parameters that may identify the non-salvageable patient

- Elevated serum potassium >10 mmol/L
- Core temperature <6–7°C
- Core temperature <15°C if there has been no circulation for >2 hours
- Venous pH <6.5—blood gas measurements should not be corrected for temperature
- Severe coagulopathy
- Clots within the heart on thoracotomy
- Failure to obtain venous return during cardiopulmonary bypass.

BIBLIOGRAPHY

1. Giesbrecht GG. Prehospital treatment of hypothermia. Wilderness and Environmental Medicine 12, 24–31 (2001).
2. Steedman D. Environmental Medical Emergencies, Oxford University Press, Oxford (1994).
3. Rogers I. Hypothermia in Textbook of Adult Emergency Medicine Ed. Cameron P, et al. Churchill Livingstone, London, 2000.

4. Resuscitation Council UK. Advanced life support course Manual 2000.
5. Alsafwah S. Electrocardiographic changes in hypothermia. Heart Lung 2001;30:161–163.
6. Olgers TJ, Ubels FL. The ECG in hypothermia: Osborn waves. Neth J Med 2006;64:350, 353.
7. Nolan J, Soar J. Images in resuscitation: the ECG in hypothermia. Resuscitation 2005;64:133–134.
8. Fauci AS, Braunwald E, Kasper DL, Hauser SL, Longo DL, Jameson JL, Loscalzo J, eds. Harrison's principles of internal medicine. 17th ed. New York, NY: McGraw-Hill; 2008.
9. Graham CA, McNaughton GW, Wyatt JP. The electrocardiogram in hypothermia. Wilderness Environ Med 2001;12:232–235.
10. Prescott LF, Peard MC, Wallace IR. Accidental hypothermia. A common condition. Br Med J. 1962 Nov 24;2 (5316):1367–1370.
11. Ledingham IM, Mone JG. Treatment of accidental hypothermia: a prospective clinical study. Br Med J. 1980 Apr 26; 280(6222):1102–1105.
12. Towne WD, Geiss WP, Yanes HO, Rahimtoola SH. Intractable ventricular fibrillation associated with profound accidental hypothermia—successful treatment with partial cardiopulmonary bypass. N Engl J Med. 1972 Nov 30;287(22): 1135–1136.
13. Wickstrom P, Ruiz E, Lija GP, Hinterkopf JP, Haglin JJ. Accidental hypothermia: core rewarming with partial bypass. Am J Surg. 1976 May;131(5):622–625.
14. Althaus U, Aeberhard P, Schüpbach P, Nachbur BH, Mühlemann W. Management of profound accidental hypothermia with cardiorespiratory arrest. Ann Surg. 1982 Apr;195(4):492–495.
15. Knowlton FP, Starling EH. The influence of variations in temperature and blood-pressure on the performance of the isolated mammalian heart. J Physiol. 1912 May 6;44(3):206–219.
16. Hegnauer AH. Lethal hypothermic temperatures for dog and man. Ann N Y Acad Sci. 1959 Sep 14;80:315–319.
17. Botterell EH, Gunton RW, Lougheed WM, Scott JW. Changes in cardiac rhythm and in the form of the electrocardiogram resulting from induced hypothermia in man. Am Heart J. 1956 Sep;52(3):419–429.
18. Swan H, Zeavin I, Holmes Jh, Montgomery V. Cessation of circulation in general hypothermia. I. Physiologic changes and their control. Ann Surg. 1953 Sep;138(3):360–376.
20. Schwab RH, Lewis DW, Killough JH, Templeton JY. 3rd Electrocardiographic Changes Occurring In Rapidly Induced Deep Hypothermia. Am J Med Sci. 1964 Sep;248:290–303.
21. Ross DN. Principles underlying the application of hypothermia to cardiac surgery. Proc R Soc Med. 1956 Jun; 49(6):365–368.
22. Osborn JJ. Experimental hypothermia; respiratory and blood pH changes in relation to cardiac function. Am J Physiol. 1953 Dec;175(3):389–398.
23. Lloyd EL, Mitchell B. Factors affecting the onset of ventricular fibrillation in hypothermia. Lancet. 1974 Nov 30;2(7892): 1294–1296.
24. Southwick FS, Dalglish PH Jr. Recovery after prolonged asystolic cardiac arrest in profound hypothermia. A case report and literature review. JAMA. 1980 Mar 28;243(12): 1250–1253.
25. Duguid H, Simpson RG, Stowers JM. Accidental hypothermia. Lancet. 1961 Dec 2;2(7214):1213–1219.
26. Hudson LD, Conn RD. Accidental hypothermia. Associated diagnoses and prognosis in a common problem. JAMA. 1974 Jan 7;227(1):37–40.
27. Weyman AE, Greenbaum DM, Grace WJ. Accidental hypothermia in an alcoholic population. Am J Med. 1974 Jan;56(1):13–21.

46 Extracorporeal Membrane Oxygenation Support in Critically Ill Children

The term extracorporeal membrane oxygenation (ECMO) was initially used to describe long-term extracorporeal support that focused on the function of oxygenation. Subsequently, in some patients, the emphasis shifted to carbon dioxide removal, and the term extracorporeal carbon dioxide removal was coined. Extracorporeal support was later used for postoperative support in patients following cardiac surgery. Other variations of its capabilities have been tested and used over the last few years, making it an important tool in the armamentarium of life and organ support measures for clinicians. With all of these uses for extracorporeal circuitry, a new term, extracorporeal life support (ECLS), has come into vogue to describe this technology.

In emergency medicine, ECMO is an extracorporeal technique of providing both cardiac and respiratory support oxygen to patients whose heart and lungs are so severely diseased or damaged that they can no longer serve their function. Initial cannulation of a patient receiving ECMO is performed by a surgeon and maintenance of the patient is the responsibility of the ECMO specialist and gives 24/7 monitoring care for the duration of the ECMO treatment.

The differences between ECMO and cardiopulmonary bypass are as follows:

- ECMO is frequently instituted using only cervical cannulation, which can be performed under local anesthesia; standard cardiopulmonary bypass is usually instituted by transthoracic cannulation under general anesthesia.
- Unlike standard cardiopulmonary bypass which is used for short-term support measured in hours, ECMO is used for longer-term support ranging from 3–10 days.
- The purpose of ECMO is to allow time for intrinsic recovery of the lungs and heart; a standard cardiopulmonary bypass provides support during various types of cardiac surgical procedures.

Types of ECMO (Figs 46.1–46.4)

1. **Venoarterial (VA)** ECMO for cardiac or respiratory failure.
2. **Venovenous (VV)** ECMO for respiratory failure.

There are several forms of ECMO, the two most common of which are VA and VV. In both modalities, blood drained from the venous system is oxygenated outside of the body. In VA-ECMO, this blood is returned to the arterial system and in VV-ECMO the blood is returned to the venous system. In VV-ECMO, no cardiac support is provided.

Venoarterial

In venoarterial ECMO - a venous cannula is usually placed in the right common femoral vein for extraction and an arterial cannula is usually placed into the right femoral artery

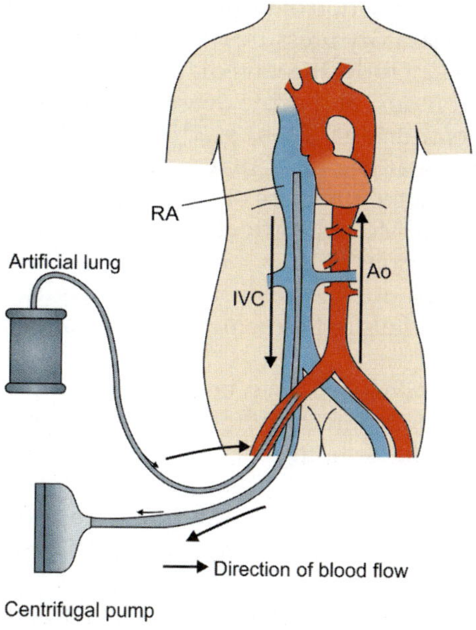

Fig. 46.1: *Diagram of ECMO system. RA, right atrium; IVC, inferior venacava; Ao, aorta*

for infusion. The tip of the femoral venous cannula should be maintained near the junction of the inferior vena cava and right atrium while the tip of the femoral arterial cannula is maintained in the iliac artery. In adults accessing, the femoral artery is preferred because the insertion is simpler.

Venovenous

In venovenous ECMO, venous cannulae are usually placed in the right common femoral vein for drainage and right internal jugular vein for infusion.

Indications for ECMO

Patients with the following two major neonatal diagnoses require the use of ECMO:

1. Primary diagnoses associated with primary pulmonary hypertension of the newborn (PPHN) including idiopathic PPHN, meconium aspiration syndrome, respiratory distress syndrome, group B streptococcal sepsis and asphyxia.
2. Congenital diaphragmatic hernia (CDH).

Selection Criteria for Neonates Include the Following

- Gestational age of 34 weeks or more
- Birth weight of 2,000 g or higher
- No significant coagulopathy or uncontrolled bleeding
- No major intracranial hemorrhage (grade 1 intracranial hemorrhage)
- Mechanical ventilation for 10–14 days or less
- Reversible lung injury
- No lethal malformations
- No major untreatable cardiac malformation
- Failure of maximal medical therapy.

Failure to meet these criteria is a relative contraindication for ECMO.

Qualifying patient criteria for ECMO are applied only when the infant has reached maximal ventilatory support of 100% oxygen [fraction of inspired oxygen (FiO_2) equals 1] with peak inspiratory pressures (PIP) often as high as 35 cm water. They include the alveolar-arterial gradient, the oxygenation index, and acute deterioration.

The alveolar-arterial (A-a) gradient of 600–624 mmHg for 4–12 hours at sea level may be computed as follows (where 47 = partial pressure of water vapor):

Pediatric ECMO is indicated or considered in the following situations:

- Low cardiac output resulting from right, left, and biventricular failure following repair of congenital heart defect
- Pulmonary vasoreactive crisis following repair of congenital heart defect leading to severe hypoxemia, low cardiac output, or both
- Rarely, as a bridge to cardiac surgery in patients with serious end-organ damage resulting from profound low cardiac output related to congenital heart disease
- As a bridge to cardiac transplant
- Possibly, as a bridge to recovery in temporary cardiomyopathy secondary to renal failure, myocarditis, and burns.

Today, other indications or less strict selection of patients in certain institutions have made the use of this technology more diverse, not only in acute cardiac problems but also in primary pulmonary diseases.

The clinical outcomes of patients undergoing ECMO can be categorized according to the indication for the ECMO: severe acute respiratory failure or cardiac failure.

Acute Respiratory Failure

With acute respiratory failure use of ECMO has been shown to improve survival rates. Survival rates from 50–70% have been reported in observational and uncontrolled clinical trials. The survival rates reported are better than historical survival rates.

Cardiac Failure

Venoarterial ECMO can provide acute support in cardiogenic shock or cardiac arrest in adults. Assuming that the brain function is normal or only minimally impaired, ECMO is provided until the patient recovers or receives a long-term ventricular assist device as a bridge to cardiac transplantation.

Indications of ECMO in Adults

Guidelines that describe the indications and practice of ECMO are published by the Extracorporeal Life Support Organization (ELSO). Criteria for the initiation of ECMO include acute severe cardiac or pulmonary failure that is potentially reversible and unresponsive to conventional management. Examples of clinical situations that may prompt the initiation of ECMO include the following:

Techniques Employed in ECMO (Figs 46.1 and 46.2)

ECMO currently comes in two varieties: (1) VA and (2) VV. VA-ECMO takes deoxygenated blood from a central vein or the right atrium, pumps it past the oxygenator, and then returns the oxygenated blood, under pressure, to the arterial side of the circulation (typically to the aorta). This form of ECMO partially supports the cardiac output as the flow through the ECMO circuit is in addition to the normal cardiac output. VV ECMO takes blood from a large vein and returns oxygenated blood back to a large vein. VV-ECMO does not support the circulation. VA-ECMO helps support the cardiac output and delivers higher levels of oxygenation support than does VV-ECMO. VA-ECMO carries a higher risk of systemic emboli than does VV. VV-ECMO systems may actually recirculate previously oxygenated blood depending on the placement of the inflow and outflow catheters. Another variant of VV-ECMO is extracorporeal CO_2 removal ($ECCO_2R$). With this mode of support, oxygenation is provided by slow ventilation of the native lungs while CO_2 removal is accomplished by the ECMO circuit. In all forms of ECMO, CO_2 removal is more efficient than O_2 addition because of the solubility and diffusion properties of CO_2 relative to O_2. In fact, CO_2 normally has to be added to ECMO circuits to offset this efficiency at CO_2 removal. The flow through the ECMO circuit is typically on the order of 100 mL/kg/minute. This

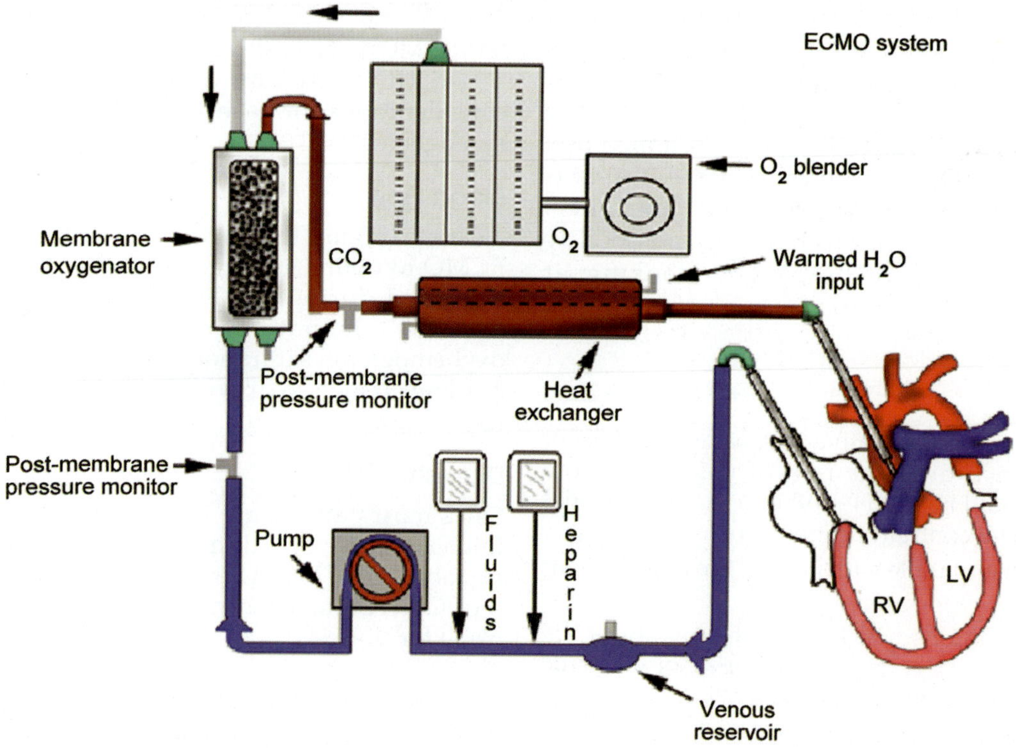

Fig. 46.2: *Extracorporeal membrane oxygenation (ECMO) system*

would be from 25–75% of the cardiac output. This high flow requires the placement of large catheters into the circulation. For adults, the intravascular catheters may be 20 Fr or larger while 14 Fr catheters might be used in infants. These are generally placed by cut-down. Current circuits require the use of systemic anticoagulation with heparin to keep the systems patent. This anticoagulation is, in large part, responsible for bleeding complications that can be seen with the use of ECMO. Bleeding may occur either at the site of catheter insertion or at remote sites such as intracranial or the gastrointestinal tract. Future catheters with inpregnated heparin may obviate the need for systemic anticoagulation and would be expected to reduce bleeding complications. Once blood leaves the patient, it comes in contact with a gas-permeable membrane that allows gas exchange to occur between the blood and the gasses (oxygen and carbon dioxide) that are run into the oxygenator. Carbon dioxide levels leaving the oxygenator can be adjusted about as low as the physician wants while oxygen levels typically reach the 400–500 mmHg level. Note that CO_2 content varies fairly directly with partial pressure while O_2 content follows the shape of the oxyhemoglobin dissociation curve. Under normobaric conditions, this limits the amount of oxygen that can be loaded into blood. If you were to try to predict the final mixed arterial oxygen content or partial pressure during VA-ECMO, you would need to know the pulmonary venous oxygen content, the ECMO effluent oxygen content, and the % of cardiac output flowing through the ECMO circuit:

$$CaO_2 = (EO \times EF + NO \times NF)/(EF + NF)$$

Where EO: = ECMO oxygen content
EF: = ECMO flow
NO: = Non-ECMO oxygen content
NF: = Non-ECMO flow

Predicting final arterial content during VV-ECMO is more complex and cannot be easily calculated. During VV ECMO, the lungs may actually excrete oxygen rather than remove it from the inspired gas. Once ECMO has been started, the ventilator is typically reduced to minimal settings to prevent atelectasis and barotrauma. The FIO_2 is lowered as much as possible, perhaps to room air. The ECMO flow rate is adjusted to the minimum needed to provide for adequate gas exchange and/or circulation support in the case of VA-ECMO. ECMO is typically used for 7–12 days and is weaned when there is evidence of pulmonary improvement as indicated by compliance or radiologic appearance. ECMO can also be stopped if there are major complications or if the patient's condition is determined to be hopeless.

Types of patient selected for application of ECMO

As mentioned previously, usual ECMO criteria include patients with a severe reversible process that would result in a very high predicted mortality with conventional ventilatory support. The best candidates are those without multisystem organ failure that are otherwise considered to be salvageable. It would be expected, that once ECMO becomes safer and more accepted by physicians, that these criteria would be revised to eliminate the requirement for a very high predicted pretreatment mortality. There are several ways to evaluate patients to determine if they are "sick enough" for ECMO. APACHE and other scoring systems could be used to predict mortality. More frequently, indexes to assess refractory hypoxemia are used. The a:A ratio or A-a gradient can be used, but the oxygenation index (OI) is currently in more common use: $OI = (FIO_2)(MAP)/PaO_2$. An OI greater than 0.40–0.55 is thought to predict an 80% predicted mortality. Unfortunately, mortality predictors have been notoriously pessimistic since they are derived by looking at retrospective data and tend to do a poor job of predicting prospective results.

Contraindications

Most contraindications are relative, balancing the risks of the procedure (including the risk of using valuable resources which could be used for others) vs. the potential benefits. The relative contraindications are:

1. Conditions incompatible with normal life if the patient recovers
2. Preexisting conditions which affect the quality of life (CNS status, end stage malignancy, risk of systemic bleeding with anticoagulation)
3. Age and size of patient
4. *Futility:* Patients who are too sick, have been on conventional therapy too long, or have a fatal diagnosis.

Maintenance

Once the initial respiratory and hemodynamic goals have been achieved, the blood flow is maintained at that rate. Frequent assessment and adjustments are facilitated by continuous venous oximetry, which directly measures the oxyhemoglobin saturation of the blood in the venous limb of the ECMO circuit.

Special Considerations

VV-ECMO is typically used for respiratory failure while VA-ECMO is used for cardiac failure. There are unique considerations for each type of ECMO which influence management.

Blood Flow

Near maximum flow rates are usually desired during VV-ECMO to optimize oxygen delivery. In contrast, the flow rate used during VA-ECMO must be high enough to provide adequate perfusion pressure and venous oxyhemoglobin saturation (measured on drainage blood), but low enough to provide sufficient preload to maintain left ventricular output.

Diuresis

Since most patients are fluid overloaded when ECMO is initiated, aggressive diuresis is warranted once the patient is stable on ECMO. Ultrafiltration can be easily added to the ECMO circuit if patients are unable to produce sufficient urine for diuresis.

Left Ventricular Monitoring

Left ventricular output is rigorously monitored during VA-ECMO because left ventricular output can become worse.

Weaning and Discontinuing

For patients with respiratory failure, improvements in radiographic appearance, pulmonary compliance, and arterial oxyhemoglobin saturation indicate that the patient may be ready to be taken off of ECMO support. For patients with cardiac failure, enhanced aortic pulsatility correlates with improved left ventricular output and indicates that the patient may be ready to be taken off of ECMO support.

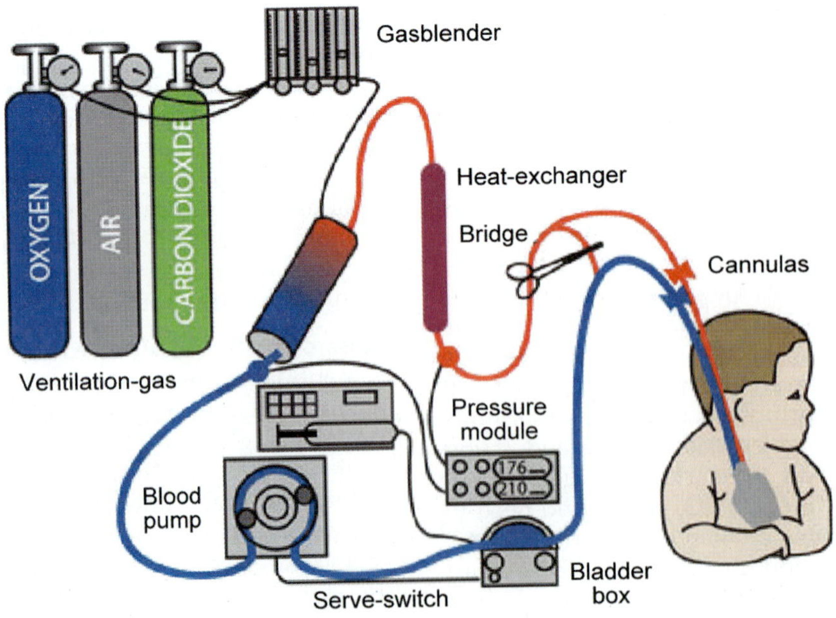

Fig. 46.3: *Application of ECMO in neonatal cardiorespiratory failure*

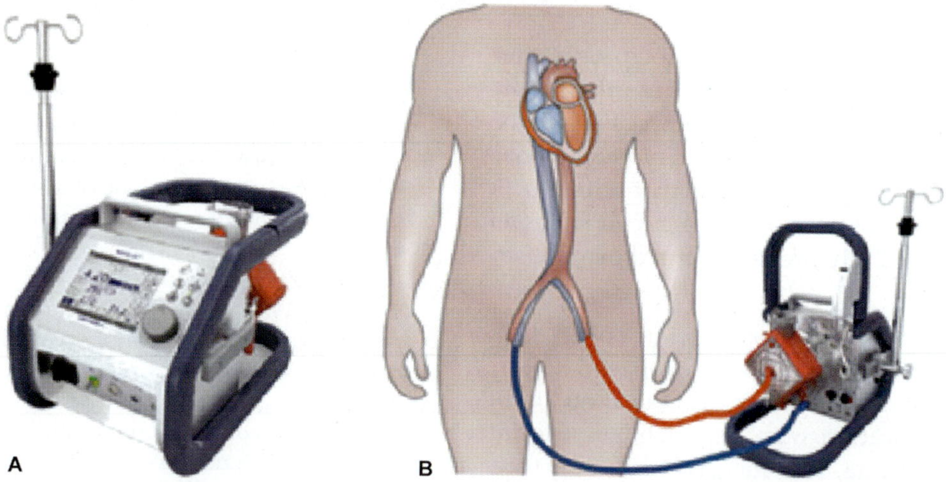

Fig. 46.4: *The device is compact and easily portable, with a total weight of only 9 kg. (A) Venoarterial extracorporeal membrane oxygenation (ECMO) is established by cannulation of a femoral vein and artery using the Seldinger technique. To expedite interhospital transfer these vessels can be located with guidewires before arrival of the outreach team. (B) The cannulas can then be inserted rapidly to begin ECMO before transport by air or ground ambulance. Images of the Cardiohelp®device courtesy of © Maquet Cardiopulmonary AG*

Once the decision has been made to discontinue ECMO, the cannulae are removed.

Complications (Fig. 46.5)

ECMO complications are those associated with cannulation (pneumothorax, vascular disruptions, bleeding, infection, emboli), those associated with systemic anticoagulation (GI bleeding, intracranial bleeding, etc.), and exsanguination resulting from circuit disruptions. These potential complications require that a trained ECMO technician be present at the bedside 24 hours per day in addition to the patient's usual nursing presence. As many as 30% of ECMO treated infants reported to the Extracorporeal Life Support Organization (ELSO) registry suffer some degree of CNS injury.

A common consequence in ECMO–treated adults is neurological injury which may include subarachnoid hemorrhage, ischemic watershed infarctions, hypoxic-ischemic encephalopathy, unexplained coma, and brain death. Fatal sepsis may occur when the large catheters inserted in the neck provide fertile field for infection Additional risks include bleeding. In adults, ECMO survival rates are around 60%. ECMO has yet to have proven survival benefit in adults with acute respiratory distress syndrome (ARDS). In VA-ECMO, patients whose cardiac function does not recover sufficiently to be weaned from ECMO may be bridged to a ventricular assist device (VAD) or transplant.

In infants aged less than 34 weeks of gestation, several physiologic systems are not well-developed, especially the cerebral vasculature and germinal matrix, resulting in high sensitivity to slight changes in pH, PaO_2, and intracranial pressure. Preterm infants are at unacceptably high risk for intraventricular hemorrhage (IVH) if administered ECMO at a gestational age less than 32 weeks. Also later, given

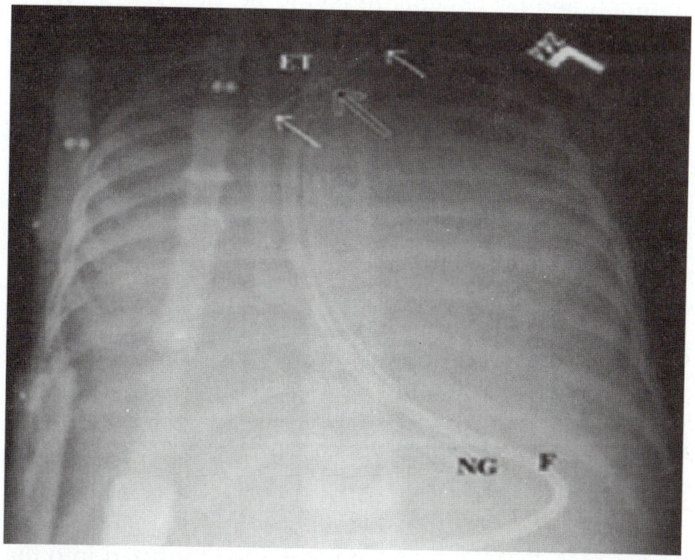

Fig. 46.5: *Portable chest radiograph of a patient undergoing extracorporeal membrane oxygenation shows pulmonary edema in the lungs and the tubing (d) going to the patient's right carotid artery and right jugular vein. Also seen are an endotracheal tube (ET), a right internal jugular vein catheter (black arrow), a left internal jugular vein catheter (white arrows), a nasogastric tube (NG), and a feeding tube (F)*

the risk of IVH, it has become standard practice to ultrasound the brain prior to administering ECMO.

Bleeding

Bleeding occurs in 30–40% of patients who receive ECMO and can be life threatening. It is due to both the necessary continuous heparin infusion and platelet dysfunction. Meticulous surgical technique, maintaining platelet counts greater than 100,000/mm^3, and maintaining the target ACT reduce the likelihood of bleeding.

Thromboembolism

Systemic thromboembolism due to thrombus formation within the extracorporeal circuit is an infrequent complication that can be devastating. Its impact is greater with VA-ECMO than VV-ECMO because infusion is into the systemic circulation. Heparin infusion that achieves its target ACT and vigilant observation of the circuit for signs of clot formation successfully prevents thromboembolism in most patients.

Cannulation-related

A variety of complications can occur during cannulation, including vessel perforation with hemorrhage, arterial dissection, distal ischemia, and incorrect location (e.g. venous cannula within the artery). These complications are rare (<5%). A skilled and experienced surgeon is important to avoid or address such complications.

Heparin-induced Thrombocytopenia

Heparin-induced thrombocytopenia (HIT) is increasingly common among patients receiving ECMO. When HIT is suspected, the heparin infusion is usually replaced by a nonheparin anticoagulant.

Venoarterial Specific Complications

Pulmonary Hemorrhage

Pulmonary hemorrhage can occur in patients who receive VA-ECMO.

Cardiac Thrombosis

There is retrograde blood flow in the ascending aorta whenever the femoral artery and vein are used for VA-ECMO. Stasis of the blood can occur if left ventricular output is not maintained which may result in thrombosis.

Coronary or Cerebral Hypoxia

During VA-ECMO, fully saturated blood infused into the femoral artery from the ECMO circuit will preferentially perfuse the lower extremities and the abdominal viscera. Blood ejected from the heart will selectively perfuse the heart, brain and upper extremities.

Future

Applications for ECMO may expand in the future to include percutaneous temporary left ventricular assistance and low flow ECMO for CO_2 removal (ECOOR). In addition, new technologies will improve the simplicity and safety of ECMO including new oxygenators, pumps, and surface coatings.

Other Uses

ECMO use on cadavers can increase the viability rate of transplanted organs.

BIBLIOGRAPHY

1. Van Meurs, K, Lally, KP, Peek, G, Zwischenberger, JB. ECMO: Extracorporeal cardiopulmonary support in critical care, Extracorporeal Life Support Organization, Ann Arbor 2005.
2. Madershahian N, Nagib R, Wippermann J, Strauch J, Wahlers T (2006). A simple technique of distal limb perfusion during prolonged femoro-femoral cannulation. J Card Surg 21 (2): 168–9.
3. Wang D, Zhou X, Liu X, Sidor B, Lynch J, Zwischenberger JB (2008). Wang-Zwische double lumen cannula-toward a percutaneous and ambulatory paracorporeal artificial lung. ASAIO J 54 (6): 606–11.
4. Peek GJ, Moore HM, Moore N, Sosnowski AW, Firmin RK (1997). Extracorporeal membrane oxygenation for adult respiratory failure. Chest 112 (3): 759–64.
5. Lewandowski K, Rossaint R, Pappert D, Gerlach H, Slama KJ, Weidemann H et al. (1997). High survival rate in 122 ARDS patients managed according to a clinical algorithm including extracorporeal membrane oxygenation. Intensive Care Med 23 (8): 819–35.
6. Hemmila MR, Rowe SA, Boules TN, Miskulin J, McGillicuddy JW, Schuerer DJ et al. (2004). Extracorporeal life support for severe acute respiratory distress syndrome in adults. Ann Surg 240 (4): 595–605.
7. Brogan TV, Thiagarajan RR, Rycus PT, Bartlett RH, Bratton SL (2009). Extracorporeal membrane oxygenation in adults with severe respiratory failure: a multi-center database. Intensive Care Med 35 (12): 2105–14.
8. Kolla S, Awad SS, Rich PB, Schreiner RJ, Hirschl RB, Bartlett RH (1997). Extracorporeal life support for 100 adult patients with severe respiratory failure. Ann Surg 226 (4): 544–64.
9. Rich PB, Awad SS, Kolla S, Annich G, Schreiner RJ, Hirschl RB et al. (1998). An approach to the treatment of severe adult respiratory failure. J Crit Care 13 (1): 26–36.
10. Ullrich R, Lorber C, Röder G, Urak G, Faryniak B, Sladen RN et al. (1999). Controlled airway pressure therapy, nitric oxide inhalation, prone position, and extracorporeal membrane oxygenation (ECMO) as components of an integrated approach to ARDS. Anesthesiology 91 (6): 1577–86.
11. Cohen G, Permut L (2005). Decision making for mechanical cardiac assist in pediatric cardiac surgery. Seminars in Thoracic and Cardiovascular Surgery. Pediatric Cardiac Surgery Annual: 41–50.
12. Vural KM (November 2008). Ventricular assist device applications. Anadolu Kardiyoloji Dergisi: AKD = the Anatolian Journal of Cardiology 8 Suppl 2: 117–30.
13. Mateen FJ, Muralidharan R, Shinohara RT, et al. Neurological Injury in Adults Treated With Extracorporeal Membrane Oxygenation Archives of Neurology 2011.
14. Groopman, Jerome (2007). How Doctors Think. Houghton Mifflin Harcourt. ISBN 978–0–618–61003–7.
15. Concepts Of Neonatal ECMO. The Internet Journal of Perfusionists. last modified on Fri, Feb 13, 9 14:01:21–0600.
16. Alan H. Jobe, MD, PhD (August 2004). Post-conceptional age and IVH in ECMO patients. Radiology Source 145 (2): A2.
17. Cornell T, Wyrick P, Fleming G, Pasko D, Han Y, Custer J et al. (2007). A case series describing the use of argatroban in patients on extracorporeal circulation. ASAIO J 53 (4): 460–3.

47 Tropical Diseases Affecting Cardiovascular System

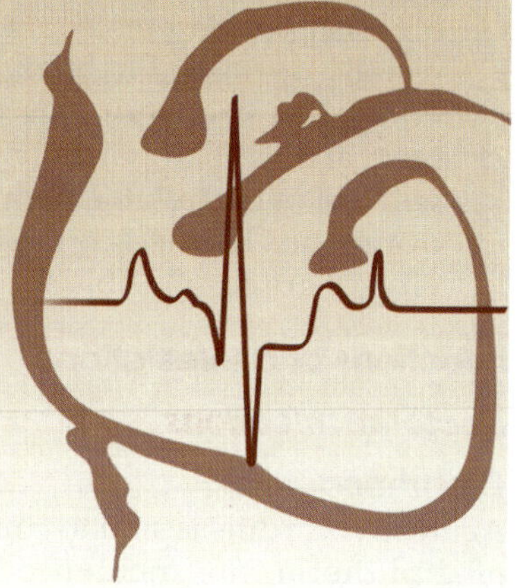

DEFINITION OF TROPICAL DISEASE

A tropical disease is any illness that is most common or only occurs (endemic) in tropical or subtropical areas. Beyond location, many have little in common with each other. They are caused by a variety of factors including viruses, bacteria, protozoa and parasitic worms (nematodes and trematodes). Some frequently cause no symptoms, while others are severe and may become fatal. The routes of transmission also range widely and include insect bites, contaminated water and food, and direct contact with an infected person. The tropics are defined by geography and climate.

They are the areas between the tropic of cancer and the tropic of capricorn (23.5 degrees of latitude north and south of the equator, respectively). In the Western Hemisphere, this includes much of the Caribbean and Mexico, Central America and much of South America. Also considered tropical are Africa between the Sahara Desert and South Africa, Southern Asia, much of India, Northern Australia and many of the Island Nations in the western Pacific Ocean. These areas have high temperatures and humidity throughout the year. Seasons are marked more by changes in rainfall than other conditions.

The subtropics are the climatic region between tropical and temperate areas. Unlike the tropics, they do not occur within defined latitudes.The reasons these diseases are geographically limited vary. Some can not develop outside the environmental conditions (e.g. temperature, humidity) provided by tropical and subtropical climates. Others require specific animal hosts that occur within this limited range. Certain diseases once had broader ranges but have been eliminated. Many of the countries in the tropics are developing nations and may not be able to afford the sanitation and medical programs required to eliminate these diseases.

The tropical diseases are largely absent naturally or as a result of eradication programs in the developed countries and other industrialized nations. Outbreaks in these countries are often linked to immigrants or travelers returning from areas where the diseases are endemic. They may occur sporadically, but are often limited by seasonal climate changes.

Types and Differences of Tropical Disease

The tropics include portions of nearly every continent and some of the world's most populous countries. The number of diseases endemic to such a large area with so many people is difficult to estimate. To better understand them, they may be categorized by the organisms. They have a more complex structure including a nucleus (the core of a cell containing chromosomes) and are often classified within the animal kingdom. Some may infect humans and cause disease. In the tropics, these diseases include:

Cardiac Involvement in Infectious Diseases

Evidence of cardiac affection in the infectious fevers may be of several different types:

1. There may be histological evidence of myocarditis in autopsied patients, in whom the cardiac diagnosis mayor may not have been suspected during life. The incidence of myocarditis in such an autopsy series would be unduly high, since patients with myocarditis are more likely to die.
2. The diagnosis of myocarditis may be based on ECG abnormalities. It is doubtful whether T wave or ST segment changes alone justify a diagnosis of myocarditis, since there is evidence that such changes can be caused by pyrexia, electrolyte imbalance or other physiological disturbances.
3. One may find definite or presumptive clinical signs of cardiac affection, such as pericardial rub, cardiac dilatation, gallop rhythm, muffling of the first heart sound, or tachycardia out of proportion to the fever. There may be ECG abnormalities such as gross conduction defects and serious arrhythmias. These

signs of carditis are superimposed and perhaps over shadowed by the other clinical manifestations of the infectious disease itself. Unexpected sudden death occurring during the course of an infectious disease is usually presumed to be due to myocarditis.

4. There is a group of cases in which pericarditis or myocarditis is apparently "idiopathic" or "isolated" with no overt involvement of any other system. Only during this last decade has it been realised that certain viruses are responsible for some of these cases.

Infections and Infestations

Bacterial Infections

Diphtheria

Acute myocarditis is said to complicate 10–25% of all cases of diphtheria, the incidence varying fromepidemic to epidemic. Histologically, fatty degeneration and necrosis of the cardiac muscle fibres are seen at the end of the first week and beginning, of the second week of the illness; interstitial inflammatory changes consisting of edema and cellular infiltrations are seen later in the second week. Fibroblasts and granulation tissue then appear and scar tissue is well formed after 3 weeks.

The clinical picture of myocarditis conforms with pathological evidence that myocarditis does not occur very early in the course of the disease. Thus cough, cyanosis and tachycardia during the first few days of the illness are usually due to the respiratory obstruction caused by the diphtheritic membrane and surrounding edema.

True cardiac manifestations usually appear at the end of the first week or during the second week, but occasionally after several weeks, particularly in cutaneous diphtheria. The onset of myocarditis in a child with diphtheria may be heralded by bradycardia. When present, a slow pulse rate mayor may not be due to AV heart block. Gallop rhythm, mufHing of the first heart sound, tic-tac rhythm and cardiac enlargement are other signs of myocarditis.The classical manifestation of of congestive heart failure such as orthopnea, hepatomegaly, pitting edema and engorged veins are the exception rather than rule. Severe diphtheritic myocarditis manifests as "cardiogenic shock" with a small thready pulse, vomiting, abdominal pain, marked apathy and severe, 4 arterial hypotension.

Electrocardiography is very useful in diagnosing myocarditis and assessing its severity, especially if serial tracings are taken. The earliest change may be slight sagging of the ST segment, and the commonest abnormality is flattening or inversion of the T wave, usually in several leads. More ominous, though less frequent, are the disturbances of impulse conduction. These include:

1. First, second and third degrees of atrioventricular block
2. Intraventricular conduction defects including bundle-branch block. If complete heart block or complete hundle-branch block is present, the mortality is from 70–100%.

Partial defects of conduction carry a somewhat better prognosis, and normal conduction is usually restored within a week (Figs 47.1 and 47.2).

Other rare cardiac complications of diphtheria are:

1. Arrhythmias such as extrasystoles, nodal rhythm, paroxysmal tachycardias, atrial flutter and fibrillation, and ventricular fibrillation.
2. Intracardiac thrombi may form which embolise to the brain, the lungs or the extremeties, causing hemiplegia, hemoptysis or gangrene of a limb respectively.

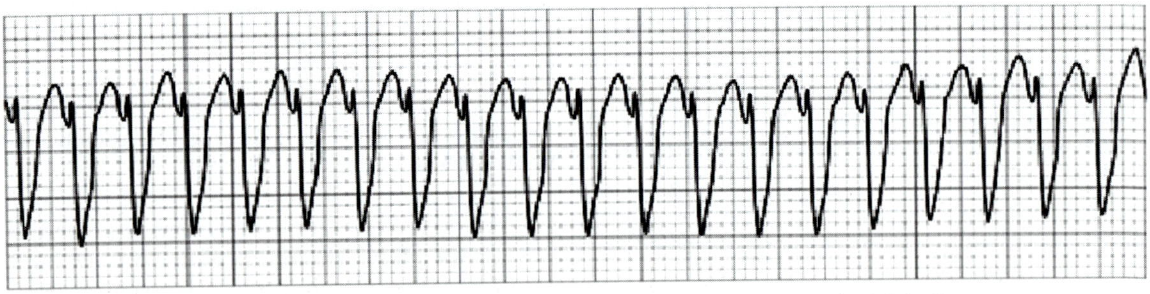

Fig. 47.1: *Ventricular tachycardia: Broad QRS complexes with no visible P waves*

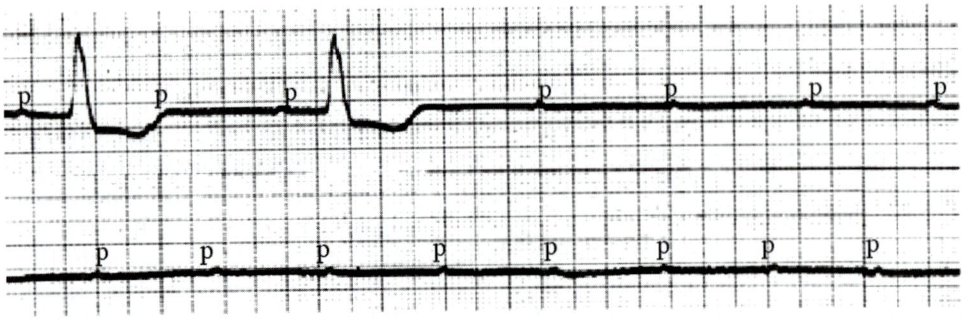

Fig. 47.2: *Extreme form of bradycardia in complete heat block in a patient who presented with stoke-Adam attacks*

3. A true bacterial endocarditis due to the diphtheria (Klebs Loeffler) bacillus has been reported.
4. Tachycardia at rest may persist for many weeks.

Prognosis

Acute myocarditis accounts for 60% of all deaths due to diphtheria. It has been estimated that the overall mortality of diphtheritic myocarditis is between 50% and 60%, being almost 100% in infants, 50% between 2 and 10 years and 25% in adults. In fatal cases death usually occurs in the first 2 weeks of the illness. It is controversial as to whether diphtheritic myocarditis ever results in permanent cardiac damage in the form of cardiac enlargement or complete heart block. Long-term follow-up studies have not shown any such persisting heart damage in individuals who have suffered from severe diphtheria in the past.

Treatment

Therapy is mainly that of diphtheria ihself with antitoxin and penicillin. Patients recovering from diphtheritic myocarditis require a longer period of bed rest than uncomplicated cases of diphtheria. Digitalis is indicated unless heart block is present.

Pneumonia (Figs 47.3 and 47.4)

In preantibiotic days, pneumococcal endocarditis to complicate 4% of all cases of lobar pneumonia. Local spread of the pneumococcus to the pericardium from the contiguous lung or pleura was also not uncommon. Acute peripheral circulatory failure is well known as a preterminal but potentially reversible complication of lobar pneumonia. Nonspecific ECG changes in the T wave and ST segment were frequently found. Pneumonia often causes rapid deterioration in patients with preexisting heart disease, especially in children suffering from congenital heart with left-to-right shunts and in adults with mitral stenosis. Unfortunately such patients are particularly prone to intercurrent respiratory infections.

Typhoid fever: Very rarely a typhoid endocarditis, pericarditis or interstitial myocarditis can occur, although nonspecific T wave changes and prolongation of the P-R interval are frequently observed.

Meningococcal infection: Meningococci can cause acute bacterial endocarditis, which is often overshadowed by the concomitant meningitis. Other rarely reported cardiac involvement in bacterial infections include pericarditis, endocarditis or myocarditis caused by brucellosis, leptospirosis or salmonellosis.

Virus Infections

Poliomyelitis: Myocardial involvement has been found in 40–90% of autopsied cases. Microscopically it is seen with focal collections of inflammatory cells in the interstitial tissue. The poliomyelitis virus has been isolated from the heart in fatal cases.

Electrocardiographic: Changes have varied from 15–45% in different series. These changes include prolonged PR interval, ST segment deviations, flattening or inversion of the T waves and prolonged QT interval. About two-thirds of patients develop hypertension, between the third and the seventh days. Subsequently, the blood pressure falls and almost always reaches normal at the end of 2 weeks. It is extremely unusual for the hypertension to persist. Viral involvement of the hypothalamus and arterial hypoxia (due to hypoventilation) may be important in the pathogenesis of hypertension. Hypertension particularly occurs in bulbar poliomyelitis (Figs 47.5 and 47.6).

A shock-like state is also seen in bulbar poliomyelitis, partly due to the myocarditis and partly to destruction of vasomotor centres in the brain sten. It is usually accompanied

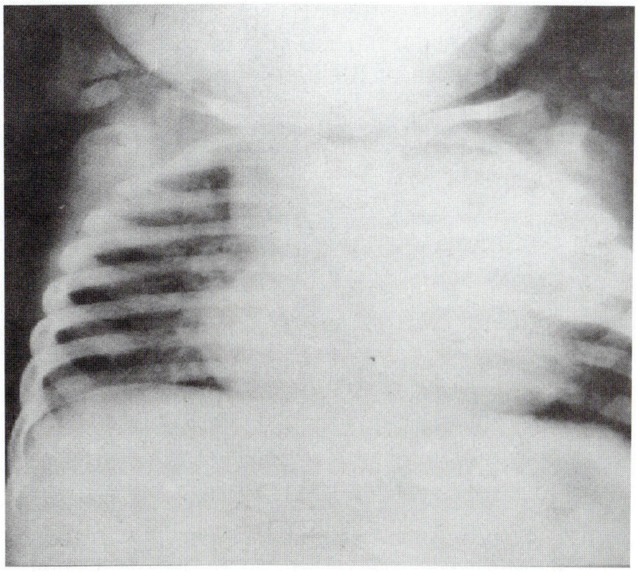

Fig. 47.3: *X-ray chest PA view showing left lung pneumonia with pulmonary arterial hypertension and acute right heart failure in 1 year-old-child with post measles infection*

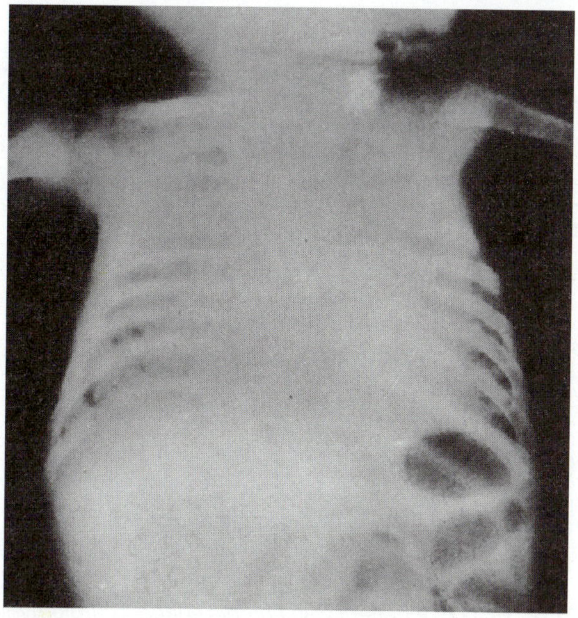

Fig. 47.4: *X-ray chest PA view showing bilateral widespread broncho-pneumonia with congestine heart failure in 2-yrs-old child with pneumococcal infection*

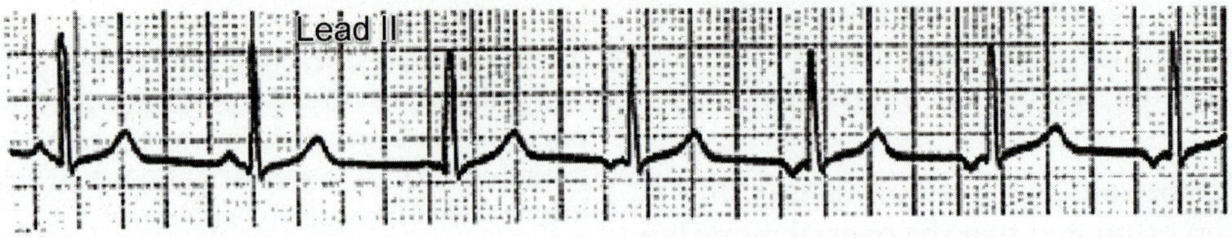

Fig. 47.5: *ECG showing ST depression in leads 11,111, aVF and varying P-R interval as a part of wandering pacemaker in 6-yrs-old boy with coxsackie virus B myopericarditis*

by hyperpyrexia and tachycardia. Pulmonary edema is often seen in the terminal stage. Inhalation of 100% oxygen or its administration by positive pressure may be valuable in such cases. Digitalis is indicated when hypertension and myocarditis are both present.

Measles: Nonspecific ECG changes occur in 20% of children suffering from measels. Measels myocarditis and pericarditis have been reported.

Influenza: During the influenza pandemic which swept the earth 16 years ago, caused by the Asian Virus (type A), myocarditis was frequently demonstrated at autopsy.

Myocarditis has been diagnosed clinically in children who have serological evidence of a recent influenza virus infection. The clinical picture was characterised by fever, a transient skin rash and severe congestive heart failure of sudden onset. The cardiac failure did not improve with routine measures, but responded dramatically to corticosteroids.

Mumps: Nonspecific ECG changes are observed in 5–15% of all patients affected by epidemic parotitis. However, mumps myocarditis severe enough to cause death is extremely rare though it undoubtedly occurs.

Coxsackie virus carditis: Much interest has been aroused in recent years by the frequent implication of coxsackie virus group B as a cause of myocarditis and pericarditis in both children and adults. It tends to occur in epidemics; outbreaks have been reported from Germany, Australia, South Africa and North America.

Infants are commonly affected. Clinically, here is a sudden onset of malaise and the infant goes off feeds; 3–10 days later high fever develops with marked tachycardia, respiratory distress, cyanosis, cardiac dilatation, gallop rhythm and hepatosplenomegaly. In severe cases, signs of aseptic meningitis or encephalomyelitis may coexist. The patient usually dies in a few days or rapidly recovers. In reported cases there has been a history of upper respiratory infections in the mother during the last weeks of pregnancy. Infection of neonatal infants with coxsackie B virus is believed to take place either transplacentally or by the oral route after birth.

In suspected cases, the diagnosis of coxsackie virus is made by isolating it from blood, faces, or throat and by demonstrating a rising titre of neutralising antibodies in the patients' blood.

Other Viral Infections

Viral myocarditis has also been reported in association with infection by ECHO viruses, adenoviruses, varicella, psittacosis, dengue, epidemic encephalits, herpes zoster, rabies and lymphocytic choriomeningitis. In addition, there is an encephalo-myocarditis family of viruses which have been shown to cause encephalitis and myocarditis in experimental animals, particularly in monkeys. There is also strong evidence of their potential pathogenecity in

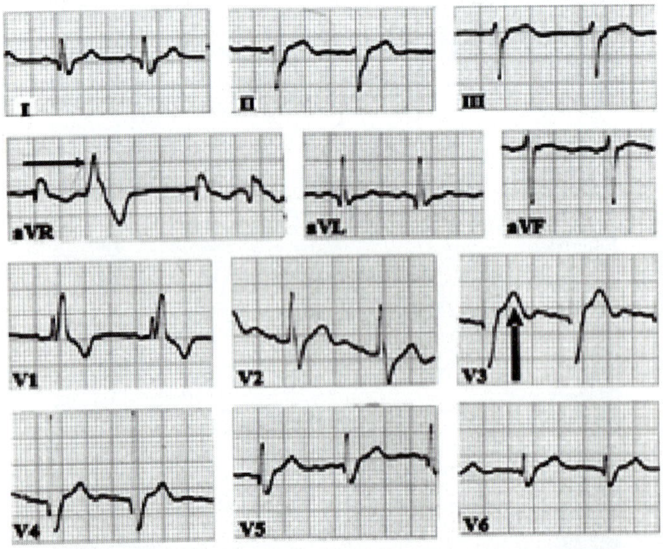

Fig. 47.6: *ECG of a patient with chronic chaga's cardiomyopathy showing the three most typical alterations: right bundle-branch block, left anterior fascicular block (large blue arrow), and ventricular extrasystole (small blue arrow)*

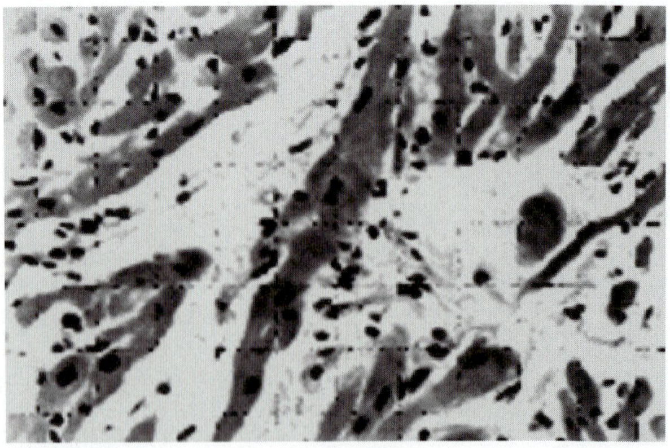

Fig. 47.7: *A biopsy specimen from the right ventricular apex of patient showed myocardial degeneration, nuclear hypertrophy, and infiltration of inflammatory cells in the interstitial tissue (hematoxylin-eosin, original magnification x 400) in one of the cases of acute viral myocarditis*

man. The theory has often been put forward that many cases of cardiomyopathy are really the end-result or burnt-out stage of viral myocarditis. Until recently, this supposition was merely a speculation not substantiated by actual proof, but recently workers in Europe and America have accumulated an impressive array of virological and autopsy evidence demonstrating that endocardial fibroelastosis is an aftermath of viral myocarditis probably caused by the coxsackie virus.

Very little is known of the prevalence of cardiac involvement in viral infections in India. Facilities for viral studies and research are extremely limited in this country. There is much scope for investigation as to whether some cases of so-called idiopathic cardiomyopathy, idiopathic myocarditis or idiopathic pericarditis are in fact related to a preceding viral infection.

Cardiac Involvement in Parasitic Diseases

Human parasitic infections are ubiquitous and affect a substantial number of individuals worldwide. Protozoan and helminth parasites can lead to a wide array of clinical manifestations during their migration inside the human body or when they reach their end organ of infection. Moreover, some parasitic infections are associated with significant morbidity and mortality in areas of high endemicity (Fig. 47.8).

The heart and the lungs are the thoracic organs more frequently affected by parasitic infections. The involvement of the heart may be part of a more generalized illness, as is the case with human African trypanosomiasis (HAT). In other situations, parasitic infections may have more direct effects on various structures of the heart (myocardium, pericardium, endocardium, or the cardiac vasculature). The involvement of the myocardium may lead to myocarditis or different types of cardiomyopathies (i.e. dilated or restrictive). When the pericardium is affected, it may lead to pericarditis, pericardial effusion, cardiac tamponade, or constrictive pericarditis. Some parasitic infections, such as schistosomiasis, may cause pulmonary hypertension in many developing tropical and subtropical settings. Latent parasitic infections may also reactivate and manifest as systemic disease, often ultimately affecting the heart, in immunosuppressive states such as organ transplantation, the use of immunosuppressive agents, or HIV/AIDS. Due to growing migration, population displacement, and travel, clinicians anywhere around the globe must be aware of the potential cardiac manifestations of parasitic diseases. In this regard, Chagas' cardiomyopathy is the hallmark of a disease that is currently considered a global parasitic disease.

In this review, we present an overview of the most frequently identified parasitic infections that affect the heart. For each topic we present a discussion of the epidemiology, pathogenesis, clinical manifestations, and treatment (Fig. 47.7).

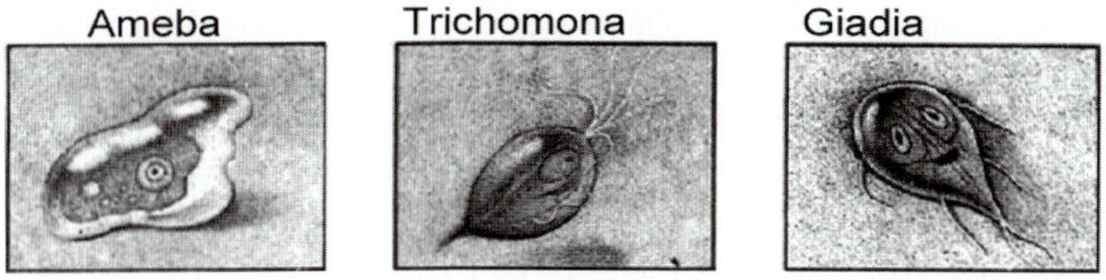

Fig. 47.8: *Photographs of morphological features of three common parasites*

Table 47.1: *Parasitic diseases affecting the heart*

Myocarditis	American trypanosomiasis African trypanosomiasis Visceral larva migrans Toxoplasmosis Trichinella spiralis Amoebiasis Echinococcus
Cardiomyopathy	Chagas' disease Toxoplasmosis
Pericarditis	Amoebiasis African trypanosomiasis Chagas disease' Toxoplasmosis Echinococcus

PARASITES THAT PREFERENTIALLY INVOLVE THE MYOCARDIUM OR CAUSE PANCARDITIS

Trypanosomes

Trypanosoma Cruzi (Chagas' Disease) (Fig. 47.9)

Chagas' disease, also known as American trypanosomiasis, is a zoonotic tropical disease caused by the flagellate protozoan parasite *Trypanosoma cruzi*. Most infections occur through vector-borne transmission by triatomine insects in areas of endemicity but can also occur through blood transfusion or organ transplantation, vertically from mother to infant, and, more rarely, by ingestion of food or liquid contaminated with *T. cruzi* or accidents among laboratory personnel who work with live parasites). Vector-borne transmission involves the transmission of the infective form

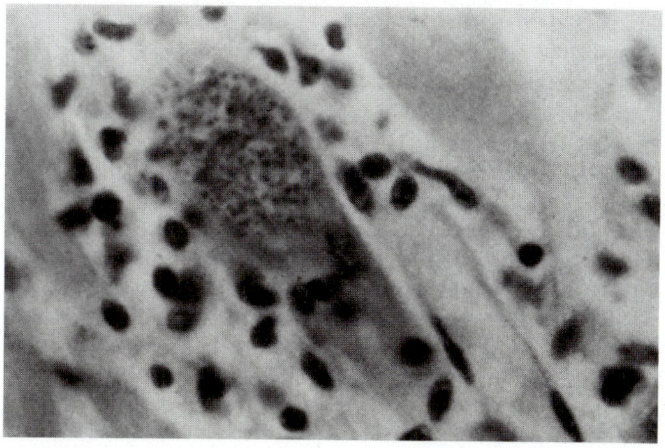

Fig. 47.9: *Myocardial invasion by Leishman-Donovan bodies causing myocarditis*

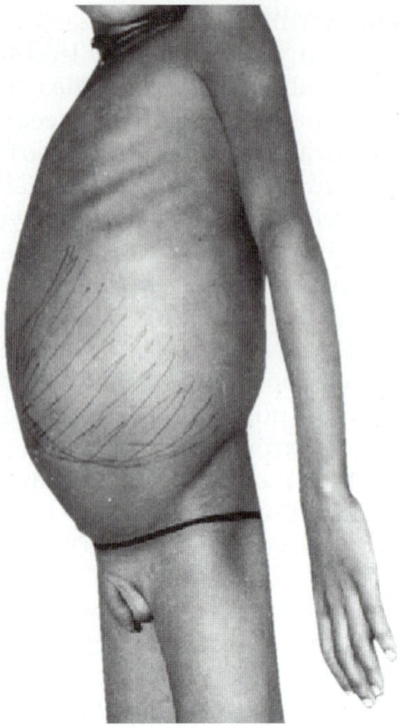

Fig. 47.10: *Tropical splenomegaly (marked) in a young patient with chronic recurrent malaria*

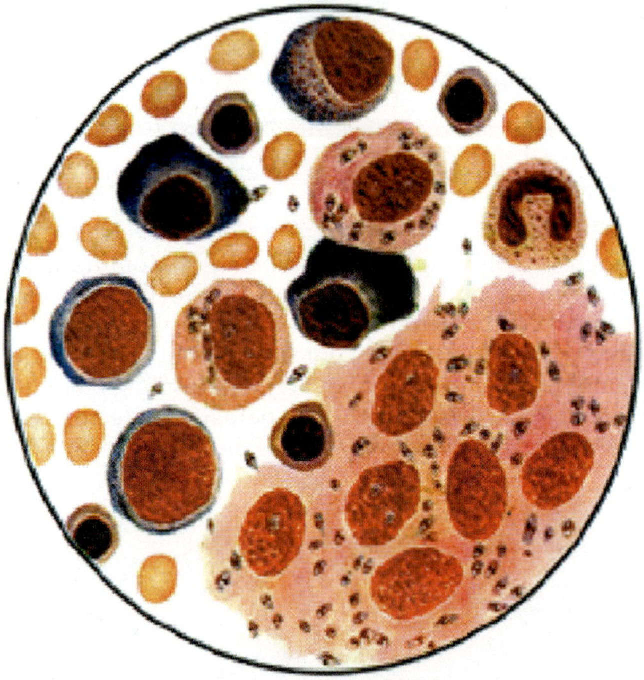

Fig. 47.11: *Microphotograph showing sternal aspirate in visceral leishmaniasis in which there is hyperplasia of reticulo-histiocystic elements which contain great numbers of leishmania parasites*

of the parasite (the metacyclic trypomastigotes) to humans by the excreta of the triatomine insect through mucous membranes or through breaks in the skin. Trypomastigotes then invade local host cells, where they differentiate into amastigotes and multiply within the cell. When the cell is swollen with amastigotes, they transform back into trypomastigotes by growing flagellae. The trypomastigotes lyse the cells, invade adjacent tissues, and spread via the lymphatics and bloodstream to distant sites. The cycle is completed when a reduviid bug becomes infected by ingesting blood from an infected host. A minority of patients will develop an acute syndrome of 4–8 weeks' duration, which invariably involves prolonged fever in addition to a variable constellation of symptoms, which include inflammation at the portal of entry, subcutaneous edema (localized or generalized), lymphadenopathy, hepatosplenomegaly, myocarditis, and, more rarely, meningoencephalitis. The manifestations of the acute phase resolve spontaneously for the vast majority of individuals even if the infection is not treated with an antiparasitic drug. About 60–70% of these patients will never develop clinically apparent diseases. They remain asymptomatic and infected life long, being recognized only if serological tests are performed (the so-called indeterminate form of chronic Chagas' disease). Roughly 30–40% of infected patients will subsequently develop the cardiac and/or digestive (megaesophagus and megacolon) form of chronic Chagas' disease, usually 10–30 years after the initial infection.

Epidemiology (Figs 47.13 and 47.14)

Trypanosoma cruzi is endemic in South America, Central America, and parts of North America (Southern United States and Mexico). Historically, the disease disproportionately affected the poor because the transmission of *T. cruzi* infection occurred mainly in rural areas where humans live in poor-quality houses and in close contact with potential vectors. However, rural-to-urban and international migrations have changed the epidemiology of Chagas' disease, affecting periurban areas, urban areas, areas of endemicity, and areas of nonendemicity alike As a result of these dynamic changes in the population and the coordinated efforts of countries where disease is endemic to interrupt vectorial and transfusional transmission, the prevalence and incidence of the disease are constantly changing. In the 1980s the overall prevalence of *T. cruzi* infection was estimated to reach 17 million cases in 18 countries where disease is endemic, with 100 million people at risk. Multinational vector control programs and compulsory blood bank screening achieved enormous success in the 1990s, decreasing the incidence of new infections (700,000 cases per year in 1983) by 70% and the number of annual deaths by approximately 50% for the whole continent and eradicating the transmission of *T. cruzi* by the main domiciliary vector species, *Triatoma infestans*, from three of the countries where *T. cruzi* is endemic (Uruguay in 1997, Chile in 1999, and Brazil in 2006). According to the most recent estimates, there are currently 7.6 million people infected with *T. cruzi* in Latin America Although precise figures documenting the total burden of cardiac involvement with *T. cruzi* are not available, it can be assumed that 20–30% of the 7.6 million infected individuals are or will potentially be developing chronic cardiac lesions. Chagas' cardiomyopathy, in turn, is thought to represent the principal cause of cardiac

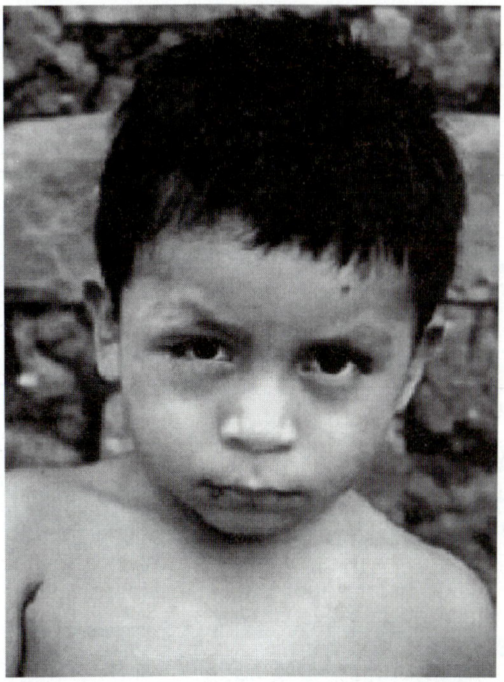

Fig. 47.12: *A young child showing swelling of right eye as one of the manifestations of the acute phase of chagas disease (Romana" sign)*

morbidity and mortality among young adults in countries where *T. cruzi* is endemic and has been estimated to result in at least 21,000 deaths each year,, Additionally, because of the constant influx of immigrants from countries where the disease is endemic, Chagas' disease is becoming an important health issue in North America (United States and Canada) and many parts of Europe, where a growing number of individuals are suspected to be infected (e.g. 300,000 individuals in the United States and 48,000–67,000 individuals in Spain (Figs 47.10 and 47.11).

Pathology and Pathophysiology of Acute Myocarditis and Chronic Cardiomyopathy

Initially, the abundance of parasites associated with the acute phase of *T. cruzi* infection argued in favor of the parasite's direct implication in the tissue damage and myocarditis observed during this stage of the disease. Shortly afterwards, a demonstration of myocytolysis of nonparasitized cardiomyocytes led to the implication of parasite-directed cellular immune-mediated inflammatory damage. This immune-mediated damage, associated with large numbers of amastigotes in cardiac myocytes, translates into the hyaline degeneration of muscle fibers, the coagulation necrosis of myocytes and surrounding tissues, as well as the involvement of the epicardium and pericardium. Cellular and, possibly, humoral immune responses elicited by the parasite eventually control the acute infection but fail to completely eliminate the parasite. A variably long asymptomatic phase then ensues, where factors such as the parasite strain, the parasite load during the acute phase, the quality of the immune response, and the presence or absence of reinfection all might influence the course of chronic disease). Regarding the pathogenesis of the interstitial fibrosis, myocytolysis, and ongoing lymphocytic infiltration observed for the chronic phase of Chagas' disease, the paucity of parasites in cardiac tissue probably reflects the use of insensitive histological techniques in past decades. In recent years, more powerful and sensitive methods of parasite detection, such as immunohistochemistry and PCR, have demonstrated a higher frequency of *T. cruzi* antigens or parasite DNA in chronic lesions). The spectrum of outcomes for patients infected with *T. cruzi* is varied and probably stems from intrinsic genetic differences of both the parasite and the host and perhaps even the likelihood of ongoing infection in areas where the disease is highly endemic. Evidence exists for multiple hypotheses to explain the etiology of chronic cardiac lesions that implicate the parasite directly, the immune reaction to the parasite, and autoimmunity elicited either directly by the parasite (mimicry) or indirectly (bystander activation). The products of these lesions are various degrees of necrosis, neuronal damage, microvascular damage, and fibrosis. The contributing role of each mechanism to the pathogenesis of Chagas' cardiomyopathy is a whole other topic of debate.

There is evidence for both functional and anatomical parasympathetic neuronal damage in Chagasic patients Patients with Chagas' disease lack the tonic inhibitory parasympathetic action on the sinus node and, thus, the chronotropic mechanism to respond to changes in blood pressure or venous return. Neuronal loss is thought to occur during the acute stage of the disease; the extent of neuronal damage, however, does not correlate with disease stage Therefore, despite possible contributions of parasympathetic impairment to the impact of Chagas' heart disease (e.g. increasing vulnerability to malignant arrhythmias and sudden death or accentuating existing contraction abnormalities that can culminate in chamber dilatation), cardiac dysautonomia is unlikely to explain the main pathogenic mechanism underlying Chagas' cardiomyopathy.

In addition to the neuronal damage, microcirculatory changes leading to ischemia have also been implicated in the pathogenesis of chronic Chagas' cardiomyopathy. A diffuse collapse of intramyocardial arterioles in the hearts of chronically infected patients has been observed Occlusive platelet thrombi in small epicardial and intramural coronary arteries and increased production of cytokines and mediators that promote vasospasm and platelet aggregation have been demonstrated with experimental models of Chagas' disease, Clinically, despite consistently normal epicardial coronary arteries upon coronary angiography, reversible perfusion defects upon stress-induced myocardial perfusion scintigraphy that correlate with ischemia and abnormal coronary flow regulation have been shown for patients with chronic Chagas' cardiomyopathy.

As mentioned above, tissue damage caused directly by the parasite or, more likely, by the immune response elicited by it has been postulated to underlie and potentiate the aggression to cardiac myocytes and neurons. The inflammatory infiltrate in chronic Chagas' cardiomyopathy

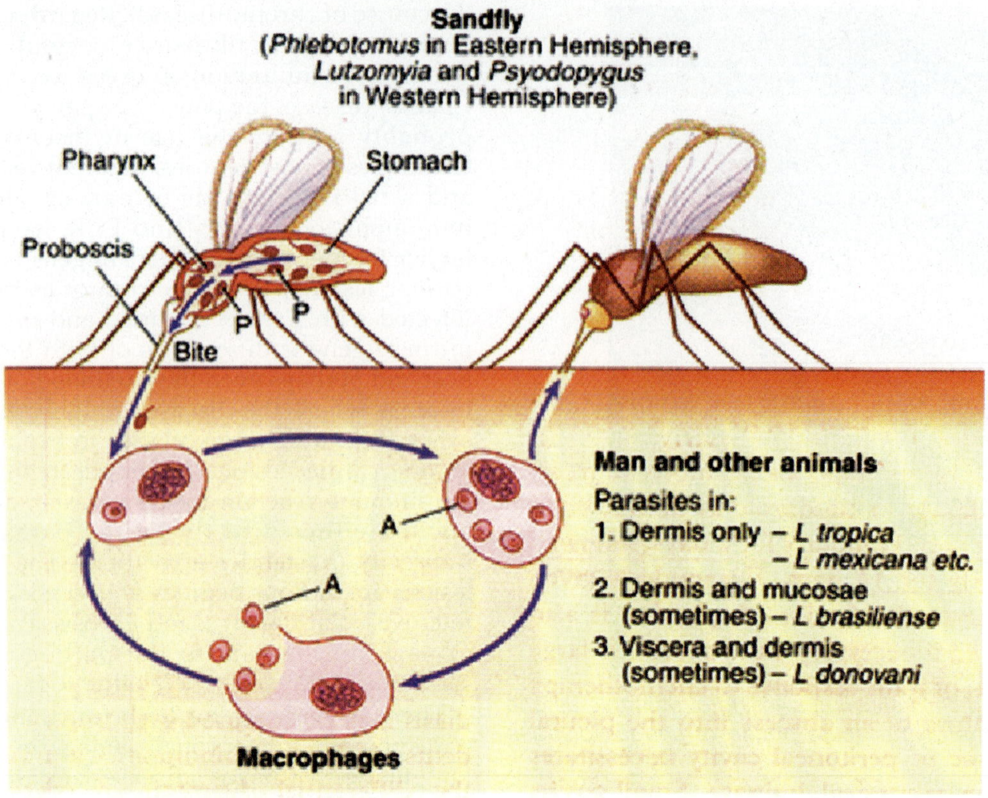

Fig. 47.13: *How sand fly is busy introducing the organisms in human and other animals in the process of disease*

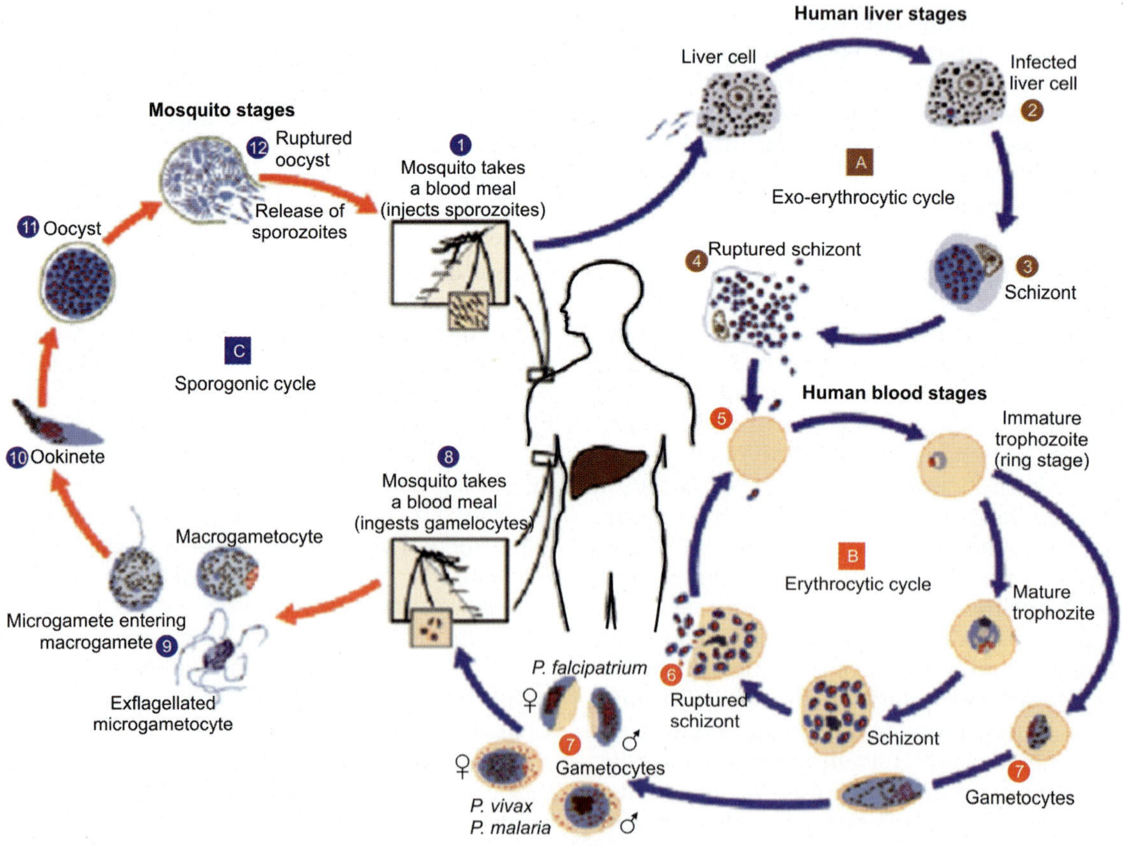

Fig. 47.14: *Life cycle of Trypanosoma cruzi in human body in the causation of Chaga's disease*

involves a predominance of macrophages, $CD8^+$ and $CD4^+$ lymphocytes (in a 2:1 ratio), and in some instances has been shown to correlate with more advanced stages of the disease. The persistence of parasites and antigens is thought to be involved in the recruitment of *T. cruzi*-specific $CD8^+$ T lymphocytes, which predominate in the myocardial infiltrate in cases of chronic Chagas' myocarditis. The cytokine profile associated with this myocarditis is also shifted toward Th1 cytokines, so elevated gamma interferon (IFN-β) levels and decreased interleukin-10 (IL-10) levels may potentially perpetuate an existent, ongoing inflammatory process. However, the exact mechanism responsible for the turning point from immunoprotection to immune-mediated aggression leading to irreversible tissue damage remains elusive: not only is parasite persistence true for both symptomatic and asymptomatic patients, but the presence of the parasite in heart tissue does not always correlate with inflammation.

Autoimmunity has also been postulated to be a plausible etiology for the chronic myocarditis observed for *T. cruzi*-infected patients. Several *T. cruzi* antigens that cross-react with cardiac and noncardiac host components have been identified, but only some have been shown to have functional activity. Among these, attention has focused on antibodies that cross-react with cardiac myosin and the immunodominant *T. cruzi* antigen B13 initially, because they were detected in 100% of patients with chronic Chagas' cardiomyopathy, in contrast to 14% of asymptomatic infected individuals and later because T-cell clones derived from lesions of patients with chronic Chagas' cardiomyopathy were found to be simultaneously reactive to cardiac myosin heavy chain and the B13 *T. cruzi* protein. Opponents of the molecular mimicry theory with specific relevance to anti-B13-cardiac myosin cross-reactive antibodies and derived cellular autoimmunity contend that these antibodies do not bind to intact myocytes, are not unique to *T. cruzi* infection, and are present in asymptomatic patients without heart lesions and that myosin autoimmunity is not essential for cardiac inflammation in experimental models. Arguing against autoimmunity developing as a result of parasite-specific immune responses, antigen exposure after tissue damage may also sensitize autoreactive T cells to self-antigens given a proinflammatory environment. The question, therefore, is not whether autoimmunity is present but whether it is a primary cause of or merely a contributing factor to the pathogenesis of chronic Chagas' myocarditis. As proposed by Kierszenbaum, this question remains to be answered by experiments that prove a clear association between the development of similar cardiac lesions with the transfer of autoantibodies and/or autoreactive cells to susceptible hosts.

To synthesize, although the effects of both autonomic and microvascular disturbances in Chagas' cardiomyopathy may play an important role in potentiating and perpetuating cardiac muscle damage, persistent inflammation in the setting of continuous antigenic stimulation is perhaps the common pathway for tissue damage. Multiple mechanisms seem to explain this chronic inflammation (mainly antiparasite immunity and, possibly, autoimmunity), which are not necessarily mutually exclusive. The course of progression to chronic Chagas' cardiomyopathy and other forms of the disease was suggested to be related to genetic properties of both the host and the parasite. However, the molecular mechanisms underlying tissue tropism and the initial trigger or determinant of the course of chronic disease are not yet known.

Table 47.2: *Hallmarks of chronic Chagas' cardiomyopathy*[a]

Arrhythmias
- Ventricular extrasystoles
- Nonsustained and sustained ventricular tachycardia
- Bradyarrhythmias
- Ventricular fibrillation
- Atrial fibrillation/flutter
- Conduction abnormalities
- Sick sinus syndrome
- Complete and incomplete right bundle-branch block
- Left anterior fascicle block
- Bifascicular and trifascicular blocks
- 1st, 2nd and 3rd degree AV blocks

Thromboembolic phenomena
- Brain (most frequent)
- Lungs, kidneys, spleen

Cardiac failure
- Diastolic dysfunction initially
- Isolated left heart failure in the early stage of cardiac decompensation
- Biventricular with a predominance of right-sided failure

Clinical Manifestations of Heart Involvement (Fig. 47.12)

a. *Myocarditis during the acute phase*: Acute myocarditis as evidenced by autopsy studies probably happens in close to 100% of patients with acute Chagas' disease. However, there is an enormous discrepancy between autopsy findings and clinical data: first because acute infection is asymptomatic for approximately 90–95% of cases and

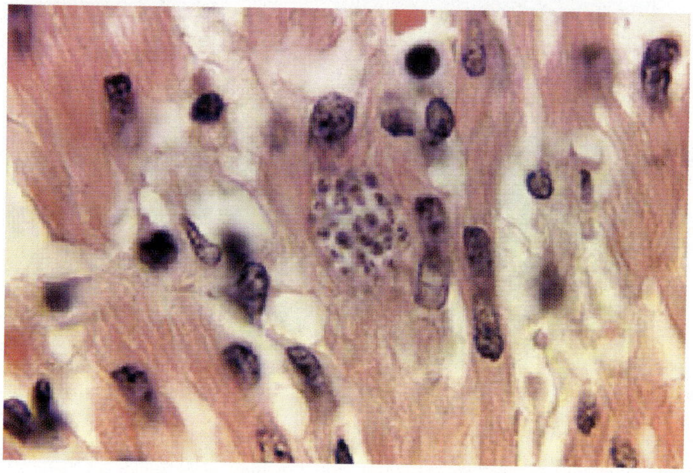

Fig. 47.15: *Photomicrograph of stained Trypanosoma cruzi found in the myocardium of the patient with Chaga's disease*

second because even for symptomatic patients, acute Chagasic myocarditis is diagnosed for only 1–40% of them findings upon cardiac auscultation may include tachycardia (not always proportional to the degree of fever), cardiac murmurs and muffled heart sounds. The principal electrocardiographic (ECG) alterations are first-degree atrioventricular (AV) block, low Q-R-S (Q-R-S interval of the ECG) voltage, and primary T-wave changes. A chest radiograph may show variable degrees of cardiomegaly, and pericardial effusion is the most frequently reported echocardiographic abnormality. Death in the acute phase occurs occasionally (for 5–10% of symptomatic patients) as a result of congestive heart failure (due to severe myocarditis) and/or meningoencephalitis. After the acute phase most patients return to a normal or near-normal myocardial status, but some patients (30%) then chronically develop fibrosing myocarditis.

Among immunosuppressed hosts such as HIV-infected individuals and transplant recipients, reactivation of infection and *de novo* infection (including transmission with transplanted organs among transplant patients) have been reported. With reactivation in HIV-positive patients, myocarditis has been reported for up to 45% of cases. Reactivation of Chagas' disease among heart transplant patients has been estimated to occur in approximately 30% of cases however, not all these cases are accompanied by florid symptoms or diagnosed by endomyocardial biopsy, and therefore, the true incidence of myocarditis with reactivation is difficult to estimate. Acute *T. cruzi* infection can also result as a consequence of donor-related transmission, which has been reported after kidney, heart, liver, and multiorgan transplants Involvement in this setting can range from asymptomatic parasitemia that easily responds to treatment without further complications to severe, fulminant disease despite therapy (including death directly attributable to Chagasic myocarditis. In congenitally infected infants, the most common symptoms, which may be apparent at birth or develop within weeks after delivery, are hipotonicity, fever, hepatosplenomegaly and anemia. Other findings include prematurity and low birth weight). *In utero* infections are also associated with abortion and placentitis. Serious manifestations including myocarditis, meningoencephalitis and pneumonitis, are uncommon but carry a high risk of death.

b. *Chronic Chagas' cardiomyopathy*: Cardiac involvement is the most frequent and most severe manifestation of chronic Chagas' disease. Transition from the indeterminate form to the cardiac form of chronic Chagas' disease is usually manifested by the appearance of ECG changes such as incomplete or complete right bundle-branch block (RBBB), left anterior fascicular block (LAFB), minimal ST-T (ST-to-T interval of the ECG) changes, and monomorphic premature ventricular contractions (PVCs), mostly in asymptomatic or oligosymptomatic patients. As the disease advances, associated intraventricular conduction defects (usually RBBB with LAFB), polymorphic PVCs bradyarrhythmias, high-grade atrioventricular blocks, Q waves, nonsustained or sustained ventricular tachycardia, and, ultimately, atrial flutter or fibrillation may ensue. Symptoms like palpitations, atypical chest pain, presyncope, syncope, dyspnea upon exertion, and edema are usually observed throughout the course of chronic Chagas' cardiomyopathy (CCC). Findings upon physical examination vary according to the stage of the disease and the presence of conduction system abnormalities. These findings include cardiac rhythm irregularities, a displaced point of maximal impulse, gallop rhythms, a loud second heart

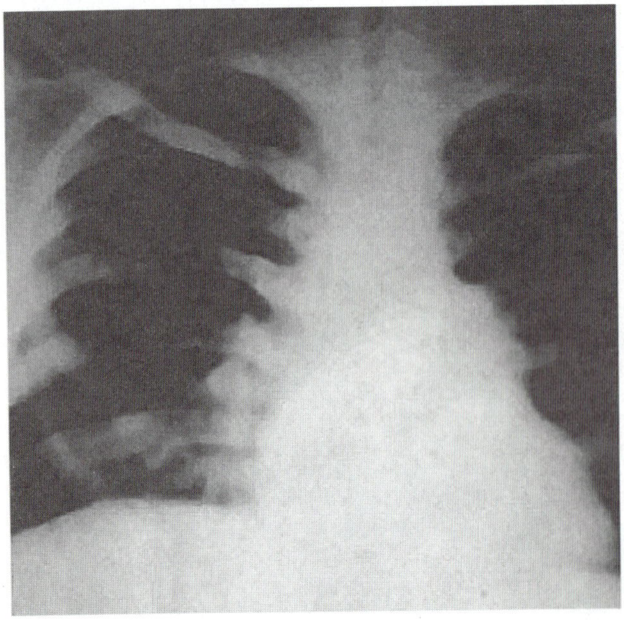

Fig. 47.16: *Chest X-ray (PA view) showing pulmonary hypertension in patient with Chagas disease*

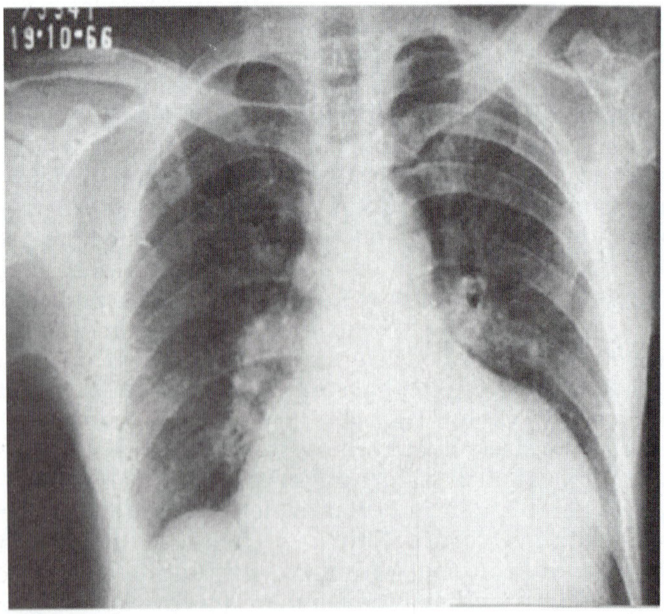

Fig. 47.17: *Chest X-ray (PA view) showing cardiomegaly in patient with Chagas disease*

sound implying pulmonary hypertension, mitral or tricuspid regurgitation murmurs, an increase in the systemic venous pressure with liver enlargement and edema, and a borderline low systolic blood pressure with a reduced radial pulse implying systolic dysfunction Upon echocardiogram, diastolic dysfunction usually precedes systolic dysfunction, potentially allowing the early detection of cardiac involvement in Chagas' disease (Characteristic echocardiographic findings include apical aneurysms (Fig. which are reported for 8.5–55% of cases (depending on the stage of the disease and the method of detection, i.e. if postmortem or at echocardiography or angiography); segmental left ventricular (LV) contractile abnormalities (more commonly at the posteroinferior wall); and reduced LV systolic function. Echocardiographic evidence of impaired LV function, as characterized by increased LV systolic dimension, reduced LV ejection fraction, or the presence of segmental or global LV wall motion abnormality and/or an LV aneurysm, is the most common and consistent independent predictor of death. Other important clinical and noninvasive adverse prognostic indicators, which not surprisingly reflect and parallel the degree of myocardial dysfunction, include advanced functional class [New York Heart Association (NYHA) classification III/IV], cardiomegaly, and nonsustained ventricular tachycardia upon 24-h ECG monitoring (Fig. 47.19).

The clinical course of CCC is diverse and difficult to predict, with some patients remaining asymptomatic life long despite electrocardiographic and/or echocardiographic evidence of the disease, some presenting with signs, symptoms, and complications of progressive heart failure or advanced cardiac arrhythmias, and others dying unexpectedly without prior symptoms. Currently, several staging systems are available. These staging systems can help to identify patients at different degrees of risk, facilitate choices among treatment alternatives, and aid patient counseling. Most systems classify patients into four or five stages based on their functional capacity, ECG findings, and the presence or absence of heart enlargement and/or systolic dysfunction upon echocardiogram. The progression of disease to more advanced stages has been estimated to occur for 10% of patients over a follow-up period of 3–10 years. Another important aspect of staging is derived from its prognostic information: the rate of mortality for individuals at early stages of CCC is not significantly different from that of the general population). However, the life expectancy of patients with symptomatic and advanced CCC stages (involving systolic dysfunction and/or cardiomegaly) is less than 30% at 5 years and their overall prognosis is worse than that of patients with dilated cardiomyopathies of other etiologies Systemic and pulmonary embolisms arising from mural thrombi in the cardiac chambers are relatively Although the brain is by

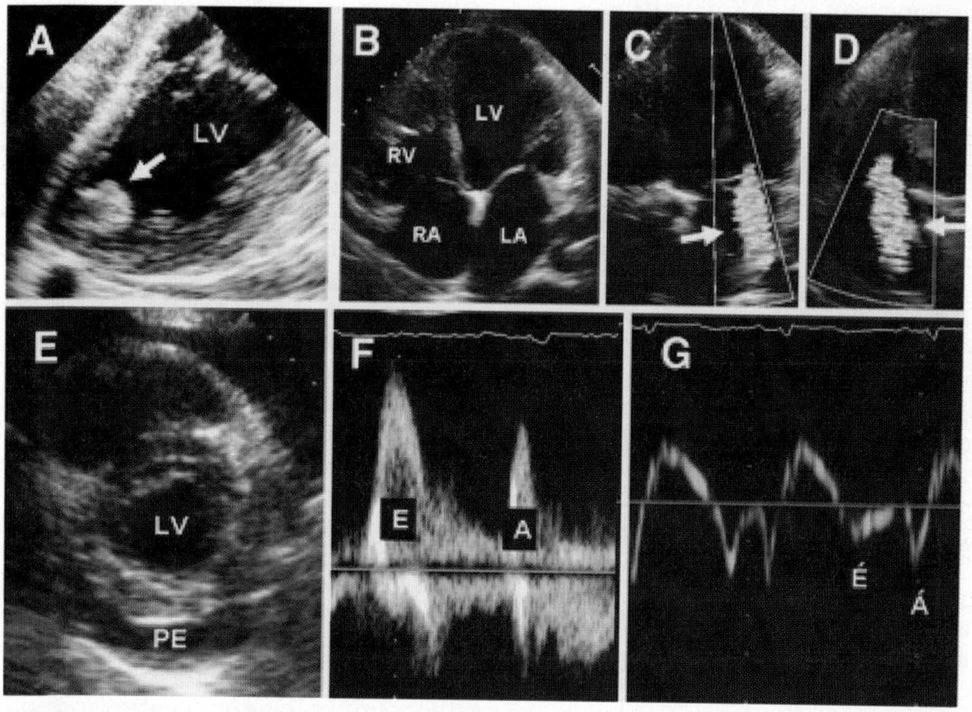

Fig. 47.18(A to G): *(A) Transesophageal echocardiography demonstrating an apical aneurysm containing a large, round, and protruding thrombus (arrow). (B to D) Transthoracic apical 4-chamber views of the heart showing dilated cardiac chambers (B) and functional mitral (C) and tricuspid (D) regurgitation (arrows). (E) Parasternal short-axis view of the heart showing a large pericardial effusion (PE). (F and G) Transmitral pulsed-Doppler (F) and lateral annulus tissue Doppler (G) demonstrating apparently normal peak early (E) and late (A) transmitral velocities, E/A ratio, and E-wave deceleration time (F) but abnormal early (E') and late (A') velocities (G) consistent with advanced diastolic dysfunctionin a patient with Chagas Disease LA, left atrium; LV, left ventricle; PE, pericardial effusion; RA, right atrium*

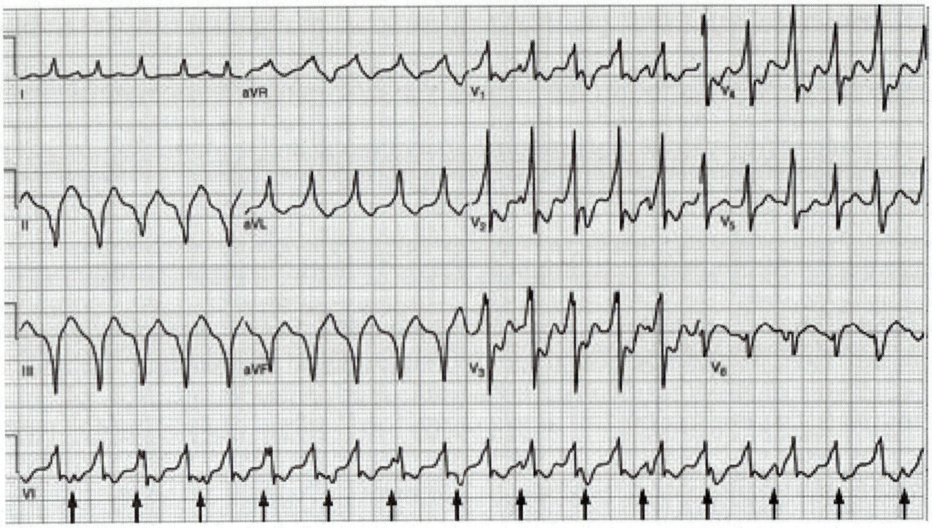

Fig. 47.19: *ECG showing AV dissociation (arrows mark P waves), wide QRS >200 ms, superior frontal plane axis, slurring of the initial portion of the QRS, and large S wave in V6—all clues to the diagnosis of ventricular tachycardia in a patient with Chaga's myocarditis*

far the most common clinically recognized site of embolisms (followed by limbs and lungs), at necropsy, embolisms are found more frequently in the lungs, kidneys, and spleen. Chagas' disease is an independent risk factor for stroke in areas where the disease is endemic. Mortality in CCC is due to sudden cardiac arrest in 55–65% of patients, congestive heart failure in 25–30% of patients, and thromboembolic phenomena in 10–15% of patients.

Diagnosis (Figs 47.16–47.18 and 47.20)

Diagnosis of acute Chagas' myocarditis relies on the demonstration of the parasite and/or anti-*T. cruzi* IgM is in a patient with the correct epidemiological background and clinical picture. IgM serology assays are not widely available in developing countries and not standardized, so diagnosis is usually performed by visualizing the trypomastigotes in fresh blood smears, thick drop preparations, or buffy coat smears. The level of parasitemia diminishes to almost undetectable levels by the 6th to 10th weeks of infection, making parasite identification in peripheral blood extremely difficult at this time. Diagnosis could also be attempted by hemoculture on specialized medium (which has improved sensitivity over direct examination) or xenodiagnosis (which involves detecting the parasite by infecting laboratory-reared triatomine bugs directly or indirectly with the patient's blood. However, even considering only congenital Chagas' disease, hemoculture is rarely performed for the diagnosis of acute infection since it requires a specialized laboratory and trained personnel and is usually not widely available. Indirect parasitological tests are of limited value in the diagnosis of acute Chagas' disease, as they can take more than 1 month to obtain results (retarding the beginning of trypanocidal therapy).

A diagnosis of CCC should be suspected for young or middle-aged patients who present with a segmental or dilated cardiomyopathy of unknown etiology if within areas of endemicity or within the right epidemiological context. It should be remembered that CCC presents years after the initial infection, and therefore, patients who migrated to areas where the disease is not endemic are still at risk of developing cardiac compromise. Given the low and probably intermittent parasitemia in the chronic phase, diagnosis relies on serological methods by detecting IgG that binds to *T. cruzi* antigens. Enzyme-linked immunosorbent assay (ELISA), indirect immunofluorescence (IIF), and indirect hemagglutination (IHA) methods are most commonly employed. Two positive tests using any of the three conventional techniques are recommended for a final diagnosis. Identification of the parasite by hemoculture or xenodiagnosis in the chronic phase of the disease is hampered by the low sensitivity of the methods, which is dependent directly on the level of parasitemia. However, these methods may have a role in confirming the diagnosis in rare cases of serologically doubtful results or in evaluating treatment failures at specialized centers.

PCR-based methods using one of two target sequences (the variable region of the minicircle kinetoplast DNA and a 195-bp reiterated DNA sequence of the parasite) have achieved higher sensitivities than those of xenodiagnosis and hemoculture). The major problems with PCR-based techniques are the lack of standardization and commercial availability of assays for *T. cruzi*, the high level of complexity required, and the reliance of their sensitivity on the level of parasitemia (which is low, by definition, in chronic disease PCR is therefore still considered among nonconventional methods and is recommended only as an adjunct in specialized centers to confirm parasitemia in congenital *T. cruzi* infection (since in this context, its sensitivity seems to be greater than that of microscopic examination) or for the evaluation of antiparasitic drug therapy. However, a single or even repeated negative posttreatment PCR results do not necessarily mean parasitological cure. The negative results are indicative only

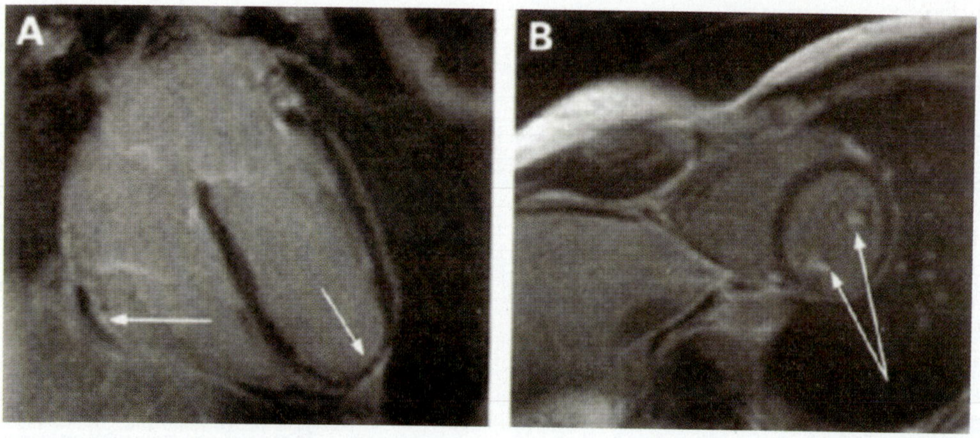

Fig. 47.20: *Contrast-enhanced magnetic resonance imaging of endomyocardial fibrosis secondary to Bancroftian filariasis. The left ventricle has an elongated appearance and there is a small posterior mitral valve leaflet with two regurgitant jets into a normal left atrium. Delayed imaging performed 10 minutes after intravenous contrast injection (0.2 mmol/ kg Gd-DTPA) showed subendocardial hyperenhancement of the left ventricular apex, both papillary muscles and the basal right ventricle (panels A and B). Contrast-enhallfed magnetic resonance imaging has noninvasively confirmed endomyocardial fibrosis as a complication of filariasis. In addition, this case is an example of non-ischaemic subendocardial delayed hyperenhancemen. A midnight blood sample was checked for microfilaria and identified as Wuchereria bancrofti. At echocardiography there was mild mitral regurgitation and pulmonary hypertension. At cardiac catheterisation the left ventricular ejection fraction was 65%, the end-diastolic pressure was raised and coronary arteries normal. Right ventricular endomyocardial biopsy showedendocardial and interstitial fibrosis. The diagnosis of filariasis with hypereosinophilia complicated by endomyocardial fibrosis was made.He was treated with ivermectin and mebendazole with steroid cover and lisinopril. The patient made an excellent recovery with gradual normalisation of the eosinophil count. At follow-up she remains clinically stable and echocardiography has shown no change in left ventricular ejection fraction or mitral regurgitation*

of the absence of parasite DNA at those moments. The value of PCR lies mainly in the positive results that they yield, which usually reflect treatment failure. Whether assessments of parasite load by quantitative real-time. PCR will correlate with the impact of trypanocidal treatment on parasitological cure or resistance, as well as on disease evolution, should be a matter for further investigation.

The initial evaluation of the newly diagnosed patient with chronic *T. cruzi* infection includes a complete medical history and physical examination and a resting 12-lead electrocardiogram. Asymptomatic patients with a normal ECG have a favorable prognosis and should be followed up only annually or biannually. Patients with ECG changes consistent with CCC should undergo a routine cardiac evaluation including ambulatory 24-h Holter monitoring (complemented with an exercise test whenever possible) to detect arrhythmias and assess functional capacity, chest radiography and two-dimensional (2D) echocardiography to assess ventricular function, and other cardiologic tests as indicated. Based on the results of these tests, it is possible to stratify individual patients by risk and implement appropriate therapy.

Treatment and Preventive Measures

a. *Etiological treatment*: Only two drugs, benznidazole and nifurtimox, are recommended for the treatment of Chagas' disease. Of the two, benznidazole (a nitroimidazole derivative) has been more extensively investigated in clinical studies and is better tolerated overall. Adverse reactions such as generalized or sometimes localized allergic dermatitis occur in approximately 20–30% of patients and consist of pruritic and nonbullous polymorphous erythematous rashes, often followed by desquamation. Severe exfoliative dermatitis can occur and should lead to a prompt discontinuation of treatment. Another adverse effect that occurs in approximately 5–10% of patients, most commonly late in the treatment course, is a dose-dependent peripheral sensitive neuropathy affecting mainly the distal parts of the lower limbs; it also should prompt the cessation of treatment. Rare serious adverse events include leukopenia with granulocytopenia or agranulocytosis (sometimes followed by fever and tonsillitis) and thrombocytopenic purpura. Additional reported side effects include nausea, vomiting, anorexia, weight loss, insomnia, loss of taste, and onycholysis. Nifurtimox, a nitrofuran compound, has been associated with gastrointestinal side effects in 30–70% of patients as well as central and peripheral nervous system toxicity. Both compounds are better tolerated by children, allowing increased dosage regimens. Children should be treated with 10 mg/kg of body weight of benznidazole per day in two divided doses for 30–90 days or 15–20 mg/kg of nifurtimox per day in four divided doses for 90–120 days. Adults should be treated with 5–7 mg/kg of benznidazole per day in two divided doses for 30–60 days or 8–10 mg/kg of nifurtimox per day in three to four divided doses for 90–120 days.
Treatment has been recommended for all cases of acute and congenital infection, reactivated infection, and early chronic Chagas' disease (particularly children/ adolescents 18 years of age) based on evidence of the

shortening of the disease's clinical course, cure of infection, or reduction in numbers of parasites. For infected adults without advanced cardiomyopathy up to the age of 50 years, etiological treatment should generally also be offered. The rationale for these recommendations stems from evidence of a slowing of the progression of cardiomyopathy. In a recent observational trial, 566 chronically infected adults (30–50 years of age) without heart failure were assigned, in alternating sequences, to benznidazole or no treatment After a median follow-up period of 9.8 years, fewer treated patients had a progression of disease or developed ECG abnormalities. Negative seroconversion was more frequent for treated patients. Another recently published controlled study, including 111 patients (17–46 years of age) with chronic Chagas' disease and a normal electrocardiogram, showed similar favorable results with benznidazole over a mean follow-up period of 21 years. For those patients over the age of 50 years, etiological treatment is considered optional because of the lack of any available data. A multicenter, randomized, placebo-controlled trial of benznidazole enrolling 3,000 patients with mild to moderate CCC who were 18–75 years of age is currently under way and should help to clarify treatment decisions for this population.

In contrast, etiological treatment is contraindicated during pregnancy and for patients with severe renal or hepatic insufficiency, and it should generally not be offered to patients with advanced Chagasic cardiomyopathy or megaesophagus with significant impairment of swallowing. A more controversial issue is prophylactic treatment for transplant patients: some authors have recommended it for patients with Chagasic cardiomyopathy who undergo cardiac transplantation to prevent disease reactivation. While others recommend it for all infected donors pretransplant and for their respective recipients posttransplant. For chronic Chagas' disease, cure is documented when previously positive serological tests are negative, usually years or decades after treatment.

b. *Symptomatic treatment*: Medical treatment of heart failure for patients with CCC should follow specific treatments targeted at each stage according to current guidelines for heart failure of other etiologies. An important exception is the use of beta-blockers, which should be used with caution for CCC due to a higher incidence of atrioventricular conduction defects and associated bradyarrhythmias. Cardiac transplantation has been performed with good results for patients with advanced CCC but may not be available or accessible in all countries where this disease is endemic. Although not tested in randomized controlled clinical trials, amiodarone has been associated with a survival advantage in case-control studies among patients with ventricular tachycardia and has therefore been proposed for the management of patients with sustained and nonsustained ventricular tachycardia. However, treatment with amiodarone has been associated with pulmonary, cardiac, thyroid, liver, ocular, skin, central nervous system (CNS), and genitourinary toxicities, so treatment needs to be individualized. Pacemaker implantation is the recommended treatment for severe bradyarrhythmias and advanced conduction abnormalities. The roles of cardioverter-defibrillator implantation and cardiac resynchronization, however, are not well established for CCC. Finally, anticoagulation has been advocated for patients with atrial fibrillation, previous thromboembolic phenomena, or an LV aneurysm with thrombus.

c. *Preventive measures*: Most *T. cruzi* infections can be prevented by decreasing vectorial transmission, improving blood product screening, and detecting and treating transplacental transmission. Multinational programs involving countries where the disease is endemic have achieved enormous success in decreasing both the prevalence and incidence of Chagas' disease by following several operational stages. The tools for interrupting transmission are based on the implementation of vector control activities such as insecticide spraying, housing improvements, and education as well as the strengthening of the implementation of policy for use and screening of blood products for transfusion. Since the end of January 2007, the American Red Cross and other blood collection agencies in the United States began screening blood donations for antibodies to *T. cruzi* donations with the approved ELISA (referred to as universal testing). All initially reactive donations are retested in duplicate by using the same screening test; donations testing repeatedly reactive undergo confirmatory testing by the radioimmunoprecipitation assay (RIPA). Continued surveillance is also important to consolidate and maintain the success achieved.

For persons traveling to areas of endemicity, compliance with general food and water precautions is advised to prevent the extremely rare occurrence of food-borne Chagas' disease. More importantly, travelers should avoid sleeping in poorly constructed houses or else consider sleeping in insecticide-impregnated bed nets. However, the protective efficacy of insecticide-treated materials in reducing Chagas' disease transmission and eliminating the vector population has yet to be demonstrated. Finally, no vaccine for Chagas' disease is available.

Other Parasites

Toxoplasmosis

Epidemiology

Toxoplasma gondii is a worldwide zoonosis capable of causing several distinct clinical syndromes in immunocompetent and immunocompromised individuals. *T. gondii* is a parasite of members of the cat family, with humans and other warm-blooded animals serving as intermediate hosts.Humans become infected by either the eating of undercooked meat, ingestion of contaminated water, fecal-oral transmission from feline feces, congenitally through transplacental transmission, blood transfusion, or transplantation. Meat for human consumption is not routinely inspected for *T. gondii* infection in the United

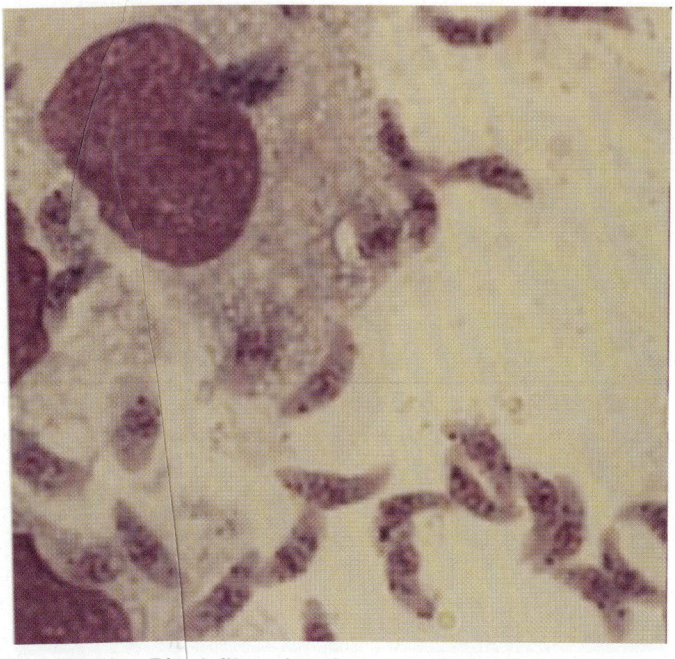

Fig. 47.21: *Blood film showing morphological features of Toxoplasma gondi*

States or elsewhere in the world. Human-to-human transmission does not occur, with the exception of mother-to-fetus transmission. The incidence of *T. gondii* antibodies increases with increasing age but does not vary between sexes. The prevalences of antibody titers vary considerably among geographic regions and within a given population. The overall seroprevalence among adolescents and adults in the United States was found to be 22.5%, with a seroprevalence among women of childbearing age (15–44 years) of 15%, using specimens collected by the third National Health and Nutrition Examination Survey (NHANES) III between 1988 and 1994. In the United States, *T. gondii* seropositivity among HIV-infected individuals varies from 10% to 45% and correlates with seropositivity in the non-HIV-infected population. In Western Europe and Africa, the seroprevalence among HIV-infected populations is approximately 50% to 78%.

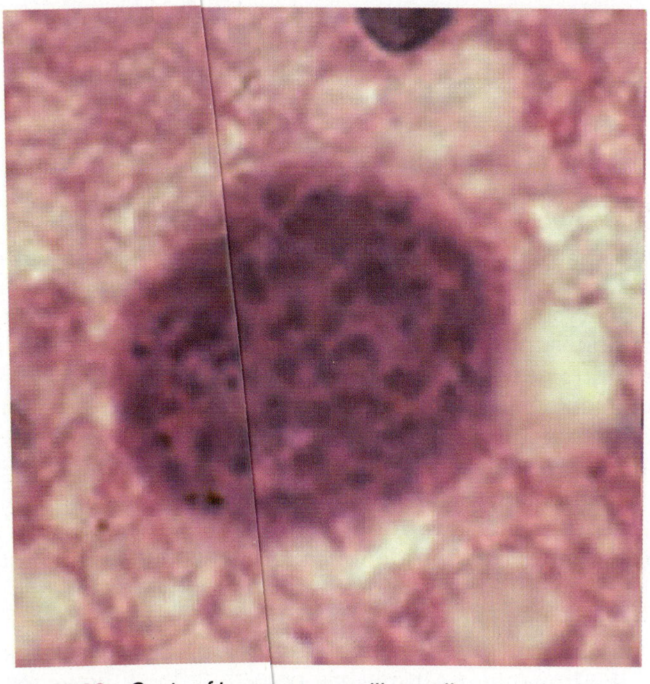

Fig. 47.22: *Cysts of toxoplasma gondii usually range in size from 5–50 µm in diameter. Cysts are usually spherical in the brain but more elongated in cardiac and skeletal muscles. They may be found in various sites throughout the body of the host, but are most common in the brain and skeletal and cardiac muscles*

Pathophysiology

Toxoplasma gondii multiplies intracellularly at the site of invasion and may spread to distant organs by the invasion of lymphatics and blood. Tissue cyst formation occurs within the first week of infection and is responsible for latent infection. *T. gondii* resides intracellularly in phagosomes within macrophages and myocardial cells. The parasite is propelled by an actin-myosin-dependent gliding-motility mechanism and establishes intracellular vacuoles. This remodeling prevents lysosome fusion, which leads to the intracellular survival of the parasite. The immune competency of the individual is the determining factor in the recrudescence of latent infection. Immunity in the immunocompetent individual persists for life. T cells, macrophages, and type 1 cytokines are crucial for the control of *T. gondii* infection. Defective production of IFN-β and interleukin-12, possibly mediated by CD40 ligand, may play a role in the lack of containment of the infection. Cytokine stimulation of macrophage production of reactive nitrogen intermediates was hypothesized to assist in the host control of established infection. Both host and parasitic genetics appear to be important for disease pathogenesis. Associations of HLA-DQ3 with the development of toxoplasmic encephalitis and the possible protective role of HLA-DQ1 suggest that host genetic factors contribute to the development of disease. In addition, population genetic analysis of *T. gondii* suggests clonal expansion, which may identify clinically relevant biological differences (Figs 47.21 and 47.28).

Clinical manifestations

The clinical expression of toxoplasmosis depends on the level of immunity in the human host. In immunocompetent patients, acute toxoplasmosis is most often asymptomatic, but latent infection can persist for life. Latent infection is due to cyst formation and may subsequently reactivate in immunocompromised persons. Among these populations, toxoplasmosis often presents in the form of encephalitis or chorioretinitis. Myocarditis has rarely been reported as a manifestation of acute toxoplasmosis. This manifestation may occur in isolation or as part of a broader clinical spectrum of illness. Pericardial effusion, constrictive pericarditis, arrhythmias, and congestive heart failure in patients with *T. gondii* myocarditis have been described. In patients with AIDS, the heart is the second most commonly affected organ after the brain.Prevalences vary according to various studies, and diagnosis is usually made postmortem since cardiac involvement is usually clinically silent or dominated by CNS manifestations. Approximately 12–22% of AIDS patients had evidence of endomyocardial involvement by *T. gondii* at autopsy. The prevalence of cardiac toxoplasmosis confirmed at autopsy in the era of highly active antiretroviral therapy has been reported to be less than 10%. *Toxoplasma gondii*-associated myocarditis can also occur in transplant patients due either to reactivation or to *de novo* infection from a seropositive donor to a seronegative recipient. Indeed, toxoplasmosis is the most commonly reported parasitic disease occurring after heart transplantation and may simulate organ rejection. Disseminated toxoplasmosis with associated myocarditis can lead to a fatal outcome if no prior prophylaxis is given to transplant patients. The prevention of toxoplasmosis relies on the serological screening of donors and recipients before transplantation to identify patients at a higher risk of toxoplasmosis, i.e. seropositive hematopoietic stem cell transplant recipients and mismatched (seropositive donor/seronegative recipients) solid-organ transplant recipients. Prevention in those patients presently relies on prophylaxis, usually with cotrimoxazole.

Diagnosis (Figs 47.21–47.24)

Test essentially rules out prior or recent infection of an immunocompetent host IgM antibodies may persist for years after infection and should not be used as the sole diagnostic criteria for recent infection. Antibody avidity testing has proven very useful.

The diagnosis of toxoplasmosis relies on serology or the identification of tachyzoites in myocardial tissue. There is considerable variation in the sensitivities and specificities of commercially available serological assays. IgG antibodies appear early, peak within 6 months of infection, and remain detectable for life. A negative IgG antibody marker of the timing of infection. The presence of a high avidity indicates that the infection occurred at least 3–5 months earlier. This test is most helpful during pregnancy, where additional evaluation and treatment depend on the timing of infection relative to pregnancy. No single serological test is sufficient to support the diagnosis of acute or chronic toxoplasmosis, and the use of a reference laboratory is often required. Patients may have slight lymphocytosis, and hepatic transaminase levels may be slightly elevated. Otherwise, laboratory findings are not specific. Kean and Grocott first described a toxoplasmosis-like cysts in the myocardium in 1945, and Adams subsequently described fluctuating S-T (S-to-T interval tracing of the ECG) changes in a 15-year-old boy with glandular-type toxoplasmosis. Endomyocardial biopsy has successfully identified the organism in heart transplant patients. Although uncommonly reported, the benefit of early and specific diagnosis with endomyocardial biopsy in the setting of heart transplantation likely outweighs the potential risks. Local necrosis with edema and an inflammatory infiltrate upon biopsy are typical. Myocardial abscesses have also been reported; however, abscesses are not common pathological features of toxoplasmosis. Parasites may also be detected by using DNA amplification techniques. The sensitivity with whole blood or buffy coat is 15–85% and appears most

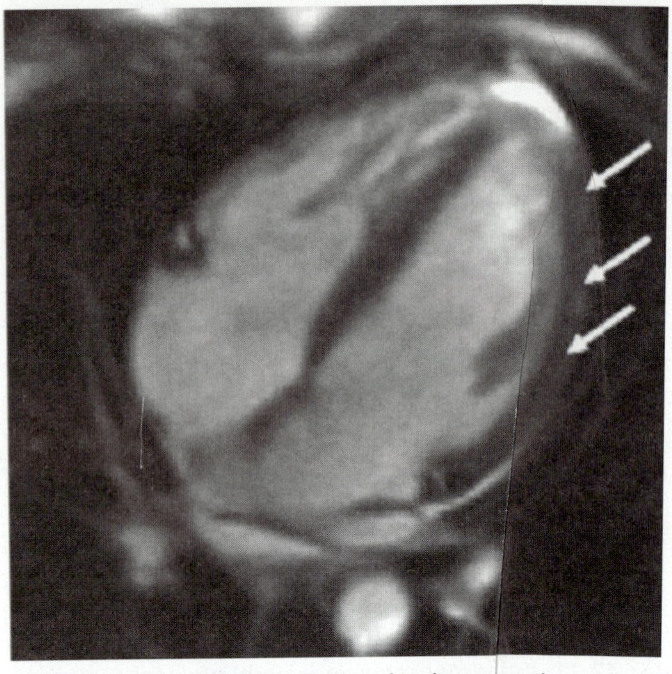

Fig. 47.23: *Cardiac MRI. Delayed-enhancement sequences performed after perfusion of gadolinium demonstrated a diffuse lumpy subepicardial enhancement (white arrows) in a patient with toxoplasminosis causing acute myopericarditis*

valuable for disseminated disease. Performance characteristics vary by the timing of testing in relation to therapy, gene target, primers, and sample preparation. PCR has been reported to diagnose *Toxoplasma* more frequently than histology of cardiac biopsy specimen samples in the transplant setting. PCR assays can be valuable in making this difficult diagnosis, and reference laboratories with experience with these assays should be utilized.

Treatment

The treatment of choice is based on a combination of pyrimethamine and sulfadiazine or pyrimethamine and clindamycin. Leucovorin should be given to all patients taking pyrimethamine. Combination of pyrimethamine and azithromycin or atovaquone may be considered for patients intolerant to other regimens based on data from immunosuppressed patients. The combination of primethamine and sulfadiazine is also a first-line treatment regimen during pregnancy. However alternatives exist for those concerned about potential toxicity and teratogenicity, and treatment choice is influenced by the duration of pregnancy and documentation of fetal infection. Serological screening of organ donors and recipients before transplantation allows the identification of patients at the highest risk of toxoplasmosis and provision of prophylaxis for these individuals. The optimal schedule for the provision of trimethoprim (TMP)-sulfamethoxazole (SMZ) prophylaxis in the transplant setting has not been defined; however, this drug is often administered daily or three times a week. Prevention is important for seronegative pregnant women and immunodeficient patients. Prevention is accomplished through physician-patient education and prophylaxis

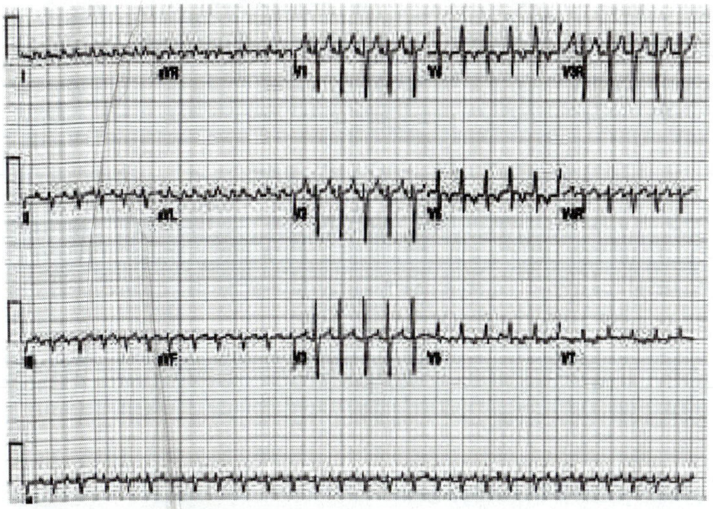

Fig. 47.24: *Electrocardiographic features showing generalised ST depression indicating myocarditis caused by Trichinella spiralis*

prescription, where appropriate. Educational efforts should focus on the avoidance of contact with materials potentially contaminated with cat feces, the use of gloves when handling cat litter or gardening, washing of hands thoroughly after contact with raw meat, cooking of meat until "well done", and washing of fruits and vegetables before consumption.

Cysticercosis

Epidemiology

Cysticercosis is a consequence of the ingestion of the eggs of the pork tapeworm *Taenia solium*. Cerebral cysticercosis is considered the most serious complication. The condition can also present as ocular, spinal, cutaneous, muscular, or cardiac lesions. The prevalence of cysticercosis varies in countries where cysticercosis is endemic and is often increased in regions where pigs are raised and sanitary conditions are lacking. Few cases are acquired in the United States, and travel to areas of endemicity may pose a small risk to travelers.

Pathophysiology

Following egg ingestion, oncospheres invade the bowel wall and disseminate to the brain, striated muscles, and other tissues. Cysticerci can remain quiescent for many years in a state of immune tolerance. Poorly understood metacestode-elaborated substances divert the complement pathway and inhibit normal cellular immune responses including macrophage function and lymphocyte proliferation. The ability of the cyst to moderate the host immune response may be lost with time.

Clinical Manifestations

Clinical manifestations often develop at the time of cyst degeneration. The trigger for this event is unknown. The myocardial inflammatory response is variable, resulting in granuloma formation and fibrosis, which subsequently leads to arrhythmias and conduction abnormalities either spontaneously or during treatment. Cardiac involvement in cysticercosis was thought to be rare, but autopsy studies have shown a prevalence of 20–25% in patients with concomitant documented neurocysticercosis. Cardiac cysticercosis is often asymptomatic and discovered during cardiac surgery or at autopsy. Cysticerci are usually multiple and randomly distributed in cardiac tissues, including the subpericardium, subendocardium, and myocardium. Rarely, a single cardiac cyst may be present.

Diagnosis

The diagnosis is based on suggestive epidemiology and serology. The extent of diagnostic evaluation depends on the severity of clinical presentation. Routine blood tests may reveal marked peripheral eosinophilia only in the case of a leaking cyst. The sensitivity and specificity of serology vary with the site and stage of infection. An enzyme-linked immunoelectrotransfer blot assay is the test of choice for the detection of antibodies. PCR-based tests have an emerging role in the epidemiological investigation of taeniasis and are available for the diagnosis of cysticercosis. Most individuals with cysticercosis do not have viable *T. solium* in their intestines. Echocardiography may play some role in identifying cardiac cysts and occasionally identifies cardiac cysts consistent with cysticercosis upon routine screening for other purposes. Cardiac magnetic resonance imaging (MRI) may also demonstrate cystic lesions, which are hypointense on T1-weighted images and hyperintense on T2-weighted images. Rounded scolices, when seen, are of intermediate to low signal intensity on T2-weighted images and of intermediate to hyperintense signal intensity within the low-signal fluid on T1-weighted images.

Treatment

Patients with extraneural cysticercosis should be evaluated with brain imaging for possible neurocysticercosis. Asymptomatic extraneural cysts may not require specific surgical or antihelminthic therapy. The role of albendazole and praziquantel or surgery in cardiac cysticercosis is unclear and has not been directly investigated; however, these therapies are likely to be effective given their efficacy at other sites. Adjunctive corticosteroids are sometimes administered during therapy for neurocysticercosis. The potential benefit of decreasing treatment-related inflammation in cardiac cysticercosis has not been defined but remains theoretically possible.

Trichinellosis

Epidemiology

Trichinellosis is caused by the nematode *Trichinella spiralis* and other *Trichinella* species and is common worldwide. Humans become infected when eating undercooked meat contaminated with cysts of *Trichinella* larvae. Approximately 15 cases of trichinellosis are reported annually in the United States.Wild carnivorous animals perpetuate infections in a sylvatic cycle, and wild-game meat is emerging as a source of infection.

Pathogenesis

Trichinella larvae excyst and cross the small intestine where they travel through lymphatics and the bloodstream until finally encysting in striated muscle tissue. The striated muscle cell is induced to transform into a nurse cell, which supports the long-term viability of the encysted larvae. The process of encystment and nurse cell formation is unique to skeletal muscle and does not take place within the heart. *Trichinella spiralis*-associated myocarditis is not caused by the direct larval invasion of the myocardium with encystation but is likely induced by an eosinophil-enriched inflammatory response resulting in eosinophilic myocarditis similar to the pathogenic process associated with tropical endomyocardial fibrosis. Some patients with trichinellosis develop organ-specific autoantibodies, whose role in pathogenesis remains unclear.

Clinical Manifestations

The clinical picture of trichinellosis is proportional to the number of larvae ingested and manifests with two clinical stages: the intestinal stage and the muscular stage). Larval migration into the muscles can cause periorbital and facial edema; subungal, conjunctival, and retinal hemorrhages; myalgias; weakness and fever. The tropism of *T. spiralis* for striated muscle may involve the myocardium in 21–75% of infected patients. Myocarditis is a consequence of migrating larvae and the resulting inflammatory response and typically occurs in the third week of infection. Trichinosis myocarditis may initially manifest with chest pain and mimic an acute myocardial infarction. Reports suggest that ECG evidence of myocardial involvement may be found for up to 75% of patients. Complications such cardiac arrhythmias are considered the most common cause of death associated with trichinellosis. In addition, pericardial effusions have also been reported during *T. spiralis* infection.

Diagnosis

The clinical suspicion of trichinellosis is based on suggestive epidemiology associated with the typical clinical presentation and the presence of eosinophilia during the second to fourth week of the muscle stage. There is no direct relationship between the severity of eosinophilia and clinical course. Confirmation is based on serology and muscle biopsy specimens. Serology is generally reliable and first becomes positive about 3 weeks after infection. Antibody levels may remain positive for longer than a year after clinical resolution. For patients without obvious myocardial involvement, some researchers have recommended screening with troponin to detect asymptomatic myocarditis. The finding of larvae in a muscle biopsy specimen provides a definitive diagnosis; however, biopsy is rarely necessary. ECG findings are considered nonspecific. In a study of 154 cases of trichinellosis, 56% of the patients had ECG abnormalities, most commonly nonspecific repolarization changes without an association with poor prognosis. One study reported pericardial effusion as the most common cardiac manifestation of trichinosis, affecting 10% of patients. Cardiac MRI may provide supportive evidence of myocardial involvement, although the MRI findings are not specific to trichinellosis.

Treatment

Treatment consists of the administration of albendazole or mebendazole in conjunction with steroids for severe cases. Although albendazole and mebendazole are relatively contraindicated in pregnancy, both have been used in patients without adverse fetal effects. Adjunctive steroids are commonly utilized for 10–15 days.

PARASITES THAT OCCASIONALLY INVOLVE THE PERICARDIUM

Entamoeba Histolytica

Epidemiology

Amebic pericarditis is caused by the protozoon *Entamoeba histolytica*, which is transmitted by the fecal-oral route. It has a worldwide distribution but is found mainly in developing countries in the tropics. In the United States, amebiasis is seen in immigrants and travelers returning from countries where the disease is endemic. Following malaria and schistosomiasis, amebiasis is the third most common cause of parasitic death. Particular high-risk groups include children, pregnant women, and malnourished individuals. Invasive amebiasis may be more common among HIV/AIDS patients, prompting some to call for routine HIV testing of those diagnosed with the disease.

Pathophysiology

The ability of *Entamoeba histolytica* to invade tissues distinguishes it from the morphologically identical *Entamoeba dispar*. The parasite causes acute inflammation and ulceration of the colonic mucosa. Adherence to colonic epithelial cells using the Gal/GalNAc lectin is essential for amebic survival and pathogenicity. Mucosal IgA immunity to this lectin has been associated with protection from *Entamoeba* infection and disease in Bangladeshi children. The trophozoite utilizes the secretion of proteinases for the dissolution of the extracellular matrix and the formation of amebepores resulting in target cell cytolysis, among other mechanisms, to establish its pathogenic niche.

Clinical Manifestations

Extraintestinal amebic disease is localized mainly to the liver. The involvement of the pericardium is very rare but is a serious complication of amebiasis. Amebic pericarditis may present as either a pericardial rub with electrocardiographic changes associated with an abscess of the left lobe or purulent pericarditis from the perforation of the abscess into the pericardium. Amebic abscesses in the right lobe of the liver have also been reported to communicate with the pericardium. The presenting clinical syndrome is usually one of two forms: (i) sudden onset as cardiac tamponade with chest pain, shortness of breath, and shock or

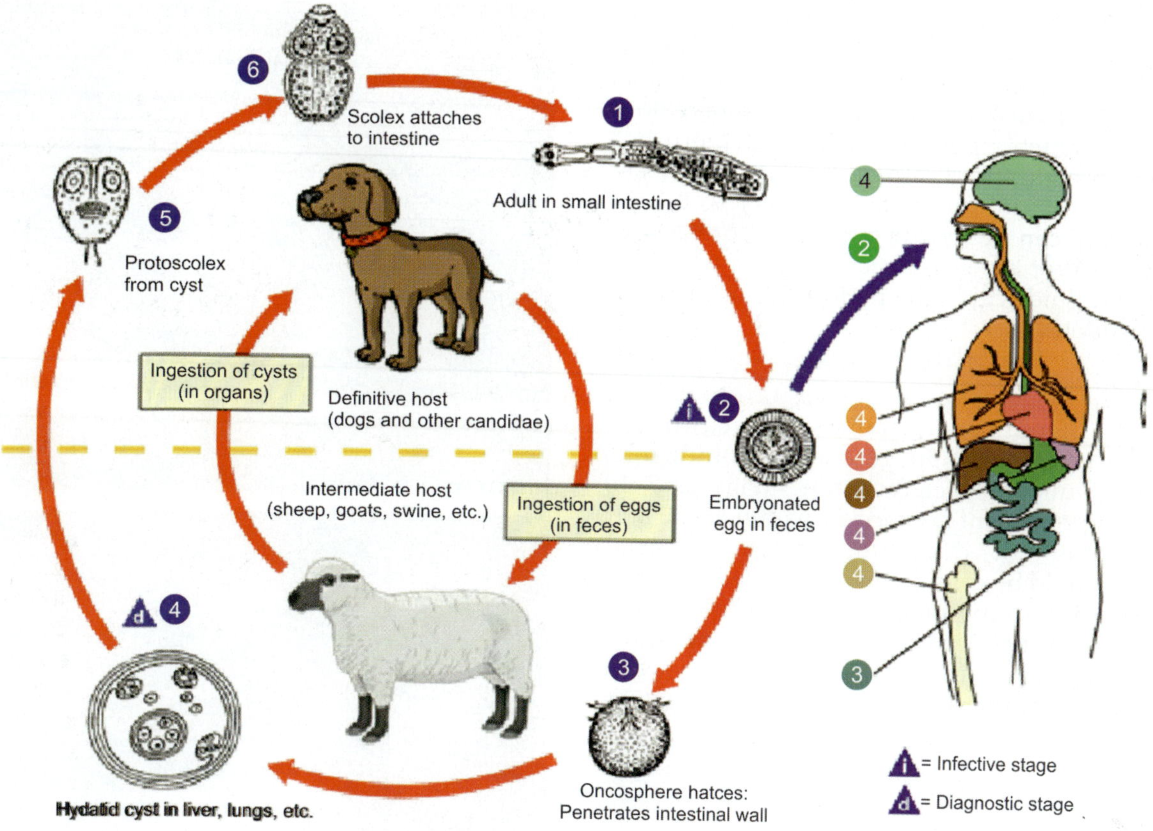

Fig. 47.25: *Life cycle of a echinococcus parasite*

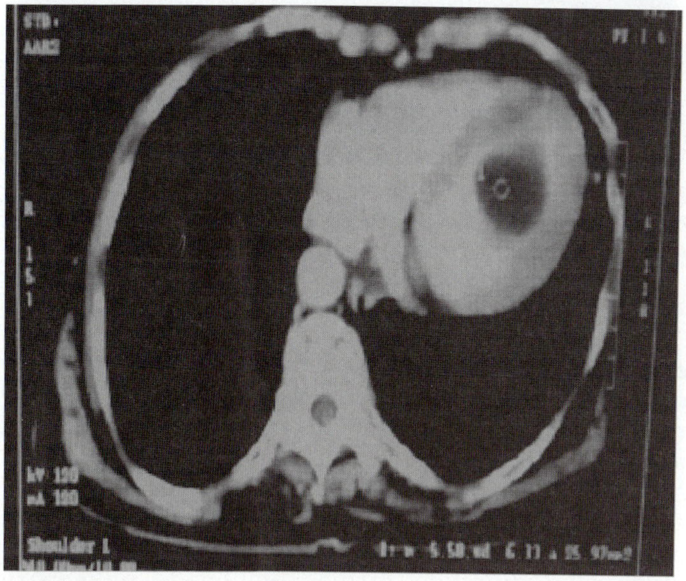

Fig. 47.26: *MRI scan showing myocardial cyst echinococcosis (hydatid cyst disease) in left ventricular cavity*

(ii) progressive effusion with a slower course to develop fever, dyspnea and pain. Amebic pericarditis has been more frequently described for pediatric populations in which the association of concomitant intestinal amebiasis may be as high as 20%.

Diagnosis

Diagnosis is usually established by serology, which has a sensitivity of about 90%. Infection with *E. histolytica* results in the development of antibodies while infection with *E. dispar* does not. Positive serology does not distinguish between acute and past infections. For this reason, serum antigen tests are often used to complement diagnosis. The galactose lectin serum antigen is present in 75% of individuals with amebic liver abscesses. Peripheral eosinophilia is not particularly common stool microscopy has limited value for the diagnosis of extraintestinal amebiasis. Amebic cysts or trophozoites are detected in the stool only 15–33% of the time. In addition, the presence of amebic cysts or trophozoites determined by stool microscopy does not definitively indicate that the extraintestinal focus is secondary to the identified intestinal parasite because both pathogenic and nonpathogenic *Entamoeba* may be present in the gut. However, an ELISA method can differentiate pathogenic from nonpathogenic *Entamoeba* in stool samples. DNA amplification techniques for the rapid and specific identification of *E. histolytica* are in development. Aspirated pus is usually sterile, and diagnosis should not be excluded based on its gross characteristics. Given the limitations of serology in the diagnosis of invasive amebiasis, PCR-based diagnostic methods have become an invaluable sensitive and specific tool for the diagnosis of intestinal and extraintestinal amebiasis and are available from many reference laboratories. The suppurative feature of amebic pericarditis may also cause it to be confused with tuberculous pericarditis. A distinguishing factor between tuberculous pericarditis and amebic pericarditis is that there is a predominance of neutrophils in patients with amebiasis. Imaging with chest computed tomography (CT) and echocardiography can be useful given the potential to demonstrate a liver abscess in continuity with the pericardium and fluid within the pericardial sac, with or without the fistulous tract.

Treatment

The treatment of pericardial amebiasis requires a combination of surgical drainage and metronidazole. Metronidazole should be given three times daily for 7–10 days. Clinical improvement is expected within 48–72 h. If clinical improvement does not occur, bacterial superinfection should be considered and treated if found, and metronidazole therapy may be prolonged. Metronidazole resistance has not been reported.Treatment with a luminal agent to is required following therapy with metronidazole, even if prior stool examination was negative.

Echinococcosis

Epidemiology

Human infection with the metacestode form of one of the four species of the tapeworm *Echinococcus* (*E. granulosus*, *E. multilocularis*, *E. vogeli*, or *E. oligarthrus*) may result in echinococcal disease. *Echinococcus* species have a worldwide distribution. *Echinococcus granulosus* causes cystic echinococcosis, the form most frequently encountered. Humans become accidental intermediate hosts when they ingest eggs from the feces of infected dogs or other canids. Direct transmission from human to human does not occur.

Pathophysiology

After the ingestion of the eggs by an intermediate host, the eggs hatch and release oncospheres, which cross the small intestine and spread to encyst in various visceral organs. Both humoral and cellular immune responses to the presence of the oncospheres and metacestodes develop. The parasite evades the host immune response by using a number of mechanisms including the cyst-laminated cuticle as a barrier to host cells, polyclonal activation of lymphocytes by parasite soluble antigens, and depression of host cell immune responses. For instance, chronic stimulation of the host by cyst fluid antigens leads to increased levels of specific IgG4 production, which is suggestive of host response immunomodulation. Th1 cell activation appears critical for protective immunity while a Th2 response is correlated with progressive disease.

Clinical Manifestations

Hydatid cysts develop over months to years. Most of them will remain asymptomatic, but some of them become large

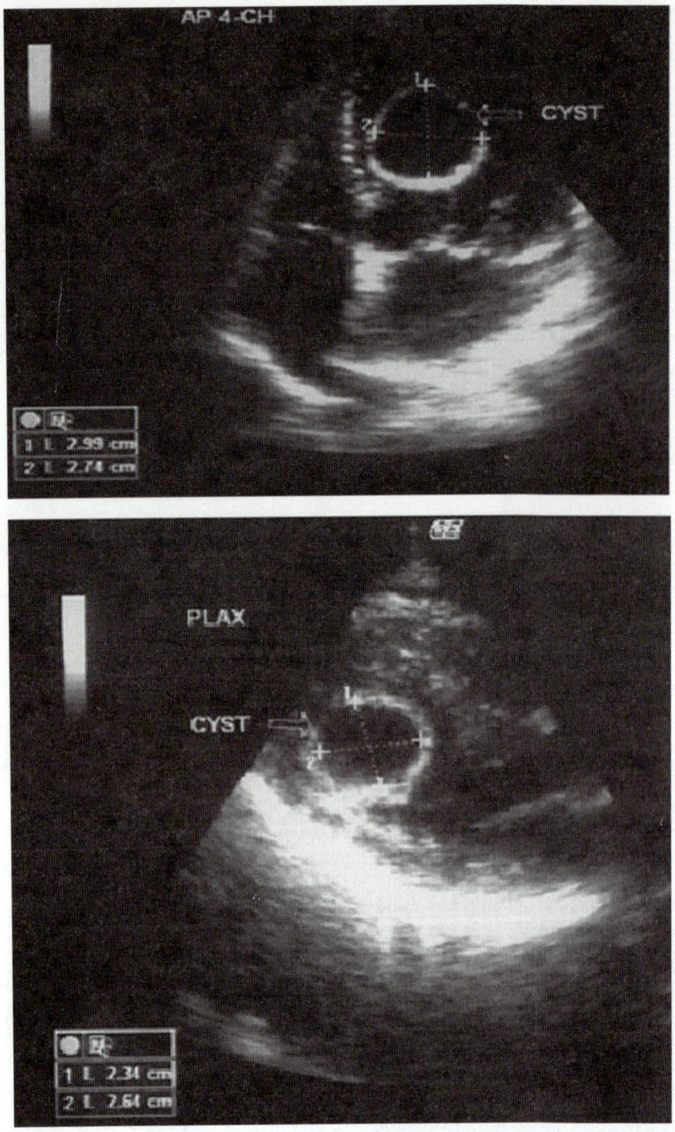

Fig. 47.27: *Upper and lower panels showing left ventricular myocardial invasion by echinococcosis (hydatid cyst disease) as marked by circle*

enough to cause symptoms. Echinococcal disease is often diagnosed as an incidental finding during imaging for other reasons. Cysts are located mainly in the liver and the lung, and only 10% can occur in the rest of the body. Cardiac hydatid cysts have been described for 0.5–3% of echinococcosis cases and are usually univesicular. Clinical presentations of cardiac echinococcosis include arrhythmias, myocardial infarction, cardiac tamponade, pulmonary hypertension syncope, purulent pericarditis, and sudden cardiac death. Isolated cardiac hydatid cysts without liver involvement are uncommon. Hydatid cysts can even mimic ST segment elevation myocardial infarction upon electrocardiography. Most cases of pericardial echinococcosis may be due to spread from an initial location at the liver dome. Rarely, an atrial or ventricular thrombus may mimic a hydatid cyst.

Diagnosis (Figs 47.25 and 47.26)

Diagnosis relies on positive serological testing and radiographic findings.The sensitivity and specificity of serology in those patients with liver involvement are greater than 80% but less sensitive when echinococcal disease is isolated at other sites. Children and pregnant women more often have negative serology than other populations. The identification of antigens in cyst fluid or serum may also assist in diagnosis. Fewer than 15% of cases have peripheral eosinophilia. DNA amplifications tests are not currently available outside the research setting. Echocardiography is the most appropriate imaging test to evaluate potential myocardial or pericardial hydatid cysts. CT imaging and MRI may also demonstrate specific signs including the calcification of the cysts' walls, the presence of daughter cysts, and membrane detachment.

Treatment

The drug of choice for the treatment of echinococcosis is albendazole or mebendazole. Mebendazole is usually continued for 3–6 months. Albendazole is preferred and is also used for 3–6 months. Antiparasitic therapy should be started at least 4 days before surgery and be continued for at least 1 month (albendazole) or 3 months (mebendazole) after surgery. Surgery, when feasible, is the most common form of treatment of echinococcosis. According to the WHO, surgery is not recommended for pregnant women, those with multiple or difficult-to-access cysts, or patients with dead or totally calcified cysts. Asymptomatic cysts, if heavily calcified and presumed nonviable, may be monitored without specific therapy. The routine use of a protoscolicidal agent during surgery is not necessary.The puncture, aspiration, injection and respiration (PAIR) technique is an option for inoperable cysts. Patients should be on antiparasitic therapy prior to this procedure to reduce the risk of cyst dissemination. The response to specific therapy may be monitored with serology and imaging.

MISCELLANEOUS SYNDROMES

Schistosomiasis

Myocardial or pericardial involvement by *Schistosoma* species is a rare event and is due to the accumulation of *Schistosoma* eggs, which induce a local granulomatous response. However, chronic schistosomiasis may lead to severe liver fibrosis secondary to hepatosplenic involvement. This process involving portal hypertension may produce a hepatopulmonary syndrome manifested as dyspnea upon exertion, right ventricular hypertrophy, and, ultimately, *cor pulmonale*. In addition, endothelial damage to the pulmonary circulation results from the shunting of *Schistosoma* eggs through portosystemic shunts. The ability of *Schistosoma mansoni* to survive during its residence in the pulmonary circulation is due to molecular masking by coating with ABO blood group glycolipids and major histocompatibility complex (MHC) molecules derived from the human host. *Schistosoma*-induced pulmonary hypertension carries a grave prognosis since it usually denotes an advanced stage of hepatosplenic schistosomiasis. Thrombosis *in situ*, particularly of the right pulmonary artery, as well as cardiac arrhythmias and sudden cardiac death syndromes may occur. The treatment of schistosomiasis (all species) is praziquantel or, alternatively, oxamniquine for *S. mansoni*.

Myocarditis Associated with *Naegleria fowleri*

Naegleria fowleri is a free-living amoeba, which is well known to cause an acute, purulent, primary amoebic meningoencephalitis (PAM), often in previously healthy young individuals with a recent history of water-sport activity in rivers, lakes or ponds. The disease process is usually confined to the central nervous system. One report in the literature, which reexamined an earlier case report of disseminated amebiasis, provided evidence of possible disseminated *N. fowleri*. Several authors have described the pathological recognition of PAM-associated diffuse or focal myocarditis. In the reported cases of associated myocarditis, clinical cardiac manifestations have been nearly universally absent. Additionally, amoebas have not been found in the heart tissue, making causal conclusions speculative. The diagnosis of PAM, when made premortem, is typically accomplished by direct wet-mount examination of the cerebral spinal fluid for trophozoite forms. *Naegleria fowleri* can be grown on agar plates coated with Gram-negative bacteria. Serological tests are not useful in the acute clinical setting given the delay in the mounting of a detectable immune response. A real-time PCR assay has been developed for *N. fowleri* identification and could become useful for fast laboratory diagnosis of PAM. To date, there are no reports of the use of this assay on myocardial specimens. Additionally, PCR-based diagnosis has been evaluated with formalin-fixed and paraffin-embedded brain sections. Amphotericin B remains the backbone of PAM therapy, and *N. fowleri* is highly susceptible to this drug *in vitro*. Successful therapy has been rare, and when reported, amphotericin B is usually part of the therapy. In a mouse model of PAM, azithromycin and amphotericin B have demonstrated synergistic success and may hold promise as combination therapy.

Zoonotic Filariasis

Dirofilaria immitis, a common parasite of dogs and other canids, is prevalent in many areas of the world and can occasionally affect humans. In the dog, the parasite undergoes its early development in the subcutaneous tissues for about 3 months before migrating to the right side of the heart. Once deposited by a mosquito vector, the adult worms live in vascular beds and can induce myocarditis. Although adult *D. immitis* worms have been found in the heart and major vessels of humans at autopsy on several occasions. The usual finding is for immature worms to be located in partially or completely occluded small pulmonary arteries, where the obstruction has produced a distal pneumonitis followed by granuloma formation, resulting in a well-circumscribed coin lesion containing the parasite. These lesions are usually identified in asymptomatic individuals undergoing routine chest radiographs. No worms have been identified by echocardiography or angiography during premortem evaluation. Other filarial species, such as lymphatic-dwelling human filariae (*Wuchereria* spp. and *Brugia* spp.), may also be identified as pulmonary nodules. The occurrence of severe, and occasionally lethal, myocardial involvement that often occurs in dogs and other canids has not been described for humans.

Tropical Pulmonary Eosinophilia

Tropical pulmonary eosinophilia is a syndrome caused by a hypersensitivity response to microfilariae of the lymphatic-dwelling filariae *Wuchereria bancrofti* and *Brugia malayi*. This process, manifested as chronic pulmonary infiltrates with eosinophilia, may result in permanent deficits in pulmonary function. Clinical symptoms usually include cough, dyspnea, and nocturnal wheezing. Eosinophils located in the lung, as a response to the presence of filariae in the pulmonary circulation, degranulate and lead to the production of toxic oxygen radicals that contribute to a chronic pulmonary inflammatory process.These restrictive pulmonary function deficits may result in pulmonary hypertension that subsequently contributes to *cor pulmonale*. The treatment of choice recommended by the WHO is the oral antifilarial drug diethylcarbamazine (DEC) for 3 weeks.

ENDOMYOCARDIAL FIBROSIS

Endomyocardial fibrosis (EMF) is an idiopathic disorder of the tropical and subtropical regions of the world that is characterized by the development of restrictive cardiomyopathy.

The nosology of EMF coincides with some related disorders. EMF is sometimes considered part of a spectrum of a single disease process that includes Löffler endocarditis (nontropical eosinophilic endomyocardial fibrosis or fibroplastic parietal endocarditis with eosinophilia).

Tropical EMF and Löffler endocarditis should be distinguished from endocardial fibroelastosis, which is characterized by cartilaginous thickening of the mural endocardium, chiefly of the left ventricle. This disease is most common in the first 2 years of life and, in some patients, appears to be an inherited disorder that is associated with congenital cardiac malformations.

Pathophysiology

In EMF, the underlying process produces patchy fibrosis of the endocardial surface of the heart, leading to reduced compliance and, ultimately, restrictive physiology as the endomyocardial surface becomes more generally involved. Endocardial fibrosis principally involves the inflow tracts of the right and left ventricles and may affect the atrioventricular valves, leading to tricuspid and mitral regurgitation.

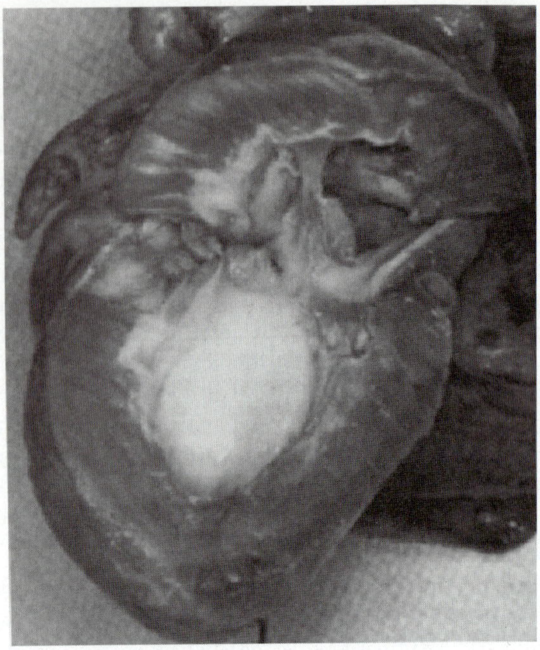

Fig. 47.28: *Morbid features of LV in a younger patient with endomyocardial fibroelastosis*

The earliest changes of EMF are not well described because most patients do not present with symptoms until relatively late in the clinical course. Olsen described 3 phases of EMF. The first phase involves eosinophilic infiltration of the myocardium with necrosis of the subendocardium and a pathologic picture consistent with acute myocarditis. This is reportedly present in the first 5 weeks of the illness. The second stage, typically observed after 10 months, is associated with thrombus formation over the initial lesions, with a decrement in the amount of inflammatory activity present. Ultimately, after several years of disease activity, the fibrotic phase is reached, when the endocardium is replaced by collagenous fibrosis. Extensive calcification is rarely associated with fibrosis. This pathomorphologic schema is not observed uniformly and has not been consistently supported by other investigators.

The etiology of EMF remains unclear. Hypotheses include infectious, inflammatory and nutritional processes. EMF is frequently associated with concomitant parasitic infections (e.g. helminths) and their attendant eosinophilia, although the role of parasitic infections and/or the eosinophil remains speculative. The development of EMF as a sequela to toxoplasma-related myocarditis has also been described, as has a relationship of malarial infection to development of EMF. However, no specific organism has been consistently associated with EMF.

The role of the eosinophil in the pathogenesis of EMF is controversial. Whether the eosinophil actually induces myocardial necrosis and subsequent fibrosis or is attracted to the endocardial surface as a result of the initial insult is unknown. The eosinophil is not present as frequently in cases of tropical EMF as in Löffler endocarditis; thus, the role of the eosinophil in the tropical disease is likely less significant.

EMF is most frequently observed in the socially disadvantaged and in children and young women. These groups frequently have malnutrition, and in regions of sub-Saharan Africa where the disease is most prevalent, the typical diet is high in a tuber called cassava, which contains relatively high concentrations of the rare earth element cerium (Ce). The combination of high Ce levels and hypomagnesemia has been shown to produce EMF-like lesions in laboratory animals. A familial tendency has rarely been noted in Uganda and Zambia.

Incidence

EMF is rarely encountered in patients who have not traveled from the subtropical regions of Africa and tropical and subtropical regions elsewhere in the world including areas in India and South America that are within 15° of the equator. Löffler endocarditis (also called nontropical eosinophilic endocarditis) is a related condition that is observed in the United States and is considered by some authors to be a different stage of a similar process related to eosinophilia.

EMF occurs primarily in the subtropical regions of Africa but is also encountered in tropical and subtropical regions elsewhere in the world including areas in India and South America that are within 15° of the equator.

More than 90% of reported cases of EMF have occurred in geographic locations that are within 15° of the equator. In equatorial African nations, such as Nigeria, EMF is the fourth most common cause of cardiac disease in adults, and EMF accounts for 22% of cases of heart failure in Nigerian children. EMF is the most common type of restrictive cardiomyopathy in tropical countries.

Mortality/Morbidity

The overall prognosis of patients with EMF is poor and depends on the extent and distribution of disease within the various chambers and valves of the heart.

Most patients have extensive disease at the time of presentation; therefore, survival after diagnosis is relatively brief. In one study, 95% of a group of patients had died at 2 years. In a second study, 44% of patients died within 1 year after the onset of symptoms, and another 40% of patients died 1–3 years after onset. EMF is most commonly reported in individuals living in Nigeria and Uganda. Women of reproductive age and children are more commonly affected than men.

Age Distribution

EMF is not generally observed in children younger than 4 years, although the typical pathology for EMF has recently been described in a 4-month-old infant with left ventricular inflow tract obstruction. The people most commonly affected are older children (aged 5–15 years) and young adults, but cases have been reported in individuals aged 70 years.

History

Typically, endomyocardial fibrosis (EMF) has an insidious onset, and symptoms relate to the specific chambers and valves where the disease is most extensive. When right ventricular involvement or tricuspid regurgitation predominates, lower extremity swelling, increasing abdominal girth, and nausea may be expected. With left ventricular involvement, dyspnea is the predominant symptom, especially exertional dyspnea. Additionally, fatigue, paroxysmal nocturnal dyspnea, and orthopnea may be present.

Thromboembolic complications may occur in EMF. Rarely, patients may present early in the course of the disease with an acute febrile illness with symptoms of cardiac insufficiency mimicking myocarditis. Recently, anginalike chest pain and syncope were reported in a patient with EMF involving the left ventricle.

Physical

Physical findings are also dependent on the extent and distribution of disease. In those with right ventricular

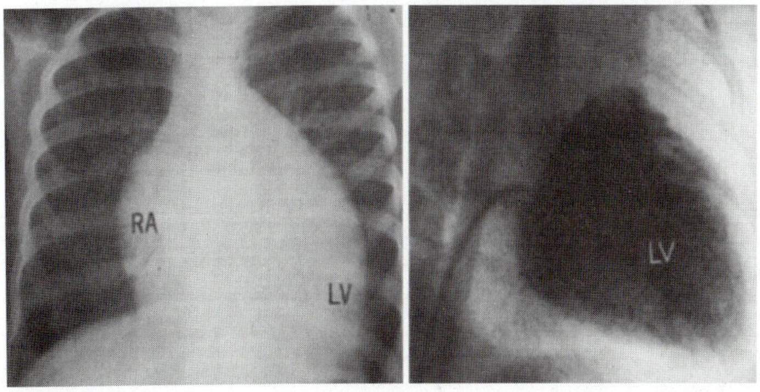

Fig. 47.29: *Photograph X-ray chest PA view (left) showing diffuse cardiomegaly with congested lung fields and hugely dilated and akinetic LV as seen on LV angiography (right) in a young patient with endocardial fibroelastosis*

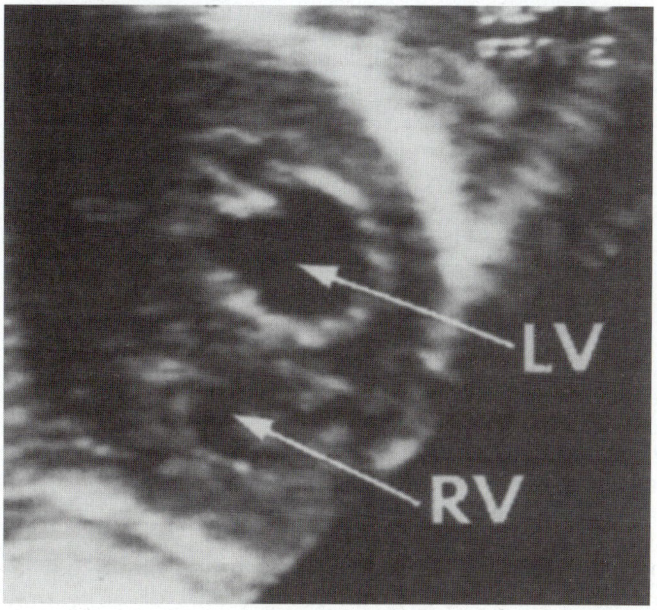

Fig. 47.30: *Echocardiogaph showing dilated LV as compared to right ventricle (RV) in patient with endocardial fibroelastosis*

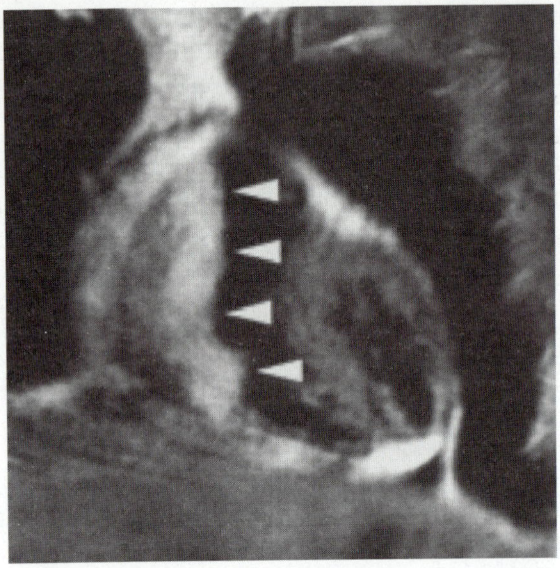

Fig. 47.31: *T1-weighted MR images after administration of gadopentetate dimeglumine show homogeneous enhancement of right ventricular mass (arrow heads). Mass is attached to free wall of right ventricle, extending from lateral tricuspid valve annulus to right ventricular outflow tract without involvement of apical portion. Mass protrudes toward right ventricular cavity with broad base on right ventricular free wall. Signal intensity of mass was intermediate on T1-weighted images and high on T2-weighted images (not shown). Note dilatation of right atrium in a patient with EMF*

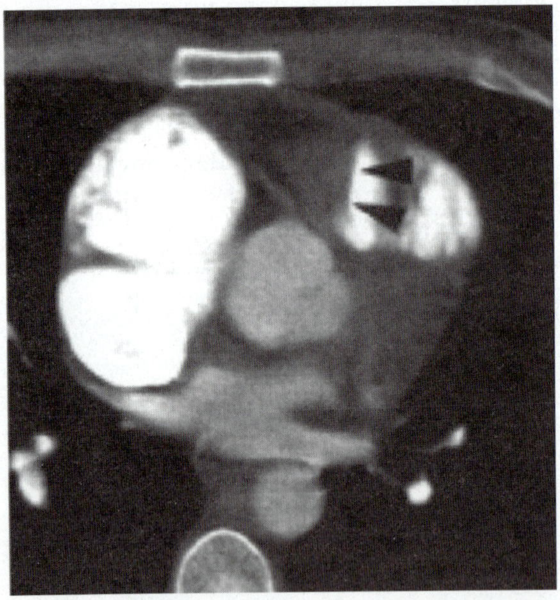

Fig. 47.32: *Follow-up contrast-enhanced CT scans obtained 3 years after reveal larger right ventricular mass (arrow heads), contributing to stenosis of right ventricular outflow tract. Mass shows homogeneous low attenuation, probably because CT was performed during arterial phase of contrast enhancement. Size of right atrium has also increased in a patient with EMF*

involvement, jugular venous pressure elevation, ascites, and edema may be present. The presence of ascites may appear out of proportion to the amount of peripheral edema. This may occur because of the cocomitant presence of a protein-losing enteropathy and subsequent hypoalbuminemia. Patients with tricuspid regurgitation may have giant V waves observed in the jugular venous pulsations. A third or fourth heart sound and tachycardia may be present. Signs of pulmonary congestion are present in patients with left-sided disease.

Causes

A specific single etiology of EMF has not been established. Suggested potential causes include the following:

Infectious causes

Parasites (e.g. helminths)
Protozoans (e.g. toxoplasmosis, malaria)

- Inflammatory causes (eosinophilia)
- Nutritional causes
  - General malnutrition
  - High-tuber diet
  - Ce toxicity
  - Hypomagnesemia
- Other problems to be considered
  - Anthracycline toxicity
  - Carcinoid heart disease
  - Drug-induced cardiotoxicity (e.g. serotonin, methysergide, ergotamine, mercurial agents, busulfan)
- Fabry disease
- Fatty infiltration
- Gaucher disease
- Glycogen storage disease
- Hurler disease
- Idiopathic cardiomyopathy
- Metastatic cancers
- Radiation
- Rheumatic heart disease
- Occasionally, a mass-like lesion seen in endomyocardial fibrosis masquerades as an intracardiac tumor.

Laboratory Studies

Complete blood cell count may show anemia and eosinophilia.

Imaging Studies

Chest Radiography (Fig. 47.33)

The cardiac silhouette in endomyocardial fibrosis (EMF) may be normal in size, and generalized cardiomegalyis unusual because the ventricles are not typically dilated.

The roentgenographic image may exhibit significant enlargement of the atria, and significant right atrial enlargement creates a cardiac silhouette in the shape of the African continent, which is a specific heart shadow sign that has been termed the heart of Africa.

Echocardiography

Echocardiography is a useful tool when making the diagnosis of EMF and has been demonstrated to successfully differentiate EMF and other processes such as rheumatic heart disease and congenital heart disease. The presence and location of fibrosis as determined by echocardiography correlates well with autopsy findings. Findings include thickening of the inferior and basal left ventricular wall, apical obliteration, thrombi adherent to endocardial surface, mitral regurgitation, and tricuspid regurgitation. A pericardial effusion is frequently present and may be large. While parameters of diastolic function by Doppler echocardiography tend to correlate with the functional status of the patient, because most patients present with later stages of EMF, a restrictive filling pattern in the left ventricular outflow tract is most common.

Recently, decreased flow propagation velocity (Vp) has been demonstrated in a large percentage of patients with EMF. Color-flow imaging frequently exhibits tricuspid and mitral regurgitation. Spectral Doppler analysis of tricuspid regurgitation frequently reflects an increased pulmonary artery systolic pressure.

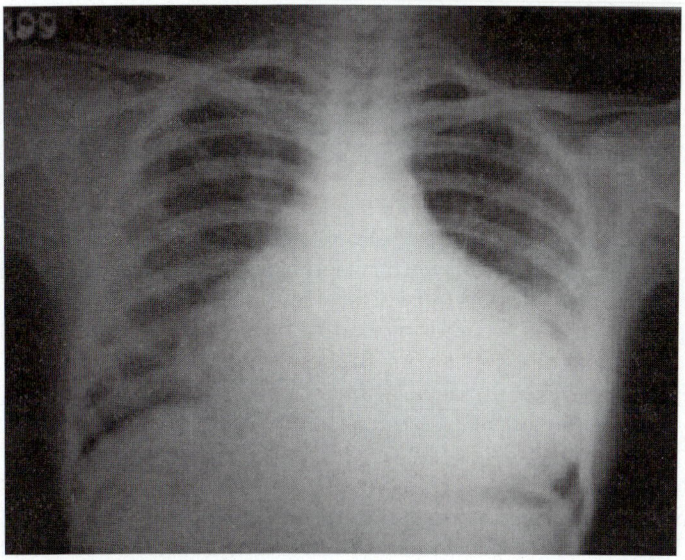

Fig. 47.33: *Photograph of X-ray chest PA showing cardiomegaly in a young child with endomyocardial fibrosis (EMF)*

Angiography

Traditionally, angiography has been considered the criterion standard when making the diagnosis of EMF.

Left and right ventriculography exhibits distortion of chamber morphology by fibrosis and obliteration and variable degrees of mitral and tricuspid regurgitation.

The mushroom sign has been used to describe the shape of the affected ventricle when the apex is obliterated completely by fibrosis.

Electron Beam Computed Tomography Scanning

Features of EMF observed with this modality were described in the mid 1990s. The fibrotic process is delineated as a band of low attenuation within the endocardium. Obliteration of the apex and inflow tract, when present, is also demonstrated. This method reportedly assists in distinguishing EMF from constrictive pericarditis (Fig. 47.32).

Cardiovascular Magnetic Resonance Imaging

Recently, the use of cardiovascular magnetic resonance imaging has been shown to demonstrate obliterative changes in the ventricles, atrial dilation, and regurgitant atrioventricular valve lesions in patients with EMF.

However, the use of contrast-enhanced imaging was not able to demonstrate fibrosis within the ventricles of these patients (Fig. 47.31).

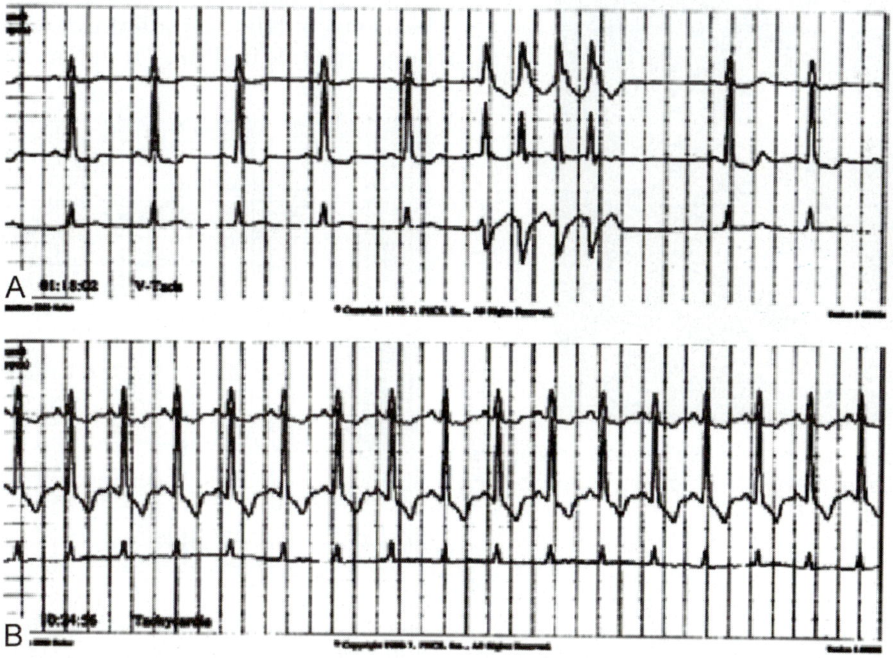

Fig. 47.34: *Holter graph showing ventricular tachycardia at 01;18;02 hrs (A) and SVT at 10;24;56 hrs (B) in patient with recurrent palpitation as a result of endocardial fibroclastosis (EFE)*

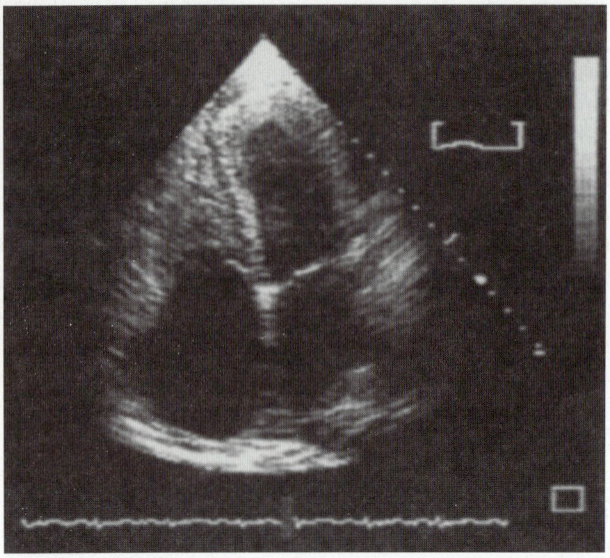

Fig. 47.35: *Apical four chamber echocardiographic image from an individual with cardiomyopathy associated with hypereosinophilic syndrome in a patient with EFE showing soft tissue thrombus deposition within the left and right ventricular apices. Right atrial deposition is also present*

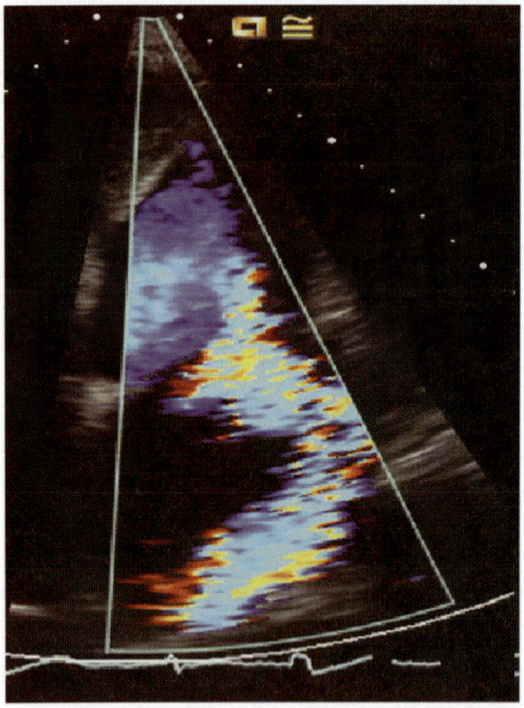

Fig. 47.36: *Colour-Doppler imaging from the patient showing the extent of mitral regurgitation. Calculated regurgitant volume 35 mL (moderate) in a patient with EFE*

Other Tests

Electrocardiography

- Atrial fibrillation
- Low QRS voltage
- First-degree atrioventricular block in up to 44% of patients
- Incomplete right bundle-branch block in up to 30% of patients
- Left atrial enlargement.

Procedures

Cardiac catheterization likely exhibits hemodynamic findings consistent with restrictive cardiomyopathy. Findings from endomyocardial biopsy may be diagnostic, but this procedure is typically not needed.

Biopsy findings may be nondiagnostic when the disease is patchy and sampling sites do not correlate with areas of disease. Because biopsy (especially from the left ventricle) carries some risk, reserve the use of this technique until other diagnostic approaches have been used.

Histologic findings: The heart size is not usually enlarged in EMF. The ventricular cavities are frequently laden with thrombi and, in severe cases, may be nearly totally obliterated by endocardial thickening and thrombosis. The histologic findings of EMF are characterized by reactive fibrosis associated with a selective increase in type I collagen deposition, subendocardial infarction and fibrosis, and thrombus formation. Additionally, specific features of other diseases, such as those associated with hemochromatosis or glycogen storage disease, are notably absent.

Medical Care

In general, the response to medical therapy is poor and unproven. Because most patients with endomyocardial fibrosis (EMF) present long after any possible period of early active myocarditis may have existed, little, if any, role exists for immunosuppressive therapy as is used in some patients with Löffler disease.

Symptomatic therapy with diuretics has been shown to be useful, but digoxin, afterload reducers, and beta-blockers have little role in EMF. For patients with severe symptoms,

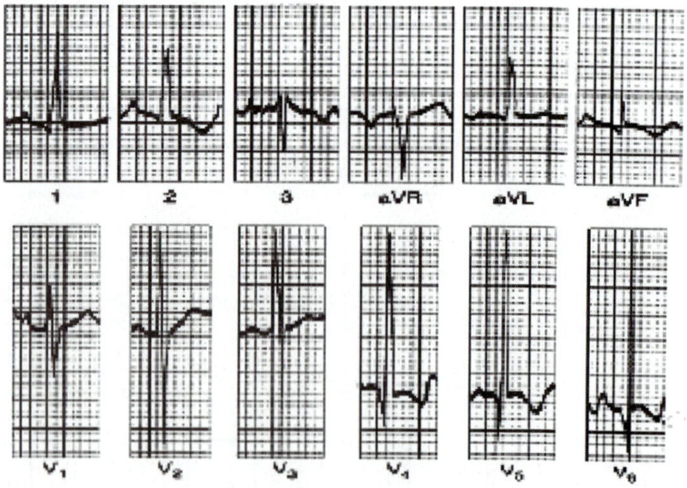

Fig. 47.37: *ECG showing tall R waves in left precordial leads with T wave inversion in leads 11,111 aVF, V5 and V6 with voltage criteria of left ventricular hypertrophy in patient with endocardial fibroelastosis*

consider surgical therapy because the prognosis for these patients with continued medical therapy alone is dismal. Because the rate of thromboembolism is low among patients with EMF and the patient population affected is not typically compliant with anticoagulation regimens, most authors do not recommend anticoagulant therapy.

Surgical Care

Surgical therapy by endocardial decortication seems to be beneficial for many patients with advanced disease who are in functional-therapeutic class III or IV. The operative mortality rate is high (15–20%), but successful surgery has a clear benefit on symptoms and seems to favorably affect survival as well. The most commonly used approach is endocardiectomy, combined with mitral and/or tricuspid repair or replacement (when indicated), using a midline thoracotomy and cardiopulmonary bypass.

Depending on the location of the disease (right or left ventricle, apex or inflow tract), a transapical or transventricular approach can be used. Because a well-defined plane of cleavage usually exists between the endocardium and myocardium, endocardiectomy is most frequently feasible. Because the myocardium is not usually affected, the severe hemodynamic derangement associated with EMF is relieved with successful resection of the endocardium. Common postoperative complications include low cardiac output, heart block, and ventricular arrhythmias.

Diet

No specific diet is recommended for this condition. No activity restrictions are recommended because activity restrictions have not been proven to alter the prognosis of this condition.

ENDOCARDIAL FIBROELASTOSIS (EFE)

The term endocardial fibroelastosis (EFE) was introduced by Weinberg and Himmelfarb in 1943. EFE refers to a pronounced, diffuse thickening of the ventricular endocardium and presents as unexplained heart failure in infants and children. The disease can be primary or secondary to various congenital heart diseases, most notably hypoplastic left heart syndrome, aortic stenosis, or atresia. The two pathologic forms of primary EFE include dilated, which is most common, and contracted. Primary EFE is not associated with any significant structural anomaly of the heart. Secondary EFE is associated with other congenital heart diseases. Once regarded as a common cause of unexplained heart failure, EFE is now considered rare.

Pathophysiology

EFE is characterized by diffuse endocardial thickening and myocardial dysfunction. The endocardial thickening is believed to be caused by persistent and increased wall tension in the ventricles, possibly secondary to damaged myocardium, mitral regurgitation, or both. However, EFE changes are progressive with age. The disease is usually sporadic, but familial cases have been reported (10%).

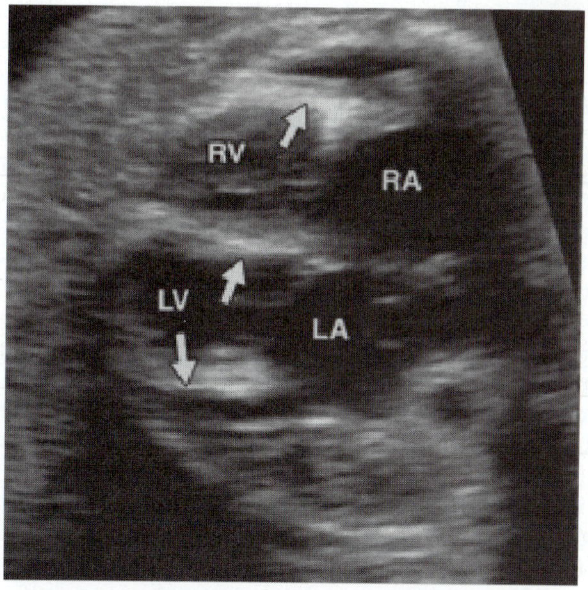

Fig. 47.38: *Endocardial fibroelastosis. Four chamber views show increased echogenicty (arrows) within myocardium of left ventricle (LV) and right ventricle (RV) in patient with endocardial fibroelastosis. LA, left atrium, RA, right atrium*

Observations that favor a viral etiology include a clinical presentation similar to that of chronic myocarditis, findings of myocarditis or myocardial fibrosis in affected patients, a higher incidence following epidemics of coxsackie virus B infection, demonstration of persistent viral infection with molecular studies, and experimental production of the disease in animal models by viral infections of the myocardium. A phenotypic resemblance to dilated cardiomyopathy has been noted. Dilated EFE is characterized by a markedly enlarged globular heart, mainly involving the left ventricle (LV) and left atrium (LA). The LV endocardium is opaque, glistening, milky white, and diffusely thickened to about 1–2 mm. The thickening is most marked in the outflow tract. Papillary muscles arise more superiorly on the ventricular wall with thickened and shortened chordae tendineae, the characteristic rolled-free edge of mitral leaflets. Papillary muscles and trabeculae carneae are flattened and partially incorporated in the fibrotic process, giving a smooth appearance to the lining of the cavity; thus, the papillary muscles exert an undesirable lateral traction on the chordae tendineae and mitral cusps, leading to faulty leaflet opposition.

Although the endocardium is thickened, the ventricular wall (myocardium) thickness is within the reference range. Endocardial thickening extends to the LA, right ventricle, and right atrium. Microthrombi may adhere to the endocardium. The right ventricle is anteriorly displaced to the right, and its cavity is usually flattened. The pulmonary artery may be enlarged, but the aorta and coronary arteries appear normal in caliber. In approximately 50% of patients, the mitral and aortic valves are involved, often producing marked deformity and either valvar regurgitation or stenosis.

The less common contracted type of primary EFE is associated with a relatively hypoplastic or normal LV size. The right and left atria and the right ventricle are markedly enlarged and hypertrophied, with minimal or no endocardial sclerosis. An early event in fetal life is believed to result in dilated EFE, which later morphoses into a contracted type. This suggests that the dilated type could appear as two different diseases while remaining a single disease. Secondary EFE, associated with cardiac malformations, is attributed to the cardiac hypertrophy and consequent imbalance in the myocardial oxygen supply-demand relationship. Resultant fibroelastotic thickening is often focal and less severe.

Acute congestive heart failure (CHF) becomes progressive CHF that results in death within weeks, usually within the first 6 months of life. In a subgroup of individuals who survive from a few months to several years, a more chronic course is common. Such patients respond to medications used to treat CHF. A variable cyclical clinical course ensues, with CHF recurrences related to respiratory or other intercurrent infections or to progression of disease. Remissions can occur with intensification of medical therapy.

History

Symptoms include feeding difficulty, excessive sweating, breathlessness, failure to thrive, and wheezing. Onset may acute enough to produce cardiogenic shock or sudden death; it is a recognized cause of sudden death in infancy.

- Approximately 20% of patients have a history of frequent or recent respiratory tract infections.
- Episodes of severe sudden abdominal pain may indicate coronary insufficiency.

The contracted form of endocardial fibroelastosis (EFE) presents with features of left-sided obstructive disease and acute LV failure. EFE is one of the recognized causes of nonimmune hydrops fetalis.

Physical

- EFE manifests as the classic features of heart failure. Tachypnea during feeding and grunting respirations with subcostal or intercostal retractions have been reported. Fine expiratory wheezes or rales in the lung bases are common. The following may be present upon admission:
  - Pallor
  - Peripheral cyanosis
  - Fever
  - Leukocytosis
  - Anemia
  - Rash.

Thromboembolic episodes may lead to sudden death, myocardial infarction, cerebrovascular events, or even pulmonary embolism. The usual physical findings are as follows:

- Cardiomegaly with normal-to-faint first and second heart sounds, a gallop rhythm with an audible third heart sound, apical pansystolic murmur of mitral regurgitation, and hepatosplenomegaly.
- Clinically detectable pleural or pericardial effusions (rare).

Causes

Possible causative factors include intrauterine viral infection (mumps, coxsackievirus B), subendocardial ischemia, impaired lymphatic drainage of the heart, and systemic carnitine deficiency. Using polymerase chain reaction (PCR) analysis, Ni et al reported that the mumps viral genome persisted in the myocardium of children with EFE; however, this requires further study. The authors suggested cause and effect and speculated that the disease disappeared after the initiation of the measles-mumps-rubella (MMR) vaccination.

- Nine patients with familial EFE were reported in 4 families, and inheritance patterns included X-linked recessive, autosomal dominant and autosomal recessive.

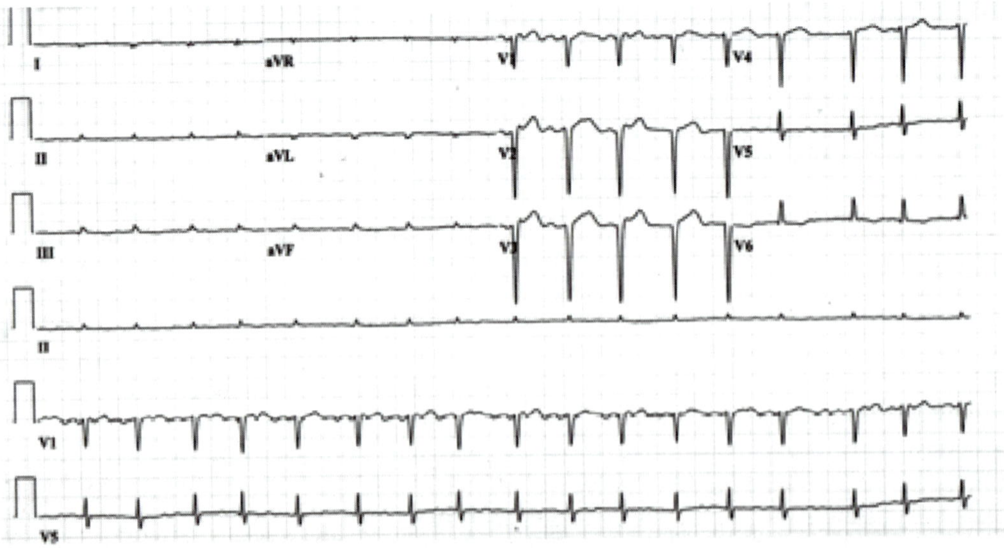

Fig. 47.39: *Twelve-lead ECG recording from a patient with amyloid infiltration of the heart. Note the low voltage in the precordial leads and a prolonged PR interval at 20 ms*

- Recently, mutation of the gene G4.5 (tafazzin) has been associated with familial X-linked EFE and Barth syndrome and has been reported to result in morphologic changes in the fetal heart as early as 18 weeks' gestation. Dilated (primary) EFE occurs when the heart is otherwise normal and no other cause of unexplained heart failure, including systemic carnitine deficiency, is demonstrable. Dilated EFE (secondary) is associated with aortic stenosis or atresia and includes coarctation of the aorta, ventricular septal defect, anomalous origin of left coronary artery from the pulmonary artery, myocardial injury from any cause, and metabolic or carnitine deficiency. Contracted EFE (secondary) is associated with hypoplastic left heart syndrome.

Lab Studies

Blood Tests Include the following:

- Serum electrolyte levels
- BUN and creatinine levels
- CBC count
- Blood culture tests indicated for management of acute episodes
- Autoantibody profile including anti-Ro and anti-La.

Imaging Studies

Chest radiography: Cardiomegaly and cardiothoracic ratios exceed 0.65 in 50% of patients. CE is present in some patients at birth. In others, the heart size is normal during the first few weeks to the first few months of life, but CE subsequently develops.

The shape of the cardiac silhouette varies although it is often globular. Pulmonary venous congestion is common. Left lower lobe atelectasis secondary to dilated LA is found in 25% of patients (Fig. 47.29).

Echocardiography (Fig. 47.30, 47.35 and 47.36)

LA and LV Dimensions are Increased

LV, septal, and posterior wall (PW) excursions are reduced The ejection fraction (EF) is reduced. Mitral valve (MV) motion is abnormal. Echogenicity along the endocardium of the LV (diagnostic clue) is dense.

Suggestive indicators include increased endocardial echo brightness and globular shape of the LV. The echocardiograph may depict a normalization of the shortening fraction and the LV dimensions when the clinical condition improves following medical therapy.

A varying degree of mitral regurgitation is common.

Fetal Echocardiography (Fig. 47.38)

This is a valuable tool for early identification, particularly of the secondary type.

One of the congenital malformations (e.g. aortic stenosis) is often demonstrated at the initial study. The EFE becomes obvious in repeat studies.

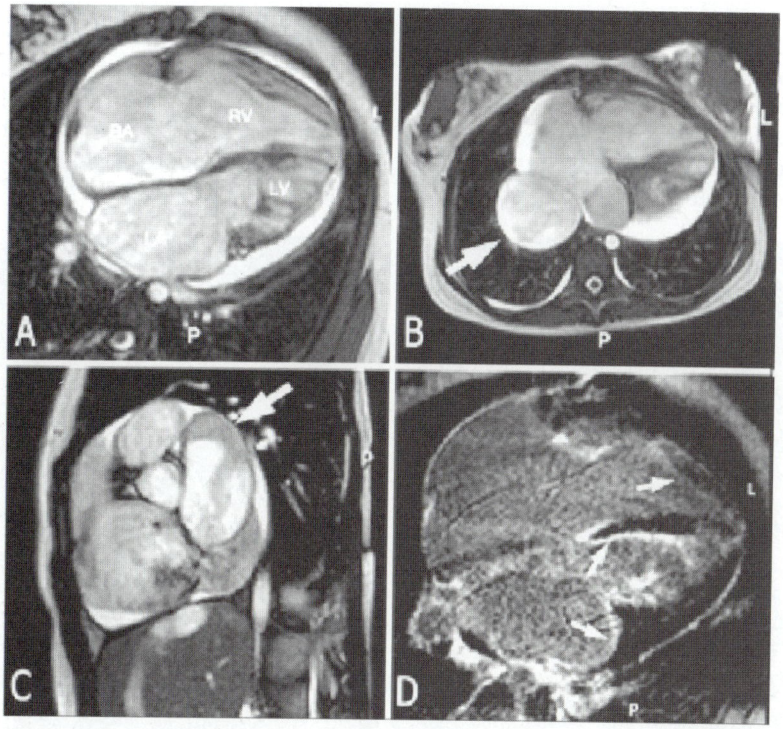

Fig. 47.40: *(A) Four chamber cine image demonstrating biatrial dilation, right ventricular hypertrophy, a small left ventricular cavity and pericardial effusion. (B) Cine image demonstrating dilation of the inferior vena cava (arrow). (C) Short-axis cine image demonstrating thrombus (arrow) extending from the left atrial appendage into the left atrium. (D) Four-chamber late gadolinium hyperenhancement image demonstrating high-signal intensity in the atrial and ventricular endocardium (arrows) in a patient with EFE. L, left; LA, left atrium; LV, left ventricle; P, posterior; RA, right atrium; RV, right ventricle*

- Recently, electron beam CT has been reported to be useful in the early diagnosis of EFE because of its demonstration of calcification and fibrosis of the ventricles, especially at the apex.
- Myocardial delayed-enhancement MRI has been reported to assist in delineation of the extent of endocardial fibroelastosis (Fig. 47.40).

Other Tests

The 24-hour Holter ECG is **useful in documenting ambient arrhythmias.**

Electrocardiography: Tall R waves, deep Q waves, and T-wave inversion or flattening in the left precordial or inferior lead have been reported. Findings depict LV hypertrophy in more than 75% of patients. In the first few weeks of life, right-axis deviation and isolated right ventricular hypertrophy are more common. Pulmonary hypertension may develop in patients who survive for a long period and appears as biventricular hypertrophy on electrocardiography. Patterns of left, right, or biatrial enlargement are evident in 50% of patients. Conduction or rhythm abnormalities include Wolff-Parkinson-White syndrome, left bundle-branch block, supraventricular and ventricular arrhythmias, and varying degrees of atrioventricular block. Low-voltage tracings in the initial stage of heart failure and in the terminal phase are noted in 5% of patients. Occasionally, an infarct pattern appears, pointing to extensive myocardial fibrosis and necrosis (Figs 47.34, 47.37 and 47.39).

Procedures

Cardiac catheterization: Cardiac chambers and pulmonary arteries contain elevated pressures consistent with heart failure. Generally, systolic pulmonary artery pressure is not more than 50% of systemic pressure. Marked pulmonary hypertension may be seen in older children (Fig. 47.29).

The constrictive type of EFE is rare and is associated with a left-sided atrioventricular obstructive pattern, with very high LA pressures from an early age. A diastolic gradient can be detected across the MV. Pulmonary artery pressure is elevated and often reaches systemic levels in this type of EFE.

Postcatheterization precautions include hemorrhage, vascular disruption after balloon dilation, pain, nausea and vomiting, and arterial or venous obstruction due to thrombosis or spasm.

Complications may include blood vessel rupture, tachyarrhythmias, bradyarrhythmias, and vascular occlusion. Angiocardiographic findings:

- Marked dilation of the LV cavity
- Reduced EF with little or no LV wall thickening
- Dyskinetic LV contraction
- Mitral regurgitation (common)

In the contracted type, dilated right ventricle, right atrium, and pulmonary artery with slow clearance of the contrast from the left side of the heart.

Digital subtraction angiography **may demonstrate** an avascular rim between the opacified LV cavity and the ventricular walls perfused by the coronary arteries. The contrast void rim can be identified even in ordinary cineangiographic films. In cases in which the diagnosis is unclear, myocardial biopsy can be helpful (Fig. 47.40).

Medical Care

The treatment of endocardial fibroelastosis (EFE) is essentially the same as that of chronic cardiac failure; its acute exacerbations are often precipitated by respiratory infections. Early and prolonged treatment with digoxin is suggested. Continue therapy for several years after the symptoms disappear; cessation of drug administration may result in acute cardiac failure, even when heart size has returned to normal.

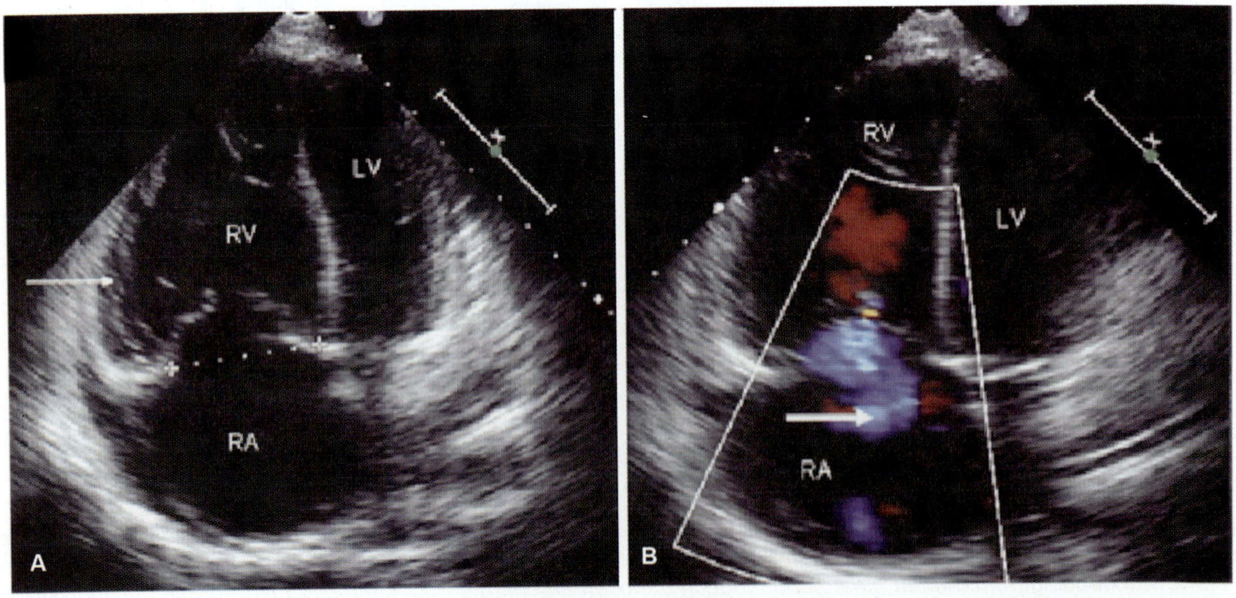

Fig. 47.41: *(A) Apical four chamber view shows right heart chamber dilatation and right ventricular hypertrophy (arrow). (B) Showing tricuspid regurgitation in color Doppler mode of echocardiography in a patient with acute congestive heart failure*

Other measures for acute failure and exacerbations of failure may be required, and precipitating factors, such as infection and anemia, require attention. Anticoagulation may be required in the presence of thromboembolic complications. Case reports in the literature cite resolution of antenatally diagnosed EFE associated with positive anti-Ro and anti-La antibodies with corticosteroid therapy.

Surgical Care

Both pericardial poudrage and MV replacement have had disappointing results.

Cardiac transplantation may be recommended for patients with end-stage disease.

Medication

If the patient is asymptomatic and his or her heart size is normal, provide early, adequate, and prolonged therapy with digitalis and diuretics for at least 2–3 years, with gradual discontinuation.

Early and prolonged treatment with digoxin is suggested. Anticoagulants may be required in the presence of thromboembolic complications.

Antibiotics for endocarditis prophylaxis are administered to patients with certain cardiac conditions, such as endocardial fibroelastosis, before procedures that may cause bacteremia are performed.

Complications

- Resistant cardiac failure
- Recurrent chest infections
- Severe failure to thrive
- Cardiac cirrhosis
- Cerebral, coronary, and pulmonary thromboembolism
- Persistent collapse of left lower lobe or entire left lung

Prognosis

- Primary endocardial fibroelastosis (EFE) prognosis is relatively poor, although the condition is not universally fatal. The prognosis is worse if onset of heart failure occurs earlier.

CONGESTIVE HEART FAILURE

Acute CHF becomes progressive CHF and terminates in death within weeks, usually within the first 6 months of life. In patients who survive from a few months to several years, a more chronic course is common. Such patients respond to medications for CHF. A variable cyclical clinical course ensues, with CHF recurrence related to respiratory or other intercurrent infections or to progression of disease. Remissions can occur through intensification of medical therapy (Fig. 47.41).

Progressive CHF causes deteriorating conditions that lead to death in one-third of patients. One-third of the patients survive and may experience persistent symptoms or show residual ECG abnormalities or evidence of cardiomegaly. Some believe that approximately one-third of patients completely recover, although others are skeptical.

Early diagnosis and prompt persistent administration of digitalis may result in clinical improvement and reversion of the ECG and CE to normal.

Poor prognostic signs of CHF include (1) presentation in the newborn period and (2) recurrent episodes of CHF despite adequate therapy, especially if episodes recur more than 6 months after initial onset of symptoms.

CARDIOVASCULAR SYSTEM IN HIV

Cardiovascular manifestations of HIV infection have been observed for more than 15 years and finally prospective data substantiates this association. Studies published over the past 2–3 years have tracked the incidence and course of HIV infection in relation to cardiac illness in both children and adults. These recent studies show that subclinical echocardiographic abnormalities independently predict adverse outcomes and identify high-risk groups to target for early intervention and treatment. The introduction of highly active antiretroviral therapy (HAART) regimens has significantly modified the course of HIV disease, with longer survival rates and improvement of life quality in HIV infected subjects expected. However, early data raised concerns about HAART being associated with an increase in both peripheral and coronary arterial diseases.

Understanding the effects of HAART on the cardiovascular system is only possible by understanding the effects of HIV coinfections first. HAART is only available to a minority of HIV infected individuals worldwide and studies before HAART remain globally applicable. UNAIDS estimates that 36.1 million people were living with HIV infection at the end of the year 2000. If 8–10% of patients develop symptomatic heart failure over a 2–5 year period, then three million cases of HIV related heart failure will have presented in that time period. Dilated cardiomyopathy, coronary artery disease, endocarditis, and pericardial effusion related to HIV infection will be reviewed here.

DILATED CARDIOMYOPATHY (Figs 47.42–47.50)

HIV disease is recognised as an important cause of dilated cardiomyopathy, with a prevalence reported at 3.6% among cardiomyopathy patients, increasing as patients with HIV infection live longer. Compared to patients with idiopathic dilated cardiomyopathy, those with HIV infection and dilated cardiomyopathy have greatly reduced survival and a hazard ratio of death of 4.0.3. The importance of cardiac dysfunction is demonstrated by a reported median survival to AIDS related death which is 101 days in patients with left ventricular dysfunction and 472 days in patients with a normal heart by echocardiography at similar infection stage.

Myocarditis still represents the best studied cause of dilated cardiomyopathy in HIV disease. HIV virions appear to infect myocardial cells in patchy distributions without a clear direct association between HIV and cardiac myocyte dysfunction. It is unclear how virus enters CD4 receptor negative cells such as myocytes. Reservoir cells (for example, dendritic cells) may play a pathogenic role in the

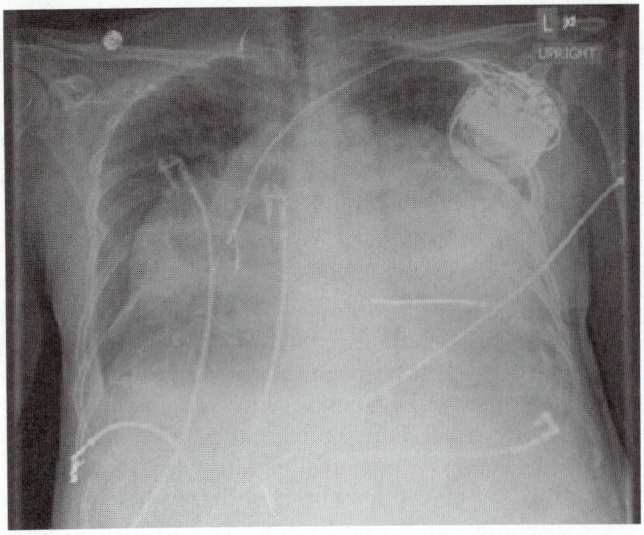

Fig. 47.42: *X-ray chest PA view shows grossly dilated heart with implanted pacemaker in patient with dilated cardiomyopathy in HIV infection*

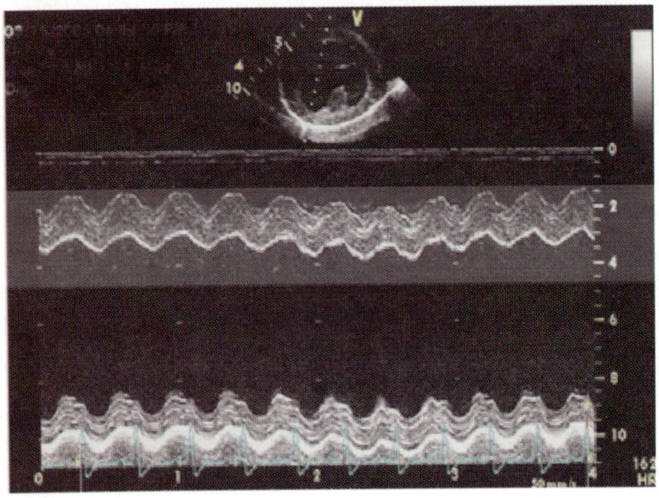

Fig. 47.43: *M-mode echo scan shows dilated LV cavity in dilated cardiomyopathy in HIV infection*

interaction between HIV and the myocyte and in the activation of multifunctional cytokines that contribute to progressive and late tissue damage. Asymptomatic left ventricular dysfunction and increased left ventricular mass independently predict accelerated mortality in both adults and children infected with HIV. Treatment for dilated cardiomyopathy associated with HIV infection is generally similar to treatment for nonischaemic cardiomyopathy. Angiotensin-converting enzyme inhibitors are recommended based on general heart failure studies, but may be poorly tolerated because of low systemic vascular resistance from diarrhoeal disease, infection, or dehydration. No studies have investigated the efficacy of specific therapeutic regimens, including HAART, other than intravenous immunoglobulin. The apparent efficacy of immunoglobulin treatment may be the result of immunoglobulins inhibiting cardiac autoantibodies by competing for Fc receptors or dampening the secretion or effects of cytokines and cellular growth factors.

Encephalopathy influences negatively the clinical course of dilated cardiomyopathy in HIV disease. HIV may persist in reservoir cells in the myocardium and the cerebral cortex even after antiretroviral treatment. The reservoir cells may hold HIV-1 on their surfaces for extended time periods and may chronically release cytotoxic cytokines [tumour necrosis factor (TNF), interleukin-6 (IL-6), endothelin-1 (ET-1)] contributing to progressive and late tissue damage in both systems independently of HAART.

CORONARY ARTERY DISEASE (Fig. 47.44)

Accelerated coronary artery disease in HIV infected patients may result from atherogenesis stimulated by virus infected monocyte-macrophages, possibly caused by altered leucocyte adhesion or arteritis. Coronary artery disease is observed with increasing frequency among HIV patients receiving protease inhibitors in the ambit of HAART. Despite the clinical benefits of protease inhibitors, complications such as lipodystrophy, insulin resistance, and high concentrations of low-density lipoprotein and triglycerides have been described in up to 60% of patients treated with HAART regimens. In 10–20% of patients, these alterations of metabolism have severe manifestations. Effects of preexisting cardiovascular risk factors combined with atherogenic effects of current drug treatments for HIV infection appear to result in an increase in acute coronary syndromes, even in young HIV infected individuals. It may be important to consider traditional coronary risk profiles and to alter those that can be modified in the evaluation and continued treatment of patients for HAART. Diet and exercise should not be overlooked, because both can be effective in managing these complications without causing further side effects. Fibric acid derivatives and statins can lower HIV associated cholesterol and triglyceride

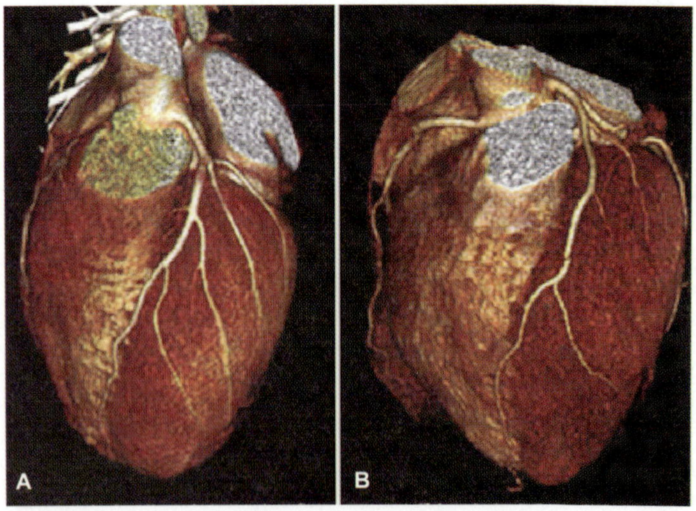

Fig. 47.44: *Multislice CT reconstructions of (A) a control heart and (B) a heart affected by DCM in HIV infection showing marked epicardial coronary artery mismatch for left ventricular mass and side-branch reduction. Abbreviation: DCM, dilated cardiomyopathy*

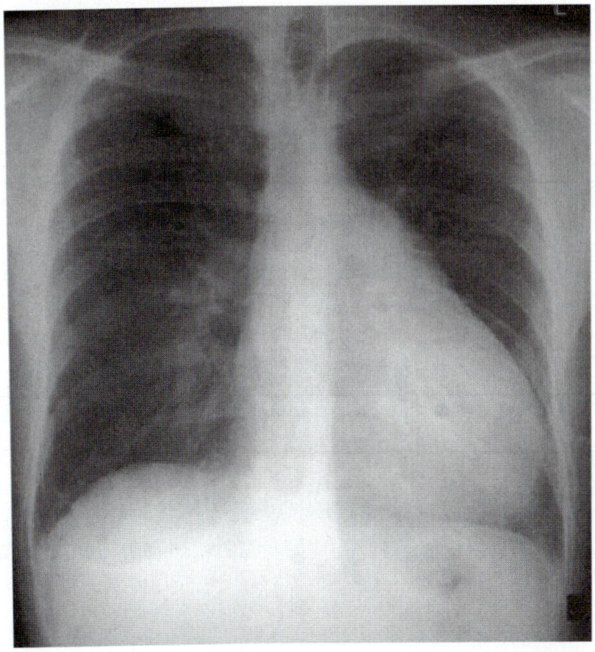

Fig. 47.45: *Chest radiograph of a patient with primary pulmonary hypertension. Note the enlarged proximal pulmonary arteries*

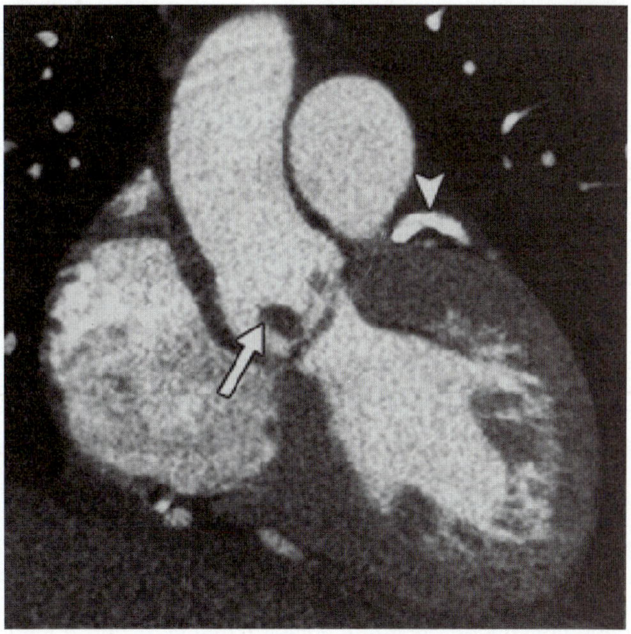

Fig. 47.46: *A patient with HIV infection, endocarditis, and coronary artery disease who had history of IV drug abuse and highly active antiretroviral therapy. Coronal multiplanar reformatted contrast-enhanced CT image shows vegetation (arrow) adjacent to aortic valve and calcified plaques (arrowhead) in left anterior descending artery (LAD)*

concentrations, although further data are needed on interactions between statins and protease inhibitors. Lovastatin should be avoided in patients receiving concomitant drugs that may potentiate skeletal muscle toxicity with this agent. Hypoglycaemic agents may have some role in managing glucose abnormalities, although troglitazone cannot be recommended for fat abnormalities alone and metformin may cause lactic acidosis. Perhaps a better understanding of protease inhibitors' effects on lipid and metabolic pathways will lead to a new generation of drug treatments without metabolic alterations. This understanding may also lead to new treatments for dyslipidaemias and alterations of metabolism unrelated to HIV infection.

HIV Associated Pulmonary Hypertension and Right Ventricular Dysfunction (Figs 47.45 and 47.47)

The incidence of HIV associated pulmonary hypertension is estimated to be 1/200, much higher than the 1/200,000 found in the general population. Primary pulmonary hypertension is estimated to occur in about 0.5% of hospitalized AIDS patients and is a cause of severe cardiac impairment with associated cor pulmonale and death. The pathogenesis is multifactorial and poorly understood. HIV may cause endothelial damage and mediator related

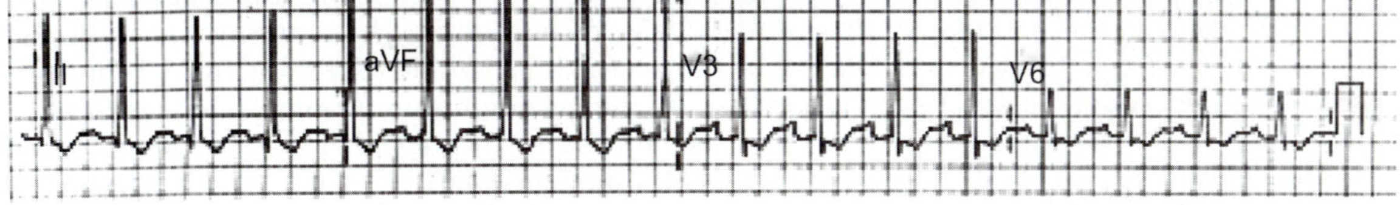

Fig. 47.47: *Showing dilated cardiomyopathy as seen in HIV infection. * There is marked LVH (S wave in V2 > 35 mm) with dominant S waves in V1-4 * Right axis deviation suggests associated right ventricular hypertrophy (i.e. biventricular enlargement).* There is evidence of left atrial enlargement (deep, wide terminal portion of the P wave in V1).* There are peaked P waves in lead II suggestive of right atrial hypertrophy (not quite 2.5 mm in height)*

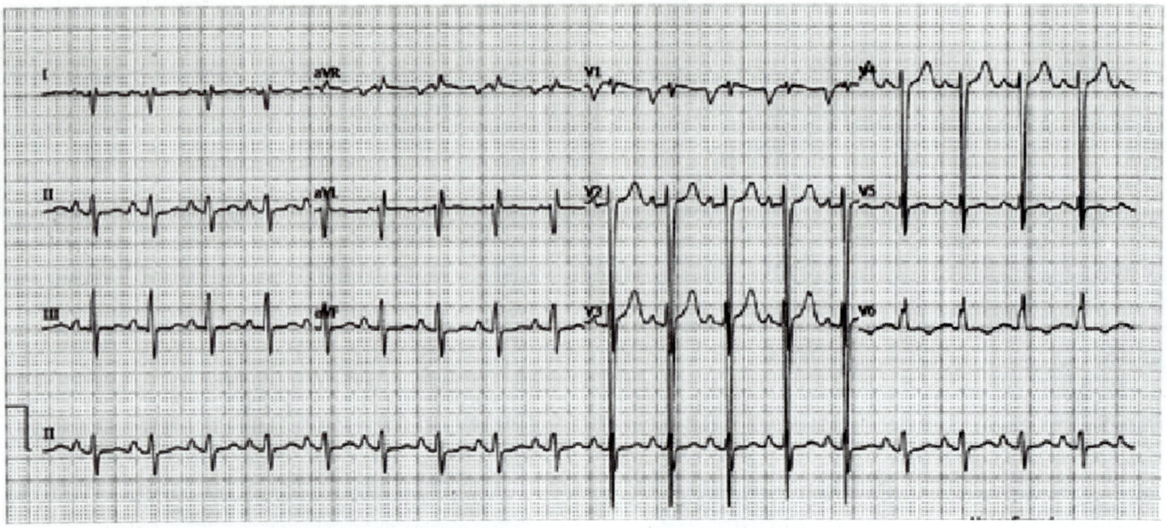

Fig. 47.48: *Showing dilated cardiomyopathy as seen in HIV infection. * There is marked LVH (S wave in V2 > 35 mm) with dominant S waves in V1-4 * Right-axis deviation suggests associated right ventricular hypertrophy (i.e. biventricular enlargement).* There is evidence of left atrial enlargement (deep, wide terminal portion of the P wave in V1).* There are peaked P waves in lead II suggestive of right atrial hypertrophy (not quite 2.5 mm in height)*

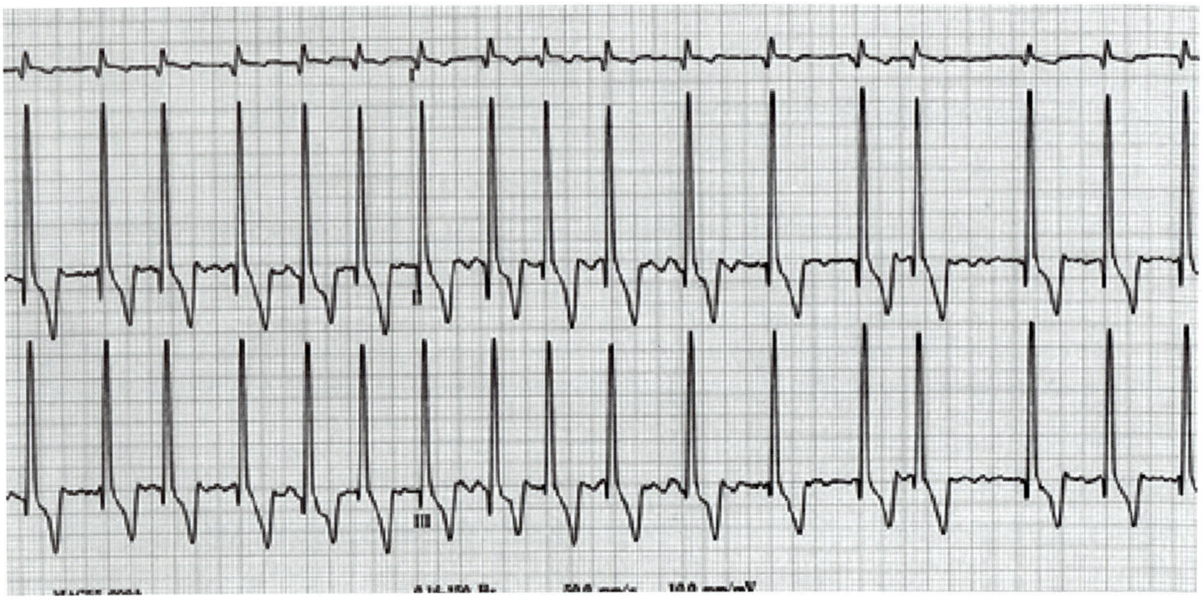

Fig. 47.49: *Atrial fibrillation with fast ventricular rate in dilated cardiomyopathy in HIV infection*

vasoconstriction through stimulation by the envelope glycoprotein including direct release and pulmonary vasoconstrictor effects of ET-1, IL-6 and TNF-β. HIV is frequently identified in alveolar macrophages on histology. These macrophages release TNF, oxide anions, and proteolytic enzymes in response to infection. Effects of HAART on pulmonary artery endothelial cells are unknown.

Endocarditis (Fig. 47.46)

The prevalence of infective endocarditis in HIV infected patients is similar to that of patients of similar behaviour risk—that is, intravenous drug use. Estimates of endocarditis occurrence vary from 6.3–34% of HIV infected patients who use intravenous drugs. Right-sided valves are predominantly affected. Patients with and without HIV generally have similar presentation and survival rates from infective endocarditis. However, patients with late stage HIV disease have higher mortality from infective endocarditis than do asymptomatic HIV infected patients. As the autoimmune response to bacterial endocarditis is often largely responsible for associated valvar destruction, HIV infected patients may have an altered course. For example, HIV infected patients have a higher risk of developing salmonella endocarditis than immunocompetent patients because they are more likely to develop salmonella bacteraemia during salmonella infection.

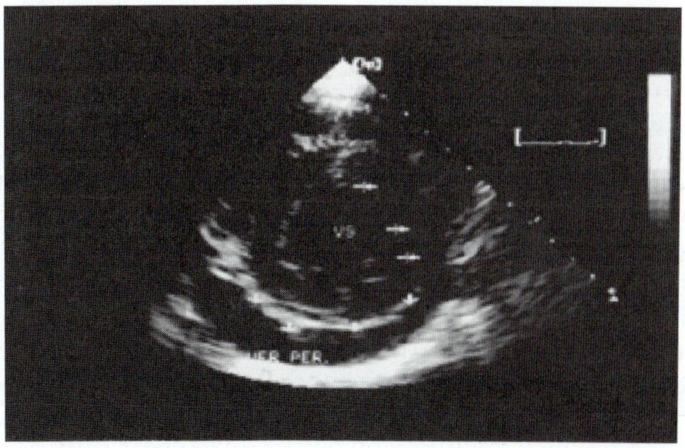

Fig. 47.50: *Circumferential pericardial effusion (arrows) in HIV infected patients induced Mycobacterium avium intracellulare infection (parasternal short-axis view)*

However, they respond better to antibiotic treatment and may be less likely to sustain valvar damage because of impaired immune function.

Necropsy finding of Candida albicans endocarditis in an AIDS intravenous heroin users. Note the thrombotic formation on the closing edge of the posterior leaflet of the tricuspid valve (arrow) going down to the right ventricular cavity and involving the chordae tendineae.

Pericardial Effusion (Fig. 47.50)

The prevalence of pericardial effusion in asymptomatic HIV infected patients is estimated at 22%. Pericardial effusion in HIV disease may be related to opportunistic infections or to malignacy, but most often a clear etiology is not found. The effusion may be part of a generalized serous effusive process also involving pleural and peritoneal surfaces. This "capillary leak" syndrome is likely related to enhanced cytokine expression in the later stages of HIV disease. Pericardial effusion spontaneously resolves in up to 42% of patients. Mortality remains increased in HIV infected patients who develop an effusion, even if the effusion resolves over time. Pericardiocentesis is currently recommended only in large or poorly tolerated effusions, for diagnostic evaluation of systemic illness, or in the presence of cardiac tamponade. The effects of HAART on pericardial effusion are largely unexplored.

Circumferential pericardial effusion (arrows) in HIV infected patients induced *Mycobacterium avium* intracellulare infection (parasternal short-axis view).

Conclusion

Cardiovascular complications of HIV infection are generally late disease manifestations. Often symptoms of congestive heart failure or pericardial effusion in HIV infected patients are nonspecific and may be attributed to generalized illness or coinfection. Echocardiographic screening noninvasively and accurately aids diagnosis during any change in clinical status and directs treatment. Patients will usually respond to early treatment for left ventricular dysfunction and increased left ventricular mass. Treatment based on these findings may prolong the quality and duration of life, and direct further patient evaluation. The role of the cardiologist in the evaluation and treatment of patients with HIV infection should therefore be expanded to include patients who are being evaluated for or who are receiving HAART regimens, especially those with underlying cardiovascular risk. HIV associated heart disease may be an important model for etiologic mechanisms of dilated cardiomyopathy with important implications in non-HIV related cardiovascular diseases. The role of infection and inflammation in many other cardiovascular diseases is beginning to be recognized, and discovering the molecular mechanisms of HIV related heart disease may provide the basis for rational therapeutic strategies and improved care.

PROTEIN ENERGY MALNUTRITION (PEM)

The World Health Organization defines malnutrition as the cellular imbalance between supply of nutrients and energy and the body's demand for them to ensure growth, maintenance, and specific functions. Malnutrition is globally the most important risk factor for illness and death, contributing to more than half of deaths in children worldwide. Protein-energy malnutrition (PEM), first described in the 1920s, is observed most frequently in developing countries but has been described with increasing frequency in hospitalized and chronically ill children in the United States.

Kwashiorkor and marasmus are two forms of PEM that have been described. The distinction between the 2 foms of PEM is based on the presence (kwashiorkor) ereas kwashiorkor represents a dysadaptation to starvationntries,

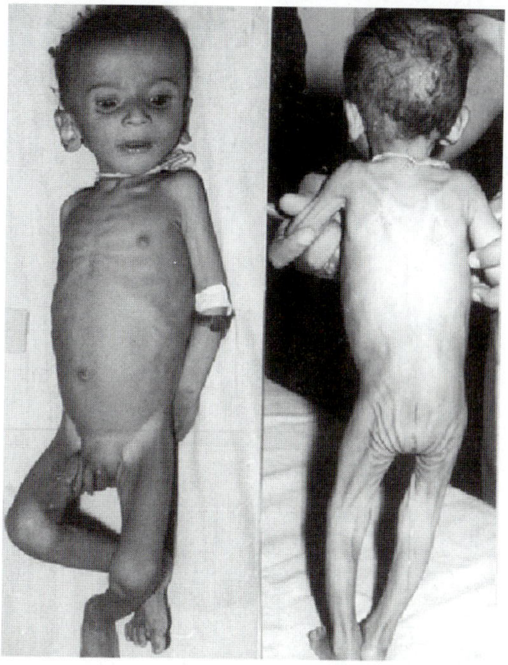

Fig. 47.51: *Stunted physical growth, anemia waisting of muscles and loss of subcutaneous fat in a 2-yrs-old child with marasmus type of PEM*

while deficiencies of vitamin C, B, and D have improved in recent years. Micronutrient deficiencies and protein and calorie deficiencies must be addressed for optimal growth and development to be attained in these individuals.

Pathophysiology

Malnutrition affects virtually every organ system. Dietary protein is needed to provide amino acids for synthesis of body proteins and other compounds that have a variety of functional roles. Energy is essential for all biochemical and physiologic functions in the body. Furthermore, micronutrients are essential in many metabolic functions in the body as components and cofactors in enzymatic processes.

In addition to the impairment of physical growth and of cognitive and other physiologic functions, immune response changes occur early in the course of significant malnutrition in a child. These immune response changes correlate with poor outcomes and mimic the changed observed in children with acquired immune deficiency syndrome (AIDS). Loss of delayed hypersensitivity, fewer T lymphocytes, impaired lymphocyte response, impaired phagocytosis secondary to decreased complement and certain cytokines, and decreased secretory immunoglobulin A (IgA) are some changes that may occur. These immune changes predispose children to severe and chronic infections, most commonly, infectious diarrhea, which further compromises nutrition causing anorexia, decreased nutrient absorption, increased metabolic needs, and direct nutrient losses.

Early studies of malnourished children showed changes in the developing brain, including, a slowed rate of growth of the brain, lower brain weight, thinner cerebral cortex, decreased number of neurons, insufficient myelinization, and changes in the dendritic spines. More recently, neuroimaging studies have found severe alterations in the

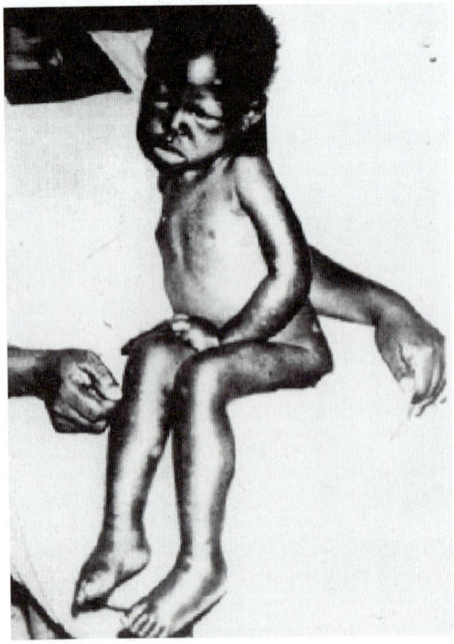

Fig. 47.52: *Generalised edema anemia, puffiness of face and stunted physical growth in a 2yrs-old child with kwashiorkor*

dendritic spine apparatus of cortical neurons in infants with severe protein-calorie malnutritary hyperaldosteronism.

Mortality/Morbidity than 5 years in developing countries and contributes indirectly to over half the deaths in worldwide of immunologic functions in these children mimics those observed in children infections. Children who are chronically malnourished exhibit behavioral changes including irritability, apathy and decreased social responsiveness, anxiety, and attention deficits. In addition, infants and young children who have malnutrition frequently demonstrate developmental delay or permanent cognitive deficits. The degree of delay and deficit depends on the severity and duration of nutritional compromise and the age at which malnutrition occurs. In general, nutritional insults at younger ages will have worse outcomes.

Although death from malnutrition in the United States is rare, in developing countries, more than 50% of the 10 million deaths each year are either directly or indirectly secondary to malnutrition in children younger than 5 years.

Age

Children are most vulnerable to the effects of malnutrition in infancy and early childhood. Premature infants have special nutritional needs that are not met with traditional feeding recommendations; they require fortified human milk or specially designed preterm formula until later in infancy. Children are susceptible to malnutrition for differing reasons. During adolescence, self-imposed dietary restrictions contribute to the incidence of nutritional deficiencies.

History

Clinical signs and symptoms of PEM include the following:
- Poor weight gain
- Slowing of linear growth
- *Behavioral changes:* Irritability, apathy, decreased social responsiveness, anxiety and attention deficits.

Clinical signs and symptoms of micronutrient deficiencies: Some of the clinical signs and symptoms of specific micronutrient deficiencies may closely resemble those observed in PEM. Deficiencies of micronutrients including vitamins, minerals, and trace elements have been well described. The most common and clinically significant deficiencies include the following:
- *Iron:* Fatigue, anemia, decreased cognitive function, headache, glossitis and nail changes
- *Iodine:* Goiter, developmental delay and mental retardation
- *Vitamin D:* Poor growth, rickets and hypocalcemia
- *Vitamin A:* Night blindness, xerophthalmia, poor growth and hair changes
- *Folate:* Glossitis, anemia (megaloblastic), and neural tube defects (in fetuses of women without folate supplementation)
- *Zinc:* Anemia, dwarfism, hepatosplenomegaly, hyperpigmentation and hypogonadism, acrodermatitis enteropathica, diminished immune response, poor wound healing.

Physical (Figs 47.51–47.53)

- Physical findings that are associated with PEM include the following:
  Decreased subcutaneous tissue: Areas that are most affected are the legs, arms, buttocks and face.
- *Edema:* Areas that are most affected are the distal extremities and anasarca (generalized edema).
- Oral changes
- Cheilosis
- Angular stomatitis
- Papillar atrophy
- Abdominal findings
- Abdominal distension secondary to poor abdominal musculature
- Hepatomegaly secondary to fatty infiltration
- Skin changes
- Dry peeling skin with raw exposed areas
- Hyperpigmented plaques over areas of trauma
- *Nail changes:* Nails become fissured or ridged
- *Hair changes:* Hair is thin, sparse, brittle, easily pulled out, and turns a dull- brown or reddish color.

Causes

- Inadequate food intake is the most common cause of malnutrition worldwide. In developing countries, inadequate food intake is secondary to insufficient or inappropriate food supplies or early cessation of breastfeeding. In some areas, cultural and religious food customs may play a role. Inadequate sanitation further endangers children by increasing the risk of infectious diseases that increase nutritional losses and alters metabolic demands.
- In developed countries, inadequate food intake is a less common cause of malnutrition. Instead, diseases and, in particular, chronic illnesses play an important role in the etiology of malnutrition. Children with chronic illness are at risk for nutritional problems for several reasons, including the following:
  - Children with chronic illnesses frequently have anorexia, which leads to inadequate food intake.
  - Increased inflammatory burden and increased metabolic demands can increase caloric need.
  - Any chronic illness that involves the liver or small bowel affects nutrition adversely by impairing digestive and absorptive functions.
- Chronic illnesses that commonly are associated with nutritional deficiencies include the following:
  - Cystic fibrosis
  - Chronic renal failure
  - Childhood malignancies
  - Congenital heart disease
  - Neuromuscular diseases
  - Chronic inflammatory bowel diseases
- In addition, the following conditions place children at significant risk for the development of nutritional deficiencies:
  - Prematurity
  - Developmental delay
  - In utero toxin exposure (i.e. fetal alcohol exposure)
- Children with multiple food allergies present a special nutritional challenge because of severe dietary restrictions. Patients with active allergic symptoms may have increased calorie and protein needs.

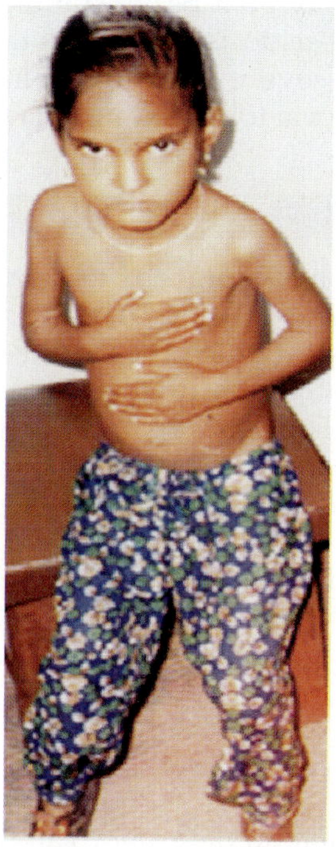

Fig. 47.53: *Stunted physical growth, anemias edema feet and dyscolouration of hair in a 6-yrs-old child with kwashiorkor*

Laboratory Studies

- The most helpful laboratory studies in assessing the nutritional status of a child are hematological studies and laboratory studies evaluating protein status.
- Hematological studies should include a complete blood count (CBC) with red blood cell indices and a peripheral smear. This could also help to exclude anemias from nutritional deficiencies such as iron, folate, and vitamin B_{12} deficiencies.
- Measures of protein nutritional status include serum albumin, retinol-binding protein, prealbumin, transferrin, creatinine, and BUN levels. Retinol-binding protein, prealbumin, and transferrin determinations are much better short-term indicators of protein status than albumin. However, in the field, a better measure of long-term malnutrition is serum albumin because of its longer half-life.
- Additional diagnostic evaluation
- In children who have a history of adequate food intake and signs/symptoms of malnutrition, focus on identifying the cause of malnutrition. Perform laboratory studies based on information from a complete history and physical examination.
- Initial diagnostic laboratory studies include a CBC, sedimentation rate, serum electrolytes, and urinalysis and culture. Stool specimens should be obtained if the child has a history of abnormal stools or stooling patterns or if the family uses an unreliable or questionable source of water.

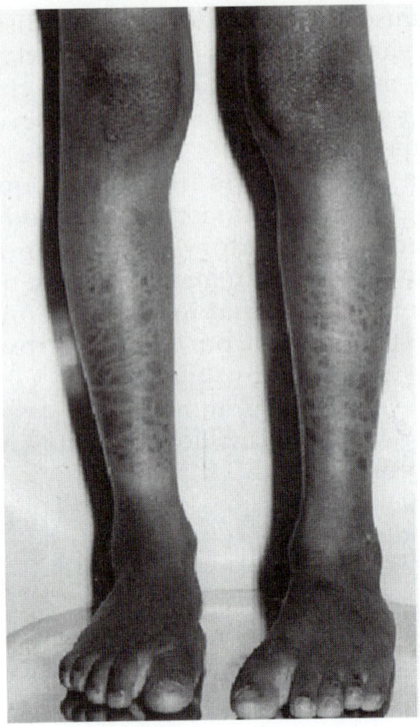

Fig. 47.54: *Edema of legs and feet with mixed picture of malnutrition in older boy with chronic wet beri -beri who was suffering from malabsorption syndrome*

- Additional studies may focus on thyroid functions or sweat chloride tests, particularly if height velocity is abnormal. Further diagnostic studies should be determined as dictated by the history and physical examination. For example, laboratory tests evaluating renal function, such as phosphorus and calcium, should be obtained in the presence of renal symptoms. Children with suspected liver disease should have triglyceride and vitamin levels obtained, while zinc levels should be obtained in patients with chronic diarrhea.
- Celiac serology is a useful screening test and should be considered, especially if there is a family history of celiac disease or if other autoimmune diseases, such as type I diabetes mellitus, are present.
- Other tests
- Practical nutritional assessment
- Complete history, including a detailed dietary history
- Growth measurements including weight and length/height; head circumference in children younger than 3 years
- Complete physical examination.

Sensitive measures of nutritional status

- Height-for-age or weight-for-height measurements greater than two standard deviations below the mean for age
- Height-for-age or weight-for-height measurements more than two standard deviations less than the mean for age
- Height-for-age measurements less than 95% of expected value
- Weight-for-height measurements less than 90% of expected value
- Less than 5 cm/y of growth in children older than 2 years
- Body mass index (BMI) (although not established by the CDC as a criteria for failure to thrive).

Treatment

Medical Care

Following evaluation of the child's nutritional status and identification of the underlying etiology of the malnutrition, dietary intervention in collaboration with a dietitian or other nutritional professionals should be initiated. Children with edema must be assessed carefully for actual nutritional status because edema may mask the severity of malnutrition. Children with chronic malnutrition may require caloric intakes more than 120–150 kcal/kg/d to achieve appropriate weight gain. The formula for determining adequate caloric intake is: kcal/kg = (RDA for age X ideal weight)/actual weight.

- Additionally, any micronutrient deficiencies must be corrected for the child to attain appropriate growth and development. Most children with mild malnutrition respond to increased oral caloric intake and supplementation with vitamin, iron, and folate supplements. The requirement for increased protein is met typically by increasing the food intake, which, in turn, increases both protein and caloric intake. Adequacy of intake is determined by monitoring weight gain.
- In mild-to-moderate cases of malnutrition, initial assessment and nutritional intervention may be done in the outpatient setting. A patient with malnutrition may require hospitalization based on the severity and instability of the clinical situation. Hospitalization of patients with suspected malnutrition secondary to neglect allows observation of the interactions between parent/caregiver and child and documentation of actual intake and feeding difficulties. It may also be warranted in cases where dehydration and acidosis complicate the clinical picture. In moderate-to-severe cases of malnutrition, enteral supplementation via tube feedings may be necessary.

BERIBERI

In 1630 a Dutch physician, Jacobus Bonitus, observed in Java, "a very troublesome affliction, called by the inhabitants Beri-beri (which means sheep), those, whom this same disease attacks, with their knees shaking and the legs raised up, walk like sheep".

In the last 100 years, the cause of beriberi was determined to be deficiency of thiamine (vitamin B_1), a water-soluble and heat-labile vitamin required for carbohydrate metabolism. Thiamine is essential for most vertebrates and some microorganisms. Beriberi has two main forms in humans, depending on the system of maximum involvement: wet beriberi (edematous cardiovascular dysfunction) and dry beri-beri (multifocal peripheral and/or central neurologic dysfunction). Often times, patients present with features of both.

How a single vitamin deficiency can have such diverse patterns of presentation is not fully understood. Possible explanations include the coexistence of other vitamin or

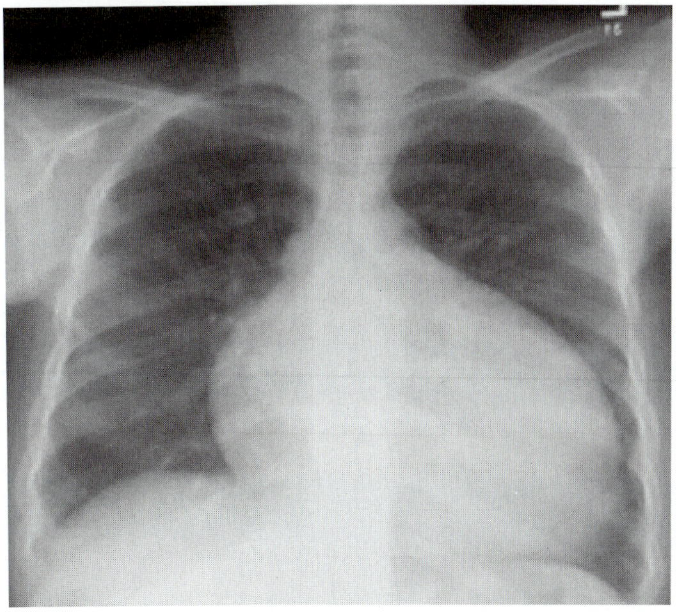

Fig. 47.55: *Cardiomegaly in wet beri-beri (B_1, thiamine deficiency)*

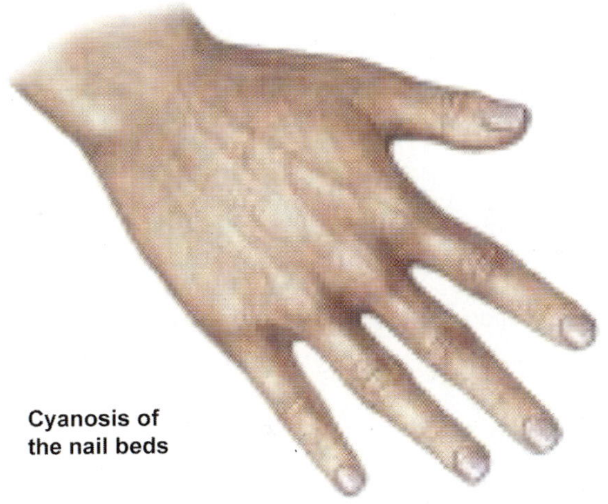

Fig. 47.56: *Cyanosis in hand nails in beri-beri disease*

dietary deficiencies; simultaneous comorbidities, simultaneous stressors, or both; individual genetic differences among the various enzymes that have thiamine as their cofactor; and variations in tissue stores or turnover of the vitamin.

In the Western world, beri-beri is usually seen in patients in defined situations outside of the normal protective measures of modern society. Also, unusual physiologic conditions in which beri-beri could have been predicted are recognized. Finally, chance circumstances in which thiamine deficiency is fully unanticipated are also recognized. Dietary thiamine deficiency can be caused by an overall poor nutritional intake, by dietary customs that rely heavily on inadequate food sources (e.g. milled rice), and, rarely, by consuming foods that contain thiaminases or antithiamine compounds. A cohort at particularly high risk are individuals with alcoholism with poor nutrition because alcohol also impairs thiamine absorption.

In 1998, the Institute of Medicine of the National Academies published the recommended dietary intake of thiamine and other vitamins B for males and females (from infants to the elderly). Also, a comprehensive monograph on beriberi was commissioned by the World Health Organization; it recommends that the term beri-beri be replaced by thiamine deficiency. For more information regarding the cardiovascular and neurologic manifestations encountered in adult patients.

Pathophysiology

Thiamine mainly functions as thiamine pyrophosphate (TPP), which serves as a prosthetic group or cofactor for several enzymes in carbohydrate metabolism. These enzymes all use thiamine's thiazole ring to activate and transfer a 2-carbon unit (aldehyde). They catalyze decarboxylation of pyruvate, ketoglutarate, and the transketolation reaction in the pentose phosphate pathway. Thiamine is also believed to have a role in nerve conduction through the synthesis of acetylcholine. An impairment in the decarboxylation pathway causes a decrease in ATP (energy) synthesis. A reduction of transketolase activity compromises the hexose monophosphate shunt and yields decreases in nicotinamide adenine dinucleotide phosphate (NADPH) formation, in electron transport, and in ATP synthesis.

Impaired energy production, increased manufacturing of free radicals, and possible *N*-methyl-D-aspartate (NMDA) receptor-mediated toxicity have been hypothesized to yield neuronal injury (dry beri-beri). The exact biochemical defect responsible for the clinical manifestations of cardiac beri-beri (wet beri-beri) or its acute form, Shoshin beri-beri (from the Japanese, meaning "sudden collapse"), is not yet fully elucidated. Cardiac dysfunction may simply be compromised by myocardial tissue edema and energy depletion.

Thiamine is not widely distributed in high concentrations; consequently, many foods are now routinely fortified with it. Rich natural sources include whole grains, lean pork, peas, spinach and legumes. Very little thiamine is present in fats, oils, and refined sugars. It is destroyed by heat, pasteurization, and ionizing radiation. Freezing does not affect the bioavailability of thiamine; however, it is insoluble in alcohol. The risk of beri-beri increases in individuals who consume a diet high in thiaminase rich foods (e.g. raw freshwater fish or shellfish, ferns), a diet high in antithiamine factors (e.g. tea, coffee, betel nuts), or both.

Deficiency of thiamine affects the cardiovascular, muscular, nervous, and GI systems. The body stores of thiamine are minimal, and the duration of thiamine reserves is unknown. In one study, deficiency was detected after approximately 6 weeks without thiamine. In another study of healthy young men who consumed less than 0.2 mg of thiamine daily, urinary excretion of thiamine stopped within 18 days. Case studies have suggested that fatal deficiency can develop in as little as 3 weeks without

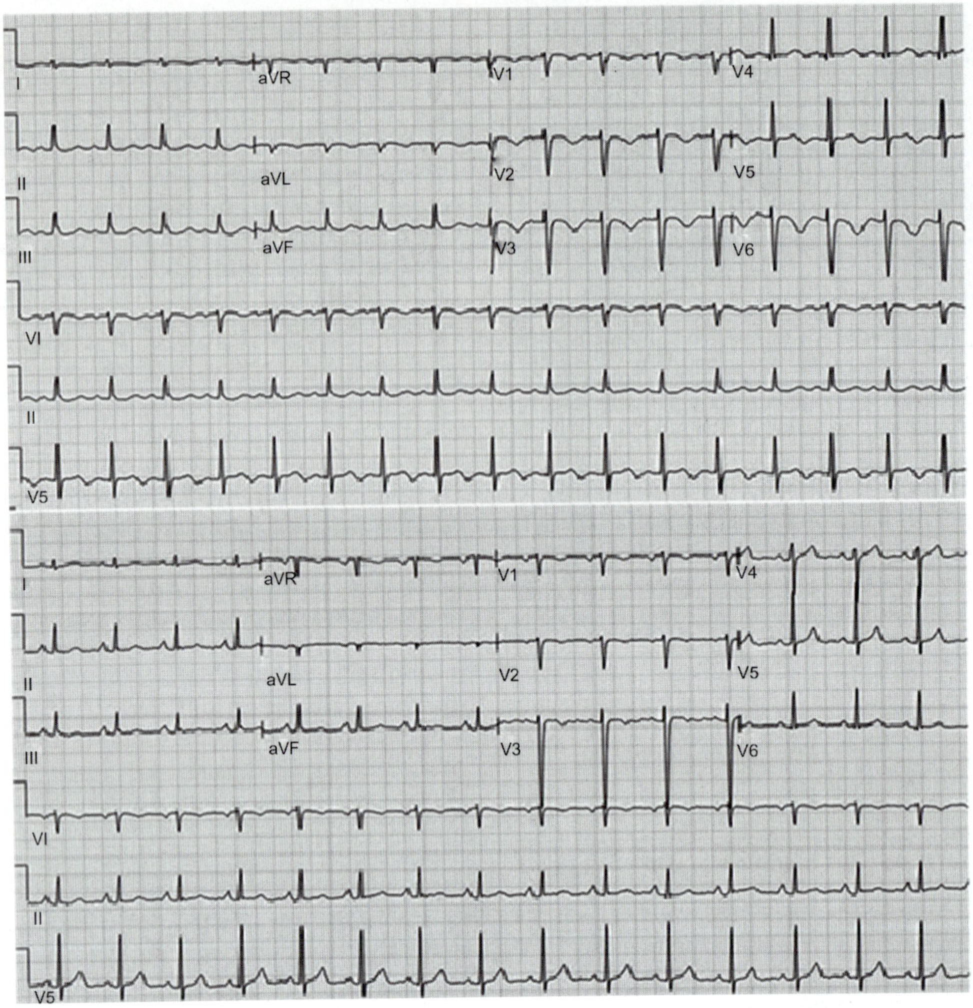

Fig. 47.57: *(Top) The electrocardiogram showed diffuse disturbances of repolarisation (ST-depression and negative T-wave). (Bottom) Showed disappearance of changes after therapeutic doses of B1*

thiamine intake. Despite the widespread fortification of many foods and infant formulas with thiamine, clinicians must remain aware of the signs and symptoms of beri-beri, a life-threatening, but rapidly reversible, condition.

Mortality/Morbidity

Mortality is rare and is usually restricted to wet beri-beri (cardiac) that goes undiagnosed for too long and, hence, can not be treated. Morbidity is also rare and is usually seen in dry beri-beri (neurologic) that is treated so late in the course of the illness that some residual neurologic deficits remain. In both situations, the timely recognition of the signs and symptoms of beri-beri can result in thiamine replacement, which rapidly reverses the cardiovascular and neurologic dysfunction.

The prevalence is highest in cultures that depend on a high proportion of their calories from foods that have poor thiamine content, such as milled rice.

Beriberi can affect both genders, although alcoholism (a major risk factor) is more prevalent in males.

Beri-beri is predominantly observed in adults and infants aged 124 months (infantile beri-beri).

Wet Beri-beri (Figs 47.54–47.59)

Clinical Examination

History

Thiamine deficiency has a wide range of clinical presentations. Although clinical overlap is common, the basic phenotypes are as follows:

This phenotype affects the cardiovascular system and is divided into acute and chronic forms.

- In acute wet beri-beri or Shoshin beri-beri, the predominant injury is to the heart, and rapid deterioration occurs because of the heart's inability to maintain function. Presenting symptoms include tachycardia, low diastolic pressure, cardiomegaly, pulmonary edema and cyanosis. Wet beriberi is characterized by elevated lactic acid levels. This condition can be readily reversed with thiamine infusion if administered early.
- *Chronic wet beri-beri with high-output cardiac failure has three stages.*

  Initially, peripheral vasodilatation occurs, yielding high-output cardiac failure.

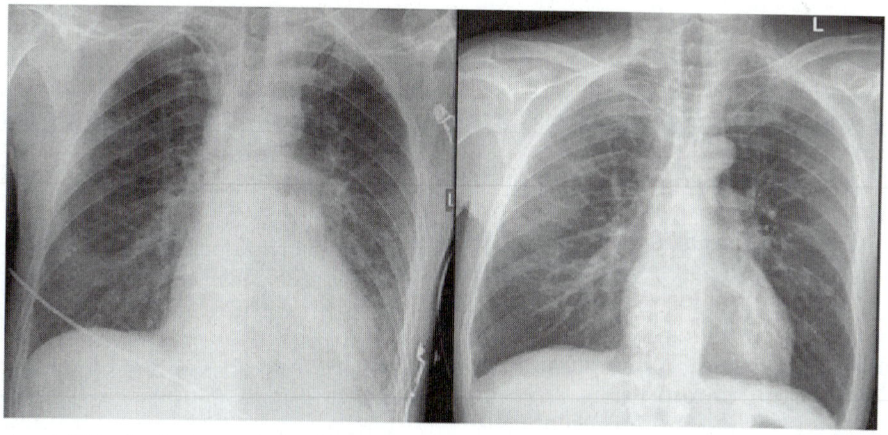

Fig. 47.58: *(Left) X-ray chest (PA view) showed significant cardiomegaly due to heart failure. (Right) showed normal sized heart after therapeutic doses of B1*

- Then, the progression of vasodilatation is perceived by the kidney as a relative loss of volume. The ensuing activation of the renin angiotensin system produces greater salt and water retention.
- Consequently, further fluid overload results in peripheral edema and pulmonary effusions.
- Cardiac overuse injury that occurs in the above setting results in tachycardia, hypertension and chest pain.
- Thyrotoxicosis, a more common cause of high-output cardiac failure, is always among the differential diagnoses.

Dry Beri-beri

- This phenotype affects the neuromuscular system.
- Polyneuritis and symmetric, ascending paralysis of the peripheral nerve systems predominate.
- The sensory system is affected first, followed by the motor and autonomic systems.
- Typically, tactile sensation is the first to be lost, followed by pain, and, finally, temperature.
- Paresthesia and hyperesthesia usually begin with the lower extremities and gradually involve the upper extremities and perioral area.
- Deep tendon reflexes are lost, calf muscles become painful, and foot drop and, eventually, wrist dropoccur.
- If untreated, progressive weakness, wasting of muscles, and, ultimately, complete paralysis occur.
- Encephalopathy is an alternative mode of presentation, with vomiting, disorientation, horizontal nystagmus, palsies of the eye movements (ophthalmoplegia), ataxia, and progressive mental impairment.
- Korsakoff syndrome is a more ominous condition that usually precludes complete recovery. Confusion is followed by the loss of recent memory and confabulation, which is the creation of accounts of events to cover up the loss of memory.

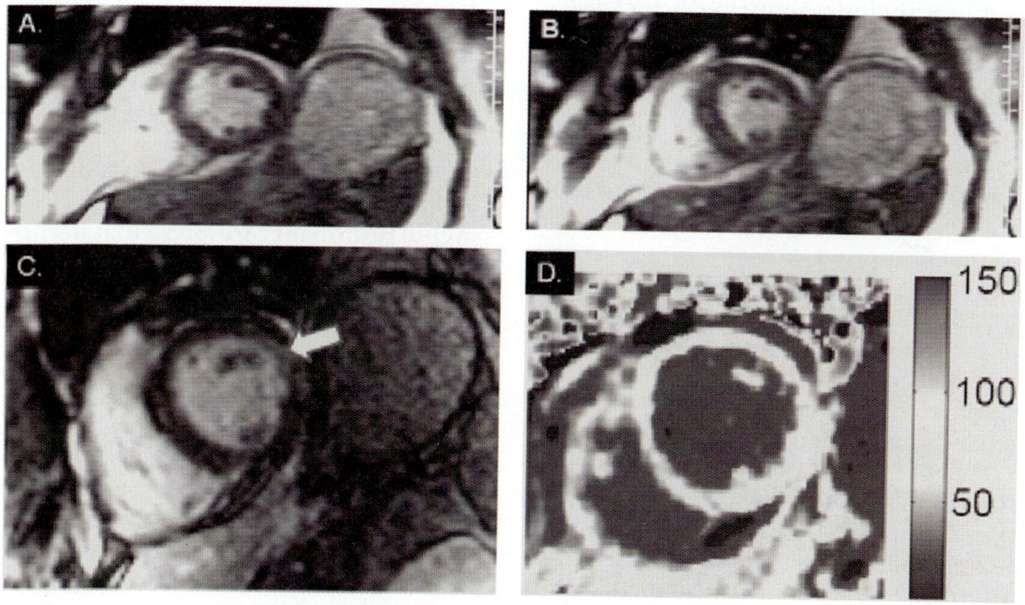

Fig. 47.59: *CMR findings in wet beri-beri. End-diastolic (A) and end-systolic (B) frames from short-axis cine imaging demonstrate global hypokinesis of the left ventricle. (C) LGE image shows borderline hyperenhancement of the basal lateral wall (arrow). (D) T2 mapping demonstrates significantly elevated myocardial T2 values suggestive of diffuse edemain a patient with beri-beri heart disease*

- **Infantile thiamine deficiency**
  This occurs in various forms and typically affects breastfed infants whose mothers had beri-beri.
- Early on, the infant is constipated, crying, restless, and has emesis. Three forms are recognized.
- The pure cardiologic or pernicious form is common in infants aged 1–3 months. They present with cyanosis and features of acute cardiac failure. Infants usually die within 2–4 hours, but this type of deficiency responds very rapidly to thiamine.
- The aphonic form is seen in infants aged 4–6 months. This milder form causes loss of voice due to paralysis of the vocal cords. The pseudomeningitic form is encountered in infants aged 7–9 months. It presents with clinical signs of meningitis, but cerebrospinal fluid findings exclude infection. Vomiting, sweating, and seizures may be present.

Wernicke-Korsakoff Syndrome

- This is an autosomal recessive genetic disease seen most often in Europeans.
- Affected patients have transketolases that bind thiamine pyrophosphate 10 times less frequently than normal. Patients with Wernicke-Korsakoff are much more sensitive to less severe thiamine deficiency.
- This syndrome occurs most often in individuals with alcoholism who are malnourished. It is often precipitated by administration of glucose because excessive carbohydrate metabolism exacerbates a subclinical thiamine deficiency. Clinically, it combines features of both Wernicke encephalopathy and Korsakoff psychosis.

Subclinical Thiamine Deficiency

- This deficiency is seen in people with high carbohydrate intake and low thiamine intake.
- Other at-risk groups include those with increased thiamine requirements because of raised physiological or metabolic demands. Clinical scenarios include pregnancy and lactation, heavy physical exertion, intercurrent illness (e.g. cancer, liver diseases, infections, hyperthyroidism) and surgery.
- This deficiency is rarely encountered in patients with increased losses, such as those seen with dialysis, chronic diuretic use, and malabsorption.
- Symptoms are usually mild, with anorexia often the presenting symptom. Anorexia is regarded to be a protective phenomenon because continued intake of a high-carbohydrate diet could be detrimental.
- Other early symptoms include weakness, aching, burning sensation in the hands and feet, indigestion, irritability, and depression. After 6–8 weeks, the only objective signs at rest may be a slight fall in blood pressure and moderate weight loss. After 2-3 months, apathy and weakness become extreme and calf muscle tenderness develops. Also, loss of recent memory, confusion, ataxia, and sometimes, persistent vomiting occur.
- Pediatric associations include growth restriction and sudden infant death syndrome (SIDS).

Causes

- Beri-beri is caused by thiamine deficiency, which can be the result of different physiologic, dietary, and environmental factors. Frequently, more than one risk factor is present.

Laboratory Studies

- The most rapid, and thus the best diagnostic test in urgent situations, is observing a clinical response to administration of intravenous thiamine (few hours duration). The most reliable in vitro laboratory tests involve measurement of whole blood or erythrocyte transketolase activity. An enhancement of enzymatic activity from the in vitro addition of TPP is referred to as the TPP effect.
- An increase in the enzymatic activity of more than 15% strongly supports the diagnosis of thiamine deficiency.
- A depressed blood level of thiamine can be seen.
- Elevated measurements of the following substances are characteristically noted because their metabolism depends on enzymes that have thiamine as their cofactors:
- Pyruvate
- Alpha-ketoglutarate
- Lactate
- Glycosylate
- Physical

Wet Beri-beri (Cardiac) (Fig. 47.54)

- Edema
- Waxy skin (Fig. 47.56)
- Vomiting
- Widened pulse pressure
- Systolic flow murmur
- Gallop rhythm (third heart sound); best heard in left-lateral position during inspiration
- Jugular venous distension
- Tachycardia
- Cardiomegaly (Fig. 47.55 and 47.58)
- Pallor
- **ECG changes** (prolonged QT, T-wave inversion, low voltage) (Fig. 47.57)
- **Acute fulminant cardiovascular beri-beri (shoshin beri-beri or occidental beri-beri)**
- Breathlessness, cyanosis
- Wet crackles in lower lung fields
- Classic heart failure
- **Dry beri-beri (paralytic or nervous)**
- Pallor
- Wasting
- Listlessness
- Tachycardia
- Hepatomegaly
- Symmetric peripheral neuropathy
- Symmetric paresthesias, especially of the distal extremities, with diminished touch sensation
- Weakness (starting with feet)

- Loss of ankle and knee reflexes
- Normal vibration and pain sensation
- Wernicke disease
- Irritability, forgetfulness
- Ataxia
- Mental confusion
- Nystagmus (horizontal more common than vertical)
- Ptosis
- Ophthalmoplegia
- Delirium
- Coma
- Korsakoff psychosis
- Retrograde amnesia
- Inability to learn
- Confabulation
- Wernicke-Korsakoff syndrome—combined features of both Wernicke disease and Korsokoff disease

Korsakoff Psychosis

- Infantile beri-beri
- Physical findings depend on the form but usually begin with nonspecific early findings including the following:
- Fatigue
- Anorexia
- Headaches
- Irritability, fatigue
- The physical findings in acute cardiac infantile beri-beri are similar to those found in Shoshin beri-beri, often with cyanosis.

The physical findings in aphonic infantile beri-beri include hoarseness that progresses to a complete loss of crying. The physical findings in pseudomeningeal infantile beri-beri include nystagmus, muscle twitching, bulging fontanelle, convulsions and coma.

Additional investigations that have been proposed as diagnostic tests include the following:

- Urinary thiamine
- Thiamine metabolites (thiazole or pyrimidine)
- Methylglyoxal values
- Unexplained lactic acidosis that persists after fluid bolus should prompt consideration of beri-beri.

Imaging Studies (Fig. 47.59)

- In infants, thiamine deficiency is characterized by involvement of the frontal lobes and basal ganglia, in addition to lesions present in the periaqueductal region, thalami, and the mammillary bodies that have been described in adults.
- MR spectroscopy (MRS) reveals a characteristic lactate peak
- Other tests
- Diffuse slowing of the EEG can be observed.

Procedures

- An intravenous push of thiamine is recommended in a deteriorating patient who has features suggestive of beri-beri.

Histologic Findings

- The histologic lesions of wet beri-beri have been reported to be due to degeneration of myelin in the muscular sheaths without inflammation.

Treatment

Medical Care

- Monitor patients with cardiac failure in an intensive care unit. Because beri-beri often presents with other vitamin B deficiencies, administer a complete vitamin B complex. After the high-output state has been addressed with thiamine, patients can go into standard congestive heart failure and, thus, may require ongoing cardiology consultation, possibly remaining in an intensive care unit.

Consultations

- Cardiologic evaluation with two dimensional echocardiography is necessary.
- Essential for diagnosis and management of beri-beri
- Reveals congestive heart failure and the poor ventricular function observed in beri-beri
- Assists in cardiac dysfunction that remains after thiamine administration.
- Neurologic and psychiatric consultations are usually necessary. If dry beri-beri has progressed, ongoing care is required.

  Nutritional consultation should be aimed at preventing a recurrence of the deficiency.
- For psychosocial causes, support counseling is essential to avoid recurrence. Specialized multidisciplinary teams are advisable for patients with chronic alcoholism to monitor their future course. Comprehensive follow-up programs are necessary to minimize recidivism in most cases of nutritional beri-beri.

Diet

- Patients with lethargy, confusion, and severe heart failure need to be kept on a diet of nothing by mouth (NPO) to prevent aspiration.
- Dietary sources of thiamine must be emphasized along with ongoing supplementation.

ACTIVITY

Patients who present with congestive heart failure should have activity restricted.

The treatment of choice is thiamine hydrochloride (i.e. aneurine hydrochloride, vitamin B_1). In a prospective study of the safety of thiamine hydrochloride, Wrenn et al evaluated 989 patients (1,070 doses of 100 mg). A total of 12 adverse reactions (1.1%) were reported. Minor reactions consisting of transient local irritation were observed in 11 patients (1.02%), and only one major reaction occurred (0.093%), consisting of generalized pruritus. Several thiamine derivatives [e.g. thiamine propyl disulfide (TPD), thiamine tetrahydrofurfuryl disulfide (TTFD)] have also been used to treat beri-beri. These compounds are barely soluble in water. Even when orally administered, TPD and

TTFD produce a higher thiamine level in the blood than thiamine hydrochloride.

If beriberi occurs in a breastfed infant, both the mother and child should be treated with thiamine. The physician should also be aware that thiamine deficiency can occur concurrently with other water soluble vitamin deficiencies.

Drug Vitamins

These agents are organic substances required by the body in small amounts for various metabolic processes. Vitamins may be synthesized in small or insufficient amounts in the body or may not be synthesized at all, thus requiring supplementation.

Complications

- GI complaints including constipation and colicky abdominal pain
- Muscle wasting
- Vision or hearing impairment
- Complete paralysis
- Ataxia
- Profound loss of recent memory with active imagination
- Delirium
- Death.

Prognosis

- In patients with wet beri-beri, improvement is observed in the first 6–24 hours after thiamine administration.
- Cyanosis disappears
- The heart rate reduces
- The respiratory rate reduces
- Diuresis and reduction in heart size may be apparent within 1–2 days.
- In patients with dry beri-beri, the complete resolution of the peripheral neurologic symptoms can take weeks to months. In patients with Wernicke encephalopathy, the ocular symptoms resolve within hours to days, and the confusional state subsides in days to weeks. Korsakoff syndrome resolves over months, and residual deficits are often reported.

RICKETS (VITAMIN D-DEFICIENCY)

Rickets is a disease of growing bone that is unique to children and adolescents. It is caused by a failure of osteoid to calcify in a growing person. Failure of osteoid to calcify in adults is called osteomalacia. Vitamin D deficiency rickets occurs when the metabolites of vitamin D are deficient. Less commonly, a dietary deficiency of calcium or phosphorus may also produce rickets. Vitamin D_3 (cholecalciferol) is formed in the skin from a derivative of cholesterol under the stimulus of ultraviolet-B light. Ultraviolet light or cod liver oil was the only significant source of vitamin D until early in the 20th century when ergosterol (vitamin D_2) was synthesized from irradiated plant steroids.

During the Industrial Revolution, rickets appeared in epidemic form in temperate zones where the pollution from factories blocked the sun's ultraviolet rays. Thus, rickets was probably the first childhood disease caused by environmental pollution.

Natural nutritional sources of vitamin D are limited primarily to fatty, ocean-going fish. In the United States, dairy milk is fortified with vitamin D (400 IU/L). Human milk contains little vitamin D, generally less than 20–40 IU/L. Therefore, infants who are breastfed are at risk for rickets, especially those who receive no oral supplementation and those who have darkly pigmented skin, which blocks penetration of ultraviolet light (Fig. 47.60).

Pathophysiology (Fig. 47.61)

Cholecalciferol (i.e. vitamin D_3) is formed in the skin from 5-dihydrotachysterol. This steroid undergoes hydroxylation in 2 steps. The first hydroxylation occurs at position 25 in the liver, producing calcidiol (25-hydroxycholecalciferol), which circulates in the plasma as the most abundant of the vitamin D metabolites and is thought to be a good indicator of overall vitamin D status. The second hydroxylation step occurs in the kidney at the 1 position, where it undergoes hydroxylation to the active metabolite calcitriol (1,25-dihydroxycholecalciferol). This cholecalciferol is not technically a vitamin but a hormone.

Calcitriol acts at 3 known sites to tightly regulate calcium metabolism. Calcitriol promotes absorption of calcium and phosphorus from the intestine, increases reabsorption of phosphate in the kidney, and acts on bone to release calcium and phosphate. Calcitriol may also directly facilitate calcification. These actions increase the concentrations of calcium and phosphorus in extracellular fluid. The increase of calcium and phosphorus in extracellular fluid, in turn, leads to the calcification of osteoid, primarily at the metaphyseal growing ends of bones but also throughout all osteoid in the skeleton. Parathyroid hormone facilitates the 1-hydroxylation step in vitamin D metabolism.

In the vitamin D deficiency state, hypocalcemia develops, which stimulates excess parathyroid hormone, which stimulates renal phosphorus loss, further reducing deposition of calcium in the bone. Excess parathyroid hormone also produces changes in the bone similar to those occurring in hyperparathyroidism. Early in the course of rickets, the calcium concentration in the serum decreases. After the parathyroid response, the calcium concentration usually returns to the reference range though phosphorus levels remain low. Alkaline phosphatase, which is produced by overactive osteoblast cells, leaks to the extracellular fluids so that its concentration rises to anywhere from moderate elevation to very high levels.

Intestinal malabsorption of fat and diseases of the liver or kidney may produce the clinical and secondary biochemical picture of nutritional rickets. Anticonvulsant drugs (e.g. phenobarbital, phenytoin) accelerate metabolism of calcidiol, which may lead to insufficiency and rickets, particularly in children who are kept indoors in institutions.

Calcium and vitamin D intakes are low in infants who are fed vegan diets, particularly lactovegans, and monitoring of their vitamin D status is essential.

Incidence

In the United States, vitamin D deficiency rickets does not occur in formula-fed infants because formula and milk sold in the United States contains 400 IU of vitamin D per liter. Except in pediatric patients with chronic malabsorption syndromes or end-stage renal disease, nearly all cases of rickets occur in breastfed infants who have dark skin and receive no vitamin D supplementation. Incidence in Europe is similar to that in the United States. In sunny areas, such as in the Middle East, rickets may occur when infants are bundled in clothing and are not exposed to sunlight. In some parts of Africa, deficiency of calcium, phosphorus, or both in the diet may also lead to rickets, especially in societies were corn is predominant in the diet.

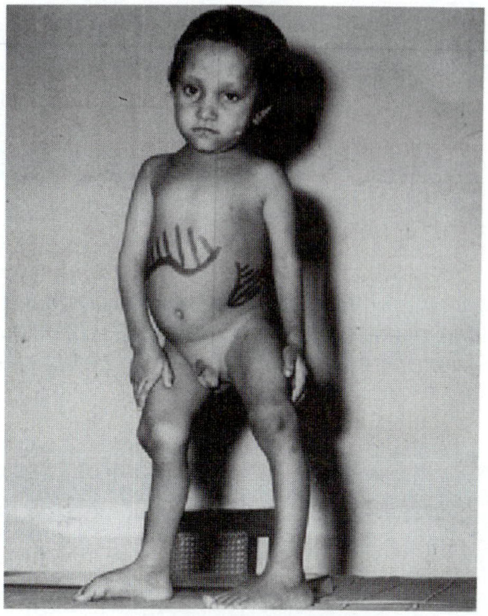

Fig. 47.60: *Bony deformities of lower legs with widening of the bony ends in a 6-yrs-old boy with clinical rickets*

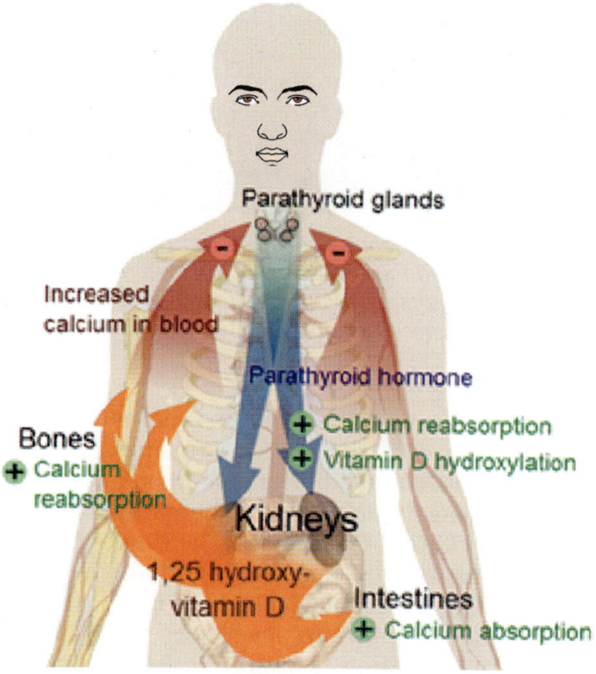

Fig. 47.61: *Calcium regulation from different organs of the body*

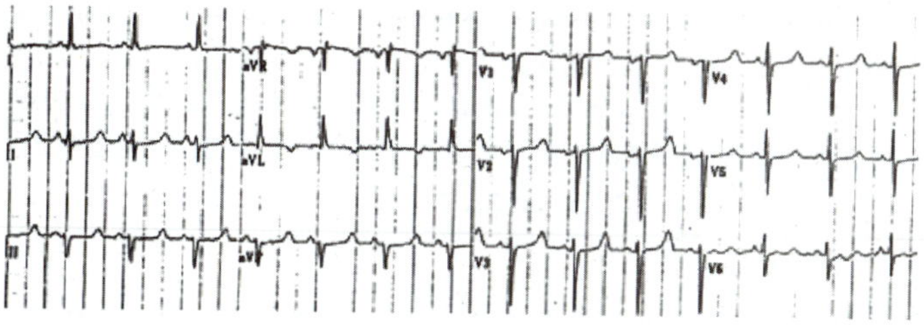

Fig. 47.62: *ECG showing prolonged QTc 510 ms due to hypocalcaemia*

Mortality/Morbidity

Skeletal deformity and short stature may occur. Severe rickets has been associated with respiratory failure in children, and resulting pelvic distortion in females may lead to problems with vaginal delivery later in life.

Race

Individuals with dark skin are at increased risk for vitamin D deficiency rickets.

Sex

No sexual predilection is noted.

Age

By definition, rickets is observed only in growing children although the effects may be observed later in life.

History

- Generalized muscular hypotonia of an unknown mechanism is observed in most patients with clinical (as opposed to biochemical and radiographic) signs of rickets. Craniotabes manifests early in infants with vitamin D deficiency, although this feature may be normal in infants, especially for those born prematurely.
- If rickets occurs at a later age, thickening of the skull develops. This produces frontal bossing and delays the closure of the anterior fontanelle. In the long bones, laying down of uncalcified osteoid at the metaphases leads to spreading of those areas, producing knobby deformity, which is visualized on radiography as cupping and flaring of the metaphyses.
- Weight bearing produces deformities such as bowlegs and knock-knees.
- In the chest, knobby deformities results in the rachitic rosary along the costochondral junctions. The weakened ribs pulled by muscles also produce flaring over the diaphragm, which is known as Harrison groove. The sternum may be pulled into a pigeon-breast deformity.
- In more severe instances in children older than 2 years, vertebral softening leads to kyphoscoliosis. The ends of

the long bones demonstrate that same knobby thickening. At the ankle, palpation of the tibial malleolus gives the impression of a double epiphysis (Marfan sign). Because the softened long bones may bend, they may fracture one side of the cortex (i.e. greenstick fracture).

Lab Studies

- Early on in the disease course, the calcium (ionized fraction) is low; however it is often within the reference range at the time of diagnosis as parathyroid hormone levels increase.
- Calcidiol (25-hydroxy vitamin D) levels are low, and parathyroid hormone levels are elevated; however, determining calcidiol and parathyroid hormone levels is typically not necessary. Calcitriol levels maybe normal or elevated because of increased parathyroid activity.
- The phosphorus level is invariably low for age unless recent partial treatment or recent exposure to sunlight has occurred.
- Alkaline phosphatase levels are elevated.
- A generalized aminoaciduria occurs from the parathyroid activity; aminoaciduria does not occur in familial hypophosphatemia rickets (FHR).

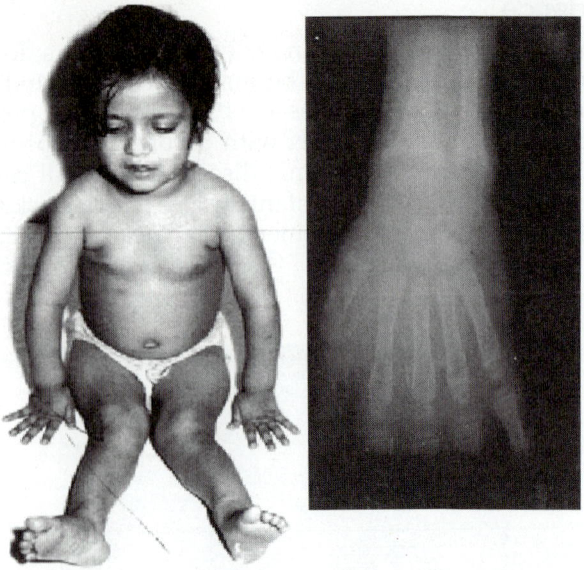

Fig. 47.63: *Bony deformities of lower legs with genu valgum (left) and radiological features of active rickets with cupping, fraying and increased distance between epiphysis and metaphysis in hand bone (right) in a 6-yrs-old boy with clinical rickets*

Imaging Studies (Figs 47.62–47.64)

- The best single radiographic view for infants and children younger than 3 years is an anterior view of the knee that reveals the metaphyseal end and epiphysis of the femur and tibia. This site is best because growth is most rapid in this location, thus the changes are accentuated.

The metaphyses exhibit widening and cupping because of their exaggerated normal concavity and irregular calcification. Because calcified osteoid is abundant, the provisional calcification zone of the metaphysis is much more distant from the calcification center of the epiphysis than is normal for age. Along the shaft, the uncalcified osteoid causes the periosteum to appear separated from the diaphysis. Generalized osteomalacia occurs (observed as osteopenia), with visible coarsening of trabeculae in contrast to the ground-glass osteopenia of scurvy.

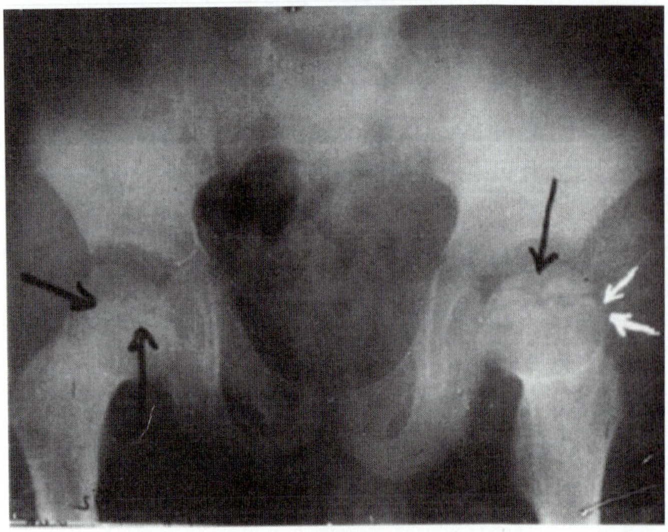

Fig. 47.64: *X-ray leg bones at the region of hip joints showing bony deformities of bones with radiological features of active ricket with epiphysiseal dysgenesis and rarefaction (arrows) in a 10-yrs-old boy with clinical rickets*

Other Tests

- Serum measurements include calcium, phosphorus, alkaline phosphatase, parathyroid hormone, 25-hydroxy vitamin D, and 1,25-dihydroxy vitamin D.

Treatment

- Treatment for rickets may be gradually administered over several months or in a single-day dose of 15,000 mcg (600,000 U) of vitamin D. If the gradual method is chosen, 125–250 mcg (5000–10,000 U) is given daily for 2–3 months until healing is well established and the alkaline phosphatase concentration is approaching the reference range. Because this method requires daily treatment, success depends on compliance.
- If the vitamin D dose is administered in a single day, it is usually divided into 4 or 6 oral doses. An intramuscular injection is also available. Vitamin D is well stored in the body and is gradually released over many weeks. Because both calcitriol and calcidiol have short half-lives, they are unsuitable; they would bypass the natural physiologic controls of vitamin D synthesis. The single-day therapy avoids problems with compliance and may be helpful in differentiating nutritional rickets from FHR. In nutritional rickets, the phosphorous level rises in 96 hours and radiographic healing is visible in 6–7 days. Neither happens with FHR.

- If severe deformities have occurred, orthopedic correction may be required after healing. Most of the deformities correct with growth.

Drug Category: Vitamin D

Fat-soluble vitamin used to treat vitamin D deficiency or for prophylaxis of deficiency.

Drug: Cholecalciferol (Delta-D)

Description: Vitamin D_3. 1 mg provides 40000 IU vitamin D activity.

Pediatric dose: Single-day dose method: 15,000 mcg (600,000 U) PO qd divided in 4–6 doses for 1 d. Gradual method: 125–250 mcg (5,000–10,000 U) qd for 2–3 months.

Clinical Implications

The possibility of a causal link between vitamin D deficiency and cardiovascular disease is supported by biological plausibility, the demonstration of a temporal association, and the finding of a dose response between 25-OH D deficiency and risk. These data raise the possibility that treatment of vitamin D deficiency, via supplementation or lifestyle measures, could reduce cardiovascular risk. However, treatment strategies suggested by observational data are not always borne out by randomized trials, as evidenced by studies of hormone replacement therapy and B vitamins for homocysteine lowering. Problems related to the use of observational data include indication bias, confounding, and reverse causation. Several features of the study design suggest that the present data may be less susceptible to these problems. First, we used a direct, objective measure of vitamin D status (25-OH D levels) rather than relying on self-reported vitamin D intake or sunlight exposure. Second, 25-OH D levels were assessed on blood samples drawn at baseline, years before the acute cardiovascular events. Third, cardiovascular risk factors and comorbid diagnoses are well characterized in the Framingham Offspring cohort, which has been followed for >3 decades.

In small clinical trials, vitamin D supplementation has promoted reductions in blood pressure, left ventricular hypertrophy, and inflammatory cytokines. On the other hand, Hsia and colleagues recently reported that use of calcium and vitamin D supplements was not associated with a reduction in cardiovascular events in the Women's Health Initiative. These apparently discrepant findings could be attributable to several factors. First, the Women's Health Initiative was a fracture-prevention trial and was not designed to evaluate cardiovascular risk. Second, the dose of vitamin D in the treatment arm (400 IU/d) was far below the amount necessary to correct vitamin D deficiency (>800 IU/d) or doses used in previous cardiovascular studies. Third, patients in the placebo arm were allowed to take vitamin D supplements, which resulted in a mean consumption of vitamin D in the placebo arm of nearly 400 IU/d. Lastly, baseline 25-OH D levels were not measured in the Women's Health Initiative; thus, the trial did not address whether vitamin D supplementation benefited individuals with vitamin D deficiency, because enrollment was performed irrespective of vitamin D status. It is noteworthy that vitamin D did appear to reduce cardiovascular risk in obese individuals, who are prone to endogenous vitamin D deficiency, and also in those with multiple coronary risk factors. The mean body mass index among individuals with vitamin D deficiency in the present study was >30 kg/m^2, in the overweight-to-obese range.

The present data, although observational, permit an assessment of cardiovascular risk across a broad range of baseline 25-OH D levels and could motivate additional prospective or interventional studies. Still, barriers to future trials of vitamin D for cardiovascular prevention exist. A primary prevention trial would require a very large sample and may be hampered by the perception that it would be unethical to randomize individuals with moderate vitamin D deficiency to placebo therapy. In this regard, additional observational studies could be used to identify surrogate end points or subgroups most likely to benefit from vitamin D supplementation, which may facilitate smaller trials.

SCURVY (DEFICIENCY OF VITAMIN C) (Fig. 47.65)

Scurvy, a state of dietary deficiency of vitamin C (ascorbic acid) is an ancient disease. Egyptians recorded its symptoms as early as 1550 BC. Scurvy was the scourge of the sea explorers of the Renaissance era (16th–18th centuries). In 1746, James Lind, a British naval surgeon, established the fact that oranges and lemons were effective in curing scurvy. The incidence of scurvy among the British sailors sharply declined upon routine provision of lemon juice on board. During the 19th century, people who experienced the Great Potato Famine, armies of the Crimean War and American Civil War, Arctic explorers, and California Gold Rush communities were prominent victims of "land" scurvy. Francis Glisson is credited with the earliest description of infantile scurvy. In 1650, Glisson observed the co-occurrence of scurvy in infants with rickets. After Glisson's description, infantile scurvy was not reported for another 200 years. By the end of the 19th century, infantile scurvy was readily recognized and frequently observed in Britain and the United States. The increased incidence of infantile scurvy during this era was attributed to the consumption of heated milk and proprietary foods deficient in vitamin C.

In 1912, Holst and Frolisch induced and cured scurvy in guinea pigs through dietary modification. Utilization of an animal model for induction and treatment of scurvy was a major advance. Soon, human experiments followed. In 1914, Alfred Hess, a pediatrician practicing at the Hebrew Asylum in New York, observed an increase in scurvy among the infants at the asylum. This increase in scurvy coincided with the introduction of pasteurized milk and exclusion of orange juice from the infants' diet (Fig. 47.65).

Modifying the infants' diet, with the provision of raw milk or orange juice or potatoes, Hess reversed the scurvy and effected a cure. Hess had demonstrated that pasteurization results in the loss of vitamin C. He recommended the provision of fresh fruit or vegetable juice for the prevention of scurvy in infants fed on heated

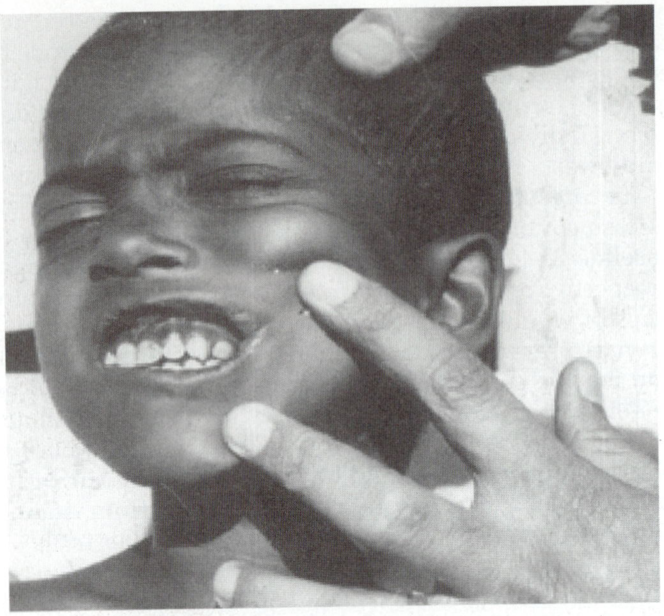

Fig. 47.65: *Gingival hypertrophy and bleeding, anemia with other physical and radiological signs of scurvy in a 7-yrs-old boy who did not consume vegetables or citrous fruits till date of examination*

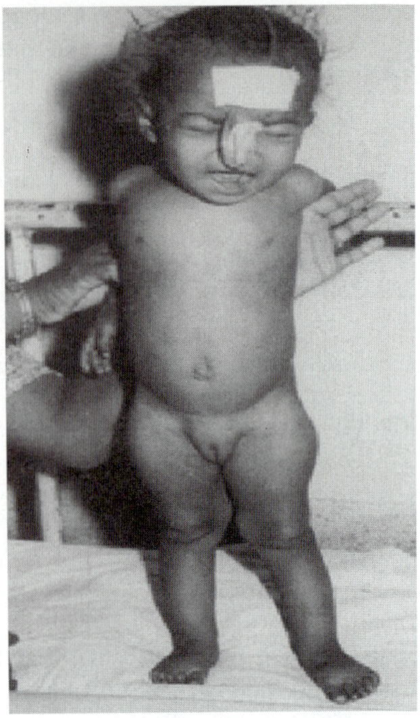

Fig. 47.67: *Stunted physical growth, anemia and edema feet with bloody diarrhoea with other physical and radiological signs in a 3-yrs-girl with clinical scurvy*

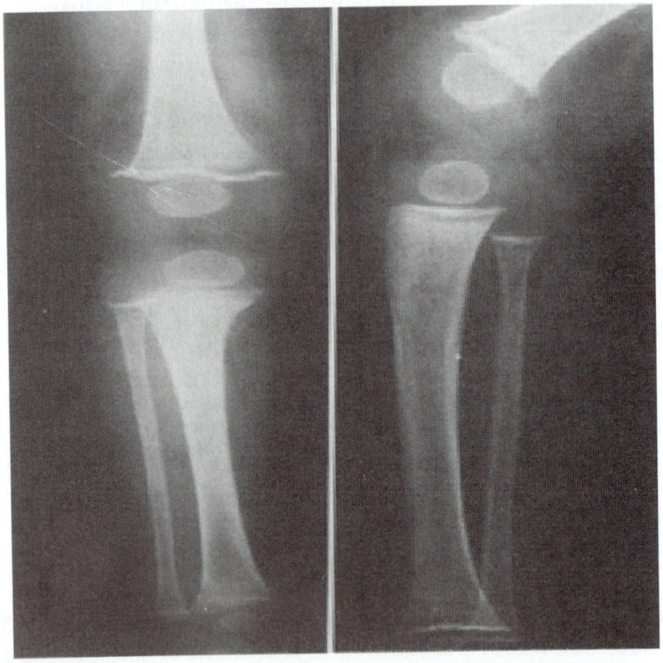

Fig. 47.66: *X-ray leg bones at the region of knee joint showing white line of Frankel, corner sign and spur formation in a young child with scurvy*

formulas. This practice of supplementing the diet of infants receiving heated formulas with fresh fruit or vegetable juices eventually led to the eradication of infantile scurvy in the United States.

The human body lacks the ability to synthesize and make vitamin C and therefore depends on exogenous dietary sources to meet vitamin C needs. Consumption of fruits and vegetables or diets fortified with vitamin C are essential to avoid ascorbic acid deficiency. Even though scurvy is uncommon, it still occurs and can affect adults and children who have chronic dietary vitamin C deficiency.

Pathophysiology

Vitamin C is functionally most relevant for collagen synthesis, and a vitamin C deficiency results in impaired collagen synthesis. The typical pathologic manifestations of vitamin C deficiency are noted in collagen-containing tissues and in organs and tissues such as skin, cartilage, dentine, osteoid and capillary blood vessels. Pathologic changes are a function of the rate of growth of the affected tissues; hence, the bone changes are often observed only in infants during periods of rapid bone growth.

Defective collagen synthesis leads to defective dentine formation, hemorrhaging into the gums, and loss of teeth. Hemorrhaging is a hallmark feature of scurvy and can occur in any organ. Hair follicles are one of the common sites of cutaneous bleeding.

Bone involvement is typical for infantile scurvy. The bony changes occur at the junction between the end of the diaphysis and growth cartilage. Osteoblasts fail to form osteoid (bone matrix), resulting in cessation of endochondral bone formation. Calcification of the growth cartilage at the end of the long bones continues, leading to the thickening of the growth plate. The typical invasion of the growth cartilage by the capillaries does not occur. Preexisting bone becomes brittle and undergoes resorption at a normal rate, resulting in microscopic fractures of the spicules between the shaft and calcified cartilage. With these fractures, the periosteum becomes loosened, resulting

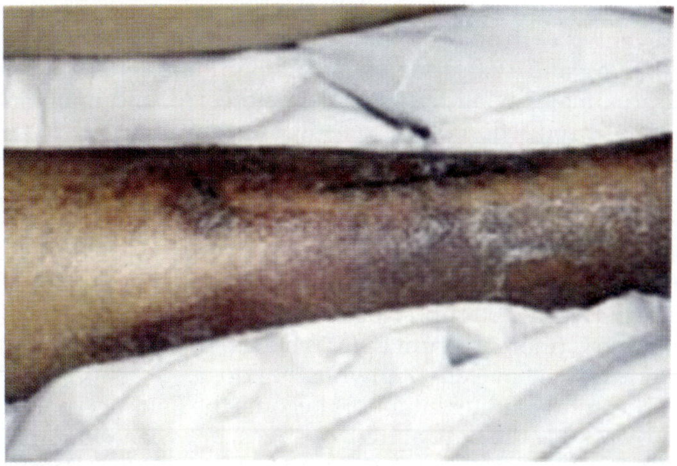

Fig. 47.68: *Lower extremity abnormalities in scurvy. The patient had xerosis, accompanied by ecchymoses and increased pigmentation from repeated cutaneous hemorrhages. A linear superficial wound covered with hemorrhagic crust has been present for an extended period, indicating impaired wound healing*

in the classic subperiosteal hemorrhage at the ends of the long bones. Intraarticular hemorrhage is rare because the periosteal attachment to the growth plate is very firm.

Cardiovascular Diseases and Vitamin C

Besides being essential for collagen synthesis, ascorbic acid is important for biosynthesis of carnitine and neurotransmitters and in hematopoiesis by promoting iron absorption.

Those few species that fail to synthesize ascorbic acid (vitamin C) are prone to a form of heart disease? That is not prevalent in other species. The theory that Cardiovascular Disease (CVD) is related to a deficiency of vitamin C was first proposed by the Canadian Physician G. C. Willis in 1953. He found that atherosclerotic plaques form over vitamin-C-starved vascular tissues in both guinea pigs and human beings. In 1989, after the discoveries of the Lp(a) cholesterol molecule (circa 1964) and its lysine binding sites (circa 1987), ***Linus Pauling and his associate Matthias Rath*** formulated a unified theory of heart disease and invented a cure. Vitamin C and lysine (and proline) in large amounts become Lp(a) binding inhibitors that restore vascular health and are patented to destroy atherosclerotic plaques.

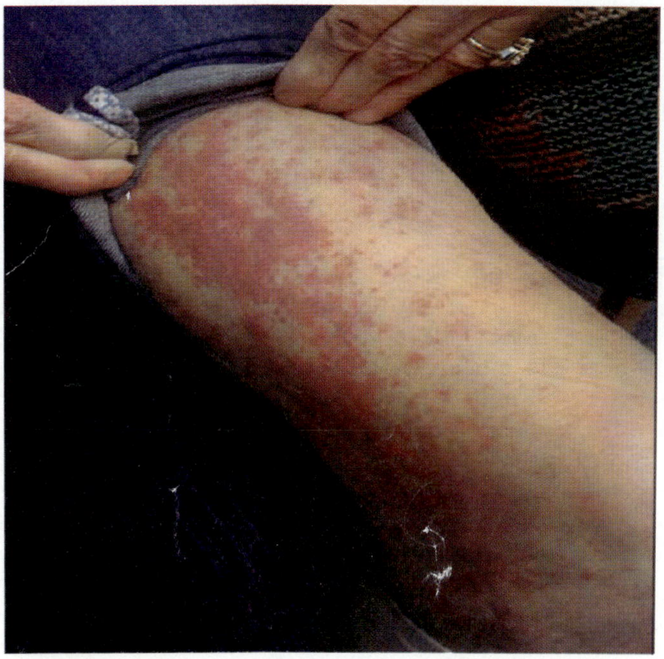

Fig. 47.69: *Perifollicular hemorrhage in scurvy*

Chronic scurvy: Heart disease is a misnomer; the underlying disease process reduces the supply of blood to the heart and other organs leading to angina ("heart cramp"), heart attack and stroke. The disease is characterized by scab-like build-ups that grow on the walls of blood vessels. The correct terminology for this disease process is chronic scurvy, a slower form of the classic vitamin C deficiency disease.

The hypothesis that CVD is an ascorbic acid (vitamin C) deficiency disease was first conceived and tested in Canada. Willis devised a method of photographing plaques with X-rays and observed that atherosclerotic plaques were not uniformly distributed throughout the vascular system; rather these "blockages" are concentrated near the heart, where arteries are constantly bent or squeezed.

Another Canadian, Paterson, had found that the tissues of heart patients were generally depleted of vitamin C, and it was well known that vitamin C is required for strong and healthy arteries. Willis reasoned that only the mechanical stress caused by the pulse could explain the typical pattern of atherosclerosis. To Willis, the body was laying down plaque precisely where it was needed in order to stabilize the vascular system.

By the late 1980s, medical researchers had made several intriguing discoveries.

First came the discovery that heart disease begins with a lesion, a crack or stress fracture, in the arterial wall. The question became, and remains, as to the cause of these lesions in human beings since they do not arise in most other animals. Then a variant of the so-called "bad" LDL cholesterol called lipoprotein(a), or Lp(a) for short, was studied and found to be really bad. Lp(a) is sticky because of receptors on the surface of the molecule called lysine binding sites. Work that led to the 1987 Nobel prize in medicine discovered that lysine (and proline) binding sites cause the formation of atherosclerotic plaques. Then, Beisiegel et al in Germany examined plaques post mortem and found only Lp(a), not ordinary LDL cholesterol.

Lp(a) was the genetic difference between beings that suffer cardiovascular disease and those that do not. Lp(a) had evolved only in species that do not make their own vitamin C (e.g. humans and guinea pigs).

Pauling and Rath repeated the earlier Willis experiments, but this time they monitored Lp(a). They discovered that it becomes elevated in guinea pigs deprived of vitamin C,

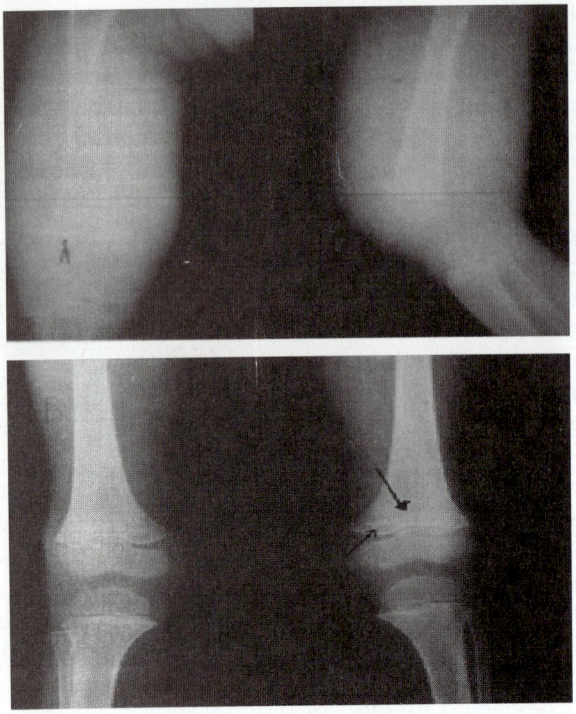

Fig. 47.70: *X-ray leg bones at the region of knee joint showing boggy swelling of the thigh (upper) rarefaction of the bones at metaphysis ans epiphysis with white line of Frankel (lower) in clinical scurvy*

but not in the controls. These experiments connected elevated-Lp(a) with low serum vitamin C. They realized that in most species, sufficient ascorbic acid will prevent stress fractures, but in those species that suffer chronic scurvy, Lp(a) had evolved to patch cracked blood vessels. As chronic scurvy progresses, the liver produces more Lp(a) molecules. As the number of Lp(a) molecules increases, they tend to deposit on top of existing plaque formations. When the healing process overshoots, the arteries narrow and the flow of blood is reduced.

This problem has a solution. The Lp(a) molecule has a finite number of lysine binding sites—points of attachment to lysine. Pauling's invention—the cure for heart disease—is to increase the serum concentration of the amino acid lysine enough to make the Lp(a) unattractive. As more lysine enters the blood stream, the probability increases that floating Lp(a) molecules will bind with it (rather than with the patches of plaques growing on the arterial walls). After all the Lp(a) molecules binding receptors are filled with the free lysine floating in the blood, the Lp(a) molecule becomes as harmless as ordinary LDL cholesterol.

Pauling and Rath called the substances that treat chronic scurvy and destroy existing plaques Lp(a) binding inhibitors. Vitamin C, to increase collagen production and to improve the health and strength of arteries, and lysine, to prevent and to dissolve Lp(a) plaques, are the primary binding inhibitors. These substances taken together are clinically effective.

Linus Pauling believed that chronic scurvy can be prevented with an orthomolecular daily intake of between 3,000 mg and 10,000 mg or more vitamin C. This amount approximates what the animals synthesize, and matching animal production is the reason Pauling ingested 18,000 mg daily.

Pauling and Rath's invention for destroying existing atherosclerotic plaques is the large amount of another essential nutrient, the amino acid lysine. Pauling filmed a video lecture in which he recommended that heart patients take between 2,000 and 6,000 mg of lysine daily with their vitamin C (more if serum Lp(a) is elevated). Neither vitamin C nor lysine have any known lethal dose.

The Lp(a) binding inhibitors become the Pauling Therapy for heart disease only at high dosages, between vitamin 3–18 g ascorbic acid and 3–6 g lysine. In his video, Pauling recounts the first cases where his high vitamin C and lysine therapy quickly resolved advanced cardiovascular disease in humans. The effect is so pronounced, and the inhibitors are so nontoxic, that Pauling doubted a clinical study was even necessary.

Recently, the amino acid proline was found to be an even more effective Lp(a) binding inhibitor than lysine in vitro. Adding between 5 g and 2 g proline may be of significant additional benefit. When serum Lp(a) is elevated, Lp(a) binding inhibitors can profoundly interfere with the disease process. Binding inhibitor formulas that include proline have been documented to lower Lp(a) in 6–14 months. In cases where Lp(a) is not reduced, binding inhibitors become even more important to neutralize Lp(a) regardless of their effect on serum Lp(a).

Recently a reevaluation of the Framingham Heart Study that Lp(a) and not ordinary LDL is highly predictive of CVD and Oxford found that elevated Lp(a) increases the risk of heart attack and stroke by 70%.

Incidence

Currently, scurvy occurs very rarely in the United States. Patients who are elderly or alcoholic and who subsist on diets devoid of fresh fruits and vegetables are vulnerable. Infants and children on restrictive diets because of medical, economic, or social reasons are at risk for scurvy. Occurrence of scurvy is uncommon in those younger than 7 months.

Global Occurance

International occurrence is unknown. A case series from Thailand reviewed 28 cases of scurvy in infants and children (10 mo to 9 y and 7 mo; median age, 29 mo) hospitalized over a 7-year period (1995–2002) and noted prolonged consumption of heated milk [ultra-high temperature (UHT) milk] and inadequate intake of vegetables and fruits as the risk factors for the development of scurvy. Epidemic scurvy has been reported among refugee populations.

Mortality/Morbidity

Sudden death due to cardiac failure is reported in infants and adults.

Predominant morbidity is a result of hemorrhage into various tissues. Subperiosteal hemorrhage in the tibia and femur causes excruciating pain.

Race

No racial predilection exists.

Sex

No sexual preponderance exists.

Age

Scurvy can occur at any age. Most cases of infantile scurvy occur when the infant is aged 6–24 months. Scurvy is uncommon in the neonatal period.

Clinical

History

Initial symptoms are nonspecific and include the following:
- Loss of appetite
- Peevishness
- Poor weight gain
- Diarrhea
- Tachypnea
- Fever

Specific symptoms include the following:
- Irritability
- Pain and tenderness of the legs
- Pseudoparalysis
- Swelling over the long bones
- Hemorrhage.

Physical (Figs 47.65, 47.67–47.69)

The infant is apprehensive, anxious, and progressively irritable. Upon handling and changing of diapers, severe tenderness over the thighs is present. The excruciating pain results in pseudoparalysis. The infant assumes the frog leg posture (i.e. keeping hips and knees slightly flexed and externally rotated) for comfort.
- Hemorrhages of the gums usually involve the tissue around the upper incisors. The gums have a bluish-purple hue and feel spongy. Gum hemorrhage occurs only if teeth have erupted.
- Subperiosteal hemorrhage is a typical finding of infantile scurvy. The lower ends of the femur and tibia are the most frequently involved sites. The subperiosteal hemorrhage is often palpable and tender in the acute phase.
  Petechial hemorrhage of the skin and mucous membranes can occur. Rarely, hematuria, hematochezia, and melena are noted.
- Proptosis of the eyeball secondary to orbital hemorrhage is a sign of scurvy.
- Costochondral beading or scorbutic rosary is a common finding. The scorbutic rosary is distinguished from rickety rosary (which is knobby and nodular) by being more angular and having a step-off at the costochondral junction. The sternum is typically depressed.
- Low-grade fever, anemia, and poor wound healing are signs of scurvy.
- Hyperkeratosis, corkscrew hair, and sicca syndrome are typically observed in adult scurvy but rarely occur in infantile scurvy.

Causes

- Inadequate intake of vitamin C
- Long sea voyages (historically)
- Famines
- Food faddism
- Ignorance (e.g. boiling of fruit juices)
- Neglect (e.g. self-imposed restrictive diets in anorexia nervosa)
- Restrictive diets imposed by food allergies
- Neurodevelopmental disabilities associated with compromised oral intake of foods.

Laboratory Studies

- Laboratory tests are usually not helpful to ascertain a diagnosis of scurvy. Presentation of an infant with the typical clinical and radiologic picture of scurvy, along with a supportive history of dietary deficiency of vitamin C, is often sufficient to diagnose infantile scurvy.
- Serum ascorbic acid levels
- A fasting serum ascorbic acid level greater than 0.6 mg/dL rules out scurvy.
- Serum ascorbic acid levels of 0.2 mg/dL or greater are considered nutritionally acceptable.
- Levels of 0.10–0.19 mg/dL are considered low.
- Levels less than 0.10 mg/dL are considered deficient. White blood cell ascorbic acid concentration is a more accurate measure of a vitamin C nutritional state.
- A level of zero indicates latent scurvy.
- Levels greater than 15 mg/dL reflect a state of nutritional adequacy.
- Levels of 8–15 mg/dL are considered low.
- Levels of 0–7 mg/dL reflect a state of deficiency.

Imaging Studies

- Radiologic findings in infantile scurvy are diagnostic. The characteristic radiologic changes occur at the growth cartilage-shaft junction of bones with rapid growth. The knee joint, wrist, and sternal ends of the ribs are typical sites of involvement (Figs 47.66 and 47.71).
- Radiologic diagnosis of scurvy is based on the following specific changes: In the early phase of scurvy, the cortex becomes thin and the trabecular structure of the medulla atrophies and develops a ground-glass appearance. The zone of provisional calcification becomes dense and widened, and this zone is referred to as the white line of Fränkel. The epiphysis also shows cortical thinning and the ground-glass appearance.

As scurvy becomes advanced, a zone of rarefaction occurs at the metaphysis under the white line. The zone of rarefaction typically involves the lateral aspects of the white line, resulting in triangular defects called the corner sign of Park. This area has multiple microscopic fractures and

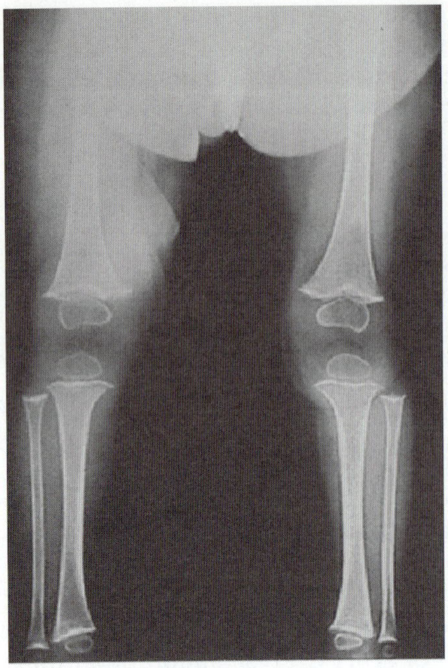

Fig. 47.71: *Radiograph of the lower extremities shows ground-glass osteopenia, a characteristic of scurvy*

may collapse with impaction of the calcified cartilage onto the shaft. The lateral aspect of the calcified cartilage can project as a spur. Subperiosteal hemorrhages are not visualized in the active phase. With healing, they become calcified and are readily observed.

Medical Care

- Vitamin C administered by mouth or the parenteral route is effective in curing infantile scurvy.
- Orange juice is an effective dietary remedy for curing infantile scurvy and was the standard treatment before the discovery of vitamin C.
- Upon instituting dietary or pharmacologic treatment, the clinical recovery is impressive. The appetite of the infant is recovered within 24–48 hours. The symptoms of irritability, fever, tenderness upon palpation, and hemorrhage generally resolve within 7 days.

Diet

A diet adequate in vitamin C can prevent the development of scurvy. The dietary requirements of vitamin C sufficient to prevent deficiency vary with the age of the individual. The following are the Food and Nutrition Board of the National Academy of Sciences, National Research Council's minimum recommended daily dietary allowances of vitamin C:

- Infants: 30–40 mg
- Children and adults: 45–60 mg
- Pregnant women: 70 mg
- Lactating mothers: 90–95 mg
- Food sources rich in vitamin C include the following:
  - Citrus fruits
  - Berries
  - Cantaloupe
  - Broccoli
  - Cauliflower
  - Cabbage
  - Spinach
  - Potatoes
  - Tomatoes.

Drug Therapy

Vitamins

Vitamins are organic substances required by the body in small amounts for various metabolic processes. Vitamins may be synthesized in small or insufficient amounts in the body or not synthesized at all, thus requiring supplementation. They are classified as either fat soluble or water soluble. Vitamins A, D, E and K are fat soluble whereas biotin, folic acid, niacin, pantothenic acid, B vitamins (i.e. B_1, B_2, B_6, B_{12}), and vitamin C are generally water soluble.

Vitamin deficiency may result from an inadequate diet, from increased requirements (e.g. pregnancy, lactation), or secondary to disease or drugs. Vitamin supplements are used clinically for the prevention and treatment of specific vitamin-deficiency states.

Drug: Ascorbic acid (Cecon, Ce-Vi-Sol, Dull-C)

Ascorbic acid (vitamin C) administered by mouth or parenterally effectively cures infantile and adult scurvy. Used by the body for collagen synthesis and tissue repair

Adult dose: 100–200 mg PO q6h for 1 wk

Pediatric dose: 25 mg PO q6h for 1 wk.

Complications

- Scurvy, if left untreated, can be fatal and has been associated with sudden death.
- Lethargy, fatigue, and hemorrhagic manifestations of impaired collagen synthesis affecting oral, ophthalmic, musculoskeletal, cardiac, and gastrointestinal structures and functions may occur.
- Cerebral hemorrhage or hemopericardium are potential complications that may lead to death.

Morbidity associated with hemorrhages depends on the site of involvement. Subperiosteal hemorrhages cause pain and tenderness resulting in pseudoparalysis. Loss of function at the site of the hemorrhage and anemia are typical sequelae of the hemorrhages observed in scurvy.

Prognosis

Typically, scurvy carries an excellent prognosis if diagnosed and treated appropriately.

ANEMIA AND HEART DISEASE

Blood is the body's delivery system. It carries oxygen and other nutrients around the body, delivering them to the cells that need them. At the same time, the blood picks up and takes away the waste products. One of the most important things the blood does is carry oxygen from the lungs to every cell, of every muscle and organ. Without that oxygen, cells could not operate properly. Hemoglobin is the part of the red blood cells that carry the oxygen.

Anemia, one of the more common blood disorders, occurs when the number of healthy red blood cells decreases in the body. The disc-shaped red blood cells contain hemoglobin, a unique molecule that carries oxygen to the body's tissues (Fig. 47.72).

Anemia is a below-normal level of hemoglobin or hematocrit. Hemoglobin is the substance in red blood cells that carries oxygen to all parts of your body. Anemia can be temporary or it can be along-term disease/illness. People with mild anemia may not have any symptoms or may have only mild symptoms. People withsevere anemia can feel tired, get short of breath with activity, and have problems doing the things they usually do.

Anemia Occurs Due to Various Reasons

Anemia occurs for different reasons

These include: Increased destruction (break-down) of red blood cells (RBCs) increased blood loss from the body inadequate production of red blood cells by the bone marrow.

In some cases, anemia results from an inherited disorder whereas in other cases the condition is caused by something in a person's environment, such as a nutritional problem, infection, or exposure to a drug or toxin.

How common is anemia in people with heart disease? Many large studies have shown anemia is common in 17% to 48% of people with heart failure. One study showed that 43% of people who were hospitalized after a heart attack had anemia.

Relationship Between Anemia and Heart Disease

Anemia occurs when your body has a below-normal level of hemoglobin, which in turn prevents your body from getting enough oxygen. In certain cases, this lowers level of oxygen causes your heart to work harder. These effects on your heart can make you susceptible to heart disease or worsen existing heart disease (Figs 47.73–47.77).

What are the effects of untreated anemia in heart disease?

With anemia, the heart is forced to work harder to deliver oxygen-rich blood, yet does not receive enough oxygen to support the body's normal functions, resulting in extensive tissue damage and death.

Anemia can lead to severe chest pain because parts of the heart are not getting enough oxygen. As the heart works harder due to lack of oxygen, the muscles in the left lower chamber can get too thick. This can result in a condition called left ventricular hypertrophy, which can worsen heart disease and increase the chance of heart failure.

In a study of people who initially had no heart disease, people with anemia were 41% more likely than those without anemia to have a heart attack, need an artery-clearing procedure, or die of heart disease within 6 years. Another study showed that anemia increases the chance of artery blockages in the arteries of the neck, a problem

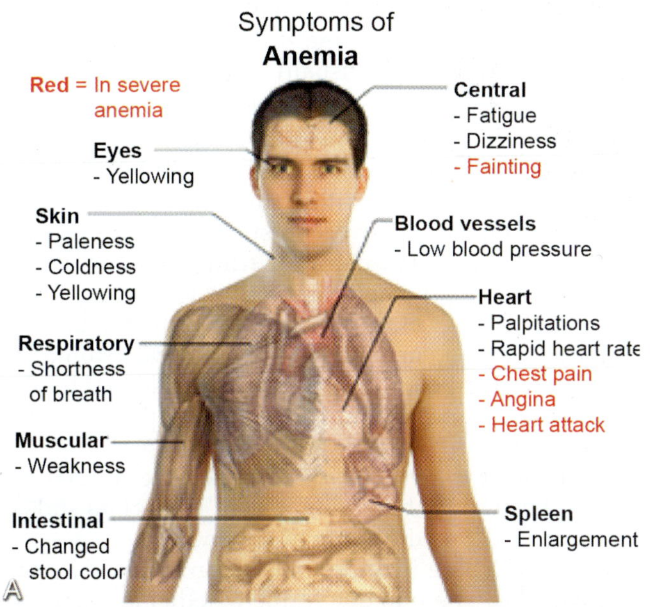

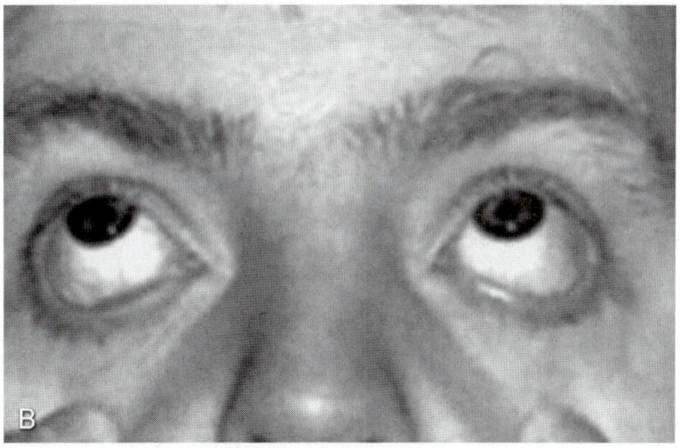

Fig. 47.72: *(A) Various symptoms of anemia (B). Examining of anemia by pulling down both the lower lids of the eyes for pallor*

that can result in a stroke. The presence of anemia increases the death rate in people with heart failure and those who have had a heart attack. The death rate is especially high in anemic people with heart failure who also have kidney disease and/or diabetes.

These studies do not guarantee you will live longer if the anemia is corrected, but they do show how important it is to pay attention to anemia.

Signs and Symptoms of Anemia

Most people do not realize they are anemic until a blood test shows a low hemoglobin or hematocrit. Symptoms and signs usually develop when anemia is moderate to severe, and can include fatigue, weakness, pale skin, chest pain, dizziness, irritability, numbness or coldness in your hands and feet, trouble breathing, a fast heartbeat, and headache. It is important to see your doctor on a regular basis in order to be tested possible anemia.

The most common sign of iron deficiency and other types of nutritional anemia is mild paleness of the skin, along with decreased pinkness of the lips, the lining of the eyelids, and the nail beds. A friend or relative who sees your child only occasionally may be more likely to notice this than you because the changes usually happen so gradually.

Other common signs of anemia may include:
- Irritability fatigue
- Dizziness, light headedness, and a rapid heartbeat

Depending on the condition causing the anemia, other signs and symptoms may occur, such as jaundice (yellow-tinged skin), dark tea-colored urine, easy bruising or bleeding, and enlargement of the spleen or liver.

In many cases, doctors don't discover anemia until they run blood tests as part of a routine physical examination. A complete blood count (CBC) may indicate that there are fewer red blood cells than normal. Other diagnostic tests may include:

Blood smear examination: Microscopic examination of red blood cells after blood is smeared on a glass slide can sometimes indicate the cause of the anemia.

Iron tests: These include total serum iron and ferritin tests, which can help to determine whether anemia is due to iron deficiency.

Sinus Tachycardia

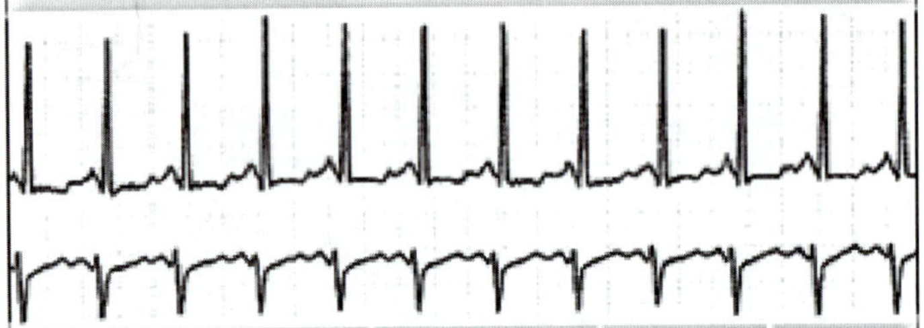

Heart rate	Rhythm	P wave	PR interval (in seconds)	QRS (in seconds)
> 100 bpm	Regular	Before each QRS, identical	.12 to .20	<.12

Fig. 47.73: *ECG showing sinus tachycardia in patient with severe anemia*

Hemoglobin electrophoresis: This test identifies various abnormal hemoglobin in the blood and is used to diagnose sickle cell anemia and the thalassemias.

Bone marrow aspiration and biopsy: This test can help to determine whether cell production is happening normally in the bone marrow. It's the only way to diagnose aplastic anemia definitively and is also used if it is suspected that a disease affecting the bone marrow (such as leukemia) could be the cause for the anemia.

Normal Laboratory Values

- Normal hemoglobin
  - >12 g/dL for women
  - >14 g/dL for men
- Normal hematocrit
  - >36% for women
  - >42% for men.

Treat of anemia: The treatment of anemia varies greatly depending on the type. Your physician will help you determine the best treatment options, such as diet modification, or nutritional supplements, or medication if needed. Close communication with your doctor will ensure you will receive the best anemia treatment available. Treating anemia is not only vital to prevent the development of severe, possibly life-threatening complications, but to improve a patient's quality of life. Patients with serious illnesses such as CKD, diabetes, cancer, heart disease and rheumatoid arthritis are at the greatest risk for developing anemia.

Treatment is based on: your age, overall health, and medical history extent of the disease your tolerance for specific medications, procedures, or therapies expectations for the course of the disease your opinion or preference *Treatment may include:* Treatment of the causative disease vitamin and mineral supplements change in diet medication blood transfusion bone marrow transplant

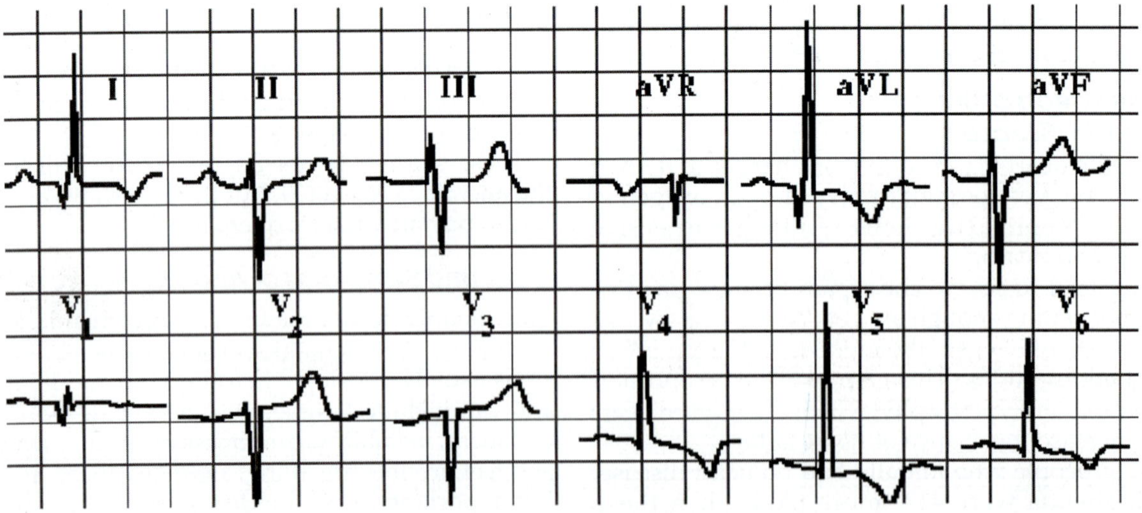

Fig. 47.74: *Left ventricular hypertrophy—12-lead ECG demonstrating NSR with LVH. The ST segment depression in the lateral leads (I, aVl, V5 and V6) is seen in approximately 70% of patients with electrocardiographic LVH; such a finding has been termed the "strain pattern". While this finding may represent altered repolarisation attributable to the presence of LVH, it may also be a manifestation of myocardial ischaemia*

surgery (to remove the spleen, if related to hemolytic anemia) antibiotics (if an infection is the causative agent).

ACUTE RHEUMATIC FEVER

Rheumatic fever is an autoimmune inflammatory disease which may develop after a Group A streptococcal infection (such as strep throat or scarlet fever) and can involve the heart, joints, skin and brain. It commonly appears in children ages 6 through 15.

General Information

Rheumatic fever is common worldwide and responsible for many cases of damaged heart valves. In the Western countries, it became fairly rare since the 1960s, probably due to widespread use of antibiotics to treat streptococcus infections. While it is far less common in the United States since the beginning of the 20th century, there have been a few outbreaks since the 1980s. Although the disease seldom occurs, it is serious and has a mortality of 2–5%.

Rheumatic fever primarily affects children between ages 6 and 15 years and occurs approximately 20 days after strep throat or scarlet fever. In up to a third of cases, the underlying strep infection may not have caused any symptoms (Figs 47.78 and 47.79).

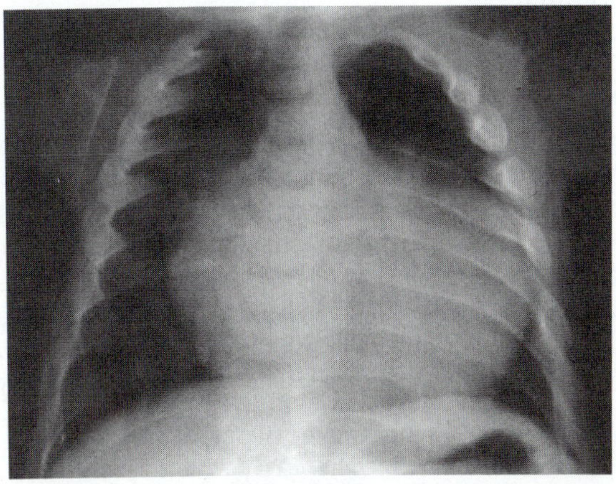

Fig. 47.75: *Chest X-ray (PA view) illustrating cardiomegaly in severe anemia in a child*

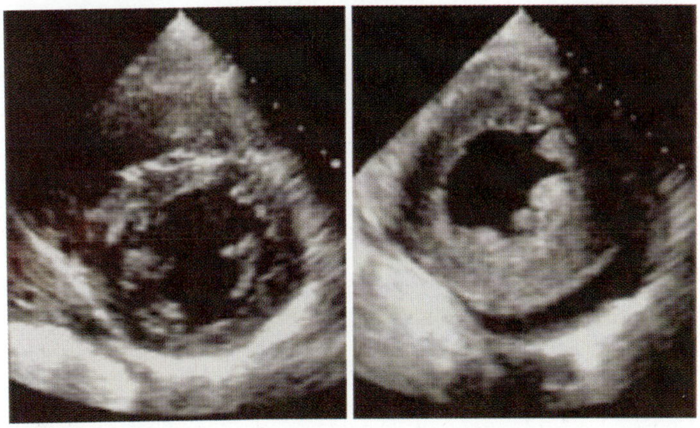

Fig. 47.76: *Echocardiography demonstrates normal LV (Left) and concenteric LVH (Right) in a child with severe anemia*

The rate of development of rheumatic fever in individuals with untreated strep infection is estimated to be 3%. The incidence of recurrence with a subsequent untreated infection is substantially greater (about 50%). The rate of development is far lower in individuals who have received antibiotic treatment. Persons who have suffered a case of rheumatic fever have a tendency to develop flare-ups with repeated strep infections. The recurrence of rheumatic fever is relatively common in the absence of maintenance of low dose antibiotics, especially during the first 3–5 years after the first episode. Heart complications may be long-term and severe, particularly if valves are involved.

Diagnosis: Modified Jones Criteria

T. Duckett Jones, MD, first published these criteria in 1944. They have been periodically revised by the American Heart Association in collaboration with other groups. **Two major criteria, or one major and two minor criteria**, when there is also evidence of a previous strep infection, support the diagnosis of rheumatic fever. Exceptions are chorea and

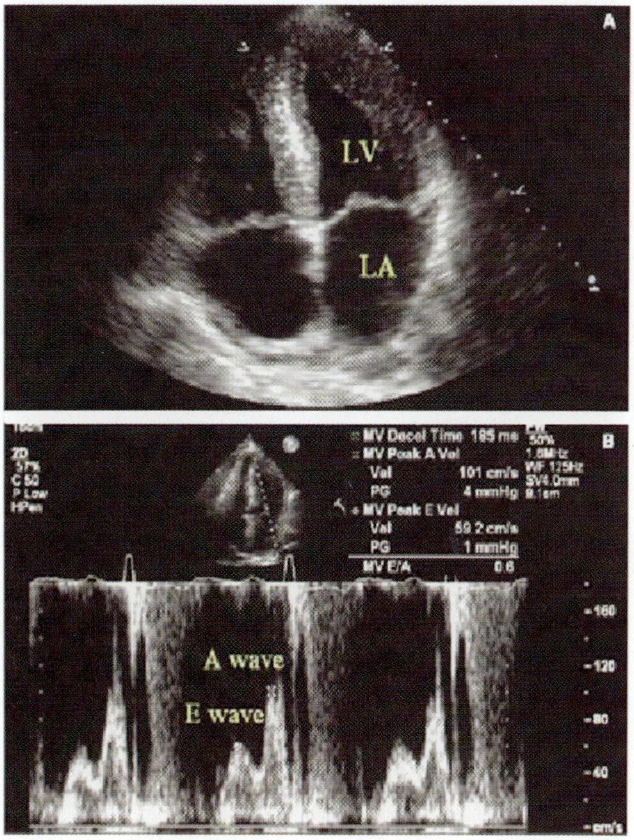

Fig. 47.77: *Severe left ventricular hypertrophy and diastolic heart failure are revealed by echocardiography. The apical four chamber view shows a thickened left ventricular wall and enlarged left atrium (A). Doppler evaluation shows impaired early diastolic relaxation (E wave) and vigorous atrial contraction (A wave) resulting in an E/A ratio of less than 0.75, which signifies early reduced left ventricular compliance (B). A normal E/A ratio is greater than 1.5, since most of the diastolic filling occurs early in a compliant left ventricle with the atrial component contributing a smaller volume at a lower velocity in an adolescent with severe anemia (LV, left ventricle; LA, left atrium)*

indolent carditis, each of which by itself can indicate rheumatic fever.

Major Criteria (Figs 47.80–47.83)

An easy way to remember the major criteria is by the **mnemonic: CANCER**

- **C:** Cardiac
- **A:** Arthritis
- **N:** Nodules (subcutaneous)
- **C:** Chorea
- **ER:** Erythema marginatum

Carditis (Figs 47.83 and 47.86): Inflammation of the heart muscle which can manifest as congestive heart failure with shortness of breath, pericarditis with a rub, or a new heart murmur.

Arthritis (migratory polyarthritis): A temporary migrating inflammation of the large joints, usually starting in the legs and migrating upwards.

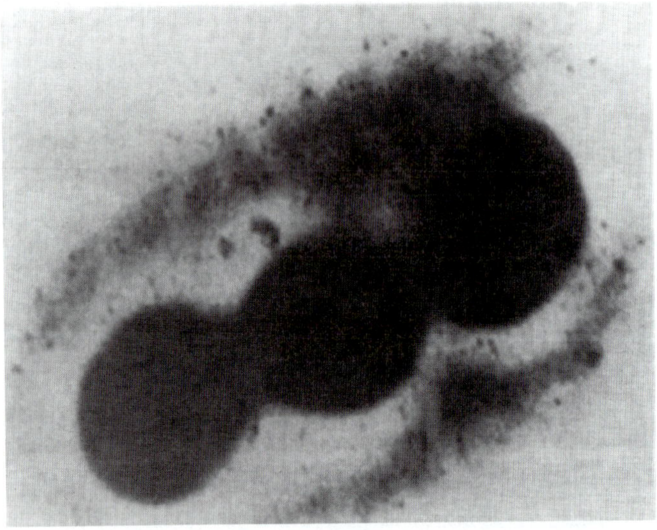

Fig. 47.78: *Electron micrograph of a chain of group A streptococci (type M-24) isolated during a rheumatic fever epidemic in a military population. The cocci are enclosed by a large hyaluronate capsule which is shadowed by type M-24 antibody precipitated on its surface. (Stollerman GH. Rheumatogenic group A streptococci and the return of rheumatic fever)*

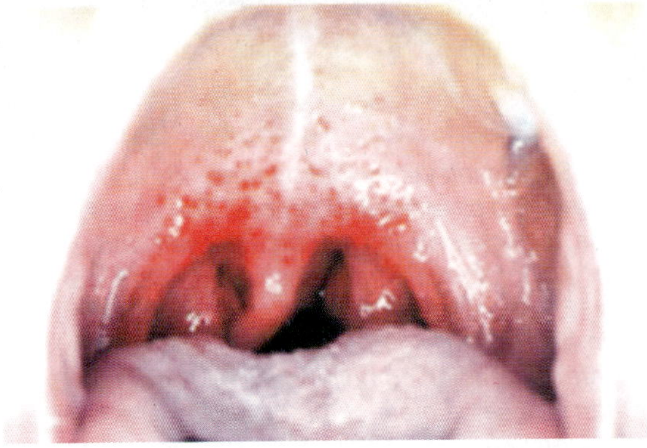

Fig. 47.79: *Acute throat infection with group A beta-hemolytic streptococcoi*

Nodules (subcutaneous nodules): A form of Aschoff bodies, painless, firm collections of collagen fibers on the back of the wrist, the outside elbow, and the front of the knees. These now occur infrequently.

Chorea

- *Sydenham's chorea (St. vitus' dance):* A characteristic series of rapid movements without purpose of the face and arms. This can occur very late in the disease.
- *Erythema marginatum:* A long lasting rash that begins on the trunk or arms as macules and spreads outwards to form a snake-like ring while clearing in the middle. This rash never starts on the face and is made worse with heat (Fig. 47.81).

Minor Criteria

- *Fever:* Temperature elevation
- *Arthralgia:* Joint pain without swelling
- *Laboratory abnormalities:* Increased erythrocyte sedimentation rate, increased C-relative protein, leukocytosis.
- Electrocardiogram abnormalities: A prolonged PR interval (Figs 47.84 and 47.85)
- Evidence of group A strep infection: Positive culture for group A strep, elevated or rising antistreptolysin O titre
- Previous rheumatic fever or inactive heart disease.

Other signs and symptoms

- Abdominal pain
- Nose bleeds.

Pathophysiology

Rheumatic fever is a systemic disease affecting the periarteriolar connective tissue and can occur after an untreated Group A streptococcal pharyngeal infection. It is believed to be caused by antibody cross-reactivity. This cross-reactivity is a type II hypersensitivity reaction and is termed *molecular mimicry*. Usually, self-reactive B cells remain anergic in the periphery without T cell co-stimulation. During a Strep, infection activated antigen presenting cells

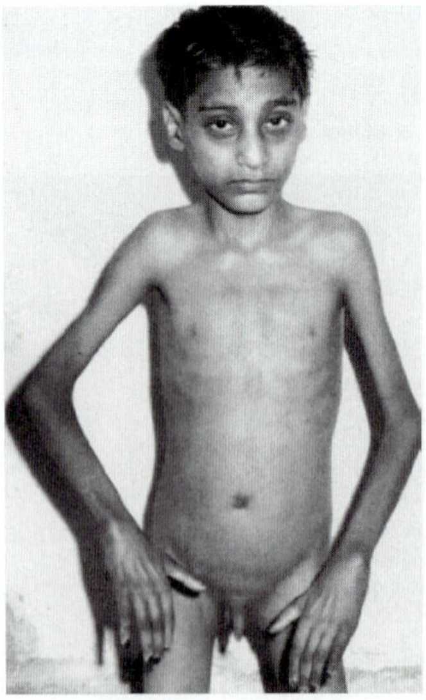

Fig. 47.80: *Subcutaneous nodules (arrows) over the writs, elbows and finger in a young child with acute rheumatic fever*

such as macrophages present the bacterial antigen to helper T cells. Helper T cells subsequently activate B cells and induce the production of antibodies against the cell wall of *Streptococcus*. However, the antibodies may also react

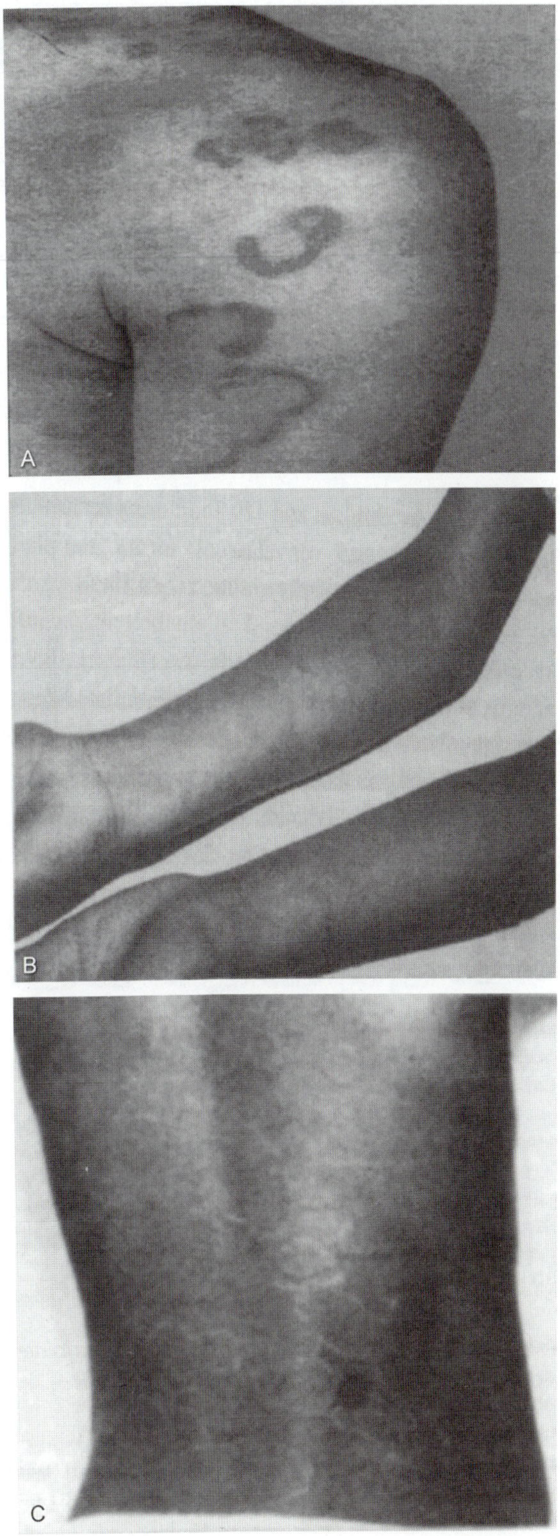

Fig. 47.81: *(Upper) shoulder and upper arm areas (Middle) Forearm and (Lower) back area erythema marginatum. The rash is classically flat to slightly elevated, erythematous and annular (ring-like) in appearance*

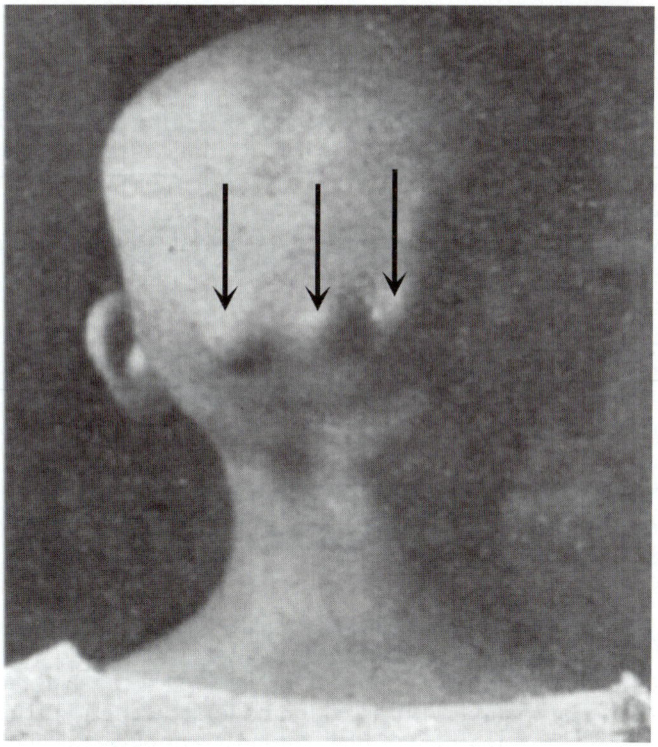

Fig. 47.82: *Rheumatic nodules over the occipit of a young child with acute rheumatic fever*

against the myocardium and joints, producing the symptoms of rheumatic fever. Group A *streptococcus pyogenes* has a cell wall composed of branched polymers which sometimes contain "*M proteins*" that are highly antigenic. The antibodies which the immune system generates against the "*M proteins*" may cross react with cardiac myofiber protein myosin and smooth muscle cells of arteries, inducing cytokine release and tissue destruction. This inflammation occurs through direct attachment of complement and Fc receptor-mediated recruitment of neutrophils and macrophages. Characteristic Aschoff bodies, composed of swollen eosinophilic collagen surrounded by lymphocytes and macrophages can be seen on light microscopy. The larger macrophages may become Aschoff giant cells. Acute rheumatic valvular lesions may also involve a cell-mediated immunity reaction as these lesions predominantly contain T-helper cells and macrophages in acute RF, these lesions can be found in any layer of the heart and is hence called pancarditis. The inflammation may cause a serofibrinous pericardial exudates described as "bread-and-butter" pericarditis, which usually resolves without sequelae. Involvement of the endocardium typically results in fibrinoid necrosis and verrucae formation along the lines of closure of the left-sided heart valves. Warty projections arise from deposition while subendothelial lesions may induce irregular thickenings called MacCallum plaques. Chronic rheumatic heart disease is characterized by repeated inflammation with fibrinous resolution. The cardinal anatomic changes of the valve include leaflet thickening, commissural fusion and shortening and thickening of the tendinous cords.

Treatment

The management of acute rheumatic fever is geared toward the reduction of inflammation with antiinflammatory medications such as aspirin or corticosteroids. Individuals with positive cultures for strep throat should also be treated with antibiotics. Aspirin is the drug of choice and should be given at high doses of 100 mg/kg/day. One should watch for side effects like gastritis, salicylate poisoning, etc. Steroids are reserved for cases where there is evidence of involvement of heart. The use of steroids may prevent further scarring of tissue and may prevent development of sequelae such as mitral stenosis. Monthly injections of long-acting penicillin must be given for a period of 5 years in patients having one attack of rheumatic fever. If there is evidence of carditis, the length of penidure therapy may be up to 40 years. Another important cornerstone in treating rheumatic fever includes the continual use of low dose antibiotics (such as penicillin, sulfadiazine, or erythromycin) to prevent recurrence.

Infection

Patients with positive cultures for *streptococcus pyogenes* should be treated with penicillin as long as allergy is not present. This treatment will not alter the course of the acute disease.

Inflammation

Patients with significant symptoms may require corticosteroids. Salicylates are useful for pain.

Heart Failure

Some patients develop significant carditis which manifests as congestive heart failure. This requires the usual treatment

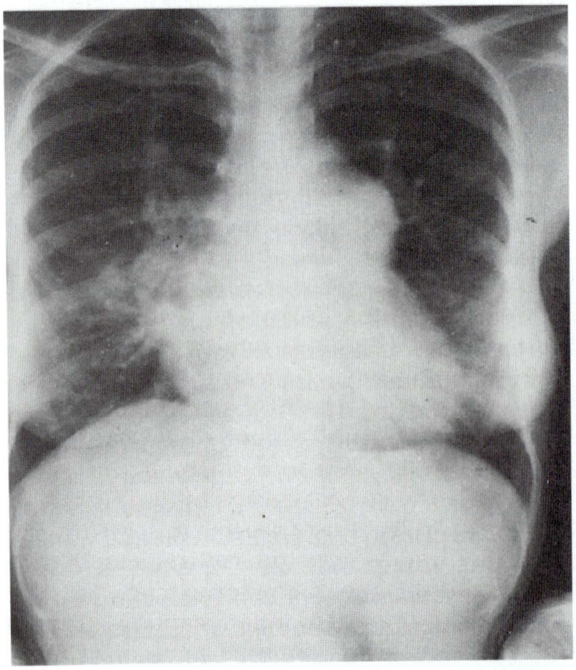

Fig. 47.83: *X-ray chest (PA view) showing cardiomegaly, prominent pulmonary artery due to acute on chronic rheumatic heart disease*

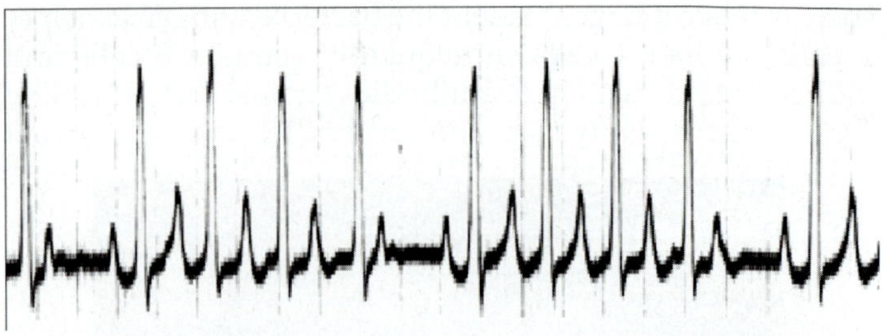

Fig. 47.84: *ECG trace shows paroxysmal atrial tachycardia with type 1 grade 2 AV block in patient with acute rheumatic fever*

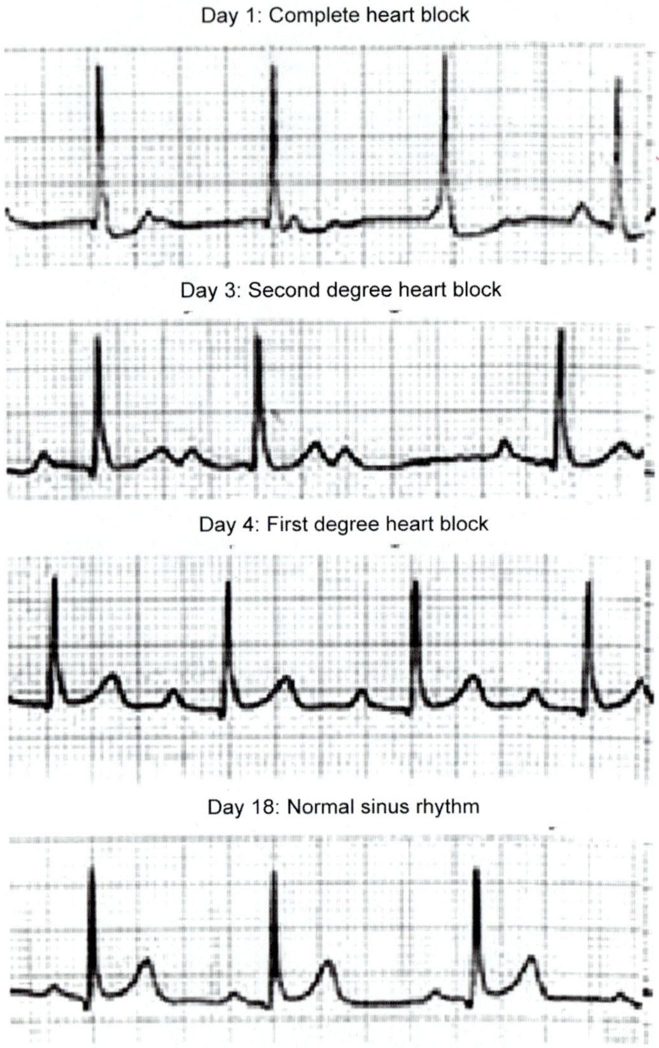

Fig. 47.85: *Regression of ECG changes from complete heart block to normal sinus rhythm in patient with ARF*

for heart failure: diuretics and digoxin. Unlike normal heart failure, rheumatic heart failure responds well to corticosteroids.

Prevention

Prevention of recurrence is achieved by eradicating the acute infection and prophylaxis with antibiotics. The

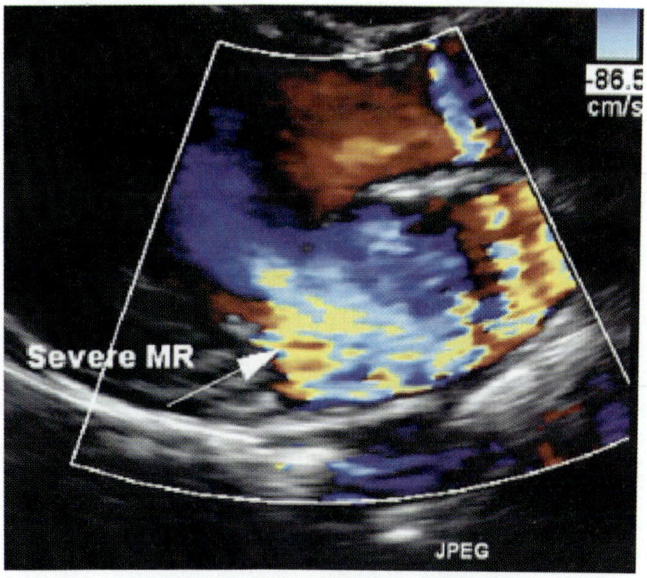

Fig. 47.86: *Color Doppler ecocardiography shows severe MR in patient with acute rheumatic fever*

American Heart Association recommends daily or monthly prophylaxis continue long-term, perhaps for life.

Nurses also have a role in prevention, primarily in screening school-aged children for sore throats that may be caused by Group A streptococci (especially Group A hemolytic *Streptococcus pyogenes*).

KAWASAKI DISEASE

Kawasaki disease, also known as lymph node syndrome, mucocutaneous node disease, infantile polyarteritis and Kawasaki syndrome, is a poorly understood self-limited vasculitis that affects many organs including the skin and mucous membranes, lymph nodes, blood vessel walls, and the heart. It does not seem to be contagious. It was first described in 1967 by Dr Tomisaku Kawasaki in Japan.

Incidence and Risk Factors

By far, the highest incidence of Kawasaki disease occurs in Japan (175 per 100,000) though its incidence in the United States is increasing. Kawasaki disease is predominantly a disease of young children, with 80% of patients younger than 5 years of age. Additional risk factors in the United States include Asian race and male sex. Approximately, 2,000 cases are identified in the United States each year.

Causes

The causative agent of Kawasaki disease is still unknown. However, current etiological theories center primarily on immunological causes for the disease. Much research is being performed to discover a definitive toxin or antigenic substance, possibly a superantigen, that is the specific cause of the disease.

An unknown virus may play a role as an inciting factor as well. An association with ITPKC has been identified.

Presentation

The cardiac complications are, by far, the most important aspect of the disease. Kawasaki disease can cause vasculitic changes (inflammation of blood vessels) in the coronary arteries and subsequent coronary artery aneurysms. These aneurysms can lead to myocardial infarction (heart attack) even in young children. Overall, about 10–18% of children with Kawasaki disease develop coronary artery aneurysms Kawasaki syndrome and risk factors for coronary artery abnormalities: United States, 1994–2003 with much higher prevalence among patients who are not treated early in the course of illness. Kawasaki disease and rheumatic fever are most common causes of acquired heart disease among children in the United States.

Symptoms (Figs 47.87 and 47.88)

Kawasaki disease often begins with a high and persistent fever that is not very responsive to normal doses of paracetamol (acetaminophen) or ibuprofen. The fever may persist steadily for up to 2 weeks and is normally accompanied by irritability. Affected children develop red eyes, red mucous membranes in the mouth, red cracked lips, a "strawberry tongue", iritis, keratic precipitates (detectable by an ophthalmologist but usually too small to be seen by the unaided eye), and swollen lymph nodes. Skin rashes occur early in the disease, and peeling of the skin in the genital area, hands, and feet (especially around the nails and on the palms and soles) may occur in later phases. Some of these symptoms may come and go during the course of the illness. If left untreated, the symptoms will eventually relent, but coronary artery aneurysms will not improve, resulting in a significant risk of death or disability due to myocardial infarction (heart attack). If treated in a timely fashion, this risk can be mostly avoided and the course of illness cut short.

- High-grade fever (greater than 39°C or 102°F; often as high as 40°C or 104°F) that normally lasts for more than a week if left untreated.
- Red eyes (conjunctivitis) without pus or drainage, also known as "conjunctival injection"
- Bright red, chapped, or cracked lips
- Red mucous membranes in the mouth
- Strawberry tongue, white coating on the tongue or prominent red bumps (papillae) on the back of the tongue
- Red palms of the hands and the soles of the feet
- Swollen hands and feet
- Rash which may take many forms, but not vesicular (blister-like), on the trunk
- Swollen lymph nodes (frequently only one lymph node is swollen), particularly in the neck area
- Joint pain (arthralgia) and swelling, frequently symmetrical Irritability, tachycardia (rapid heart beat)
- Peeling (desquamation) palms and soles (later in the illness); peeling may begin around the nails
- Beaus lines (transverse grooves on nails)

Blood Tests

Complete blood count (CBC) may reveal normocytic anemia and eventually thrombocytosis.

- **Erythrocyte sedimentation rate (ESR)** will be elevated
- **C-reactive protein (CRP)** will be elevated
- **Liver function tests** may show evidence of hepatic inflammation and low serum albumi.

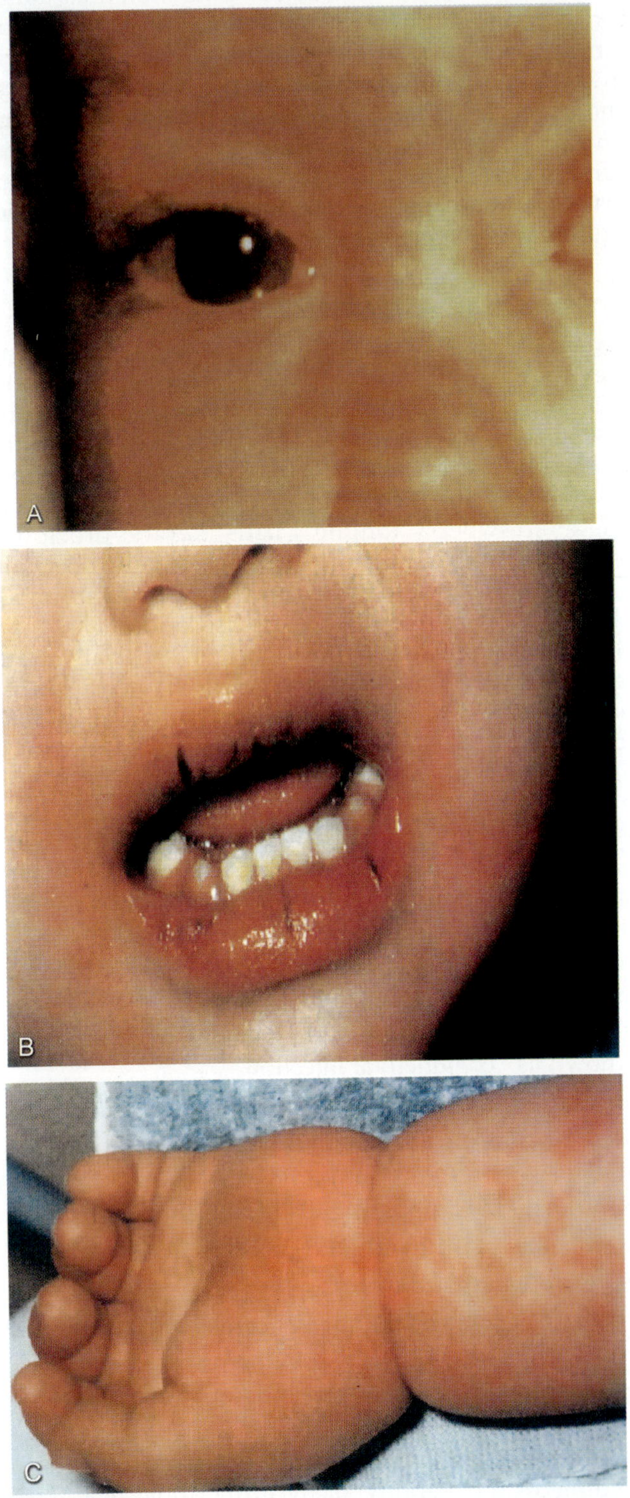

Fig. 47.87(A to C): *Different manifestations of Kawasaki's disease. (Upper) redness of conjuntiva with facial rash. (middle) red fissured lips and strawberry tongue (lower) redness of the palm and edema of the hand with induration*

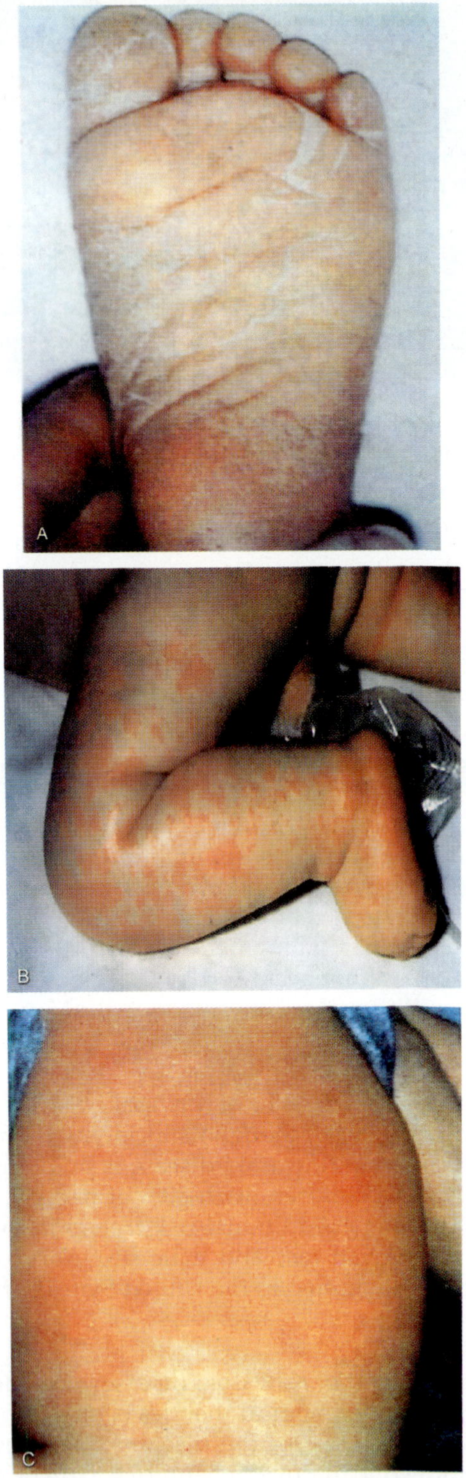

Fig. 47.88(A to C): *Different manifestations of Kawasaki's disease (upper) desquammation of the foot in the subacute phase (middle) Skin rash with edema and redness of the foot (lower) erythema and induration around a BCG vaccination site*

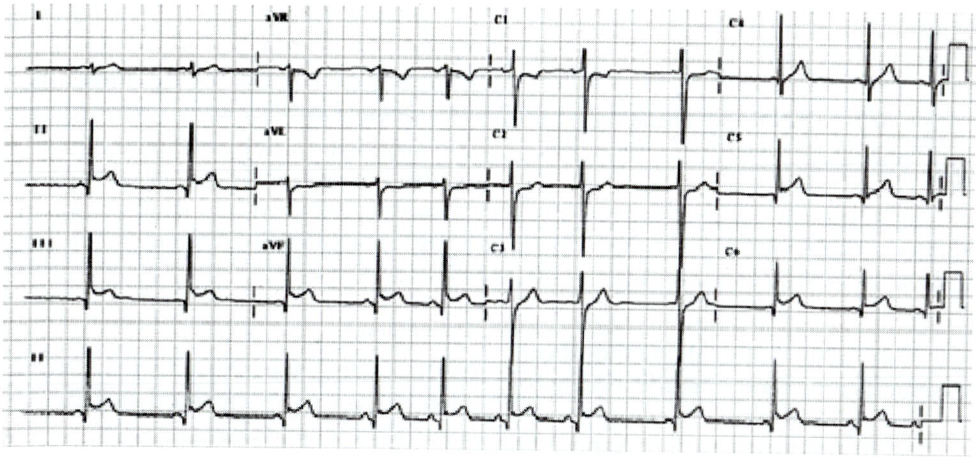

Fig. 47.89: *Twelve-lead ECG from 12-months-old girl with kawasaki disease. The ECG showing ST elevation in leads 11,111,aVF and V4-V6 as acute coronary syndrome*

Other tests (may or may not be performed)

Electrocardiogram may show evidence of ventricular dysfunction or, occasionally, arrhythmia due to myocarditis (Figs 47.89 and 47.90).

Echocardiogram may show subtle coronary artery changes or, later, true aneurysms.

Ultrasound or computerized tomography may show hydrops (enlargement) of the gallbladder.

- Urinalysis may show white blood cells and protein in the urine (pyuria and proteinuria) without evidence of bacterial growth lumbar puncture may show evidence of aseptic meningitis.

Angiography was historically used to detect coronary artery aneurysms and remains the gold standard for their detection, but is rarely used today unless coronary artery aneurysms have already been detected by echocardiography. If not treated in time it can cause many heart problems (Fig. 49.91).

Diagnosis

Kawasaki disease can only be diagnosed clinically (by medical signs and symptoms), as there exists no specific laboratory test that can tell if someone has it. It is normally difficult to establish the diagnosis, especially early in the course of illness, and frequently children are not diagnosed until they have seen their doctor several times, or visited a number of different health care providers. Many other serious illnesses can cause similar symptoms, and must be considered in the differential diagnosis including scarlet fever, toxic shock syndrome, and juvenile idiopathic arthritis.

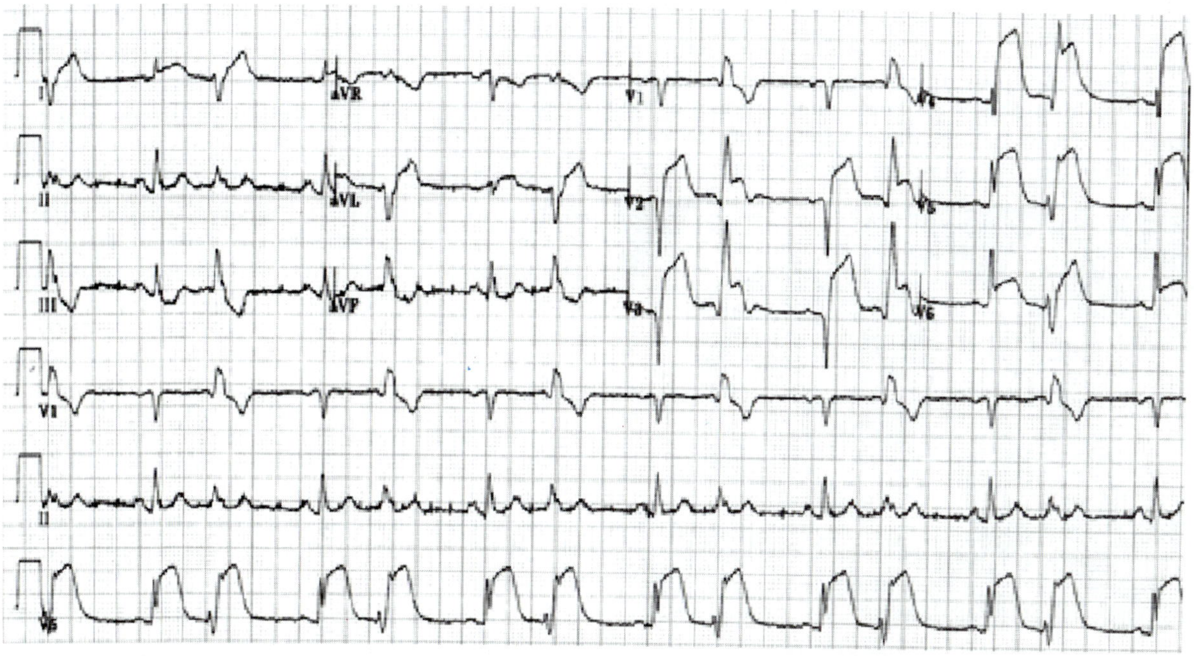

Fig. 47.90: *12-lead ECG acute ST elevation infarction with delayed presentation (ST elevation and Q waves present in a patient with Kawasaki disease)*

Classically, 5 days of fever plus 4–5 diagnostic criteria must be met in order to establish the diagnosis. The criteria are:

1. Erythema of the lips or oral cavity or cracking of the lips
2. Rash on the trunk
3. Swelling or erythema of the hands or feet
4. Red eyes (conjunctival injection)
5. Swollen lymph node in the neck of at least 15 millimeters.

Many children, especially infants, eventually diagnosed with Kawasaki disease do not exhibit all of the above criteria. In fact, many experts now recommend treating for Kawasaki disease even if only 3 days of fever have passed and at least three diagnostic criteria are present, especially if other tests reveal abnormalities consistent with Kawasaki disease. In addition, the diagnosis can be made purely by the detection of coronary artery aneurysms in the proper clinical setting.

Treatment

Children with Kawasaki disease should be hospitalized and cared for by a physician who has experience with this disease. When in an academic medical center, care is often shared between pediatric cardiology and pediatric infectious disease specialists although no infectious agent has been demonstrated. It is imperative that treatment be started as soon as the diagnosis is made to prevent damage to the coronary arteries. Intravenous immunoglobulin (IVIG) is the standard treatment for Kawasaki disease and is administered in high doses with marked improvement usually noted within 24 hours. If the fever does not respond, an additional dose may have to be considered. IVIG by itself is most useful within the first 7 days of onset of fever, in terms of preventing coronary artery aneurysm.

Salicylate therapy, particularly aspirin, remains an important part of the treatment (though questioned by some) but salicylates alone are not as effective as Intravenous immunoglobulin. Aspirin therapy is started at high doses until the fever subsides, and then is continued at a low dose when the patient returns home, usually for 2 months to prevent blood clots from forming. Except for Kawasaki disease and a few other indications, aspirin is otherwise normally not recommended for children due to its association with Reye's syndrome.

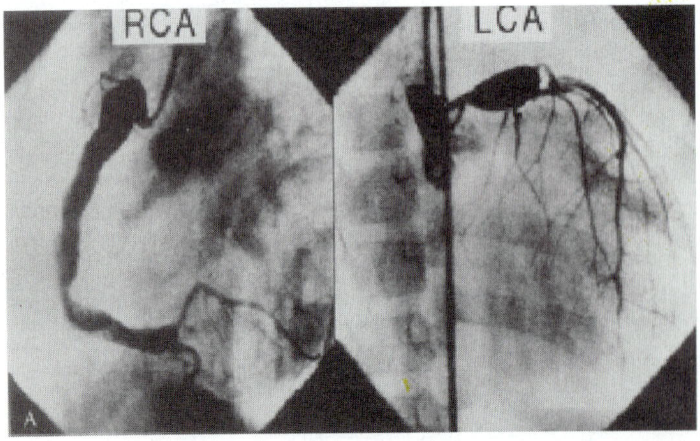

Fig. 47.91: *Coronary angiography showing longitudinal dilatation (RCA) and saccular aneurysm at proximal site of (LCA) in a young patient of 5 yrs with Kawasaki disease*

Corticosteroids have also been used, especially when other treatments fail or symptoms recur, but in a randomized controlled trial, the addition of corticosteroid to immune globulin and aspirin did not improve outcome. There are also treatments for iritis and other eye symptoms.

Prognosis

With early treatment, rapid recovery from the acute symptoms can be expected and the risk of coronary artery aneurysms greatly reduced. Untreated, the acute symptoms of Kawasaki disease are self-limited (i.e. the patient will recover eventually), but the risk of coronary artery involvement is much greater. Overall, about 2% of patients die from complications of coronary vasculitis. Patients who have had Kawasaki disease should have an echocardiogram initially every few weeks, and then every 1–2 years to screen for progression of cardiac involvement. It is also not uncommon that a relapse of symptoms may occur soon after initial treatment with IVIG. This usually requires re-hospitalization and retreatment. Treatment with IVIG can cause allergic and nonallergic acute reactions, aseptic meningitis, fluid overload and, rarely, other serious reactions. Aspirin may increase the risk of bleeding from other causes and may be associated with Reye's syndrome. Overall, life-threatening complications resulting from therapy for Kawasaki disease are exceedingly rare, especially compared with the risk of nontreatment.

TYPHOID FEVER

Typhoid fever, also known as enteric fever, is a systemic infection by *Salmonella typhi* or by the related but less virulent *Salmonella paratyphi*. Since ancient times, these bacteria have thrived during wartime and during the breakdown of basic sanitation. Archeologists have found *S. typhi* in Athenian mass graves from the era of the Peloponnesian wars, implicating it as the cause of the Great Plague of Athens. *S. typhi* persists mostly in developing nations where sanitation is generally poor. Although sporadic outbreaks occur in developed nations, most individuals with typhoid fever in such areas have recently returned from travel to an endemic region.

Of all *Salmonella* serotypes, only *S. typhi* and *S. paratyphi* are pathogenic exclusively in humans. Typhoid fever is a severe multisystemic illness characterized by the classic prolonged fever, sustained bacteremia without endothelial or endocardial involvement, agative, enteric, rond bacterial invasion of and multiplication within the mononuclear phagocytic cells of the liver, spleen, lymph nodes, and Peyer patches. Typhoid fever is potentially fatal if untreated. People are typically infected with *S. typhi* and *S. paratyphi* through food and beverages contaminated by a chronic stool carrier. Less commonly, carriers may shed the bacteria in urine. Individuals may also be infected by drinking sewage-contaminated water or by eating contaminated shellfish or faultily canned meat.

Salmonella is a genus in the family *Enterobacteriaceae* that has more than 2,300 serotypes previously described in the Kauffman-White schema. Salmonellae are gram-negative, flagellate, nonsporulating, facultative anaerobic bacilli that ferment glucose, reduce nitrate to nitrite, and synthesize peritrichous flagella when motile. All but *S. typhi* produce gas upon sugar fermentation.

Salmonellae are grouped based on the somatic O antigen and further divided into serotypes based on flagellar H and surface virulence (Vi) antigens. In particular, *S. typhi*, the cause of typhoid fever, has O and H antigens, an envelope (K) antigen, and a lipopolysaccharide macromolecular complex called endotoxin that forms the outer portion of the cell wall. *S. typhi, S. paratyphi C*, and *Salmonella dublin* are the only *Salmonella* serotypes that carry Vi antigen. Based on DNA studies, all salmonellae are now considered one of two species: *Salmonella enterica* (formerly called *Salmonella choleraesuis*) and *Salmonella bongori*. *S. enterica* has six subspecies (I, II, IIIa, IIIb, IV, VI); *S. bongori* has one (V). *S. typhi* and *S. paratyphi* are *S. enterica* I subspecies, serotypes *typhi* and *paratyphi*.

Pathophysiology: After ingestion by the host, *S. typhi* invades through the gut and multiplies within the mononuclear phagocytic cells in the liver, spleen, lymph nodes, and Peyer patches of the ileum.

In studies of healthy, previously unvaccinated men, ingestion of 10^7 *S. typhi* bacilli caused disease in 50% of volunteers. Investigations of outbreaks seem to indicate that an inoculum of as few as 200 organisms may lead to the disease. Perhaps such a discrepancy exists because many who ingest *S. typhi* are not healthy men and have any one of a number of risk factors (*see* below). As the number of organisms increases, the incubation period decreases. The number of bacilli ingested does not change the subsequent clinical syndrome.

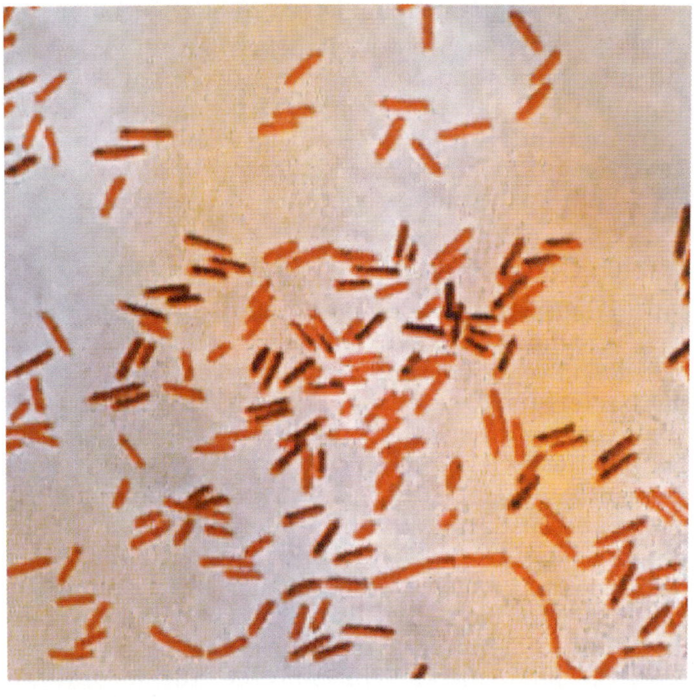

Fig. 47.92: *Microscopic features of Salmonella typhi, the agent of typhoid, Gram stain (CDC)*

After successfully passing through the stomach, any *Salmonella* subspecies may be phagocytized by the gut's intraluminal dendritic cells, causing inflammation that leads to diarrhea. Only the subspecies *S. enterica* causes severe disease in the rest of the body. Its specialized fimbriae adhere to the epithelium that overlies Peyer patches. Peyer patches are grossly visible aggregates of 5–100 lymphoid follicles in the small bowel submucosa; these patches are larger and more numerous distally. They are the primary mechanism for sampling antigens in the gut and initiating response. *S. enterica* enters them via 1 of 3 pathways.

Intraluminal dendritic cells may infiltrate through the gut epithelium while carrying the bacterium. M cells may transport it as well. Immobile and interspersed among regular enterocytes in Peyer patches, M cells are epithelial cells that mature into professional phagocytes. They phagocytize bacteria such as *S. enterica* and present them to macrophages and T cells in the lamina propria. Most interestingly, *S. enterica* may convert normally nonphagocytic epithelial cells into bacterially-mediated endocytosis (BME).

In BME, *Salmonella* uses a type III secretion system—macromolecular channels that Gram-negative bacteria such as *Salmonella* insert into eukaryotic cells and intracellular membranes to inject virulence proteins—to inject proteins SipA and SipC into the epithelial cell. These disrupt the normal brush border and force the cell to form membrane ruffles. The ruffles engulf the bacilli and create vesicles that carry them across the epithelial cell cytoplasm and the basolateral membrane. *Salmonella* pathogenicity island 1 (SPI-1) in the genome encodes the elements of BME.

In the submucosa, *Salmonella* enters macrophages via bacteria-triggered pinocytosis or via macrophage receptor-mediated phagocytosis. The intravacuolar environment activates the PhoP/PhoQ regulon, leading to modification of protein and lipopolysaccharide elements of the bacterial inner and outer membranes. Thus, *Salmonella* resists lysis and decreases host proinflammatory signaling. The bacterium also produces homocysteine to inactivate nitric oxide and enzymes against other microbicides. Finally, with the Vi antigen, a polysaccharide capsule, *S. typhi* and *S. paratyphi* further protect themselves from lysis within the macrophage and from neutrophils and complement without. The newly described *Salmonella* pathogenicity island 2 (SPI-2) encodes a type III secretion system that carries bacterial proteins across the vacuole membrane and into the cytosol. Other virulence factors from SPI-2 prevent or alter fusion of the *Salmonella*-containing vacuole with other intracellular compartments, rearrange the actin cytoskeleton around the vacuole, and may prevent the implantation of nicotinamide adenine dinucleotide

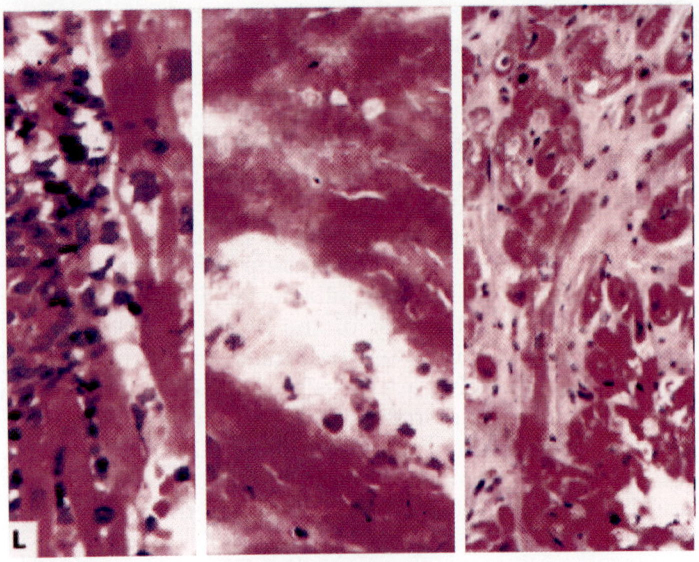

Fig. 47.93: *Serial biopsy samples taken from the patient with toxic typhoid myocarditis showing from left to right: acute myocarditis and healing myocarditis. All sections have the same magnification with haematoxylin and eosin stain*

phosphate (NADPH) oxidase and nitric oxide synthase into the vacuole membrane.

The infected macrophage provides *Salmonella* a vehicle safe from other elements of the immune system and in which it can multiply and travel. It passes through the mesenteric lymph nodes into the thoracic duct and the lymphatics beyond to seed the reticuloendothelial tissues—liver, spleen, bone marrow and lymph nodes. In these havens, it multiplies until some critical density is reached. It causes the apoptosis in the macrophages and enters the bloodstream to attack the rest of the body. At this stage, the Vi antigen comes into play. It forms a capsule to protect the bacterium from complement and from phagocytic immune cells.

From blood or from the liver via bile ducts, it infects the gallbladder and reenters the gastrointestinal tract in the bile, spreading to other hosts via stool. In addition, it occasionally invades the urinary tract and spreads via urine. After primary intestinal infection, further seeding of the Peyer patches occurs through infected bile. They may become hyperplastic and necrotic with infiltration of mononuclear cells and neutrophils, forming ulcers that may hemorrhage through eroded blood vessels or perforate the bowel wall, causing peritonitis.

The host recognizes the invader with toll-like receptors 2, 4 and 5. These induce cytokines such as interferon alpha, interleukin (IL)–12, and tumor necrosis factor-alpha, which recruit macrophages and cause the high fevers of the disease. Macrophages and neutrophils suppress the active infection. Later, humoral and CD4 T-cell-mediated immunity clears it.

Physical: The classic signs of enteric fever include fever, toxemia, delirium, abdominal pain, constipation, and hepatosplenomegaly.

Fever occurs in 75–85% of patients in the first week and is often initially remittent but becomes steady. The individual's temperature often rises to as high as 103–104°F (39–40°C) by the beginning of week 2. Constipation often develops early and is likely due to obstruction at the ileocecal valve by swollen Peyer patches. It may last for the entire duration of illness.

At approximately the end of the first week of illness, about a third of patients develop bacterial emboli to the skin known as rose spots. These are considered a classic symptom in typhoid fever, but they occasionally appear in shigellosis and nontyphoidal salmonellosis. Rose spots constitute a subtle, extremely sparse (often $\leq$5 spots), salmon-colored, blanching, truncal, maculopapular rash with 1 to 4 cm lesions that generally resolve within 2–5 days. Relative bradycardia and a dicrotic pulse are also common during this stage of illness.

During the second week of illness, the patient is toxic-appearing and apathetic with sustained fever. The abdomen is slightly distended, and soft splenomegaly is common.

In the third week, the patient grows more toxic and anorexic with significant weight loss. The patient may have a thready pulse, tachypnea, conjunctivitis, and crackles over the lung bases. Pyrexia persists. The patient may enter into a typhoid state of apathy, confusion, and even psychosis. Patients may develop polyneuropathy. Abnormal cerebrospinal fluid should prompt a search for a different cause. Meanwhile, the patient commonly has pronounced abdominal distension. Some individuals may produce liquid, foul, green-yellow diarrhea (pea soup diarrhea). At this stage, the patient may die from overwhelming toxemia, myocarditis, intestinal hemorrhage, or perforation due to necrotic Peyer patches. Rare complications of enteric fever include pancreatitis, meningitis, orchitis and osteomyelitis.

During the fourth week, the fever, mental state, and abdominal distension slowly improve over a few days, but intestinal complications may still occur in surviving untreated individuals. Weight loss and debilitating weakness last months. Relapses occur in 10% of patients, mostly during the first 2–3 weeks of convalescence.

Chronic Carrier State

One to four percent of untreated patients become chronic carriers, defined as individuals who excrete *Salmonella* for more than 1 year. Some individuals may continue to excrete the bacterium for decades. Bladder infection with *Schistosoma haematobium* predisposes to urinary carriage. The parasite itself becomes a carrier. Stool carriage is more frequent in people with preexisting biliary abnormalities, perhaps because S. *enterica* survives in gallstones, and these people have a greater incidence of cholecystitis. Chronic carriers have a greater risk for carcinoma of the gallbladder and other gastrointestinal malignancies; chronic carriers had a sixfold increase in the risk of death due to hepatobiliary cancer. This may be due to chronic inflammation caused by the bacterium.

Causes: *S. typhi* and *S. paratyphi* cause typhoid fever.

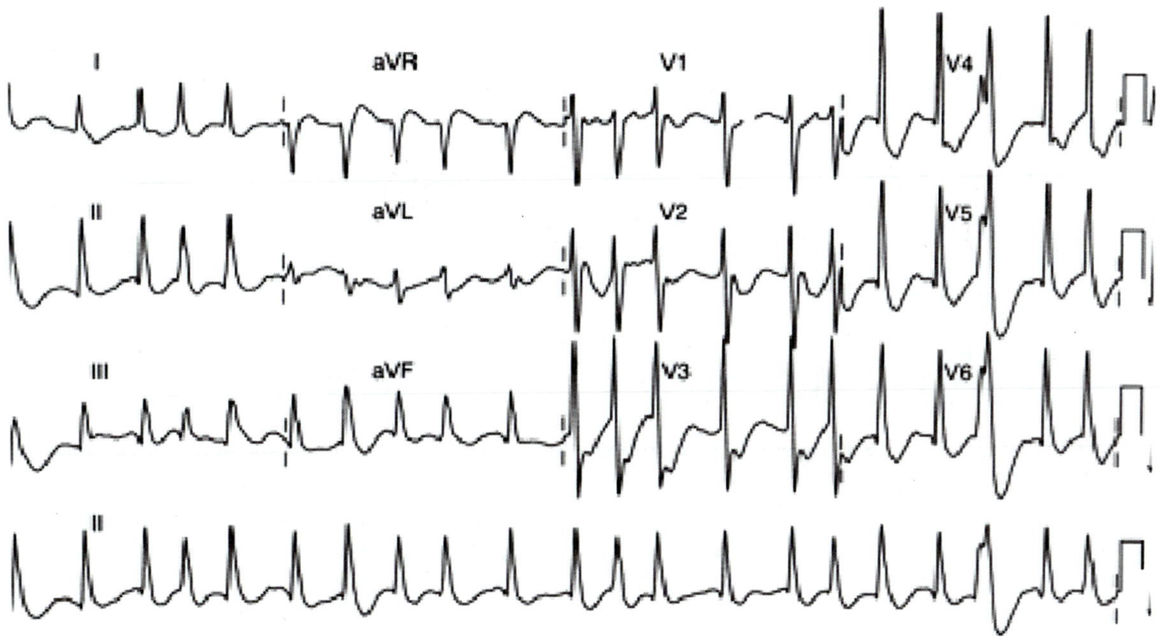

Fig. 47.94: *ECG showing irregular broad complex tachycardia as a part of typhoid toxic myocarditis*

Laboratory Studies (Figs 47.92 and 47.93)

- Typhoid fever causes various abnormalities in standard laboratory tests. Serological tests and cultures are the mainstay of diagnosis. DNA probes are used by researchers and are available to patients in well-funded facilities. The diagnosis is suggested by assays that identify *Salmonella* antibodies and antigens and is then confirmed by isolation of the organism.
- ***Standard laboratory tests:*** Most patients are moderately anemic, have an elevated erythrocyte sedimentation rate, thrombocytopenia, and relative lymphopenia. Most also have a slightly elevated prothrombin time (PT) and activated partial thromboplastin time, decreased fibrinogen levels, and levels of circulating fibrin degradation products that commonly rise to subclinical disseminated intravascular coagulation levels. Liver transaminase values and serum bilirubin levels are usually elevated to twice the reference range. Mild hyponatremia and hypokalemia are common.
- **Specific serological tests**
- Assays that identify *Salmonella* antibodies or antigens support the diagnosis but should be confirmed with cultures or DNA evidence.
- **The widal test** is more than a century old and was the standard serologic test for typhoid fever diagnosis for decades. Now, it is mostly of historical interest. It produces false-negative results in a significant proportion of patients who do not mount a detectable antibody response. It is highly nonspecific, especially in endemic areas where cross-reacting antigens from similar organisms are common. ***The Widal test measures agglutinating antibodies against H and O antigens of S. typhi.***
- In acute infection, O antibody appears first, rising progressively, later falling, and often disappearing within a few months. H antibody appears slightly later but persists longer and can be used to distinguish between various types of enteric fever.
- Indirect hemagglutination, indirect fluorescent Vi antibody, and indirect enzyme-linked immunosorbent assay for immunoglobulin M (IgM) and IgG antibodies to *S. typhi* polysaccharide are available. Monoclonal antibodies against *S. typhi* flagellin are promising developments.
- **Culture**

Definitive diagnosis of typhoid fever generally requires isolation of the organism from blood, bone marrow, vomitus, fresh stool, or urine. A bone marrow aspirate (BMA) culture is the most sensitive method of isolating *S. typhi*. The sensitivity is 90% at any point in the disease course for as long as 5 days after the initiation of antibiotics. The test is extremely painful. Clinicians should try to establish the diagnosis with less traumatic means.

If patients present within the first week of the disease, blood, intestinal secretions, and stool culture results are usually positive in approximately 85–90% of patients with typhoid fever. They decline to 20–30% later in the course of the disease. In particular, stool culture results may be positive for several days after *S. typhi* ingestion. This is because of inflammation from the intraluminal dendritic cells. Later in the illness, bacteria shed through the gallbladder again cause positive stool culture results. Multiple positive blood culture results are 73–97% specific for typhoid fever. Large-volume blood culture and clot culture after serum removal increase sensitivity. Stool culture alone is less than 50% sensitive, and urine even less so. Cultures of punch biopsy samples of rose spots reportedly have a sensitivity of 63% and may show positive results even after antibiotics. A single rectal swab culture at hospital admission can be expected to detect

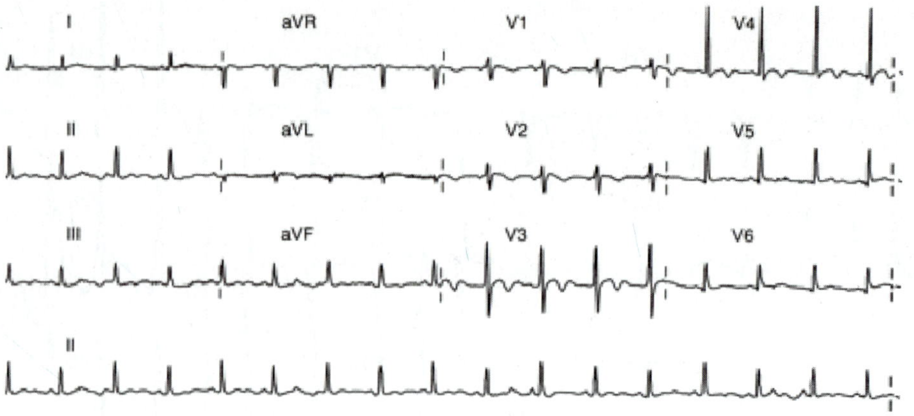

Fig. 47.95: *ECG showing T wave abnormalities in chest leads. Subsequent biopsy showed healing myocarditis*

S. typhi in 30–40% of patients. *S. typhi* has also been isolated from the cerebrospinal fluid, peritoneal fluid, mesenteric lymph nodes, resected intestine, pharynx, tonsils, abscess, bone, and urine, among others. After disease resolution, three stool cultures one month apart should be taken to rule out carrier state.

BMA and blood are cultured in a selective medium, such as 10% aqueous oxgall, or a nutritious medium, such as tryptic soy broth, and are incubated at 37°C for at least 7 days. Subcultures are made daily to one selective medium, such as MacConkey agar, and one inhibitory medium, such as *Salmonella-Shigella* agar. These conventional culture techniques usually take 48–72 hours from acquisition until the organism is identified.

- ***DNA testing:*** Polymerase chain reaction assays for identifying *S. typhi* are available in some areas. However, this is used mostly for research since the test is generally too expensive for patients in developing countries.

Imaging Studies

Radiography of the kidneys, ureters, and bladder (KUB) are useful if the clinician suspects bowel perforation. CT scanning or MRI may be warranted to investigate abscesses that may occur in, among other sites, the liver or bones.

Procedures

The most sensitive method of isolating *S. typhi* is obtaining a BMA culture.

Histologic findings: The hallmark histologic finding in typhoid fever is infiltration of tissues by macrophages (typhoid cells) that contain bacteria, erythrocytes, and degenerated lymphocytes. Aggregates of these macrophages are called typhoid nodules, which are found most commonly in the intestine, mesenteric lymph nodes, spleen, liver, and bone marrow but may be found in the kidneys, testes, and parotid glands. In the intestines, four classic pathologic stages occur in the course of infection: (1) hyperplastic changes, (2) necrosis of the intestinal mucosa, (3) sloughing of the mucosa and (4) the development of ulcers. The ulcers may perforate into the peritoneal cavity.

In the mesenteric lymph nodes, the sinusoids are enlarged and distended by large collections of macrophages and reticuloendothelial cells. The spleen is enlarged, red, soft, and congested; its serosal surface may have a fibrinous exudate. Microscopically, the red pulp is congested and contains typhoid nodules. The gallbladder is hyperemic and may show evidence of cholecystitis. A liver biopsy specimen from a person with typhoid often shows cloudy swelling, balloon degeneration with vacuolation of hepatocytes, moderate fatty change, and focal typhoid nodules. Intact typhoid bacilli can be observed at these sites.

Complications

- ***Intestinal manifestations:*** The two most common complications of enteric fever are intestinal hemorrhage (12% in one British series) and perforation (3–4.6% of hospitalized patients).
  From 1884–1909 (i.e. preantibiotic era), the mortality rate in patients with intestinal perforation in typhoid fever was 66–90% but now is significantly lower. Approximately 75% of patients have guarding, rebound tenderness, and rigidity, particularly in the right lower quadrant.
  Diagnosis is particularly difficult in the approximately 25% of patients with perforation and peritonitis who do not have the classic physical findings. Often, the discovery of free intraabdominal fluid may be the only sign of perforation.
- ***Hepatobiliary manifestations:*** Mild elevation of transaminases without symptoms is common in persons with typhoid fever.
  Jaundice may occur in persons with enteric fever and may be due to hepatitis, cholangitis, cholecystitis, or hemolysis.
  Pancreatitis and simultaneous acute renal failure and hepatitis with hepatomegaly have been reported.

Cardiopulmonary

Nonspecific electrocardiographic changes occur in 10–15% of patients with typhoid. Toxic myocarditis occurs in 1–5% of persons with typhoid and is a significant cause of death in disease-endemic countries.

Toxic myocarditis occurs in patients who are severely ill and toxemic and is characterized by tachycardia, weak pulse and heart sounds, hypotension, and **electrocardiographic abnormalities** (Figs 47.94 and 47.95).

- Pericarditis rarely occurs, but peripheral vascular collapse without other cardiac findings is increasingly described. Pulmonary manifestations have also been reported in patients with typhoid fever.
- **Neuropsychiatric manifestations:** In the past 2 decades, reports from the disease-endemic areas have documented a wide spectrum of neuropsychiatric manifestations of typhoid fever.
  A toxic confusional state, characterized by disorientation, delirium, and restlessness, is characteristic of late-stage typhoid. Occasionally, these and other neuropsychiatric features may dominate the clinical picture at an early stage. Facial twitching or convulsions may be the presenting feature; sometimes, paranoid psychosis or catatonia may develop during convalescence. Meningismus is not uncommon, but frank meningitis is rare. Encephalomyelitis may develop, and the underlying pathology may be that of demyelinating leukoencephalopathy. Rarely, transverse myelitis, polyneuropathy, or cranial mononeuropathy may develop.
  Other less commonly reported events are spastic paraplegia, peripheral or cranial neuritis, Guillain-Barré syndrome, schizophrenialike illness, mania, and depression.
- ***Hematologic manifestations:*** Subclinical disseminated intravascular coagulation occurs commonly in persons with typhoid fever.
  Hemolytic-uremic syndrome is rare.
  Hemolysis may also be associated with glucose-6-phosphate dehydrogenase deficiency.
- ***Genitourinary manifestations:*** Approximately 25% of patients excrete *S. typhi* in their urine at some point during their illness.
  Immune complex glomerulitis and proteinuria have been reported, and IgM, C3 antigen, and *S. typhi* antigen can be demonstrated in the glomerular capillary wall.
  Nephritic syndrome may complicate chronic *S. typhi* bacteremia associated with urinary schistosomiasis.
- ***Musculoskeletal manifestations:*** Skeletal muscle characteristically shows Zenker degeneration, particularly affecting the abdominal wall and thigh muscles.

Clinically evident polymyositis may occur.

CNS Manifestations

- Focal intracranial infections are uncommon.
- Recently, multiple brain abscesses have been reported.

Prognosis

The prognosis depends on the geographical area and its demographics. Generally, the mortality rate in untreated disease is 10–20%. In properly treated disease, it is less than 1%.

Between 10% and 20% of patients treated with antibiotics have a relapse after initial recovery. A relapse typically occurs approximately 1 week after therapy is discontinued, but relapse after 70 days has been reported. The blood culture results are again positive, and high serum levels of H, O, and Vi antibodies and rose spots may reappear. A relapse generally is milder and shorter than the initial illness. Rarely, second or even third relapses may occur. Notably, the relapse rate is much lower following treatment with the new quinolone drugs, which have effective intracellular penetration.

Medical care: Health care workers caring for patients with typhoid fever should pay strict attention to adequate hand washing and safe disposal of feces and urine. Antibiotic therapy is essential and should begin empirically if the clinical evidence is strong. Patients must receive adequate fluids, electrolytes and nutrition. Antimicrobials shorten the course, reduce the rate of complications if begun early, and drastically reduce the case-fatality rate.

Surgical care: Surgery is usually indicated in cases of intestinal perforation. Most surgeons prefer simple closure of the perforation with drainage of the peritoneum. Small bowel resection is indicated for patients with multiple perforations.

If antibiotic treatment fails to eradicate the hepatobiliary carriage, the gallbladder should be resected. Cholecystectomy is not always successful in eradicating the carrier state because of persisting hepatic infection.

Physicians should consult an infectious disease specialist: Consultation with a surgeon is indicated upon suspected gastrointestinal perforation, serious gastrointestinal hemorrhage, cholecystitis, or extraintestinal complications (arteritis, endocarditis, organ abscesses).

Antibiotics should be started empirically while the results of confirmatory tests are pending. The literature describes varying medication recommendations. The regional sensitivity profiles in the antibiotic sensitivity of typhoid vary; thus, the authors' opinion is that these should be taken into account in the initial choice of treatment. Final sensitivity results should be used to determine the definitive treatment.

In absolute numbers, most patients in the United States with typhoid fever were infected in Latin America. However, the greatest risk of infection is travel to India and Pakistan. Because *S. typhi* and *S. paratyphi* rarely develop antibiotic resistance during treatment, patients who relapse may be given the same drug. However, relapse should dictate a search for anatomical, pathological, or genetic predispositions.

Drug therapy—Chloramphenicol was introduced in 1948 and was once the mainstay of treatment. By the 1970s, widespread resistance to the drug developed. Ampicillin and cotrimoxazole became treatments of choice. However, in the late 1980s, some *S. typhi* strains developed simultaneous plasmid-mediated resistance to all three drugs. Fluoroquinolones and third-generation cephalosporins have filled the breach, but some resistance exists to both.

Resistance to ciprofloxacin is increasing. Up to 50% of the isolates from Finns with typhoid fever returning from Southeast Asia had reduced susceptibility to ciprofloxacin, with a minimum inhibitory concentration (MIC) of 0.125-

0.250—a ninefold increase. For therapeutic purposes, intermediate susceptibility should be regarded as full resistance. Ciprofloxacin is no longer a good first-line treatment for *S. typhi* infection that arises in Southeast Asia. When last evaluated, the rate of intermediate sensitivity in strains was 3.7% in the Americas ($P = 0.132$), 4.7% ($P = 0.144$) in Sub-Saharan Africa, and 10.8% ($P = 0.706$) in the Middle East.

Uncomplicated typhoid fever from the Western hemisphere should be treated empirically with ciprofloxacin for 7 days. The treatment for cases from Southeast Asia is controversial. Some authorities recommend high-dose ciprofloxacin in patients from areas with typhoid fever that is resistant to nalidixic acid. (Nalidixic acid is not used clinically but as an in vitro stand-in for measuring fluoroquinolone resistance.) The authors consider this inadequate, as reports of treatment failure under those conditions have increased. The authors recommend empiric first-line therapy with trimethoprim/sulfamethoxazole and second-line therapy with ampicillin or chloramphenicol. Resistance to these agents in Southeast Asia has declined to 5–10%.

Resistance to ceftriaxone is only sporadic in Southeast Asia and elsewhere. Ceftriaxone should be the first-line empiric treatment for severe typhoid fever, and the course should last 10–14 days.

Clinicians should consider a 48-hour course of dexamethasone if the patient has shock or altered mental status. This may reduce the mortality risk from 56% to 10%. Corticosteroids are reserved for the only the most ill patients because they may increase the risk of relapse.

THYROID HORMONAL DISORDERS AFFECTING

Cardiovascular System

Increased or reduced action of thyroid hormone on certain molecular pathways in the heart and vasculature causes relevant cardiovascular derangements. It is well established that overt hyperthyroidism induces a hyperdynamic cardiovascular state (high cardiac output with low systemic vascular resistance), which is associated with a faster heart rate, enhanced left ventricular (LV) systolic and diastolic function, and increased prevalence of supraventricular tachyarrhythmias—namely, atrial fibrillation—whereas overt hypothyroidism is characterized by the opposite changes. However, whether changes in cardiac performance associated with overt thyroid dysfunction are due mainly to alterations of myocardial contractility or to loading conditions remains unclear. Extensive evidence indicates that the cardiovascular system responds to the minimal but persistent changes in circulating thyroid hormone levels, which are typical of individuals with subclinical thyroid dysfunction.

Subclinical hyperthyroidism is associated with increased heart rate, atrial arrhythmias, increased LV mass, impaired ventricular relaxation, reduced exercise performance, and increased risk of cardiovascular mortality. Subclinical hypothyroidism is associated with impaired LV diastolic function and subtle systolic dysfunction and an enhanced risk for atherosclerosis and myocardial infarction. Because all cardiovascular abnormalities are reversed by restoration of euthyroidism ("subclinical hypothyroidism") or blunted by β-blockade and L-thyroxine (L-T4) dose tailoring ("subclinical hyperthyroidism"), timely treatment is advisable in an attempt to avoid adverse cardiovascular effects. Interestingly, some data indicate that patients with acute and chronic cardiovascular disorders and those undergoing cardiac surgery may have altered peripheral thyroid hormone metabolism that, in turn, may contribute to altered cardiac function. Preliminary clinical investigations suggest that administration of thyroid hormone or its analogue 3,5-diiodothyropropionic acid greatly benefits these patients, highlighting the potential role of thyroid hormone treatment in patients with acute and chronic cardiovascular disease.

Thyroid hormone has relevant effects on the cardiovascular system (Klein and Ojamaa, 2001). Many symptoms and signs recognized in patients with overt hyperthyroidism and hypothyroidism are due to the increased or reduced action of thyroid hormone on the heart and the vascular system, respectively, and the related hemodynamic derangements. In recent decades, it has emerged that subclinical thyroid dysfunction may affect the cardiovascular system, which may increase cardiovascular

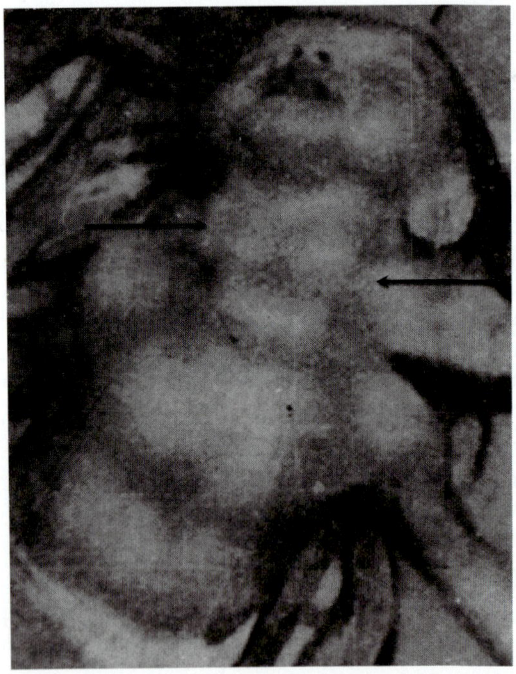

Fig. 47.96: *Photograph of a 12 hours newborn baby with goitrous hypothyroidim with the a history of mother consuming 0.8 g of pottassium iodide for many years in asthma mixture which she was prescribed by the physician. The baby had significant goitre (arrows), marked dyspnoea and huge cardiomegaly and signs of biventricular failure. The baby expired 12 hrs after birth before further measures could be initiated. (This case was later published by Dr KC Verma and Girja Dhar in journal of the Indian Medical Asoociation. Feb 16,1977)*

Table 47.3: *Normal range of TSH, T4 and T3 values in infancy and childhood*

	TSH (mIU/mL)	*T4 (g/dL)*	*T3 (ng/dL)*
Cord blood	3–12	8–13	30–70
Newborn	3–18	11–24	75–260
1–5 yrs	2–10	7–15	100–260
5–10 yrs	2–10	6–13	90–240
10–16 yrs	2–10	5–12	80–110
Thereafter	2–10	5–12	115–190

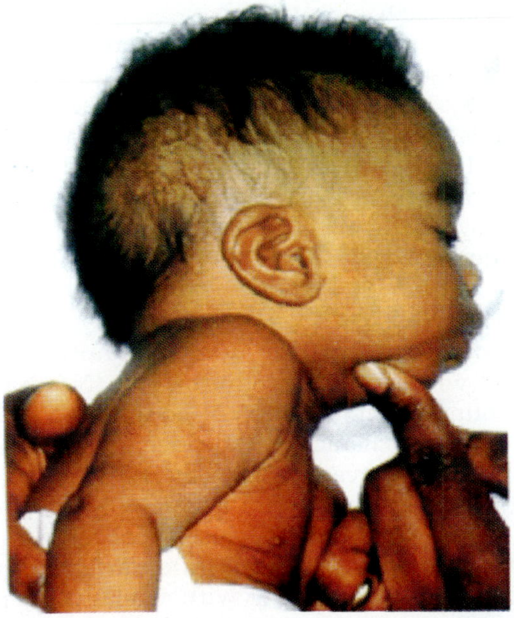

Fig. 47.97: *Photograph showing rough, dry skin, facial puffiness and alopecia in a child with congenital hypothyroidism*

risk. It is becoming increasingly apparent that acute and chronic cardiovascular disease may alter thyroid hormone metabolism and contribute to cardiovascular impairment. This chapter will provide an overview of the basic mechanisms underlying the effects of thyroid hormone on the cardiovascular system and their clinical correlates, then address the potential benefit of thyroid hormone treatment in patients with cardiovascular disorders (Tables 47.3 and 47.4).

Most of the molecular and cellular mechanisms responsible for the cardiovascular effects of thyroid hormone have been clarified. Thyroid hormone may exert both genomic and nongenomic effects on cardiac myocytes. The genomic effects of thyroid hormone are mediated by the transcriptional activation or repression of specific target genes that encode both structural and functional proteins (Dillmann, 1990). This process begins with the entry of triiodothyronine (T3), the biologically active thyroid hormone, into the cardiomyocyte through specific transport proteins located within the cell membrane (Everts et al., 1996). To date, there is no clear evidence of a biologically relevant conversion of thyroxine (T4) to T3 in cardiomyocytes (Everts et al. 1996). Once in the cardiomyocyte, T3 enters the nucleus and interacts with specific transcriptional activators (nuclear receptor alpha-1) or repressors (nuclear receptor alpha-2). Occupancy of these receptors by T3, in combination with recruited cofactors, allows the thyroid hormone-receptor complex to bind (nuclear receptor alpha-1) or release (nuclear receptor alpha-2) specific sequences of DNA (thyroid-responsive elements) that, in turn, by acting as cis- or transregulators, modify the rate of transcription of specific target genes (Brent, among various proteins whose expression is modulated at transcriptional level the most-extensively characterized are myosin heavy chains (Morkin, 1993; Ojamaa et al. 1996b) and the sarcoplasmic reticulum protein involved in the regulation of intracellular calcium handling, namely, calcium-activated ATPase and its inhibitory cofactor, phospholamban (Dillmann, 1990; Kiss et al. 1994). Many studies in vitro and in experimental rats incontrovertibly show that thyroid hormone upregulates the expression of the alpha-isoform of the myosin heavy chain in cardiomyocytes, while it downregulates the β-isoform (Morkin, 1993; Ojamaa et al. 1996b). There is some evidence that this regulation also occurs in humans (Ladenson et al., 1992). However, the magnitude of this phenomenon is certainly less pronounced than in rodents—a finding that fuels uncertainties about the functional correlate of this molecular effect. In humans, the β-isoform of the myosin heavy chain is more prevalent than the alphaisoform (Magner et al. 1988; Ladenson et al. 1992) and the ratio is only marginally modified by thyroid hormone (Ladenson et al. 1992).

In contrast, several lines of evidence suggest that some abnormalities of cardiac function in patients with thyroid dysfunction directly reflect the effects of thyroid hormone on calcium-activated ATPase and phospholamban, which

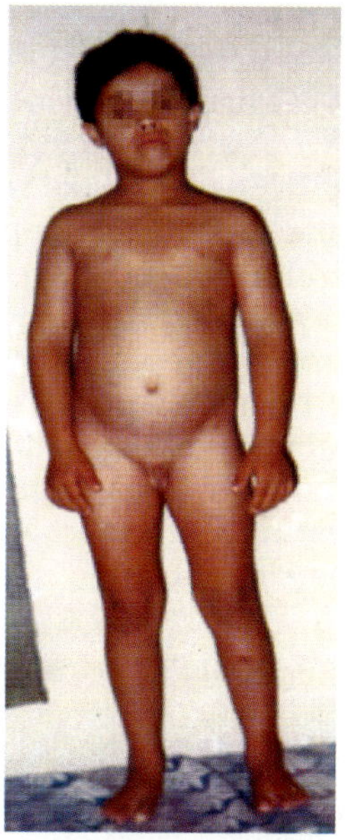

Fig. 47.98: *Physical features of mongolism associated with VSD and subclinical hypothyroidiism which was treated fully after hormone replacement therapy*

are involved primarily in the regulation of systodiastolic calcium concentrations in cardiomyocytes (Dillmann, 1990; Kiss et al. 1994). Sarcoplasmic reticulum calcium-activated ATPase is responsible for the rate of calcium reuptake into the lumen of the sarcoplasmic reticulum during diastole that, in turn, is a major determinant of the velocity of myocardial relaxation after contraction (Dillmann, 1990; Kiss et al. 1994). However, the performance of sarcoplasmic reticulum calcium-activated ATPase is influenced by the level of expression of phospholamban: the higher the phospholamban expression, the lower the sarcoplasmic reticulum calcium-activated ATPase activity (Kiss et al. 1994). In this regard, it has been extensively demonstrated that thyroid hormone upregulates expression of the sarcoplasmic reticulum calcium-activated ATPase and downregulates expression of phospholamban, thereby enhancing myocardial relaxation (Dillmann, 1990; Kiss et al. 1994). Indeed, the improved calcium reuptake during diastole may favorably affect myocardial contractility. In fact, the greater reduction in cytoplasmatic concentration of calcium at end-diastole increases the magnitude of the systolic transient of calcium that, in turn, augments its availability for activation of tropo-myosin units. In fact, in phospholamban-deficient mice, cardiac contractility was found to be increased, with no further increase after thyroid hormone treatment (Kiss et al. 1998). This finding strongly supports the key role of sarcoplasmic reticulum proteins and their effects on intracellular calcium handling in thyroid hormone-mediated changes in systo-diastolic cardiac function in patients with thyroid dysfunction. In this context, it is important to recognize that thyroid hormone also modifies the expression of other ion channels, such as Na^+/K^+-activated ATPase, Na^+/Ca^{++} exchanger, and some voltage-gated K^+ channels (Kv1.5, Kv4.2, Kv4.3), thereby coordinating the electrochemical and mechanical responses of the myocardium (Gick et al. 1990; Ojamaa et al. 1999).

In addition to these genomic effects, thyroid hormone produces changes in cardiac inotropism and chronotropism more rapidly than would be expected from regulation of gene expression, which usually take minutes to hours to be phenotypically and functionally appreciable. This calls into question the involvement of nongenomic mechanisms (Davis and Davis, 1993; Walker et al. 1994). Some evidence indicates that thyroid hormone promotes the acute phosphorylation of phospholamban and that this action attenuates the inhibitory effect of phospholamban on sarcoplasmic reticulum calcium-activated ATPase (Ojamaa et al. 2002). Interestingly, the fact that this process is mediated at least in part by the activation of intracellular kinase pathways involved in signal transduction of the adrenergic stimulus (Ojamaa et al. 2002) may help to explain functional analogies between the cardiovascular effects of thyroid hormone and those promoted by the adrenergic system (Levey and Klein, 1990). Indeed, although most of the cardiovascular manifestations associated with hyperthyroidism and hypothyroidism mimic a condition of increased and reduced adrenergic activity, respectively, the sensitivity of the cardiovascular system to adrenergic stimulation does not seem to be substantially altered in these conditions (Hoit et al. 1997; Ojamaa et al. 2000).

Thyroid hormone also exerts an important effect on the vascular system. It acutely reduces peripheral vascular resistance by promoting relaxation in vascular smooth-muscle cells (Klemperer et al. 1995; Ojamaa et al. 1996a; Park et al. 1997). A single study has reported that chronic thyroid hormone excess exerts profound effects on vascular reactivity by improving both endothelium-dependent and -independent mechanisms (Napoli et al. 2001).

Overt Hyperthyroidism (Fig. 47.103)

Palpitation is one of the most-common symptoms associated with overt hyperthyroidism (Nordyke et al. 1988). Continuous, ambulatory, 24-hour electrocardiogram (ECG) monitoring characteristically demonstrates that heart rate is constantly increased during the day and exaggerated in response to exercise, although its circadian rhythm usually is preserved (von Olshausen et al. 1989; Cacciatori et al. 1996). Analysis of heart rate variability reveals sympatho-vagal unbalancing with a relative increase in sympathetic tone (Cacciatori et al. 1996). In this respect, although β-adrenergic blockade usually attenuates tachycardia in patients with overt hyperthyroidism, heart rates remain slightly higher, in comparison with euthyroid controls. This supports the notion that thyroid hormone is able to directly affect sinus node firing (Sun et al., 2001). About 5–10% of overt hyperthyroid patients have atrial fibrillation, which may be the presenting problem (Sawin et al. 1994; Auer et al. 2001). Atrial fibrillation usually reverts to sinus rhythm with achievement of euthyroidism (Nakazawa et al. 1982), the reversion rate decreasing with age and duration of arrhythmia (Nakazawa et al., 1982; Nordyke et al. 1988). Therefore, achievement of the euthyroid state should be the primary treatment strategy of atrial fibrillation associated with overt hyperthyroidism. β-adrenergic blockade may be used effectively to control the ventricular rate. In all instances, electrical or

Table 47.4: *Severity of hypothyroidism in relation to thyroid hormone deficiency*

Iodine deficiency	*None*	*Mild*	*Moderate*	*Severe*
Median urine iodine, mcg/L	>100	50–99	20–49	<20
Goiter prevalence	<5%	5–20%	20–30%	>30%
Neonatal thyroid stimulating hormone (TSH) >5 IU/mL whole blood	<3%	3–20%	20–40%	>40%
Cretinism	0	0	+	+

Table 47.4: *Cardiovascular changes — hyperthyrodium/ hypothyroidism*

Symptoms palpitations
Exertional dyspnoea
Angina exercise intolerance
Cold intolerance
Physical signs systolic hypertension
Peripheral oedema
Arrhythmia low-volume pulse
Narrow pulse pressure
Peripheral oedema
ECG sinus tachycardia (most common)
Atrial flutter/fibrillation
Left ventricular hypertrophy bradycardia
Prolonged PR/QT intervals
Second/third degree heart block
T wave abnormalitues
Low-voltage ECG (pericardial effusion)
Blood test: Increased serum cholestrol; increased CRP
Increased CRP

pharmacological cardioversion should be an option only after achievement of euthyroidism. In this context, it remains controversial whether overt hyperthyroid patients with atrial fibrillation should receive anticoagulant therapy. In general, the risk of bleeding with anticoagulant therapy always should be weighed against the risk of systemic embolization (Gilligan et al. 1996) and the decision made on a case-by-case basis. In general, it would be appropriate to administer anticoagulant agents to older patients with known or suspected heart disease or with atrial fibrillation of longer duration (Petersen and Hansen, 1988; Gilligan et al. 1996) (Table 47.5).

Systolic arterial pressure is almost invariably increased and diastolic arterial pressure decreased in subjects with overt hyperthyroidism, so that pulse pressure is characteristically wider and mean arterial pressure is only marginally decreased (Graettinger et al., 1959; Theilen and Wilson, 1967; DeGroot and Leonard, 1970). These hemodynamic changes are associated with a remarkable increase in cardiac output and a notable reduction in peripheral vascular resistance, thereby resulting in the classic hyperdynamic cardiovascular state (Graettinger et al. 1959; Theilen and Wilson, 1967; DeGroot and Leonard, 1970).

The main determinants of increased at-rest left ventricular (LV) performance in patients with overt hyperthyroidism have not been definitively established (Biondi et al. 2002a). The high cardiac output state results from a remarkably faster heart rate and a slightly augmented stroke volume that, in turn, is associated with normal or marginally enlarged LV end-diastolic size and normal or marginally decreased LV end-systolic size (Biondi et al. 2002a). As a result, LV ejection fraction, an index of overall systolic chamber function, characteristically is increased in overt hyperthyroid subjects (Biondi et al. 2002a). Whether this process is sustained mainly by a true enhancement of myocardial contractility or by the interaction of hemodynamic factors is unclear (Biondi et al., 2002a). Studies by Merillon and colleagues (1981) and by Feldman and coworkers (1986) are emblematic of the controversy surrounding this argument.

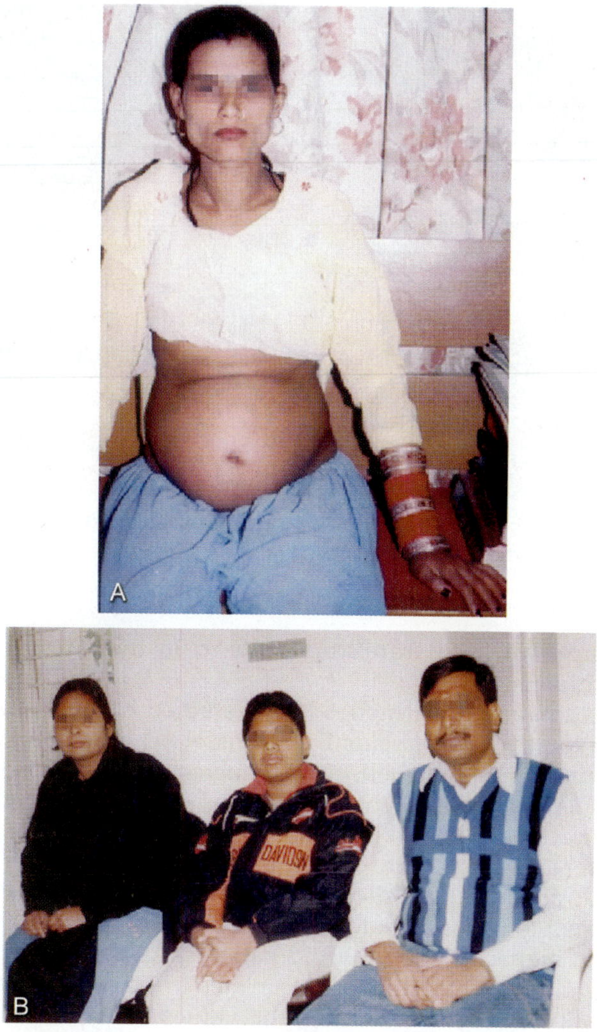

Fig. 47.99: *(A) Showing pregnant young lady with hyperthyroidism under treatment (B) a family of hypothyroidism (husband, wife and their child)*

Merillon and coworkers (1981) assessed LV function in seven overt thyrotoxic subjects by cardiac catheterization, compared with 11 euthyroid controls atrially paced at a near-identical heart rate. They found no differences between the two groups in such parameters of contractile performance as LV ejection fraction, rate of rise of LV pressure as a proportion of the total pressure, velocity of circumferential fiber shortening, and ratio of LV end-systolic pressure to end-systolic volume. Conversely, it was noted that atrial pacing, but not hyperthyroidism, was accompanied by a marked reduction in both end-diastolic volume and pressure and by a significant increase in systemic vascular resistance and mean aortic pressure. As expected, cardiac performance was not increased in atrially paced subjects. Although atrial pacing and hyperthyroidism are not strictly comparable (acute vs. chronic condition), the authors concluded that there was no realistic increase in the true level of myocardial contractility independent of

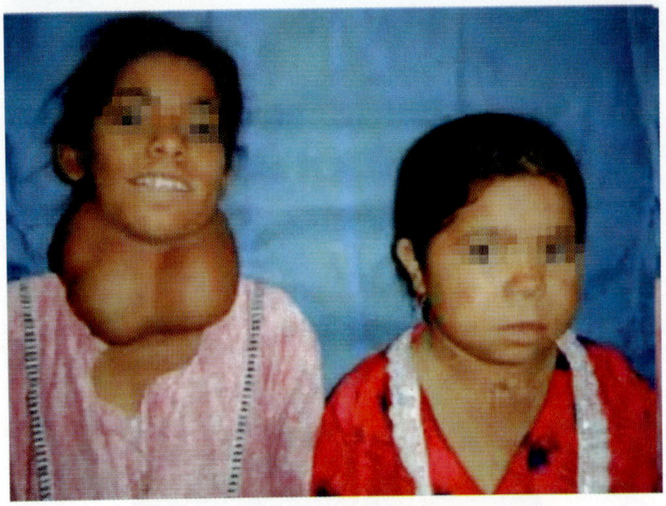

Fig. 47.100: *Two children showing multinodular thyroid goitor (left) and hypothyroidism without goitor (right)*

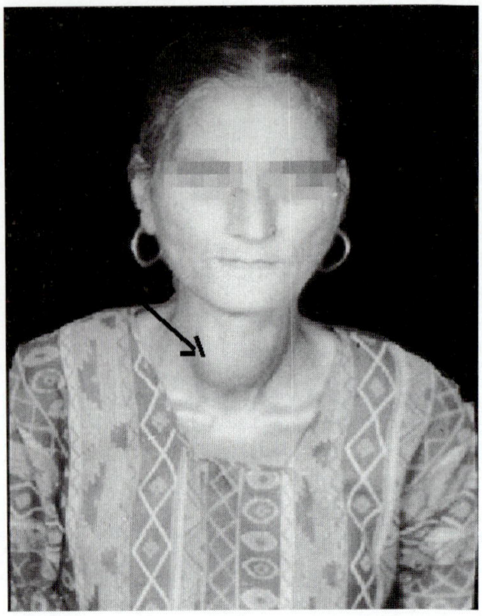

Fig. 47.101: *Enlargement of thyroid gland, mild exophthalmos, thin physique in 40-yrs-old female suffering from hyperthyroidism who clinically presented with atrial fibrrilation and cardiomegaly*

changes in heart rate and preload in human hyperthyroidism.

Feldman and colleagues (1986) studied LV function in 11 hyperthyroid patients by means of echocardiography and in 11 age-matched normal subjects. They found no differences between the two groups in LV end-diastolic diameter or in end-systolic meridional wall stress. Differently, the rate-corrected mean velocity of circumferential fiber shortening (a measure of LV function claimed to be independent of preload and heart rate) was much higher in hyperthyroid patients. As a result, when LV end-systolic wall stress was related to the rate-corrected velocity of fiber shortening, the values of hyperthyroid patients were above the mean regression line for normal subjects, reflecting the presence of an increased contractile state. The authors, however, did not consider that the normal end-diastolic dimension, despite the augmented heart rate in their patients, corresponded to an effective increase in preload, given the inverse relationship between the two variables. Furthermore, the noninvasive method of assessing myocardial contractility by relating the rate-corrected circumferential fiber-shortening velocity to meridional LV end-systolic wall stress may overestimate myocardial performance in pathophysiological states characterized by simultaneous increases in preload and heart rate.

Based on these remarks, it may be assumed that the notably faster heart rate in hyperthyroid patients masks the actual increase in cardiac preload, leading to an underestimation of the extent to which the Frank-Starling mechanism contributes to improving cardiac performance (Biondi et al. 2002a). Indeed, there is evidence that cardiac preload is increased in overt hyperthyroidism. Some studies have demonstrated clearly that blood volume is enlarged in patients with overt hyperthyroidism (Gibson and Harris, 1939; Anthonisen et al. 1960). Other studies showed that the renin-angiotensin-aldosterone system is activated in hyperthyroid patients (Resnick and Laragh, 1982). In addition, thyroid hormone has been shown to upregulate erythropoietin secretion and, in turn, red blood cell mass, which may also contribute to the increase in total blood volume (Gibson and Harris, 1939; Graettinger et al.

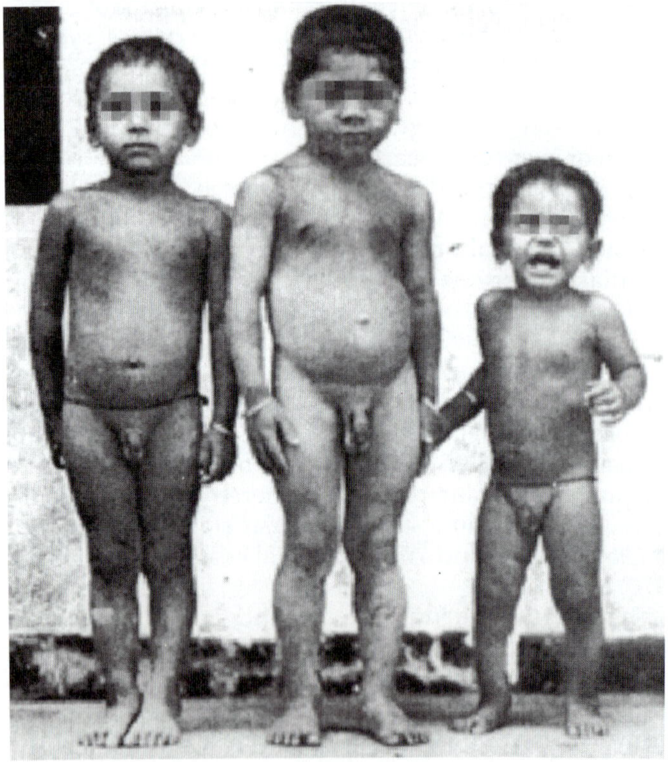

Fig. 47.102: *Three children showing rough, dry skin, facial puffiness and calf muscle hypertrophy with hypothyroidism (Kocker -Debrie-semilangene syndrome)*

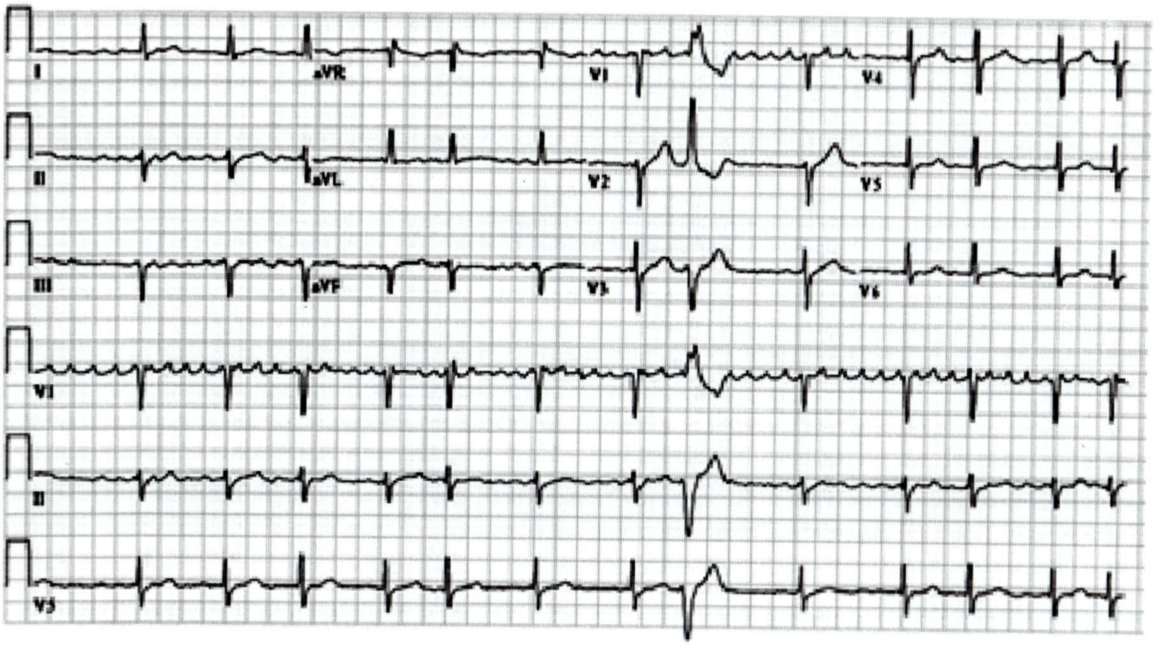

Fig. 47.103: *Electrocardiogram showing atrial fibrillation. P waves are absent and replaced by irregular electrical activity. The ventricular rate is irregular and chaotic in a patient with hyperthyroidism*

1959; Klein and Levey, 1984). Moreover, the analysis of LV diastolic function in different investigations has almost invariably revealed an increase in indices of early LV filling and a faster LV relaxation independent of the effect of heart rate (Lewis et al. 1979; Friedman et al. 1982; Mintz et al. 1991; Kahaly et al. 1999). This pattern of diastolic function is consistent with a greater venous return and enhanced ventricular suction, suggesting that the improvement in diastolic function would allow the increased venous return to be accommodated without relevant changes in filling pressure. This interpretation is supported by the observation of comparable values of LV end-diastolic volume and pressure in hyperthyroid patients and normal subjects (Merillon et al. 1981).

It is, therefore, conceivable that the hyperthyroid heart increases its performance through the advantageous modulation of hemodynamic loads, rather than through recourse to its inotropic reserve (Biondi et al. 2002a). In this regard, it is important to underline that the mechanisms that utilize myocardial contractility involve an ever and necessarily greater myocardial metabolic demand. On the contrary, recourse to the hemodynamic loads to improve cardiac performance is an energetically favorable mechanism. Indeed, recourse to the latter mechanism optimizes the cardiac mechanic-energetic utilization in a condition such as hyperthyroidism, in which a clear increase of myocardial energetic consumption is already present (Bengel et al. 2000).

The complicated and delicate interaction between the different factors determining cardiac function in the patient with overt hyperthyroidism may explain, at least in part, two clinical observations. The first, and more frequent, is reduced exercise tolerance (Kahaly et al. 1998, 1999); the second–less frequently encountered than in the past—is development of congestive heart failure (CHF) (Magner et al. 1988). On the one hand, reduced exercise tolerance of hyperthyroid patients may result from their reduced cardiovascular reserve (Kahaly et al. 1998, 1999). In fact, the mechanisms used by the cardiovascular system during exercise are almost largely used at rest. On the other hand, CHF may be precipitated by the occurrence of atrial fibrillation. The loss of atrial contribution to ventricular filling and the reduced diastolic time may severely compromise diastolic dynamics, increasing end-diastolic pressure and promoting systemic congestion. Occasionally, CHF may develop as a result of the so-called "rate-related cardiomyopathy" (Magner et al. 1988).

Subclinical Hyperthyroidism

Subclinical hyperthyroidism is characterized by subnormal or suppressed thyrotropin (TSH) serum levels in the presence of circulating thyroid hormones in the normal range for the general population (Biondi et al. 2002c). It may be due to an intrinsic pathology of the thyroid gland (endogenous subclinical hyperthyroidism) but, more often, is the consequence of suppressive or replacement L-thyroxine (L-T4) therapy (exogenous subclinical hyperthyroidism) (Biondi et al. 2002c). Exogenous subclinical hyperthyroidism is the condition more-frequently seen in clinical practice (Biondi et al. 2002c).

Over past decades, a number of studies have investigated the effects of subclinical hyperthyroidism on the heart, showing that this condition may be associated with important abnormalities of cardiac structure and function (Biondi et al. 2002c). The more-consistent abnormalities found in patients with subclinical hyperthyroidism are increased heart rate and prevalence of supraventricular

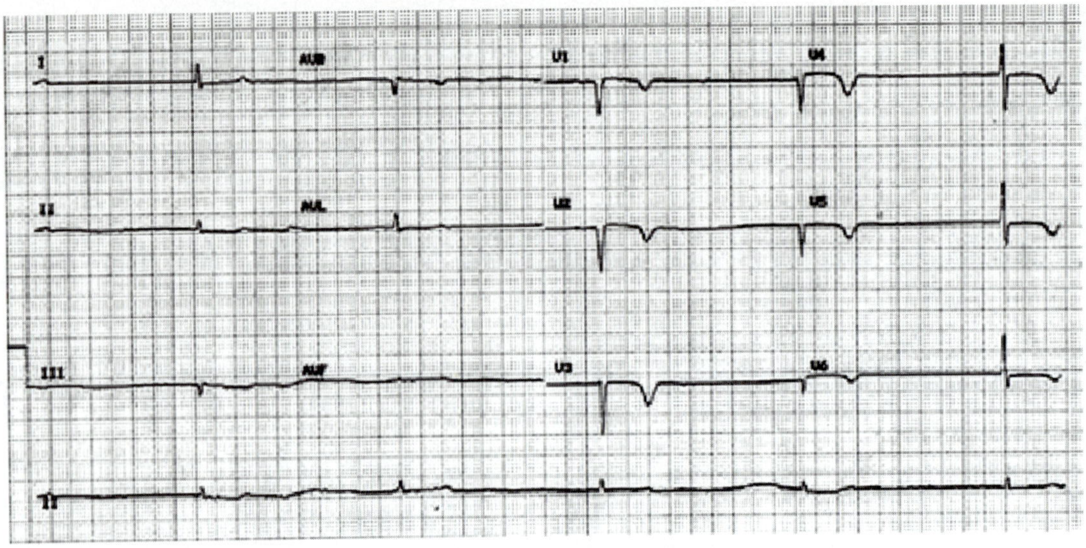

Fig. 47.104: *ECG shows marked bradycardia (30 bpm) with low QRS voltages (especially in the limb leads) and widespread T-wave inversions, typical of severe myxoedema*

arrhythmias and enhanced LV mass (Biondi et al. 1993, 1994, 1996, 1999b, 2000; Fazio et al. 1995; Ching et al. 1996; Shapiro et al., 1997; Mercuro et al. 2000). The latter feature often is associated with slightly enhanced systolic function and almost always with impaired diastolic function due to slowed myocardial relaxation (Biondi et al. 1993, 1994, 1996, 1999b, 2000; Fazio et al. 1995; Ching et al. 1996; Shapiro et al. 1997; Mercuro et al., 2000). The increase in LV mass is due to increased wall thickness without changes of cavity dimension ("concentric remodeling"). It rarely corresponds to an actual LV hypertrophy and is related to the duration of subclinical hyperthyroidism rather than to circulating thyroid hormone levels. The mechanism responsible for the increase in LV mass has not been completely clarified. In general, it is assumed to develop in response to a chronic hemodynamic overload due to the mild hyperkinetic cardiovascular state (Klein, 1988; Fazio et al. 1995). In fact, as happens with classic models of overload-induced cardiac hypertrophy, the increase of LV mass observed in patients with subclinical hyperthyroidism is associated with slowed myocardial relaxation and impaired ventricular filling. It has been suggested that this diastolic dysfunction results from altered intracellular calcium handling due to reduced expression of sarcoplasmic reticulum calcium ATPase and/ or increased expression of phospholamban, with the consequent delayed sarcoplasmic reuptake of calcium. However, this view would contrast with the well-known effects of thyroid hormone on such genes (Dillmann, 1990; Kiss et al. 1994). Therefore, it may be hypothesized that, in the long-term, the effects of chronically increased cardiac workload on calcium metabolism would prevail on those promoted by thyroid hormone. Be that as it may, abnormalities of LV morphology and function promptly normalize with achievement of euthyroidism and are effectively attenuated by β-blocking drugs (Biondi et al. 1994, 1995, 1999b, 2000). This supports the concept that cardiac involvement in subclinical hyperthyroidism is reversible and mostly determined by functional mechanisms.

Importantly, compelling evidence exists that subclinical hyperthyroidism is associated with increased cardiovascular mortality (Parle et al. 2001). Although the mechanism responsible for this association remains obscure, several factors may contribute to this phenomenon (Biondi et al. 2002b). There are indications that patients with subclinical hyperthyroidism, particularly the elderly, have an increased risk of atrial fibrillation (Sawin et al. 1994; Auer et al. 2001), which may enhance the incidence of thromboembolic events (Petersen and Hansen 1988; Ladenson 1993). It has been shown that the increase of LV mass per se, even in the absence of a clear LV hypertrophy, and of heart rate are associated with an increased risk of sudden death (Haider et al., 1998; Greenland et al., 1999). Moreover, it is well-recognized that diastolic dysfunction may precede development of more-severe LV dysfunction. Indeed, especially in the elderly, it may precipitate cardiac decompensation and CHF. Therefore, the current opinion is to avoid or correct subclinical hyperthyroidism in all patients affected with benign thyroid disease (Biondi et al., 2002c). On the contrary, when subclinical hyperthyroidism is a therapeutic indication (e.g. in patients with differentiated thyroid cancer), L-T4 should be administered at the lowest dose sufficient to achieve a stable TSH suppression, eventually associated with chronic β-blockade (Biondi et al. 2002c). Contextually, subclinical hyperthyroidism should be suspected in all subjects with a history of atrial fibrillation, especially in the elderly and in those with underlying cardiac disease who complain of worsening of angina pectoris or cardiac decompensation.

Overt Hypothyroidism (Figs 47.96–47.102)

The cardiovascular effects of thyroid hormone deficiency are opposite to those caused by thyroid hormone excess.

However, the clinical presentation of overt hypothyroidism is not obvious and most patients have few symptoms and signs (Klein and Ojamaa, 2000). Bradycardia and systemic hypertension, with narrow pulse pressure and slightly increased mean arterial pressure, and some degree of exercise impairment are the most-common findings in patients with overt hypothyroidism (McAllister et al. 1995; Klein and Ojamaa, 2000).

Many patients with overt hypothyroidism have abnormal standard ECG, including QT interval lengthening and flattening or inversion of the T wave (Fredlund and Olsson, 1983; Klein and Ojamaa, 2000), which reflects the prolonged cardiac action potential (Ojamaa et al. 1999). In addition, overt hypothyroid patients are more prone to ventricular arrhythmias, particularly in the presence of an underlying ischemic heart disease, due to increased electrical dispersion in the myocardium (Fredlund and Olsson, 1983; Klein and Ojamaa, 2000).

The prevalence of systemic hypertension is nearly threefold higher in patients with overt hyperthyroidism than in euthyroid subjects. In addition, in patients with systemic hypertension, overt hypothyroidism is associated with higher blood pressure (Endo et al. 1979; Saito et al. 1983; Streeten et al. 1988; Klein, 1989; Fletcher and Weetman, 1998; Fommei and Iervasi, 2002). Two factors contribute to systemic hypertension in overt hypothyroidism. The first, and certainly the most-widely recognized, is the remarkable increase in peripheral vascular resistance (Klein and Ojamaa, 2000). The second, and more-recently documented, is the increase in arterial stiffness, which likely results from myxedema of the arterial wall (Dernellis and Panaretou, 2002; Obuobie et al. 2002). In general, systemic hypertension associated with overt hypothyroidism is poorly controlled by conventional treatments, whereas it promptly improves with achievement of euthyroidism (Dernellis and Panaretou, 2002). This finding would encourage the routine assessment of thyroid function in all patients with preexisting systemic hypertension that becomes resistant to pharmacological treatment.

The most-consistent cardiac abnormality recognized in patients with overt hypothyroidism is impairment of LV diastolic function, which is characterized by slowed myocardial relaxation and impaired early ventricular filling (Crowley et al. 1977; Wieshammer et al. 1989). LV systolic function usually is only marginally subnormal, as demonstrated by slightly reduced values of ejection fraction and stroke volume (Crowley et al. 1977; Wieshammer et al. 1989). On the one hand, the reduced cardiac preload, in combination with bradycardia and slightly depressed myocardial contractility, accounts for a subnormal cardiac output in overt hypothyroidism (Crowley et al. 1977; Wieshammer et al. 1989). On the other hand, the lower cardiac performance and the abnormalities in peripheral and proximal vascular function may contribute to the poor exercise tolerance in overt hypothyroidism (McAllister et al. 1995).

Occasionally, cardiac function may be further compromised by the development of pericardial effusion, which occurs with severe, long-standing overt hypothyroidism (Ladenson et al. 1992). In addition, overt hypothyroidism may be associated with some increase in LV mass. However, as shown by necropsy and ultrasound investigations, the increase in LV mass does not correspond to myocardial hypertrophy sensu strictu but rather to interstitial myxedema (Aber, 1964). By increasing wall stiffness, cardiac myxedema may further compromise LV mechanics, contributing to reduced cardiac output.

In this context, it is important to recall that although overt hypothyroidism is associated with a lower myocardial oxygen demand, myocardial mechanical work efficiency is worse than in euthyroid controls and improves with achievement of euthyroidism (Bengel et al. 2000). The increase in peripheral vascular resistance and arterial stiffness in overt hypothyroidism contributes to increased cardiac afterload, one of the major factors determining myocardial oxygen consumption (Bengel et al. 2000). The disproportionate increase in myocardial oxygen uptake with respect to the level of cardiac performance may, therefore, explain at least in part why overt hypothyroidism may precipitate or worsen angina in patients with suspected or known ischemic heart disease (Keating et al. 1960) and why some of these patients have an improvement in anginal symptoms after thyroid hormone replacement is initiated.

Overt hypothyroidism may be particularly hazardous in the elderly, independent of the presence of underlying cardiovascular disease. Aging is accompanied by the development of cardiac hypertrophy and interstitial fibrosis, which may be responsible per se for diastolic dysfunction and reduced cardiovascular performance. Therefore, the onset of overt hypothyroidism in this vulnerable population occasionally may precipitate cardiac decompensation and CHF. In a single study, it was estimated that approximately 30–50% of elderly subjects with heart failure have normal values of ejection fraction (diastolic heart failure) (McDermott et al. 1995). Noteworthy, diastolic heart failure was strongly associated with hypothyroidism and was more prevalent in women (McDermott et al. 1995). Therefore, thyroid function should be routinely assessed in older patients with newly diagnosed or worsening heart failure.

Subclinical Hypothyroidism (Figs 47.104 and 47.105)

Subclinical hypothyroidism (SH), defined by elevated serum TSH level in the presence of normal levels of free thyroid hormones, is common in the adult population, especially among women above 60 years of age (Tunbridge et al. 1977; Canaris et al. 2000). Up to two-thirds of patients have serum TSH between 5–10 mU/L and thyroid autoantibodies (Tunbridge et al. 1977; Canaris et al. 2000). Almost half of these individuals may progress to overt thyroid failure (Vanderpump et al. 1995; Huber et al. 2002). Striking evidence indicates that elevated TSH levels in SH patients do not reflect pituitary compensation to maintain euthyroidism but mild tissue hypothyroidism sensu strictu (Andersen et al. 2002). Several changes in metabolic and organ function indexes have been reported in most clinical investigations of patients with persistent SH (Biondi et al. 2002c). Deviation from normality progressively increases with serum TSH level ("dosage effect" phenomenon) (Lekakis et al. 1997; Bindels et al. 1999; Faber et al. 2002). In general, resting heart rate and blood pressure are normal in SH subjects (Biondi et al. 1999a; Monzani et al. 2001; Di Bello et al. 2002; Vitale et al. 2002). However, significant hypofunctional abnormalities in the parasympathetic nervous system and an increased prevalence of systemic hypertension have been reported in patients with SH (Kahaly, 2000; Luboshitzky et al. 2002).

The most-consistent cardiac abnormality recognized in SH patients is LV diastolic dysfunction, characterized by slowed myocardial relaxation and impaired early ventricular filling, both at rest and with exercise (Biondi et al. 1999a; Monzani et al. 2001; Di Bello et al. 2002; Vitale et al. 2002; Brenta et al. 2003). Often, this is associated with a variable impairment in LV systolic function at rest (Biondi et al. 1999a; Monzani et al. 2001; Di Bello et al. 2002; Vitale et al. 2002), which becomes more consistent on exercise (Foldes et al. 1987; Kahaly, 2000; Brenta et al. 2003). In a comprehensive study of exercise capacity, it was reported that SH is associated with impairment of several exercise-related cardiopulmonary responses, resulting in some degree of exercise impairment (Kahaly, 2000).

Recently, a strong association between SH and atherosclerotic cardiovascular disease, independent of the traditional risk factors (i.e. hypercholesterolemia, hypertension, smoking, diabetes mellitus), was noted in a large cross-sectional survey of postmenopausal women (the Rotterdam Study) (Hak et al. 2000). Although the mechanism responsible for this association remains to be clarified, compelling evidence indicates that SH is associated with an atherogenic lipid profile, characterized by increased circulating levels of total and low-density cholesterol and increased levels of oxidized low-density lipoproteins (Duntas, 2002; Duntas et al. 2002). It has been reported that SH may affect the hemostatic profile, thereby promoting a hypercoagulable state (Müller et al. 2001). Moreover, a reduced endothelium-dependent, flow-mediated vasodilation, which is an early marker of atherosclerosis, has been reported in patients with SH (Lekakis et al. 1997).

Importantly, when SH patients are treated with L-T4, most metabolic and cardiovascular abnormalities improve or even normalize (Danese et al. 2000; Biondi et al. 2002c). However, whether patients with SH should be treated remains the subject of disagreement (Chu and Crapo, 2001; McDermott and Ridgway, 2001).

Amiodarone and Thyroid Disease

Amiodarone, a class III antiarrhythmic agent, is widely used in atrial and ventricular rhythm disturbances. The high iodine content of amiodarone (3 mg iodine per 100 mg amiodarone) can result in hypothyroidism (5–25% of treated patients) or hyperthyroidism (2–10%).

The baseline serum TSH, free T4 and T3, and antithyroid antibodies should be measured before starting amiodarone and monitored every 6 months.

Amiodarone-induced hyperthyroidism is described as type-1 in patients with existing thyroid disease or goitre and type-2 in euthyroid patients. Hypothyroidism should be treated with thyroxine replacement.

Treatment of both types of amiodarone-induced hyperthyroidism is more difficult. It is relatively resistant to the thioureas owing to high intrathyroid iodine content, and the effect of radioactive iodine is poor because iodine uptake by the thyroid is reduced.

A pragmatic approach is to treat patients with high-dose carbimazole. Resistance to carbimazole should raise the possibility of type-2 disease.

Treatment with potassium perchlorate, with or without oral prednisolone 30–40 mg per day, should be considered. Refractory cases may need thyroidectomy.

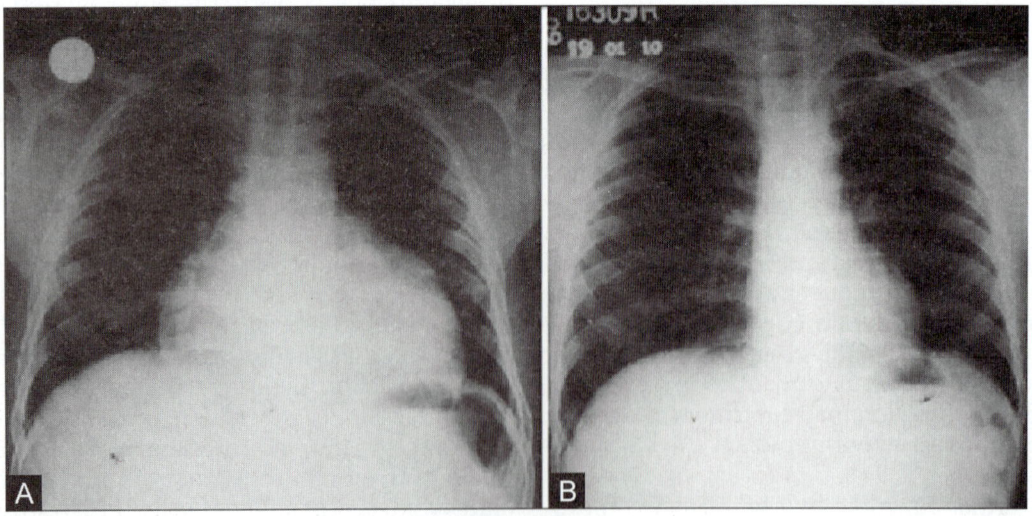

Fig. 47.105: *(A) Chest X-ray PA view showing cardiomegaly before treatment. (B) Chest X-ray PA view showing resolution of cardiac enlargement after thyroxine supplementation at follow-up (8 months)*

Conclusion

Thyroid dysfunction causes remarkable cardiovascular derangements. Because signs and symptoms referable to the cardiovascular system may be the only manifestations of overt thyroid dysfunction and because persistent subclinical thyroid dysfunction may notably increase the cardiovascular risk, thyroid status should be systematically investigated in all patients with newly diagnosed or worsening cardiovascular disease, especially the elderly. In addition, patients with acute or chronic cardiovascular disorders have abnormalities in peripheral thyroid hormone metabolism that may alter cardiac function. The finding that administration of thyroid hormone or its analog 3,5-diiodothyropropionic acid may greatly benefit these patients should foster further investigation in this area.

THALASSEMIAS AND HEART DISEASE

Thalassemia (British spelling, "thalassaemia") is an inherited autosomal recessive blood disease. In thalassemia, the genetic defect results in reduced rate of synthesis of one of the globin chains that make up hemoglobin. Reduced synthesis of one of the globin chains can cause the formation of abnormal haemoglobin molecules, and this in turn causes the anemia which is the characteristic presenting symptom of the thalassemias.

Thalassemia is a quantitative problem of too few globins synthesized, whereas sickle-cell disease (a haemoglobinopathy) is a qualitative problem of synthesis of an incorrectly functioning globin (Figs 47.106–108).

Thalassemias usually result in under production of normal globin proteins, often through mutations in regulatory genes. Hemoglobinopathies imply structural abnormalities in the globin proteins themselves. The two conditions may overlap, however, since some conditions which cause abnormalities in globin proteins (hemoglobinopathy) also affect their production (thalassemia). Thus, some thalassemias are hemoglobinopathies, but most are not. Either or both of these conditions may cause anemia. The disease is particularly prevalent among Mediterranean peoples, and this geographical association was response between ble for its naming: Thalassa (èÜëáóóá) is Greek for the sea, Haema is Greek for blood. In Europe, the highest concentrations of the disease are found in Greece including the Greek islands; in parts of Italy, in particular, the lower Po valley; in Southern Italy; and in the Italian islands. Sicily, Sardinia (Italian islands), Corsica (French island) and Cyprus and Crete (Greek islands) are heavily affected in particular; the higher incidence in these islands likely is because of the higher inbreeding that occurs in isolated populations. But Asia now has even greater prevalence with the highest concentration of carriers (18% of the population) in the Maldives.

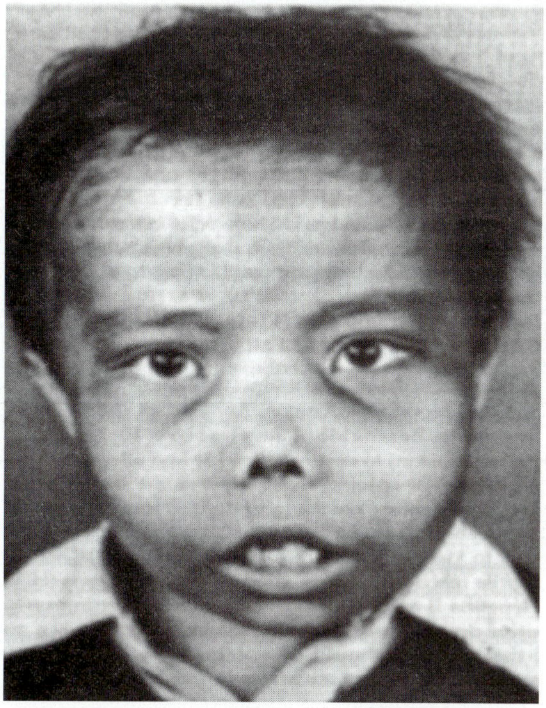

Fig. 47.106: *Prominence of frontal, parietal, and maxillary bones due to bone marrow hypertrophy ,depressed bridge of nose and typical pallor giving an impression of 'mongoloid facies' in a young patient with thalassemia major*

Prevalence

Generally, thalassemias are prevalent in populations that evolved in humid climates where malaria was endemic, but affects all races. Thalassemias are particularly associated with Arabs, people of Mediterranean origin, and Asians. The Maldives has the highest incidence of Thalassemia in the world with a carrier rate of 18% of the population. The estimated prevalence is 16% in people from Cyprus, 3–14% in Thailand, and 3–8% in populations from Bangladesh, China, India, Malaysia and Pakistan. There are also prevalences in descendants of people from Latin America and Mediterranean countries (e.g. Greece, Italy, Portugal, Spain and others). A very low prevalence has been reported from people in northern Europe (0.1%) and Africa (0.9%), with those in Northern Africa having the highest prevalence. Ancient Egyptians suffered from Thalassemia and it was particularly common in populations of indigenous ethnic minorities such as the Beja, Hadendoa, Saiddi and Siwans.

Pathophysiology

The thalassemias are classified according to which chain of the hemoglobin molecule is affected (*see* hemoglobin for a description of the chains). In α thalassemias, production of the α globin chain is affected, while in α thalassemia production of the α globin chain is affected.

Thalassemia produces a deficiency of β or α globin, unlike sickle-cell disease which produces a specific mutant form of α globin. α globin chains are encoded by a single gene on chromosome 11; α globin chains are encoded by two closely linked genes on chromosome 16. Thus in a normal person with two copies of each chromosome, there are two loci encoding the β chain, and four loci encoding the β chain.

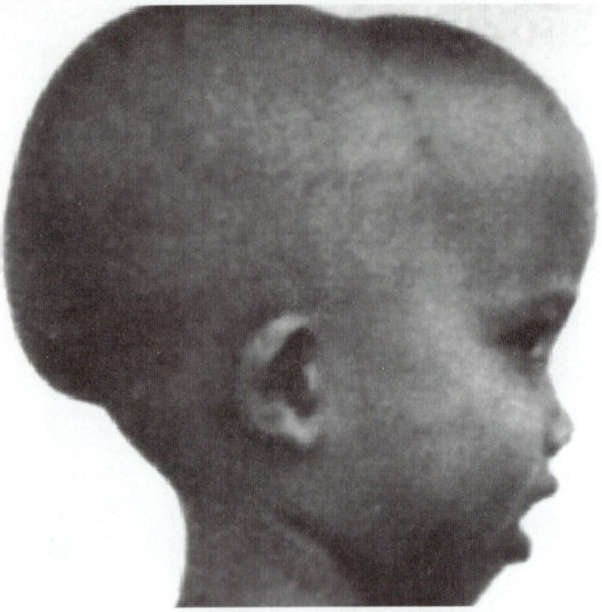

Fig. 47.107: *Enlargement of skull bones in a child with long-standing beta-thalassemia*

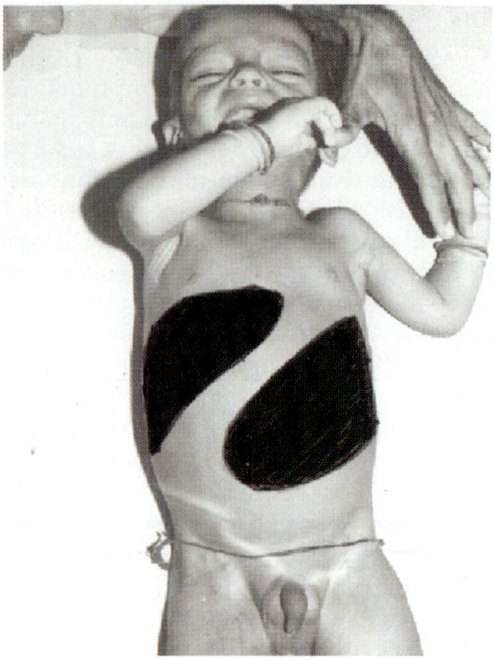

Fig. 47.108: *Splenohepatomegaly in a young child with thalassemia*

Deletion of one of the α loci has a high prevalence in people of African-American or Asian descent, making them more likely to develop α thalassemias. α-thalassemias are common in African-Americans, but also in Greeks and Italians.

Alpha (α) Thalassemias

The α thalassemias involve the genes HBA1 [Online 'Mendelian Inheritance in Man' (OMIM) 141800] and HBA2 [Online 'Mendelian Inheritance in Man' (OMIM) 141850], inherited in a Mendelian recessive fashion. It is also connected to the deletion of the 16p chromosome. α thalassemias result in decreased alpha-globin production, therefore fewer alpha-globin chains are produced, resulting in an excess of β chains in adults and excess β chains in newborns. The excess β chains form unstable tetramers (called Hemoglobin H or HbH of 4 beta chains) which have abnormal oxygen dissociation curves.

There are four genetic loci for α globin, two of which are maternal in origin and two of which are paternal in origin. The severity of the á thalassemias is correlated with the number of affected á globin loci: the greater the number of affected loci, the more severe will be the manifestations of the disease.

- If one of the four α loci is affected, there is minimal effect. Three α-globin loci are enough to permit normal hemoglobin production, and there are no clinical symptoms. They have been called silent carriers. They may have a slightly reduced mean corpuscular volume and mean corpuscular hemoglobin.

If two of the four α loci are affected, the condition is called alpha thalassemia trait. Two α loci permit nearly normal erythropoiesis, but there is a mild microcytic hypochromic anemia. The disease in this form can be mistaken for iron deficiency anemia and treated inappropriately with iron. Alpha thalassemia trait can exist in two forms: one form, associated with Asians, involves cis deletion of two alpha loci on the same chromosome; the other, associated with Blacks, involves trans deletion of alpha loci on different (homologous) chromosomes.

- If three loci are affected, the condition is called hemoglobin H disease. Two unstable hemoglobins are present in the blood: hemoglobin Barts (tetrameric γ chains) and Hemoglobin H (tetrameric β chains). Both of these unstable hemoglobins have a higher affinity for oxygen than normal hemoglobin, resulting in poor oxygen delivery to tissues. There is a microcytic hypochromic anemia with target cells and Heinz bodies (precipitated

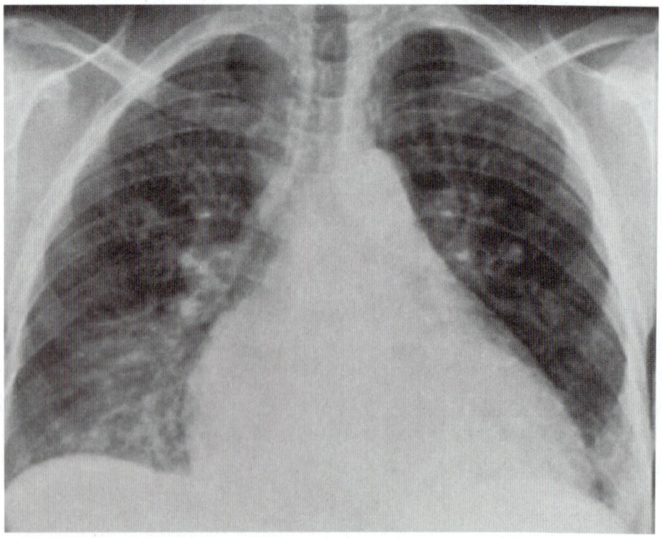

Fig. 47.109: *Cardiomegaly and pulmonary congestion due to heart failure in patient with long-standing beta-thalassemia*

HbH) on the peripheral blood smear, as well as splenomegaly. The disease may first be noticed in childhood or in early adult life when the anemia and splenomegaly are noted.

- If all *four* loci are affected, the fetus cannot live once outside the uterus and may not survive gestation: most such infants are dead at birth with *hydrops fetalis*, and those who are born alive die shortly after birth. They are edematous and have little circulating hemoglobin, and the hemoglobin that is present is all tetrameric ã chains (hemoglobin Barts).

Beta (β) Thalassemias (Fig. 47.110)

Beta thalassemias are due to mutations in the HBB gene on chromosome 11 [Online "Mendelian Inheritance in Man" (OMIM) 141900], also inherited in an autosomal-recessive fashion. The severity of the disease depends on the nature of the mutation. Mutations are characterized as (β^o) if they prevent any formation of β chains; they are characterized as (β^+) if they allow some β chain formation to occur. In either case there is a relative excess of β chains, but these do not form tetramers: rather, they bind to the red blood cell membranes, producing membrane damage, and at high concentrations they form toxic aggregates. Any given individual has two α globin alleles.

- If only *one* α-globin allele bears a mutation, the disease is called **α-thalassemia minor** (or sometimes called **β–thalassemia trait**). This is a mild microcytic anemia. In most cases β-thalassemia minor is asymptomatic, and many affected people are unaware of the disorder. Detection usually involves measuring the mean corpuscular volume (size of red blood cells) and noticing a slightly decreased mean volume than normal. The patient will have an increased fraction of hemoglobin A2 (>2.5%) and a decreased fraction of hemoglobin A (<97.5%).

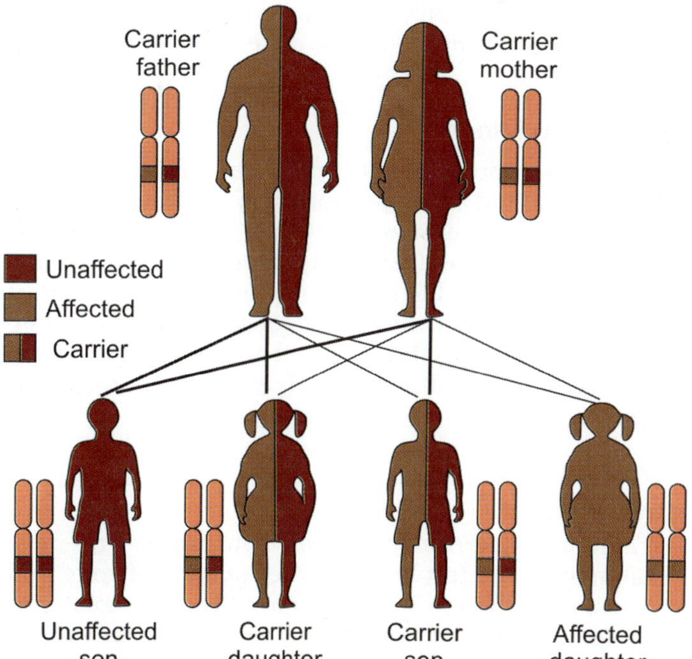

Fig. 47.110: *Genetic transmission of beta -thalassemia*

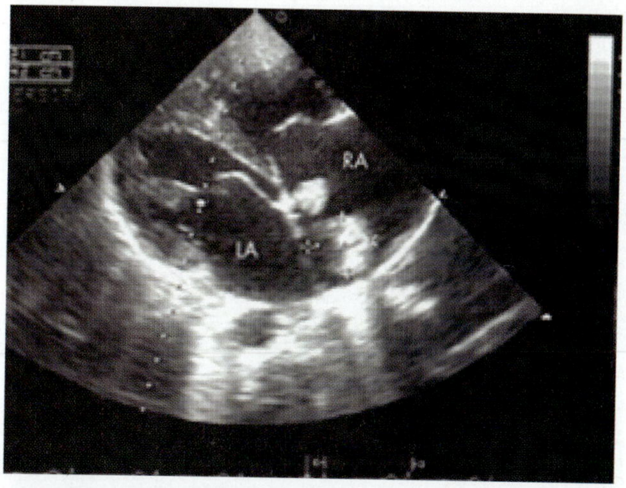

Fig. 47.111: *Transthoracic echocardiographic examination revealed two mobile, homogenous masses suggesting thrombus or myxoma at two separate locations in the right atria. Both atrial and ventricular dimensions and functions were normal. A transoesophageal echocardiogram confirmed the presence of the two masses*

If *both* alleles have thalassemia mutations, the disease is called **β-thalassemia major** or **Cooley's anemia**. This is a severe microcytic, hypochromic anemia. Untreated, this progresses to death before age 20 years. Treatment consists of periodic blood transfusion; splenectomy if splenomegaly is present, and treatment of transfusion-caused iron overload. Cure is possible by bone marrow transplantation.

Thalassemia intermedia is a condition intermediate between the major and the minor forms. Affected individuals can often manage a normal life but may need occasional transfusions, e.g. at times of illness or pregnancy, depending on the severity of their anemia.

The genetic mutations present in α–thalassemias are very diverse, and a number of different mutations can cause reduced or absent β globin synthesis. Two major groups of mutations can be distinguished.

Nondeletion forms: These defects generally involve a single base substitution or small deletion or inserts near or upstream of the β globin gene. Most commonly, mutations occur in the promoter regions preceding the beta-globin genes. Less often, abnormal splice variants are believed to contribute to the disease.

Deletion forms: Deletions of different sizes involving the a globin gene produce different syndromes such as (b^o) or hereditary persistence of fetal hemoglobin syndromes.

Delta (δ) Thalassemia

As well as alpha and beta chains being present in hemoglobin about 3% of adult hemoglobin is made of alpha and delta chains. Just as with beta-thalassemia, mutations can occur which affect the ability of this gene to produce delta chains. A mutation that prevents formation of any delta chains is termed a delta$^+$ mutation, whereas one that

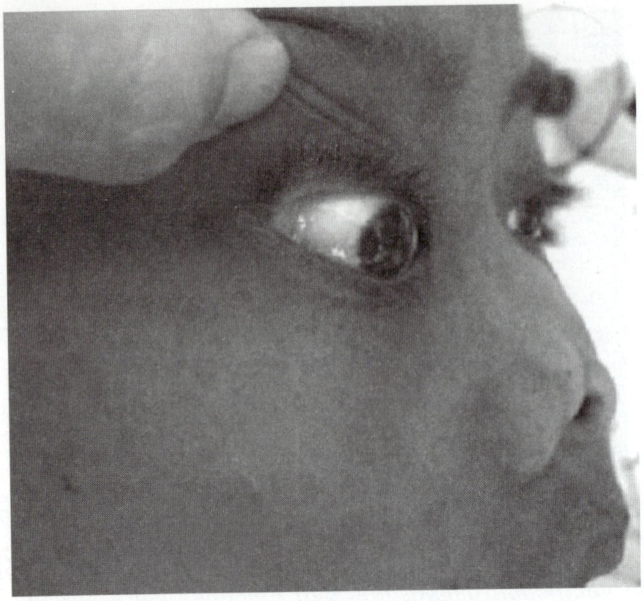

Fig. 47.112: *Follow-up examination of eyes after blood transfusion therapy in patient with beta-thalassemia*

decreases but does not eliminate production of delta chain is termed a delta$^+$ mutation. When one inherits two delta^0 mutations, no hemoglobin A2 (alpha2, delta2) can be formed. Hematologically, however, this is innocuous because only 2–3% of normal adult hemoglobin is hemoglobin A2. The individual will have normal hematological parameters (erythrocyte count, total hemoglobin, mean corpuscular volume, red cell distribution width). Individuals who inherit only one delta-thalassemia mutation gene will have a decreased hemoglobin A2, but also no hematological consequences. The importance of recognizing the existence of delta-thalassemia is seen best in cases where it may mask the diagnosis of beta-thalassemia trait. In beta thalassemia, there is an increase in hemoglobin A2, typically in the range of 4–6% (normal is 2–3%). However, the coexistence of a delta-thalassemia mutation will decrease the value of the hemoglobin A2 into the normal range, thereby obscuring the diagnosis of beta thalassemia trait. This can be important in genetic counseling, because a child who is the product of parents each of whom has $\beta°$-thalassemia trait has a one in four chance of having $\beta°$-thalassemia major. In combination with other hemoglobinopathies

Thalassemia can coexist with other hemoglobinopathies. The most common of these are:

- Hemoglobin E/thalassemia: Common in Cambodia, Thailand, and parts of India; clinically similar to α–thalassemia major or thalassemia intermedia. Hemoglobin S/thalassemia, common in African and Mediterranean populations; clinically similar to sickle cell anemia, with the additional feature of splenomegaly.
- Hemoglobin C/thalassemia: Common in Mediterranean and African populations, hemoglobin C/α^o thalassemia causes a moderately severe hemolytic anemia with splenomegaly; hemoglobin C/α^+-thalassemia produces a milder disease.

Treatment and Complications

Anyone with thalassemia should consult a properly qualified hematologist. Thalassemias may co-exist with other deficiencies such as folic acid (or folate, a B-complex vitamin) and iron deficiency (only in thalassemia minor).

Thalassemia Major and Intermedia

Thalassemia major patients receive frequent blood transfusions that lead to iron overload. Iron chelation treatment is necessary to prevent iron overload damage to the internal organs in patients with thalassemia major. Because of recent advances in iron chelation treatments, patients with thalassemia major can live long lives if they have access to proper treatment. Popular chelators include deferoxamine and deferiprone. Of the two, deferoxamine is preferred; it is more effective and is associated with fewer side-effects.

The most common complaint by patients receiving deferoxamine is that it is difficult to comply with the intravenous chelation treatments because they are painful and inconvenient. The oral chelator deferasirox (marketed as Exjade by Novartis) was approved for use in 2005 in some countries. It offers some hope with compliance but is very expensive, and has been associated with deaths from toxicity.

Untreated thalassemia major eventually leads to death usually by heart failure, therefore birth screening is very important. In recent years, bone marrow transplant has shown promise with some patients of thalassemia major. Successful transplant can eliminate the patients dependencies in transfusions.

All thalassemia patients are susceptible to health complications that involve the spleen (which is often enlarged and frequently removed) and gall stones. These complications are mostly prevalent to thalassemia major and intermedia patients. Thalassemia intermedia patients vary a lot in their treatment needs depending on the severity of their anemia.

Thalassemia Minor

Contrary to popular belief, thalassemia minor patients should not avoid iron-rich foods by default. A serum ferritin test can determine what their iron levels are and guide them to further treatment if necessary. Thalassemia minor, although not life threatening on its own, can affect quality of life due to the effects of a mild to moderate anemia. Studies have shown that thalassemia minor often coexists with other diseases such as asthma, and mood disorders.

Complications

- Iron overload
- Traditionally, ferritin level assessment has been the most commonly used test for indirect evaluation of body iron stores, even though it reflects only 1% of the total iron storage pool. The test is not perfect or accurate, as various conditions complicate the interpretation of its values. For this reason, reliance on serum ferritin assessment alone

can lead to an inaccurate assessment of body iron stores in patients with iron overload who have been transfused heavily and who have levels in excess of the upper limit for the physiologic ferritin synthesis (400 mcg/L). At high levels, the test loses its clinical relevance since ferritin can be released from damaged cells in certain pathologic conditions.

Furthermore, certain drugs and clinical conditions such as ascorbate deficiency, fever, acute and chronic infections, and hemolysis may influence the ferritin level, producing misleading values. Despite its deficiencies, and for lack of a better practical, noninvasive test, ferritin assessment continues to be the most commonly used tool to diagnose and to monitor iron overload.

MRI or CT scanning is used to assess liver iron levels as a measure of total body iron load.

Liver biopsy may be performed to assess liver iron concentration, which is considered the most sensitive method to assess body iron burden. Again, this procedure is an invasive one and not without complications. Furthermore, because iron distribution in the thalassemic liver is uneven and could be affected by fibrosis, one can expect conflicting and inaccurate results in some patients. Grading of stainable iron or measuring parenchymal iron by atomic absorption spectroscopy has been helpful in measuring tissue iron levels, with good correlation to calculated body iron burden.

Cardiac Complications (Figs 47.109, 47.111, 47.114–47.115)

- Most deaths in patients with thalassemia are due to cardiac involvement. These complications range from constrictive pericarditis to heart failure and arrhythmias.
- Transfusional hemosiderosis has been classified into 3 stages based on the number of blood units given. The higher the number of PRBC units given, the more advanced the stage. Advanced stage is associated with more severe clinical symptoms and more abnormal findings on cardiac function studies.
- Cardiac hemosiderosis does not occur without significant accumulation of iron in other tissues.
- Chelation therapy has shown promising results in patients with cardiac symptoms due to iron overload.
- Ventricular myocardium is the first site of cardiac iron deposition while the conduction system is usually the last to be affected. The value of endomyocardial biopsy, which has been used to evaluate iron deposits in the heart, has been questioned. Iron has been reported as absent from the right ventricular subendocardium in some patients with cardiac iron overload.

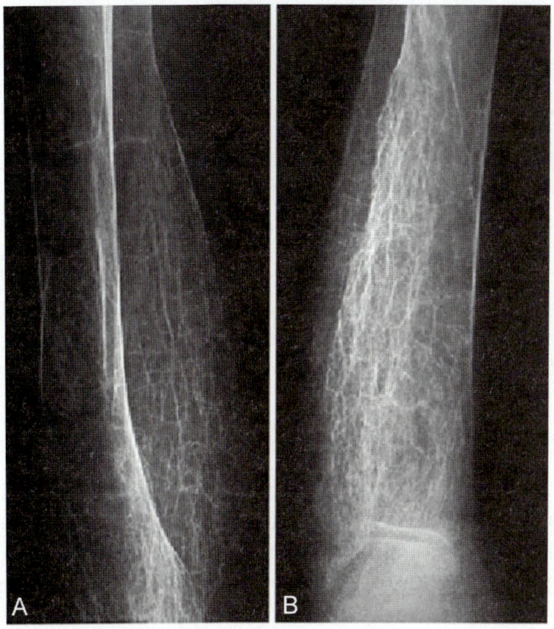

Fig. 47.113: *A cobwebbing trabecular pattern of long bones in patient with long-standing beta-thalassemia*

Echocardiography,radionuclide cineangiogrphy, **and 24-hour ECG** are to be used to monitor these patients (Fig. 47.115).

Hepatic Complications

Patients who have received regular blood transfusions for some time develop liver enlargement due to swelling of the phagocytic and parenchymal cells from the deposition of hemosiderin.

- Liver enzyme levels are not typically elevated unless hemosiderin deposition is associated with hepatitis.
- Chelation therapy may prevent or delay progressive liver disease, which may end in cirrhosis.

Long-Term Therapy Complications

Because of improved medical care, patients with thalassemia are surviving their disease longer and reaching old age. With this longer survival comes new issues related to complications that need to be addressed.

HCV has emerged as the paramount risk in patients who have been receiving blood transfusions all their lives. HCV screening was initiated in 1990. Since then, according to the registry of the TCRN, the incidence rate of HCV has dropped significantly. The current prevalence of HCV in patients with thalassemia older than 25 years is 70%, as opposed to only 5% in those with thalassemia aged 15 years or younger.

Unfortunately, a high incidence rate of HCV continues in developing countries, leading to an increased incidence of fibrosis, cirrhosis, and hepatocellular carcinoma (HCC), especially in the presence of a second risk factor such as iron overload. For this reason, many centers advocate screening patients with HCV every 6 months by obtaining a fetoprotein (AFP) and an ultrasound of the liver. According to the TCRN, approximately 33% of patients with thalassemia major who are also HCV positive develop a spontaneous clearance of the HCV. Two-thirds of patients with β-thalassemia major have multiple calcified bilirubin stones by age 15 years.

Hematologic Complications

Recently, thrombosis was encountered in relatively significant numbers of patients with thalassemia. In a study of 83 patients with thalassemia intermedia, a 26% incidence

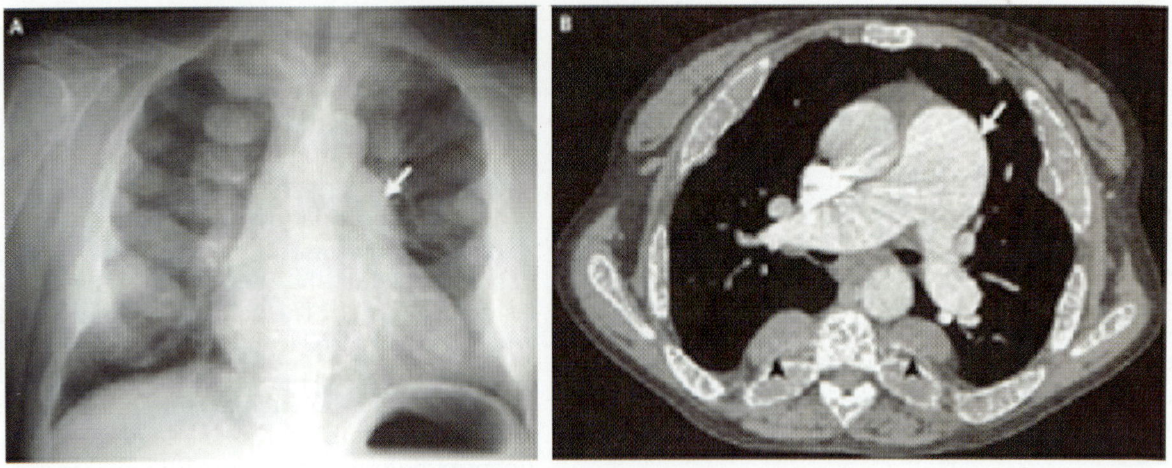

Fig. 47.114: *Chest radiography (Panel A, arrow) and computed tomography (Panel B, arrow) show enlarged central pulmonary arteries owing to pulmonary arterial hypertension. In patients with thalassemia, such enlargement is thought to arise from chronic anemia, hemolysis, and an increased tendency for microscopic thrombi to form within the pulmonary vasculature. Bilateral paravertebral soft-tissue masses (Panel B, arrowheads), as well as marked medullary expansion of the bony structures (with the ribs showing the most pronounced involvement), were also present, findings that are associated with compensatory extramedullary hematopoiesis*

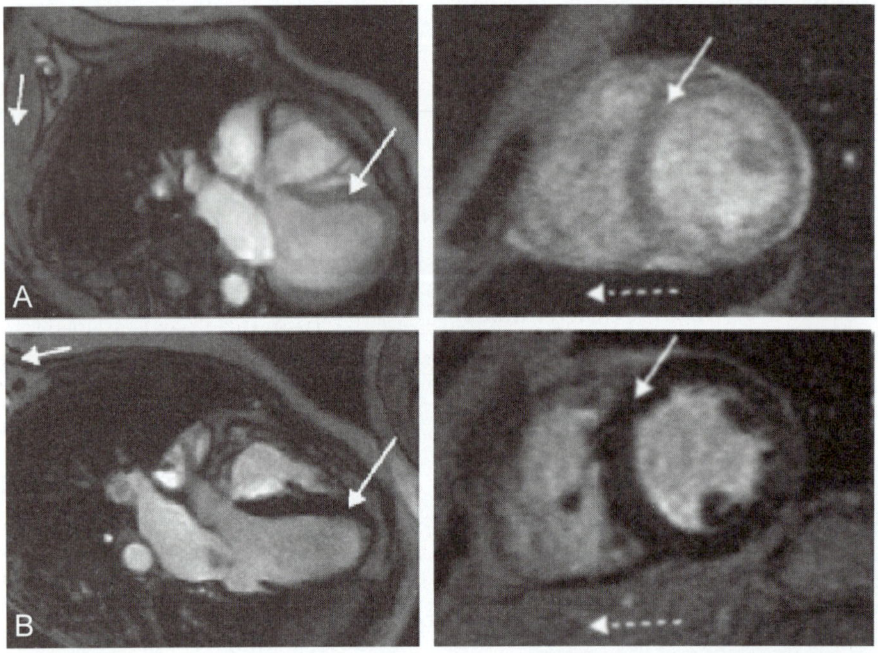

Fig. 47.115: *Magnetic resonance scans in patients with thalassemia major. Left scans are horizontal long axis, the right ones mid-short axis. (A) Low myocardial iron deposition. The left ventricular volumes are normal, and myocardial signal intensity (long arrow) is similar to that arising from skeletal muscle (short arrow). Left ventricular ejection fraction was 70%. In this case, the liver is very dark (dotted arrow), indicating heavy hepatic iron deposition despite the normal myocardial appearances. (B) Severe myocardial iron overload. The myocardial signal intensity is dark (long arrow) compared with skeletal muscle (short arrow). The ventricle is dilated and thickened. Cine imaging showed greatly reduced systolic function (left ventricular ejection fraction 39%) with a restrictive filling pattern. Liver signal in this case is well preserved (dotted arrow)*

rate of VTEs was encountered while only 2% of 65 patients with thalassemia major developed VTE.

- One study determined that most of the patients with thalassemia intermedia who developed VTE had been splenectomized. Based on this fact, several centers recommend some type of prophylactic therapy to prevent thrombosis in such patients. Short-term antithrombotic therapy, both perioperatively and in the presence of thrombotic risk factors, is recommended. Patients who have undergone splenectomy and have a platelet count in excess of 600,000/μL receive low-dose daily aspirin. Development of pulmonary hypertension in such patients as a result of small pulmonary thrombi represents a significant indication of the increased risk for clotting. Based on the observation of hypercoagulable state in patients with thalassemia, exaggerated by splenectomy, the role of such a procedure in patients with thalassemia needs to be reconsidered.

Endocrine Complications

People with thalassemia major frequently exhibit features of diabetes mellitus; 50% or more exhibit clinical or subclinical diabetes. This is believed to be due to defective pancreatic production of insulin, but insulin resistance also has been implicated.

Glucose intolerance encountered in these patients usually correlates with the numbers of transfusions received and the patient's age and genetic background.

A recent study compared the incidence of endocrinopathy in patients with thalassemia with the incidence in patients with sickle cell disease and a similar iron overload due to transfusion. The study also compared patients with sickle cell disease who received transfusion with those who did not receive transfusion. The study showed that patients with thalassemia are far more prone to develop various endocrinopathies than patients with sickle cell disease. Furthermore, the incidence did not differ between patients with sickle cell disease who received transfusion and those who did not. However, the duration of transfusion was found to be a significant predictor. Thus, the underlying disease may modulate iron-related endocrine injury.

Growth Retardation

Growth retardation is frequently severe in patients with thalassemia. This retardation is caused, in part, by the diversion of caloric resources for erythropoiesis, as well as by the chronic anemia, since hypertransfusion usually restores normal growth. Unless chelation therapy is initiated early in life, patients rarely grow normally. Excessive chelation with DFO may also cause growth retardation.

The direct cause of growth retardation in these patients is thought to be an impaired growth hormone production or deficiency in production of somatomedin by the hemosiderotic liver. Involvement of the adrenal glands or the thyroid gland may also contribute to growth failure.

Fertility and Pregnancy Complications

Adult patients with thalassemia major are known to have low fertility; this is attributed to the commonly encountered hypogonadotrophic hypogonadism.

Both primary and secondary sexual characteristics are usually delayed in both males and females.

Females are frequently oligomenorrheic or amenorrheic. Pregnancy complications are also seen frequently and are likely due to endocrinologic and cardiac complications. Case reports demonstrated, however, that successful pregnancy and delivery of healthy babies is possible in women with thalassemia major.

Early intervention with hormonal therapy and aggressive chelation to prevent permanent damage may help to preserve fertility.

Transfusion complications: The most common complications of blood transfusion.

Chelation Therapy Complications

These complications and the specific adverse effects of DFO

Viral hepatitis: Viral hepatitis has been reported in nontransfused patients with iron overload, suggesting that iron overload predisposes patients to viral hepatitis, as was stated above.

Prognosis

The prognosis depends on the type and severity of thalassemia. As stated above, the clinical course of thalassemia varies greatly from mild or even asymptomatic to severe and life-threatening.

Prevention

Screening and Prevention

In persons with b thalassemia trait, confirming the diagnosis is usually easy. In such situations, genetic counseling is necessary, and, if both parents are carriers, a detailed discussion with the couple should include all possible outcomes. These include the 1 in 4 chance of having a severely affected or completely healthy child and a 1 in 2 chance of having a child with heterozygous thalassemia.

For a thalassemia carriers, confirmation is not that simple. Hb electrophoresis is usually not informative. For this reason, more sophisticated studies are warranted if confirmation is critical. Genetic counseling should be provided for patients with b thalassemia if a sibling or a family member is known to be affected.

Prenatal DNA testing has been available for several years. The decision to perform prenatal diagnosis in parents known to be at risk for having a child with thalassemia is complex and is usually influenced by several factors, such as religion, culture, education, and the number of children in the family. Genetic counseling by professionals that addresses the details of both the genetic risks and the testing risks involved is expected to help the parents make an informed and intelligent decision concerning the procedure. Unfortunately, such tests are not available in certain areas of the world where they are needed most. Extensive screening programs and prenatal diagnosis has resulted in a significant decline in the incidence of β-thalassemia in some of the high-risk Mediterranean countries.

Successful prevention programs in different parts of the world have resulted in an impressive decline in the number of patients with severe forms of thalassemia. Ferrara, Cyprus, Sardinia, Greece, and the United Kingdom were among the first to report a significant decline in the birth rate of children with thalassemia major. Many other regions with more limited resources are following their steps with remarkable success. In addition to the effective prenatal diagnosis adopted in the countries mentioned, other measures such as premarital screening programs, genetic counseling, and restrictions on issuing marriage certificates and licenses also proved to be effective. Because many of the countries where thalassemia prevails are poor and cannot afford sophisticated preventive programs, more practical approaches are clearly needed.

Screening of children, pregnant women, and individuals visiting public health facilities is effective in identifying individuals at risk who require further testing. A simple CBC count, with emphasis on the RBC counts and indices, including the MCV, MCH, and RDW, is the main component of such screening processes. Persons suspected to be positive for thalassemia are checked for elevated levels of Hb A_2, Hb F, or both for confirmation. In some situations, this simple method is not adequate, and further testing including analyses of globin chain synthesis, must be performed to reach a final diagnosis.

Prenatal Diagnosis

Globin chain synthesis, which was once used in postnatal diagnosis, was also used on fetal cells obtained by fetoscopy to screen the fetus. This test reveals imbalanced production of certain globin chains that are diagnostic of thalassemia.

Since polymerase chain reaction (PCR) techniques have become available, several new methods are now in use to identify affected babies or carrier individuals accurately and quickly. The DNA material is obtained by chorionic villus sampling (CVS), and mutations that change restriction enzyme cutting sites can be identified. Because many of the mutations that cause α and β thalassemia have become known in recent years, identifying such mutations on the amplified β-globin gene region is now possible with specific labeled oligonucleotide probes. Some of the new techniques can give accurate results in less than 3 hours.

IDIOPATHIC DILATED CARDIOMYOPATHY (DCM)

Idiopathic dilated cardiomyopathy (DCM) refers to congestive cardiac failure secondary to dilatation and systolic dysfunction (with or without diastolic dysfunction) of the ventricles (predominantly left) in the absence of congenital, valvular, or coronary artery disease or any systemic disease known to cause myocardial dysfunction. DCM is the most common type of heart muscle disease in children.

All 4 cardiac chambers are dilated and are sometimes hypertrophied. Dilation is more pronounced than hypertrophy, and the left ventricle is affected more often than the right ventricle. The cardiac valves are intrinsically normal, although the mitral and tricuspid valve rings are dilated, and the valve leaflets do not appose each other in systole, giving rise to varying degrees of mitral regurgitation, tricuspid regurgitation or both. Persistent mitral regurgitation leads to thickening of the mitral valve leaflets, and, at times, distinguishing this thickening from other causes of mitral regurgitation is difficult. Thrombus formation (secondary to the low-flow cardiac output state) is often seen in the left ventricular apex and, at times, is seen in the atria. Occasionally, the right ventricle is preferentially involved in the cardiomyopathic process; this often indicates a familial basis.

Pathophysiology

Injury to the myocardial cell is the initiating factor that leads to cell death. If considerable cell loss occurs, the myocardium fails to generate enough contractile force to produce adequate cardiac output. This results in the activation of compensatory mechanisms including the renin-angiotensin-aldosterone system, sympathetic stimulation, antidiuretic hormone production, release of atrial natriuretic peptide, tumor necrosis factor (TNF)-α, and mechanical factors, such as increased end-diastolic stretch on the ventricle.

These compensatory mechanisms help to maintain cardiac output in the initial phase; however, as myocardial damage progresses, persistent and excessive activation can be detrimental to cardiac function, leading to overt congestive heart failure. Over-stretching of the ventricles causes myocardial thinning, cavity dilation, secondary valvular regurgitation, and compromised myocardial

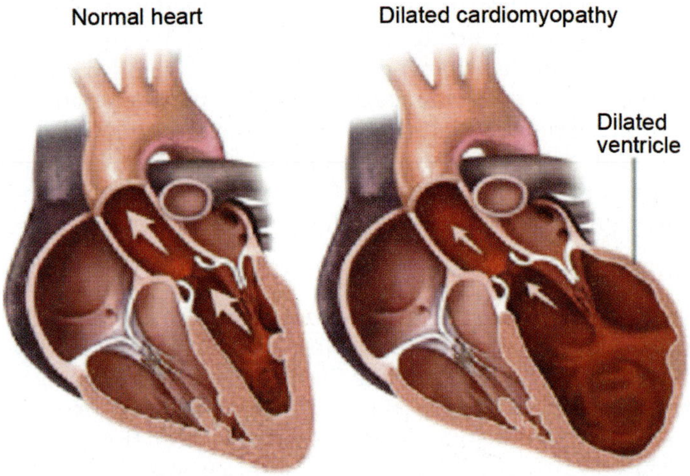

Fig. 47.116: *A comparison in the cross-section between a normal heart and a heart affected by DCM*

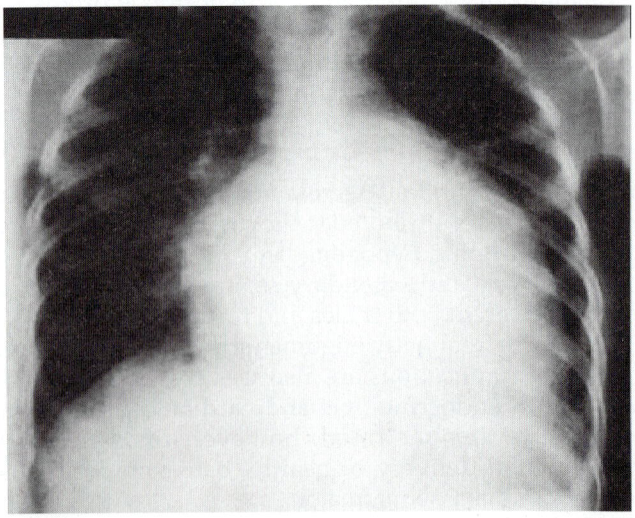

Fig. 47.117: *X-ray chest PA view showing massive cardiomegaly involving almost all chambers of the heart in Idiopathic dilated cardiomyopathy*

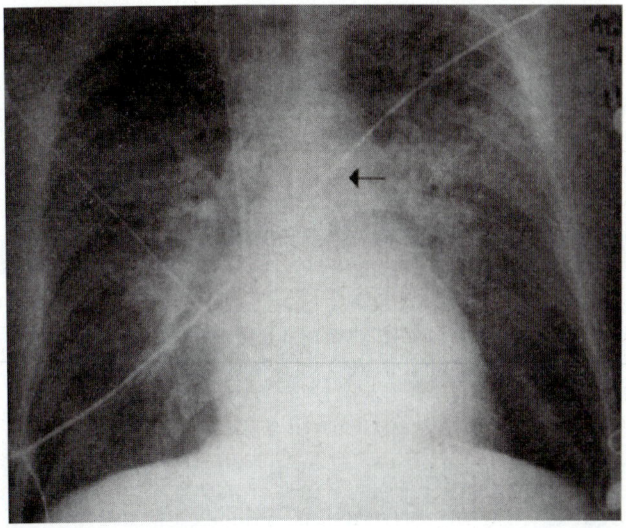

Fig. 47.118: *Cardiogenic alveolar oedema. Symmetrical air space opacity with perihilar predominance is one characteristic pattern produced by dilated cardiomyopathy*

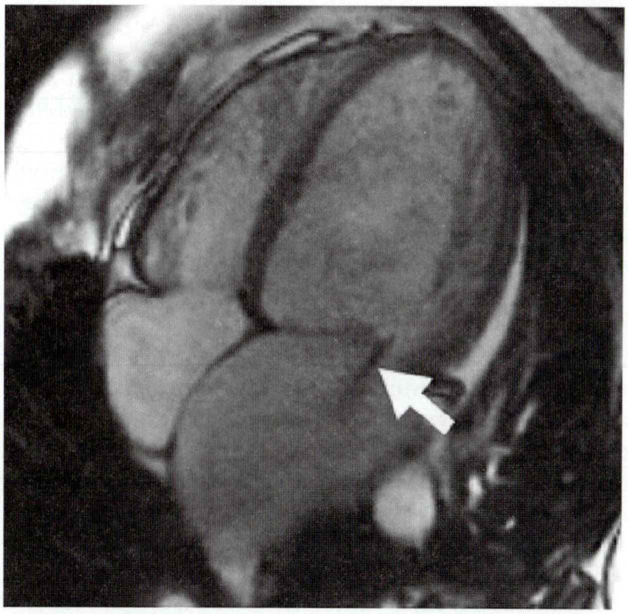

Fig. 47.119: *Idiopathic dilated cardiomyopathy in a 18-year-old girl with shortness of breath. Four chamber steady-state free-precession MR image shows marked dilation of LV, which measures 68 mm. Note black jet (arrow) from mitral regurgitation, a common finding in dilated cardiomyopathy*

perfusion. The resulting subendocardial ischemia perpetuates myocyte damage. Myocardial remodeling is an important contributor to worsening heart failure. Lost myocyte cells are replaced with fibrous tissue, thereby decreasing the compliance of one or more ventricles and adversely affecting performance. Aldosterone, angiotensin II, catecholamines, endothelins, and mechanical factors, such as excessive myocardial stretch and ischemia, have been identified as mediators of remodeling. Apoptosis is a process of programmed cell death and is now believed to play a role in the continuing loss of myocardial cells in chronic heart failure. Overloading of myocytes possibly triggers apoptosis without fibrosis.

Heightened peripheral vasoconstriction, abnormal and excessive remodeling of the peripheral vasculature, and abnormalities in endothelium-dependent vasodilation contribute to the progression of heart failure. Abnormal responses to muscarinic stimulation along with a defect in the endothelial nitric oxide pathway have been suggested as the potential underlying mechanisms.

Altered gene expressions resulting in calcium-handling abnormalities, down regulation of myosin or conversion to the less-active beta isoform, and abnormal beta-receptor signal transduction have all been identified at the molecular level in the chronically failing heart.

Incidence

The reported incidence rate is 0.57 cases per 100,000 children. The incidence rate in Finland is 2.6 cases per 100,000 children. No reliable figures are available for the rest of the world.

- Genetic causes account for more than 30% of DCM.

Mortality/Morbidity

Mortality and morbidity have greatly decreased because of advances in medical management. Studies from 1975-1990 reported 70% survival at 2 years and 52% survival at 11.5 years of follow-up. Studies from 1992–1997 document more than 85% survival at 5 years. In general, approximately one-third of patients die from the disease, one-third of patients continue to have chronic heart failure requiring therapy, and one-third of patients experience improvement in their condition.

Causes of death include heart failure, ventricular arrhythmias, and transplantation-related complications (less common).

Gender Distribution

DCM is reportedly more common in boys than in girls, and some forms are clearly X-linked.

Age Distribution

All age groups are affected. However, studies suggest that DCM is more common in infancy age (fetal presentation is uncommon).

History

- Onset is usually insidious but may be acute in as many as 25% of patients, especially if exacerbated by a complicating lower respiratory infection.
- Cough, poor feeding, irritability, and shortness of breath are usually the initial presenting symptoms.
- Pallor, sweating, easy fatigability, failure to gain weight, and decreased urine output may be observed.
- Wheezing may be an important clinical sign, suggesting congestive heart failure manifestation in infants.
- Chest pain, palpitations, orthopnea, hemoptysis, frothy sputum, sudden death, abdominal pain, syncope, and

neurologic deficit are other symptoms at presentation (20%).

- Cardiomegaly that is incidentally detected on a chest radiograph or an arrhythmia that is incidentally detected on an ECG may be the basis for initial cardiac referral.
- Approximately 50% of patients with dilated cardiomyopathy (DCM) have a history of preceding viral illness. A detailed family history for familial cardiomyopathy is revealing in as many as 25% of cases.

Physical Examination

In a patient with established disease, features of congestive heart failure are dominant.

The infant or young child with the disease is often tachypneic, tachycardic with weak peripheral pulses, and has cool extremities and hepatomegaly. Blood pressure is low with a decreased pulse pressure. In extreme cases, patients may present in shock.

Older children may show dependent edema, elevated jugular venous pulses, and fine basal crepitations in the lungs.

Major cardiac findings include cardiomegaly, quiet precordium, tachycardia, gallop rhythm (S_3 and/or S_4), accentuated P-2, and murmurs of mitral and tricuspid regurgitation. Murmurs may be inconspicuous initially if the patient presents with acute heart failure.

Infants often present with predominantly respiratory signs and, in the absence of a precordial heave or prominent murmur, the underlying cardiac disease may remain undiagnosed until cardiomegaly is detected on a chest radiograph.

Causes

Various factors have been identified as causes of myocardial damage. However, in the vast majority of patients, no specific etiology is demonstrable (idiopathic). Systemic carnitine deficiency and anthracycline-induced cardiomyopathy are notable exceptions.

Three major factors have been implicated in the pathogenesis of myocardial damage in DCM: preceding viral myocarditis, autoimmunity, and underlying genetic predisposition.

VIRAL MYOCARDITIS

Currently, no methods can be used to distinguish cardiovirulent strains of enteroviruses from those that are not virulent. Furthermore, the presence of a virus a patient with DCM does not necessarily establish a causal relationship. Demonstration of viral DNA or RNA by polymerase chain reaction (PCR) is a more reliable method for revealing viral myocarditis. Unfortunately, obtaining myocardial tissue is invasive. The exact mechanism of myocardial damage (rapid destruction or a long-term slowing of cardiomyocyte function) also remains unclear.

Autoimmunity

Animal studies have shown that DCM is an autoimmune disease in genetically predisposed strains of mice. Approximately 30–40% of adult patients with DCM have organ-specific and disease-specific autoantibodies. The absence of these antibodies in the remaining patients may be related to the stage of disease progression. The notion that an insult such as viral myocarditis initiates an autoimmune process with superantigen-triggered immune responses, resulting in massive T-lymphocyte activation and myocardial damage, has been postulated.

Genetic Predisposition

Genetic causes account for 25–50% of DCM cases.

The role of genetic factors is exemplified by the studies on familial DCM.

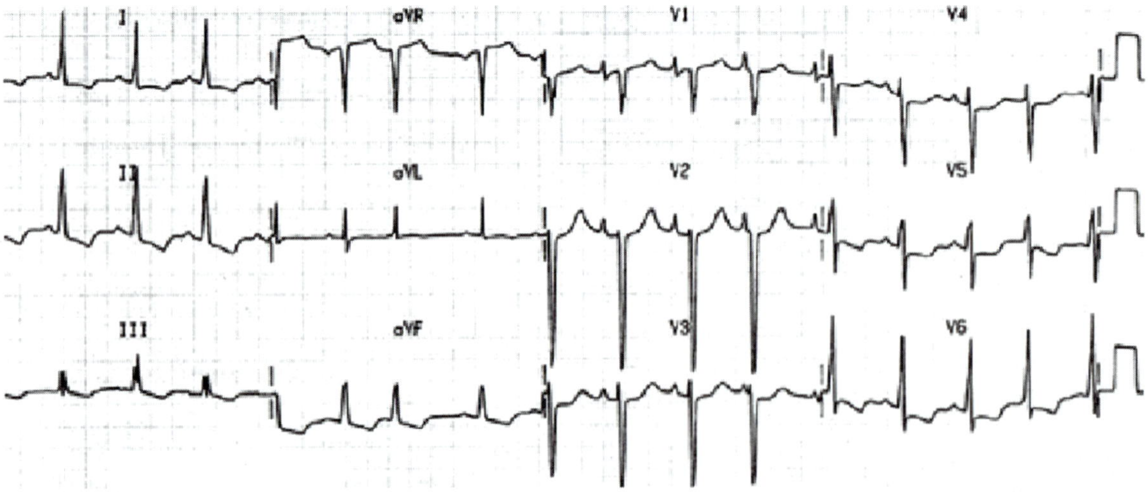

Fig. 47.120: *Idiopathic dilated cardiomyopathy: there is evidence of left ventricular hypertrophy with large precordial voltages and an LV strain pattern in leads with a dominant R wave (I, II, V6). There is also evidence of biatrial enlargement in V1 with a peaked initial portion of the P wave (RAE) followed by a deep terminal negative portion (LAE). The changes of right ventricular hypertrophy are masked by left ventricular dominance; however, this patient had four chamber dilatation on echocardiography*

Patients with familial DCM have an increased frequency of human leukocyte antigen (HLA)-DR4. The frequency of HLA-DQA1 0501 alleles has been reported to be significantly higher in patients with idiopathic DCM.

Autosomal dominant and recessive inheritance, X-linked transmission, and polygenic and mitochondrial inheritance have all been documented.

Mutation analysis: Mutation screening of the exons that code for actin, α myosin heavy chain (MYH7 gene), cardiac troponin T (TNNT2 gene), phospholamban (PLN gene), titin, αβ-crystallin, and the cardiospecific exon of metavinculin (VCL gene) could be helpful in detecting some forms of familial DCM.

- **Anthracyclines and cardiomyopathy:** Anthracyclines, which are widely used in the management of childhood malignancies, account for as many as 30% of cases of DCM in the United States and a lesser percentage in other countries. Besides DCM, the other manifestations of anthracycline cardiotoxicity include restrictive cardiomyopathy (symptomatic and asymptomatic), asymptomatic left ventricular enlargement, and more subtle changes of cardiac function. Early diagnosis requires periodic Doppler echocardiography studies during therapy and for several years after cessation of treatment. It also requires more widespread use of load-independent measurements of cardiac contractility (like stress velocity index) which incorporate measurements of contractility, afterload and preload.

Cardiotoxicity has two types: early onset and late onset. The early onset type may be acute nonprogressive orchronically progressive.

Acute-onset type is defined as left ventricular dysfunction during or immediately following infusion of anthracycline and is attenuated by discontinuation of therapy. With use of low-dose regimens, this type is becoming rare. ECG changes include nonspecific ST segment and T wave changes, decreased QRS voltage, prolonged QT interval, and sinus tachycardia. Less commonly, ventricular, junctional, or supraventricular tachycardia or atrioventricular and bundle-branch blocks. Blood levels of cardiac troponin T (cTnT) are a specific marker of this type of injury.

Early onset chronically progressive toxicity presents within 1 year of completion of therapy and persists or progresses even after discontinuation of therapy. Clinical features are similar to any other type of cardiomyopathy and include ECG changes, left ventricular dysfunction, arrhythmias, reduced exercise-stress capacity, and even overt signs of heart failure. Blood levels of cTnT are elevated. Presence of early onset cardiotoxicity is believed to be a harbinger of poor patient outcome.

Late-onset toxicity clinically manifests after a latent period of 1 or more years following completion of therapy. This type of manifestation is presumably due to diminished left ventricular contractility and an inappropriately thin left ventricular wall, resulting in elevated wall stress and progressive left ventricular dysfunction. Myocyte loss underlies all these sequelae, and alteration of myocellular protein transcription by anthracyclines may contribute. Thus, the latent period is not latent at all, and more sensitive markers may be abe to detect the changes earlier. Late-onset asymptomatic toxicity has also been reported, but more detailed questioning often reveals easy fatigability or dyspnea in many of these patients.

Risk factors contributing to the development of cardiotoxicity include the following: (1) the total cumulative dose of the drug received (20% mortality with cumulative dose >550 mg/m^2, 65% frequency of subtle echo changes with dose >400 mg/m^2, and histologic evidence of toxicity with >240 mg/m^2), (2) female sex (higher cellular concentrations because of higher body fat percentage), (3) young children, (4) rate of drug administration (maximum risk with doses >50 mg/m^2/dose), (5) concomitant cardiac radiation exposure or use of amsacrine, (6) black race, and (7) trisomy 21.

Laboratory Studies

Full blood counts, erythrocyte sedimentation rate, and C-reactive proteins may show evidence of acute inflammation in the presence of active myocarditis.

Similarly, creatine kinase-myocardial fraction may be elevated.

Rising titers of specific viral-neutralizing antibodies in the serum and positive viral cultures from nasopharyngeal or stool swabs may suggest a viral etiology; however, this does not necessarily mean a cause-and-effect relationship. Serum carnitine levels (total and free) are low when the disease is due to systemic carnitine deficiency.

Arterial blood gas (ABG) analysis reveals early stages of mild respiratory alkalosis and, later, mild hypoxemia secondary to pulmonary edema. In advanced disease, mixed acid-base disturbances with metabolic acidosis indicate the need for intravenous inotropes and ventilatory assistance.

Imaging Studies

Chest radiography: Chest radiography reveals cardiomegaly with a prominent left ventricular apex and prominent pulmonary artery segment. Elevation of left main bronchus reflects dilation of the left atrium. This can result in compression of the left lower lobe bronchus when combined with a dilated pulmonary artery, leading to collapse of the left lower lobe of the lung (Figs 47.117, 47.118 and 47.121).

Pulmonary venous congestion and frank pulmonary edema are often evident. When present, pleural effusion is better appreciated in the erect and lateral decubitus films. Massive cardiomegaly resembling pericardial effusion is the hallmark of established disease.

Rarely, in fulminant cases, cardiomegaly may not be prominent because the ventricle has not had time to dilate despite the presence of features of pulmonary edema.

Echocardiography and Doppler studies: These form the basis for the diagnosis of dilated cardiomyopathy (DCM) in most patients. Marked dilation of the left ventricle with global hypokinesia is the hallmark of the disease. Left

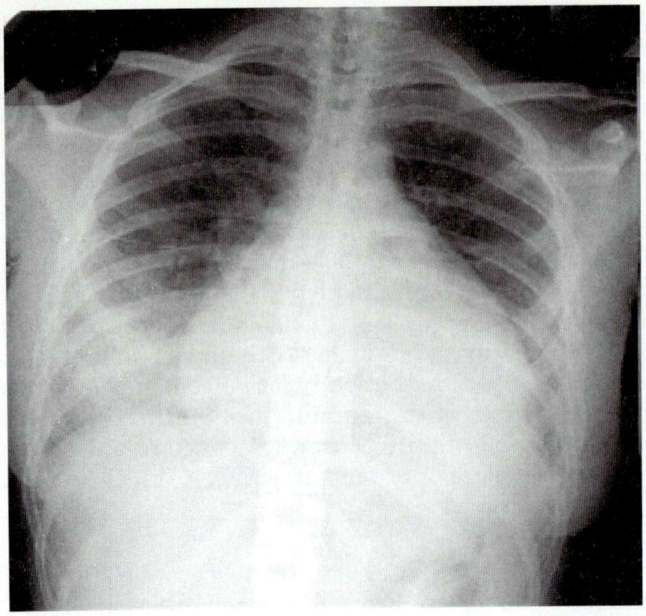

Fig. 47.121: *X-ray chest PA view demonstrates cardiomegaly, pulmonary edema and pleural effusions as a result of congestive heart failure due to viral myocarditis*

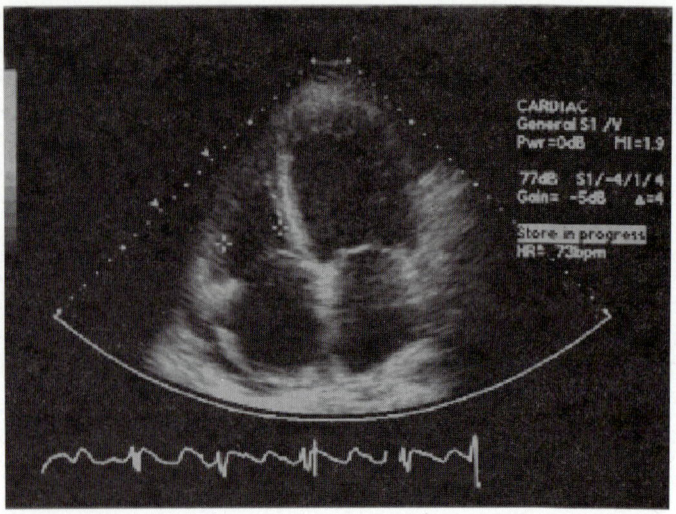

Fig. 47.122: *Two dimensional echo-cardiogram. Four-chamber view shows atrial and ventricular dilatation in viral myocarditis*

ventricular fractional shortening is usually less than 25% (ejection fraction Doppler studies show varying degrees of mitral regurgitation secondary to left ventricular dilation and possible papillary muscle dysfunction. Mitral regurgitation is more prominent in follow-up studies after commencing therapy when the cardiac output has improved. Left ventricular ejection parameters show decrease in peak velocity and peak acceleration, prolongation of the pre-ejection period, and decrease in ejection time. These flow measurements are dependent on loading conditions. The dilatation of the mitral valve ring and the altered shape of the left ventricle cavity, which leads to change in the direction of the papillary muscles, are used to explain the secondary mitral regurgitation seen in a large proportion of children with DCM. Tissue Doppler studies have recently been reported in children with DCM (Fig. 47.122).

Parameters of diastolic dysfunction are not reliable in the presence of established systolic dysfunction and mitral regurgitation; however, they may be useful in the early stages of the disease. Diastolic dysfunction is not as typical or as pronounced as it is in hypertrophic cardiomyopathy. Long-standing cases show evidence of pulmonary hypertension in the form of right ventricular dilation and hypertrophy and tricuspid regurgitation. Tricuspid regurgitation and pulmonary regurgitation velocities give an estimate of the pulmonary artery systolic and diastolic pressures respectively. In severe cases, swirling echodensity (smoke or spontaneous echocardiographic contrast) can be observed along the outer ventricular wall, moving from the mitral valve towards the aortic valve. Occasionally, thrombi can be visualized in the left ventricular apex and in the left atrium. Pericardial effusion also may be present. Echocardiography can exclude other heart diseases, both congenital and acquired. Cardiomyopathy secondary to severe aortic stenosis, coarctation of aorta or congenital mitral valve dysplasia, and anomalous left coronary artery arising from pulmonary artery (ALCAPA) are the major differential diagnoses. At times, identifying cardiomyopathy secondary to congenital mitral regurgitation (dysplastic mitral valve without stenosis) is difficult, but the abnormal anatomy of the mitral valve leaflets should help. The echo-dense papillary muscles and the dilated proximal right coronary artery and continuous retrograde flow of blood into the origin of pulmonary artery all direct the attention of the cardiologist to ALCAPA, a potentially treatable that mimics DCM (Fig. 47.122).

Radionuclide imaging: First-pass test and multiple gated acquisition (MUGA) scans help to measure the left and right ventricular stroke volumes and cardiac outputs. They are also helpful in documenting dyskinetic segments in the ventricular walls. Although theoretically superior to echocardiographic measurements, their practical application is limited because of a lack of standardization and because of nonreproducibility, especially in children. Thallium studies can identify areas of decreased myocardial perfusion, although this is seldom required.

Gallium citrate Ga 67 scintigraphy and indium In-111 altumomab pentetate antimyosin antibody cardiac imaging have been suggested to help identify ongoing inflammation noninvasively. They may be used to identify patients who might benefit from myocardial biopsy (Figs 47.119 and 47.125).

Other Tests

Electrocardiography (Figs 47.120 and 47.123)

ECG changes are usually nonspecific. Some patients have sinus tachycardia, downward frontal plane QRS axis, left atrial enlargement, left ventricular hypertrophy, deep Q waves with ST segment depression, and tall T waves in leads I, aVL, V_5, V_6 (the latter reflect left ventricular volume overload). In more advanced disease, right-axis deviation, right atrial enlargement, and right ventricular hypertrophy are seen (because of pulmonary hypertension).

The main role of ECG is to detect evidence of myocardial ischemia (pathologic Q waves with ST elevation and T-wave inversion in leads I, aVL, V_5, V_6) that might point to anomalous coronary artery as the etiology of the cardiomyopathy. A segmental myocarditis may result in ECG features of myocardial infarction.

Cardiac arrhythmias, such as supraventricular/ventricular ectopy or tachycardia, may be revealed. These might indicate an underlying myocarditis or cardiomyopathy; wever, if sustained, the arrhythmia may be the cause of the cardiomyopathy rather than the result (i.e. tachycardia-mediated cardiomyopathy).

Procedures

Cardiac catheterization and angiography: Children with DCM are at a particular risk for complications during cardiac catheter studies and angiography. Should be performed by experienced pediatric cardiologists and only when absolutely essential.

At present, preparation for cardiac transplant and need for myocardial biopsy are the main indications for performing the procedure.

Patients should be under optimum medical therapy and kept hemodynamically stable before and after catheterization. Careful observation is required during the procedure for ventricular arrhythmias and hemodynamic deterioration.

Echocardiography should be considered after catheterization to identify any pericardial effusion secondary to subclinical perforation of the myocardium, especially if a biopsy has also been performed.

Aortography may be performed to identify a coronary artery anatomy, and left ventricular angiography may be performed to assess mitral valve function. The number of biopsy specimens collected should be limited to the minimum required (usually 4–8). Usual findings include elevated filling pressures in all the cardiac chambers (especially the left ventricle), pulmonary wedge pressure, and reduced cardiac output and stroke volume. Mixed venous oxygen saturation and reduced arterial saturation reflect low cardiac output and pulmonary edema. Pulmonary and systemic vascular resistances are elevated. With end-stage disease, the peak systolic left ventricular and aortic pressures drop.

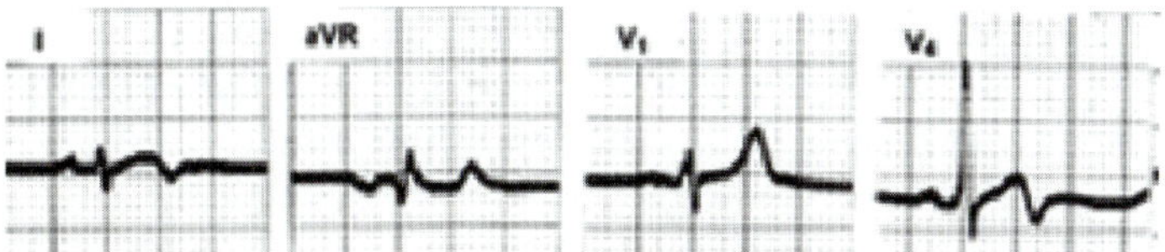

Fig. 47.123: *Abnormal ECG with nondiagnostic ST-T wave abnormalities. The T waves are deeply and symmetrically inverted in I, II, III, and V4-6, suggesting a diffuse myocardial process*

Myocardial Biopsy (Fig. 47.124)

At present, preparation for cardiac transplant and post-transplant follow-up monitoring for rejection are the main indications for biopsy. If facilities are available, molecular or metabolic studies can be additional indications for academic and research purposes. Rarely, suspected metabolic diseases (isolated myocardial carnitine deficiency, rare forms of glycogen storage disease, fatty acid oxidation defects) or persistent myocarditis might require biopsy for confirmation. Specimens should be subjected to both light and electron microscopy. PCR and metabolic studies should be performed when indicated. The most important aspect is the availability of a sufficient level of expertise for interpretation of the findings. PCR has been used to aid the detection of viral antigens in myocardial tissue in patients with DCM. Studies have revealed an association between viral antigens and DCM. However, a proportion of the studies gave negative results. A recently published meta-analysis of the studies on DCM gave an odds ratio of 3.8 to the association between presence of viral antigens in DCM. The results are influenced by factors like contamination from the reference strain used in the laboratory and choice of the controls. It also is not clear whether these positive cases among DCM actually represented acute myocarditis rather than DCM.

Medical care: Perform general supportive measures during acute-stage management including endotracheal intubation and mechanical ventilation, vasoactive infusions, and fluid/acid-base management. Treat chest infections appropriately. Treat anemia appropriately.

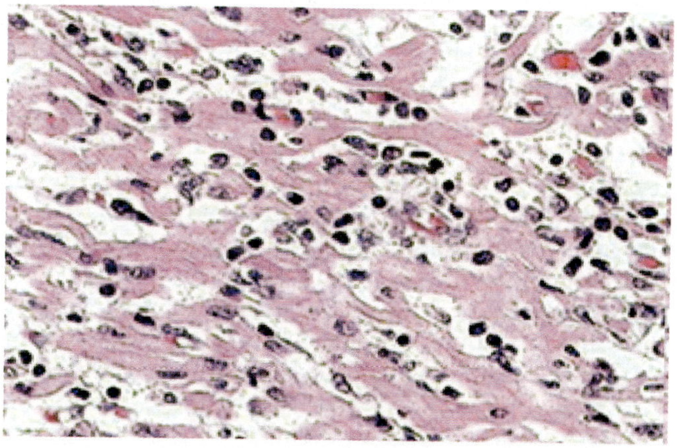

Fig. 47.124: *There is myocyte necrosis along with inflammation consisting of mononuclear cells, typical for a viral myocarditis*

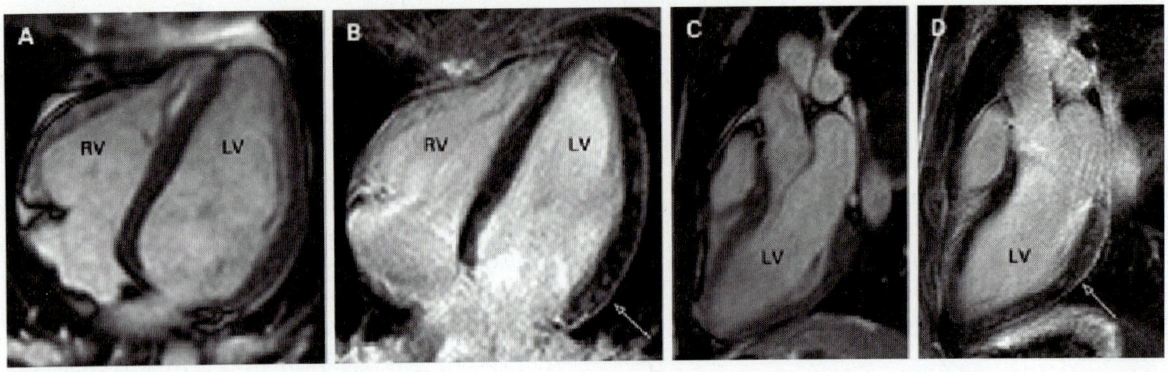

Fig. 47.125: *There is myocyte necrosis along with inflammation consisting of mononuclear cells, typical for a viral myocarditis*

- Oxygen inhalation is of benefit only in the presence of hypoxia (as with pneumonia or pulmonary edema).
- Carnitine supplements (100 mg/kg IV infusion over 30 min, followed by 100 mg/kg/d as continuous infusion for 24–72 h; 25–50 mg/kg/dose PO bid/tid, not to exceed 200 mg/kg/d) reverse the myocardial dysfunction in most patients affected by systemic carnitine deficiency.
- Coenzyme Q10 has also been used in children with dilated cardiomyopathy (DCM), with variable results.

Decreased serum levels of growth hormone (GH), which acts on cardiac myocytes primarily through insulin-like growth factor (IGF)-1, are associated with impaired myocardial growth and function, which can be improved with the restoration of GH/IGF-1 homeostasis. Based on this hypothesis and on observation of benefits in animal models, GH therapy has been used in children with DCM, but the results have not been conclusive.

Surgical Care

Cardiac transplantation is currently the optimal treatment for DCM-induced resistant chronic congestive heart failure in children.

- Limiting factors include availability of a suitable donor, complications of rejection, and lifelong immunosuppression. Survival rates of as much as 92% at 5 years have been reported.
- Palliative surgical measures are associated with significant mortality and morbidity rates despite advances. Resection of a large segment of the hypertrophied ventricular muscle **(Batista procedure)** and repair or replacement of mitral valve to minimize volume overload of left ventricle have been used as palliative measures. Cardiomyoplasty is the transposition of electrically transformed skeletal muscle to provide systolic and diastolic augmentation to the native heart.
- **Implantable mechanical support devices,** modified for used in infants and children, have been introduced to support the failing heart until a suitable donor is available for transplantation (bridge to transplant). Major limitations include infection, thromboembolism, disturbance from noise, and the need to recharge batteries frequently.
- **Cardiac resynchronization therapy** using a biventricular pacemaker has been shown to be effective in adults with DCM. In addition, these devices are available with defibrillator backup for patients at risk for ventricular arrhythmias. They are being used in children with DCM, with early favorable results.
- Prolonged support of left ventricular function with these devices has shown restoration of the native cardiac function, enabling removal of the device in a few cases. This raises the possibility that mechanical intervention at an earlier stage in viral myocarditis and DCM might prevent the deterioration of cardiac function. Recent adult studies have documented myocardial recovery and successful explantation of the left ventricular assist system, even after they were on the device for a year. A lesser degree of fibrotic changes in the left ventricle could predict better chances of recovery.

Diet

- Dietary requirements are high because of the catabolic state, recurrent infections, increased muscle activity, and need for rapid growth.
- Dietary intake may be inadequate consequent to the anorexia, dietary restrictions, malabsorption, diarrhea, and frequent exacerbations of heart failure.
- Ensuring an appropriate and palatable diet is a challenge.
- Temporary nasogastric tube feedings may be required for sick and severely anorectic children.
- Powerful diuretics have largely obviated the need for stringent restrictions on salt and fluid intake.

Activity

- Enforced bed rest is impractical and probably unnecessary.
- Often, restriction of physical activity is self-enforced.
- Infants might need intravenous alimentation for relief from feeding activity.
- Apart from the above, activity to the limit of tolerance should be allowed and encouraged.
- In patients with chronic illness, regular graded exercise has been shown to improve effort tolerance and quality of life.
- All feasible support should be provided for peer interaction and participation in normal life activities. Restricted life activities, frequent diagnostic and therapeutic interventions, and an uncertain prognosis make these children prone to psychological problems that may significantly influence prognosis and outcome.

Among the described abnormalities are inhibition of emotions, marked anxiety, depressive reaction with loneliness, low self-esteem, feelings of inadequacy, emotional lability, impulsiveness, and weakness of self-identity.

Medical therapy is largely directed at the symptoms and is aimed at the underlying heart failure. Diuretics, angiotensin-converting enzyme (ACE) inhibitors, and beta-blockers form the initial therapy. Diuretics may provide an improvement in symptoms, whereas ACE inhibitors appear to prolong survival. Beta-blockers also have a long-term positive effect on outcome. Intravenous infusions of vasoactive agents may be required in patients with resistant heart failure. Recently, the use of beta-blockers has become more extensive in childhood dilated cardiomyopathy (DCM) drug therapy.

Antibiotics for endocarditis prophylaxis are administered to patients with certain cardiac conditions, such as DCM, before performing procedures that may cause bacteremia.

Complications

Congestive heart failure

- Pneumonia
- Cardiac arrhythmias (supraventricular and ventricular)
- Infective endocarditis
- Thromboembolism
- Venous thrombosis
- Cardiac cirrhosis
- Posttransplant complications
- Sudden, unexplained death.

Prognosis

- If a treatable cause is discovered, prognosis is better.
- Prognosis is worst for cardiomyopathy secondary to storage diseases that do not have effective therapy.
- History of viral illness in the 3 months before onset may suggest a better prognosis.
- In DCM with no obvious detectable etiology, outcome depends on severity of myocardial dysfunction, improvement during the first year after onset, compliance to therapy, and availability of timely transplant.
- Degree of depression of fractional shortening or ejection fraction at time of initial echocardiography, elevation of left ventricular end diastolic pressure, and cardiothoracic ratio have all been applied as predictors of outcome, although they are not often predictive. Other possible prognostic factors include age at onset (better for infants), presence of symptomatic arrhythmias, and thromboembolic episodes.
- Arrhythmic death can occur even after the left ventricular ejection fraction has returned to normal.
- Following cardiac transplant, survival rates of as much as 77% at 1 year and as much as 65% at 5 years have been reported in children.
- School teachers should be informed of the child's condition. Teachers and other caregivers should be adequately trained for first aid and cardiopulmonary resuscitation (CPR).
- Family members should be screened with ECG and echocardiography to detect asymptomatic cases.
- Pregnancy imposes special demands on the cardiac reserve, and the decision to have children has to be individualized, depending mainly on the degree of exercise tolerance and the severity of ventricular dysfunction and cardiomyopathy.

ACUTE AND CHRONIC PERICARDITIS

Pericarditis is inflammation of the pericardium, often with fluid accumulation. Pericarditis may be caused by many disorders (e.g. infection, MI, trauma, tumors, metabolic disorders) but is often idiopathic. Symptoms include chest pain or tightness, often worsened by deep breathing. Cardiac output may be greatly reduced. Diagnosis is based on symptoms, a friction rub, ECG changes, and evidence of pericardial fluid accumulation on X-ray or echocardiogram. Finding the cause requires further evaluation. Treatment depends on the cause, but general measures include analgesics, antiinflammatory drugs, and sometimes surgery. Pericarditis is the most common pericardial disorder. Congenital pericardial disorders are rare.

Anatomy and Pathophysiology (Fig. 47.126)

The pericardium has two layers. The visceral pericardium is a single layer of mesothelial cells that is attached to the myocardium, folds back (reflects) on itself over the origin of the great vessels, and joins with a tough, fibrous layer to envelop the heart as the parietal pericardium. The sac created by these layers contains a small amount of fluid (< 25–50 mL), composed mostly of an ultrafiltrate of plasma. The pericardium limits distention of the cardiac chambers and increases the heart's efficiency. The pericardium is richly innervated with sympathetic and somatic afferents. Stretch-sensitive mechanoreceptors sense changes in cardiac volume and tension and may be responsible for transmitting pericardial pain. The phrenic nerves are embedded in the parietal pericardium and are vulnerable to injury during surgery on the pericardium. Pericarditis may be acute or chronic. Acute pericarditis develops quickly, producing an inflammatory reaction. Chronic pericarditis (defined as persisting > 6 mo) develops more slowly; its prominent feature is effusion. Acute disease may become chronic. Adverse hemodynamic effects and rhythm disturbance are rare, although cardiac tamponade is possible. Occasionally, pericarditis produces a marked thickening and stiffening of the pericardium (constrictive pericarditis). Pericarditis can lead to inflammation of the epicardial myocardium.

Pericardial effusion is accumulation of fluid in the pericardium. The fluid may be serous fluid (sometimes with fibrin strands), serosanguineous fluid, blood, pus, or chyle.

Cardiac tamponade occurs when a large pericardial effusion impairs cardiac filling, leading to low cardiac output and sometimes shock and death. If fluid (usually blood) accumulates rapidly, even small amounts (e.g. 150 mL) may produce tamponade because the pericardium

Heart in the pericardial sac

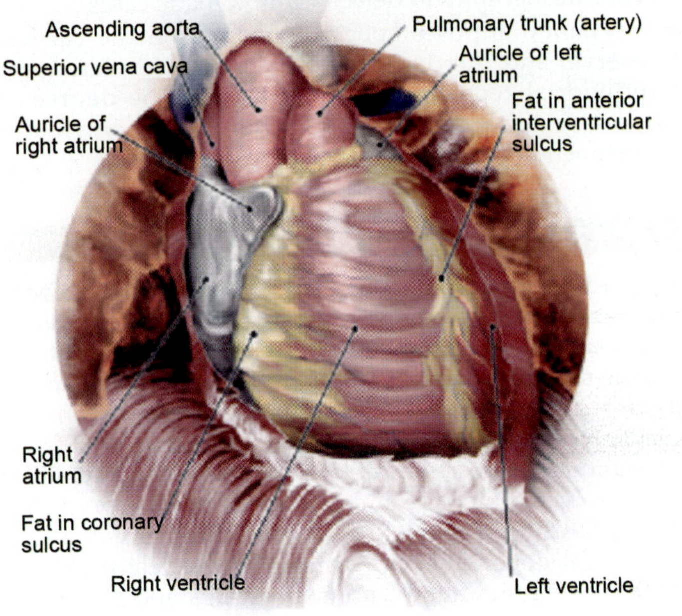

Fig. 47.126: *Anatomy of sac after exposing two layers of pericardium*

Table 47.3: *Causes of acute pericarditis*

- Idiopathic
- Viral infections (echovirus, influenza virus, coxsackie B virus, HIV*)
- Bacterial infections† (streptococci; staphylococci; Gram-negative bacilli; in children, *Haemophilus influenzae*)
- Fungal infections (histoplasmosis, coccidioidomycosis, candidiasis, blastomycosis)
- Parasitic infections (toxoplasmosis, amebiasis, echinococcosis)
- Autoimmune disorders (RA, SLE, scleroderma)
- Inflammatory disorders (amyloidosis, inflammatory bowel disease, sarcoidosis)
- Uremia
- Trauma
- Post-MI (Dressler's) syndrome
- Postpericardiotomy
- Drugs (e.g. hydralazine, isoniazid, methysergide, phenytoin, procainamide)

* If patients with AIDS develop lymphoma, Kaposi's sarcoma, or certain infections (i.e. *Mycobacterium avium, M. tuberculosis, Nocardia*, other fungal or viral infections), pericarditis may follow.

† Tuberculous pericarditis accounts for < 5% of cases of acute or subacute pericarditis in the US but the majority of cases in some areas of India and Africa.

cannot stretch quickly enough to accommodate it. Slow accumulation of up to 1,500 mL may not produce tamponade. Loculated effusion may produce localized tamponade on the right or left side of the heart.

Constrictive pericarditis, which is uncommon, results from marked inflammatory, fibrotic thickening of the pericardium. Sometimes, the visceral and parietal layers adhere to each other or to the myocardium. The fibrotic tissue often contains Ca deposits. The stiff, thickened pericardium markedly impairs ventricular filling, decreasing stroke volume and cardiac output. Significant pericardial fluid accumulation is rare. Rhythm disturbance is common. The diastolic pressures in the ventricles, atria, and venous beds become virtually the same. Systemic venous congestion occurs, causing considerable transudation of fluid from systemic capillaries, with dependent edema and, later, ascites. Chronic elevation of systemic venous and hepatic venous pressure may lead to cardiac cirrhosis. Constriction of the left atrium, the left ventricle, or both may elevate pulmonary venous pressure etiology.

Acute pericarditis may result from infection, autoimmune and inflammatory disorders, uremia, trauma, MI, or certain drugs.

Pericarditis (Table 47.3)

Causes of Acute Pericarditis

Infectious pericarditis is most often viral. Purulent bacterial pericarditis is uncommon but may follow infective endocarditis, pneumonia, septicemia, penetrating trauma, or cardiac surgery. Often, the cause cannot be identified (called nonspecific or idiopathic pericarditis), but many of these cases are probably viral. Overall, the most common causes are viral and idiopathic. Acute MI causes 10–15% of cases of acute pericarditis. Post-MI syndrome (Dressler's syndrome) is a less common cause now, occurring mainly when reperfusion with percutaneous transluminal coronary angioplasty (PTCA) or thrombolytic drugs is ineffective in patients with transmural infarction. Pericarditis occurs after pericardiotomy (called postpericardiotomy syndrome) in 5–30% of cardiac operations.

Myocardial Infarction

- Post-MI (Dressler's) syndrome
- Post pericardiotomy
- Drugs (e.g. hydralazine, isoniazid, methysergide, phenytoin, procainamide)

***If patients with AIDS develop lymphoma, Kaposi's sarcoma, or certain infections** (i.e. *Mycobacterium avium, M. tuberculosis, Nocardia*, other fungal or viral infections), may follow.

Tuberculous pericarditis accounts for < 5% of cases of acute or subacute pericarditis in the US but the majority of cases in some areas of India and Africa. Chronic pericardial effusion or constrictive pericarditis may follow almost any disorder that causes acute pericarditis, as well as TB, tumor, irradiation, rheumatoid disease, and cardiac surgery. Sometimes, no cause of chronic pericarditis is identified. Pericarditis with large effusion (serous, serosanguineous, or bloody) is most commonly caused by metastatic tumors, most often by lung or breast carcinoma, sarcoma (especially melanoma), leukemia, or lymphoma. Fibrosis of the pericardium may follow purulent pericarditis or myocardial infection (myocarditis—a common cause in young people) or accompany a connective tissue disorder.

In elderly patients, common causes are malignant tumors, MI, and TB. Hemopericardium (accumulation of blood within the pericardium) may lead to pericarditis or pericardial fibrosis; common causes include chest trauma, iatrogenic injury (e.g. from cardiac catheterization, pacemaker insertion, or central venous line placement), and rupture of a thoracic aortic aneurysm (Fig. 47.128).

Symptoms, Signs and Diagnosis

Some patients present with symptoms and signs of inflammation (acute pericarditis); others present with those of fluid accumulation (pericardial effusion). Symptoms and signs vary depending on the severity of inflammation and the amount and rate of fluid accumulation. Even a large amount of pericardial fluid may be asymptomatic if it develops slowly (e.g. over months).

Acute Pericarditis

Acute pericarditis tends to cause chest pain and a pericardial rub, sometimes with dyspnea. The first evidence can be tamponade, with hypotension, shock, or pulmonary edema. Because the innervation of the pericardium and myocardium is the same, the chest pain of pericarditis is sometimes similar to that of myocardial inflammation or ischemia: Dull or sharp precordial or substernal pain may radiate to the neck, trapezius ridge (especially the left), or shoulders. Pain ranges from mildespecially the left), or shoulders. Pain ranges from mild to severe. Unlike ischemic chest pain, pain due to pericarditis is usually aggravated by thoracic motion, cough, breathing, or swallowing food; it may be relieved by sitting up and leaning forward. Tachypnea and nonproductive cough may be present; fever, chills, and weakness are common. In 15–25% of patients with idiopathic pericarditis, symptoms recur intermittently for months or years. The most important physical finding is a triphasic or a systolic and diastolic precordial friction rub. However, the rub is often intermittent and evanescent; it may be present only during systole or, less frequently, only during diastole. If no rub is heard with the patient seated and leaning forward, auscultation may be attempted with the patient on all fours and listening with the diaphragm of the stethoscope. Sometimes, a pleural component to the rub is noted during breathing, which is due to inflammation of the pleura adjacent to the pericardium. Considerable amounts of pericardial fluid may muffle heart sounds, increase the area of cardiac dullness, and change the size and shape of the cardiac silhouette. If acute pericarditis is suspected, hospitalization is sometimes required for initial evaluation. ECG and chest X-ray are done. If symptoms or signs of elevated right-sided pressure, tamponade, or an enlarged cardiac silhouette are present, echocardiography to check for effusion and cardiac filling abnormalities is also done. Blood tests may detect leukocytosis and an elevated ESR, but these findings are nonspecific. The diagnosis is based on the presence of typical clinical findings.

ECG abnormalities: Serial ECGs may be needed to show abnormalities. The ECG in acute pericarditis may show abnormalities confined to ST segments and T waves, usually in most leads peri carditis: acute pericarditis: stage

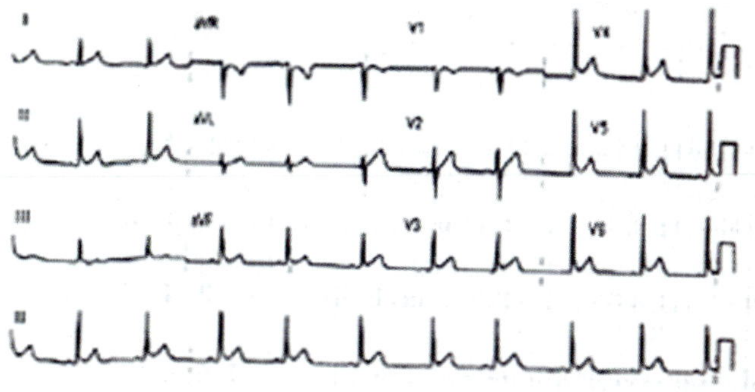

Fig. 47.127: *ECG in acute pericarditis showing wide spread concave ST elevation and depression of PR segment*

1 ECG.). The ST segments in 2 or 3 of the standard leads become elevated but subsequently return to baseline. Unlike MI, acute pericarditis does not cause reciprocal depression in ST segments (except in leads aVR and V_1), and there are no pathologic Q waves. The PR segment may be depressed. After several days or longer, T waves may become flattened and then inverted throughout the ECG, except in lead aVR; T-wave inversion occurs after the ST segment has returned to baseline and thus differs from the pattern of acute ischemia or MI (Fig. 47.131).

Acute Pericarditis

Stage 1 ECG (Fig. 47.127)

J points, except aVR and V_1, are elevated. T waves are essentially normal. PR segments, except aVR and V_1, are depressed. PR deviations are commonly absent in one limb

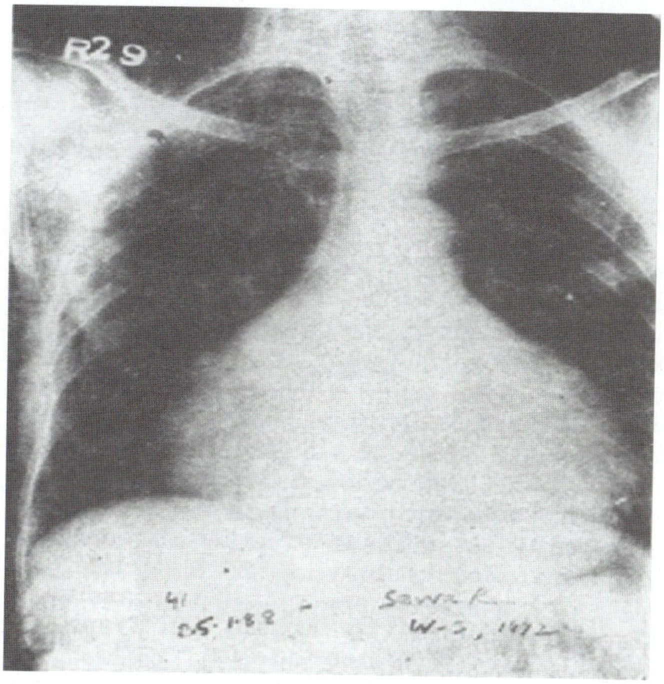

Fig. 47.128: *X-ray chest showing money bag appearance of cardiac silhoute in patient with moderate pericardial effusion*

lead (here, aVL). Because the pain of pericarditis may resemble that of acute MI or pulmonary infarction, additional tests (e.g. serum cardiac marker measurement, lung scan) may be required if the history and ECG findings are atypical for pericarditis. Troponin is almost always elevated in acute pericarditis due to epicardial inflammation so it cannot discriminate between acute infarction and pulmonary embolism. The CPK level is usually normal in acute pericarditis unless myocarditis is also present. Postpericardiotomy and post-MI syndromes may be difficult to identify and must be distinguished from recent MI, pulmonary embolism, and pericardial infection after surgery. Pain, friction rub, and fever appearing 2 wk to several months after surgery and a rapid response to aspirin, NSAIDs, or corticosteroids aid diagnosis.

Tuberculoma of Left Ventricle (Fig. 47.129)

It may be seen as a part of wide spread systemic tuberculosis or rarely as an independant pathology.

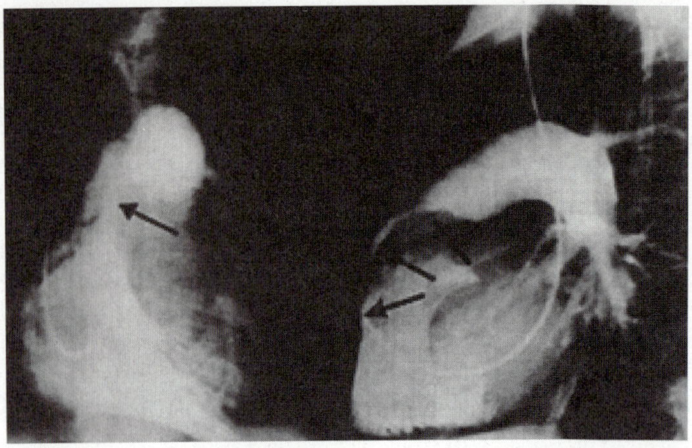

Fig. 47.129: *Angiocardiography LV showing tuberculama of LV as shown with arrows*

Pericardial effusion: Pericardial effusion is often painless, but when it occurs with acute pericarditis, pain may be present. Typically, heart sounds are muffled. A pericardial rub may be heard. With large effusions, compression of the base of the left lung can decrease breath sounds (heard near the left scapula) and produce crackles (rales). Arterial pulse, jugular venous pulse, and BP are normal unless intrapericardial pressure increases substantially, causing tamponade. In the post-MI syndrome, pericardial effusion can occur with fever, friction rub, pleurisy, pleural effusions and joint pain. This syndrome usually occurs within 10 days to 2 mo after MI. It is usually mild but may be severe. Occasionally, the heart ruptures post-MI, causing hemopericardium and tamponade, usually 1–10 days post-MI and more commonly in women. Diagnosis is suggested by clinical findings but often is suspected only after finding an enlarged cardiac silhouette on chest X-ray. On ECG, QRS voltage is often decreased, and sinus rhythm remains in about 90% of patients. With large, chronic effusions, the ECG may show electrical alternans (i.e. P, QRS, or T wave amplitude increases and decreases on alternate beats). Electrical alternans is associated with variation in cardiac position (swinging heart). Echocardiography has a high degree of sensitivity and specificity for detecting pericardial fluid. Patients with a normal ECG, small (< 0.5 L) effusion, and no suspicious findings from the history and examination may be observed with serial examination and echocardiography. Other patients must be evaluated further to determine etiology. Cardiac tamponade the clinical findings are similar to those of cardiogenic shock: decreased cardiac output, low systemic arterial pressure, tachycardia and dyspnea. Neck veins are markedly dilated. Severe cardiac tamponade is nearly always accompanied by a fall of > 10 mmHg in systolic BP during inspiration (pulsus paradoxus—*see* Approach to the Cardiac Patient: Pulsus paradoxus). In advanced cases, pulse may disappear during inspiration. (However, pulsus paradoxus can also occur in COPD, bronchial asthma, pulmonary embolism, right ventricular infarction, and noncardiogenic shock.) Heart sounds are muffled unless the effusion is small. Low voltage and electrical alternans on the ECG suggest cardiac tamponade, but these findings lack sensitivity and specificity. When tamponade is suspected, echocardiography is done unless even a brief delay might be life-threatening. Then pericardiocentesis is done immediately for diagnosis and treatment. On an echocardiogram, respiratory variation of transvalvular and venous flows and compression or collapse of right cardiac chambers in the presence of a pericardial effusion support the diagnosis. If tamponade is suspected, right heart (Swan-Ganz) catheterization may be done. In cardiac tamponade, there is no early diastolic dip in the ventricular pressure record.

In the atrial pressure curve, x descent is preserved and y descent is lost. In contrast, in severe congestive states due to dilated cardiomyopathy, pulmonary artery occlusion or left ventricular diastolic pressure usually exceeds right atrial mean pressure and right ventricular diastolic pressure by ≥ 4 mmHg. Constrictive pericarditis Fibrosis or calcification rarely produces symptoms unless constrictive pericarditis develops. The only early abnormalities may be elevated ventricular diastolic, atrial, pulmonary, and systemic venous pressures. Symptoms and signs of peripheral venous congestion (e.g. peripheral edema, neck vein distention, hepatomegaly) may appear with an early diastolic sound (pericardial knock), often best heard during inspiration. This sound is due to abrupt slowing of diastolic ventricular filling by the rigid pericardium. Ventricular systolic function (based on ejection fraction) is usually preserved. Prolonged elevation of pulmonary venous pressure results in dyspnea (particularly during exertion) and orthopnea. Fatigue may be severe. Distention of neck veins with a rise in venous pressure during inspiration (Kussmaul's sign) is present; it is absent in tamponade. Pulsus paradoxus is rare and is usually less severe than in tamponade. Lungs are not congested unless severe left ventricular constriction develops. Diagnosis may be suspected based on ECG, chest X-ray, and Doppler echocardiography findings, but cardiac catheterization and CT (or MRI) are usually required. Because ventricular filling is restricted, ventricular pressure tracings show a sudden

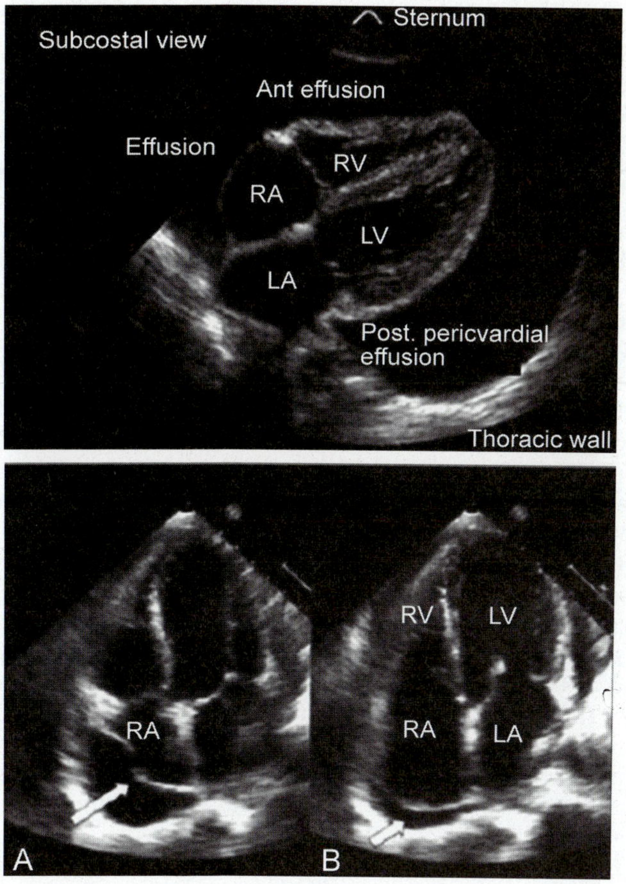

Fig. 47.130: *(Upper) Echocardiogram showing anterior and posterior pericardial effusion in the pericardial sac surrounding the heart (Bottom) (A) Apical 4C View showing pericardial effusion (arrow) with collapse of right atrium during diastole. (B) Circumferential small effusion surrounding the right atrium (arrow)*

dip followed by a plateau (resembling a square root sign) in early diastole. Rarely, right heart biopsy is needed to exclude restrictive cardiomyopathy. ECG changes are nonspecific. QRS voltage is usually low. T waves are usually nonspecifically abnormal. Atrial fibrillation occurs in about $^1D_3$ of patients; atrial flutter is less common. Lateral chest X-rays often show pericardial calcification best, but the finding is nonspecific. The changes on echocardiogram are also nonspecific. When the right and left ventricular filling pressures are equally elevated, Doppler echocardiography helps distinguish constrictive pericarditis from restrictive cardiomyopathy. During inspiration, mitral diastolic flow velocity usually falls > 25% in constrictive pericarditis but < 15% in restrictive cardiomyopathy. In constrictive pericarditis, inspiratory tricuspid flow velocity increases more than it normally does, but it does not do so in restrictive cardiomyopathy. Determining tissue velocities at the mitral annulus may be helpful when excessively high left atrial pressure blunts respiratory variation in transvalvular velocities. If clinical and echocardiographic findings suggest constrictive pericarditis, right heart cardiac catheterization is done. It helps to confirm and quantify the abnormal hemodynamics that define constrictive pericarditis: mean pulmonary artery occlusion pressure (pulmonary capillary wedge pressure), pulmonary artery diastolic pressure, right ventricular end-diastolic pressure, and mean right atrial pressure are all at about 10–30 mmHg. The pulmonary artery and right ventricular systolic pressures are normal or modestly elevated, so that pulse pressures are small. In the atrial pressure curve, x and y descents are typically accentuated; in the ventricular pressure curve, a diastolic dip occurs at the time of rapid ventricular filling. These changes almost always occur with significant constrictive pericarditis. Right ventricular systolic pressure of > 50 mmHg often occurs in restrictive cardiomyopathy but less often in constrictive

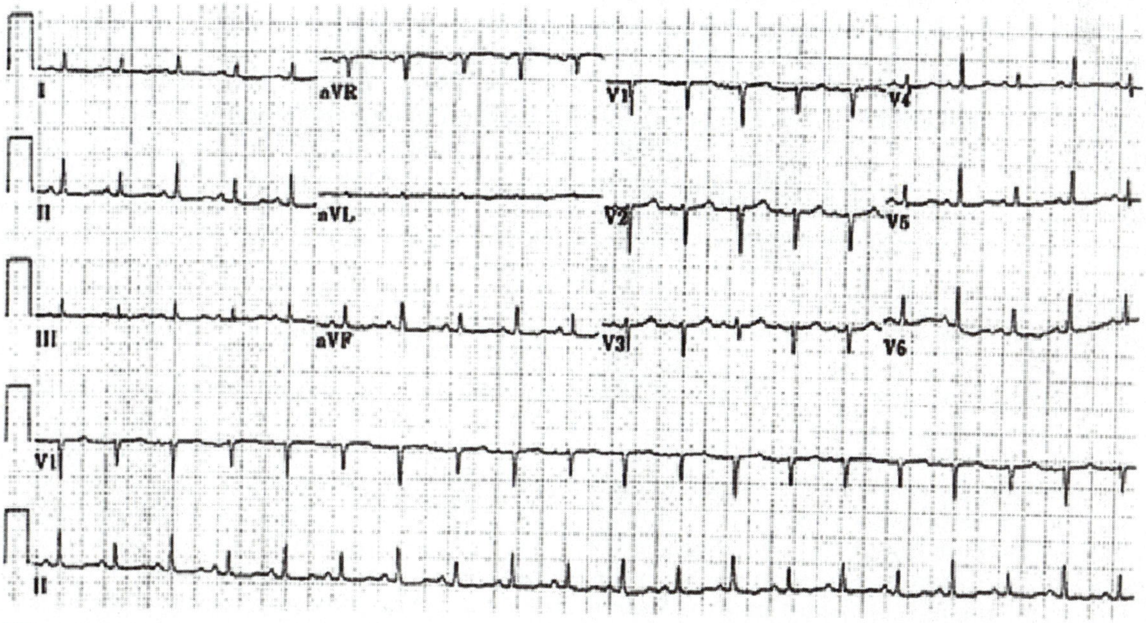

Fig. 47.131: *ECG showing low voltage graph with electrical alternans in massive pericardial effusion (cardiac tamponade)*

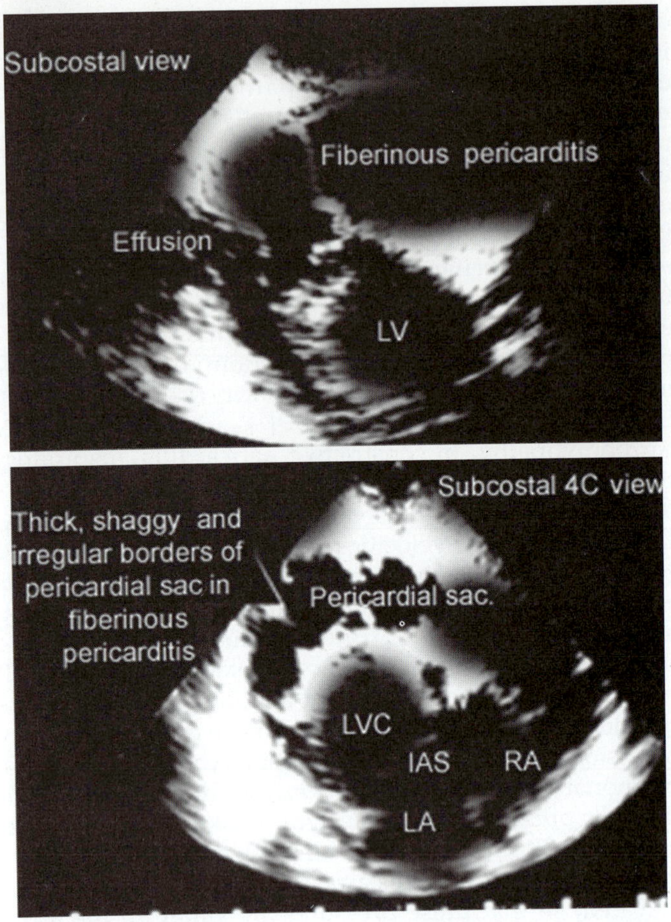

Fig. 47.132: *(Top and bottom) echocardiographic scans show fibrous strands in pericardial sac in a patient with fibrinous pericarditis*

pericarditis. When the pulmonary artery occlusion pressure equals the right atrial mean pressure and an early diastolic dip in the ventricular pressure curve occurs with large x and y waves in the right atrial curve, either disorder may be present. CT or MRI can identify pericardial thickening > 5 mm. Such thickening with typical hemodynamic changes can confirm a diagnosis of constrictive pericarditis. When no pericardial thickening or fluid is seen, the diagnosis of restrictive cardiomyopathy is favored but not proved; a normal pericardial thickness does not exclude the diagnosis of constrictive pericarditis. Diagnosis of cause After pericarditis is diagnosed, tests to determine etiology and the effect on cardiac function are done. In a young, previously healthy adult who presents with a viral infection and pericarditis, an extensive evaluation is usually unnecessary. Differentiating viral from idiopathic pericarditis is difficult, expensive, and generally of little practical importance. A biopsy of pericardial tissue or aspiration of pericardial fluid may be needed to establish a diagnosis. Acid-fast stains and cultures of pericardial fluid help to identify infectious causes. Samples are examined for malignant cells. However, complete drainage of a newly identified pericardial effusion is usually unnecessary for diagnosis. Persistent (usually > 3 mo) or progressive effusion, particularly when the etiology is uncertain, also warrants pericardiocentesis. The choice between needle pericardiocentesis and surgical drainage depends on institutional resources and physician experience, the etiology of the effusion, the need for diagnostic tissue samples, and the prognosis of the patient. Needle pericardiocentesis is often best when the etiology is known or the presence of tamponade is in question. Surgical drainage is best when the presence of tamponade is certain but the etiology is unclear. Laboratory tests of pericardial fluid other than culture and cytology are usually nonspecific. But, specific diagnoses are sometimes possible using newer visual, cytologic, and immunologic analysis of fluid obtained via pericardioscopic-guided biopsy. Cardiac catheterization is useful for evaluating pericarditis and identifying the cause of reduced cardiac function. CT or MRI can help to identify metastases although echocardiography is usually sufficient. Other tests include CBC, acute-phase reactants, routine chemistries, cultures, autoimmune tests, and, when appropriate, tests for HIV, histoplasmosis complement fixation (in endemic areas), streptozyme, and neutralizing antibodies for coxsackievirus, influenza virus, and echovirus. Anti-DNA and anti-RNA antibody tests may be useful. A PPD skin test is done. Treatment hospitalization to watch for complications is usually advisable. Possible causative drugs (e.g. anticoagulants, procainamide, phenytoin) are stopped. For cardiac tamponade, immediate pericardiocentesis is done.

Echocardiography may be used to guide the needle as agitated saline is injected through it. Once in place, the needle should be clamped next to the skin to prevent it from entering further than necessary and possibly puncturing the heart or injuring a coronary vessel.

ECG monitoring is essential for detecting arrhythmias produced when the myocardium is touched or punctured. As a rule, right atrial pressure and pulmonary artery occlusion pressure (pulmonary capillary wedge pressure) are monitored. Fluid is withdrawn until intrapericardial pressure falls below right atrial pressure, usually to subatmospheric levels. If continued drainage is needed, a plastic catheter may be passed through the needle into the pericardium and the needle withdrawn. The catheter may be left in place for 2–4 days. Pain can usually be controlled with aspirin 325–650 mg po q 4 to 6 h or other NSAIDs (e.g. ibuprofen 600–800 mg po q 6 to 8 h) for 1–4 days; duration of therapy varies, and patients should be treated until an effusion if present, has resolved. Colchicine 1 mg/day, added to NSAIDs or given alone, is effective for the initial episode of pericarditis and helps prevent recurrences. The intensity of therapy is dictated by the patient's distress. Severe pain may require opioids and corticosteroids (e.g. prednisone 60–80 mg po once/day for 1 wk, followed by rapid tapering of the dose). Corticosteroids are particularly useful in acute pericarditis due to uremia or a connective tissue disorder, but tuberculous and pyogenic pericarditis should be excluded before corticosteroid therapy is initiated. Intrapericardial instillation of triamcinolone (300 mg/m^2) avoids systemic adverse effects and is highly effective. Anticoagulants are usually contraindicated in acute pericarditis because they may cause intrapericardial bleeding and even fatal tamponade; however, they can be given in early pericarditis complicating acute MI. Uncommonly, pericardial resection is required. Infections are treated with specific antimicrobial drugs. Complete drainage is often necessary. In postpericardiotomy syndrome, post-MI syndrome, or idiopathic pericarditis, antibiotics are not indicated. An NSAID at full doses may control pain and effusion. When required to control pain, fever, and effusion, prednisone 20–60 mg po once/day may be given for 3–4 days. If the response is satisfactory, the dose is gradually reduced, and the drug may be stopped in 7–14 days. But sometimes, many months of treatment are needed. For pericarditis due to rheumatic fever, another connective tissue disorder, or tumor, therapy is directed at the underlying process. For pericardial effusion due to trauma, surgery is sometimes required to repair the injury and evacuate blood from the pericardium. Pericarditis due to uremia may respond to increased frequency of hemodialysis, aspiration, or systemic or intrapericardial adrenal corticosteroids. Intrapericardial triamcinolone may be useful. Chronic effusions are best treated by treating the cause, if known. Recurrent or persistent symptomatic effusions may be treated with balloon pericardiotomy, a surgical pericardial window, or sclerosing drugs (e.g. tetracycline). Recurrent effusion due to malignant tumor invasion may be treated with sclerosing drugs. Asymptomatic effusions of unknown cause may require only observation. Congestion in chronic constrictive pericarditis may be alleviated with bed rest, salt restriction, and diuretics. Digoxin is indicated only if atrial arrhythmias or ventricular systolic dysfunction is present. Symptomatic constrictive pericarditis usually requires pericardial resection. However, patients with mild symptoms, heavy calcification, or extensive myocardial damage may be poor surgical candidates. The mortality rate for pericardial resection may approach 40% in New York Heart Association (NYHA) functional class IV patients. Patients who have constrictive pericarditis due to irradiation or a connective tissue disorder are especially likely to have severe myocardial damage and may not benefit from pericardial resection.

Complications

Most cases of acute idiopathic pericarditis resolve without complications or recurrence. Complications may include:

Pericardial effusion

- Constrictive pericarditis
- Cardiac tamponade
- Fibrinous pericarditis.

Fibrinous pericarditis is an exudative inflammation.

The pericardium is infiltrated by the fibrinous exudate. This consists of fibrin strands and leukocytes. Fibrin describes an amorphous, eosinophilic (pink) network. Leukocytes (mainly neutrophils) are found within the fibrin deposits and intrapericardic. Vascular congestion is also present. The myocardium has no changes. Sometimes referred to as having "Bread and Butter Appearance".

Pericarditis Due to Tuberculosis

Pericarditis caused by tuberculosis is difficult to diagnose, because definitive diagnosis requires culturing *Mycobacterium tuberculosis* from aspirated pericardial fluid or pericardial biopsy, which requires high technical skill and is often not diagnostic (the yield from culture is low even with optimum specimens). The Tygerberg scoring system helps the clinician to decide whether pericarditis is due to tuberculosis or whether it is due to another cause: night sweats (1 point), weight loss (1 point), fever (2 point), serum globulin > 40 g/L (3 points), blood total leucocyte count <10 × 10^9/L (3 points); a total score of 6 or more is highly suggestive of tuberculous pericarditis. Pericardial fluid with an interferon-level greater than 50 pg/mL is highly specific for tuberculous pericarditis.

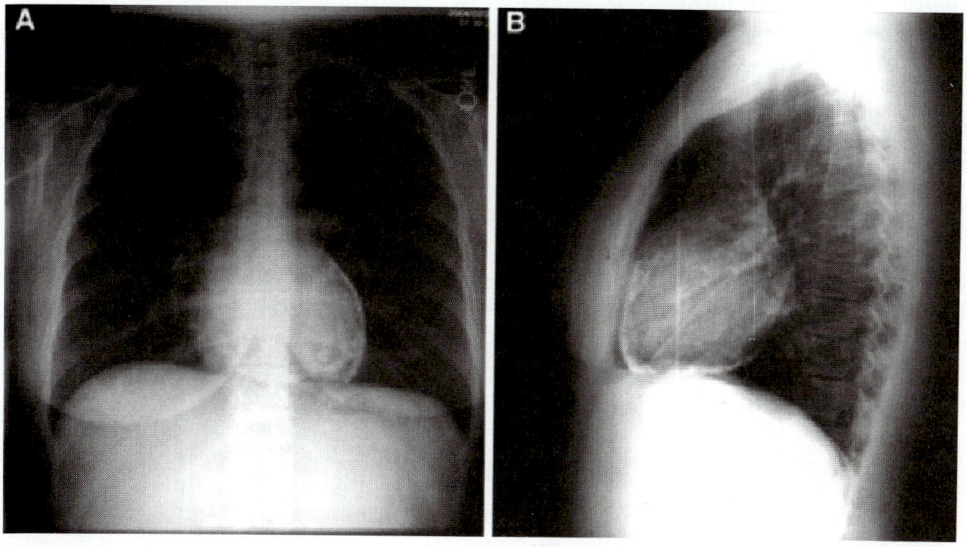

Fig. 47.133: *Chest X-ray [PA (A) and lateral views (B)] obtained on initial presentation showing dense circumferential calcification of pericardium in patient with chronic pericarditis*

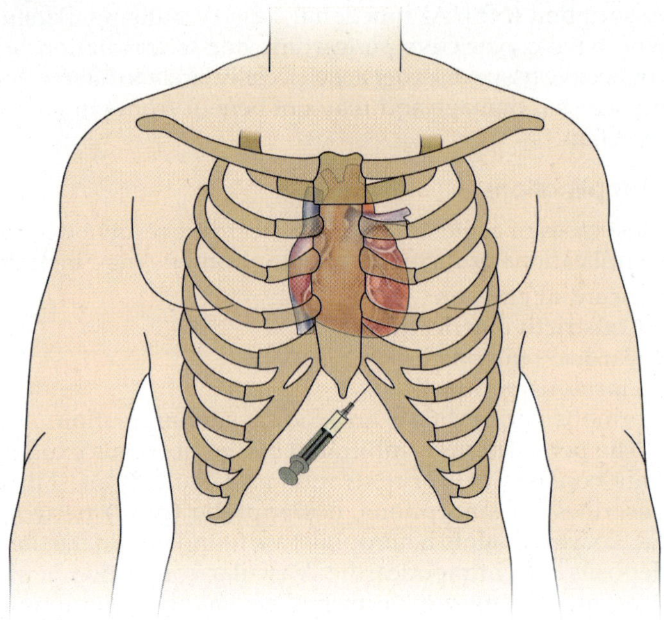

Fig. 47.134: *Placement and angle at which the fluid aspirating needle should be directed in the procedure of pericardiocentesis*

Treatment

The treatment in viral or idiopathic pericarditis is with non-steroidal antiinflammatory drugs. Severe cases may require: pericardiocentesis

- Antibiotics
- Steroids
- Colchicine
- Surgery.

Pericardiocentesis (Fig. 47.134)

Except in emergencies (e.g. cardiac tamponade), pericardiocentesis, a potentially lethal procedure, should be done using echocardiographic guidance in a cardiac catheterization laboratory and should be supervised by a cardiologist or thoracic surgeon if possible. Resuscitation equipment must be at hand. IV sedation (e.g. morphine 0.1 mg/kg or meperidine 1 mg/kg plus midazolam 3–5 mg) is desirable. The patient should be recumbent, with the head elevated 30° from the horizontal. Under aseptic conditions, the skin and subcutaneous tissues are infiltrated with lidocaine. A 75 mm short-beveled, 16-gauge needle is attached via a 3-way stopcock to a 30 or 50 mL syringe. The pericardium may be entered via the right or left xiphocostal angle or from the tip of the xiphoid process with the needle directed inward, upward, and close to the chest wall. The needle is advanced with constant suction applied to the syringe.

BIBLIOGRAPHY

1. Abd-Alla MD, TF Jackson, V Gathiram, AM el-Hawey, and JI Ravdin. 1993. Differentiation of pathogenic Entamoeba histolytica infections from nonpathogenic infections by detection of galactose-inhibitable adherence protein antigen in sera and feces. J. Clin. Microbiol. 31:2845–2850.
2. Acquatella H. 2007. Echocardiography in Chagas heart disease. Circulation 115:1124–1131.
3. Adair OV, N Randive, and N Krasnow. 1989. Isolated toxoplasma myocarditis in acquired immune deficiency syndrome. Am. Heart J. 118:856–857.
4. Adams JH, L Haller, FY Boa, F Doua, A Dago, and K Konian. 1986. Human African trypanosomiasis (T. b. gambiense): a study of 16 fatal cases of sleeping sickness with some observations on acute reactive arsenical encephalopathy. Neuropathol. Appl. Neurobiol. 12:81–94.
5. Adams JL. 1962. Acute toxoplasmosis with involvement of the heart. N. Z. Med. J. 61:20.
6. Adkins RB, Jr., and AH Dao. 1984. Pulmonary dirofilariasis: a diagnostic challenge. South. Med. J. 77:372–374.
7. Aerts D, P Truc, L Penchenier, Y Claes, and D Le Ray. 1992. A kit for in vitro isolation of trypanosomes in the field: first trial with sleeping sickness patients in the Congo Republic. Trans. R. Soc. Trop. Med. Hyg. 86:394–395.
8. Aikat BK, SR Bhusnurmath, AK Pal, PN Chhuttani, and D V Datta. 1978. Amoebic liver abscess—a clinicopathological study. Indian J. Med. Res. 67:381–391.
9. Ammann RW, and J Eckert. 1996. Cestodes. Echinococcus. Gastroenterol. Clin. North Am. 25:655–689.
10. Amorim DS, and JA Marin Neto. 1995. Functional alterations in the autonomic nervous system in Chagas' heart disease. Sao Paulo Med. J. 113:772–784.
11. Ancelle T, A De Bruyne, D Poisson, and J Dupouy-Camet. 2005. Outbreak of trichinellosis due to consumption of bear meat from Canada, France, September 2005. Euro Surveill. 10:E051013.3.
12. Anderson SE, and JS Remington. 1975. The diagnosis of toxoplasmosis. South. Med. J. 68:1433–1443.
13. Andrade LO, and NW Andrews. 2005. The Trypanosoma cruzi-host-cell interplay: location, invasion, retention. Nat. Rev. Microbiol. 3:819–823.
14. Andrade ZA. 1999. Immunopathology of Chagas disease. Mem. Inst. Oswaldo Cruz 94(Suppl. 1):71–80.
15. Andy JJ, JP O'Connell, R. C. Daddario, and W. C. Roberts. 1977. Trichinosis causing extensive ventricular mural endocarditis with superimposed thrombosis. Evidence that severe eosinophilia damages endocardium. Am. J. Med. 63:824–829.
16. Angel SO, M Matrajt, J Margarit, M Nigro, E Illescas, V Pszenny, MR Amendoeira, E Guarnera, and JC Garberi. 1997. Screening for active toxoplasmosis in patients by DNA hybridization with the ABGTg7 probe in blood samples. J. Clin. Microbiol. 35:591–595.
17. Arness MK, JD Brown, JP Dubey, RC Neafie, and DE Granstrom. 1999. An outbreak of acute eosinophilic myositis attributed to human Sarcocystis parasitism. Am. J. Trop. Med. Hyg. 61:548–553.
18. Bailey JW, and DH. Smith. 1994. The quantitative buffy coat for the diagnosis of trypanosomes. Trop. Doct. 24:54–56.
19. Balasegaram MH. Young F. Chappuis G. Priotto ME. Raguenaud, and F Checchi. 2009. Effectiveness of melarsoprol and eflornithine as first-line regimens for gambiense sleeping sickness in nine Medecins Sans Frontieres programmes. Trans. R. Soc. Trop. Med. Hyg. 103:280–290.

20. Barnard PM, LA MacGregor, and HF Weich. 1989. Primary echinococcus cyst of the heart. A case report. S. Afr. Med. J. 76:275–277.
21. Barry JD. 1997. The relative significance of mechanisms of antigenic variation in African trypanosomes. Parasitol. Today 13:212–218.
22. Barsoum RS. 2004. Parasitic infections in organ transplantation. Exp. Clin. Transplant. 2:258–267.
23. Bastien P. 2002. Molecular diagnosis of toxoplasmosis. Trans. R. Soc. Trop. Med. Hyg. 96(Suppl. 1):S205–S215.
24. Beaver P, R Jung, and E Cupp. 1984. Clinical parasitology. Lea and Febiger, Philadelphia, PA.
25. Berensztein CS, D Pineiro, M Marcotegui, R Brunoldi, MV Blanco, and J Lerman. 2000. Usefulness of echocardiography and Doppler echocardiography in endomyocardial fibrosis. J. Am. Soc. Echocardiogr. 13:385–392.
26. Berger PB, J Duffy, GS Reeder, BL Karon, and WD Edwards. 1994. Restrictive cardiomyopathy associated with the eosinophilia-myalgia syndrome. Mayo Clin. Proc. 69:162-165.
27. Bern C, and SP Montgomery. 2009. An estimate of the burden of Chagas disease in the United States. Clin. Infect. Dis. 49:e52-e54.
28. Bern C, SP Montgomery, BL Herwaldt, A Rassi, Jr. JA. Marin-Neto RO. Dantas JH. Maguire H. Acquatella C. Morillo L. V Kirchhoff, RH Gilman, PA Reyes, R Salvatella, and AC. Moore. 2007. Evaluation and treatment of Chagas disease in the United States: a systematic review. JAMA 298:2171–2181.
29. Bern C, SP Montgomery, L Katz, S Caglioti, and SL Stramer. 2008. Chagas disease and the US blood supply. Curr. Opin. Infect. Dis. 21:476–482.
30. Bertrand E, F Serie, I Kone, J Rive, P Campaore, L Sentilhes, and J Philippe. 1973. Symptomatologie generale de la trypanosomiase humaine Africaine au moment du depistage. Med. d'Afrique Noire 20:303–314.
31. Bertrand E, F Serie, J Rive, and I Kone. 1973. La symptomatologie cardio-vasculaire dans la trypanosomiase humaine Africaine a Trypanosoma gambiense. Med. d'Afrique Noire 20:327–339.
32. Bhalla A, A Sood, and A. Sachdev. 2008. Heart involvement in disseminated cysticercosis—a case report and review of literature. Indian Heart J. 60:260–262.
33. Bhatia G. 1997. Echinococcus. Semin. Respir. Infect. 12:171-186.
34. Biava MF, A Dao, and B Fortier. 2001. Laboratory diagnosis of cystic hydatic disease. World J. Surg. 25:10–14.
35. Bisser S, V Lejon, PM Preux, B. Bouteille, A. Stanghellini, M. O. Jauberteau, P. Buscher, and M. Dumas. 2002. Blood-cerebrospinal fluid barrier and intrathecal immunoglobulins compared to field diagnosis of central nervous system involvement in sleeping sickness. J. Neurol. Sci. 193:127-135.
36. Bittencourt AL. 1976. Congenital Chagas disease. Am. J. Dis. Child. 130:97–103.
37. Blessmann J, H Buss, PA. Nu, BT Dinh, QT Ngo, A. L. Van, M. D. Alla, T. F. Jackson, J. I. Ravdin, and E. Tannich. 2002. Real-time PCR for detection and differentiation of Entamoeba histolytica and Entamoeba dispar in fecal samples. J. Clin. Microbiol. 40:4413–17.
38. Blum J, C Schmid, and C Burri. 2006. Clinical aspects of 2541 patients with second stage human African trypanosomiasis. Acta Trop. 97:55–64.
39. Blum JA, C Burri, C Hatz, L. Kazumba, P. Mangoni, and M. J. Zellweger. 2007. Sleeping hearts: the role of the heart in sleeping sickness (human African trypanosomiasis). Trop. Med. Int. Health 12:1422–1432.
40. Bobic B, D Sibalic, and O Djurkovic-Djakovic. 1991. High levels of IgM antibodies specific for Toxoplasma gondii in pregnancy 12 years after primary toxoplasma infection. Case report. Gynecol. Obstet. Invest. 31:182–184.
41. Bocchi EA, and A Fiorelli. 2001. The paradox of survival results after heart transplantation for cardiomyopathy caused by Trypanosoma cruzi. First Guidelines Group for Heart Transplantation of the Brazilian Society of Cardiology. Ann. Thorac. Surg. 71:1833–1838.
42. Boggild AK, JS Keystone, and KC Kain. 2004. Tropical pulmonary eosinophilia: a case series in a setting of nonendemicity. Clin. Infect. Dis. 39:1123–1128.
43. Bohne W, J Heesemann, and U Gross. 1994. Reduced replication of Toxoplasma gondii is necessary for induction of bradyzoite-specific antigens: a possible role for nitric oxide in triggering stage conversion. Infect. Immun. 62:1761–1767.
44. Borst P, and S Ulbert. 2001. Control of VSG gene expression sites. Mol. Biochem. Parasitol. 114:17–27.
45. Boschetti A, and J Kasznica. 1995. Visceral larva migrans induced eosinophilic cardiac pseudotumor: a cause of sudden death in a child. J. Forensic Sci. 40:1097–1099.
46. Botero D, HB Tanowitz, LM Weiss, and M. Wittner. 1993. Taeniasis and cysticercosis. Infect. Dis. Clin. North Am. 7:683–697.
47. Bouraoui H, B Trimeche, A Mahdhaoui, A Majdoub, J Zaaraoui, SH Ernez, J Gouider, and H Ammar. 2005. Echinococcosis of the heart: clinical and echocardiographic features in 12 patients. Acta Cardiol. 60:39–41.
48. Bracha R, LS Diamond, JP Ackers, GD Burchard, and D Mirelman. 1990. Differentiation of clinical isolates of Entamoeba histolytica by using specific DNA probes. J. Clin. Microbiol. 28:680–684.
49. Britto CC. 2009. Usefulness of PCR-based assays to assess drug efficacy in Chagas disease chemotherapy: value and limitations. Mem. Inst. Oswaldo Cruz 104(Suppl. 1):122–135.
50. Brown CR, and R McLeod. 1990. Class I MHC genes and CD8+ T cells determine cyst number in Toxoplasma gondii infection. J. Immunol. 145:3438–3441.
51. Brown RL. 1991. Successful treatment of primary amebic meningoencephalitis. Arch. Intern. Med. 151:1201–1202.
52. Bustamante JM, HW Rivarola, AR Fernandez, JE Enders, R Fretes, JA Palma, and PA. Paglini-Oliva. 2003. Indeterminate Chagas' disease: Trypanosoma cruzi strain and re-infection are factors involved in the progression of cardiopathy. Clin. Sci. (Lond.) 104:415–420.
53. Cameron EW. 1978. The treatment of pleuropulmonary amebiasis with metronidazole. Chest 73:647–650.
54. Campbell D, and K Chadee. 1997. Survival strategies of Entamoeba histolytica: modulation of cell-mediated immune responses. Parasitol. Today 13:184–190.
55. Candolfi E, R Pastor, R Huber, D Filisetti, and O Villard. 2007. IgG avidity assay firms up the diagnosis of acute toxoplasmosis on the first serum sample in immuno-competent pregnant women. Diagn. Microbiol. Infect. Dis. 58:83–88.

56. Carod-Artal FJ, AP Vargas, TA Horan, and LG Nunes. 2005. Chagasic cardiomyopathy is independently associated with ischemic stroke in Chagas disease. Stroke 36:965–970.
57. Carrasco HA, JS Barboza, G Inglessis, A Fuenmayor, and C Molina. 1982. Left ventricular cineangiography in Chagas' disease: detection of early myocardial damage. Am. Heart J. 104:595–602.
58. Carrasco HA, H Parada, L Guerrero, M Duque, D Duran, and C Molina. 1994. Prognostic implications of clinical, electrocardiographic and hemodynamic findings in chronic Chagas' disease. Int. J. Cardiol. 43:27–38.
59. Carter RF. 1972. Primary amoebic meningo-encephalitis. An appraisal of present knowledge. Trans. R. Soc. Trop. Med. Hyg. 66:193–213.
60. Castro AM, AO Luquetti, A Rassi, GG Rassi, E Chiari, and LM Galvao. 2002. Blood culture and polymerase chain reaction for the diagnosis of the chronic phase of human infection with Trypanosoma cruzi. Parasitol. Res. 88:894–900.
61. Castro JA, MM de Mecca, and L. C. Bartel. 2006. Toxic side effects of drugs used to treat Chagas' disease (American trypanosomiasis). Hum. Exp. Toxicol. 25:471–479.
62. CDC. 2004. Trichinellosis associated with bear meat—New York and Tennessee, 2003. MMWR Morb. Mortal. Wkly. Rep. 53:606–610.
63. Chappuis F, L Loutan, P Simarro, V Lejon, and P Buscher. 2005. Options for field diagnosis of human African trypanosomiasis. Clin. Microbiol. Rev. 18:133–146.
64. Chappuis F, N Udayraj, K Stietenroth, A Meussen, and PA Bovier. 2005. Eflornithine is safer than melarsoprol for the treatment of second-stage Trypanosoma brucei gambiense human African trypanosomiasis. Clin. Infect. Dis. 41:748–751.
65. Checchi F, JA Filipe, MP Barrett, and D Chandramohan. 2008. The natural progression of gambiense sleeping sickness: what is the evidence? PLoS Negl. Trop. Dis. 2:e303.
66. Cheever AW, IA Kamel, AM Elwi, JE Mosimann, R Danner, and JE Sippel. 1978. Schistosoma mansoni and S haematobium infections in Egypt. III. Extrahepatic pathology. Am. J. Trop. Med. Hyg. 27:55275.
67. Chen Y, Y Zhang, B Yang, T Qi, H Lu, X Cheng, and H. Tachibana. 2007. Seroprevalence of Entamoeba histolytica infection in HIV-infected patients in China. Am. J. Trop. Med. Hyg. 77:825–828.
68. Cheung YY, S Steinbaum, WT Yuh, and L Chiu. 1987. MR findings in extracranial cysticercosis. J Comput. Assist. Tomogr. 11:179–181.
69. Clumeck N. 1991. Some aspects of the epidemiology of toxoplasmosis and pneumocystosis in AIDS in Europe. Eur. J. Clin. Microbiol. Infect. Dis. 10:177–178.
70. Collomb H, and D Bartoli. The heart in human African trypanosomiasis caused by Trypanosoma gambiense. Bull. Soc. Pathol. Exot. Filiales 1967;60:142–156.
71. Compton SJ, CL Celum, C Lee, D Thompson, SM Sumi, TR Fritsche, and RW Coombs. 1993. Trichinosis with ventilatory failure and persistent myocarditis. Clin. Infect. Dis. 16:500–504.
72. Conter RL, HA Pitt, RK Tompkins, and WP Longmire, Jr. 1986. Differentiation of pyogenic from amebic hepatic abscesses. Surg. Gynecol. Obstet. 162:114–120.
73. Cordon-Obras C, P Berzosa, N Ndong-Mabale, L Bobuakasi, JN. Buatiche P. Ndongo-Asumu, A Benito, and J Cano. 2009. Trypanosoma brucei gambiense in domestic livestock of Kogo and Mbini foci (Equatorial Guinea). Trop. Med. Int. Health 14:535–541.
74. Cunha-Neto E, AM Bilate, KV Hyland, SG Fonseca, J Kalil, and DM Engman. 2006. Induction of cardiac autoimmunity in Chagas heart disease: a case for molecular mimicry. Autoimmunity 39:41–54.
75. Cunha-Neto E, V Coelho, L Guilherme, A Fiorelli, N Stolf, and J Kalil. 1996. Autoimmunity in Chagas' disease. Identification of cardiac myosin-B13 Trypanosoma cruzi protein crossreactive T cell clones in heart lesions of a chronic Chagas' cardiomyopathy patient. J. Clin. Invest. 98:1709–1712.
76. Cunha-Neto E, M Duranti, A Gruber, B Zingales, I De Messias, N Stolf, G. Bellotti, M. E. Patarroyo, F. Pilleggi, and J. Kalil. 1995. Autoimmunity in Chagas disease cardiopathy: biological relevance of a cardiac myosin-specific epitope crossreactive to an immunodominant Trypanosoma cruzi antigen. Proc. Natl. Acad. Sci. USA. 92:3541–3545.
77. Dannemann BR, DM Israelski, GS Leoung, T McGraw, J Mills, and JS Remington. 1991. Toxoplasma serology, parasitemia and antigenemia in patients at risk for toxoplasmic encephalitis. AIDS 5:1363–1365.
78. Dao AH, and R Virmani. 1986. Visceral larva migrans involving the myocardium: report of two cases and review of literature. Pediatr. Pathol. 6:449–456.
79. de Carvalho VB, EF Sousa, JH Vila, JP da Silva, MR Caiado, SR Araujo, R Macruz, and EJ Zerbini. 1996. Heart transplantation in Chagas' disease. 10 years after the initial experience. Circulation 94:1815–1817.
80. de Cleva R, P Herman, V Pugliese, B Zilberstein, WA Saad, JJ Rodrigues, and AA Laudanna. 2003. Prevalence of pulmonary hypertension in patients with hepatosplenic Mansonic schistosomiasis—prospective study. Hepatogastroenterology 50:2028–2030.
81. De Cock C, J Lemaitre, and FE Deuvaert. 1998. Loeffler endomyocarditis: a clinical presentation as right ventricular tumor. J. Heart Valve Dis. 7:668–671.
82. deGhetaldi LD, RM Norman, and AW Douville, Jr. 1983. Cerebral cysticercosis treated biphasically with dexamethasone and praziquantel. Ann. Intern. Med. 99:179–181.
83. Dempsey WL, and JM Mansfield. 1983. Lymphocyte function in experimental African trypanosomiasis. V. Role of antibody and the mononuclear phagocyte system in variant-specific immunity. J. Immunol. 130:405–411.
84. Denie C, F Vachiery, A Elman, T Soupison, A Gadano, R Moreau, and D Lebrec. 1996. Systemic and splanchnic hemodynamic changes in patients with hepatic schistosomiasis. Liver 16:309–312.
85. de Raadt P, and JW Koten. 1968. Myocarditis in rhodesiense trypanosomiasis. East Afr. Med. J. 45:128–132.
86. Derouin F, and H Pelloux. 2008. Prevention of toxoplasmosis in transplant patients. Clin. Microbiol. Infect. 14:1089–1101.
87. Derrick EH. 1948. A fatal case of generalized amoebiasis due to a protozoan closely resembling, if not identical with Iodamoeba butschlii. Trans. R. Soc. Trop. Med. Hyg. 42:191–198.
88. Despommier DD. 1998. How does Trichinella spiralis make itself at home? Parasitol. Today 14:318–323.
89. Dubey JP, HR Gamble, D Hill, C Sreekumar, S Romand, and P. Thuilliez. 2002. High prevalence of viable Toxoplasma

gondii infection in market weight pigs from a farm in Massachusetts. J. Parasitol. 88:1234–1238.

90. Dubey JP, DS Lindsay, and CA Speer. 1998. Structures of Toxoplasma gondii tachyzoites, bradyzoites, and sporozoites and biology and development of tissue cysts. Clin. Microbiol. Rev. 11:267–299.
91. Duma RJ, HW Ferrell, EC Nelson, and MM Jones. 1969. Primary amebic meningoencephalitis. N. Engl. J. Med. 281:1315–1323.
92. Dupouy-Camet J. 2008. Presidential address of ICT12 Conference: "Trichinella and trichinellosis—a never ending story." Vet. Parasitol. 159:194-196.
93. Dupouy-Camet J, SL de Souza, C Maslo, A Paugam, AG Saimot, R Benarous, C Tourte-Schaefer, and F Derouin. 1993. Detection of Toxoplasma gondii in venous blood from AIDS patients by polymerase chain reaction. J. Clin. Microbiol. 31:1866–1869.
94. Dursun M, E Terzibasioglu, R Yilmaz, B Cekrezi, S Olgar, K Nisli, and A Tunaci. 2008. Cardiac hydatid disease: CT and MRI findings. Am. J. Roentgenol. 190:226–232.
95. Eberly MD, EK Soh, S. P. Bannister, H. Tavaf-Motamen, and JS Scott. 2008. Isolated cardiac cysticercosis in an adolescent. Pediatr. Infect. Dis. J. 27:369–371.
96. Eckert J, and P Deplazes. 2004. Biological, epidemiological, and clinical aspects of echinococcosis, a zoonosis of increasing concern. Clin. Microbiol. Rev. 17:107–135.
97. Enanga B, RJ Burchmore, ML Stewart, and MP Barrett. 2002. Sleeping sickness and the brain. Cell. Mol. Life Sci. 59:845–858.
98. Engman DM, and JS Leon. 2002. Pathogenesis of Chagas heart disease: role of autoimmunity. Acta Trop. 81:123–132.
99. Erentug V, N Bozbuga, K Kirali, I Mataraci, C Kaymaz, M Balkanay, E Akinci, G Ipek, and C Yakut. 2004. Cardiac hydatid cysts: surgical treatment and results. J. Card. Surg. 19:358–360.
100. Hotez 2009. The unfinished public health agenda of Chagas disease in the era of globalization. PLoS Negl. Trop. Dis. 3:e470.

48 Fetal Cardiac Interventions: Overview

The potential benefits of fetal cardiac intervention (FCI) have been realized for many years. In 1975, Eibschitz et al reported intrapartum treatment of fetal ventricular tachycardia by administering propranolol to the mother, and as early as 1986, in utero pacing was attempted for complete heart block in a human fetus. Recently, however, interest in FCI has accelerated. As with other fetal interventions, FCI can only become a highly useful clinical tool if it is applied to conditions in which a feasible mode of therapy is available and either the fetus is at risk for demise as a result of the condition or intervention may alter the evolution of the condition such that the severity of the postnatal disease is substantially reduced. For conditions in which the fetus is at high risk for prenatal or neonatal death, the rationale for FCI is obvious, to improve survival. If death is not imminent but the disease is likely to have major lifelong morbidity, the rationale is that FCI will modify the course of cardiac growth, function, and/or development in utero sufficiently to alter postnatal outcome and justify the potential risks of the procedure. Prenatal intervention may also allow the fetus to recover in the supportive in utero environment during a developmental period when there is enhanced wound healing and the capacity for myocyte proliferation (Figs 48.1 and 48.2).

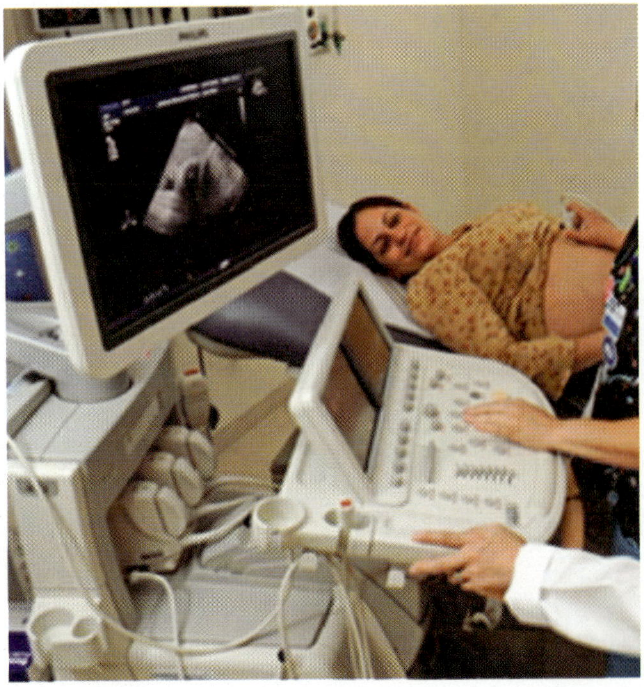

Fig. 48.1: *Doctor is performing foetal echocardiography*

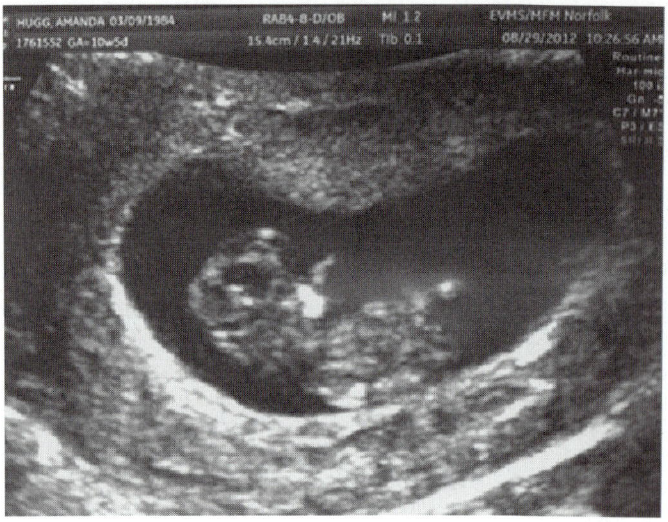

Fig. 48.2: *Abdominal ultrasound showing viable intrauterine 10 weeks old foetus*

This construct rightfully emphasizes death or significant morbidity as therapeutic targets. FCI can entail substantial short-term risk to the fetus, uncertain long-term risk to the fetus and child, and at least some risk to the mother. There are no known medical benefits to the mother. With that risk profile, FCI will not be embraced by the maternal-fetal medicine and cardiology communities unless it is used to treat serious conditions in which the potential benefits to

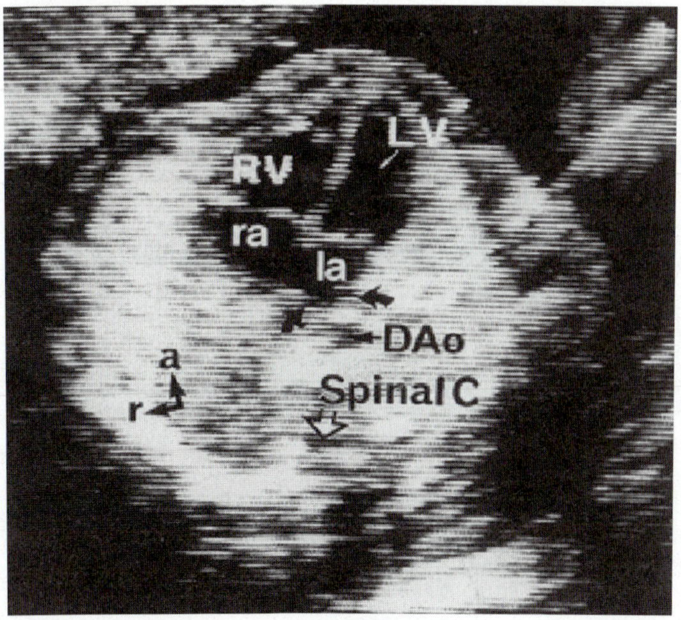

Fig. 48.3: *Foetal echocardiographic graph showing well formed four chambers of the heart with concordant A-V valves communicating through their respective chambers*

the fetus are high and can be achieved in a reasonable percentage of cases.

Although many recent publications have dealt with closed, "minimally invasive" FCI, there is a considerable body of evidence regarding pharmacological and surgical FCI as well. This review will touch on all of these topics, with a focus on the most recent literature.

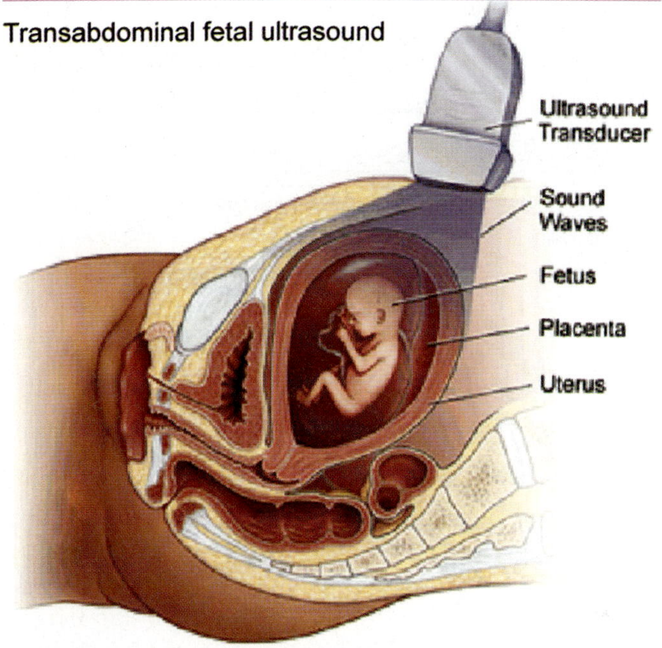

Fig. 48.4: *Illustration showing ultrasound beam striking at different parts of fetus for their identification and perfomance of selected percutaneous intervention*

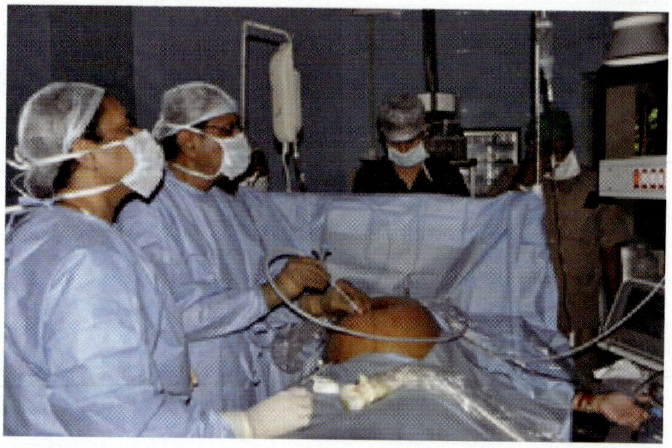

Fig. 48.5: *Photograph showing team of doctors performing fetoscopy procedure on a pregnant woman for assessment of fetal health*

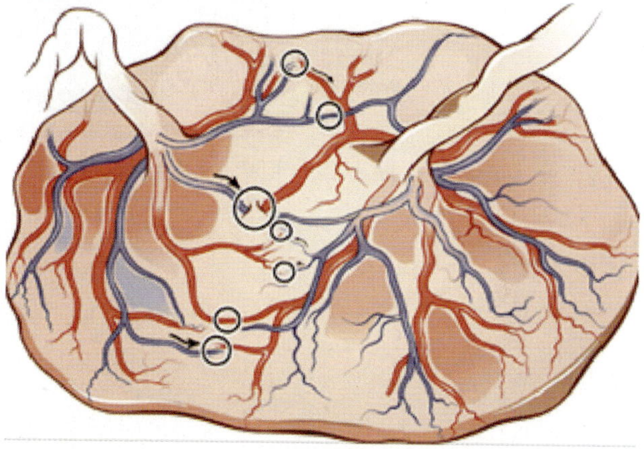

Fig. 48.6: *Drawing of the shared placenta in twin to twin transfusion syndrome multiple vessels connect both fetuses over what is called "anastomoses" (open circles). These anastomoses are the subject of laser coagulation*

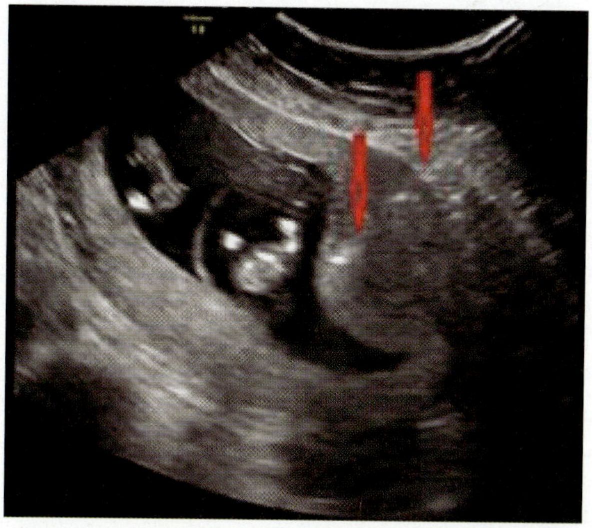

Fig. 48.7: *Fetal skin biopsy is the optimal way to evaluate ambiguity that occasionally arises in the interpretation of amniocentesis data. These biopsies are performed without a hospital stay, and under ultrasound guidance*

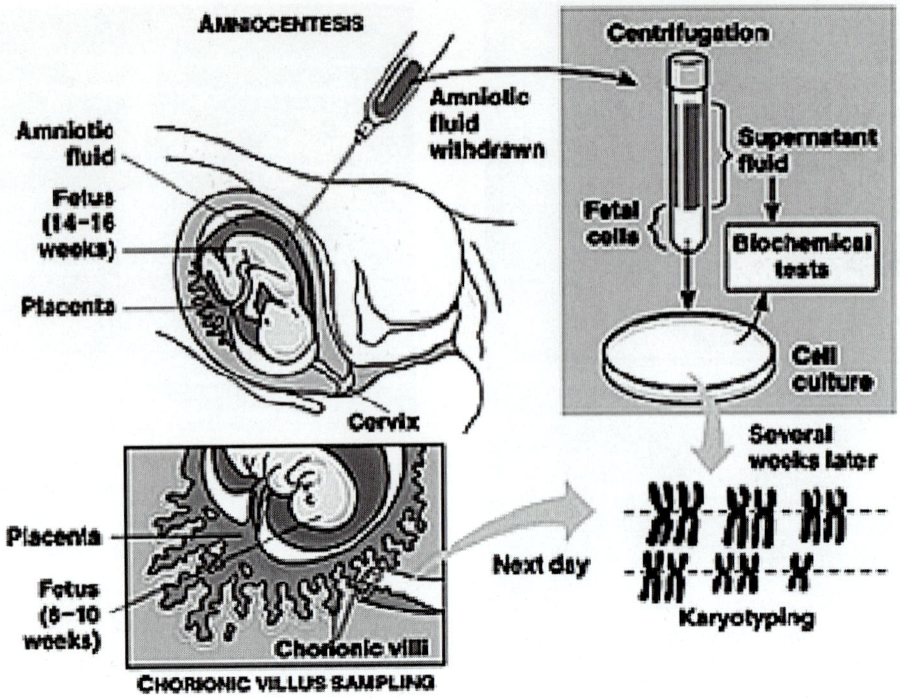

Fig. 48.8: *Illustrations show the technique of amniocentesis for identification fetal genetic disorders*

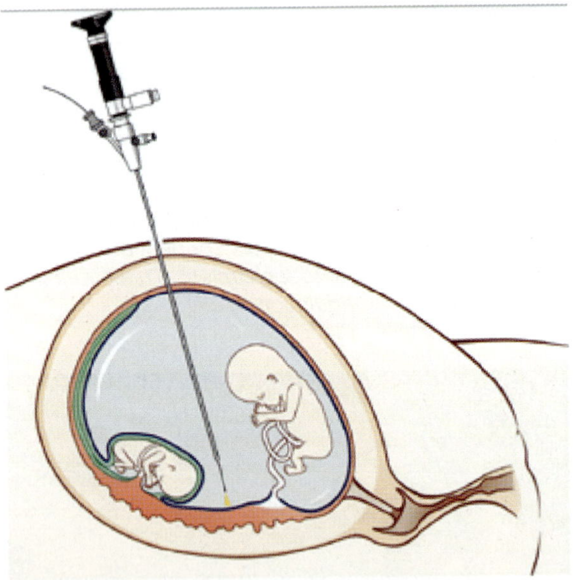

Fig. 48.9: *Illustration of a fetoscopic laser treatment. A cannula has been placed through the abdominal wall through which a scope and laser beam has been passed. The connecting vessels are identified and subsequently destroyed*

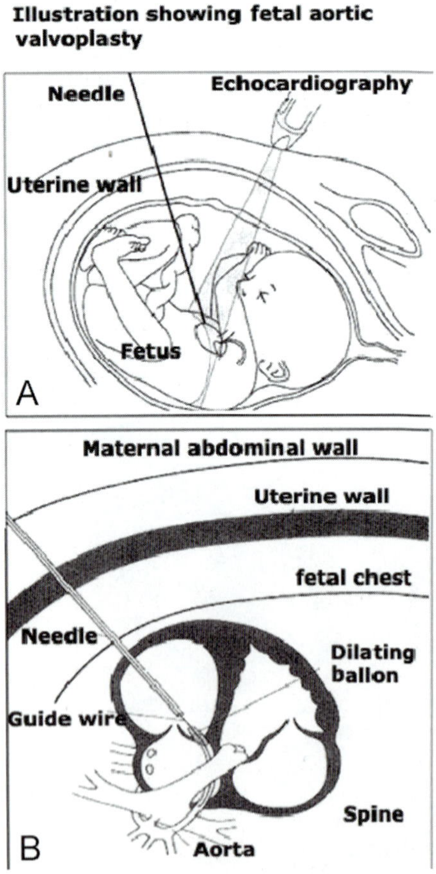

Fig. 48.10: *Ideal fetal position and cannula course. Fetal left chest is anterior, and pathway from maternal abdomen to LV apex is unobstructed. This pathway, which corresponds to cannula course, continues from LV apex to aortic valve*

Fetoscopic and Ultrasonographic Techniques in FCI

These are useful not only in diagnosis of congenital heart defects in utero but also helps in the management of critical cardiovascular disorders.

Pharmacological FCI (Table 48.1)

The first reported and most entrenched mode of FCI is pharmacological therapy, most often for fetal arrhythmia or heart block. Pharmacological FCI typically consists of medication taken orally by the mother with transplacental passage to the fetus, but it may be provided directly through

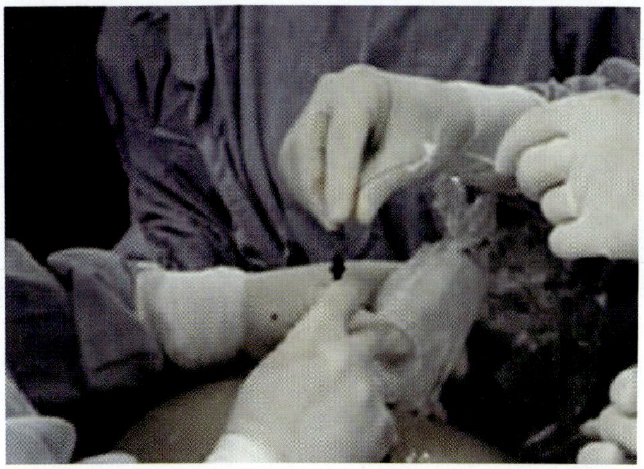

Fig. 48.11: *Experts performing aortic valvoplasty with premounted balloon in the needle that is positioned below the aortic valve with the help of maternal transabdominal ultrasound monitoring*

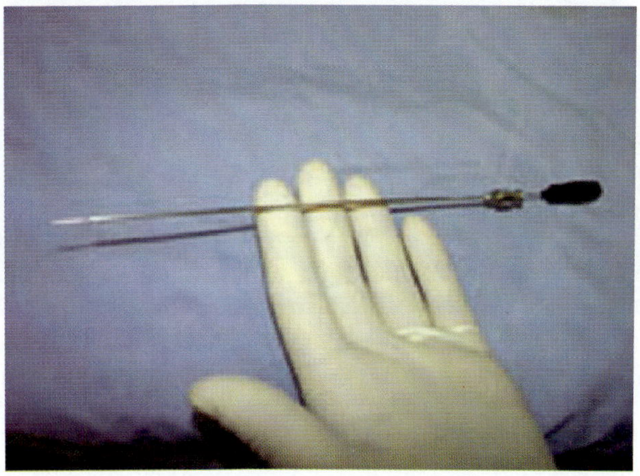

Fig. 48.12: *Features of Chiba needle used for fetal invasive procedures*

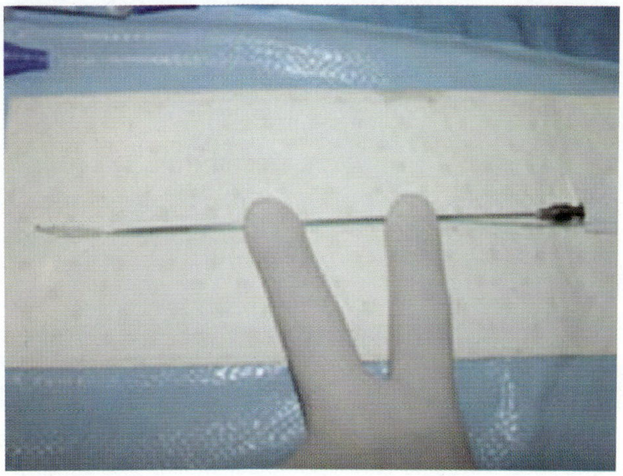

Fig. 48.13: *Balloon angioplasty preassembled on guide that will be introduced through the needle Chiba to dilate the aortic valve*

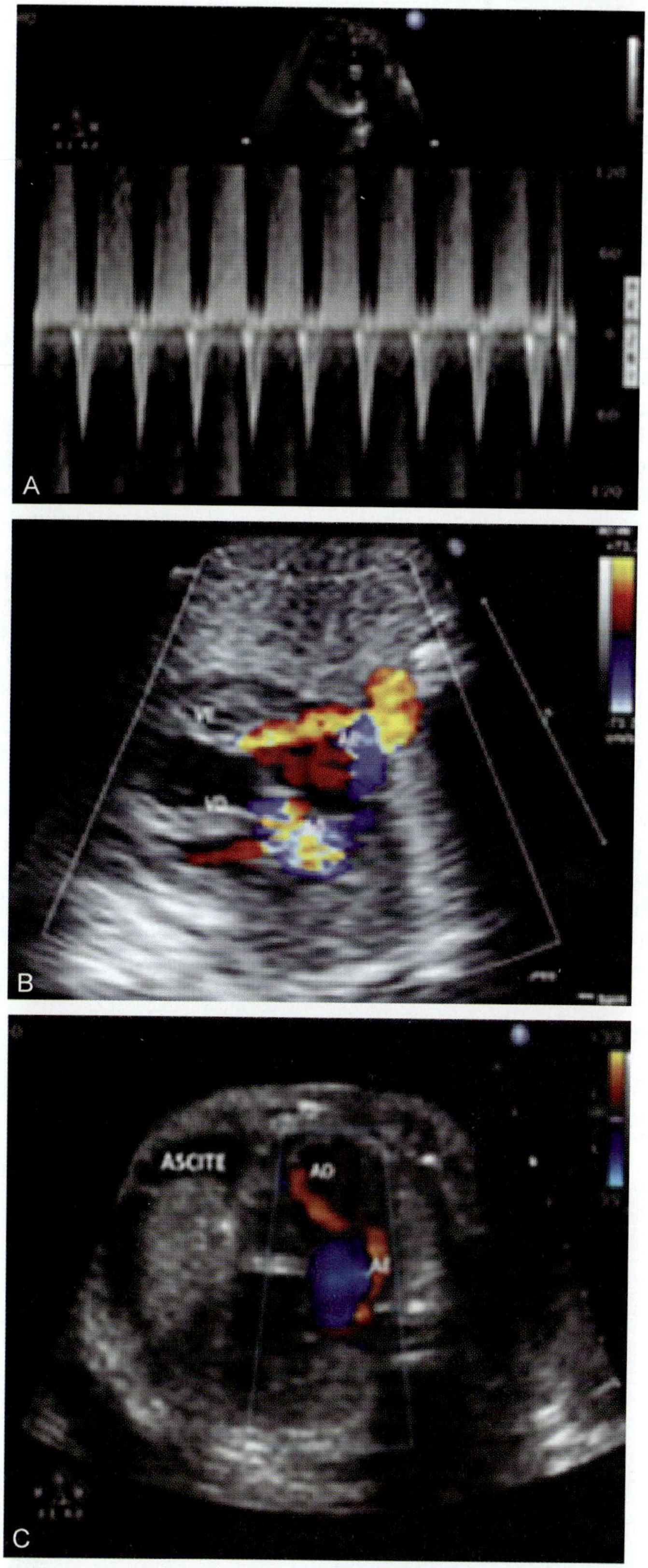

Fig. 48.14: *Echocardiographic images of fetus with aortic stenosis with parameters indicative of progression to left ventricular hypoplasia. (A) Color Doppler of the mitral valve demonstrating single-phase left ventricular filling and mitral insufficiency important. (B) Reverse flow in the ascending aorta. (C) Left-right flow through the atrial septum*

the umbilical vein or by fetal intramuscular or intravascular injection.

Fetal Tachyarrhythmias (Figs 48.22 and 48.23)

Pharmacological FCI was first described by Eibschitz et al. who treated fetal tachycardia with propranolol in 1975. Maternal digoxin was first used to treat fetal supraventricular tachycardia several years later. Fetal supraventricular tachycardia, most often atrioventricular (AV) reentry or atrial flutter, probably remains the most common indication for pharmacological FCI. Over the years, most antiarrhythmic agents have been used to treat fetal supraventricular tachycardia. Digoxin has been a mainstay of therapy; other agents have come io more common use recently including sotalol, darone, and flecainide. Transplacental therapy with first-line agents is usually effective in nonhydropic fetuses, but outcomes remain suboptimal, with fetal death in 10% of cases overall and a higher percentage of fetuses with hydrops.

The optimal therapeutic strategy for fetal supraventricular tachycardia has not been determined in a standardized trial, and practice varies. The indications for therapy may depend on fetal age and disease severity. When hydrops is present, pharmacological FCI may help as a bridge to delivery and postnatal treatment. In preterm fetuses, sustained tachycardia should probably be treated regardless of cardiac dysfunction or hydrops because these sequelae can develop rapidly. For intermittent tachycardia, treatment is generally unnecessary unless hydrops or cardiac dysfunction is evident. Transplacental delivery of some drugs is impaired in the setting of hydrops, and supraventricular tachycardia may be refractory for other reasons as well. In such circumstances, intravascular administration and/or oral agents with better placental uptake kinetics may be indicated. Direct administration, usually by percutaneous umbilical venous injection, introduces the risks of cordocentesis and is reserved for high-acuity refractory cases.

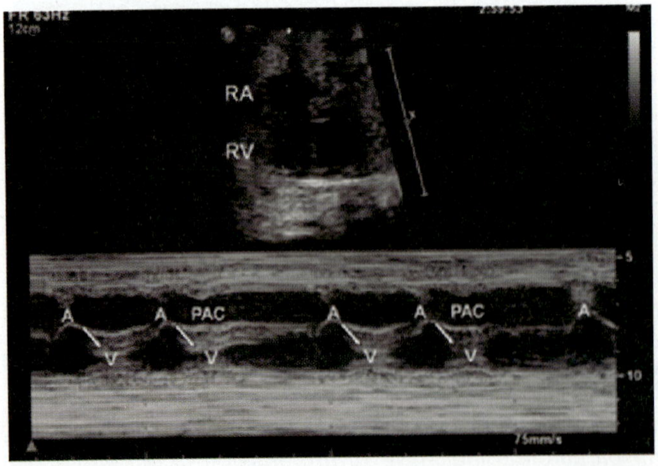

Fig. 48.15: *Blocked PAC. M-mode tracing from a four chamber view with the transducer beam through the RA and the RV. There are blocked PAC's in a trigeminy pattern. Only the normal atrial contractions (A) are followed by a ventricular contraction (V)*

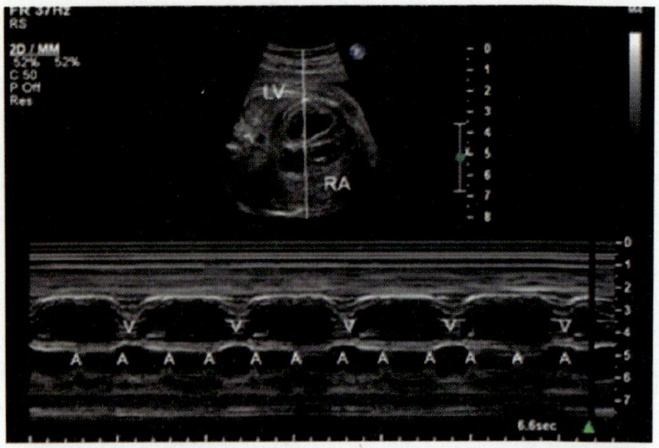

Fig. 48.16: *Complete heart block. M-mode tracing from a four chamber view with the transducer beam through the RA and the LV. There are regular atrial contractions (A) with a normal heart rate of 125 bpm and independent ventricular contractions (V) with a heart rate of 50 bpm*

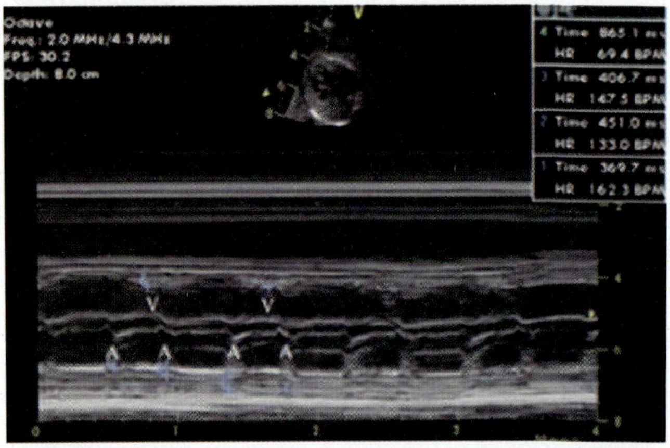

Fig. 48.17: *M-mode echocardiography at 20 weeks showing significant fetal bradycardia (V-V: 67 beats/min) related to atrial bigeminy. There is atrial beat-to-beat variation with the premature atrial beats (A-A interval: 370 ms) being blocked and the normal atrial impulses (450 ms) being conducted. A repeat echocardiogram showed normal cardiac rhythm 1 week later*

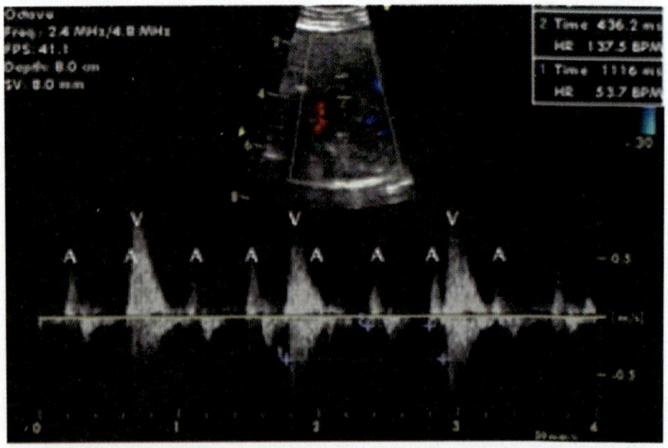

Fig. 48.18: *Simultaneous Doppler of the aorta and superior vena cava showing complete atrioventricular block. The atrial (A-A) rate was 138 beats/min (bpm) and the ventricular (V-V) rate was 54 bpm, with complete atrioventricular dissociation*

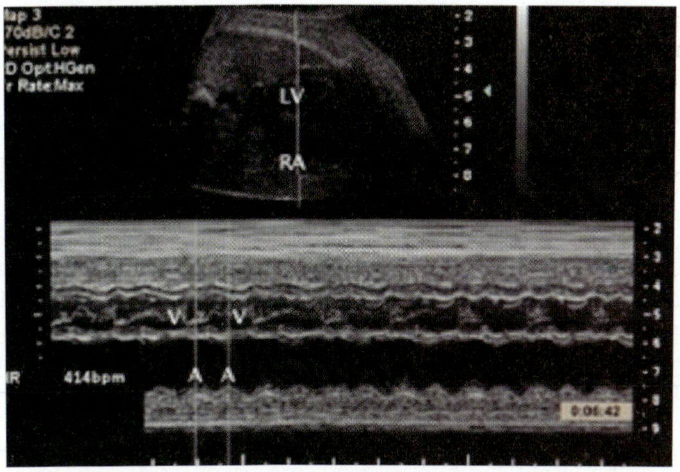

Fig. 48.19: *M-mode tracing using a four chamber view to demonstrate atrial (A) and ventricular (V) wall motions. The M-mode is directed simultaneously through the left ventricle (LV) and right atrium (RA). There is atrial flutter with an atrial rate of 414 beats/min (bpm), functional 2:1 atrioventricular block, and a regular ventricular rate of 207 bpm*

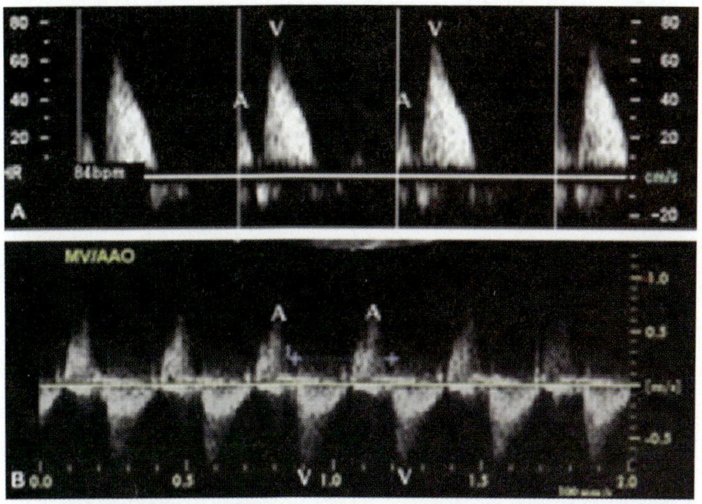

Fig. 48.20: *Pulsed Doppler flow modalities. (A) Simultaneous ascending aorta (V) and superior vena cava (A). Doppler flow recording at 20 weeks of gestation showing sinus bradycardia with normal 1:1 atrioventricular conduction. (B) Simultaneous inflow/outflow Doppler of a 19-week fetus with long ventriculo-atrial tachycardia of 190 beats/min due to fetal thyrotoxicosis. The mother had a medical history of Graves' disease for which she had been treated with propylthiouracil and radioactive iodine*

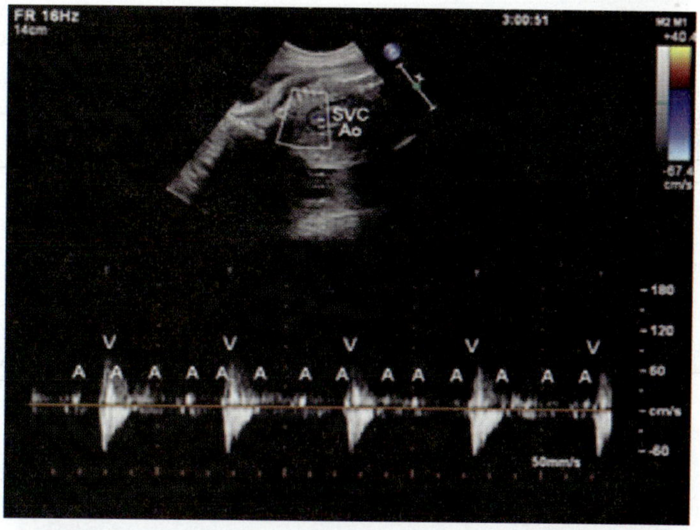

Fig. 48.21: *Simultaneous pulse wave Doppler of the aorta and vena cava superior of a fetus with complete heart block showing back flow following atrial contractions (A) in the superior vena cava with an atrial rate of 140/min (A) and in the same direction aortic outflow following ventricular contractions (V) which are independent with a regular rate of 60/min*

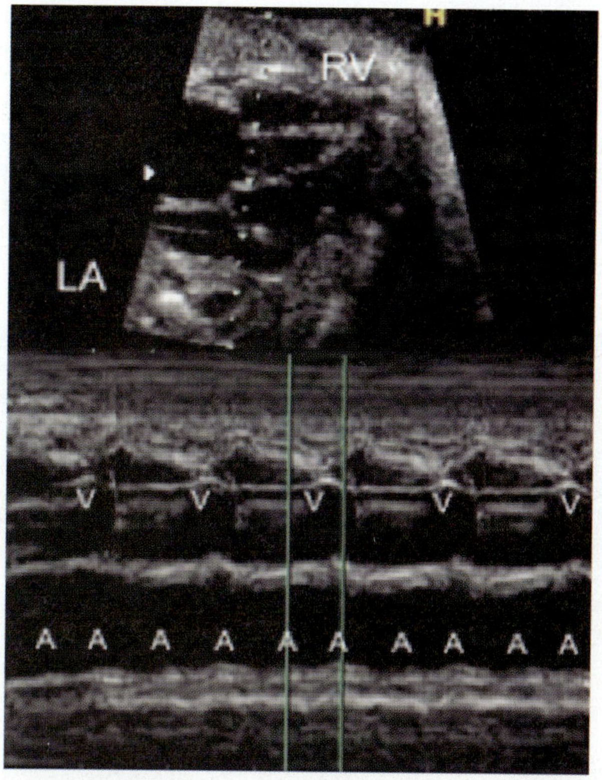

Fig. 48.22: *Atrial flutter. Simultaneous M-mode tracing to record the RV and LA free wall movements during the cardiac cycles. The atrial rate is very fast and regular at 462 bpm while the ventricular rate is 231 bpm suggesting 2:1 AV conduction*

Fetal Bradycardia (Figs 48.15–48.21)

Sustained fetal bradycardia may be caused by sinus node dysfunction, long-QT syndrome, AV block, or fetal distress with acidosis. The most common fetal bradyarrhythmia and the primary indication for FCI is high-grade AV block. The potential consequences of fetal AV block are cardiomyopathy and hydrops. AV block in the fetus generally occurs in association with either maternal autoimmune disease, malformation syndromes such as heterotaxy, or L-loop transposition of the great arteries.

Autoimmune fetal AV block can be treated with maternal administration of dexamethasone and/or sympathomimetic agents. Several recent multicenter studies found that transplacental dexamethasone did not reverse high-grade

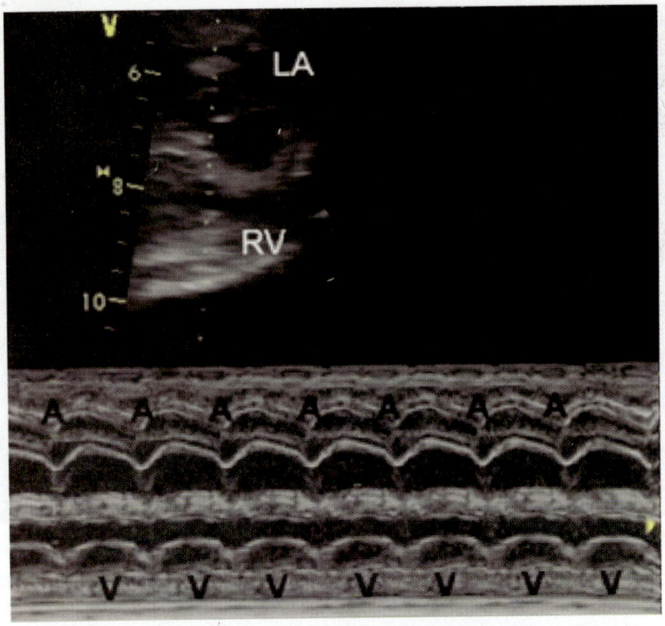

Fig. 48.23: *SVT with a heart rate of 240 bpm. M-mode tracing through the right atrium (bottom) and the right ventricle (top). There is 1:1 AV-conduction with a short AV-interval*

block, although it may have prevented the progression of first-degree block to second- or third-degree block, and it was associated with a higher risk of premature birth and growth restriction. Other studies reported that dexamethasone, typically in association with α-adrenergic agonists when significant bradycardia was present, improved the overall prognosis in fetuses with autoimmune AV block. Sympathomimetic agents may increase the heart rate in fetuses with bradycardia due to AV block or sinus node dysfunction, but they do not restore AV synchrony. It is unclear whether in utero α-adrenergic stimulation improves outcome, because the postnatal management of AV block associated with complex congenital heart disease is challenging under any circumstances.

Fetal Hydrops Due to Other Cardiac Causes

Transplacental treatment with digoxin has also been described for fetal hydrops resulting from other conditions including structural anomalies (e.g. Ebstein's anomaly, absent pulmonary valve syndrome), right heart dysfunction from left heart disease, premature closure of the ductus arteriosus, intrauterine myocardial infarction, cardiac tumor, cardiomyopathy and others. These are uncommon conditions, with published reports limited to individual cases, so the efficacy of digoxin in their management is unknown (Figs 48.29–48.34).

Maternal Hyperoxia

Maternal hyperoxia, which affects fetal vascular function and hemodynamics, has been used to assess placental function and treat intrauterine growth retardation, but its benefits have not been established. Recently, Szwast et al. reported using maternal hyperoxia to assess pulmonary vasoreactivity in fetuses with hypoplastic left heart syndrome (HLHS) and found diminution of the normal pulmonary arterial flow response to predict fetuses at high risk for critical atrial septal restriction after birth. Although not therapeutic, maternal hyperoxia in this application is a form of pharmacological transplacental FCI that may have implications for postnatal intervention and other methods of prenatal intervention.

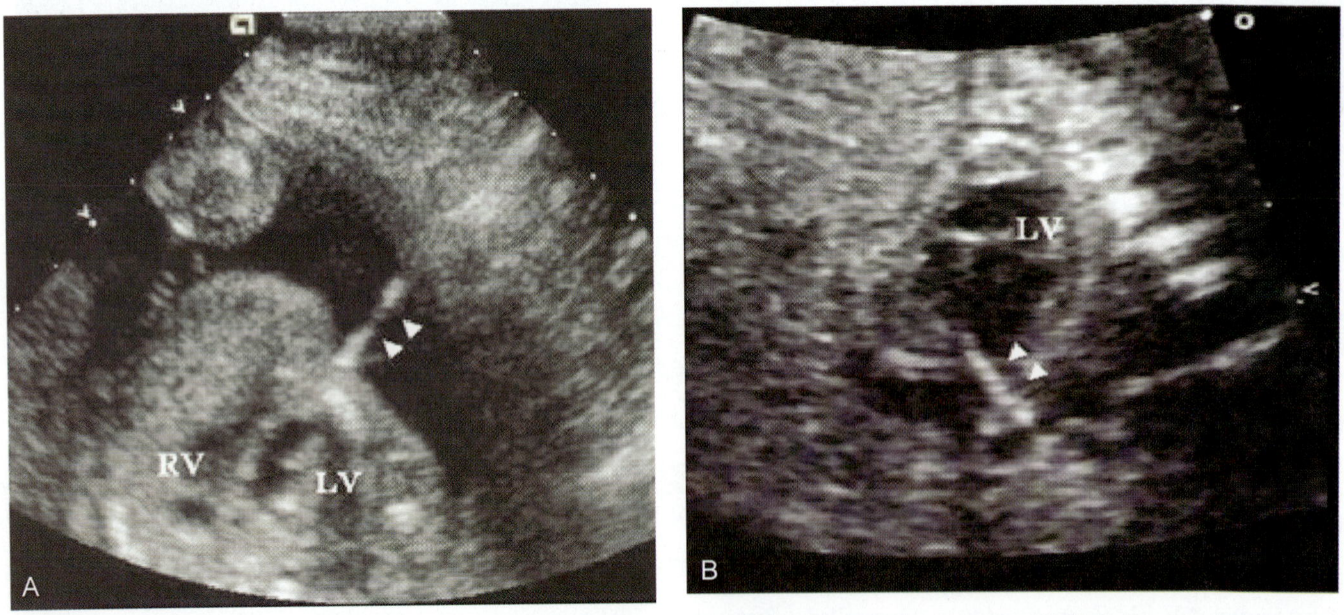

Fig. 48.24: *Fetal echocardiographic views of aortic balloon dilation in fetuses with aortic stenosis. (A) Note the needle approaching the left ventricular apex; (B) Note the wire crossing the left ventricular outflow tract; and the balloon being inflated at the level of the aortic valve. RV, right ventricle, LV, left ventricle, arrows demarcate needle, wire, or balloon during the procedure. (Images courtesy of Dr Wayne Tworetsky from Boston Children's Hospital)*

Table 48.1: *Pharmacological interventions in fetal arrhythmias*

Condition and drug	*Dose range*	*Therapeutic level and effect*	*Adverse effects*
Atrial flutter			
Digoxin	LD 1, 200 μg per 24 h IV in 3 divided doses; MD 375–750 μg daily PO in two equal daily doses	0.7–2.0 ng/mL Mild nausea, fatigue and sinus bradycardia, first-degree atrioventricular block, rare nocturnal Wenchebach atrioventricular block	Severe nausea and/or vomiting, severe sinus bradycardia or atrioventricular block, maternal and fetal proarrhythmia
Sotalol	160–480 mg daily in two equal daily doses or every 8 h PO	NA Improved survival, bradycardia, first-degree atrioventricular block, P and QRS widening, QT prolongation	Nausea and/or vomiting, dizziness, fatigue, bundle-branch block, maternal and/or fetal proarrhythmia
Supraventicular tachycardia			
Flecainide	100–300 mg daily in equal doses given every 8 h PO	0.2–0.1 μg/mL Mild IVCD headache, QT prolongation	Visual and central nervous system symptoms, bundle-branch block, QT prolongation, fetal or neonatal proarrhythmia
Amiodarone	LD 1,800–2,400 mg daily in equal doses given every 6 h for 48 h; MD 200–600 mg daily PO	0.7–2.8 μg/mL Maternal and/or fetal sinus bradycardia, first- degree atrioventricular block, P and QRS widening, QT prolongation	Nausea and/or vomiting, maternal and/or fetal thyroid dysfunction, photosensitivity rash, thrombocytopenia, bundle-branch block, proarrhythmia, torsades de pointes in fetuses with long QT syndrome
Procainamide	LD 500–600 mg over 20 min IV; MD 2–6 mg/min IV Initially 1,250 mg, followed in 1 h by 750 mg, then 250–1,000 mg every 3–6 h PO	410 μg/mL Uterine irritability, QT prolongation	Nausea and/or vomiting, hypotension, proarrhythmia, blood dyscrasias
Ventricular tachycardia‡			
Magnesium sulfate	LD 2–4 g IV followed by 1–2 g/h IV	1.5–3.0 mmol/L	Fatigue, central nervous system symptoms, stop for loss of patellar reflex at levels of 3.5–5.0 mmol/L, cardiac arrhythmias at high levels
Lidocaine	LD 1.0–1.5 mg/kg IV followed by 1–3 mg/min IV	1.5–5.0 μg/mL	Central nervous system symptoms
Propranolol	40–80 mg every 8 h PO	NA Increased uterine tone, bronchoconstriction	Fatigue, bradycardia, hypotension
Dexamethasone	LD 4–8 mg PO; MD 4 mg daily	NA Fluid retention	Similar to other corticosteroids. Short-term use preferred, fetal growth restriction
Sotalol	160–480 mg daily in two equal daily doses or every 8 h PO	NA Bradycardia, first-degree atrioventricular block, P and QRS widening, QT prolongation	Nausea and/or vomiting, dizziness, fatigue, bundle-branch block, maternal and/or fetal proarrhythmia

MD, maintenance dose; PO, orally; LD, low dose.

1. Open Fetal Cardiac Intervention

For the present review, "open FCI" denotes any intervention in which the uterus is opened surgically or accessed through a surgical trochar e"3 mm in diameter, which includes most fetoscopic techniques. This delineation is based on reports that preterm labor occurs in 80% of fetal surgical procedures in which a single 10F (3.3 mm) port is used and almost universally with larger ports or incisions.

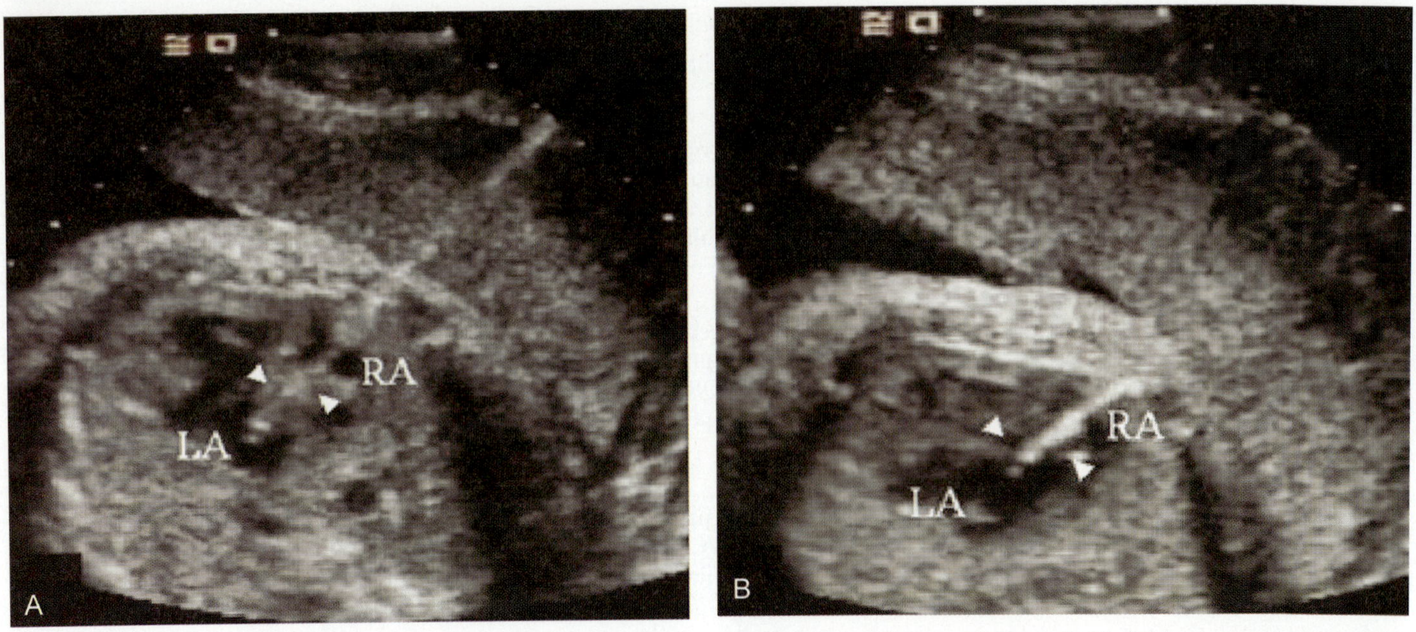

Figs 48.25A and B: *Fetal echocardiographic views of an atrial septal dilation in a fetus with hypoplastic left heart syndrome and an intact atrial septum. (A) Note the needle crossing the atrial septum; (B) Note the balloon crossing the atrial septum; RA, right atrium; LA, left atrium; arrows demarcate the needle or balloon for the procedure*

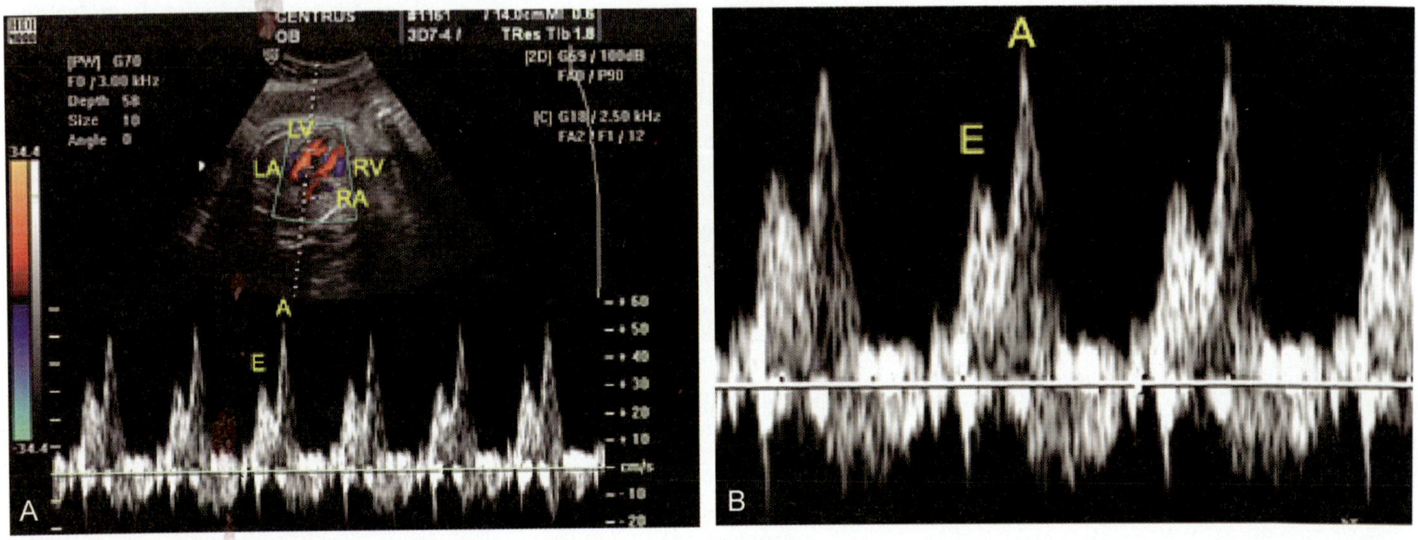

Figs 48.26 A and B: *Low velocity waveform across the tricuspid valve at 28 weeks of gestation (left). (E-wave, early ventricular filling; A-wave, atrial ventricular filling)*

Experimental Fetal Cardiac Surgery (Figs 48.22–48.67)

Research on fetal cardiac surgery has been performed for more than 25 years. The major focus of investigation has been the pathophysiology of extracorporeal circulatory bypass, which is likely to be necessary for fetal cardiac surgery. In early studies, it was shown that a 1- to 1.5-kg lamb fetus could be placed on and separated from cardiac bypass reproducibly but that postbypass fetal demise was imminent. Further work in sheep, goats, and primates has furthered our knowledge of the pathophysiology of fetal cardiac bypass and the feasibility of fetal cardiac surgery. Survival to term can now be achieved in a high percentage of cases (Table 48.2).

Cardiovascular and placental response to extracorporeal circulation

The most significant response to fetal bypass when the placenta is incorporated as the oxygenator is severe placental dysfunction characterized by increased vascular resistance, reduced blood flow, and consequent impairment in fetal gas exchange, with fetal acidosis rapidly ensuing during and after bypass. The pathophysiology of postbypass placental dysfunction is multifactorial and

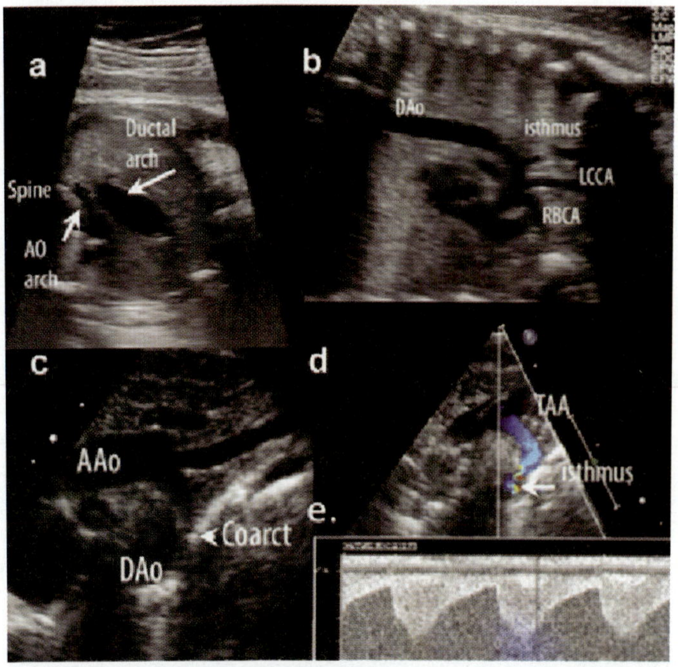

Fig. 48.27: *Images obtained from a 35 week fetus with gastroschisis and postnatal coarctation. The only cardiac finding before birth was (a) a discrepancy in the aortic and ductal arches shown in a cross-sectional view through the fetal chest and (b) mild transverse and distal arch hypoplasia. With ductus arteriosus constriction after birth there was progressive severe discrete distal arch obstruction with (c) a very small lumen (arrow) and high velocity continuous flow by (d) color and (e) CW Doppler (systolic gradient 64 mmHg) prompting surgical intervention. AO, aortic; DAo, descending aorta; RBCA, right brachiocephalic artery; LCCA, left common carotid artery; TAA, transverse aortic arch, AAo, ascending aorta; DAo, descending aorta*

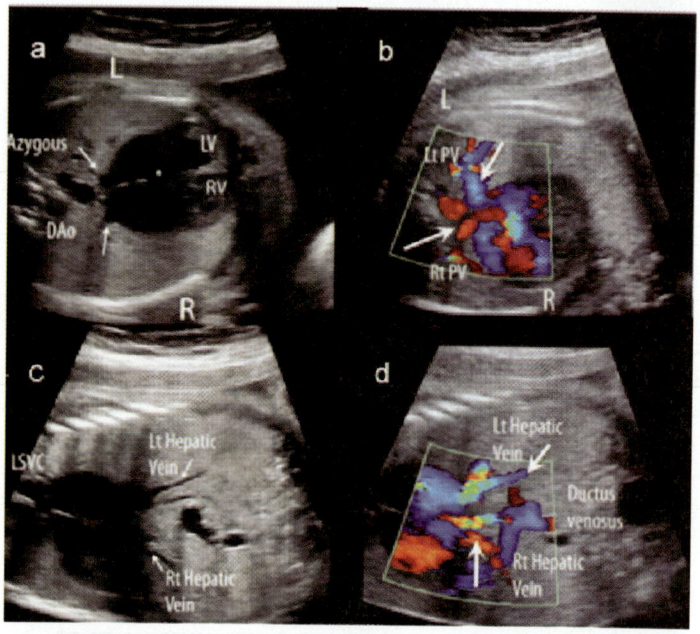

Fig. 48.28: *Images from a 30 week fetus with left atrial isomerism, mesocardia and anomalous systemic and pulmonary venous connections. Left and right pulmonary veins (A and B, arrows) and left and right hepatic veins (C and D, arrows) can be seen connecting on either side of the atrial septum by 2D and color flow map imaging. A coronary sinoseptal defect was identified (*). The dilated azygous vein connected with a left superior vena cava that drained into the left sided atrium. Surgical repair with intra-atrial baffling of systemic and pulmonary veins was used to correct this lesion at 9 months. L, left; R, right; Lt, left; Rt, right; DAo, descending aorta; RV, right ventricle; LV, left ventricle; PV, pulmonary vein; LSVC, left superior vena cava*

Table 48.2: *Congenital cardiovascular anomalies potentially amenable to FCI*

Indication for intervention and condition	*Actual or possible FCI*
• Risk of fetal or early neonatal death	
• Fetal tachycardia with hydrops	Maternal antiarrhythmic pharmacotherapy
• Structural anomalies causing hydrops	Maternal digoxin
• Congenital heart block	Pacemaker; maternal antiarrhythmic and/or adrenergic pharmacotherapy
• Severe Ebstein malformation	Tricuspid valve repair; tricuspid valve occlusion
• Severe congenital MR with AS and intact atrial septum	Balloon or surgical aortic valvuloplasty; creation of atrial septal defect
• HLHS with intact atrial septum	Creation of atrial septal defect
• Obstructed, totally a nomalous pulmonary venous return	Stenting of obstructed vertical vein/ducts venosus; surgical repair
• Fetal AS with evolving HLHs	Balloon or surgical aortic valvuloplasty; resection of endocardial fibroelastosis
• PA/IVS with evolving hypoplastic right heart	Percutaneous or open pulmonary valve perforation and dilation
• Premature closure of ductus anteriosus with evolving hypertension	Ductal stenting
• Absent pulmonary valve syndrome with evolving bronchomalacia	Pulmonary arteriop lasty and/or valvuloplasty

MR, mitral regurgitation; HLHs, hypoplastic left heart syndrome; AS, aortic stenosis; PA, pulmonary artery

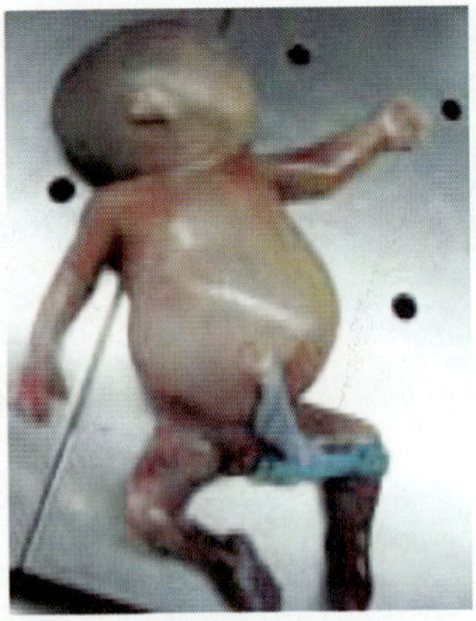

Fig. 48.29: *A 22 weeks of gestation fetus with generalized hydropic aspect. Subcutaneous edema and abdominal distention secondary to ascites*

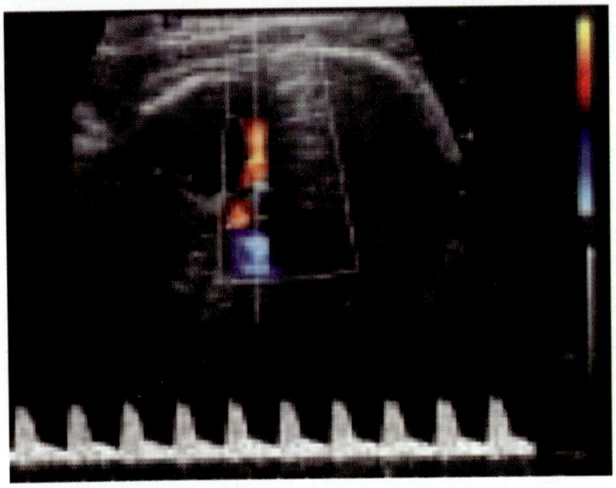

Fig. 48.30: *Hydrops. During diagnostic evaluation a meticulous ultrasound must be performed in order to detect fetal or placental malformations and to exclude fetal anemia by Doppler study of the peak systolic velocity of the middle cerebral artery*

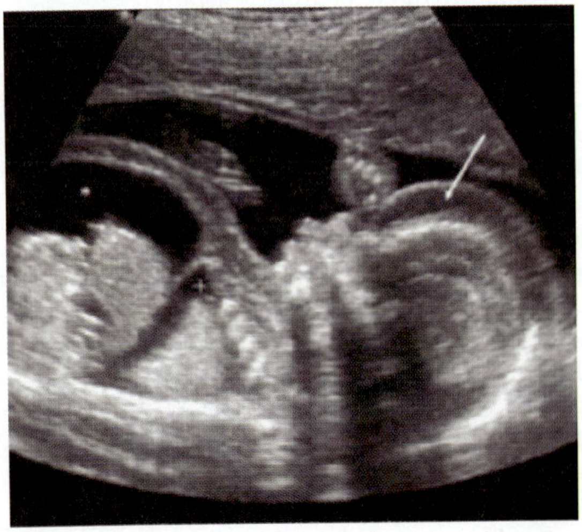

Fig. 48.31: *Hydrops. Severe ascites (*), pleural effusion (+) subcutaneous edema (white arrow)*

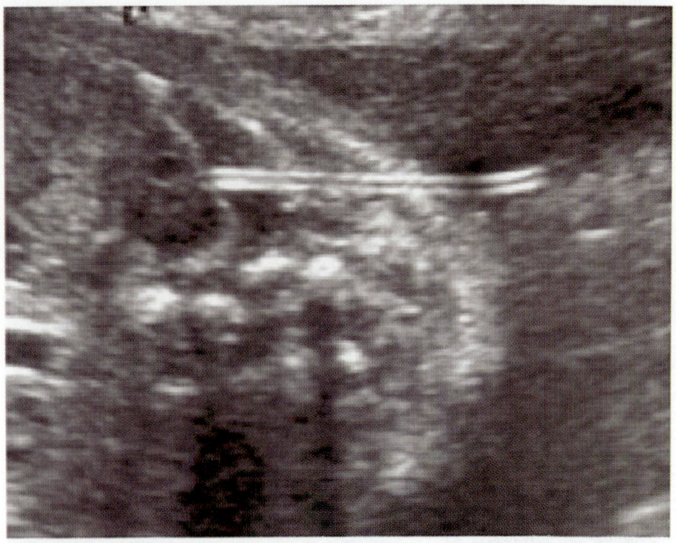

Fig. 48.32: *Placement of a catheter in one of the cysts connecting with the amniotic cavity*

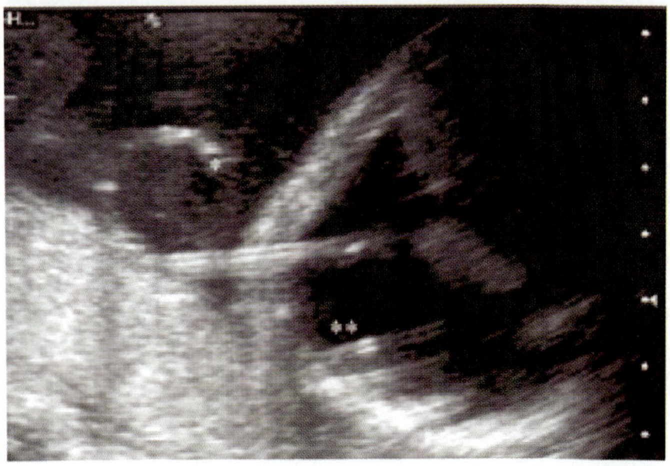

Fig. 48.33: *Left pleural effusion. Pleuroamniotic shunting (pig tail). One of the ends is within the amniotic cavity (*) the other (**) in the pleural cavity. It allows to drain the effusion, decompress the lung and prevent pulmonary hypoplasia*

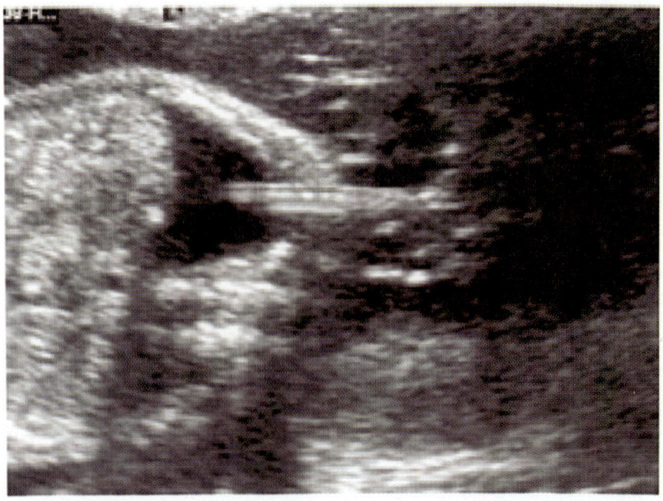

Fig. 48.34: *Ultrasound thoracoamniotic shunt*

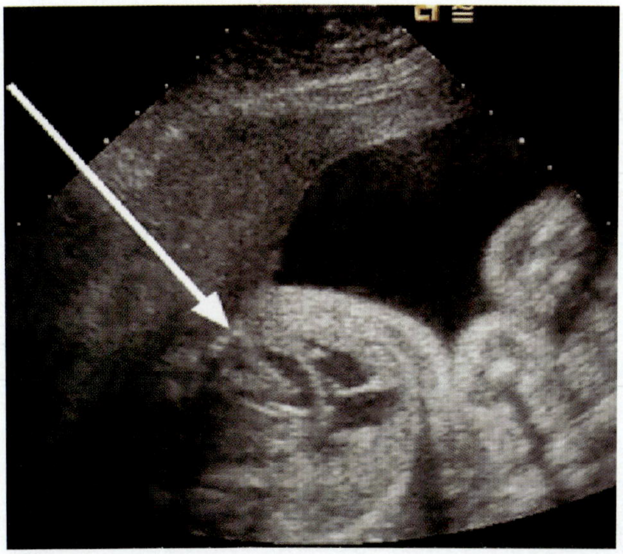

Fig. 48.35: *Fetal aortic stenosis, intraoperative image illustrating the needle trajectory that will afford access to the left ventricle and aortic valve. The initial needle course must be precised as very little manipulation is possible once the device has punctured the left ventricle*

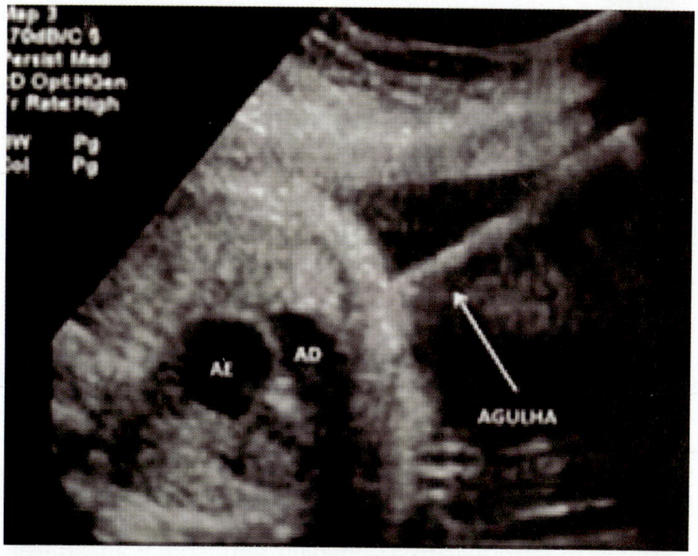

Fig. 48.36: *Ultrasound image of fetal atrioseptostomy. The balloon is being inflated at the atrial level. Note the interatrial septum tense and bulging into the right atrium due to left atrial hypertension. AD, right atrium; AE, left atrium*

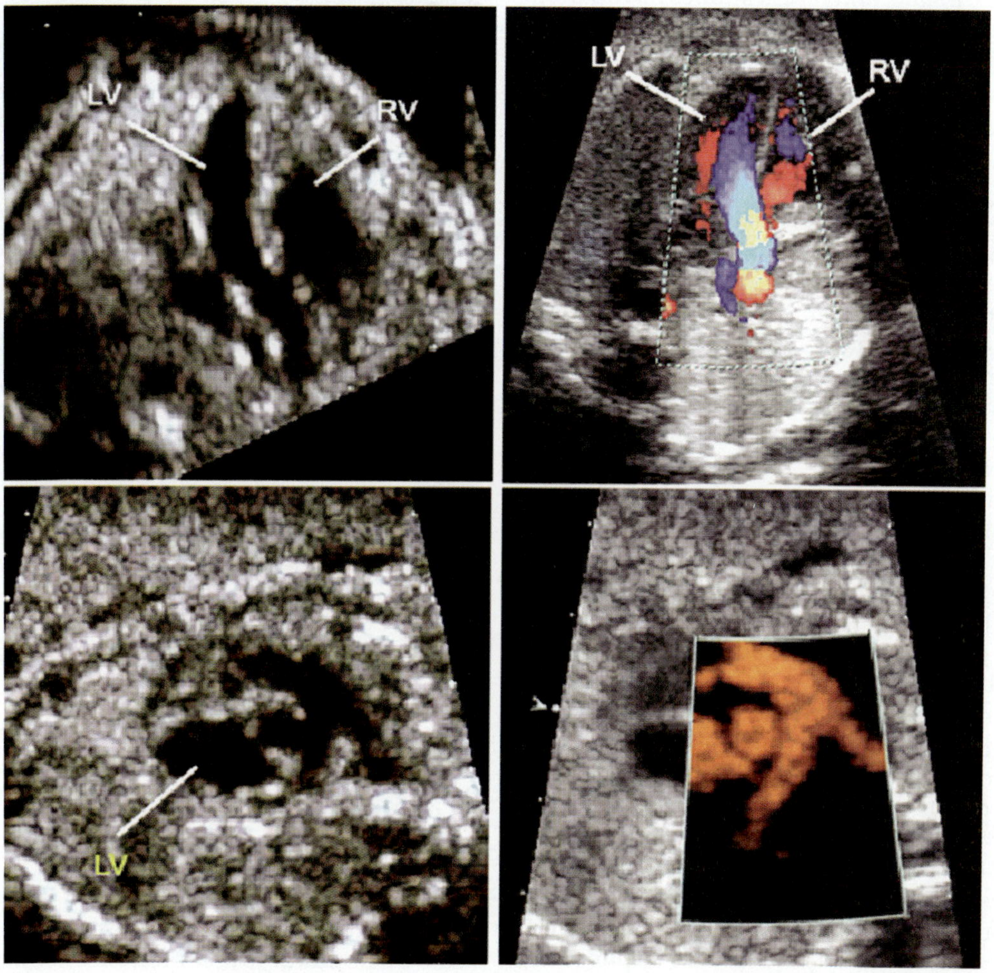

Fig. 48.37: *Five chamber view of the fetal heart with superimposed color Doppler showing the aorta (blue) originating from the left ventricle (top). Short-axis view of the fetal heart with superimposed color Doppler showing the pulmonary artery originating from the right ventricle (bottom)*

includes bypass-induced production of prostanoids, endothelial dysfunction, leukocyte and complement activation, and other endogenous vasoactive and inflammatory pathways. Fetal cardiac bypass and surgery may also lead to changes on the maternal side of the placenta, with reduction in uterine arterial flow and consequent impairment of fetoplacental gas exchange.

Fetal cardiac function and the fetal stress response

Fetal cardiac bypass and surgery induce a significant stress response that has important effects on fetal hemodynamics independent of the placental dysfunction discussed above. The stress response stimulates a rise in endogenous fetal catecholamines, which increases total vascular resistance and cardiac afterload. Because the contractile apparatus of the fetal myocardium is immature, the heart tolerates increased afterload poorly. In ovine fetal bypass studies, survival to term was first achieved with spinal anesthesia to blunt the stress response and indomethacin to block prostaglandin synthesis. More recently, it was shown that fetal bypass leads to cardiac injury, reflected in troponin elevation and increased plasma natriuretic peptides. Calcium-handling properties of the fetal myocardium differ from the more mature state, and recent studies have started to define strategies for myocardial protection during fetal open heart surgery.

Technical considerations for fetal cardiac surgery

In experimental fetal cardiac bypass, surgical exposure, intervention, and cardiac bypass have proven technically feasible. Nevertheless, successful fetal bypass requires consideration of several technical adaptations (Figs 48.1–48.13).

Placental function during fetal bypass is altered by inclusion or exclusion of the placenta in the bypass circuit. Placental inclusion obviates the need for an extracorporeal oxygenator, which decreases contact activation of inflammatory and vasoactive mediators. On the other hand, inclusion of the high-capacitance, low-resistance placenta in the circuit requires high flow rates, which can be limited by cannula size. Placental perfusion during bypass also causes placental endothelial damage and dysfunction, although these effects may be mitigated when bypass is performed with pulsatile rather than continuous flow, possibly owing to preserved nitric oxide production during the former (Figs 48.1–48.48).

The systemic effects of postnatal cardiopulmonary bypass are known to result in part from blood contact with artificial surfaces in the bypass circuit. Thus, miniaturization of the fetal bypass circuit has been a technical priority. For example, in fetuses undergoing cardiac bypass with a modified bypass circuit that uses an in-line axial flow pump and no maternal blood prime, placental function was preserved relative to control fetuses in which a conventional circuit was used. Despite these difficulties, models of congenital heart disease created in utero confirm the feasibility of operating on the heart of the lamb fetus with survival to full term.

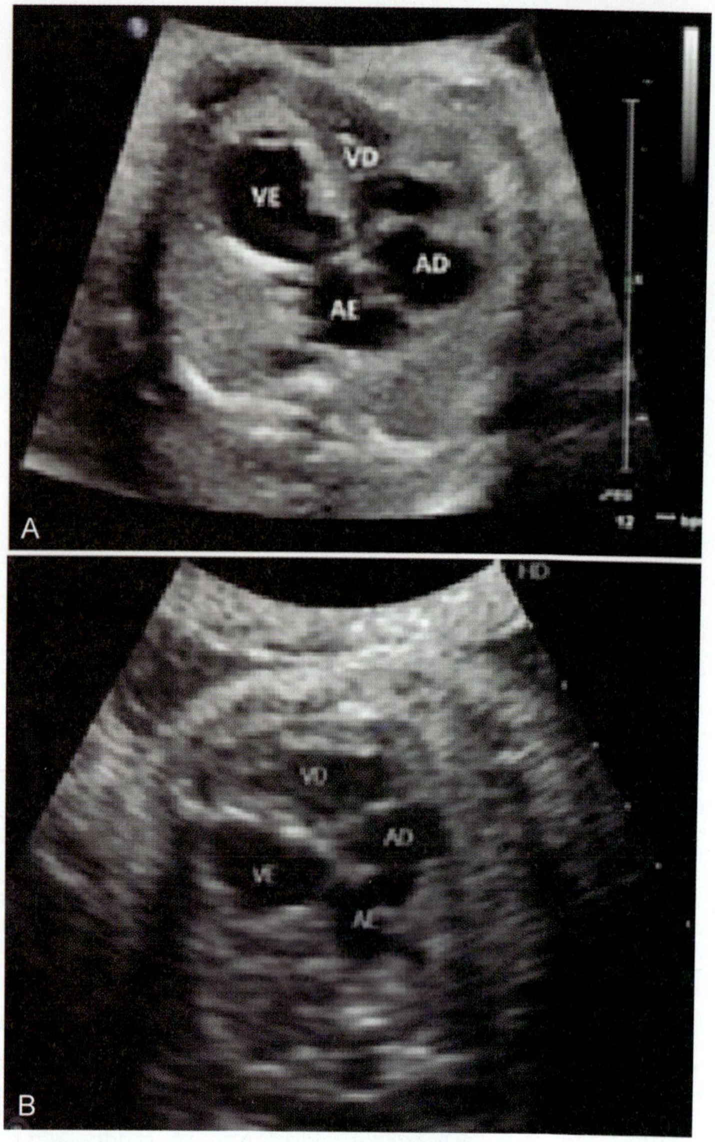

Fig. 48.38: *Fetal echocardiogram fetus with critical aortic valve stenosis. (A) The left ventricle is dilated with signs of diffuse endocardial fibroelastosis, and we note a mild pericardial effusion. (B) After the valvuloplasty; note a significant improvement in left ventricular dilatation has observed 3 days after the procedure. AD, right atrium; AE, left atrium; CEO, right ventricle*

Fetoscopic and adjunctive forms of closed FCI

Fetoscopic access has been investigated as an approach to FCI and fetal monitoring during cardiac and noncardiac interventions. Although the relative risks of percutaneous and fetoscopic access have not been assessed, port-access uterine entry for fetoscopic FCI may carry a higher risk of premature labor than percutaneous access.

Open FCI in humans

The first reported open FCI procedure in a human fetus was pacemaker placement for complete AV block. Subsequently, animal models were developed to evaluate pacing for fetal AV block, but this has not become a clinically viable treatment strategy, isolated human cases

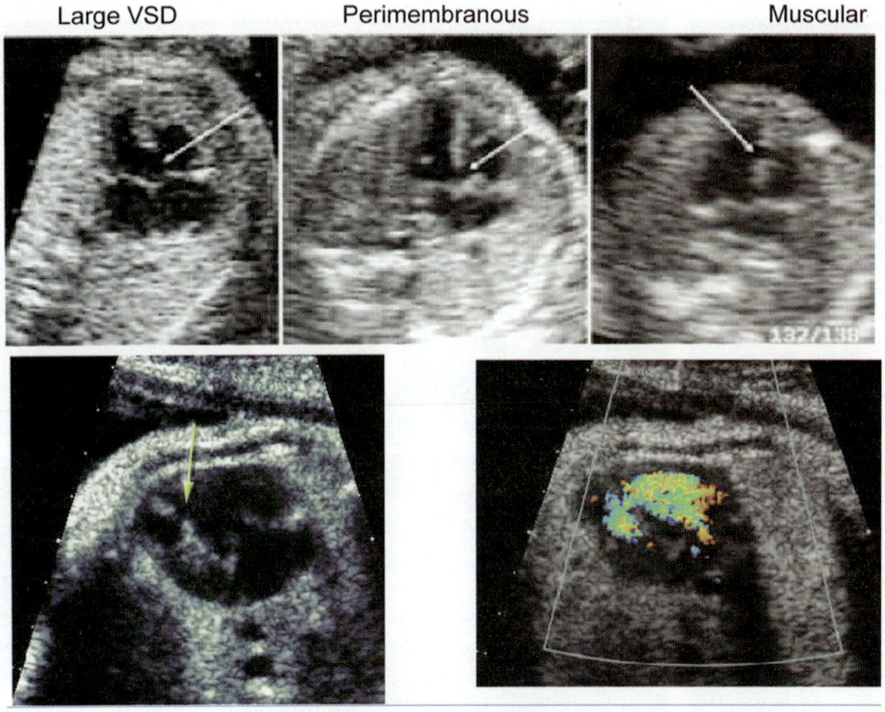

Fig. 48.39: *Foetal echocardiogram showing different types of VSD*

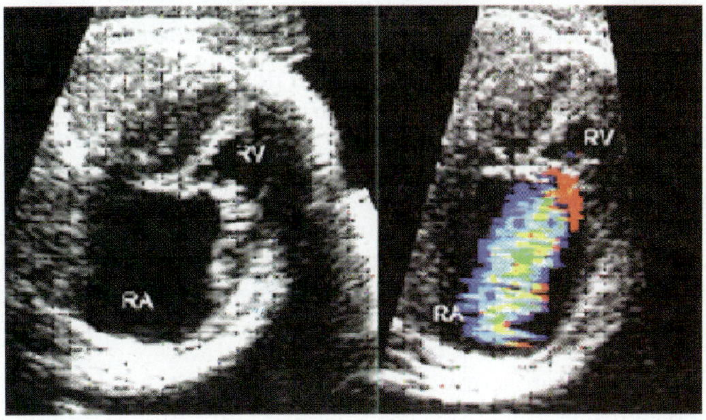

Fig. 48.40: *Foetal echocardiogram showing tricuspid valve dysplasia with severe tricuspid insufficiency and cardiomegaly. Retrograde flow from the right ventricle (RV) to the right atrium (RA) is seen in blue and turbulence is coded by green pixels*

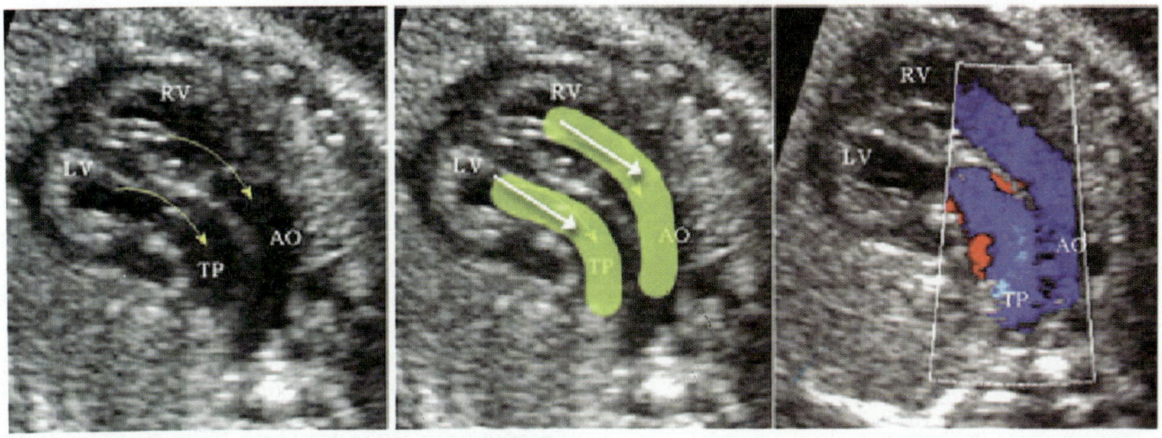

Fig. 49.41: *Fetal echocardiogram showing transposition of the great arteries demonstrating the abnormal connection of the right ventricle (RV) with the aorta (AO) and the left ventricle (LV) with the pulmonary trunk (TP). Both great arteries show a parallel course associated with tricuspid atresia*

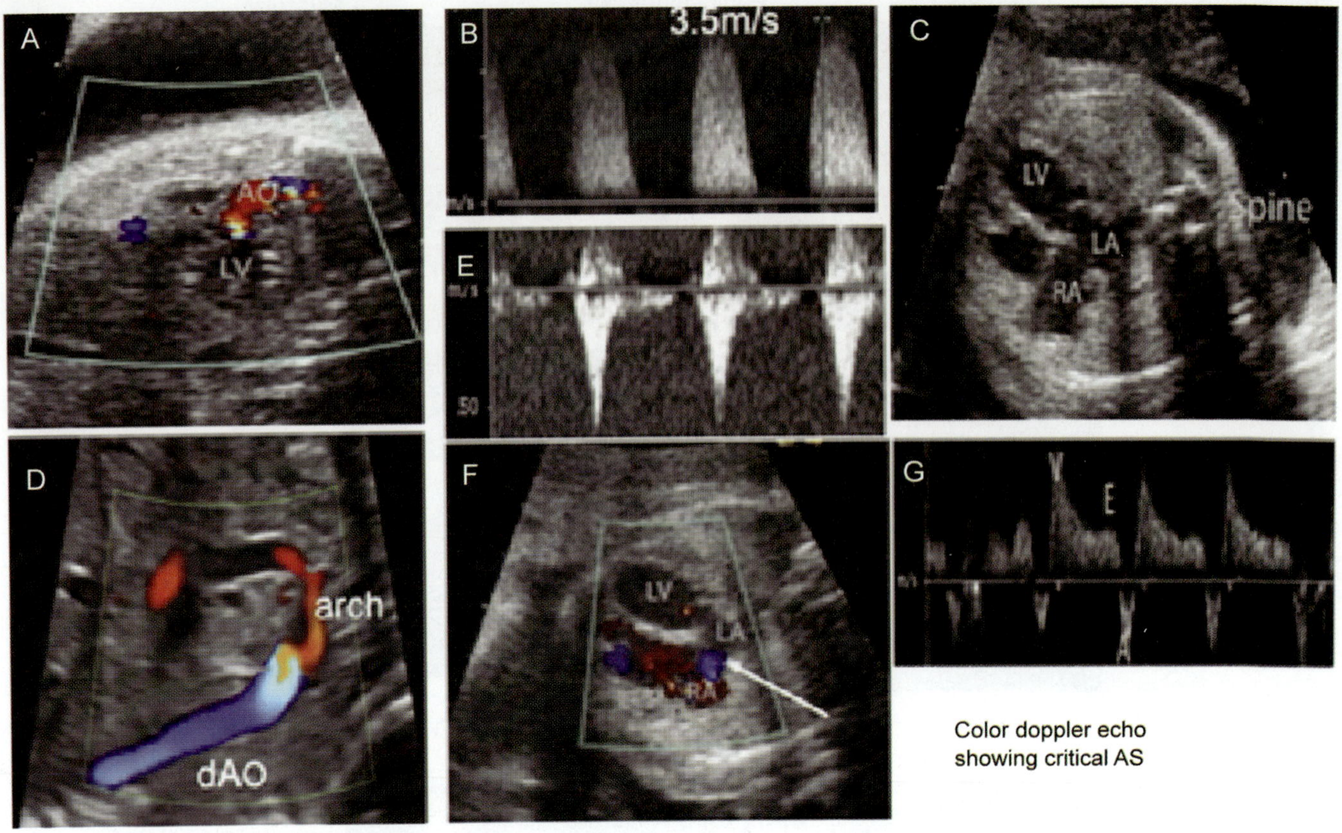

Fig. 48.42: *Critical AS encountered in a mid trimester fetus. (A) Early in gestation the left ventricle was hypertrophied and there was turbulent forward flow by color Doppler through the aortic valve. (B) CW Doppler interrogation suggested the peak aortic valve gradient was 30–35 mmHg. As the obstruction worsened, (C) the LV became dilated with reduced systolic function and (D) eventually retrograde flow was observed through the distal arch. (E) In addition to systolic dysfunction, an uniphasic rather than biphasic Doppler inflow pattern was observed suggesting reduced LV diastolic function, a feature associated with progressive LV hypoplasia. (F) Increased LV filling pressure resulted in left to right atrial level shunting (arrow). (G) As a consequence of increased left atrial pressure, there was reversal of flow during atrial systole in the pulmonary veins. A, flow in atrial systole; V, flow in ventricular systole; E, flow through the pulmonary veins in early ventricular diastole; LV, left ventricle; RA, right atrium; LA, left atrium; Ao, aorta; dAo, descending aorta*

notwithstanding. Human FCI aided by fetoscopy and cardioscopy has also been reported, with technical success and fetal survival in several cases. We are aware of 1 open heart surgery performed in a third-trimester human fetus with tricuspid valve dysplasia, severe tricuspid regurgitation, and hydrops by Dr Frank Hanley in 2003 (personal communication, June 6, 2009). Cardiopulmonary bypass was initiated and the tricuspid valve repaired successfully, but separation from bypass was prevented by anatomic pulmonary atresia (thought to be functional atresia before surgery), and the fetus died.

2. Closed Fetal Cardiac Intervention

In the present review, "closed FCI" indicates mechanical interventions in which the uterus is not opened or accessed with a port ≤ 3 mm in diameter. In practice, closed FCI consists primarily of percutaneous interventions in which an 18- to 19-gauge needle is used to gain uterine and fetal access. The first reported case of closed FCI was a balloon aortic valvuloplasty performed in 1989. Since then, FCI has been reported in human fetuses with aortic stenosis (AS), HLHS with atrial septal restriction, pulmonary atresia or stenosis, and AV block. In 2000, a program for FCI was started, initially to treat fetal AS with evolving HLHS, then expanding to include HLHS with an intact or highly restrictive atrial septum, pulmonary atresia with an intact ventricular septum (PA/IVS) and evolving hypoplastic right heart syndrome, and structural anomalies causing hydrops.

Typically, FCI is pertermed using a percutaneous ultrasound-guided approach with maternal and fetal anesthesia; in a minority of cases, laparotomy without hysterotomy is used to facilitate fetal imaging or access. All of the procedures consist of opening an atretic or restrictive valve or septum, and instrumentation is limited and simple, with an access cannula, a guidewire, an angioplasty balloon and/or stent, and sometimes an additional needle to enter the heart or perforate an atretic valve or septum. With the exception of an 18-gauge curved-tip cannula that was developed specifically for FCI.

Fetal Aortic Valvuloplasty (Figs 48.47 and 47.13)

The most common closed FCI procedure is aortic valvuloplasty, and the primary indication for fetal aortic

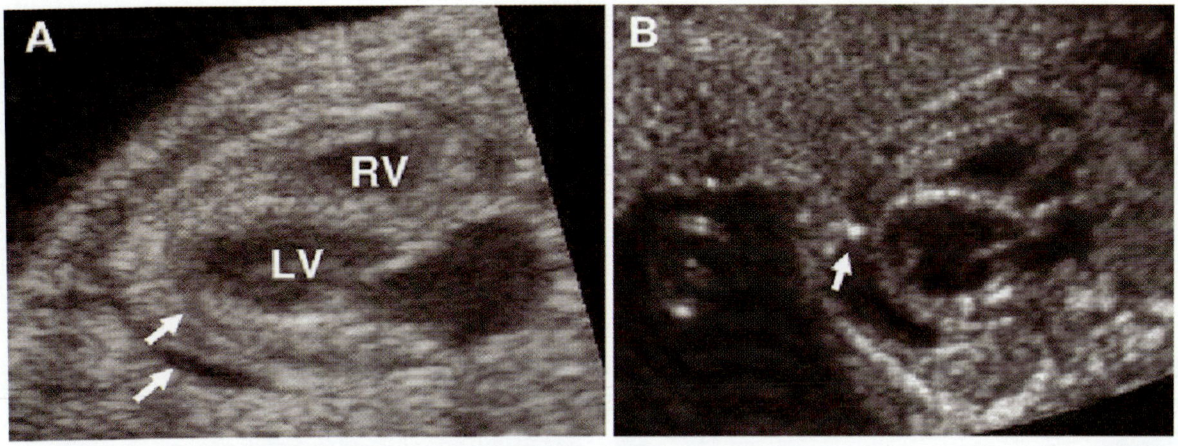

Fig. 48.43: *Long-axis echocardiograms demonstrating a partially coagulated hemopericardium after transventricular fetal aortic valvuloplasty (A) and drainage of a hemopericardium (B). (A) The pericardial space has echolucent regions consistent with liquid blood and echogenic areas consistent with thrombus; arrows demarcate the epicardial surface of the LV and the pericardium. (B) The arrow is positioned over the hemopericardium and indicates the tip of the pericardiocentesis needle*

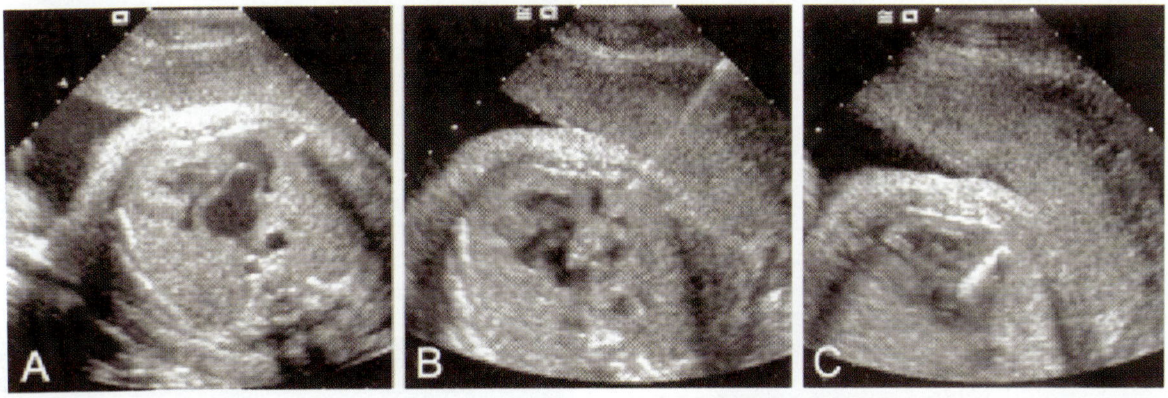

Fig. 48.44: *Creation of an atrial septal defect in utero for fetuses with hypoplastic left heart syndrome and intact or highly restrictive atrial septum. (A–C) Transabdominal ultrasound image of heart in fetus with dilated left atrium and thin, bulging atrial septum before atrial septal puncture (A), during septal puncture with Chiba needle (B), and during dilation with 3-mm coronary angioplasty balloon (C)*

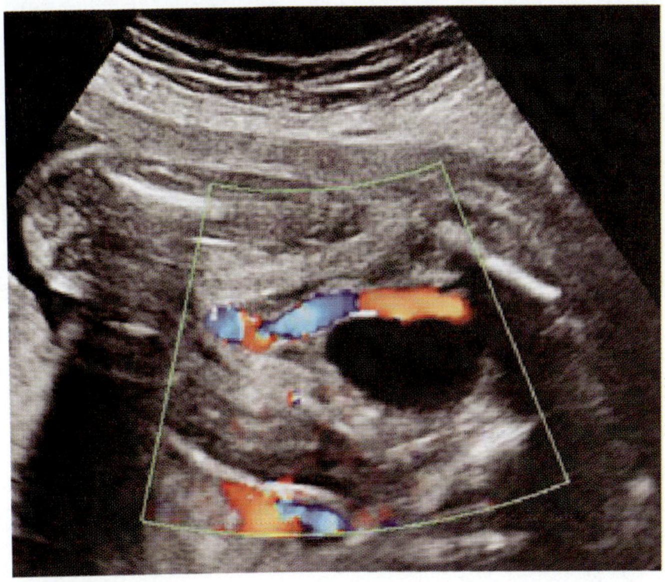

Fig. 48.45: *Color Doppler image of single umbilical artery around the fetal bladder*

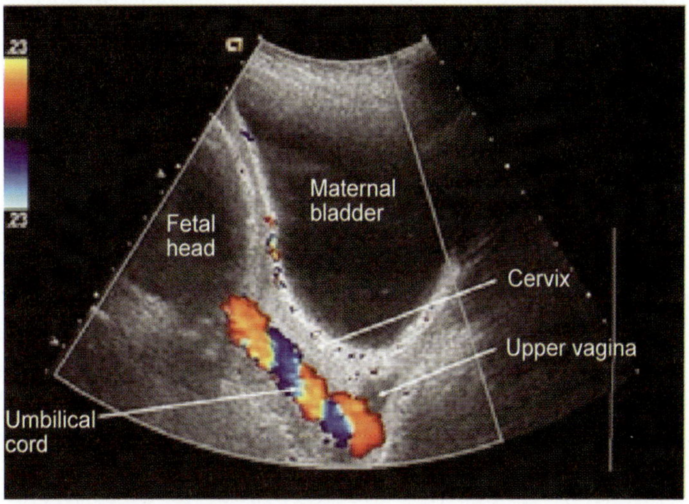

Fig. 48.46: *Fetal color Doppler echocardiography shows umbilical-cord prolapse at 29 weeks' gestation*

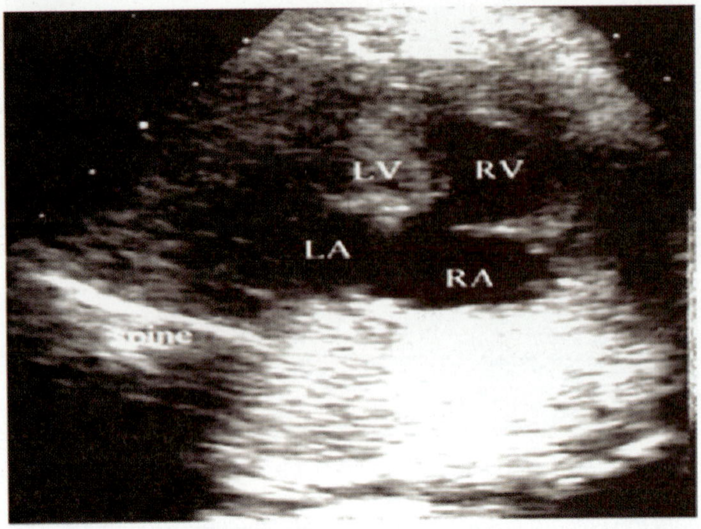

Fig. 48.47A: *Ultrasonography showing small sized left atrium, hypoplastic heart forming the apex and atresic mitral valve in an unborn baby with hypoplastic left heart syndrome*

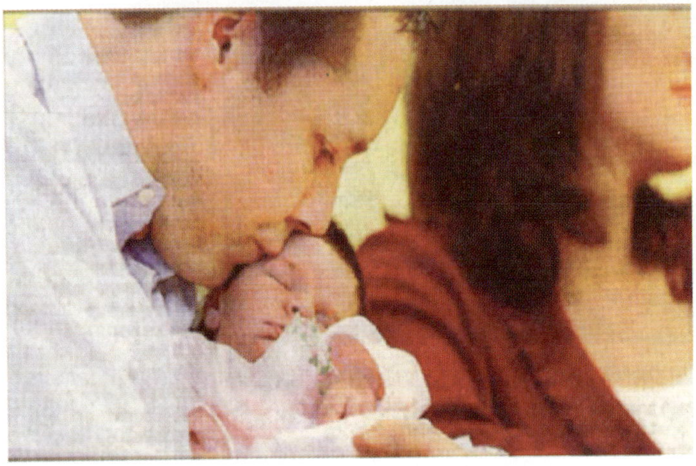

Fig. 48.47B: *Showing photograph of a newborn baby, Grace out of US national couple with mother angela VanDer-Werken of Virginia who became Worlds first baby to receive intrauterine stent for the treatment of hypoplastic left heart syndrome when this baby was 7 months old in the womb of the mother. The surgery was performed by the team of experts under chief surgeon (Dr James Lock at children hospital Boston and Brigham and women hospital, Boston)*

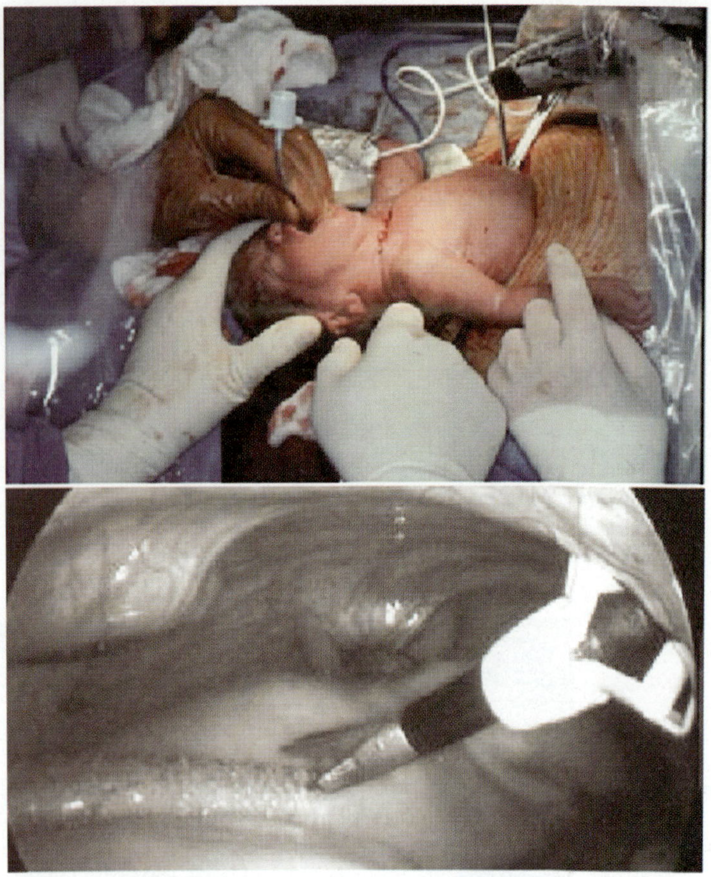

Fig. 48.48: *Fetus undergoing ex utero intrapartum treatment*

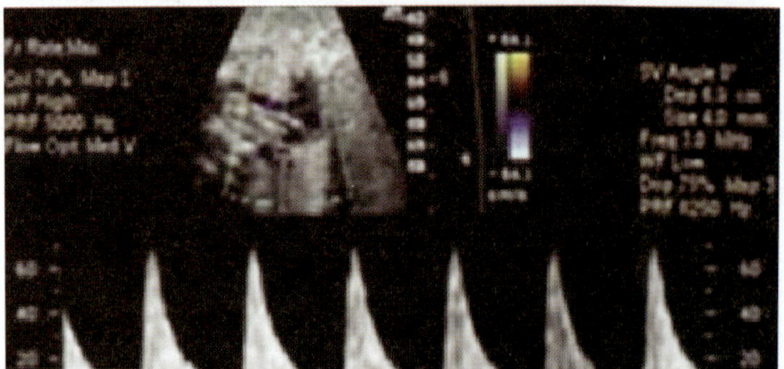

Fig. 48.49: *Pulmonary vein Doppler of fetal carrier syndrome showing hypoplasia of the left heart with critically restrictive foramen ovale. Note that the flow is bidirectional wave at the expense of the reverse flow*

valvuloplasty is to alter the in utero natural history of midgestation fetal AS with evolving HLHS. Some patients with HLHS are diagnosed during the second trimester with valvar AS and a normal-sized or dilated left ventricle (LV) and evolve to HLHS over the course of gestation. In other fetuses diagnosed with AS in midgestation, left heart growth and function will remain sufficient for a biventricular outcome. Several abnormal physiological features are associated with progression to HLHS: Retrograde flow in the transverse aortic arch, severe LV dysfunction, monophasic and short mitral valve inflow, and left-to-right flow across the foramen ovale. Thus, one can reliably predict which midgestation fetuses with AS will evolve to HLHS. The potential benefit of FCI for evolving HLHS is that decreasing LV afterload or promoting flow through the left heart may help to prevent progressive left heart dysfunction and hypoplasia over the subsequent course of gestation and, in the process, prevent evolution to HLHS.

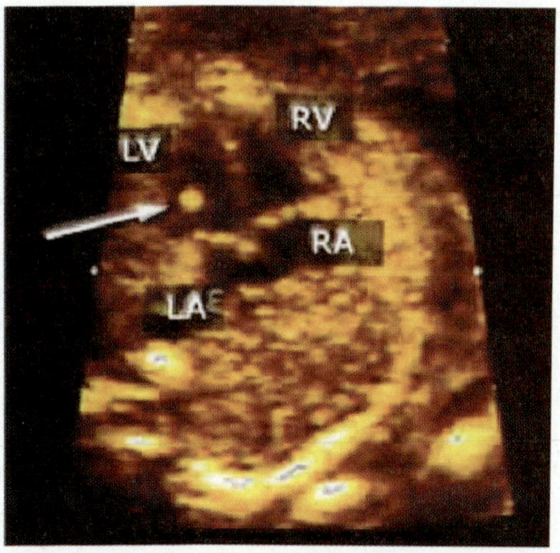

Fig. 48.50: *Four chamber view. Note the white arrow pointing the echogenic foci in the left ventricule. Echogenic foci are usually of no pathological significance and in more than 90% of cases the resolve by the third trimester or during pregnancy. However, they are sometimes associated with cardiac defects and chromosomal abnormalities. For isolated hyperechogenic foci the risk for trisomy 21 may be three-times the background maternal age and gestation related risk*

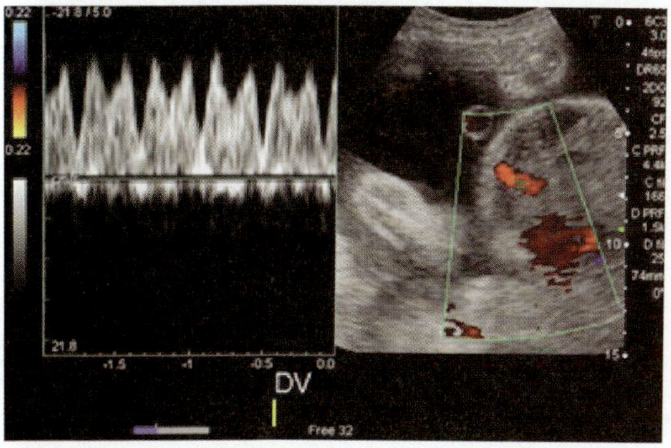

Fig. 48.51A: *Twin-twin transfusion syndrome. The ductus venosus flow in the recipient twin is still within acceptable limits though the atrial contraction "a" wave is almost reaching the baseline. Such a flow pattern needs to be monitored closely*

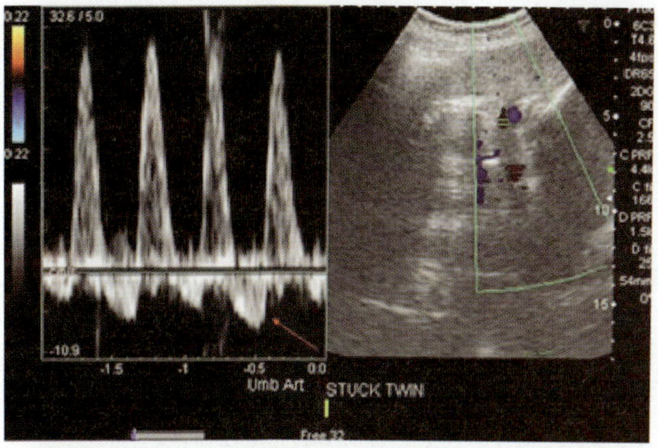

Fig. 48.51B: *Twin-twin transfusion syndrome. Umbilical artery Doppler of the donor (stuck) twin shows diastolic reversal (arrow). This is a predictor of poor outcome*

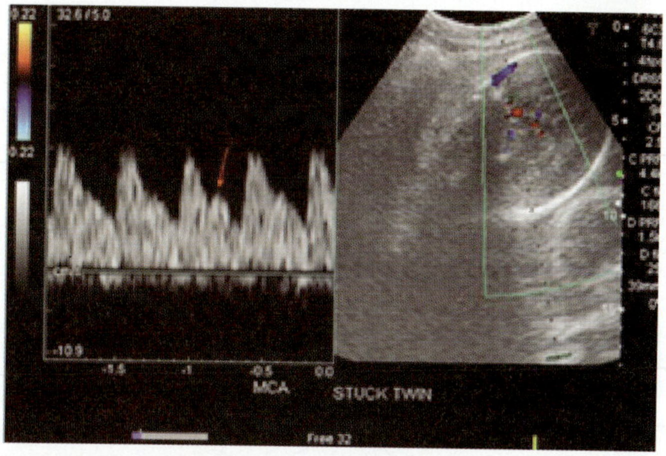

Fig. 48.51C: *Twin-twin transfusion syndrome. Middle cerebral artery Doppler of the donor (stuck) twin shows high diastolic flow (arrow), suggesting a brain-favoring effect and fetal adaptation to hypoxemia*

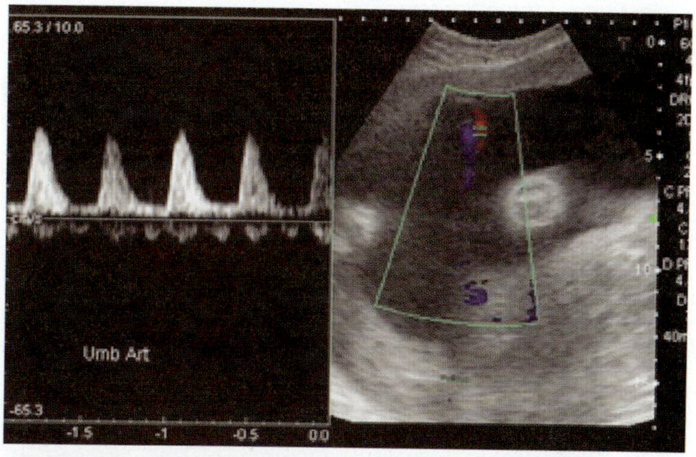

Fig. 48.51D: *Twin-twin transfusion syndrome. Umbilical artery Doppler in the recipient twin. The flow pattern is unidirectional, but the diastolic flow is very low. This is an indicator of a poor prognosis*

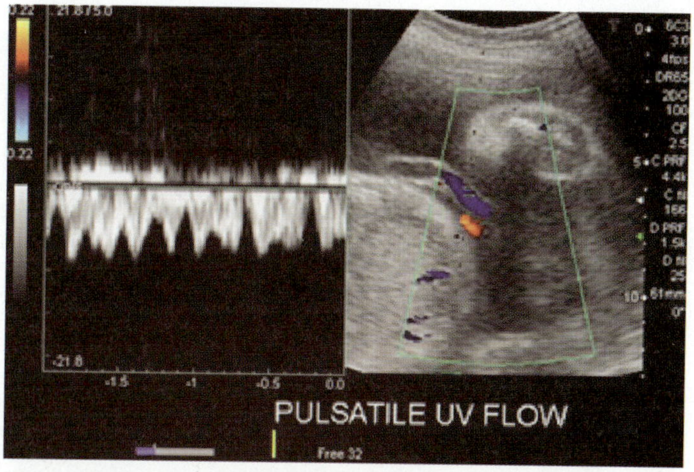

Fig. 48.51E: *Twin-twin transfusion syndrome. Pulsatile umbilical venous flow in the recipient twin suggests a critically ill fetus. Normal umbilical venous flow is continuous and nonpulsatile with phasic/respiratory variations at times*

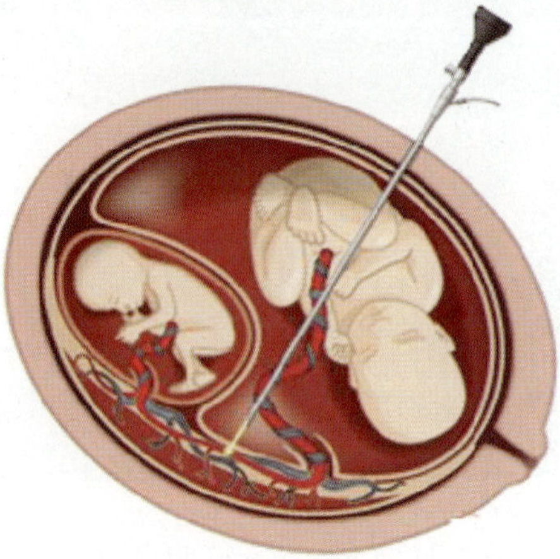

Fig. 48.51F: *Illustration shows placental vessels supply in twin to twin transfusion syndrome and applicabitity of radiofrequency ablation in coagulation of blood supply to the weeker fetus in order to save the other fetus*

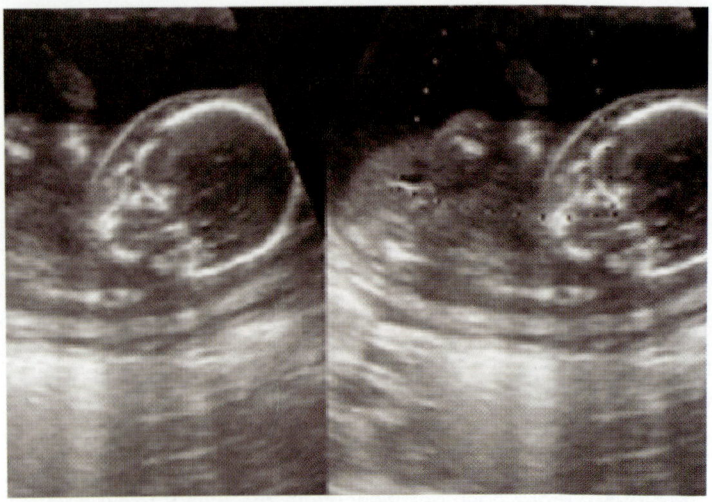

Fig. 48.51G: *Absent blood flow in the umbilical cord of the 2nd twin after radiofrequency cord ablation*

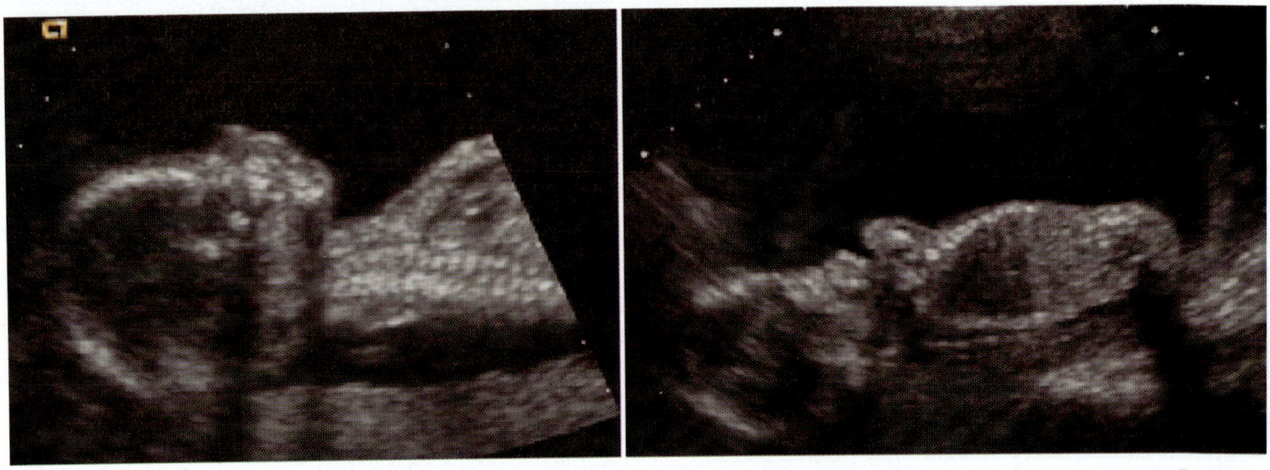

Fig. 48.52A: *Amniotic fluid volume alters imaging. The large baby on the left (recipient) has increased amniotic fluid, so a clear profile and clear imaging are obtained. The donor, on the right, is tightly wrapped in his membrane and imaging is very indistinct*

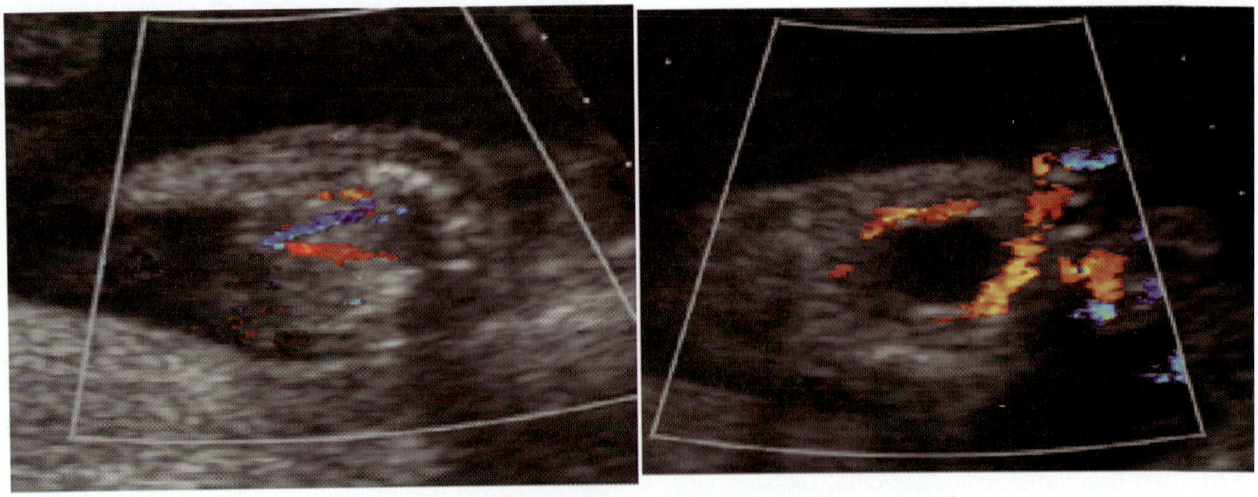

Fig. 48.52B: *The donor on the left has no visible bladder (the colored lines represent umbilical arteries, one on each side of the bladder, which is empty). The recipient on the right has a continuously over-filled bladder (the black circle in between the two arteries)*

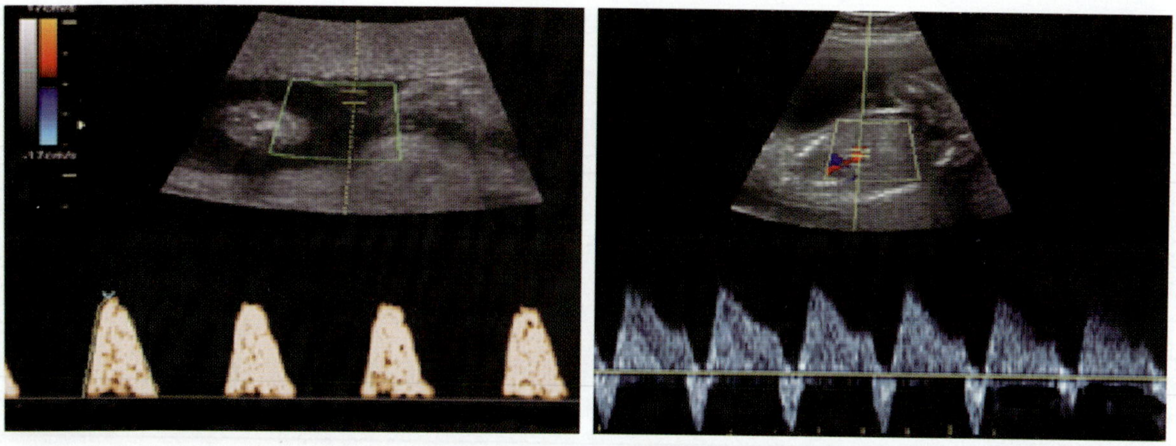

Fig. 48.52C: *Each baby has circulatory problems as twin to twin transfusion syndrome progresses. On the left, the donor has severe placental resistance and very low blood flow to the placenta. On the right, the recipient is struggling with heart failure, with blood running backward during the cardiac cycle*

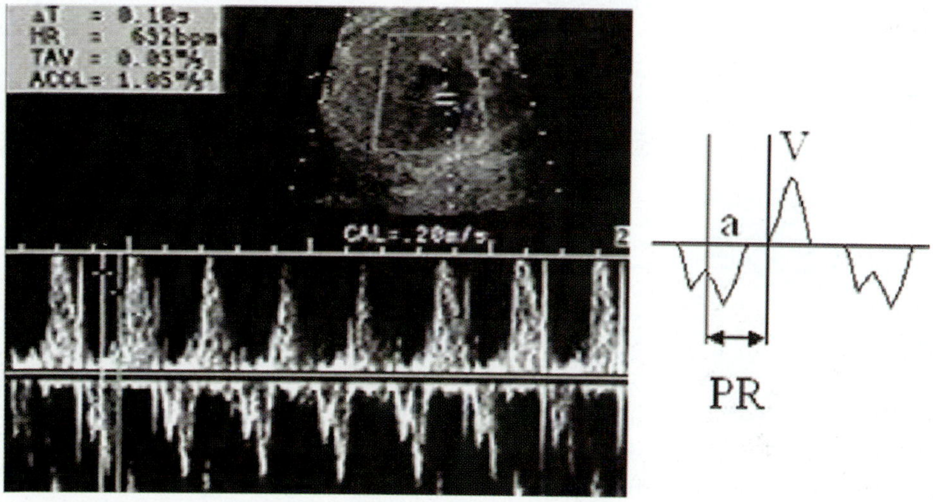

Fig. 48.53: *Mitral valve and aortic valve Doppler in a 20 week fetus. Calculation of the PR interval to assess for first degree heart block is made measuring from the onset of the mitral a wave to the onset of the aortic outflow wave. a, mitral a wave; V, aortic outflow*

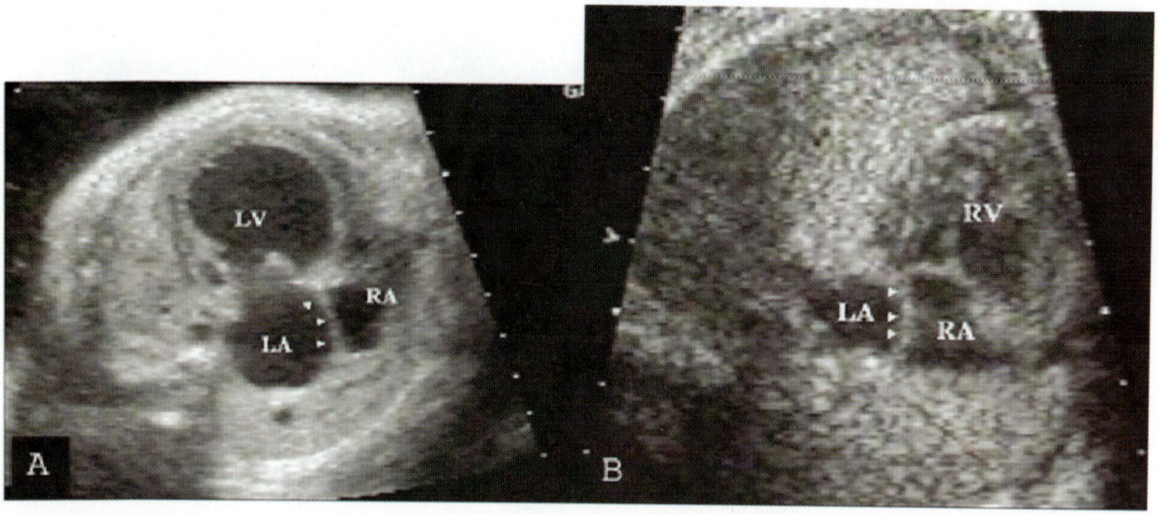

Figs 48.54A and B: *Fetal echocardiographic apical view of the heart in a fetus with foramen ovale closure and ductus arteriosus closure and transposition of the great arteries (A) and in a fetus with foramen ovale closure and hypoplastic left heart syndrome (B). RA, right atrium; RV, right ventricle; LA, left atrium; LV, left ventricle, arrows demarcate the atrial septum*

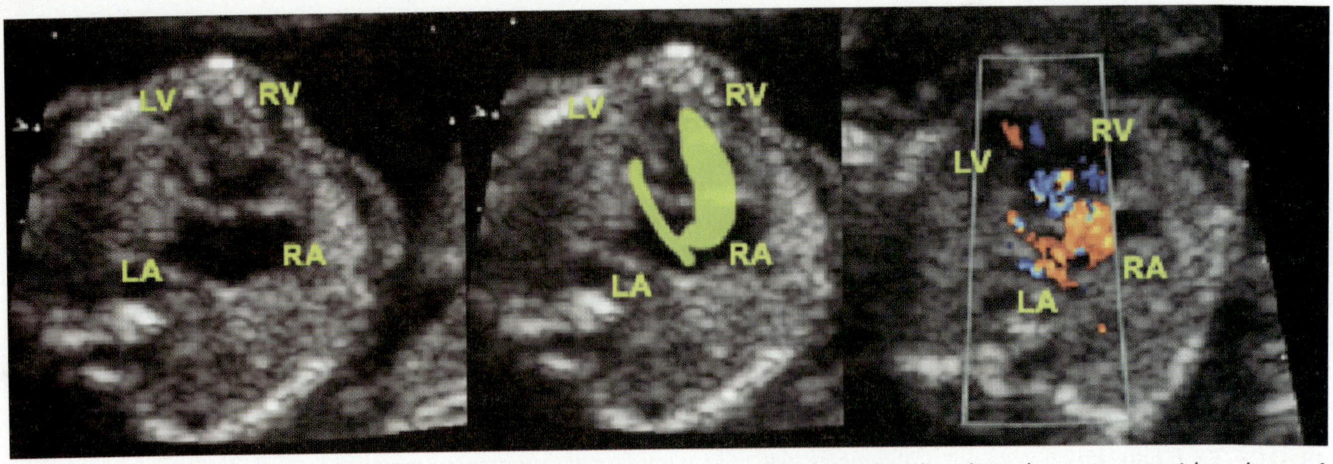

Fig. 48.55 *Hypoplastic left heart syndrome—the left ventricle diminutive, with color doppler; there is an asymmetric color perfusion of the chambers*

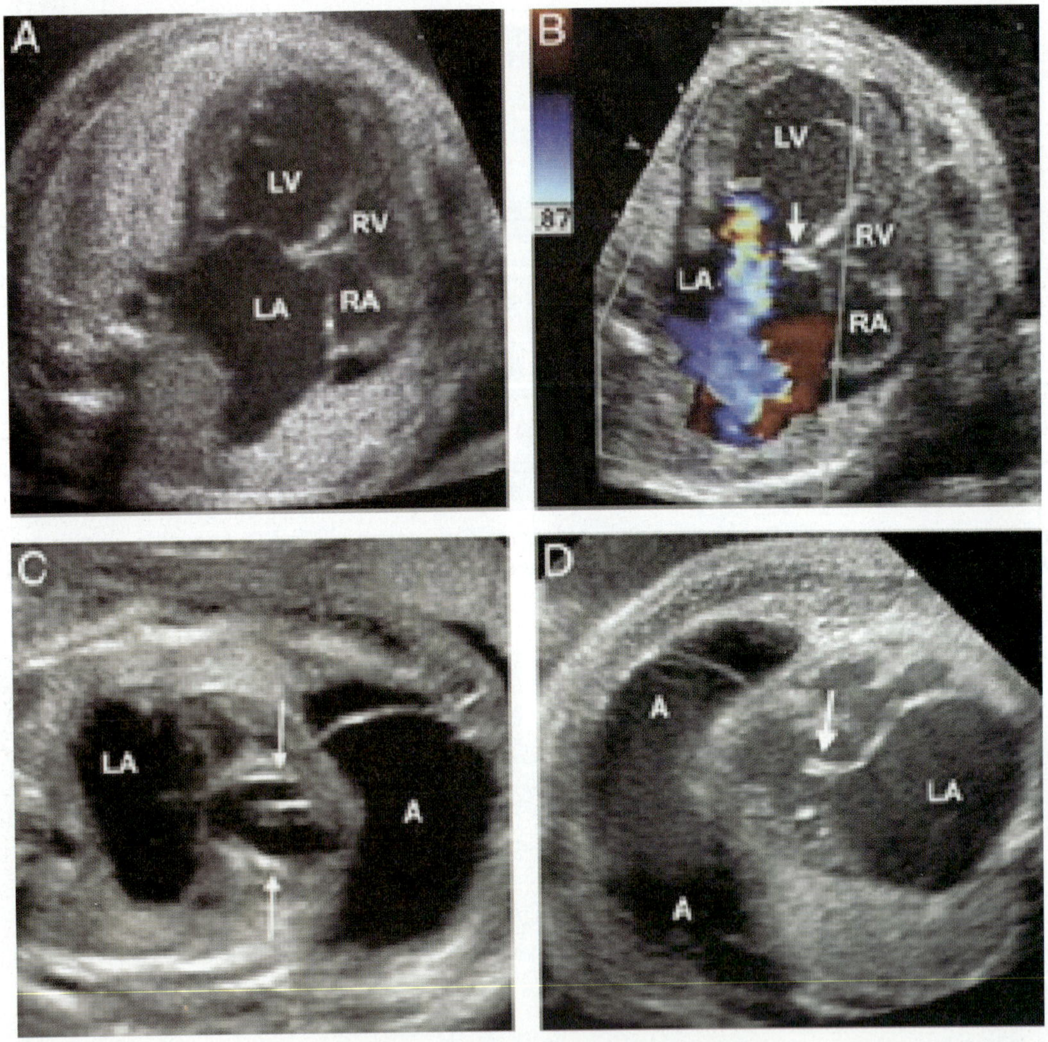

Fig. 485.56: *Fetal echocardiogram images (A) fetal echocardiogram in a four chamber view, demonstrating severe left atrial (LA) enlargement, with bowing of the atrial septum (*) into the right atrium (RA) and partial obstruction of the tricuspid valve. The right ventricle (RV) is compressed by a dilated left ventricle (LV). (B) Doppler color flow image in a four chamber view from the same fetus demonstrating severe LA and LV enlargement, severe mitral regurgitation, and an anatomically abnormal mitral valve with an echogenic anterior leaflet (arrow). There is significant compression of the RA and RV. (C and D). These oblique transverse images from a different fetus demonstrate severe LA enlargement, ascites (A), and moderate to severe LV endocardial fibroelastosis (arrows). In D, the anterior leaflet of the mitral valve (arrow) is bright and immobile*

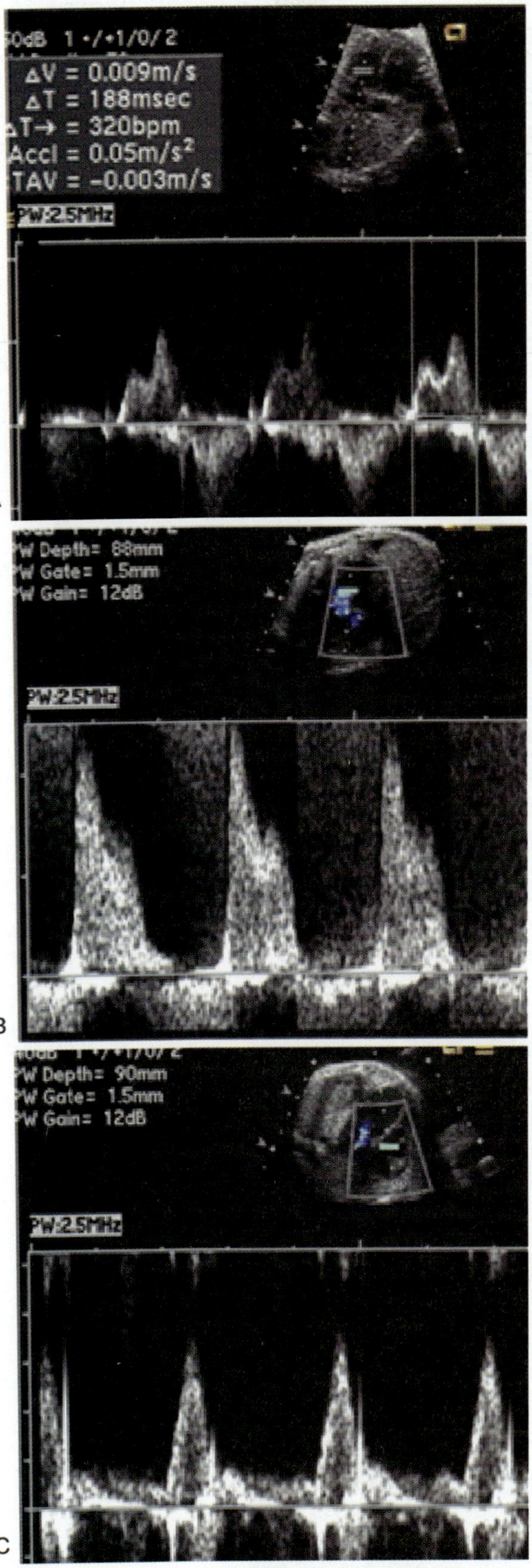

Fig. 48.57: *Mitral and tricuspid valve doppler inflow patterns (A) Normal mitral valve Doppler. (B) Abnormal Doppler with a partially fused mitral valve inflow pattern. (C) Tricuspid valve monophasic Doppler pattern*

The first known fetal aortic valvuloplasty was performed in 1989. Kohl et al reviewed the published experience with this procedure in 2000. From 1989 to 1997, 12 cases were performed in third-trimester fetuses with AS or atresia (not midgestation AS with evolving HLHS) at 6 centers. A balloon was passed across the valve and expanded in 7 of the 12 fetuses, but only 1 of these 7 survived beyond the newborn period. This early experience highlighted several important issues including the technical feasibility of third-trimester closed FCI, the importance of delivering the valvuloplasty balloon through an access cannula without a sharp edge, and the risk and potential consequences of fetal bradycardia.

After an initial learning curve, technical success has been achieved consistently in 75–80% of procedures. When the valve is dilated, there is immediate improvement in flow across the aortic valve, and there may be an obvious decrease in LV size. Moderate or severe postdilation aortic regurgitation (AR) occurs in nearly 40% of technically successful procedures. As with postnatal aortic valvuloplasty, the larger the balloon—annulus diameter ratio, the higher the likelihood of significant AR, but in contrast to neonatal aortic valvuloplasty, the target ratio is 1.1 to 1.2 instead of 0.9.

After successful fetal aortic valvuloplasty, in utero aortic and mitral valve growth are improved relative to control fetuses, but there is no difference in LV short- or long-axis growth velocity. In contrast to the modest changes in left heart growth, there are clear beneficial changes in left heart physiology after fetal aortic valvuloplasty, as reported previously—namely, after successful FCI, the left heart physiological parameters reported by Makikallio et al to predict progression to HLHS were improved in a large majority of successfully treated fetuses but not in controls that were similar before intervention. In summary, there is solid evidence that balloon dilation of the aortic valve in fetuses with AS and evolving HLHS improves left heart physiology and leads to improved growth of the aortic and mitral valves but has no apparent effect on LV growth per se.

Ultimately, the goal of FCI for AS with evolving HLHS is to alter left heart physiology and growth sufficiently to allow postnatal survival with a healthy biventricular circulation. In recently published experience, just over 30% of patients who underwent technically successful FCI for this indication had a biventricular circulation from birth, and another 8% were converted to a biventricular circulation after initial univentricular palliation. Patients with larger LV size and higher LV pressure at the time of intervention are more likely to have a biventricular outcome. Using multivariable analysis, identification of a cohort of patients with essentially no chance of biventricular outcome and modified the selection criteria to exclude patients was done who fall below a defined threshold score. It has become clear that prenatal intervention is not a stand-alone intervention. In all cases that have gone on to biventricular outcome postnatally, postnatal interventions have been required including repeat aortic valvuloplasty in most cases, temporary left atrial decompression, and

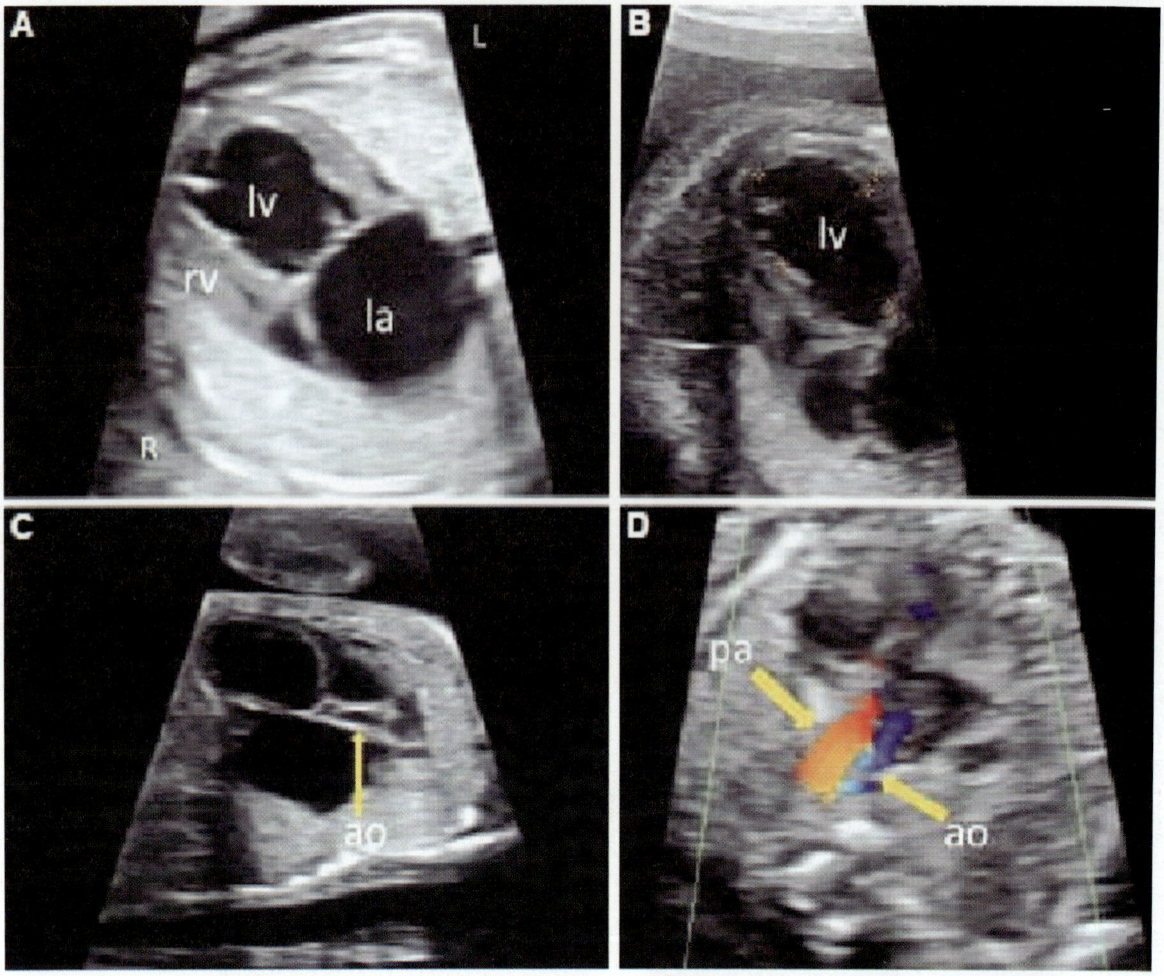

Fig. 48.58: *Echocardiographic images: (A, B) Dilated left ventricle, left atrium and compressed right ventricle. (C) Critical aortic stenosis. (D) In the three vessel and tracheal view, the aortic diameter is such smaller than the pulmonary artery with reversed flow in the aortic arch*

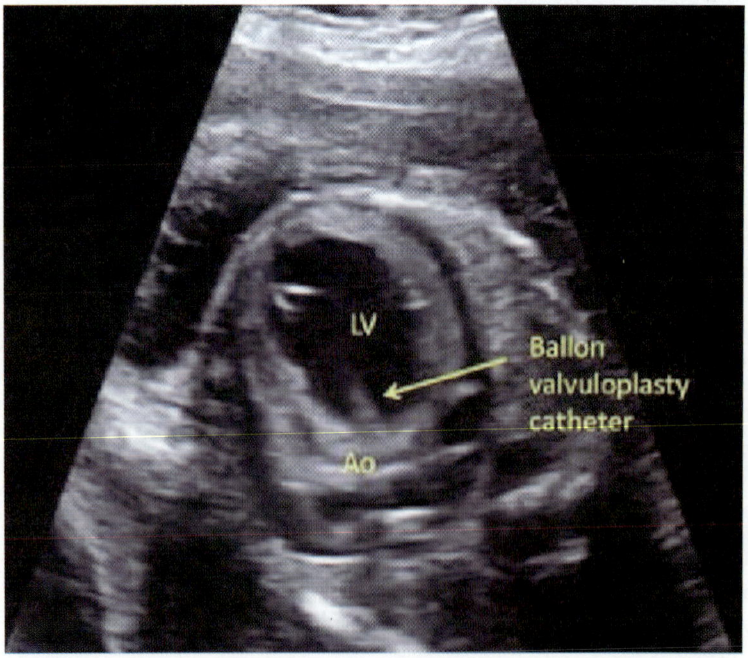

Fig. 48.59: *Echocardiographic image showing introducer cannular and ballon catheter inflation in the aortic valve*

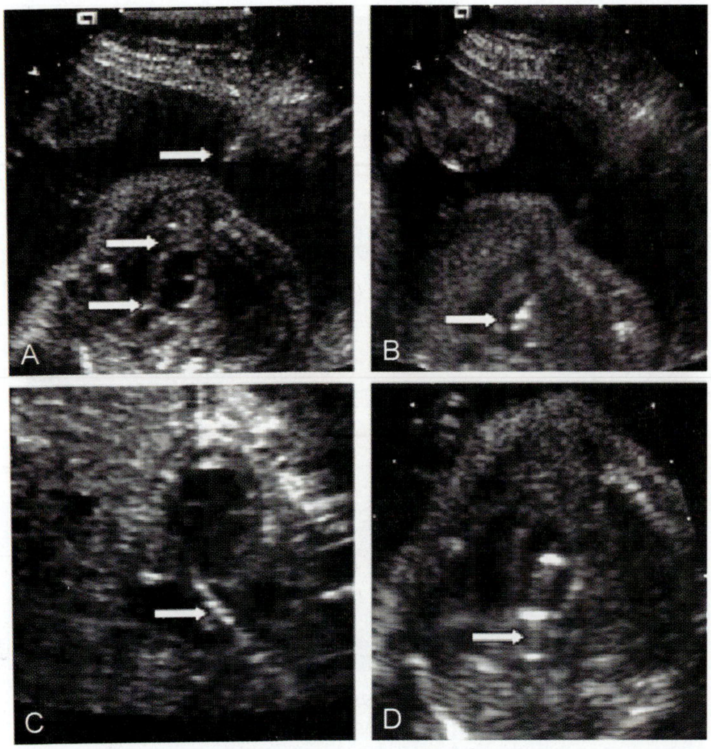

Fig. 48.60: *Ultrasound images of technically successful percutaneous in uteroaortic valvuloplasty. (A) LV before intervention. Four chamber view demonstrating echogenic LV, apex-forming RV, and alignment of needle (arrow), LV apex (arrow), aortic valve, and ascending aorta (arrow). (B) Cannula in LV. After LV puncture with cannula, LV appears smaller. Cannula can be seen as echo-bright line in LV, with its tip directed at aortic valve (arrow). (C) Guidewire across aortic valve in ascending aorta (arrow). (D) Balloon across valve. Correct position of balloon across aortic valve is confirmed by external measurements of catheter and by ultrasound imaging. Balloon inflation appears as movement of bright reflection along line of LV outflow track and across level of valve (arrow)*

frequently surgical intervention such as coarctation repair, resection of endocardial fibroelastosis, and mitral valvuloplasty.

Almost half of fetuses undergoing prenatal aortic valvuloplasty experience a combination of bradycardia and right ventricular dysfunction of variable severity. Fetal hemodynamic instability occurs almost exclusively in fetuses undergoing ventricular puncture (as opposed to atrial access) and may become evident either before the balloon is introduced into the ventricle, during dilation, or even after removal of equipment from the fetal heart. In early experience, these were treated with intramuscular or intracardiac epinephrine, but currently use a prophylactic approach, introducing epinephrine and bicarbonate through the balloon catheter at the time of intervention, regardless of whether bradycardia and right ventricular dysfunction have been identified. If subsequent treatment is necessary, intracardiac or intramuscular medication is given as well. In addition to fetal hemodynamic instability, hemopericardium is also common and may be accompanied by bradycardia. The hemopericardium is frequently small

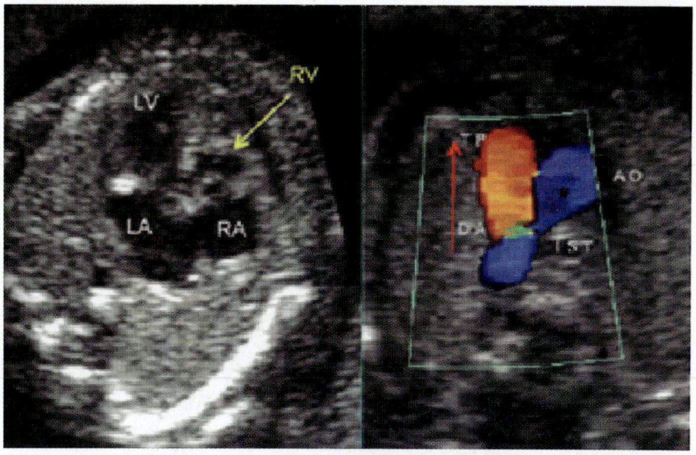

Fig. 48.61: *Hypoplastic right ventricle (arrow) in a fetus with pulmonary atresia and intact ventricular septum (a). Color doppler of the four chamber view with asymmetric flow between the left heart and right heart. Pulmonary valve atresia can be diagnosed using color Doppler by visualizing the great vessels—aorta (Ao) and pulmonary trunk (TP)—in the upper thorax and demonstrating the retrograde flow from the descending aorta across the ductus arteriosus toward the pulmonary valve*

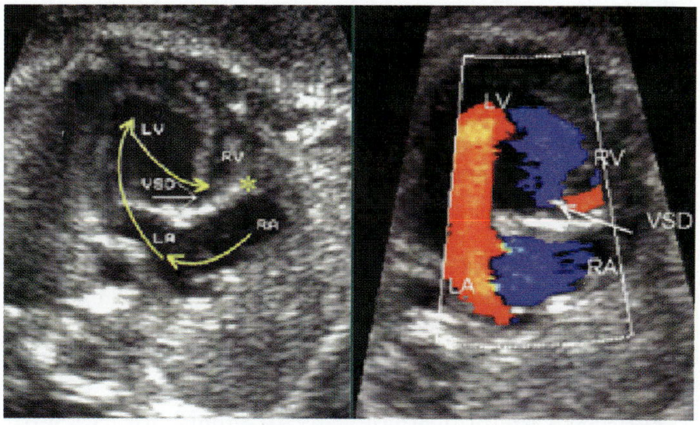

Fig. 48.62: *Tricuspid atresia (*) and ventricular septal defect (VSD). Arrows show the direction of flow; due to the atresia of the tricuspid valve, blood entering the right atrium cannot enter directly into the right ventricle and it flows to the left atrium, left ventricle and across the VSD to the hypoplastic right ventricle (right)*

(less than 1–2 mm) but may be substantially larger, in which case percutaneous drainage is attempted, usually with successful removal of fluid. In fetuses that develop hemodynamic instability or hemopericardium, treatment generally results in restoration of an adequate circulation. The pathophysiology and inciting factors for hemodynamic instability are not entirely clear but are likely the result of some combination of fetal hypoxemia and autonomic or direct response to ventricular compression and puncture.

The foundation for FCI in fetuses with AS and evolving HLHS is the belief that a biventricular circulation is superior to a univentricular circulation. Of course, this is not a simple dichotomous calculus, because all univentricular or biventricular circulations are not of equal functional quality. Although this determination is central to the debate about the practice of FCI, the details are beyond the scope of this

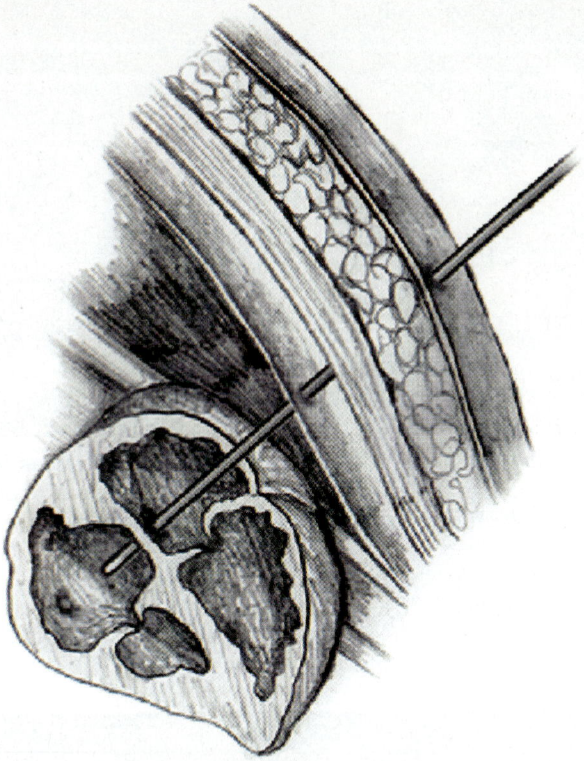

Fig. 48.63: *Illustrating optimal fetal position and needle trajectory for atrial septoplasty. The right atrium is punctured through the fetal chest and the needle advanced through the atrial septum, which is thickened and bows tensely into the right atrium*

review. Another potential benefit of FCI for AS, in the event that a biventricular circulation is not achieved, is a greater contribution of the left side of the heart to the functionally univentricular circulation, which may improve its efficiency and/or durability.

The risks of fetal aortic valvuloplasty for AS with evolving HLHS have not been defined completely.

In the final analysis, the risk-benefit analysis of FCI for evolving HLHS depends to a large extent on individual opinions about the importance of biventricular versus univentricular physiology, and it must take into account both the chronic morbidity and mortality risks of a functionally univentricular circulation and the unknown longer-term risks of a biventricular circulation after FCI. The robustness and health of a biventricular circulation can vary, and the presence of multilevel left heart disease may significantly impact the health of a biventricular circulation. Thus, any risk-benefit analysis before FCI is necessarily speculative and based on the limited available data, as well as being situated in the context of evolving management options and outcomes in patients with both univentricular and biventricular heart disease.

Fetal HLHS with intact or highly restrictive atrial septum

Although neonatal survival in infants with HLHS continues to improve, outcomes among certain subsets of patients remain poor; one of the strongest risk factors for early mortality is an intact or highly restrictive atrial septum.

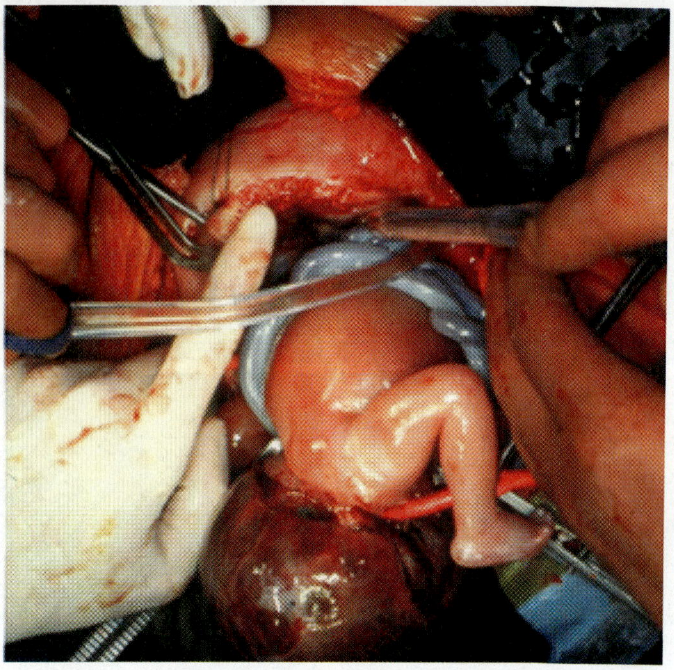

Fig. 48.64: *The first prenatal resection of SCT for fetal hydrops was performed in 1989, and despite successful resection of the mass and resolution of fetal hydrops, the baby could not be saved*

Although limited pulmonary venous egress may be well tolerated in utero, neonates with major septal restriction are at substantially higher risk of death than those without. There are two primary problems associated with this condition: (1) profound hypoxemia after birth due to restricted outflow from the pulmonary veins, which results in little effective pulmonary blood flow and (2) chronic pulmonary venous hypertension in utero due to restriction to left atrial outflow, which results in pulmonary venous thickening and perioperative morbidity and mortality. Thus, even if postnatal opening of the atrial septum is rapid and effective, damage to the pulmonary vasculature may contribute to further mortality in the first few weeks or months of life (Figs 48.47A and B).

In fetuses with HLHS and an intact atrial septum, FCI may improve both of the major problems posed by the restriction of pulmonary venous outflow. If the left atrium can be decompressed before birth, the profound perinatal hypoxemia and acidosis and their associated morbidities may be prevented. If left atrial decompression can be achieved sufficiently early in gestation, adverse pulmonary venous remodeling may also be prevented. Physiologically, the earliest possible treatment of left atrial hypertension on diagnosis of atrial septal restriction should maximize the benefit of normalizing the developmental conditions for the pulmonary vasculature.

Recently, some workers have reported their experience with FCI in 21 fetuses with HLHS and an intact or highly restrictive atrial septum. Prenatal atrial septoplasty for this condition has also been reported by others with various monitoring and interventional approaches. The atrial septum is crossed and an interatrial communication created, either

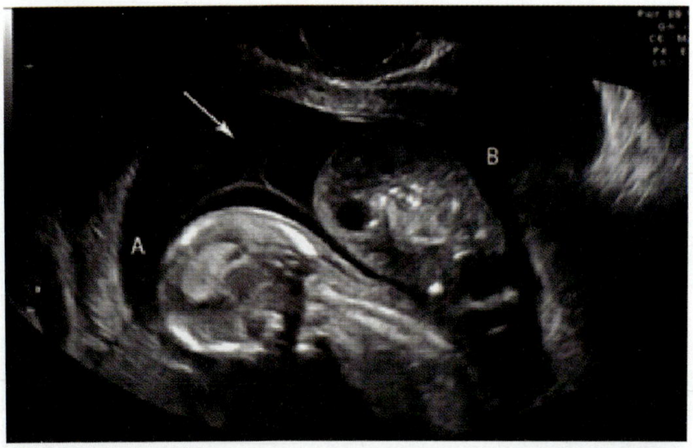

Fig. 48.65: *Two dimensional cross section at 12 postmenstrual weeks showing monochorionic-diamniotic twins. The arrow points to the dividing membranes. Note the pump twin (A) on the left and the grossly abnormal acardiac twin (B) on the right with absence of the head and heart*

with balloon dilation or placement of a stent. Among neonates delivered after FCI for HLHS with significant atrial septal restriction, surgical survival remains quite poor (58%); however, in utero creation of an atrial septal defect does appear to have some benefit in terms of preoperative management, because neonates with an interatrial defect ≤ 3 mm after FCI had higher oxygen saturation at birth and were less likely to need urgent postnatal left atrial decompression. Although assessment of any postnatal survival benefit of FCI in patients with HLHS and an intact atrial septum will require more extensive experience, the potential to avert immediate postnatal deterioration has been demonstrated, and FCI indicated for the comprehensive management of these high-risk fetuses.

Fetal Pulmonary Atresia with Intact Ventricular Septum (PA/IVS)

PA/IVS occurs as a spectrum of hypoplastic right heart disease, with cases at the mild end of the spectrum amenable to biventricular repair and those with more severe right heart hypoplasia managed with univentricular palliation or transplantation. In newborns with PA/IVS, the likelihood of a biventricular outcome can be estimated from the Z-score of the tricuspid valve annulus, with a Z-score above 3″ associated with biventricular outcome and below 3″ with univentricular palliation.

The potential role of FCI in fetuses with PA/IVS is to promote right heart growth and functional development and increase the chance of a biventricular circulation after birth. Identification of potential candidates for FCI for PA/

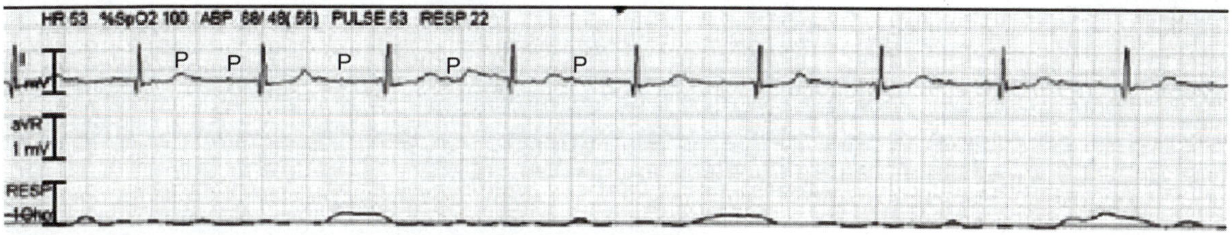

Fig. 48.66A: *Electrocardiography shows complete atrioventricular block before pacemaker implantation*

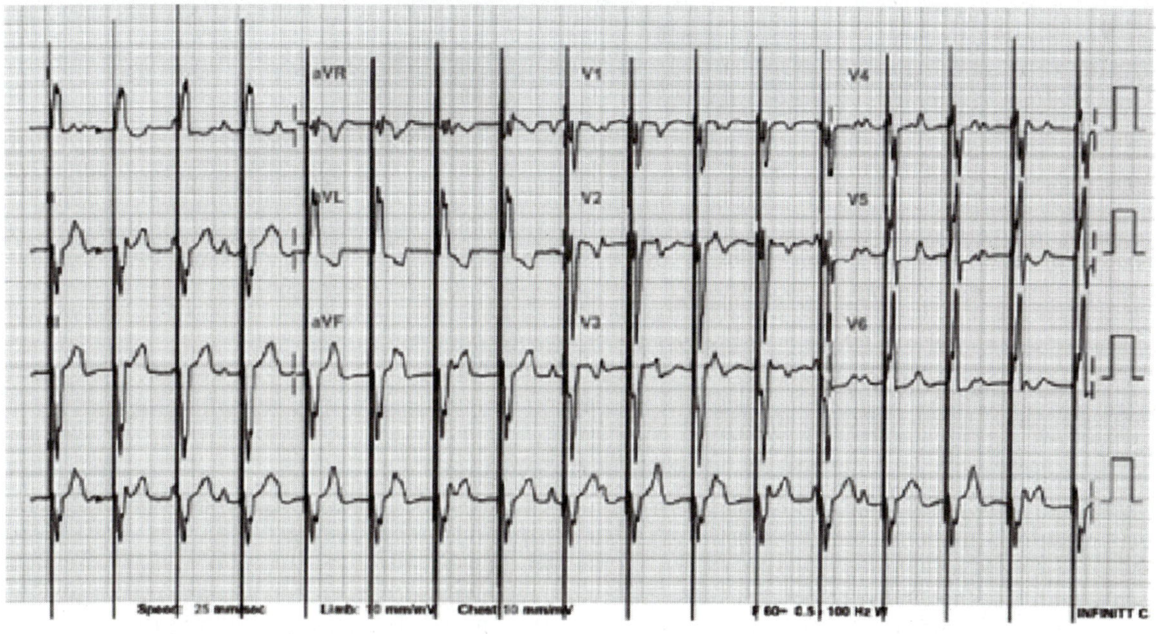

Fig. 48.66B: *Electrocardiography: regular ventricular pacing rhythm after pacemaker implantation*

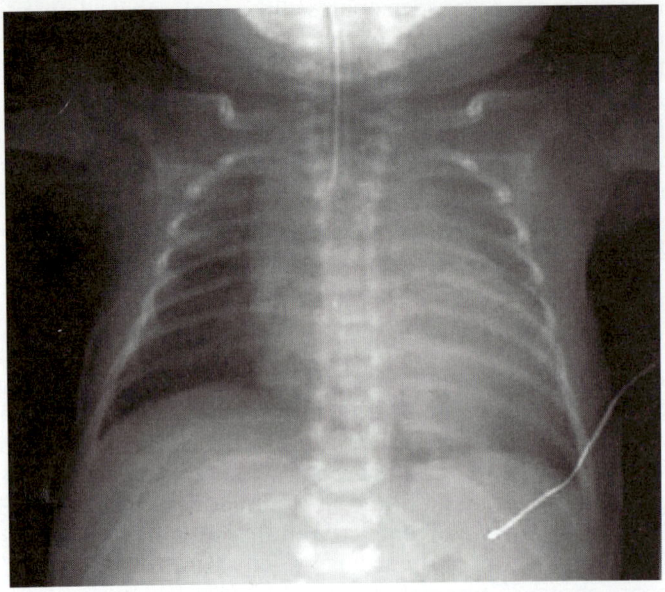

Fig. 48.66C: *Chest X-ray: cardiomegaly and impending congestive heart failure before pacemaker implantation*

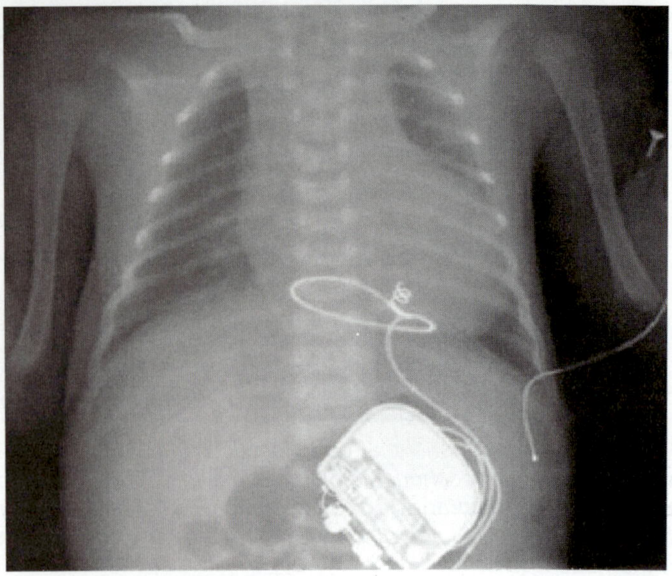

Fig. 48.66D: *Chest X-ray: normal heart size after pacemaker implantation*

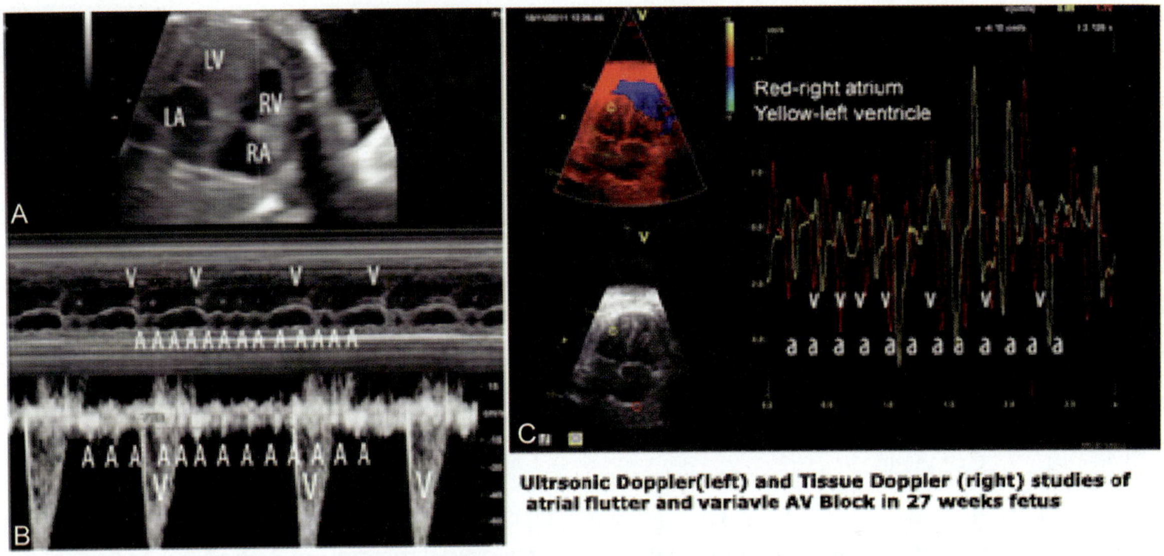

Fig. 48.67: *Assessment of a 27 week fetus with atrial flutter and variable A-V conduction. (A) M mode tracings demonstrate the timing of atrial (A) and ventricular (V) contractions. (B) Simultaneous superior vena cava and ascending aortic pulsed Doppler spectra show timing of a wave reversal in atrial systole in the superior vena cava (A) and forward flow in the aorta during ventricular systole (V). (C) Tissue color Doppler tracings also demonstrate the temporal relationship between atrial (A) and ventricular (V) contractions by changes in myocardial velocities. The atrial rate (A-atrial contraction or systolic flow) is roughly 300 bpm whereas the ventricular rates (V-ventricular contraction or systolic flow) range from 100–200 bpm. A-atrial systolic contraction or flow, V-ventricular contraction or forward aortic flow in ventricular systole. Maternal sotalol therapy successfully treated this rhythm with subsequent vaginal delivery at 40 weeks. LA, left atrium; LV, left ventricle; RA, right atrium; RV, right ventricle*

IVS should be based on the risk of progression to a functionally univentricular circulation postnatally without FCI and the possibility of altering that progression prenatally. There is limited information about predictors of postnatal outcomes in fetuses with PA/IVS. Both anatomic and physiological characteristics are likely to be important, but many patients are in the middle of the severity spectrum, and postnatal management strategy plays an important role in the ultimate outcome.

On the basis of this limited experience, it appears that prenatal pulmonary valve perforation and dilation may be performed successfully in midgestation fetuses, with maintenance of valvar patency throughout gestation and apparently improved growth of right heart structures. The effects of this strategy on right heart functional development and postnatal outcome remain to be determined. Because postnatal outcomes for the majority of patients with PA/IVS are usually favorable, it may be more of a challenge to appropriately select patients and demonstrate effectiveness than for the previously discussed anomalies (Figs 48.68 and 48.69).

Future Directions (Figs 48.9, 48.51A and 48.52B)

There is much that remains to be learned about the benefits and potential adverse effects of FCI. Although pharmacological FCI is well established in the management of fetal arrhythmias and heart block, there is room for improvement nonetheless. In addition, novel pharmacological strategies, such as maternal hyperoxia, and the prospect of other agents for other conditions will inevitably emerge. On the basis of the experimental evidence, open FCI appears feasible, although the indications for and establishment of open FCI in humans must be explored critically. There are severe congenital cardiac anomalies for which more complex interventions may be beneficial, such as severe Ebstein's malformation with fetal hydrops.

Ultimately, the utility of FCI will depend on a variety of clinical and technological factors including more frequent, earlier diagnosis of congenital heart disease in utero, characterization of prognostic features in fetuses with congenital heart disease, better understanding of the capacity and optimal gestational windows for cardiovascular remodeling after FCI, and improved and focused technology. Advances in imaging and instrumentation should facilitate greater precision and effectiveness of intervention and may open the door to procedures for more complex indications. More sophisticated image-guided or robotic interventional approaches to closed FCI are being explored and may help improve precision and success, potentially shifting the gestational horizon to allow safe intervention in younger fetuses. At the same time, as experience with FCI accumulates, risk profiles can be expected to improve, which may facilitate FCI for less severe conditions if such procedures can be expected to improve outcomes.

Fetoscopic Laser Photocoagulation of Placental Vessels

It is considered as one of future techniques in FCI where one of the fetuses dying with deprivation of blood supply from the other fetus can be saved (twin to twin transfusion syndrome) and other similar like critical fetal conditions (Figs 48.51A–G).

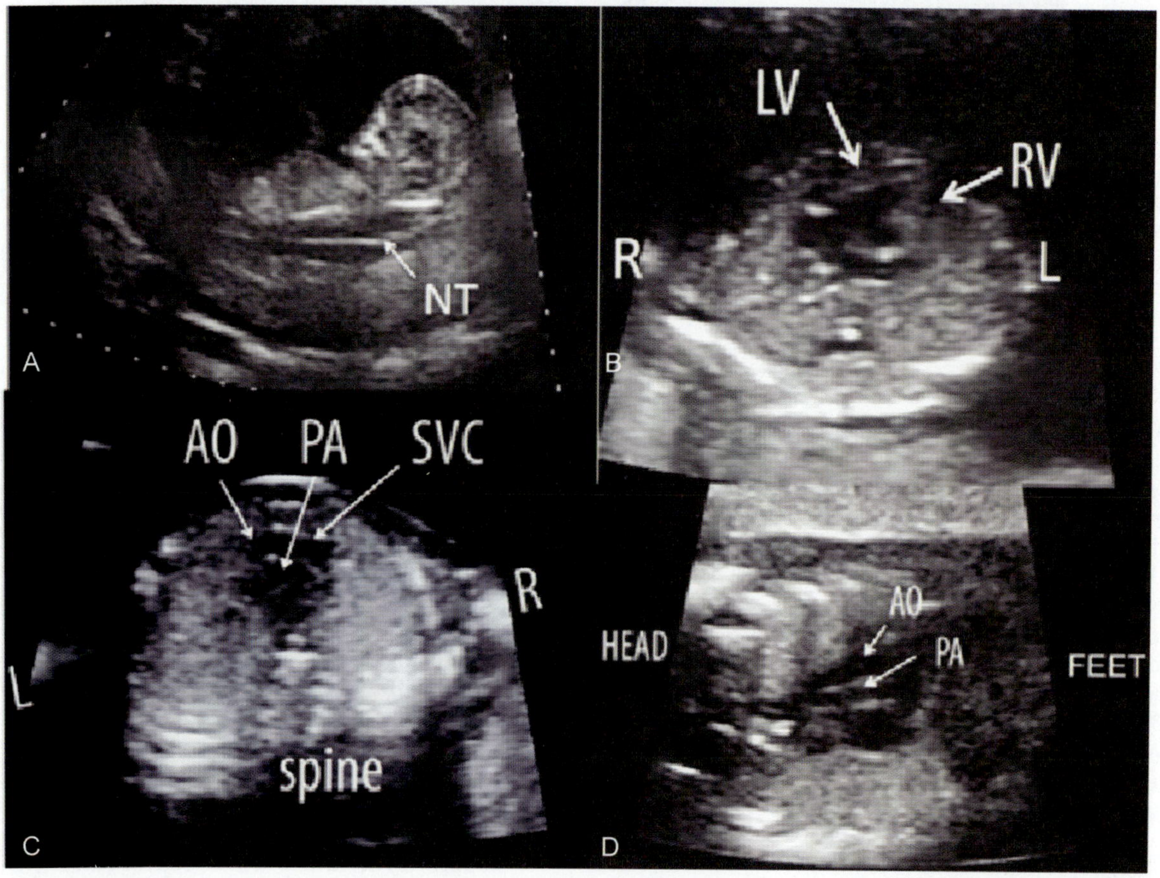

Fig. 48.68: *Echocardiographic images obtained during the intervention for patient. (A) This four chamber view demonstrates a hypoplastic RV (arrow). (B) In this oblique projection, the 19-gauge cannula can be seen passing through the uterus, amniotic cavity, and chest wall of the fetus and approaching the RV outflow tract (arrow). (C) This short-axis image demonstrates the tip of the Chiba needle in the pulmonary artery (arrow). (D) After successful valvuloplasty, color Doppler ultrasound flow imaging demonstrates an antegrade jet of flow across the patent PV (arrow)*

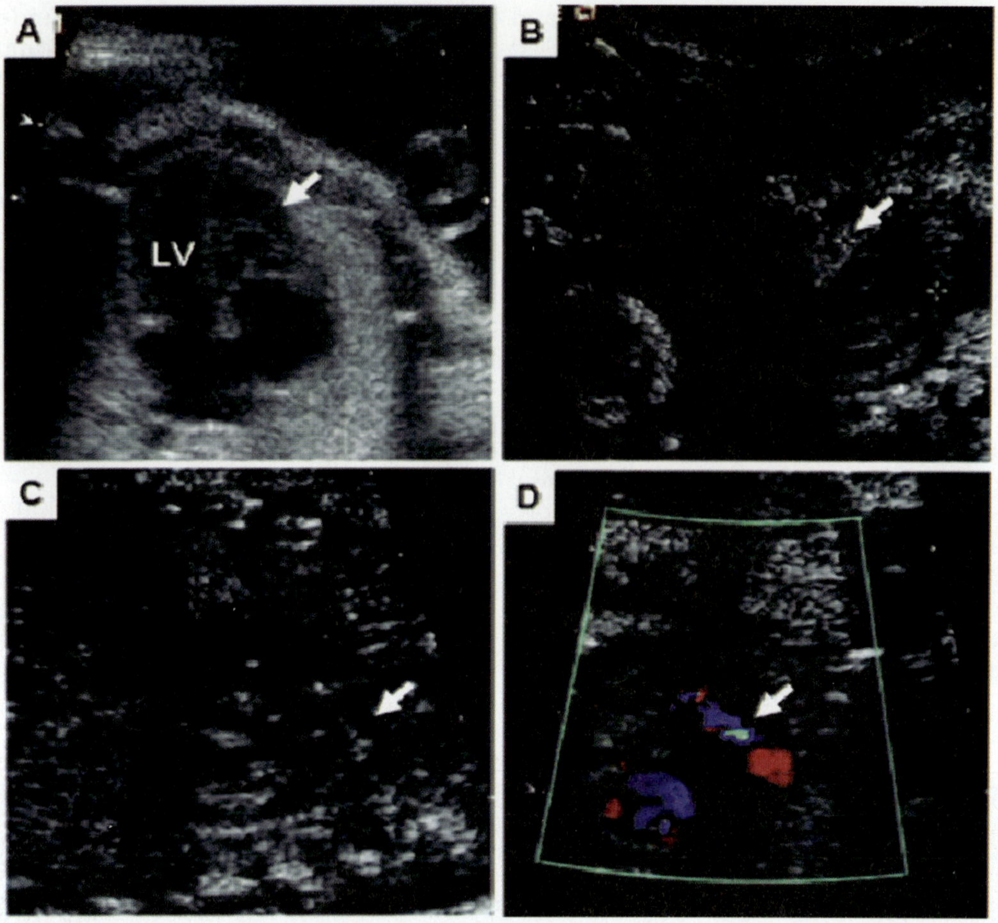

Fig. 48.69: *Echocardiographic images obtained during the intervention. (A) This four chamber view demonstrates a hypoplastic RV (arrow). (B) Oblique projection, the 19-gauge cannula can be seen passing through the uterus, amniotic cavity, and chest wall of the fetus and approaching the RV outflow tract (arrow). (C) Short-axis image demonstrates the tip of the Chiba needle in the pulmonary artery (arrow). (D) After successful valvuloplasty, color Doppler ultrasound flow imaging demonstrates an antegrade jet of flow across the patent PV (arrow)*

BIBLIOGRAPHY

1. Eibschitz I, Abinader EG, Klein A, Sharf M. Intrauterine diagnosis and control of fetal ventricular arrhythmia during labor. Am J Obstet Gynecol. 1975; 122: 597–600.
2. Carpenter R, Strasburger JF, Garson A, Smith RT, Deter RL, Englehardt H. Fetal ventricular pacing for hydrops secondary to complete atrioventricular block. J Am Coll Cardiol. 1986; 8: 1434–1436.
3. Tulzer G, Arzt W, Franklin RC, Loughna PV, Mair R, Gardiner HM. Fetal pulmonary valvuloplasty for critical pulmonary stenosis or atresia with intact septum. Lancet. 2002; 360: 1567–1568.
4. Arzt W, Tulzer G, Aigner M, Mair R, Hafner E. Invasive intrauterine treatment of pulmonary atresia/intact ventricular septum with heart failure. Ultrasound Obstet Gynecol. 2003; 21: 186–188.
5. Tworetzky W, Wilkins-Haug L, Jennings RW, van der Velde ME, Marshall AC, Marx GR, Colan SD, Benson CB, Lock JE, Perry SB. Balloon dilation of severe aortic stenosis in the fetus: potential for prevention of hypoplastic left heart syndrome: candidate selection, technique, and results of successful intervention. Circulation. 2004; 12: 2125–2131.
6. Marshall AC, van der Velde ME, Tworetzky W, Gomez CA, Wilkins-Haug L, Benson CB, Jennings RW, Lock JE. Creation of an atrial septal defect in utero for fetuses with hypoplastic left heart syndrome and intact or highly restrictive atrial septum. Circulation. 2004; 110: 253–258.
7. Mizrahi-Arnaud A, Tworetzky W, Bulich LA, Wilkins-Haug LE, Marshall AC, Benson CB, Lock JE, McElhinney DB. Pathophysiology, management, and outcomes of fetal hemodynamic instability during prenatal cardiac intervention. Pediatr Res. 2007; 62: 325–330.
8. Selamet Tierney ES, Wald RM, McElhinney DB, Marshall AC, Benson CB, Marcus EN, Marx GR, Levine JC, Wilkins-Haug L, Lock JE, Tworetzky W. Changes in left heart hemodynamics after technically successful in utero aortic valvuloplasty. Ultrasound Obstet Gynecol. 2007; 30: 715–720.
9. Marshall AC, Levine J, Morash D, Silva V, Lock JE, Benson CB, Wilkins-Haug LE, McElhinney DB, Tworetzky W. Results of in utero atrial septoplasty in fetuses with hypoplastic left heart syndrome. Prenat Diagn. 2008; 28: 1023–1028.
10. Kohl T, Müller A, Tchatcheva K, Achenbach S, Gembruch U. Fetal transesophageal echocardiography: clinical introduction as a monitoring tool during cardiac intervention

in a human fetus. Ultrasound Obstet Gynecol. 2005; 26: 780–785.

11. Quintero RA, Huhta J, Suh E, Chmait R, Romero R, Angel J. In utero cardiac fetal surgery: laser atrial septotomy in the treatment of hypoplastic left heart syndrome with intact atrial septum. Am J Obstet Gynecol. 2005; 193: 1424–1428.
12. Wilkins-Haug LE, Tworetzky W, Benson CB, Marshall AC, Jennings RW, Lock JE. Factors affecting technical success of fetal aortic valve dilation. Ultrasound Obstet Gynecol. 2006; 28: 47–52.
13. Galindo A, Gutierrez-Larraya F, Velasco JM, de la Fuente P. Pulmonary balloon valvuloplasty in a fetus with critical pulmonary stenosis/atresia with intact ventricular septum and heart failure. Fetal Diagn Ther. 2006; 21: 100–104.
14. Kohl T, Sharland G, Allan LD, Gembruch U, Chaoui R, Lopes LM, Zielinsky P, Huhta J, Silverman NH. World experience of percutaneous ultrasound-guided balloon valvuloplasty in human fetuses with severe aortic valve obstruction. Am J Cardiol. 2000; 85: 1230–1233.
15. Suh E, Quintessenza J, Huhta J, Quintero R. How to grow a heart: fibreoptic guided fetal aortic valvotomy. Cardiol Young. 2006; 16 (suppl 1): 43–46.
16. Kohl T, Breuer J, Heep A, Wenningmann I, Weinbach J, Gembruch U. Fetal transesophageal echocardiography during balloon valvuloplasty for severe aortic valve stenosis at 28+6 weeks of gestation. J Thorac Cardiovasc Surg. 2007; 134: 256–257.
17. Tworetzky W, McElhinney DB, Marx GR, Benson CB, Brusseau R, Morash D, Louise E, Wilkins-Haug LE, Lock JE, Marshall AC. In utero valvuloplasty for pulmonary valve atresia with hypoplastic right ventricle: techniques and outcomes. Pediatrics. 2009 Aug 24.
18. McElhinney DB, Marshall AC, Wilkins-Haug LE, Brown DW, Benson CB, Silva V, Marx GR, Mizrahi-Arnaud A, Lock JE, Tworetzky W. Predictors of technical success and postnatal biventricular outcome after in utero aortic valvuloplasty for aortic stenosis with evolving hypoplastic left heart syndrome. Circulation. 2009; 120: 1482–1490.
19. Kunisaki SM, Jennings RW. Fetal surgery. J Intensive Care Med. 2008; 23: 33–51.
20. Cortes RA, Farmer DL. Recent advances in fetal surgery. Semin Perinatol. 2004; 28: 199–211.
21. Gurtner GC, Werner S, Barrandon Y, Longaker MT. Wound repair and regeneration. Nature. 2008; 453: 314–321.
22. Ahuja P, Sdek P, MacLellan WR. Cardiac myocyte cell cycle control in development, disease, and regeneration. Physiol Rev. 2007; 87: 521–544.
23. Newburger JW, Keane JF. Intrauterine supraventricular tachycardia. J Pediatr. 1979; 95: 780–786.
24. Kleinman CS, Donnerstein RL, DeVore GR, Jaffe CC, Lynch DC, Berkowitz RL, Talner NS, Hobbins JC. Fetal echocardiography for evaluation of in utero congestive heart failure. N Engl J Med. 1982; 306: 568–575.
25. Schmolling J, Renke K, Richter O, Pfeiffer K, Schlebusch H, Höller T. Digoxin, flecainide, and amiodarone transfer across the placenta and the effects of an elevated umbilical venous pressure on the transfer rate. Ther Drug Monit. 2000; 22: 582–588.
26. Oudijk MA, Michon MM, Kleinman CS, Kapusta L, Stoutenbeek P, Visser GH, Meijboom EJ. Sotalol in the treatment of fetal dysrhythmias. Circulation. 2000; 101: 2721–2726.
27. van den Heuvel F, Bink-Boelkens MT, du Marchie Sarvaas GJ, Berger RM. Drug management of fetal tachyarrhythmias: are we ready for a systematic and evidence-based approach? Pacing Clin Electrophysiol. 2008; 31 (suppl 1): S54–S57.
28. Strasburger JF, Cuneo BF, Michon MM, Gotteiner NL, Deal BJ, McGregor SN, Oudijk MA, Meijboom EJ, Feinkind L, Hussey M, Parilla BV. Amiodarone therapy for drug-refractory fetal tachycardia. Circulation. 2004; 109: 375–379.
29. Friedman DM, Kim MY, Copel JA, Llanos C, Davis C, Buyon JP. Prospective evaluation of fetuses with autoimmune-associated congenital heart block followed in the PR Interval and Dexamethasone Evaluation (PRIDE) Study. Am J Cardiol. 2009; 103: 1102–1106.
30. Maeno Y, Himeno W, Saito A, Hiraishi S, Hirose O, Ikuma M, Inamura N, Kawataki M, Mizukami A, Ota M, Shiraishi H, Satomi G, Kato H. Clinical course of fetal congenital atrioventricular block in the Japanese population: a multicentre experience. Heart. 2005; 91: 1075–1079.
31. Jaeggi ET, Fouron JC, Silverman ED, Ryan G, Smallhorn J, Hornberger LK. Transplacental fetal treatment improves the outcome of prenatally diagnosed complete atrioventricular block without structural heart disease. Circulation. 2004; 110: 1542–1548.
32. Fesslova V, Vignati G, Brucato A, De Sanctis M, Butera G, Pisoni MP, Chiappa E, Acaia B, Meroni PL. The impact of treatment of the fetus by maternal therapy on the fetal and postnatal outcomes for fetuses diagnosed with isolated complete atrioventricular block. Cardiol Young. 2009; 19: 282–290.
33. Patel D, Cuneo B, Viesca R, Rassanan J, Leshko J, Huhta J. Digoxin for the treatment of fetal congestive heart failure with sinus rhythm assessed by cardiovascular profile score. J Matern Fetal Neonatal Med. 2008; 21: 477–482.
34. Almström H, Sonesson SE. Doppler echocardiographic assessment of fetal blood flow redistribution during maternal hyperoxygenation. Ultrasound Obstet Gynecol. 1996; 8: 256–261.
35. Battaglia C, Artini PG, D'Ambrogio G, Bencini S, Galli PA, Genazzani AR. Maternal hyperoxygenation in the treatment of mild intrauterine growth retardation: a pilot study. Ultrasound Obstet Gynecol. 1994; 4: 472–475.
36. Szwast A, Tian Z, McCann M, Donaghue D, Rychik J. Vasoreactive response to maternal hyperoxygenation (MH) in the fetus with hypoplastic left heart syndrome (HLHS). Circ Cardiovasc Imaging. 2009 Dec 31.
37. Pomini F, Noia G, Mancuso S. Hypothetical role of prostaglandins in the onset of preterm labor after fetal surgery. Fetal Diagn Ther. 2007; 22: 94–99.
38. Turley K, Vlahakes GJ, Harrison MR, Messina L, Hanley F, Uhlig PN, Ebert P. Intrauterine cardiothoracic surgery: the fetal lamb model. Ann Thorac Surg. 1982; 34: 422–426.
39. Richter RC, Slate RK, Rudolph AM, Turley K. Fetal blood flow during hypothermic cardiopulmonary bypass in utero. J Cardiovasc Surg. 1985; 26: 86.
40. Sabik JF, Assad RS, Hanley FL. Prostaglandin synthesis inhibition prevents placental dysfunction after fetal cardiac bypass. J Thorac Cardiovasc Surg. 1992; 103: 733–742.

41. Assad RS, Lee FY, Sabik J, Hanley FL. Tolerance of the placenta to normothermic umbilical circulatory arrest. J Matern Fetal Invest. 1992; 2: 145–150.
42. Fenton KM, Heinemann MK, Hanley FL. Exclusion of the placenta during fetal cardiac bypass allows improved systemic perfusion and provides important information about the mechanism of placental injury. J Thorac Cardiovasc Surg. 1993; 105: 502–512.
43. Fenton KN, Heinemann MK, Klautz RJM, Liddicoat JR, Hanley FL. Inhibition of fetal stress response improves cardiac output and gas exchange after fetal cardiac bypass. J Thorac Cardiovasc Surg. 1994; 107: 1416–1422.
44. Fenton KN, Zinn HE, Heinemann MK, Liddicoat JR, Hanley FL. Long-term survivors of fetal cardiac bypass in lambs. J Thorac Cardiovasc Surg. 1994; 107: 1423–1427.
45. Sabik JF, Heinemann MK, Assad RS, Hanley FL. High dose steroids prevent placental dysfunction after fetal cardiac bypass. J Thorac Cardiovasc Surg. 1994; 107: 116–125.
46. Reddy VM, McElhinney DB, Rajasinghe HA, Rodriguez JL, Hanley FL. Cytokine response to fetal cardiac bypass. J Matern Fetal Invest. 1998; 8: 46–49.
47. Reddy VM, McElhinney DB, Rajasinghe HA, Liddicoat JR, Hendricks-Munoz K, Fineman JR, Hanley FL. Role of the endothelium in placental dysfunction after fetal cardiac bypass. J Thorac Cardiovasc Surg. 1999; 117: 343–351.
48. Parry AJ, Petrossian E, McElhinney DB, Reddy VM, Hanley FL. Neutrophil degranulation and complement activation during fetal cardiac bypass. Ann Thorac Surg. 2000; 70: 582–589.
49. Reddy VM, Liddicoat JR, Klein JR, McElhinney DB, Wampler RK, Hanley FL. Fetal cardiac bypass using an in-line axial flow pump to minimize extracorporeal surface and avoid priming volume. Ann Thorac Surg. 1996; 62: 393–400.
50. Reddy VM, Liddicoat JR, Klein JR, Wampler RK, Hanley FL. Long-term fetal outcome after fetal cardiac bypass: fetal survival to full term and organ abnormalities. J Thorac Cardiovasc Surg. 1996; 111: 536–544.

49 Stem Cells and Gene Therapy in Heart Disease

SECTION 1: STEM CELL TRANSPLANTATION

Despite the development of improved therapies and the significant advances in the understanding of the basis of disease pathogenesis, millions of people all over the World are living with life-threatening cardiovascular diseases. Recent breakthroughs suggest exciting directions that are likely to produce more effective therapies for the treatment of cardiovascular disease. One such area, cell transplantation (grafting of healthy cells into the diseased heart), holds enormous potential as an approach to cardiovascular pathophysiology. Once thought to be a scientific long shot, cell transplantation is becoming recognized as a viable strategy to strengthen weak hearts and limit infarct growth. The technology could also be used for the long-term delivery of beneficial recombinant proteins to the heart, which is a strategy to complement molecular biology advances and provide an alternative strategy for gene therapy. In an attempt to reduce the invasiveness of cell transfer, catheter-based techniques have been rapidly developed. They basically rely on three routes (Fig. 49.1):

- Endoventricular
- Intracoronary
- Transvenous

The guidance of cell delivery being achieved with electromagnetic mapping, coronary angiography, and endovascular ultrasounds, respectively. In our experience, the latter technique has been found particularly user-friendly and we are currently testing its potential benefits in a sheep model of myocardial infarction. However, although these percutaneous approaches have been expeditiously applied in patients, they have actually undergone limited preclinical testing. Thus, the extent of intramyocardial cell trapping following endoventricular

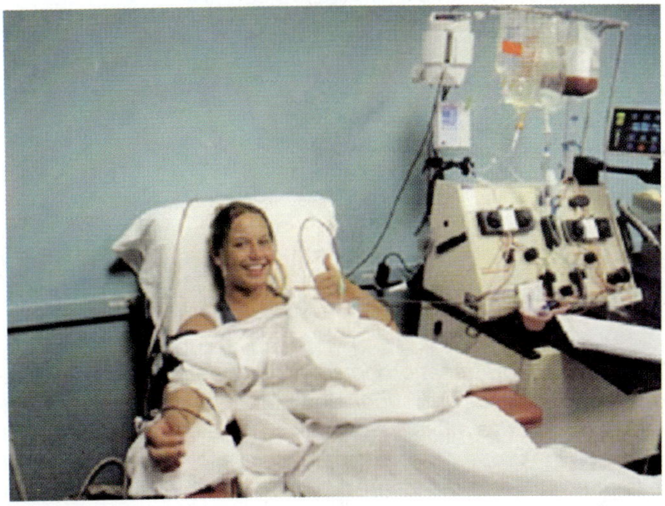

Fig. 49.1: *Transplantation (transfer of stem cell) is a safe, and usually painless procedure. It should be conducted in a sterile environment by a professional medical personnel. Usually, an ambulatory procedure, within a day the patient usually returns to normal life. Ongoing monitoring of the patient is usually carried out on an "out-patient" basis*

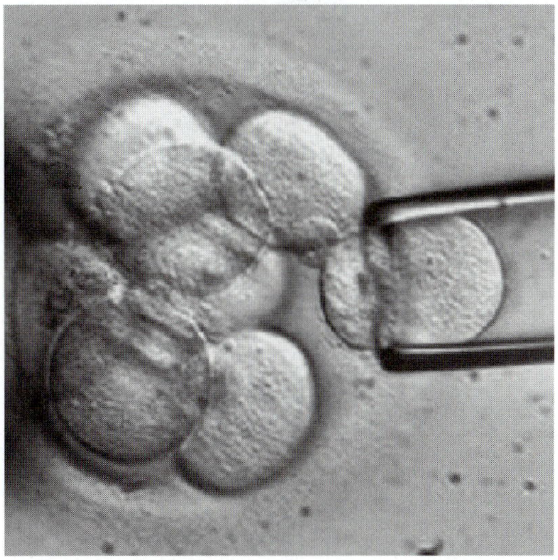

Fig. 49.2: *Histopathological photograph showing hematopoietic stem cell ready for transplantation*

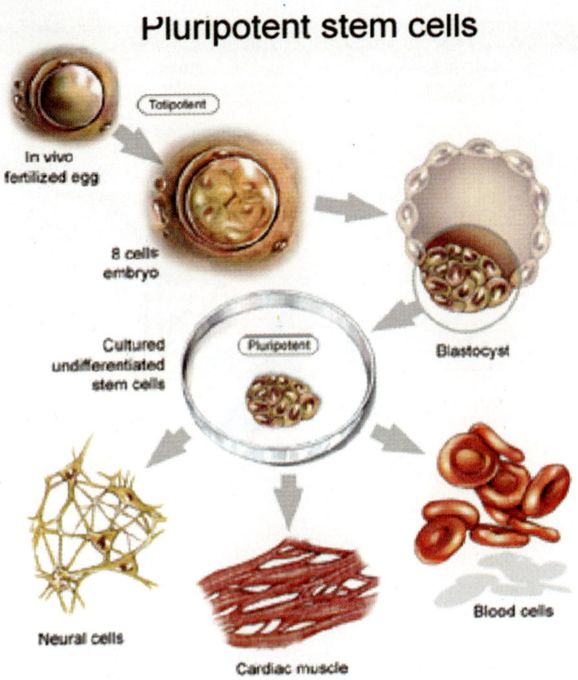

Fig. 49.3: *Diagrammatic representation of morphology of a pluripotent stem cell*

injections has not been fully investigated, nor is the ability of intracoronarily injected bone marrow cells to gain access to myocardial tissue, even if their transendothelial migration is thought to be enhanced by high-pressure infusion and angioplasty balloon inflation to prevent backflow. Indeed, viability of cells following passage through the catheters has usually been assessed but their functionality (i.e. ability of skeletal myoblasts and bone-marrow cells to differentiate into myotubes and cardiac/ vascular cells, respectively), which is an equally important end point, as well as their long-term survival have often been underlooked. For example, in a recent study follow-up of myoblasts injected through an endoventricular catheter was limited to 10 days. Likewise, there are also limited data regarding the functional efficacy of these techniques and only found one experimental study in which the effects of transen docardially injected bone marrow cells were extensively investigated. Clearly, there is still much work to be done in this area, particularly for comparing the results of percutaneous cell delivery with that of the surgical approach, which remains the benchmark against which alternate modes of cell transplantation should be tested. This remark does not only apply to percutaneous approaches but also to biografts made of bioresorbable cell-seeded scaffolds, which could represent an effective means of repairing wall defects in adult and pediatric open-heart operations (Figs 49.2–49.7).

The Problem of Cell Death

Regardless of the route of delivery, cell death remains a major problem of cell transplantation common to all cell lineages. Thus, up to 90% of transplanted cardiomyocytes have been shown to die within the first 24 hours. The mechanisms of this high death rate are multiple and include particularly physical strain during injections, ischemia due to the poor vascularity of the target scar, and apoptosis. As it is uncertain whether multiplication of surviving cells can catch up to this initially high attrition rate, the development of cell survival-enhancing strategies appears critical for

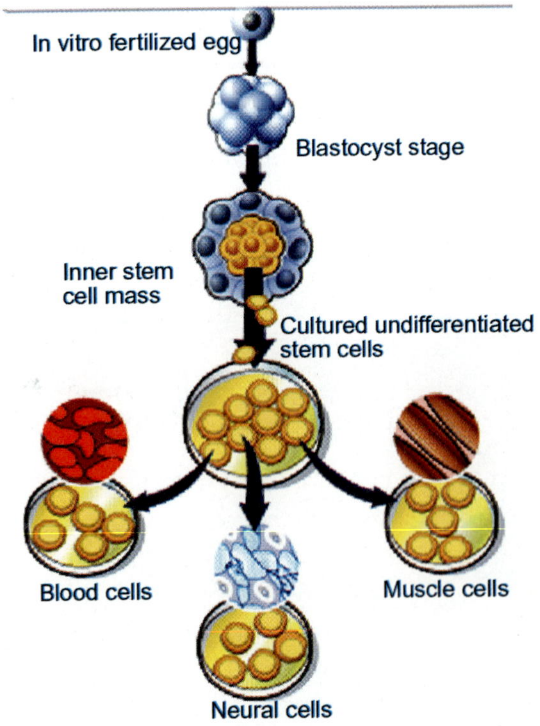

Fig. 49.4: *Diagram showing working pattern of stem cells to heal the damaged structures in the body*

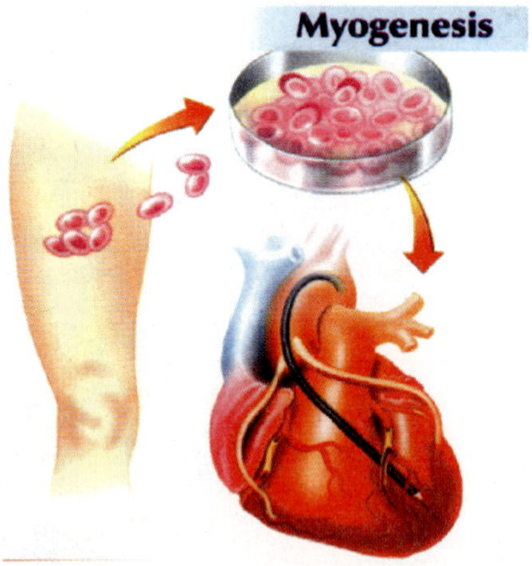

Fig. 49.5: *Diagrammatic depiction of myogenesis in the heart muscle. Myoblasts are super power house cells that originate from human bodys muscle stem cells. These cells have the ability to take on the properties of the other cells such as cardiac muscle cells that make-up the heart. Unlike cardiac muscle myoblasts can regenerate and repair themselves. The myoblasts can be transplanted from the skeletal muscles into heart and can stimulate myogenesis. A biopsy of muscle cells from patient thigh is taken and isolated and expanded in culture in a special cell laboratory for 3 weeks. These multiple cells are injected directly into the areas of heart where the muscle is damaged*

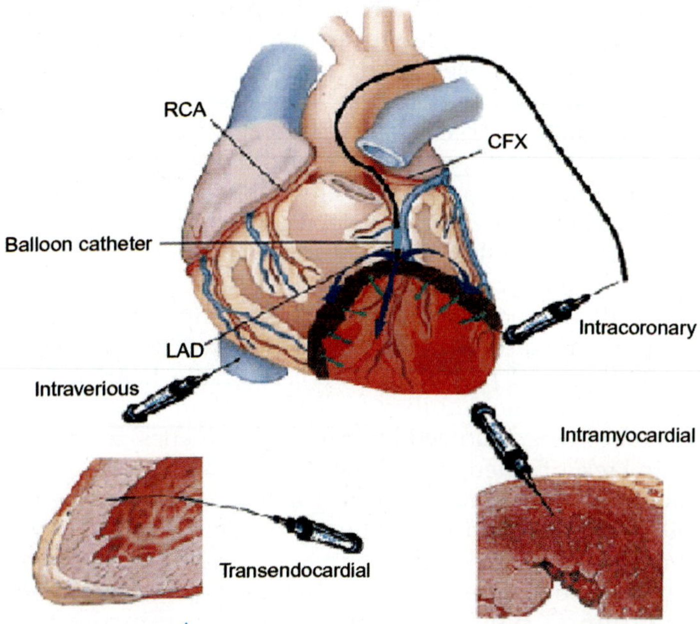

Fig. 49.6: *Showing tranfer of stem cells into damaged myocardium and obstructed coronary vessels for the treatment of damaged muscle in cardiomyopathy and ischemic heart disease*

optimizing the functional benefits of the procedure. Two of them are of potentially great clinical relevance. The first consists of enhancing angiogenesis to limit the ischemic component of cell death, an approach based on the observation that the survival of cardiomyocytes grafted into highly vascularized granulation tissue is twofold greater than that observed after grafting into acutely necrotic myocardium. In practice, increased angiogenesis can be achieved by pretransplantation transfection of cells with genes encoding vascular growth factors, direct co injection of these factors or concomitant revascularization of cell-transplanted segments (an approach which appears sound but only be confirmed when efficacy is demonstrated by ongoing randomized trials committed to avoiding bypass surgery in these segments to avoid confounding factors in the interpretation of outcome measures). The second strategy aimed at increasing the survival rate of transplanted cells relies on limitation of apoptosis, which can be successfully achieved by heat shocking cells just prior to their implantation. Finally, it is also likely that even though an immune response is unlikely to occur in the case of autologous transplantation, the inflammatory state created by needle punctures can contribute to cell damage. This mechanism is expected to be still greater if it superimposes upon the inflammation that occurs during the early phase of infarction. Conversely, late injections may equally reduce the effectiveness of the procedure if they are performed once the remodeling process has been completed. These observations suggest that there is probably an optimal time window for cell transplantation following myocardial infarction and that bracketing this time frame is another means of optimizing the benefits of the procedure.

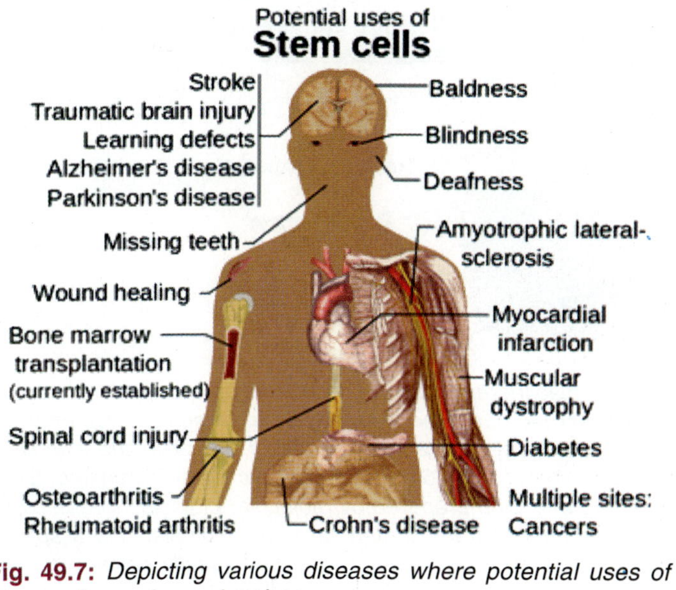

Fig. 49.7: *Depicting various diseases where potential uses of stem cells can be undertaken*

Analysis of Early Clinical Data

Skeletal Myoblasts

On June 15, 2000, the first human transplantation of autologous skeletal myoblasts was performed. The operation was uneventful, the cardiac condition markedly improved including the scarred segment which had been grafted, and the patient died 18 months later from a stroke. At autopsy, myotubes were identified in scar tissue and found to express in roughly similar proportions fast, slow, and composite (fast and slow) myosin isoforms. This operation was the first of a series of 10 designed to assess the feasibility and safety of the procedure and included patients meeting the following three criteria: (1) severe left ventricular dysfunction (ejection fraction <35%); (2) history of myocardial infarct with a residual discrete, echocardiographically akinetic (after dobutamine challenge) and,metabolically nonviable scar (as assessed by fluorodeoxyglucose positron emission tomography); and indication for concomitant coronary artery bypass grafting in remote (i.e. different from the transplanted area), ischemic myocardium. Since then, two other series have been reported, one in Poland (10 patients) and the other in the United States (16 patients). Similar to the protocol of phase I trial, all these patients underwent cell transplantation during a conventional coronary artery bypass operation, except for five of the American study who underwent placement of a left ventricular assist device at the time of cell transplantation with the objective of assessing the fate of the engrafted cells at the time of subsequent transplantation. Finally, catheter-based endoventricular or transvenous myoblast transplantations have also been performed in Europe as part of both physician driven and industry-sponsored trials and, based on the presentation made by P. Serruys at the TCT meeting in October, 2002, totalled 13 patients before the study was stopped because of serious adverse events (it has then been reinitiated after protocol changes) (Figs 49.8–49.11).

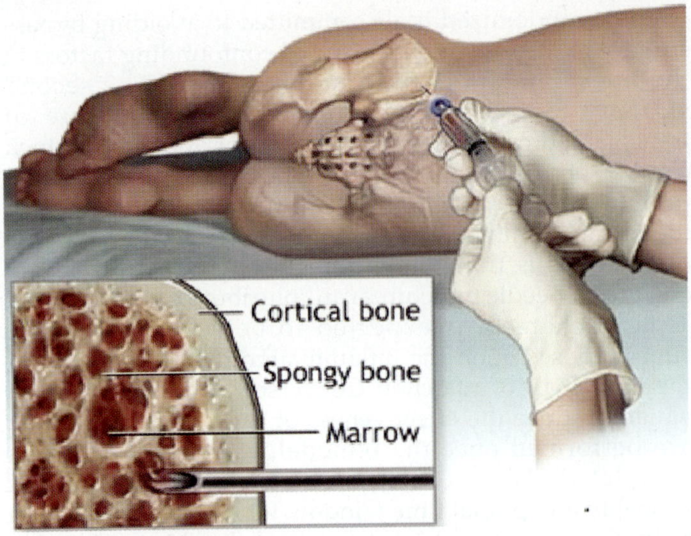

Fig. 49.8: *Technique of bone marrow aspiration. A small amount of bone marrow is removed during a bone marrow aspiration. Aspirated bone marrow contains stem cells which can be used to repair damaged myocardium or obstructed coronary artery*

The protocol of the surgical procedure that originally designed (and which has remained unchanged over time) is fairly straight forward and involves three steps: a biopsy of the ***vastus lateralis*** retrieved from the thigh under local anesthesia; a 2- to 3-week period of cell expansion and the reimplantation of the final cell yield concentrated in a small volume (5–6 mL) in and around the postinfarct scar while remote ischemic areas are revascularized by bypass grafts. Overall, these phase I trials have now established the feasibility of the procedure, i.e. the possibility of growing hundreds million of cells (an average of 871 × 106 cells were injected, of which 86% were identified as myogenic by specific antibodies and 90% were viable at the time of the final collection), in compliance with Good Medical Practice standards and within a clinically relevant time frame (2–3 weeks). The operation, by itself, has also turned out to be safe, without specific procedure-related complications, while companion experiments have documented the persisting functionality of myoblasts harvested from heart failure patients (i.e. their ability to differentiate in vitro into myotubes when allowed to grow to confluence) as well as their lack of oncogenic potential (when injected into immunodeficient mice). The only adverse event ascribed to cell transplantation is sustained ventricular tachycardia, which has occurred in some patients (and presumably caused two deaths in the catheter-based trial). These arrhythmias have been documented within the first postoperative weeks, with a seemingly low rate of late recurrences, as demonstrated by interrogation of the automatic internal cardioverter-defibrillator (AICD) implanted in these cases. The mechanism of these arrhythmias is being investigated and although the involvement of inflammatory reactions (triggered by needle punctures and cell injections) would fit their early posttransplantation timing of onset, rather favor the

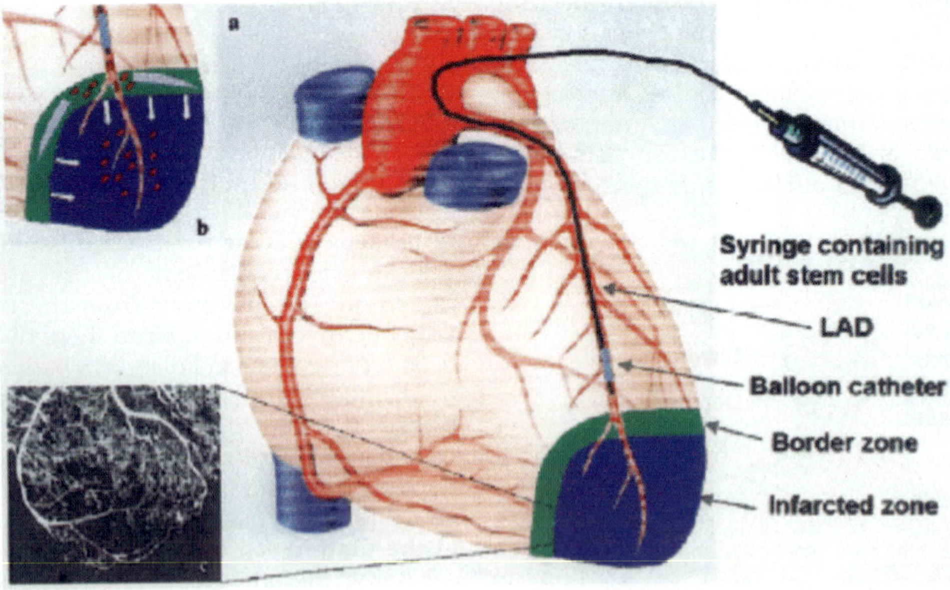

Fig. 49.9: *Cardiac stem cell therapy after a patient has obtained standard cardiac therapy (e.g. balloon dilatation of occluded coronary arteries, stent implantation), harvesting and transplantation of stem cells is carried out in the following way: during the days after the infarct, the patient obtains medication causing stem cells to be flushed out into the bloodstream. Blood tests are made and examined every day. If they indicate that the peak of stem cells in the blood is reached (after about 4-6 days), stem cells will be harvested. Stem cells are "filtered out" from the patient's blood by special dialysis equipment and then prepared by molecular biologists of the blood center. After approximately 5 hours of filtering and preparation, stem cells can be transplanted (a) by cardiologist. Via a special balloon catheter, stem cells are injected into the coronary artery supplying the infarcted zone. There, they ideally develop to new heart muscle cells and regenerate heart muscle functionality by reducing the area of the infarcted zone*

hypothesis that differences in action potential duration between engrafted myotubes and native cardiomyocytes provide a substrate for microreentry circuits. This hypothesis could account for the efficacy of amiodarone to blunt these arrhythmias since one of the mechanisms of action of this drug is to reduce repolarization dispersion. The arrhythmogenic potential of engrafted myotubes might be further enhanced by their capacity to generate depolarizing rebounds from which bursts of action potentials can be fired and interfere with those of host cardiomyocytes in areas where the two cell populations are not insulated by scar tissue but close enough (which is not unlikely given the patchy pattern of human infarcts) to allow electrotonic currents to be operative. Regardless of the mechanism, and even if data derived from phase I studies do not conclusively establish a causal relationship between cell transplantation and arrhythmias, in particular in a patient population particularly susceptible to this complication, it has been considered safe by most investigators to include implantation of AICDs in the protocol of phase II studies. In addition to providing protection against the potential pro-arrhythmic risk of cell grafting, the device may offer long-term survival benefits in this high-risk subset of heart failure patients while its interrogation should yield useful information about the true incidence of these arrhythmias by comparison with control placebo-injected groups.

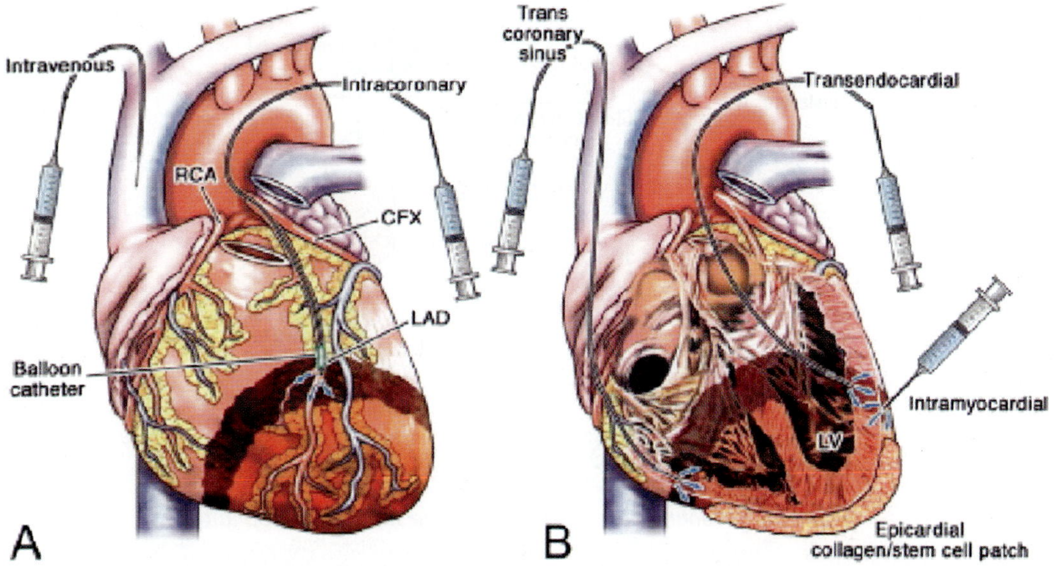

Fig. 49.10: *Various transplantation methods in heart disease (A) intracoronary and (B) intramyocardial transplantation methods in heart disease. Depicted are clinically used methods for vascular and myocardial cell delivery in cardiac intervention and cardiac surgery. CFX, circumflex artery; LAD, left anterior descending artery; LV, left ventricle; RCA, right coronary artery*

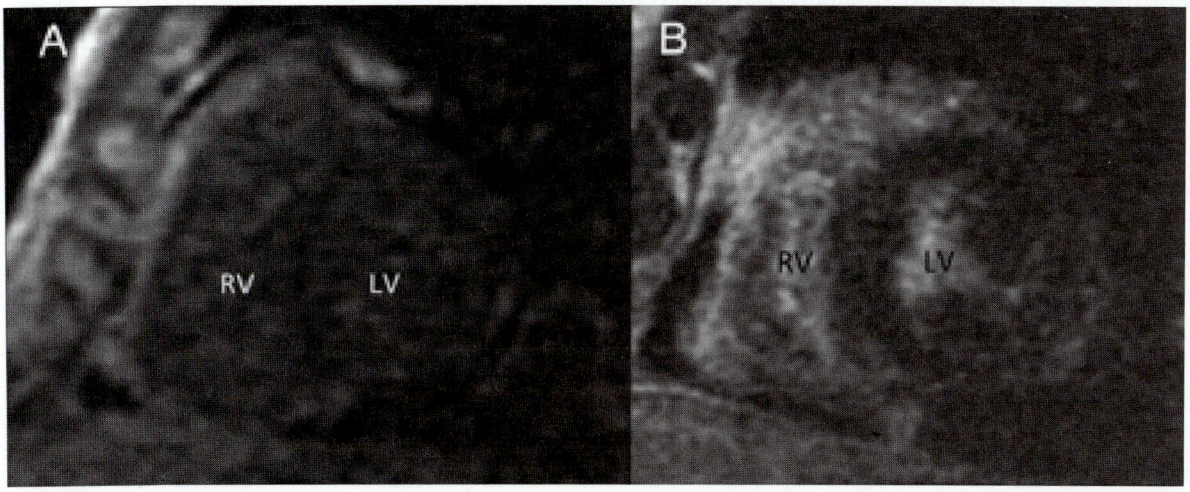

Fig. 49.11: *(A) Baseline midventricular short axis magnetic resonance imaging (MRI) obtained 10 minutes after administration of intravenous gadolinium shows diffusely abnormal nulling of the myocardium with a characteristic dark blood pool, consistent with cardiac amyloidosis. (B) Three years after stem cell transplant, postgadolinium midventricular short axis MRI image shows normal nulling of the myocardium with faint patchy areas of residual delayed enhancement. RV indicates right ventricle; LV, left ventricle*

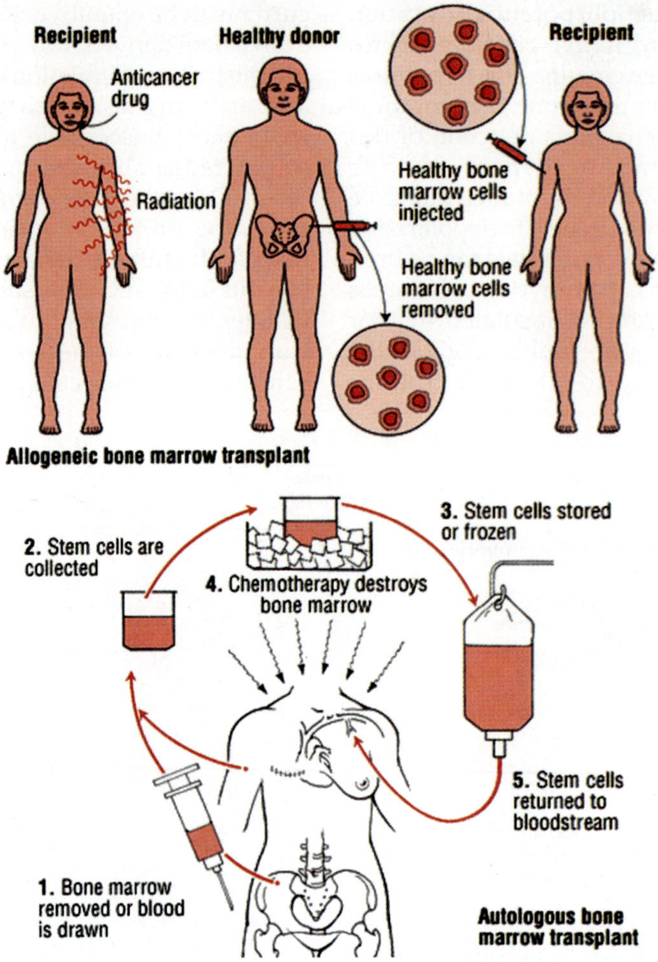

Fig. 49.12: *Technique of allogeneic bone marrow transplant*

The small number of patients operated on so far, the lack of control groups, and the confounding effect of concomitant revascularization clearly preclude any definite conclusion pertaining to the efficacy of the procedure. It is, encouraging, however, that approximately 60% of the cell-implanted scar areas demonstrated a new postoperative systolic thickening that did not deteriorate over the 1- to 2.5-year follow-up, whereas at most 10% of segments meeting their inclusion criteria (lack of contractile reserve and of metabolic viability) would have been expected to improve following bypass surgery alone. Efficacy data are more difficult to interpret in the US dose-escalating adjunct-to-bypass trial, in that the number of injected cells peaked at the relatively low value of 300 million. The same caveat applies to the series of Siminiak et al. Put together, however, these data are encouraging enough to warrant further confirmation by randomized phase II trials designed and powered so as to demonstrate efficacy if any.

Bone Marrow-Derived Cells (Figs 49.12–49.14)

The number of clinical studies of bone-marrow cell transplantation is growing tremendously, with some of them being reported in peer-reviewed journals while others are limited to isolated and anectodal cases agressively announced through Internet-mediatedpress releases. So far, surgical approaches have entailed intramyocardial implantation of bone marrow mononuclear cells or CD 133 + progenitors at the time of concomitant coronary artery bypass grafting whereas catheter-based approaches have consisted of intracoronary injections of mononuclear cells coupled with balloon angioplasty and stenting in patients with acute myocardial infarction or endoventricular stand alone injections in ischemic patients targeted for increased angiogenesis. Overall, these phase I studies should be credited for documenting the feasibility of the procedure, the apparent lack of adverse events, and the similarity of results with both blood-derived and bone marrow-derived cells. The claims for efficacy, based on improved perfusion and function, are more questionable in the absence of control randomized groups of patients, particularly if one keeps in mind the powerful placebo effect seen in end-stage ischemic heart disease-a remark equally relevant to the previously mentioned trials of skeletal myoblast transplantation. Hopefully, a forthcoming phase II trial involving intracoronary injections of bone marrow (fresh or briefly cultivated) or placebo solution in patients with acute myocardial infarction should allow more objective assessment of the expected benefits of this modality of cell therapy.

The recent observation that the majority of endothelial progenitor cells are derived from the monocyte/macrophage pathway also makes it clinically relevant to know whether injection of these cells, alone or as part of the mononuclear cell mix, carries a specific risk related to the recognized role of macrophages in atherosclerotic plaque instability and rupture.

Conclusion

Cellular transplantation appears as a promising means of "rejuvenating" infarcted myocardium through the engraftment of cells that may positively affect heart function by various mechanisms involving elastic, contractile, and paracrine effects. Although still scarce, laboratory investigations also suggest that the regenerating capacity of the transplanted cells could also be relevant to nonischemic cardiomyopathies, thereby contributing to expanding the potential for cell replacement therapy. As mentioned in this review, several basic issues remain to be addressed to better characterize the optimal cell type, define the most effective mode and timing of cell delivery, optimize graft survival and understand the mechanism(s) of action of the donor cells. In parallel, the initial encouraging efficacy data collected in a still limited number of patients need to be validated by large prospective randomized trials complying with the stringent methodologic rules commonly applied to drug trials. Only such an approach will conclusively establish whether the hopes currently raised by cellular transplantation are met, to what extent the cell-related regeneration process affects patient function and clinical outcome and, consequently, the place this novel strategy may occupy within the armamentarium of techniques designed to treat heart failure.

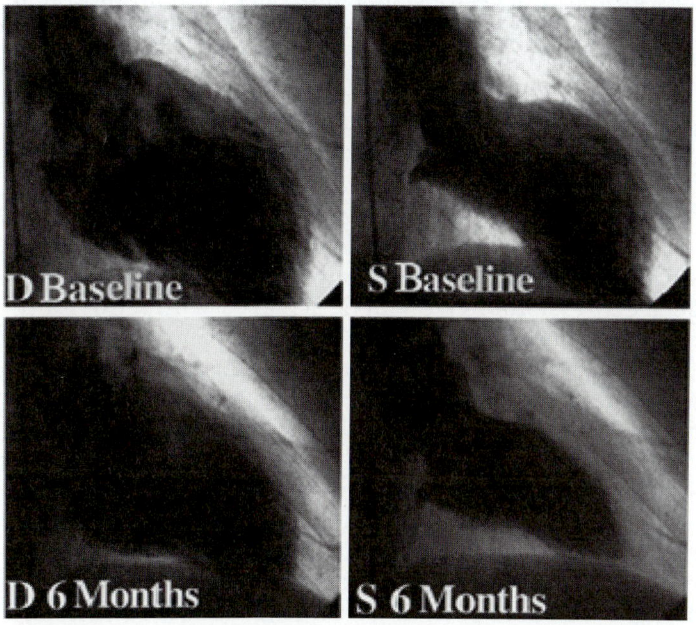

Fig. 49.13: *Ventriculography at baseline (akinesia in anterior region) and after 6 months after stem cell transplantation (with clear improvement in contractility of anterior region) for patient D indicates diastole; S, systole*

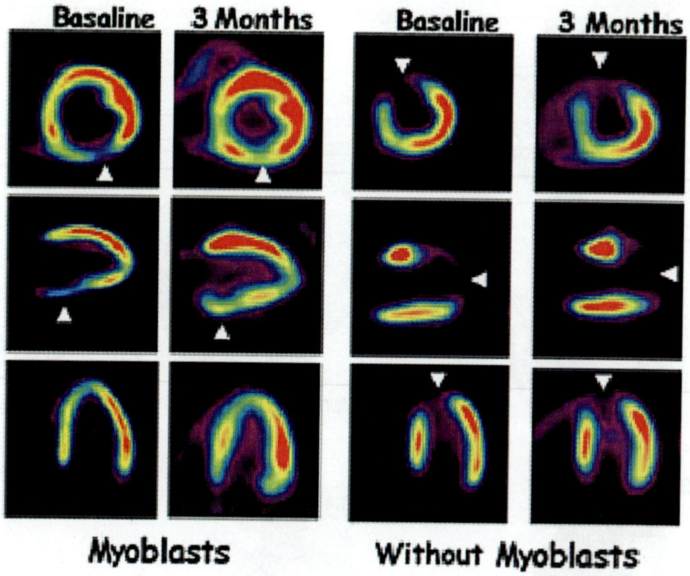

Fig. 49.14: *F-18-fluorodeoxyglucose (FDG) positron emission tomography (PET) imaging. The left-hand panel corresponds to the PET image in a postmyocardial infarction patient. The arrow heads point to a deficit of FDG uptake that would indicate an image of necrosis. At 3 months after revascularization surgery and autologous myoblasts implantation, a highly significant improvement in FDG uptake can be seen which would indicate greater viability. The right-hand panel corresponds to a patient who underwent revascularization surgery without cell transplantation and in whom improved tissue viability cannot be seen*

Three important clinical studies have been published. One entailed surgical implantation of skeletal myoblasts and reported improved functional outcomes without adverse events but interpretation of the data is confounded by the fact that the cell-transplanted segments were also concomitantly revascularized. Two other studies have looked at the effects of bone marrow derived mononuclear or mesenchymal stem cells injected directly into the coronary arteries shortly after myocardial infarction. The strength of these two trials is that they have been randomized although only the latter included a placebo-controlled group. Both have reported improvement in function and perfusion, thereby supporting the concept that these cell types may be beneficial in acutely infarcted patients undergoing concomitant revascularization of the culprit vessel. Their conclusions, however, still require validation by additional, larger-scale placebo-controlled, double-blind randomized trials.

SECTION II: GENE THERAPY FOR CARDIOVASCULAR DISEASE

The field of cardiovascular gene transfer has developed rapidly during the past 5 years. Important advances have been made in vector development, in vivo gene delivery, and definition of potential therapeutic targets. Despite substantial progress, a number of technical issues need to be addressed before gene therapy is applied safely and broadly to cardiovascular diseases. In this review, major

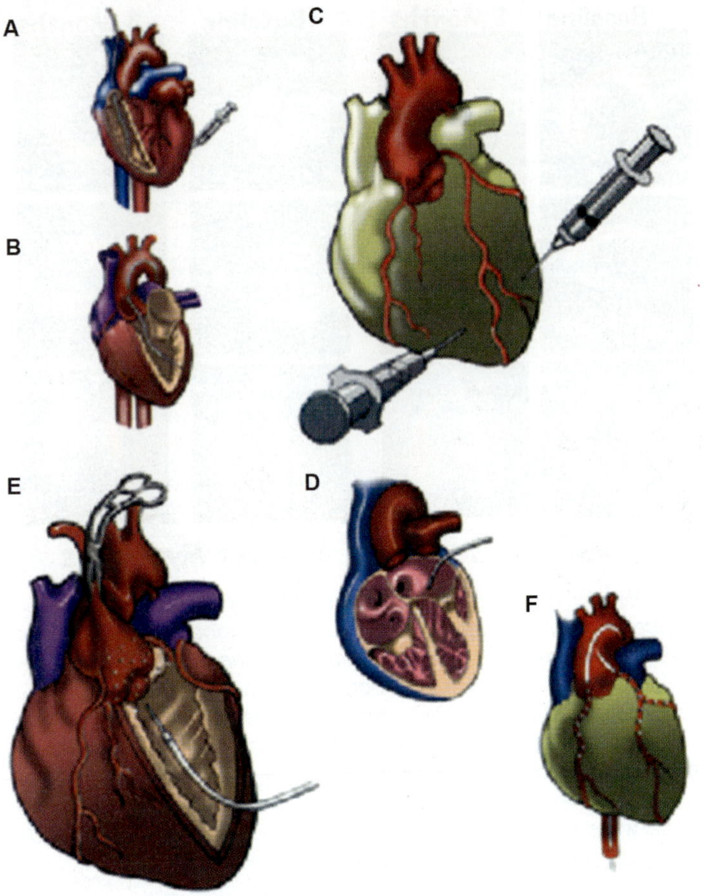

Fig. 49.15: *Direct and transvascular techniques of gene delivery. (A) Intramyocardial injection via the intracavitary catheter in right ventricle. (B) Intramyocardial injection via the intracavitary catheter in left ventricle. (C) Intramyocardial injection via the syringe. (D) Transvascular intracavitary delivery. (E) Transvascular nonselective intracoronary delivery with aortic cross-clamping. (F) Transvascular selective antegrade intracoronary delivery*

advances in cardiovascular gene transfer are summarized. In addition, technical issues required for translation of preclinical studies of gene transfer into clinical protocols are discussed (Table 49.2).

Advances in recombinant DNA technology including gene transfer, have stimulated hope that this technology can be used to improve the practice of cardiovascular medicine. Applications of this technology that affect the clinical management of patients include the development of new therapeutic products, engineered by the overexpression of genes, such as recombinant tissue-type plasminogen activator. Recombinant DNA technology has also provided techniques that have been used to create animal models of cardiovascular diseases. These models permit definition of the role of specific gene products in the pathogenesis of cardiovascular diseases. Characterization of its molecular basis has led to a more precise definition of diseases and the potential for relevant clinical treatments. The development of molecular genetic interventions to treat cardiovascular diseases depends on technical advances in the development of methods of gene delivery; achievement of long-term, highly efficient, and targeted expression to relevant cells of the cardiovascular system; and design of vectors that are safe for long-term human administration.

Methods of Gene Delivery (Figs 49.15–49.22)

The transduction and expression of genes in appropriate cell types represent important steps in the development of gene therapy. Therefore, investigations have focused on the development of methods to deliver and express genes in vascular cells and cardiac myocytes. Viral vectors (retroviruses and adenoviruses), viral conjugate vectors [adenovirus-augmented receptor-mediated vectors and hemagglutinating virus of Japan (HVJ) liposomes], and nonviral vectors (cationic liposomes, polymers, and injection of plasmid DNA) have been used. To optimize gene delivery to target cells, characteristics of the cell must be considered, such as proliferative capacity and location within the target tissue. Vascular cells (endothelial and smooth muscle cells) and cardiac myocytes differ particularly in proliferation features, and therefore different strategies have been used to transduce these cells.

Vascular Cells

Retroviral Vectors

Because vascular cells are accessible through the blood stream, percutaneous, site-specific gene delivery was developed for local arterial segments. Retroviral vectors were initially used in in vivo vascular gene transfer studies. Interest in retrovirus-mediated gene transfer was based on the use of these vectors in gene transfer to other organ systems including bone marrow stem cells, liver, and the skin, where in some target cells, these vectors transduce a large proportion of target cells. In the case of retroviral vectors, the viral vector stably integrates into chromosomal DNA of the target cell, resulting in potentially stable gene expression although integration into chromosomal DNA could potentially result in insertional mutagenesis. These vectors are most appropriate for ex vivo gene transfer for cardiovascular disease which involves removal of the relevant target cells, i.e. endothelial cells or hepatocytes from the host, transfection of the cells in vitro, and subsequent reintroduction of the modified cells into the animal or patient. It is unknown whether stable high-level gene expression in vivo will be achieved with retrovirally transduced cells (Fig. 49.17).

Several features of retroviral gene transfer may limit its application to cardiovascular medicine, particularly with respect to direct in vivo gene therapy. Replication of target cells is necessary for proviral integration. Recent studies suggest that viral integration may depend on mitosis, not just DNA synthesis. Successful retrovirus-mediated gene transfer to vascular cells may require induction of proliferation in target endothelial or smooth muscle cells, at least for short periods of time. In uninjured arteries, endothelial and smooth muscle cell proliferation occurs slowly, and therefore retroviral integration would occur at a low frequency. After vascular injury or stimulation, such as with a balloon catheter, injured vascular cells may be

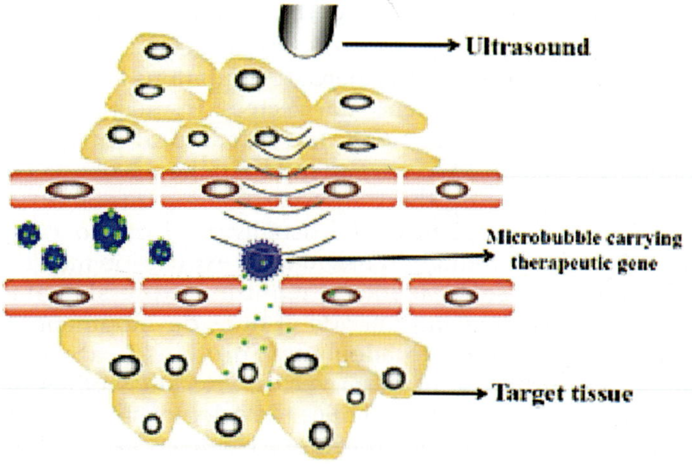

Fig. 49.16: *Schematic diagram of gene therapy mediated by UTMD. Microbubbles carrying therapeutic gene are destroyed at the site of the target tissue, resulting in sonoporation and delivery of the drug directly to the target cell. The process of sonoporation induced by ultrasound application leads to transiently holes in cell membrane and capillary, which facilitates the uptake of therapeutic gene*

transduced at higher rates. Previous studies have suggested that retroviral transduction of vascular cells can be used successfully in vivo. Limitations of this gene delivery vector include its low frequency of gene transfer and the relative lability of retroviral particles compared with other viruses. Retroviral particles are rapidly inactivated in vivo in primates, presumably by the presence of complement in serum. Because of the instability of retroviral particles and the inability of retroviruses to integrate in nonreplicating cells, retroviral vectors may have limited use for direct gene transfer in vivo although there may be a role for these vectors for ex. vivo gene transfer to vascular stents or prosthetic grafts.

Adenoviral Vectors (Table 49.1)

To improve the frequency of direct gene transfer into arteries, recent investigations have focused on adenoviral vectors. The adenovirus genome is composed of linear, double-stranded DNA of approximately 36 kb in length. The gene products are organized into early (E1–E4) and late (L1–L5) regions, based on expression before or after initiation of DNA replication. Expression of viral genes depends on cellular transcription factors and expression of the adenoviral E1 region, which encodes a transactivator of viral gene expression. The E3 region encodes viral proteins that regulate immunosurveillance in vivo. Adenoviruses have a lytic life cycle, characterized by attachment to an adenoviral glycoprotein receptor on mammalian cells and cell entry by receptor-mediated endocytosis. Adenoviruses escape degradation in lysosomes due to adenoviral capsid proteins, and viral DNA is transported to the nucleus. In the nucleus, adenoviral genome persists in an unintegrated form. During the lytic infection, viral genome replicates to several thousand copies per cell.

Adenovirus serotypes 2 (Ad-2) and 5 (Ad-5) have been developed as viral vectors for gene transfer the *E1A* and *E1B* genes from the viral genome. Vectors are produced by homologous recombination in 293 cells or any cell line that contains an integrated copy of the adenoviral *E1* gene. A foreign cDNA with eukaryotic regulatory sequences is introduced into a bacterial plasmid containing a region of the left adenoviral genome that is deleted of the *E1* gene. This plasmid is cotransfected into 293 cells with an

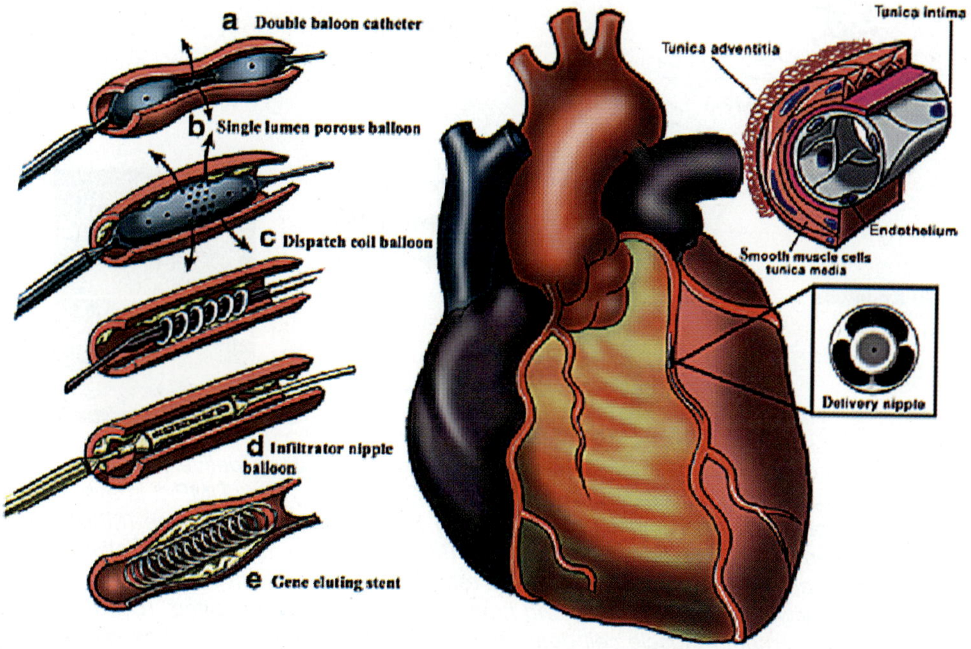

Fig. 49.17: *Different catheters and stent for transvascular intracoronary wall gene delivery*

incomplete adenoviral genome. Homologous recombination between the two DNAs generates a recombinant genome in which the *E1* gene is replaced by the foreign DNA. Viral stock is propagated in 293 cells to high titer, approximately 10 to 10 particles per milliliter.

Adenoviruses effectively infect mammalian cells including nondividing cells in vitro and in vivo. Physiological levels of recombinant proteins have been secreted into the circulation after adenoviral infection of skeletal muscle. The virus particle is relatively stable and amenable to purification and concentration at a high titer. Integration of adenoviral DNA sequences into chromosomal DNA of the target cell occurs at a low frequency, and adenoviral DNA is maintained in an extrachromosomal form. Extrachromosomal replication of the vector reduces the likelihood of mutation by random integration and dysregulation of cellular genes.

Despite these advantages, there are limitations to current, or "first-generation", adenoviral vectors. In most models, gene expression is transient after adenoviral infection, generally less than 3 weeks, and inflammation is observed in organs expressing the transgene. Gene expression in vascular cells is transient as well, usually persisting for only several weeks. Although transient gene expression may be well suited to vascular therapies requiring expression of a gene product over a short period of time, development of an immune response to adenoviral proteins is a major limitation to the use of these vectors. Recent studies in genetically defined strains of mice have demonstrated that viral proteins, expressed from the E1-deleted adenoviral

Table 49.1: *Key features of genetherapy viral vectors*

Viral vectors	*Integration*	*Long-term gene*	*Immune response*	*Comments*
Adenovirus	–	–	+	Broad tropism, easy to produce high titre stocks, widely characterised in vivo
Adeno-associated virus (AAV)	+	+	–	Limited cloning capacity, nonpathogenic, integrate randomly in the absence of the rap gene
Lentivirus	+	+	–	Retrovirus-derived, psudotyping with heterologous coat proteins improves biosafety
Retrovirus	+	+	–	Only infects dividing cells

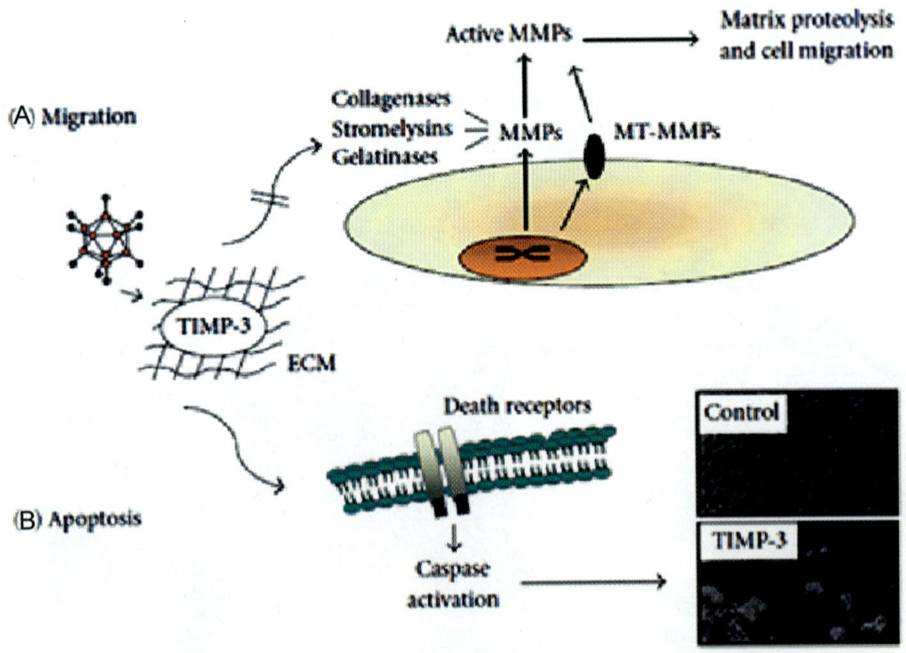

Fig. 49.18: *Gene therapy by overexpression of TIMP-3. Following Ad-mediated gene delivery to vascular smooth muscle cells, TIMP-3 is secreted and is found located with the extracellular matrix (ECM). From here, TIMP-3 is available to exert two distinctly different phenotype through its metalloproteinase inhibitory effect. (A) Matrix metalloproteinases (MMPs), including colagenases, stromelysins, gelatinases, and membrane-type metalloproteinases (MT-MMPs) are upregulated following vascular injury. TIMPs through their native MMP inhibitory activity, are able to bind to and retard pro-MMP-to-active enzyme conversion and combined with the ability to block active MMP activity, matrix proteolysis and hence cell migration is inhibited, (B) TIMP-3, uniquely amongst the TIMP family, is also able to promote smooth muscle cell death through death receptor-induced capase activation and induction of apoptosis. Micrographs courtesy of Mark Bond, Bristol heart institute, UK*

genome, are presented as foreign antigens and lead to the generation of cytolytic T lymphocytes that destroy adenovirus-infected cells. Insertion of a temperature-sensitive mutation within the E2A region of E1-deleted adenoviral vectors results in lack of expression of late viral gene products at nonpermissive temperatures, resulting in prolonged gene expression (≥ 70 days) and blunted cytolytic T-cell infiltration in mouse liver. In arterial gene transfer studies using first-generation adenoviral vectors, mononuclear cell infiltrates have been occasionally observed in the adventitia of peripheral and pulmonary arteries of pigs, but medial and intimal inflammation, necrosis, and aneurysm formation have not been observed. Further studies are required to examine the use of first-generation adenoviral vectors for vascular gene transfer studies. It is likely that further modifications in these vectors including deletions in the E2 and E4 regions and modifications in the E3 region, will diminish host immune responses.

Adenovirus-Augmented, Receptor-Mediated Gene Delivery

Viral vector conjugate systems may have application in vascular gene therapy and include adenovirus-augmented, receptor-mediated gene delivery. This vector uses inactivated adenovirus complexed to a receptor ligand to facilitate entry of DNA to a cell. This vector consists of two components. DNA condenses with polylysine, which in turn is bound to inactivated virus. The virus is coupled to a ligand such as transferrin. The transferrin ligand binds to a transferrin receptor in a cell, and the transferrin viral polylysine DNA complex enters the cell by receptor-mediated endocytosis. The inactivated adenovirus functions to disrupt lysosomes in the host cell, reducing DNA degradation and releasing DNA into the cytoplasm. The use of these vectors for vascular gene transfer is being investigated.

Cationic Liposomes

Most nonviral methods of gene transfer rely on normal mechanisms used by cells for the uptake and cellular transport of macromolecules. These methods rely on receptor-mediated endocytotic pathways or fusion of cell membranes. One example is cationic liposomes, which are positively charged artificial lipid vesicles that incorporate negatively charged DNA and deliver nucleic acid to cells through fusion with cell membranes or receptor-mediated endocytosis. Plasmid DNA is released in the cytoplasm and transported to the nucleus where it is maintained in an unintegrated form. Cationic liposomes interact spontaneously and rapidly with polyanions, such as DNA and mRNA, to form liposome complexes. Cationic liposome reagents used in vascular gene transfer studies include DOTMA/DOPE (lipofectin), DC-cholesterol, DOSPA/DOPE (lipofectamine) and DMRIE/DOPE. Expression of recombinant genes in vivo after liposomal transfection has been reported in rats, rabbits, dogs and pigs. Cationic liposomes produce more efficient gene delivery compared

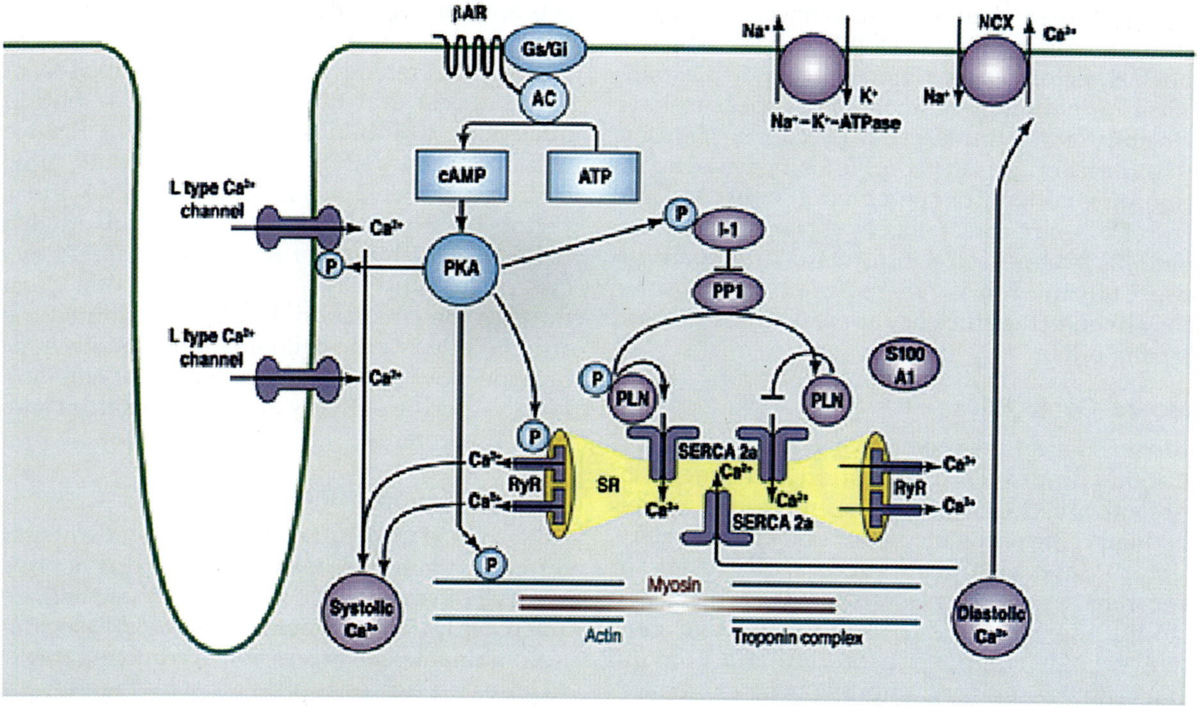

Fig. 49.19: *Excitation-contraction signaling in cardiomyocytes with emphasis on targets for gene therapy. Interplay between calcium handling (purple) and β-adrenergic (blue) systems is illustrated. AC, adenylyl cyclase; ATP, adenosine triphosphate; β-AR, beta-adrenergic receptor; I-1, (protein phosphatase) inhibitor-1; cAMP, cyclic adenosine monophosphate; Gs, stimulatory G protein; Gi, inhibitory G protein; NCX, sarcolemnal sodium/calcium exchanger; PKA, protein kinase A; PLN, phospholamban; PP, protein phosphatase; RyR, ryanodine receptor; SERCA, sarcoplasmic/endoplasmic reticulum calcium ATPase; SR, sarcoplasmic reticulum*

Table 49.2: *Gene therapy strategies for the treatment of cardiovascular disease*

Disease	*Therapeutic approach*	*Target*
Atherosclerosis	Antiatherogenic	LCAT, apoAl, apoE mRNA
Vein graft failure ischaemia, thrombosis	Diffusable/secreted gene products	VEGF, FGF, eNOS, antithrombotic agents, SOD, heme oxygenase
Vein graft failure	Inhibitors of smooth muscle cell migration/proliferation	p53, TIMPs, Rb, p21
Thrombosis	Prevention of thrombus formation	TFPI, tPA
Restenosis	Suicide genes	Tk
Hypertension	Antisene oligonucleotides	Angiotensinogen, AT_1 receptor, ACE
Vein graft failure	Decoys	Soluble VCAM, E2F
Hypertension	Reduction in blood pressure	Kallikrein, ANP, eNOS, endothelin

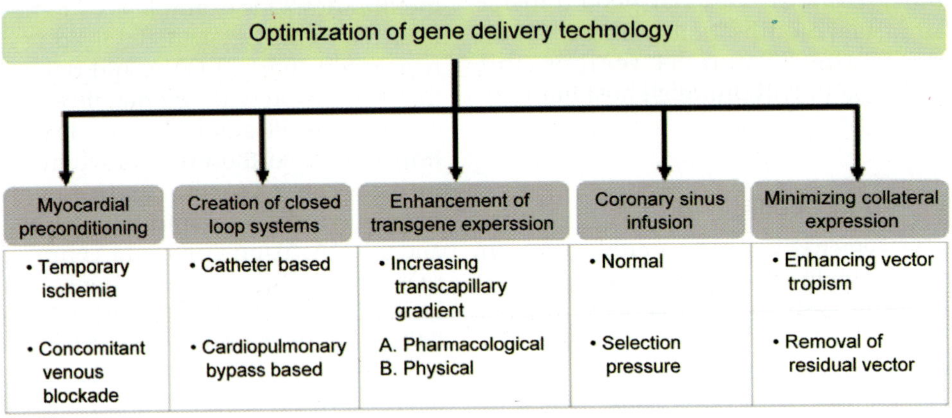

Fig. 49.20: *Optimization of gene delivery technology*

with neutrally charged or anionic liposomes, but current formulations including DOSPA/DOPE, are less efficient than adenoviral vectors. Further modifications in plasmids and chemical formulations of liposomes appear to have promise in improving transfection efficiency. Cationic liposomes have a favorable safety profile for in vivo administration. Liposome vectors contain no viral sequences, and there are no cDNA size constraints in vector construction. In addition, this vector is straightforward to prepare for clinical use. Cell division is not required for liposome transfection although the efficiency appears to be increased in proliferating cells.

HVJ Liposome Conjugates

Recent studies suggest that complexing inactivated HVJ with liposomes improves transfection efficiencies of vascular smooth muscle cells in in vitro and in vivo models of vascular injury, including the injured rat carotid artery. These vectors have also been successfully used for hepatic and renal in vivo gene transfer. It is likely that further modifications to vectors used for vascular gene transfer will include components of viral and nonviral vectors that optimize delivery, improve gene expression, and minimize toxic side effects.

Polymers

Additional strategies for the local delivery of therapeutic agents include impregnating oligonucleotides into polymer gels and applying the polymer to the external surfaces of arteries. Although pharmacokinetics of oligonucleotide delivery and retention have not been precisely defined, the data suggest that there is sufficient retention of oligonucleotide to inhibit c-*myb* and PCNA RNA expression within 24 hours after balloon injury and inhibit intimal thickening after 2 weeks. Plasmid DNA and adenoviral vectors have been applied directly to polyethylene balloons coated with a hydrogel polymer. Although there is some loss of plasmid DNA from the balloon during transit through the circulation, DNA is distributed transmurally after inflation of the balloon. Modifications in polymers to provide slow release of therapeutic agents hold promise for site-specific delivery of oligonucleotides and vectors to arterial segments.

Myocyte Gene Transfer (Fig. 49.21)

Dissection of molecular mechanisms governing myocardial differentiation has been performed in neonatal cardiac myocytes in culture, in part because these cells are relatively amenable to gene transfer with plasmid-based transfections. Recombinant gene expression in adult myocardium in vivo requires an expression vector with high-level activity in adult cardiac myocytes and a method for introducing this vector into myocardial cells. Because cardiac myocytes are terminally differentiated cells, they require a vector that is not dependent on cell replication for delivery and expression. The analysis of foreign genes within intact adult

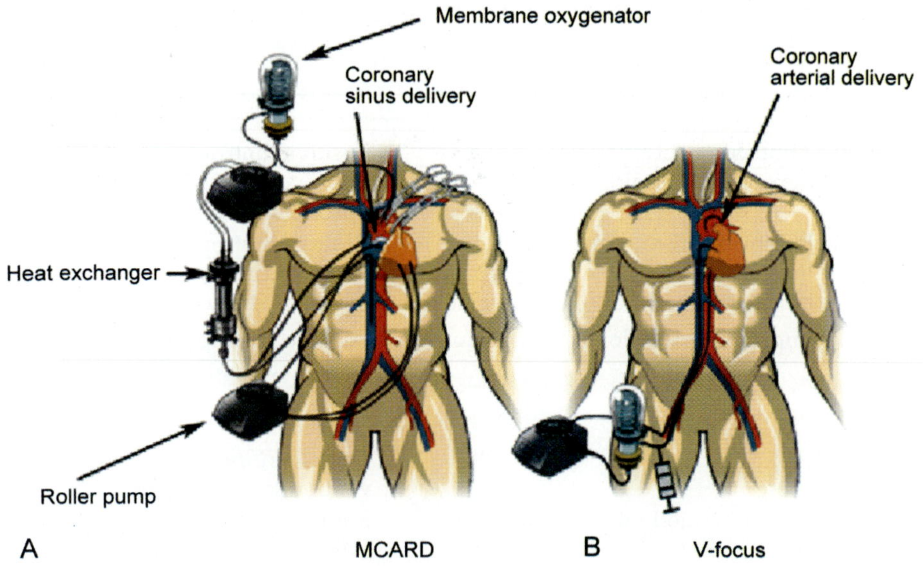

Fig. 49.21: *Closed-loop recirculatory systems. (A) Cardiopulmonary bypass-based technology e.g., molecular cardiac surgery with recirculating delivery (MCARD). After initiating systemic bypass, the vent cannulas were placed into left and right ventricles and connected to the venous limb of the circuit. The arterial limb is connected to the coronary sinus catheter. After stopping the heart with cardioplegia, recirculation commences for 20 min and then coronary circuit flashed. (B) Catheter-based technology (V-focus). Coronary venous blood was drained from the coronary sinus. Following oxygenation the blood is returned to the left main coronary artery via a roller pump. Gene of interest was delivered into the antegrade limb of the circuit. Time of recirculation is 10 min. To minimize systemic expression coronary venous blood collection continued for 2 min, and the blood was diverted to a drainage bag. Main differences between V-Focus and MCARD: (i) beating vs stopping heart; (ii) direction of recirculation (coronary arteries to coronary sinus vs coronary sinus to coronary arteries); (iii) time of recirculation (10 vs 20 min); (iv) percutaneous catheter-based methodology vs cardiopulmonary bypass-based*

myocardium has been performed by direct injection of plasmid DNA. Although direct injection of genes is a simple procedure and permits examination of the behavior of genes in vivo, this technique is limited by transfection of a small number of cells within several millimeters around the injection site. Expression of recombinant genes is temporally limited as well, with expression peaking within several weeks and declining rapidly thereafter. Episomal persistence of the introduced DNA and the postmitotic state of adult cardiac myocytes, which prevent integration of genes into chromosomes, limit stability of the transgene.

Some limitations of in vivo plasmid DNA injection have been addressed by adenoviral vectors. Adenoviruses effectively infect nonreplicating mammalian cells including skeletal and cardiac myotubes. These viruses are grown and purified in high titer. These properties result in highly efficient gene transfer into adult cardiac myocytes in vitro and in vivo. Quantitative comparisons of chloramphenicol acetyltransferase (CAT) activity resulting from injection of a CAT plasmid or an adenoviral vector encoding CAT revealed that the amount of CAT activity resulting from adenovirus infection was 10- to 100-fold higher compared with plasmid DNA. Similar findings were observed comparing adenoviral vectors and plasmids encoding *lacZ*. *Although* adenoviral vectors produce efficient gene transfer into the myocardium, expression is transient, peaking at 1–2 weeks. Acute inflammatory responses have been observed in hearts injected with adenovirus although inflammation along the injection path has also been noted after injection of plasmid DNA. Further investigations will identify factors that account for the transient nature of gene expression and will characterize potential proinflammatory effects of this vector.

Animal Models of Gene Transfer

Vascular Gene Transfer (Fig. 49.22)

In the past 5 years, there has been great interest in expressing recombinant DNA and other nucleic acids in blood vessels in vivo. The goals of these studies have been to define gene function and to develop new therapeutic strategies for vascular diseases.

The feasibility of direct gene transfer to arteries in vivo was demonstrated using viral (retrovirus) and nonviral (liposomes) vectors in several animal species, including pigs, rabbits, and dogs. These studies reported a low efficiency of gene transfer, generally 1% or less of vascular cells in vivo. More recent studies have suggested that the efficiency of gene transfer into arteries can be improved with adenoviral vectors; increased expression of reporter genes has been reported in sheep, rat, rabbit and pig vessels. Endothelial cells of normal arteries and endothelial and smooth muscle cells in injured arteries have been transduced at efficiencies approximately 10- to 100-fold higher than reported for retroviral and liposome vectors. A major limitation to adenoviral gene transfer in

Table 49.3: *Potential gene therapy targets for heart failure*

System	*Gene*	*Mechanism*	*Outcome*	*Clinical trials*
β-adrenergic system	β2–AR	Increases a denylyl cy activity	Positive inotropic effect	No
	GRK2	Abolishing GRK2 reverses agonist-dependent desnsitization of β-ARs	Positive inotropic effect and improved ventricular remodeling (inconsistent results)	No
	ACVI	Full mechanism remains unclear Increases cAMP generating capacity improves phosphorylation of cTnI	Positive inotropic effect Improved ventricular remodeling reduced apoptosis	No
Ca^{2+} cycling	SERCA2a	Improves cytosloic Ca^{2+} regulation	Positive inotropic effect Improved ventricular remodeling Decreased oxygen cost of LV contractility Decreased incidence of ischemic ventricular arrhythmias	h process
	PLN	PLN inhibition relieves inhibitory effect on SERCA2a expression	Improved systolic and diastolic function (inconsistent results)	No
	I–1	Inhibits PP1 leading to phosphorylation of PLN and increased	Positive inotropic effect improves diastolic function Ameliorates sichemia/reperfusion induced injury	No
	S100A1	Enhances the activity of ryanodine receptors and SERCA2a	Positive inotropic effect Improved ventricular remodeling	No
Cell death	Bcl-2	Enhances cell survival	Antiapoptotic and positive inotropic effect in ischemia/reperfusion	No
	I-1, S100 A1	Regulation of calcium handling and decreased endoplasmic reticulum stress	Anti-apoptotic effect	No
	β2–AR	Gi-mediated pathway	Anti-apoptotic effect	No

the vasculature has been transient expression; in most studies, expression of reporter gene has been observed for 7 to 14 days and is diminished or lost by 28 days. Lack of persistence of gene expression may result from cytolytic responses directed against infected cells. Transient gene expression, however, may be desirable for vascular diseases, like restenosis after angioplasty, which are characterized by cellular proliferation peaking in the first several weeks after arterial injury.

Several observations concerning the delivery of recombinant genes and patterns of gene expression can be drawn from these studies. Infusion of vector into normal arteries with an intact endothelium results in transfection of intimal cells (primarily endothelial cells). Injury to the vessel and/or application of pressure to the vector infusate results in delivery of DNA transmurally and gene expression in the media. Several catheters have been used in gene transfer studies including double-balloon catheters, porous balloon catheters, and hydrogel catheters, and the patterns of gene expression within an artery may differ depending on the design of the catheter, animal species, and type of artery transduced.

Direct gene transfer has been used to create somatic transgene models to define gene function in arteries. In this system, genes can be expressed within arterial segments, and their biological function can be investigated. This approach has proved useful for investigation of genes whose direct in vivo effects have been difficult to analyze. For example, transfection of a recombinant angiotensin-converting enzyme gene into rat arteries using HVJ liposomes promotes angiotensin II–mediated vascular hypertrophy. After transfer of a recombinant endothelial cell-type nitric oxide (NO) synthase (ec-NOS) gene into balloon-injured rat carotid arteries, NO production was associated with a reduction in intimal thickening. Gene transfer approaches have also proved useful in the analysis of atrial natriuretic peptide, type 2 angiotensin II receptor, and VCAM-1.

Growth factors and cytokines stimulate vascular cell proliferation and vessel formation in vivo. Although the genes encoding many factors have been cloned and their mechanism of action defined in vitro, definition of their role in vivo has been more difficult to analyze. Several recombinant growth factor genes including platelet-derived growth factor–B (PDGF-B), a secreted form of acidic fibroblast growth factor[1] (FGF-1), and an active form of transforming growth factor-$^{2}{}_{1}$ (TGF-$^{2}{}_{1}$) have been expressed by direct gene transfer in porcine arteries, and the function of these gene products has been analyzed. Expression of a PDGF-B gene in porcine arteries stimulated intimal

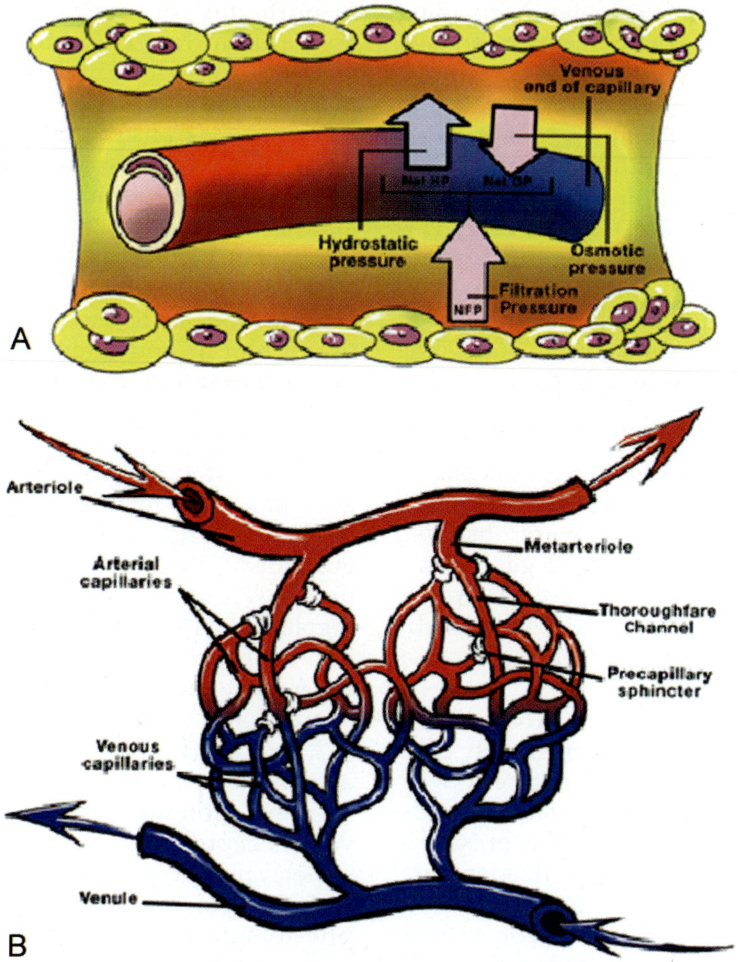

Fig. 49.22: *(A) The movement of fluid between capillaries and the interstitial fluid. The direction of fluid with vector movement across the capillary wall depends on the difference between two opposing forces: hydrostatic and osmotic pressure. With retrograde perfusion, hydrostatic pressure increases at the venous end of the capillaries and therefore gene filtration and transduction are also increased. (B) Coronary capillary net. After the tissue has been perfused through the coronary sinus, capillaries join to become arterioles and metarterioles which return blood to the aorta. A capillary net consist of two types of vessels: true capillaries which provide exchange between cells and thoroughfare (shunts) channels which directly connects the arterioles and venules. Precapillary sphincters are rings of smooth muscles at the origin of arterial capillaries that regulate blood flow through a tissue. The advantage of the retrograde delivery is its ability to overcome the resistance of precapillary sphincters proximally located on the arterial side of the capillary bed. Thus, less blood is shunted through the thoroughfare channels into the cardiac chambers*

hyperplasia characterized by smooth muscle cell proliferation. Synthesis and secretion of FGF-1 were associated with expansion of the intima as well as intimal angiogenesis. Arteries transfected with a TGF-$^{2}_{1}$ gene demonstrated increased procollagen synthesis in the intima and media as early as 4 days after gene transfer compared with control arteries transfected with a reporter gene. Although these recombinant genes stimulate vascular cell proliferation in vivo, they exert otherwise distinct effects on smooth muscle cell proliferation, angiogenesis, and extracellular matrix formation. These studies suggest that intimal thickening may represent a common response to gene expression of multiple growth factors, which in turn exert different effects on vessel repair.

Another approach to investigating the pathogenesis of vascular cell proliferation in vivo is to examine gene products that inhibit cell proliferation. Local delivery of an antiproliferative agent during the peak of smooth muscle cell proliferation or extracellular matrix synthesis after balloon injury might limit expansion of the intima. Several approaches have been explored in this setting, including recombinant chimeric toxins, antisense oligonucleotide strategies, and gene transfer.

One approach to the selective elimination of dividing cells is to express a herpes virus thymidine kinase (HSV-tk) gene in smooth muscle cells after balloon injury. Thymidine kinase, when expressed in transduced cells, converts ganciclovir, a nucleoside analogue, into an active toxic form, and subsequent incorporation of phosphorylated ganciclovir into cellular DNA induces chain termination in dividing cells, causing cell death. A bystander effect, demonstrated in smooth muscle and endothelial cells, confers susceptibility to ganciclovir in neighboring dividing cells, leading to inhibition of cell growth in nontransduced neighboring cells as well. Adenoviral vectors encoding a HSV-tk gene or no cDNA insert were introduced into porcine arteries immediately after balloon injury, and a course of ganciclovir or saline was initiated. Three weeks after balloon injury and adenoviral infection, a significant reduction in intima-to-media area ratios (54–59%) was observed. A reduction in intimal BrdC (5-bromodeoxycytosine) incorporation of 40% was observed in HSV-tk ganciclovir-treated animals compared with HSV-tk saline-treated animals 7 days after gene transfer, indicating that inhibition of smooth muscle cell proliferation contributed to this effect. A significant reduction in intima-to-media area ratios in the HSV-tk ganciclovir-treated animals was observed 6 weeks after treatment, suggesting that the decrease in intimal hyperplasia was stable. In addition, no major systemic toxicities were observed associated with adenoviral infection and ganciclovir treatment. These data suggest that expression of an enzyme that catalyzes the formation of a cytotoxic drug locally within an artery may limit smooth muscle cell proliferation after balloon injury.

In balloon-injured rat carotid arteries, introduction of adenoviral vectors encoding HSV-tk immediately after balloon injury or 7 days later and treatment with ganciclovir also result in significant reductions in intima-to-media area ratios. Reendothelialization was present in rat and porcine arteries infected with HSV-tk adenoviral vectors and treated with ganciclovir, and significant toxicities were not observed in treated arteries or systemic organs. Additional approaches to limiting smooth muscle cell proliferation after vascular injury include targeting of nuclear cell cycle regulatory pathways, including the retinoblastoma gene product (Rb). Studies in injured rat carotid and porcine femoral artery models suggest that expression of a nonphosphorylatable, constitutively active form of Rb after adenoviral infection limits intimal smooth muscle proliferation for at least 3 weeks after vascular injury.

Myocardial Gene Transfer

(Figs 49.15, 49.17 and Table 49.3)

Recent exciting developments hold promise for transduction of adult myocytes in vivo. Initial studies demonstrated the feasibility of expression of reporter genes in rat and canine myocardium by direct injection of plasmid DNA, but these studies were limited by low efficiencies that hindered investigations of gene expression in myocytes. The observation that adenoviruses infect nondividing cells has heightened interest in these vectors for gene transfer to adult myocardium. Indeed, recent studies have demonstrated higher levels of gene expression in rat myocardium after direct injection of adenovirus vectors compared with injection of plasmid DNA alone. Adult myocardium in vivo has also been transduced by intravascular administration of adenoviral vectors encoding reporter genes. Gene expression was observed in both the coronary vasculature and the adjacent myocardium. Levels of gene expression in the myocardium were 10- to 50-fold higher compared with direct DNA plasmid injection. Although adenoviral vectors provide efficient gene transfer, gene expression in the myocardium is transient. In most studies, reporter gene expression peaked at 1 week, diminished at 2 weeks, and was present at low levels after 1 month in adult myocytes. The mechanisms for loss of gene expression including immune responses, are not completely understood.

Gene transfer to the myocardium has proven to be a useful tool in understanding cardiac gene regulation in vivo. For example, transcriptional elements regulating basal and thyroid hormone-responsive cardiac ±-myosin heavy chain (±-MHC) gene expression in adult rat hearts in vivo have been studied; sequences upstream of the rat ±-MHC gene-linked to a luciferase reporter were injected into adult rat hearts, and thyroid hormone responsiveness was evaluated. The thyroid hormone-responsive element was necessary, but not sufficient, to confer positive and negative regulation of thyroid hormone. Direct injection of constructs into the myocardium is a model system for investigating DNA elements and regulatory pathways that control gene expression and growth in the heart.

An additional promising area is the direct injection of adenoviral vectors into skeletal muscle for production of secreted proteins. Myoblasts, transduced by retroviral vectors expressing human growth hormone, injected into skeletal muscle produced physiological levels of human growth hormone in the serum. Recent studies suggest that physiological levels of recombinant erythropoietin are secreted into the circulation after intramuscular injection of adenovirus into skeletal muscle of neonatal mice or adult SCID mice. Neonatal and adult SCID mice injected once with 10 to 10 plaque-forming units demonstrated significant dose-dependent elevations in serum human erythropoietin levels and increased hematocrit levels that were stable over the 4-month time course of the experiments, and no evidence of a localized inflammatory response or systemic infection was present. Intramuscular injection of adenoviral vectors may be useful for the treatment of inherited disorders of deficient serum proteins.

Lipoprotein Metabolism

Direct gene transfer has been a promising tool for investigations of hepatic regulation of lipoprotein metabolism. Initial approaches used ex vivo transduction of hepatocytes to express an LDL receptor (LDLR). Hypercholesterolemia in the Watanabe rabbit was reversed after infusion of LDLR-expressing hepatocytes into the liver. This approach has been used in a human gene therapy trial of familial hypercholesterolemia. Recently, adenoviral vectors have been used to reconstitute LDLR function in Watanabe rabbits and in homozygous mice lacking LDLRs produced by homologous recombination. In this latter study, adenoviral vectors encoding a human LDL cDNA were injected intravenously into the tail vein of mice, and the hypercholesterolemic effects of the LDLR deficiency were reversed at 4 days. Adenoviral targeting to hepatocytes has also been demonstrated in healthy mice, where transient gene expression was observed.

Hepatic chylomicron remnant uptake has been studied by adenovirus-mediated gene transfer. The hypothesis that LDLR-related protein (LRP) mediates the uptake of dietary lipoprotein into hepatocytes in concert with LDLR was tested by transferring a dominant negative regulator of LRP function into livers of homozygous mice lacking LDLR. Inhibition of LRP was associated with accumulation of chylomicron remnants in these mice, suggesting a role for LRP and LDLR in chylomicron remnant clearance. Intravenous injection of an adenoviral vector encoding an apolipoprotein A-I gene results in transient hepatic production of HDL and total cholesterol. These studies demonstrate the usefulness of genetically engineered animal models for the study of lipoprotein metabolism.

BIBLIOGRAPHY

1. Yoo KJ, Li RK, Weisel RD, Mickle DA, Jia ZQ, Kim EJ, Tomita S, Yau TM. Heart cell transplantation improves heart function in dilated cardiomyopathic hamsters. Circulation 2000; 102(suppl III):III-204–III–209.
2. Scorsin M, Hagege AA, Dolizy I, Marotte F, Mirochnik N, Copin H, Barnoux M, Ie Bert M, Samuel JL, Rappaport L, Menasche P. Can cellular transplantation improve function in doxorubicin-induced heart failure? Circulation. 1998; 98(suppl 11):11-151–11-156.
3. Herreros J, Prosper F, Perez A, Gavira JJ, Garcia-Velloso MJ, Barba J, Sanchez PL, Canizo C, Rabago G, Marti-Climent JM, Hernandez M, Lopez-Holgado N, Gonzalez-Santos JM, Martin-Luengo C, Alegria E. Autologous intramyocardial injection of cultured skeletal mus-cle-derived stem cells in patients with non-acute myocardial infarction. Eur Heart J. 2003; 24:2012–2020.
4. Wollert KC, Meyer GP, Lotz J, Ringes-Lichtenberg S, Lippolt P, Breidenbach C, Fichtner S, Korte T, Hornig B, Messinger D, Arseniev L, Hertenstein B, Ganser A, Drexler H. Intracor-onary autologous bone-marrow cell transfer after myocardial infarction: the BOOST randomi-sed controlled clinical trial. Lancet. 2004; 364:141–148.
5. Chen SL, Fang WW, Ye F, Liu YH, Qian J, Shan SJ, Zhang JJ, Chunhua RZ, Liao LM, Lin S, Sun JP. Effect on left ventricular function of intracoronary transplantation of autologous bone marrow mesenchymal stem cell in patients with acute myocardial infarction. Am J Cardiol 2004; 94:92–95.
6. Ma N, Stamm C, Kaminski A, Li W, et al. Human cord blood cells induce angiogenesis following myocardial infarction in NOD/scid-mice. Cardiovascular Research. 2005;66(1):45–54.
7. [10]Hu CH, Wu GF, Wang XO et al. Transplanted human umbilical cord blood mononuclear cells improve left ventricular function through angiogenesis in myocardial infarction. Chin Med J (Engl). 2006;119(18):1499–506.
8. Ma N. Ladilov Y, Kaminski A, Piechaczek C. Stamm C. Umbilical cord blood cell transplantation for myocardial regeneration. Transplant Proc. 2005;38(3):771–3.
9. J, Guetta E, Feinberg MS et al. Human umbilical cord blood-derived CD133+ cells enhance function and repair of the infarcted myocardium. Stem Cells. 2006;24(3):772–80.
10. Henning RJ, Abu-Ali H, Balis JU, Morgan MB, Willing AE, Sanberg PR. Human umbilical cord blood mononuclear cells for the treatment of acute myocardial infarction. Cell Transplant. 2004;13(7–8):729–39.
11. Cheng F, Zou P, Handong Y. Induced differentiation of human cord blood mesenchymal stem/progenitor cells into cardiomyocyte-like cells in vitro. J Huazong Univ Sci and Tech. 2003;23(2):154–157.
12. Nishiyama N, Miyoshi S, Hida N, et al. The significant cardiomyogenic potential of human umbilical cord blood-derived mesenchymal stem cells in vitro. Stem Cells. 2007;25(8):2017–24.
13. Bonanno G, Mariotti A, Procoli A, et al. Human cord blood CD133+ cells immunoselected by a clinical-grade apparatus differentiate in vitro into endothelial- and cardiomyocyte-like cells. Transfusion. 2007;47(2):280.
14. Yamada Y, Yokoyama S, Fukuda N, et al. A novel approach for myocardial regeneration with educated cord blood cells cocultured with cells from brown adipose tissue. Biochem Biophys Res Commun. 2007;353(1):182.
15. Nabel EG, Plautz G, Boyce FM, Stanley JC, Nabel GJ. Recombinant gene expression in vivo within endothelial cells of the arterial wall. Science.1989;244:1342–1344.
16. Wilson JM, Birinyi LK, Salomon RN, Libby P, Callow AD, Mulligan RC. Implantation of vascular grafts lined with genetically modified endothelial cells. Science. 1989;244: 1344–1346.
17. Hock RA, Miller AD. Retrovirus-mediated transfer and expression of drug resistant genes in human haematopoietic progenitor cells. Nature.1986;320:275–277.
18. Wilson JM, Jefferson DM, Chowdhury JR, Novikoff PM, Johnston DE, Mulligan RC. Retrovirus-mediated transduction of adult hepatocytes. Proc Natl Acad Sci U S A. 1988;85:3014–3018.
19. Garver RI Jr, Chytil A, Courtney M, Crystal RG. Clonal gene therapy: transplanted mouse fibroblast clones express human ±1- antitrypsin gene in vivo. Science. 1987;237:762–764.
20. Cone RD, Mulligan RC. High-efficiency gene transfer into mammalian cells: Generation of helper-free recombinant retrovirus with broad mammalian host range. Proc Natl Acad Sci U S A. 1984;81:6349–6353.
21. Grossman M, Raper SE, Kozarsky K, Stein EA, Engelhardt JF, Muller D, Lupien PJ, Wilson JM. Successful ex vivo gene therapy directed to liver in a patient with familial hypercholesterolaemia. Nat Genet. 1994;6:335–341.
22. Miller DG, Adam MA, Miller AD. Gene transfer by retrovirus vectors occurs only in cells that are actively replicating at the time of infection. Mol Cell Biol. 1990;10:4239–4242.
23. Roe TY, Reynolds TC, Yu G, Brown PO. Integration of murine leukemia virus DNA depends on mitosis. EMBO J. 1993;12:2099–2108.
24. Flugelman MY, Jaklitsch MT, Newman KD, Casscells W, Bratthauer GL, Dichek DA. Low-level in vivo gene transfer into the arterial wall through a perforated balloon catheter. Circulation. 1992;3:1110–1117.
25. Cornetta K, Moen RC, Culver K, Morgan RA, McLachlin JR, Sturm S, Selegue J. Amphotropic murine leukemia retrovirus is not an acute pathogen for primates. Hum Gene Ther. 1990;1:15–30.
26. Graham FL, Prevec L. Adenovirus-based expression vectors and recombinant vaccines. In: Ellis RW, ed. Vaccines: New

Approaches to Immunological Problems. Boston, Mass: Butterworth-Heinemann; 1992:363–390.

27. Berkner KL. Expression of heterologous sequences in adenoviral vectors. Curr Top Microbiol Immunol. 1992; 58: 39–66.
28. Tripathy SK, Goldwasser E, Lu MM, Barr E, Leiden JM. Stable delivery of physiological levels of recombinant erythropoietin to the systemic circulation by intramuscular injection of replication-defective adenovirus. Proc Natl Acad Sci USA. 1994;91:11557–11561.
29. Simon RH, Engelhardt JF, Yang Y, Zepeda M, Weber-Pendleton S, Grossman M, Wilson JM. Adenovirus-mediated transfer of the CFTR gene to lung of nonhuman primates: toxicity study. Hum Gene Ther. 1993;4:771–780.
30. Engelhardt JF, Simon RH, Yang Y, Zepeda M, Weber-Pendleton S, Doranz B, Grossman M, Wilson JM. Adenovirus-mediated transfer of the CFTR gene to lung of nonhuman primates: biological efficacy study. Hum Gene Ther.1993;4:759–769.
31. Gerard RD, Herz J. Adenovirus-mediated low density lipoprotein receptor gene transfer accelerates cholesterol clearance in normal mice. Proc Natl Acad Sci USA. 1993;90:2812–2816.
32. Zabner J, Petersen DM, Puga AP, Graham SM, Couture LA, Keyes LD, et al. Safety and efficacy of repetitive adenovirus-mediated transfer of CFTR cDNA to airway epithelia of primates and cotton rats. Nat Genet. 1994;6:75–83.
33. Lemarchand P, Jones M, Yamada I, Crystal RG. In vivo gene transfer and expression in normal uninjured blood vessels using replication-deficient recombinant adenovirus vectors. Circ Res. 1993;72:1132–1138.
34. Guzman RJ, Lemarchand P, Crystal RG, Epstein SE, Finkel T. Efficient and selective adenovirus-mediated gene transfer into vascular neointima. Circulation. 1993;88:2838–2848.
35. Lee SW, Trapnell BC, Rade JJ, Virmani R, Dichek DA. In vivo adenoviral vector-mediated gene transfer into balloon-injured rat carotid arteries. Circ Res. 1993;73:797–807.
36. Barr E, Carroll J, Kalynych AM, Tripathy SK, Kozarsky K, Wilson JM, Leiden JM. Efficient catheter-mediated gene transfer into the heart using replication-defective adenovirus. Gene Ther. 1994;1:51–58.
37. .Muller DWM, Gordon D, San H, Yang ZY, Pompili VJ, Nabel GJ, Nabel EG. Catheter-mediated pulmonary vascular gene transfer and express. Circ Res. 1994;75:1039–1049.
38. Yang Y, Nunes FA, Berencsi K, Furth EE, Gonczol E, Wilson JM. Cellular immunity to viral antigens limits E1-deleted adenoviruses for gene therapy. Proc Natl Acad Sci USA. 1994;91:4407–4411.
39. Engelhardt JF, Ye X, Doranz B, Wilson JM. Ablation of E2A in recombinant adenoviruses improves transgene persistence and decreases inflammatory response in mouse liver. Proc Natl Acad Sci USA. 1994;91:6196–6200.
40. Ohno T, Gordon D, San H, Pompili VJ, Imperiale MJ, Nabel GJ, Nabel EG. Gene therapy for vascular smooth muscle cell proliferation after arterial injury. Science. 1994;265:781–784.

50 Robotic-Assisted Cardiac Interventions

The Minimally Invasive Cardiac Surgery was invented by Francis Duhaylongsod, a Filipino heart surgeon in Hawaii. The first minimally invasive heart cardiac surgery was performed in the United States on January 21, 2005 at The Heart Institute at Staten Island University Hospital in Staten Island, New York by a team led by Dr Joseph T McGinn. This technique is an off-pump coronary artery bypass surgery. The procedure is much less invasive than traditional bypass surgery because it is performed through three small incisions rather than the traditional sternotomy. Since its first procedure, over 600 MICS-CABG procedures have been performed at The Heart Institute amongst many more around the world.

Minimally invasive heart surgery (also called keyhole surgery) is performed through small incisions, sometimes using specialized surgical instruments. The incision used for minimally invasive heart surgery is about 3–4 inches instead of the 6- to 8-inch incision required for traditional surgery.

Selection of Patients for Minimally Invasive or Robotic Surgery

Your surgeon will review the results of your diagnostic tests before your scheduled surgery to determine if you are a candidate for a minimally invasive or robotic surgery technique. The surgical team will carefully compare the advantages and disadvantages of these techniques with those of traditional surgery (Fig. 50.1).

The type of treatment recommended for your condition depends on several factors including the type and severity of heart disease, age, medical history and lifestyle.

The Procedure

MICS-CABG is performed through one window incision that stretches 5–7 cm in the 4th intercostal space (ICS). In some cases, the thoractomy may be necessary in the 5th ICS instead. A soft tissue refractor is used to allow for greater visibility and access.

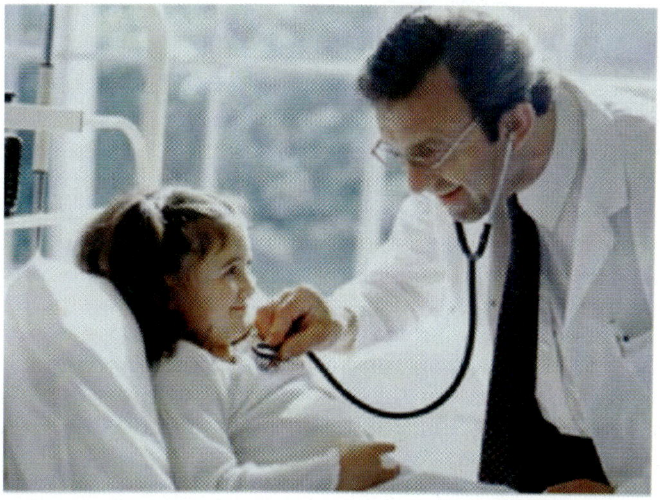

Fig. 50.1: *A young child is being examined by the cardiac surgeon for cardiovascular fitness prior to robotic heart surgery*

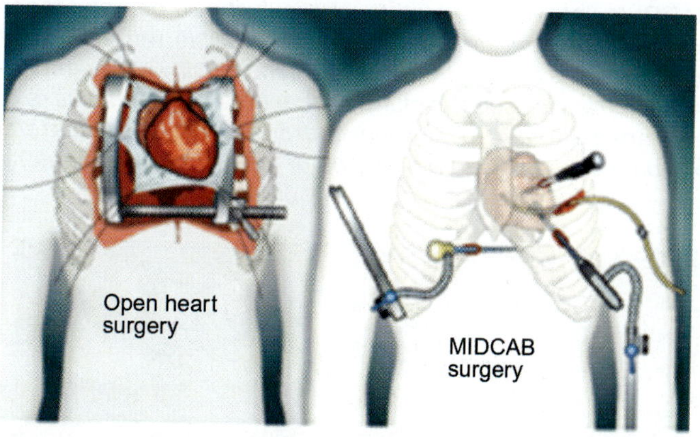

Fig. 50.2: *Cardiac surgeons are operating on the heart (right) through tiny openings in the chest, eliminating the need for sternotomy—a large incision through the breastbone (sternum). This method of surgery, called minimally invasive cardiac surgery, is a remarkable improvement over traditional, open-chest procedures (left)*

Two access incisions are also made at the 6th intercostal space and xphoid process to allow for operative Medtronic® instruments to pass through.

The McGinn Technique (Proximal Anastomoses)

(Figs 50.2–50.7)

The McGinn Proximal Technique is performed with blood pressure lowered to 90–100 systolic which reduces stress to the aorta, reducing the risk of damage. A series of tools are used to position and stabilize vessels. The technique uses devices developed by Medtronic® to support the surrounding heart tissues while vital surgery takes place. The devices are managed externally and access the heart through small incisions between the ribs.

Pump-Assisted Beating Heart Bypass

A cannula with a pump and vacuum action is fed up through an artery in the groin to reduce the stress on the heart so that it may still function during the operation. This pump flows at 2–3L per minute to support circulation and eliminates the need for a heart-lung bypass machine.

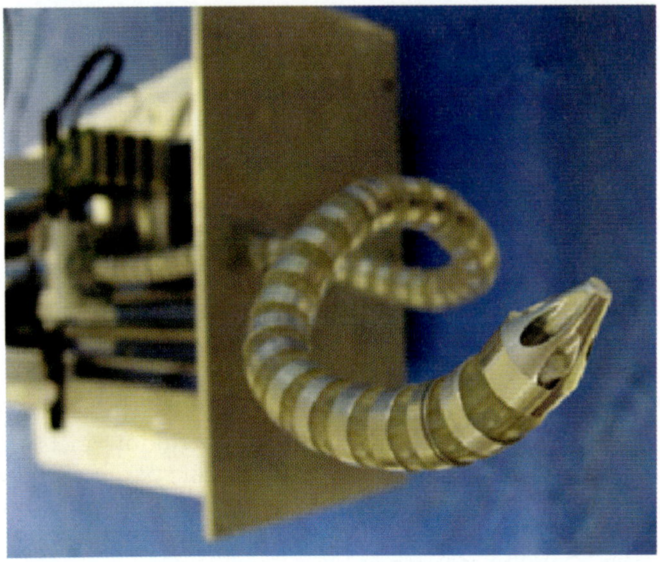

Fig. 50.3: *Serpentine robots in heart surgery. Robotic probe (HARP) to enter the thorax through a subxiphoid port and reach regions of the pericardium that are inaccessible with traditional techniques. It is believed that HARP's functionality will eventually lead to application such as multiple intrapericardial therapies (e.g. cell transplantation by intramyocardial injection, epicardial ablation, epicardial lead placement for resynchronization, etc)*

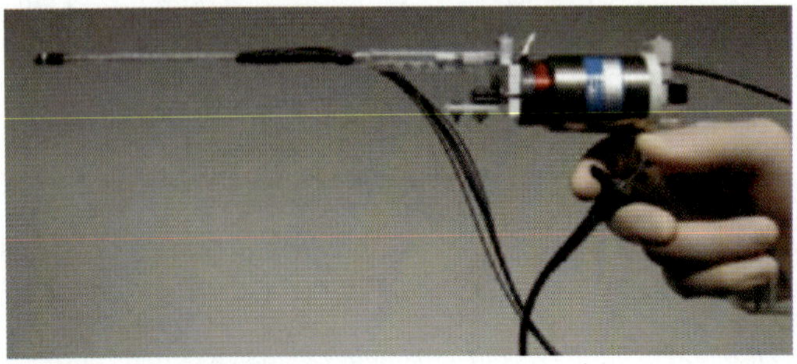

Fig. 50.4: *Biorobotics and its role in minimal-invasion cardiac surgery (Image courtesy of Harvard SEAS)*

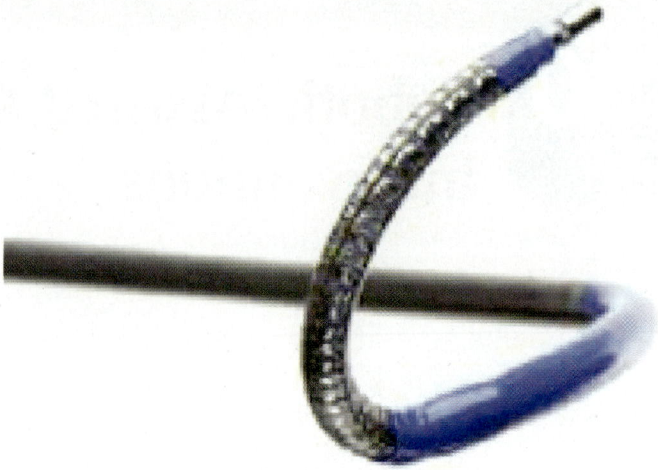

Fig. 50.5: *Hansen medical's robotic catheter control system for EP study*

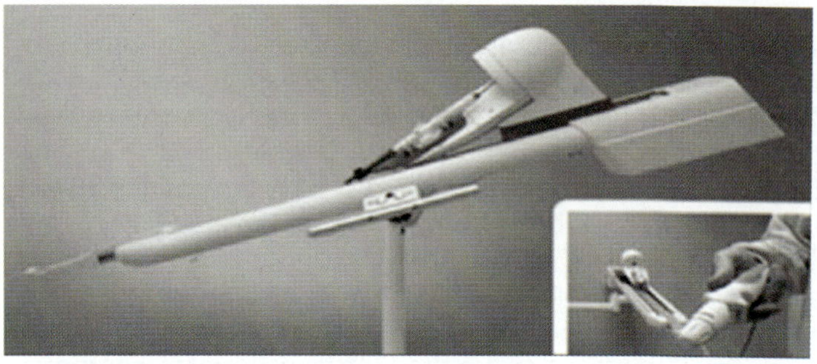

Fig. 50.6: *World's first remote heart rhythm treatment procedure using a robotic arm. The world's first remote robotic heart rhythm treatment procedure was conducted at the University Hospitals of Leicester. It was performed using the catheter robotics remote catheter manipulation system. A patient with atrial fibrillation had a catheter ablation controlled by a robotic arm while the cardiologist—sitting in a separate room—used remote control to steer the catheter endovascularly into the heart*

ROBOTICALLY ASSISTED HEART SURGERY

Robotically assisted heart surgery, also called closed-chest heart surgery, is a type of minimally invasive surgery. The cardiac surgeon uses a specially designed computer console to control surgical instruments on thin robotic arms. Robotically assisted technology allows surgeons to perform certain types of complex heart surgeries with smaller incisions and precise motion control, offering patients excellent outcomes. In robotic surgery, small incisions—less than 2 inches—are used, compared with the 3- to 4-inch incision used in traditional minimally invasive heart surgery.

Types of Robotically Assisted Heart Surgeries

1. Robotic-assisted CABG

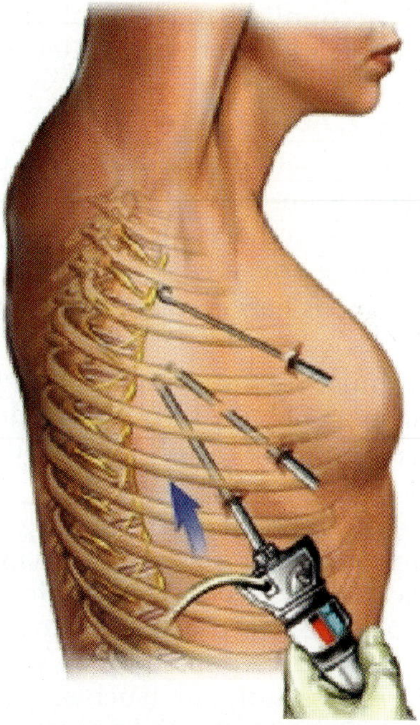

Fig. 50.7: *Sites of incisions endoscopes practiced in an operation theatre in conducting robotic valve heart surgery*

2. Robotic assisted coronary angioplasty (Fig. 50.13)
3. Mitral valve repair and replacement surgery
4. Tricuspid valve repair and replacement surgery
5. Combined mitral and tricuspid valve surgery
6. Ablation of atrial fibrillation
7. Atrial septal defect (ASD) and PFO repair
8. Removal of cardiac tumors
9. Lead placement (Figs 50.22 and 50.23)
10. Robot implant.

Benefits of Minimally Invasive Surgical Techniques

The benefits of minimally invasive and robotic heart surgery techniques include:

1. Small incisions (Figs 50.2 and 50.7)
2. Small scars
3. *Shorter hospital stay after surgery:* The average stay is 3–5 days after minimally invasive surgery, while the average stay after traditional heart surgery is 7–10 days.
4. Low risk of infection
5. Low risk of bleeding and blood transfusion
6. Shorter recovery time and faster return to normal activities/work:

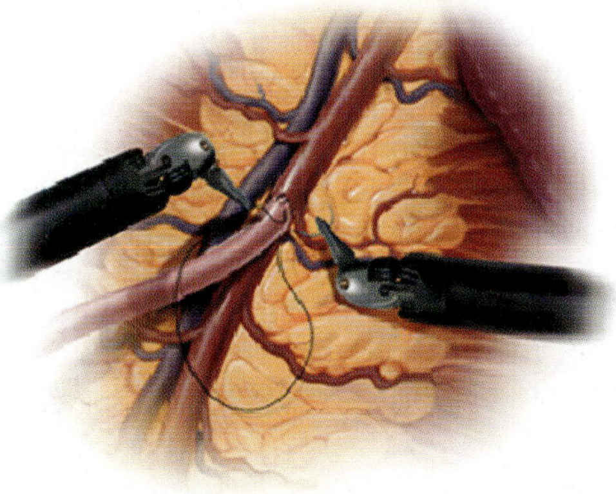

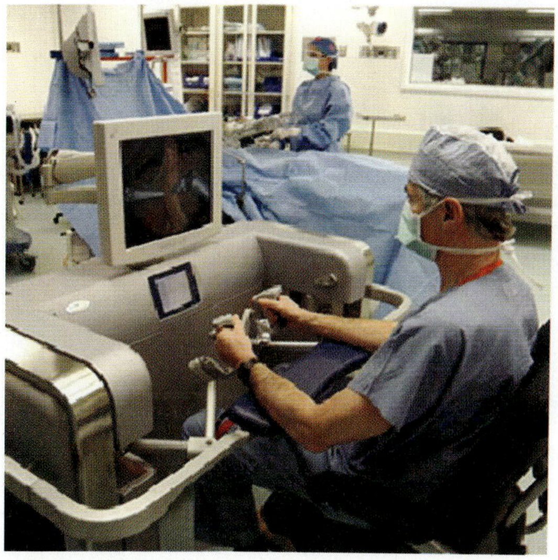

Fig. 50.8: *Robotic arms are performing coronary bypass with robot-assisted heart surgery, In this procedure, a surgeon controls small surgical instruments attached to robotic arms*

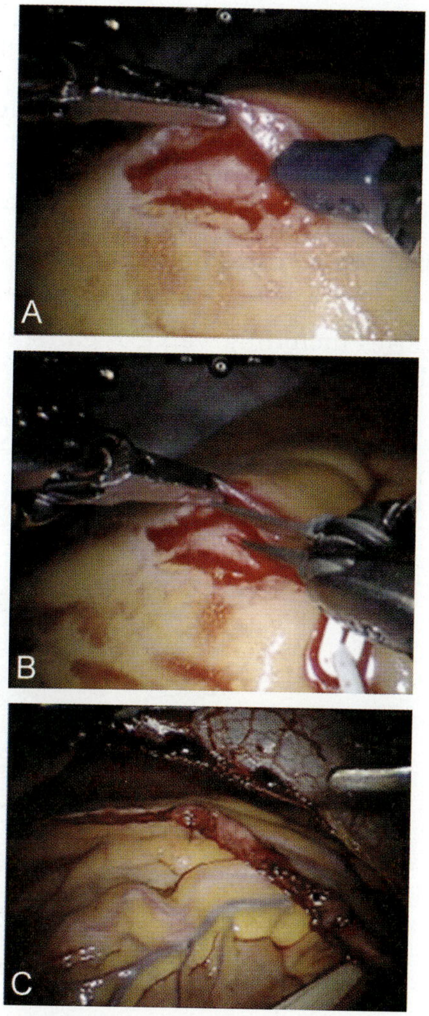

Fig. 50.9: *(A) Opening of coronary with endoscopic knife. (B) Coronary arteriotomy with endoscopic Pott scissors. (C) Final result in robotic coronary bypass surgery*

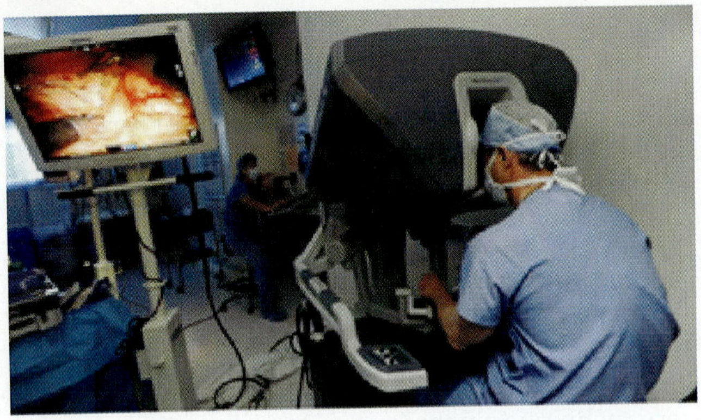

Fig. 50.10: *Surgeon is operating on patient with the help of the da Vinci's arms through the system's console (right)*

The average recovery time after minimally invasive surgery is 1–4 weeks while the average recovery time after traditional heart surgery is 6–8 weeks. The recovery time and return to regular activities is shorter for patients who undergo robotically assisted heart surgery.

Division of the breastbone is not needed for robotically assisted heart surgery.

Important note: Not everyone is a candidate for these surgical techniques. Your surgeon will review the results of your diagnostic tests before your scheduled procedure to determine if you are a candidate for minimally invasive surgery. The surgical team will carefully compare the advantages and disadvantages of minimally invasive techniques versus traditional surgery techniques.

Types of Minimally Invasive Heart Surgeries

Minimally Invasive Valve Surgery

Valve surgeries including valve repairs and valve replacements, are the most common type of minimally invasive surgery, accounting for 87% of all minimally invasive cardiac surgeries performed at Cleveland Clinic.

Minimally Invasive CABG Surgery

Minimally invasive direct coronary artery bypass graft (MIDCABG) surgery is an option for some patients who require a left internal mammary artery bypass graft to the left anterior descending artery.

Saphenous (leg) vein harvest also may be performed using small incisions.

Several techniques for minimally invasive CABG surgery are being explored at Cleveland Clinic including surgeries performed on a beating (off-pump) or nonbeating (on-pump) heart.

Off-pump/beating heart bypass surgery allows surgeons to perform surgery on the heart while it is still beating. A medication may be given to slow the heart during surgery, but the heart keeps beating during the procedure. This type of surgery may be an option for patients with single-vessel disease (such as disease of the left anterior descending artery or right coronary artery).

Traditionally, CABG surgery is performed using a heart-lung bypass machine. This machine allows the heart's beating to be stopped, so the surgeon can operate on a surface that is blood-free and still. The heart-lung bypass machine maintains life despite the lack of a heartbeat, removing carbon dioxide from the blood and replacing it with oxygen before pumping it around the body.

During off-pump/beating heart surgery, the heart-lung machine is not used. The surgeon uses advanced operating equipment to stabilize (hold) portions of the heart and bypass the blocked artery in a highly controlled operative environment. Meanwhile, the rest of the heart keeps pumping and circulating blood to the body.

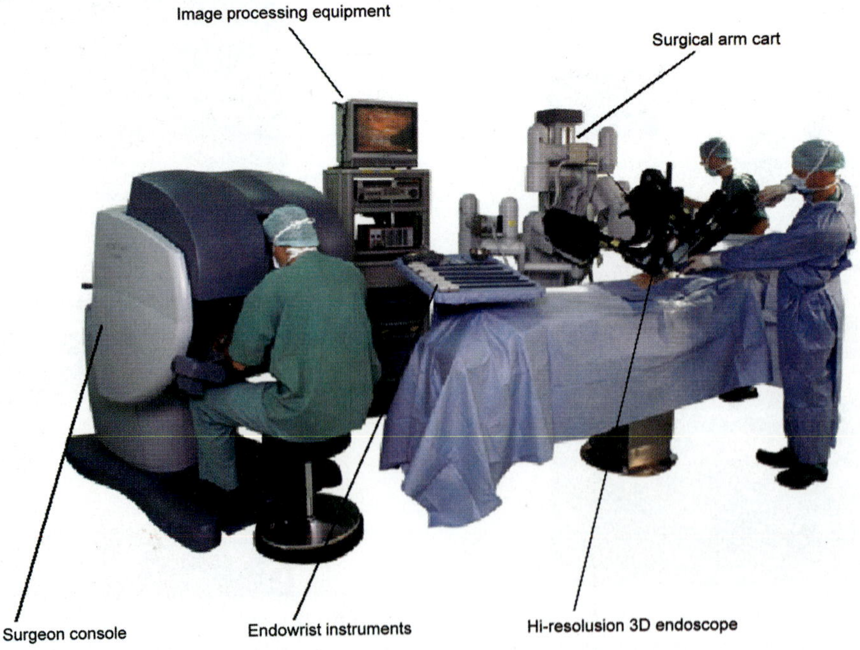

Fig. 50.11: *Different equipments in a operation theatre utilized in conducting robotic heart surgery*

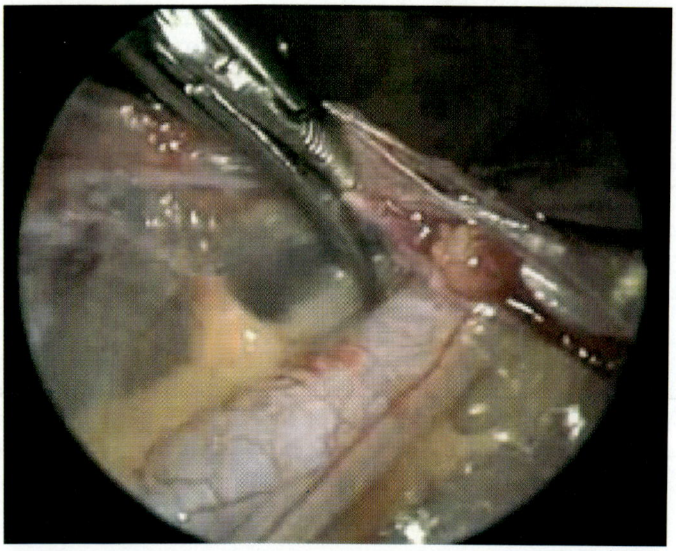

Fig. 50.12: *Videoscopic photograph taken from one of the patients undergoing robotic heart surgery*

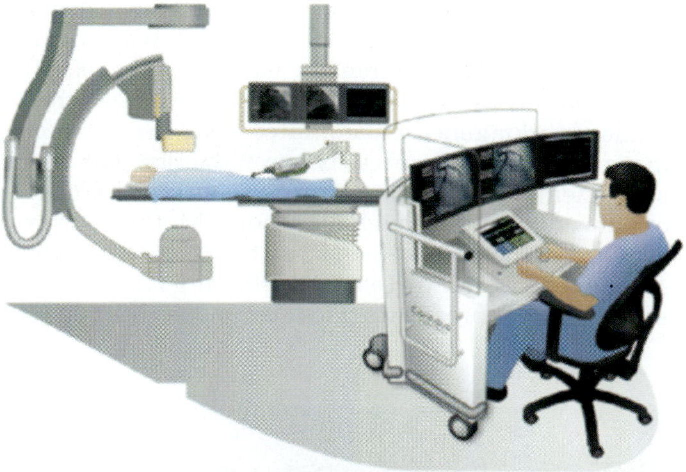

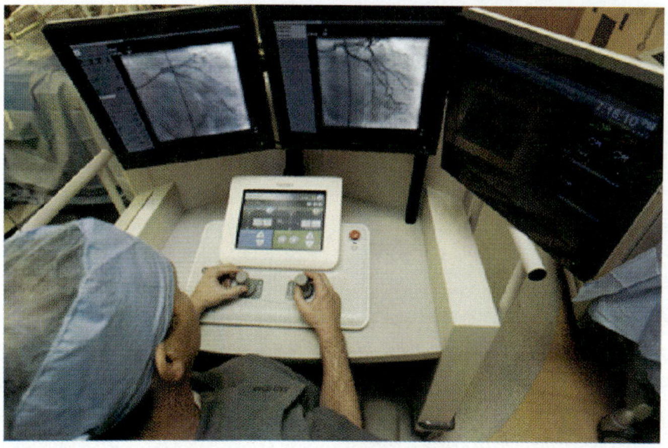

Fig. 50.13: *The method of performing robot-assisted coronary angioplasty*

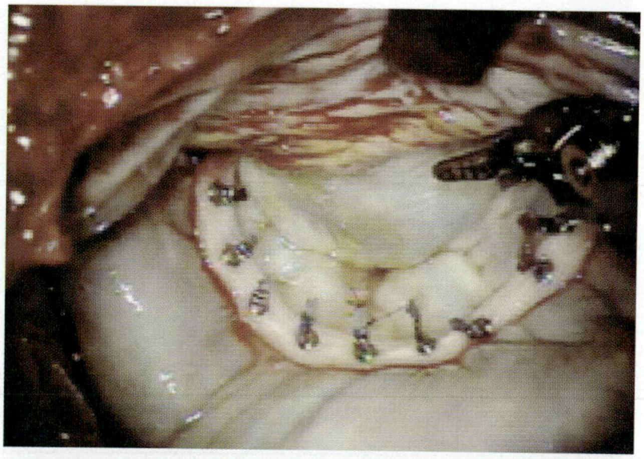

Fig. 50.14: *Intraoperative view of a competent mitral valve repaired using robotic assistance*

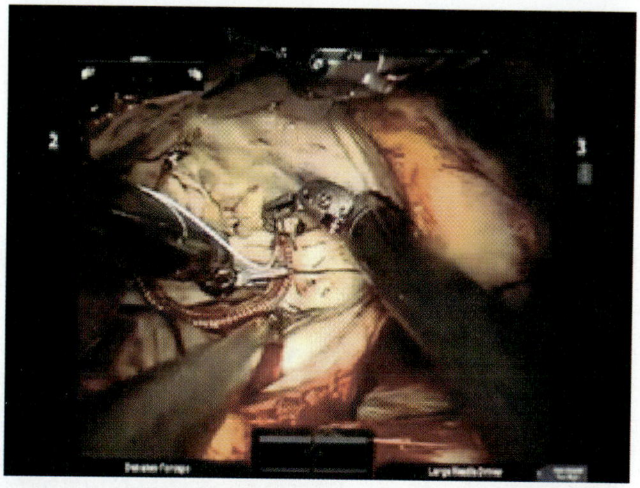

Fig. 50.15: *Robotic-assisted mitral and tricuspid valve repair*

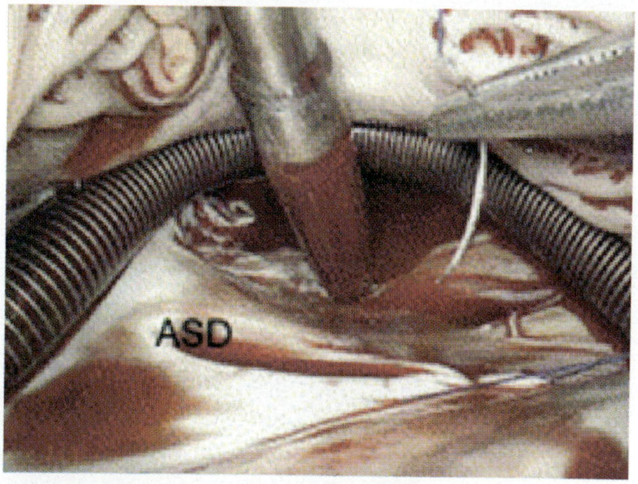

Fig. 50.16: *An intraoperative view of atrial septal defect (ASD) that was closed by sutures*

Types of Robotically Assisted Heart Surgeries

Robotically Assisted CABG Surgery (Figs 50.10–50.12)

Robotically assisted CABG surgery can be performed without opening the sternum (breastbone). Robotically

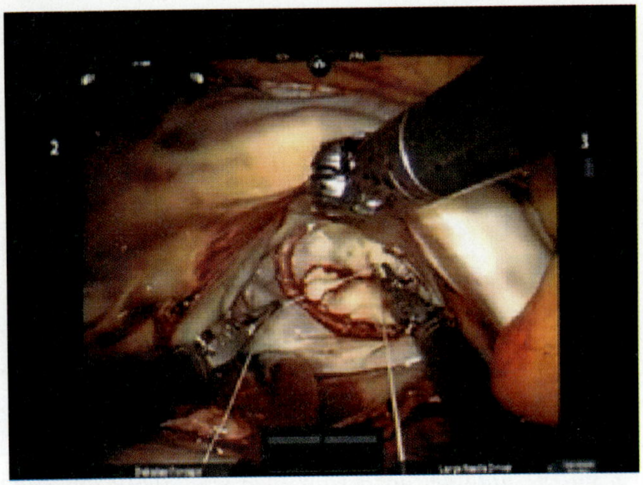

Fig. 50.17: *Robotic repair of mitral valve and PFO closure*

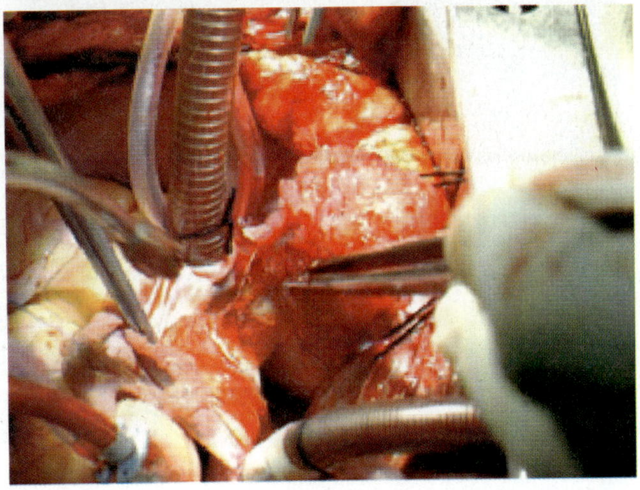

Fig. 50.18: *Intraoperative robotic surgery showing LA myxoma on stalk*

assisted CABG surgery also can be performed "off pump," which means the surgery can be performed on a beating heart, without using the heart-lung bypass machine.

Robotically Assisted Valve Surgery (Figs 50.14 and 50.15)

Robotically assisted mitral valve repair can be used to treat mitral valve regurgitation. Tricuspid valve surgery also can be performed using the robotically assisted surgical technique (Figs 50.2, 50.8, 50.9 and 50.15).

Robotically Assisted ASD and PFO Repair

Robotically assisted atrial septal defect (ASD) and patent foramen ovale (PFO) repair surgeries can be performed using a robotically assisted approach. Robotic instruments are used to harvest a small patch of pericardial tissue (the sac that surrounds the heart). The patch is then sutured (sewn) over the defect (Fig. 50.16).

Robotically Assisted Removal of Cardiac Tumors

The most common benign tumor of the heart is a myxoma, which most frequently occurs in the left atrium. This type of tumor increases the risk of stroke. Removal of these tumors almost always cures the problem and greatly reduces the risk of stroke. During the robotically assisted tumor removal procedure, the surgeon's hands control the movement and placement of the endoscopic instruments through small incisions in the chest wall, and the instruments are used to remove the tumor (Fig. 50.18).

Robotically assisted heart surgery is performed through a small working incision and three small incisions (ports) that are made in the spaces between the ribs. The surgical instruments (attached to the robotic arms) and one tiny camera are placed through these ports. Motion sensors are attached to the robotic "wrist", so the surgeon can control the movement and placement of the surgical instruments to perform the procedure (Figs 50.2 and 50.12).

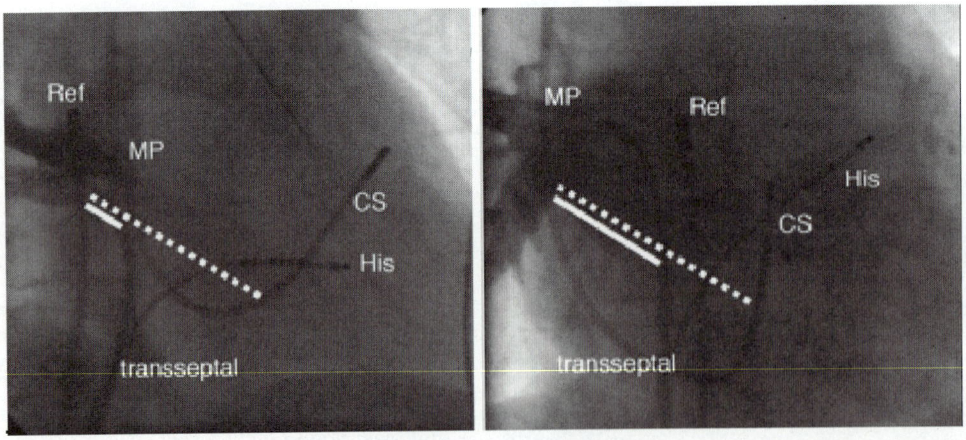

Fig. 50.19: *Remote robotic navigation and electroanatomical mapping for ablation of atrial fibrillation selective angiographies of the RIPV (RAO 30°). The distance between the anterior border of the RPV ostium and the coronary sinus catheter (dCS, dotted line) and the transseptal puncture site (dTS, full line) were measured. The left panel shows a patient with a posterior transseptal puncture (ratio dCS:dTS, 0.12). The right panel shows a patient with an anteromedial transseptal puncture (ratio dCS:dTS, 0.68). CS, coronary sinus catheter; His, multipolar catheter at the His bundle; Ref, Reference catheter on the back of the patient; MP, multi-purpose catheter for angiography*

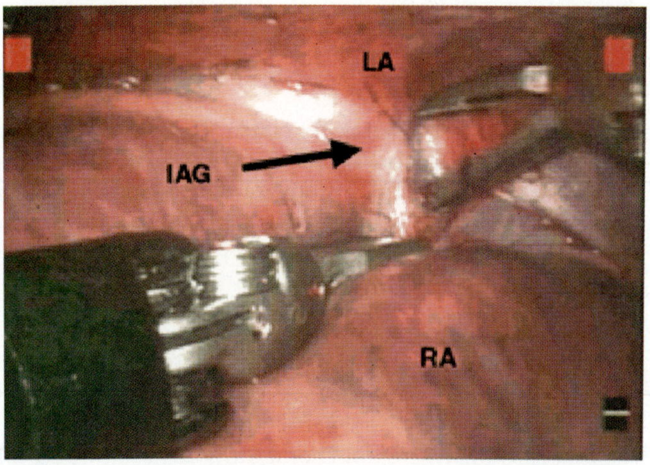

Fig. 50.20: *Atrial fibrillation. Robot-assisted ablation of the PVs Opening of the transverse and oblique sinus was performed robotically. Opening of the pericardial reflections between the superior right PV and the superior caval vein, and between the inferior right PV and the inferior caval vein, and development of the interatrial groove were also performed robotically*

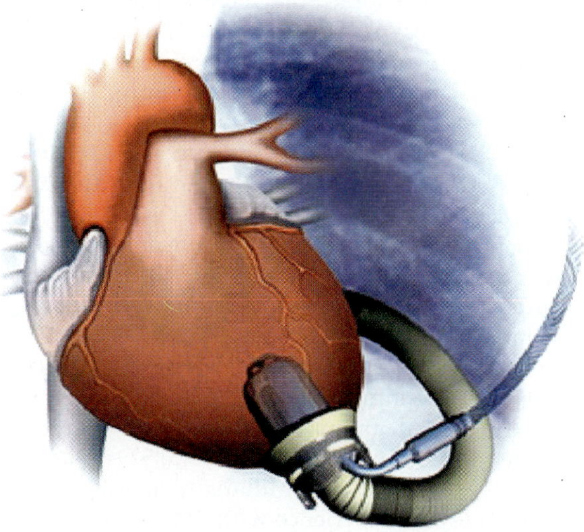

Fig. 50.21: *This type of robot implant is to be used on a permanent basis rather than a more common temporary artificial heart*

During robotically assisted surgery, the sternum (breastbone) does not need to be opened to perform the procedure. Depending on the technique, the surgeon may choose to perform surgery on a "beating heart", in which case the patient is not placed on the heart-lung bypass machine (this is called "off-pump" surgery).

In comparison, traditional valve and CABG surgery involve using the heart-lung bypass machine to circulate the patient's oxygenated blood during surgery and stopping the heart in order to stabilize the blood vessels; creating a 6- to 8-inch incision through the sternum; and spreading the ribs to view the heart.

Robotically Assisted Atrial Fibrillation Surgery

During the robotically assisted ablation procedure for atrial fibrillation (an irregular heart rhythm that begins in the upper chambers of the heart), the surgeon's hands control the movement and placement of the endoscopic instruments to open the pericardium (thin sac that surrounds the heart). The instruments are used to precisely place the catheter for ablation, in which energy is applied to correct the abnormal heart rhythm (Figs 50.19 and 50.20).

Robotically Assisted Device Implant for Heart Failure (Fig. 50.21)

During the robotically assisted biventricular pacemaker or defibrillator implant procedure, the surgeon's hands control the movement and placement of the endoscopic instruments through small incisions in the chest wall. This surgical technique can be used to place leads on the surface of the left ventricle. The leads then are attached to the biventricular device (defibrillator or pacemaker) to "resynchronize" the heartbeat and improve heart failure symptoms.

Patient's Health after Surgery

You may feel some discomfort at the incision site after surgery. You can take medications to help to relieve this discomfort. Ask your doctor which medication you should take for pain relief. If you have discomfort in your chest

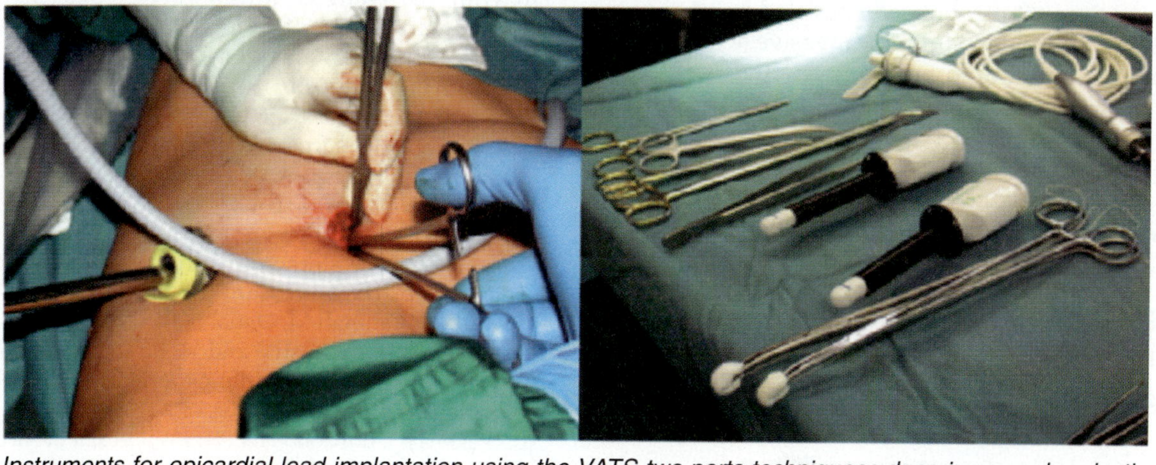

Fig. 50.22: *Instruments for epicardial lead implantation using the VATS two ports techniqueas done in resynchronization therapy in chronic heart failure*

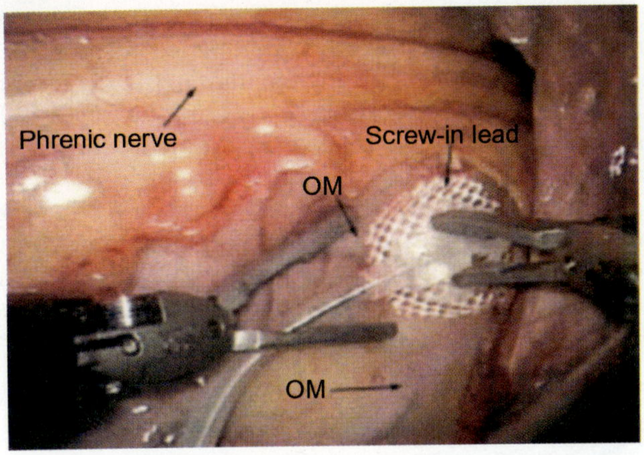

Fig. 50.23: *Robot-enhanced thoracoscopic approach may provide greater maneuverability in placement of an LV pacing lead on the lateral wall through small chest wall incisions*

that is similar to the symptoms you had before your surgery, call your doctor.

Recovery of Patient after Surgery

Patients who have minimally invasive or robotic surgery may be able to go home 2–5 days after surgery. Your healthcare team will follow your progress and help you recover as quickly as possible.

Your healthcare team will provide specific instructions for your recovery and return to work including guidelines for activity, driving, incision care and diet.

Recovery after Minimally Invasive Heart Surgery

In general, you may be able to return to work (if you have a sedentary job), resume driving and participate in most nonstrenuous activities within 1–4 weeks after traditional minimally invasive heart surgery. You can resume heavy lifting and other more strenuous activities within 5–8 weeks after surgery. Your healthcare team will provide specific guidelines based on your rate of recovery.

Recovery after Robotically Assisted Heart Surgery

The recovery time after robotically assisted heart surgery is shorter than traditional minimally invasive heart surgery. Most patients can resume normal activities, drive and return to work as soon as they feel up to it—usually within 2–4 weeks after surgery. Your healthcare team will provide specific guidelines based on your rate of recovery.

Recovery for All Patients after Heart Surgery

To maintain your cardiovascular health after surgery, we strongly encourage you to make lifestyle changes and take your medications as prescribed. Heart-healthy lifestyle changes that are important to your recovery include:

- Quitting smoking
- Treating high cholesterol
- Managing high blood pressure and diabetes
- Exercising regularly

BIBLIOGRAPHY

1. Cohn LH. Fifty years of open-heart surgery. Circulation. 2003;107(17):2168–2170.
2. Cosgrove DM, 3rd, Sabik JF, Navia JL. Minimally invasive valve operations. Ann Thorac Surg. 1998;65(6):1535–1538.
3. Kronzon I, Matros TG. Intraoperative echocardiography in minimally invasive cardiac surgery and novel cardiovascular surgical techniques. Am Heart Hosp J. 2004;2(4):198–204.
4. Gammie JS, Zhao Y, Peterson ED, O'Brien SM, Rankin JS, Griffith BP. Less-invasive mitral valve operations trends and outcomes from the society of thoracic surgeons adult cardiac surgery database. Ann Thorac Surg. 2010;90:1401–1410.
5. Iribarne A, Russo MJ, Easterwood R, et al. Minimally invasive versus sternotomy approach for mitral valve surgery: a propensity analysis. Ann Thorac Surg. 2010;90(5):1471–1477.
6. Iribarne A, Karpenko A, Russo MJ, et al. Eight-year experience with minimally invasive cardiothoracic surgery. World J Surg. 2010;34(4):611–615.
7. Schmitto JD, Mokashi SA, Cohn LH. Minimally-invasive valve surgery. J Am Coll Cardiol. 2010;56(6):455–462.
8. Navia JL, Cosgrove DM. Minimally invasive mitral valve operations. Ann Thorac Surg. 1996;62:1542–1544.
9. Gillinov AM, Cosgrove DM. Minimally invasive mitral valve surgery: mini-sternotomy with extended transseptal approach. Semin Thorac Cardiovasc Surg. 1999;11(3):206–211.
10. Loulmet DF, Carpentier A. Less invasive techniques for mitral valve surgery. J Thorac Cardiovasc Surg. 1998;115(4):772–779.
11. Svensson LG, D'Agostino RS. J incision minimal-access valve operations. Ann Thorac Surg. 1998;66(3):1110–1112.
12. Machler HE, Bergmann P. Minimally invasive versus conventional aortic valve operations: a prospective study in 120 patients. Ann Thorac Surg. 1999;67(4):1001–1005.
13. Mihaljevic T, Cohn LH, Unic D, Aranki SF, Couper GS, Byrne JG. One thousand minimally invasive valve operations: early and late results. Ann Surg. 2004;240(3):529–534.
14. Grossi EA, Galloway AC. Minimally invasive mitral valve surgery: a 6-year experience with 714 patients. Ann Thorac Surg. 2002;74(3):660–664.
15. Walther TS. Midterm results after stentless mitral valve replacement. Circulation. 2003;108(Suppl 1):II85–II89.
16. Wang D, Wang Q. Mitral valve replacement through a minimal right vertical infra-axillary thoracotomy versus standard median sternotomy. Ann Thorac Surg. 2009;87(3):704–708.
17. Cohn LH, Adams DH, Couper GS, et al. Minimally invasive cardiac valve surgery improves patient satisfaction while reducing costs of cardiac valve replacement and repair. Ann Surg. 1997;226(4):421–428.
18. Farhat F, Lu Z, Lefevre M, et al. Prospective comparison between total sternotomy and ministernotomy for aortic valve replacement. J Card Surg. 2003;18(5):396–402.
19. Corbi P, Rahmati M, Donal E, et al. Prospective comparison of minimally invasive and standard techniques for aortic valve replacement: initial experience in the first hundred patients. J Card Surg. 2003;18(2):133–139.
20. Stevens JH, Burdon TA, Peters WS, et al. Port-access coronary artery bypass grafting: a proposed surgical method. J Thorac Cardiovasc Surg. 1996;111(3):567–573.

21. Schwartz DS, Ribakove GH, Grossi EA, et al. Minimally invasive mitral valve replacement: port-access technique, feasibility, and myocardial functional preservation. J Thorac Cardiovasc Surg. 1997;113(6):1022–1030.
22. Mohr FW, Falk V, Diegeler A, Walther T, van Son JA, Autschbach R. Minimally invasive port-access mitral valve surgery. J Thorac Cardiovasc Surg. 1998;115(3):567–576.
23. Chitwood WR, Jr, Elbeery JR, Chapman WH, et al. Video-assisted minimally invasive mitral valve surgery: the 'micro-mitral' operation. J Thorac Cardiovasc Surg. 1997;113(2):413–414.
24. Carpentier A, Loulmet D, Carpentier A, et al. Open heart operation under videosurgery and minithoracotomy First case (mitral valvuloplasty) operated with success. CR Acad Sci. 1996;319(3):219–223.
25. Reichenspurner H, Boehm DH, Gulbins H, et al. Three-dimensional video and robot-assisted port-access mitral valve operation. Ann Thorac Surg. 2000;69(4):1176–1181.
26. Falk V, Walther T, Autschbach R, Diegeler A, Battellini R, Mohr FW. Robot-assisted minimally invasive solo mitral valve operation. J Thorac Cardiovasc Surg. 1998;115(2):470–471.
27. Carpentier A, Loulmet D, Aupècle B, et al. Computer assisted open heart surgery First case operated on with success. CR Acad Sci III. 1998;321:437– 42.
28. Robicsek F. Robotic cardiac surgery: time told! J Thorac Cardiovasc Surg. 2008;135(2):243–246.
29. Argenziano M, Katz M, Bonatti J, et al. Results of the prospective multicenter trial of robotically assisted totally endoscopic coronary artery bypass grafting. Ann Thorac Surg. 2006;81(5):1666–1675.
30. Chitwood WR., Jr Current status of endoscopic and robotic mitral valve surgery. Ann Thorac Surg. 2005;79(6):S2248–S2253.
31. Morgan JA, Thornton BA, Peacock JC, et al. Does robotic technology make minimally invasive cardiac surgery too expensive? A hospital cost analysis of robotic and conventional techniques. J Card Surg. 2005;20(3):246–251.
32. Srivastava S, Gadasalli S, Agusala M, et al. Use of bilateral internal thoracic arteries in CABG through lateral thoracotomy with robotic assistance in 150 patients. Ann Thorac Surg. 2006;81:800–806.
33. Chitwood WR, Jr, Elbeery JR, Moran JF. Minimally invasive mitral valve repair: using a minithoracotomy and transthoracic aortic occlusion. Ann Thorac Surg. 1997;63:1477–1479.
34. Grossi EA, LaPietra A, Ribakove GH, et al. Minimally invasive versus sternotomy approaches for mitral reconstruction: comparison of intermediate-term results. J Thorac Cardiovasc Surg. 2001;121(4):708–713.
35. Gaudiani VA, Grunkemeier GL, Castro LJ, Fisher AL, Wu Y. Mitral valve operations through standard and smaller incisions. Heart Surg Forum. 2004;7(4):E337–E342.
36. Gammie JS, Bartlett ST, Griffith BP. Small-incision mitral valve repair: safe, durable, and approaching perfection. Ann Surg. 2009;250(3):409–415.
37. de Vaumas C, Philip I, Daccache G, et al. Comparison of minithoracotomy and conventional sternotomy approaches for valve surgery. J Cardiothorac Vasc Anesth. 2003;17(3):325–328.
38. Modi P, Hassan A, Chitwood WR. Minimally invasive mitral valve surgery: a systematic review and meta-analysis. Eur J Cardiothorac Surg. 2008;34:943–952.
39. Svensson LG, Atik FA, Cosgrove DM, et al. Minimally invasive versus conventional mitral valve surgery: a propensity-matched comparison. J Thorac Cardiovasc Surg. 2010;139(4):926–932.
40. Vanermen H, Farhat F, Wellens F, et al. Minimally invasive video-assisted mitral valve surgery: from port-access towards a totally endoscopic procedure. J Card Surg. 2000;15:51–60.
41. Walther T, Falk V, Metz S, et al. Pain and quality of life after minimally invasive versus conventional cardiac surgery. Ann Thorac Surg. 1999;67:1643–1647.
42. Casselman FP, Van Slycke S, Wellens F, et al. Mitral valve surgery can now routinely be performed endoscopically. Circulation. 2003;108(Suppl 1):II48–II54.
43. Vleissis AA, Bolling SF. Mini-reoperative mitral valve surgery. J Cardiac Surg. 1998;13(6):468–470.
44. Yamada T, Ochiai R, Takeda J, Shin H, Yozu R. Comparison of early postoperative quality of life in minimally invasive versus conventional valve surgery. J Anesth. 2003;17(3):171–176
45. Galloway AC, Schwartz CF, Ribakove GH, et al. A decade of minimally invasive mitral repair: long-term outcomes. Ann Thorac Surg. 2009;88:1180–1184.
46. Iribarne A, Russo MJ, Moskowitz AJ, Ascheim DD, Brown LD, Gelijns AC. Assessing technological change in cardiothoracic surgery. Semin Thorac Cardiovasc Surg. 2009;21(1):28–34.
47. Blackstone EH. Comparing apples and oranges. JTCVS. 2002;123(1):8–15.
48. Pisano GP, Bohmer RM. Organizational differences in rates of learning: evidence from the adoption of minimally invasive cardiac surgery. Manag Sci. 2001;47(6):752–768.
49. Wong MC, Clark DJ, Horrigan MC, Grube E, Matalanis G, Farouque HM. Advances in percutaneous treatment for adult valvular heart disease. Intern Med J. 2009;39(7):465–474.
50. Lapierre H, Chan V, Ruel M. Off-pump coronary surgery through mini-incisions: is it reasonable? Curr Opin Cardiol. 2006;21(6):578–583.
51. SOS Investigators. Coronary artery bypass surgery versus percutaneous coronary intervention with stent implantation in patients with multivessel coronary artery disease (the Stent or Surgery trial), a randomized controlled trial. Lancet. 2002;360:965–970.
52. Stover EP, Siegel LC, Parks R, et al. Variability in transfusion practice for coronary artery bypass surgery persists despite national consensus guidelines: a 24-institution study Institutions of the Multicenter Study of Perioperative Ischemia Research Group. Anesthesiology. 1998;88:327–333.
53. Stamou SC, Hill PC, Dangas G, et al. Stroke after coronary artery bypass: incidence, predictors, and clinical outcome. Stroke. 2001;32:1508–1513.
54. Mathew JP, Parks R, Savino JS, et al. Atrial fibrillation following coronary artery bypass graft surgery: predictors, outcomes, and resource utilization MultiCenter Study of Perioperative Ischemia Research Group. JAMA. 1996;276:300–306.
55. Atluri P, Kozin ED, Hiesinger W, Woo YJ. Off-pump, minimally invasive and robotic coronary revascularization yield improved outcomes over traditional on-pump CABG. Int J Med Robot. 2009;5(1):1–12.
56. Sellke FW, Chu LM, Cohn WE. Current state of surgical myocardial revascularization. Circ J. 2010;74(6):1031–1037. Examines the current state of modern surgical

revascularization techniques including off-pump, limited access and robotic-assisted coronary artery bypass graft surgery.
57. Puskas J, Cheng D, Knight J, et al. Off-pump versus conventional coronary artery bypass grafting: a meta-analysis and consensus statement from the 2004 ISMICS consensus conference. Innovations. 2005;1(1):3–27.
58. Sellke FW, DiMaio JM, Caplan LR, et al. Comparing on-pump and off-pump coronary artery bypass grafting: numerous studies but few conclusions: a scientific statement from the American Heart Association council non cardiovascular surgery and anesthesia in collaboration with the interdisciplinary working group on quality of care and outcomes research. Circulation. 2005;111:2858–2864.
59. Holzhey DM, Jacobs S, Mochalski M, et al. Seven-year follow-up after minimally invasive direct coronary artery bypass: experience with more than 1300 patients. Ann Thorac Surg. 2007;83(1):108–114.
60. Shapira OM, Natarajan V, Kaushik S, et al. Off-pump versus on- pump reoperative CABG via a left thoracotomy for circumflex coronary artery revascularization. J Cardiac Surg. 2004;19(2):113–118.
61. Morishita A, Shimakura T, Miyagishima M, et al. Minimally invasive direct redo coronary artery bypass grafting. Ann Thorac Cardiovasc Surg. 2002;8(4):209–212.
62. Pascucci S, Gunkel L, Zietak T, et al. Use of MIDCAB procedure for redo coronary artery bypass. J Cardiovasc Surg. 2002;43(2):143–146.
63. Cohn WE. Advances in surgical treatment of acute and chronic coronary artery disease. Tex Heart Inst J. 2010;37(3):328–330.
64. Srivastava SP, Patel KN, Skantharaja R, et al. Off-pump complete revascularization through a left lateral thoracotomy (ThoraCAB), the first 200 cases. Ann Thorac Surg. 2003;76(1):46–49.
65. Greenspun HG, Adourian UA, Fonger JD, Fan JS. Minimally invasive direct coronary artery bypass (MIDCAB), surgical techniques and anesthetic considerations. J Cardiothorac Vasc Anesth. 1996;10:507–509.
66. Detter C, Reichenspurner H, Boehm DH, et al. Minimally invasive direct coronary artery bypass grafting (MIDCAB) and off-pump coronary artery bypass grafting (OPCAB), two techniques for beating heart surgery. Heart Surg Forum. 2002;5:157–162.
67. Subramanian VA, Patel NU. Current status of MIDCAB procedure. Curr Opin Cardiol. 2001;16:268–270.
68. Kiaii B, McClure RS, Stewart P, et al. Simultaneous integrated coronary artery revascularization with long-term angiographic follow-up. J Thorac Cardiovasc Surg. 2008;136:702–708.
69. Bonatti J, Schachner T, Bonaros N, et al. Robotic totally endoscopic double-vessel bypass grafting: a further step toward closed-chest surgical treatment of multivessel coronary artery disease. Heart Surg Forum. 2007;10:E239–E242.
70. de Canniere D, Wimmer-Greinecker G, Cichon R, et al. Feasibility, safety, and efficacy of totally endoscopic coronary artery bypass grafting: Multicenter European experience. J Thorac Cardiovasc Surg. 2007;134:710–716.
71. Novick RJ, Fox SA, Kiaii BB, et al. Analysis of the learning curve in telerobotic, beating heart coronary artery bypass grafting: a 90 patient experience. Ann Thorac Surg. 2003;76(3):749–753.
72. Bonatti J, Schachner T, Bonaros N, et al. How to improve performance of robotic totally endoscopic coronary artery bypass grafting. Am J Surg. 2008;195(5):711–716.
73. Bonatti J, Schachner T, Bernecker O, et al. Robotic totally endoscopic coronary artery bypass: program development and learning curve issues. J Thorac Cardiovasc Surg. 2004;127(2):504–510.
74. Cosgrove DM, 3rd, Sabik JF. Minimally invasive approach for aortic valve operations. Ann Thorac Surg. 1996;62(2):596–597.
75. Estrera AL, Reardon MJ. Current approaches to minimally invasive aortic valve surgery. Curr Opin Cardiol. 2000;15(2):91–95.
76. Svensson LG, D'Agostino RS. Minimal-access aortic and valvular operations, including the J/j incision. Ann Thorac Surg. 1998;66(2):431–435.
77. Korach A, Shemin RJ, Hunter CT, Bao Y, Shapira OM. Minimally invasive versus conventional aortic valve replacement: a 10-year experience. J Cardiovasc Surg (Torino) 2010;51(3):417–421.
78. Plass A, Scheffel H, Alkadhi H, et al. Aortic valve replacement through a minimally invasive approach: preoperative planning, surgical technique, and outcome. Ann Thorac Surg. 2009;88(6):1851–1856.
79. Cohn LH, Adams DH, Couper GS, Bichell DP. Minimally invasive aortic valve replacement. Semin Thorac Cardiovasc Surg. 1997;9(4):331–336.
80. Riess FC, Lower C, Bleese N. Prevention of potential complications after minimal access aortic valve replacement. Ann Thorac Surg. 1998;66(5):1866.
81. Aris A, Cámara ML, Montiel J, Delgado LJ, Galán J, Litvan H. Ministernotomy versus median sternotomy for aortic valve replacement: a prospective, randomized study. Ann Thorac Surg. 1999;67(6):1583–1588.
82. Brinkman WT, Hoffman W, Dewey TM, et al. Aortic valve replacement surgery: comparison of outcomes in matched sternotomy and PORT ACCESS groups. Ann Thorac Surg. 2010;90(1):131–135.
83. Liu J, Sidiropoulos A, Konertz W. Minimally invasive aortic valve replacement (AVR) compared to standard AVR. Eur J Cardiothorac Surg. 1999;16(Suppl 2):S80–S83.
84. Stamou SC, Kapetanakis EI, Lowery R, et al. Allogeneic blood transfusion requirements after minimally invasive versus conventional aortic valve replacement: a risk-adjusted analysis. Ann Thorac Surg. 2003;76(4):1101–1106.
85. Dake MD, Miller DC, Semba CP, Mitchell RS, Walker PJ, Liddell RP. Transluminal placement of endovascular stent-grafts for the treatment of descending thoracic aortic aneurysms. N Engl J Med. 1994;331(26):1729–1734.
86. Cheng D, Martin J, Shennib H, et al. Endovascular aortic repair versus open surgical repair for descending thoracic aortic disease a systematic review and meta-analysis of comparative studies. J Am Coll Cardiol. 2010;55(10):986–1001.
87. Ihnken K, Sze D, Dake MD, Fleischmann D, Van der Starre P, Robbins R. Successful treatment of a Stanford type A dissection by percutaneous placement of a covered stent graft in the ascending aorta. J Thorac Cardiovasc Surg. 2004;127(6):1808–1810.

88. Senay S, Alhan C, Toraman F, Karabulut H, Dagdelen S, Cagil H. Endovascular stent-graft treatment of type A dissection: case report and review of literature. Eur J Vasc Endovasc Surg. 2007;34(4):457–460.
89. Zhang H, Li M, Jin W, Wang Z. Endoluminal and surgical treatment for the management of Stanford Type A aortic dissection. Eur J Cardiothorac Surg. 2004;26(4):857–859.
90. Zimpfer D, Czerny M, Kettenbach J, et al. Treatment of acute type a dissection by percutaneous endovascular stent-graft placement. Ann Thorac Surg. 2006;82(2):747–749.
91. Chuter TA, Buck DG, Schneider DB, Reilly LM, Messina LM. Development of a branched stent-graft for endovascular repair of aortic arch aneurysms. J Endovasc Ther. 2003;10(5):940–945.
92. Chuter TA, Schneider DB, Reilly LM, Lobo EP, Messina LM. Modular branched stent graft for endovascular repair of aortic arch aneurysm and dissection. J Vasc Surg. 2003;38(4):859–863.
93. Waldenberger P, Fraedrich G, Mallouhi A, et al. Emergency endovascular treatment of traumatic aortic arch rupture with multiple arch vessel involvement. J Endovasc Ther. 2003;10(4):728–732.
94. Wolf PA, Mitchel JB, Baker CS, Kannel WB, D'Agostino RB. Impact of atrial fibrillation on mortality, stroke, and medical costs. Arch Intern Med. 1998;158:229–234.
95. Hansen ML, Sorensen R, Clausen MT, et al. Risk of bleeding with single, dual, or triple therapy with warfarin, aspirin, and clopidogrel in patients with atrial fibrillation. Arch Intern Med. 2010;170:1433–1441.
96. Shinbane JS, Wood MA, Jensen DN, Ellenbogen KA, Fitzpatrick AP, Scheinman MM. Tachycardia-induced cardiomyopathy: a review of animal models and clinical studies. J Am Coll Cardiol. 1997;29:709–715.
97. Wang TJ, Massaro JM, Levy D, et al. A risk score for predicting stroke or death in individuals with new-onset atrial fibrillation in the community: the Framingham Heart Study. JAMA. 2003;290:1049–1056.
98. Wolf PA, Abbott RD, Kannel WB. Atrial fibrillation as an independent risk factor for stroke: the Framingham Study. Stroke. 1991;22:983–988.
99. Reston JT, Shuhaiber JH. Meta-analysis of clinical outcomes of maze-related surgical procedures for medically refractory atrial fibrillation. Eur J Cardiothorac Surg. 2005;28:724–730.
100. Gaynor SL, Diodato MD, Prasad SM, et al. A prospective, single-center clinical trial of a modified Cox maze procedure with bipolar radiofrequency ablation. J Thorac Cardiovasc Surg. 2004;128:535–542.
101. Cox JL, Schuessler RB, D'Agostino HJ, Jr, et al. The surgical treatment of atrial fibrillation III: development of a definitive surgical procedure. J Thorac Cardiovasc Surg. 1991;101:569–583.
102. Suri RM, Schaff HV, Meyer SR, Hargrove WC. Thoracoscopic versus open mitral valve repair: a propensity score analysis of early outcomes. Ann Thorac Surg. 2009;88:1185–1190.
103. Sagbas E, Akpinar B, Sanisoglu I, et al. Video-assisted bilateral epicardial pulmonary vein isolation for the treatment of lone atrial fibrillation. Ann Thorac Surg. 2007;83:1724–1730.
104. Edgerton JR, McClelland JH, Duke D, et al. Minimally invasive surgical ablation of atrial fibrillation: six-month results. JTCVS. 2009;138:109–114.
105. Wudel J, Chaudhuri P, Hiller J. Video-assisted epicardial ablation and left atrial appendage exclusion for atrial fibrillatin: extended follow-up. Ann Thorac Surg. 2008;85:34–38.
106. Sirak J, Jones D, Sun B, Sai-Sudhakar C, Crestanello J, Firstenberg M. Toward a definitive, totally thoracoscopic procedure for atrial fibrillation. Ann Thorac Surg. 2008;86:1960–1964.
107. Yilmaz A, Geuzebroek G, Van Putte B, et al. Completely thoracoscopic pulmonary vein isolation with ganglionic plexus ablation and left atrial appendage amputation for treatment of atrial fibrillation. Eur J Cardiothorac Surg. 2010;38:356–360.
108. Lee A, Clark K, Bailey M, Aziz A, Schuessler R, Damiano RA. Minimally invasive coxmaze procedure: operative technique and results. Innovations. 2010;5:281–286.
109. Vanelli P, Lemma M, Antona C. Right mini-thoracotomy for left maze with transesophageal echo guidance. Int Cardiovasc Thorac Surg. 2010;10:843–846.
110. Beyer E, Lee R, Lam B. Point: minimally invasive bipolar radiofrequency ablation of lone atrial fibrillation: early multicenter results. JTCVS. 2009;137:521–526.
111. Comas GM, Imren Y, Williams MR. An overview of energy sources in clinical use for the ablation of atrial fibrillation. Semin Thorac Cardiovasc Surg. 2007;19:16–24.
112. Pruitt JC, Lazzara RR, Ebra G. Minimally invasive surgical ablation of atrial fibrillation: the thoracoscopic box lesion approach. J Interv Card Electrophysiol. 2007;20:83–87.
113. Gaynor SL, Byrd GD, Diodato MD, et al. Microwave ablation for atrial fibrillation: Dose-response curves in the cardioplegia-arrested and beating heart. Ann Thorac Surg. 2006;81:72.
114. Gaynor SL, Byrd GD, Diodato MD, et al. Dose response curves for microwave ablation in the cardioplegia-arrested porcine heart. Heart Surgery Forum. 2005;23:331–336.
115. Van Brakel TJ, Bolotin G, Salleng KJ, et al. Evaluation of epicardial microwave ablation lesions: histology versus electrophysiology. Ann Thorac Surg. 2004;78:1397–1402.
116. Lee R, Kruse J, McCarthy P. Surgery for atrial fibrillation. Nat Rev Cardiol. 2009;6:505–513.
117. Byrne JG, Leacche M, Vaughan DE, Zhao DX. Hybrid cardiovascular procedures. JACC Cardiovasc Interv. 2008;1:459–468.
118. Kim KB, Cho KR, Jeong DS. Midterm angiographic follow-up after off-pump coronary artery bypass: serial comparison using early, 1-year, and 5-year postoperative angiograms. J Thorac Cardiovasc Surg. 2008;135:300–307.
119. Hayward PA, Buxton BF. Contemporary coronary graft patency: 5-year observational data from a randomized trial of conduits. Ann Thorac Surg. 2007;84:795–799.
120. Tatoulis J, Buxton BF, Fuller JA. Patencies of 2127 arterial tocoronary conduits over 15 years. Ann Thorac Surg. 2004;77:93–101. [PubMed]
121. DeRose JJ. Current state of integrated hybrid coronary revascularization. Semin Thorac Cardiovasc Surg. 2009;21(3):229–236.
122. Murphy GJ, Bryan AJ, Angelini GD. Hybrid coronary revascularization in the era of drug-eluting stents. Ann Thorac Surg. 2004;78(5):1861–1867.
123. Edwards FH, Peterson ED, Coombs LP, et al. Prediction of operative mortality after valve replacement surgery. J Am Coll Cardiol. 2001;37:885–892.

124. Zajarias A, Cribier AG. Outcomes and safety of percutaneous aortic valve replacement. J Am Coll Cardiol. 2009;53(20):1829–1836.
125. Krishnaswamy A, Tuzcu EM, Kapadia SR. Update on transcatheter aortic valve implantation. Curr Cardiol Rep. 2010;12(5):393–403.
126. Leon MB, Smith CR, Mack M, et al. PARTNER Trial Investi8gators: Transcatheter aortic-valve implantation for aortic stenosis in patients who cannot undergo surgery. N Engl J Med. 2010;363(17):1597–1607.
127. Ye J, Cheung A, Lichtenstein SV, et al. Six month outcome of transapical transcatheter aortic valve implantation in the initial seven patients. Eur J Cardiothorac Surg. 2007;31:16–21.
128. Lichtenstein SV, Cheung A, Ye J, et al. Transapical transcatheter aortic valve implantation in humans: initial clinical experience. Circulation. 2006;114:591–596.
129. Walther T, Simon P, Dewey T, et al. Transapical minimally invasive aortic valve implantation Multicenter experience. Circulation. 2007;116(Suppl 1):I240–I245.
130. Chandrashekhar Y, Westaby S, Narula J. Mitral stenosis. Lancet. 2009;374:1271–1283.
131. Goldberg SL, Feldman T. Percutaneous mitral valve interventions: overview of new approaches. Curr Cardiol Rep. 2010;12(5):404–412.
132. Percutaneous Mitral Valve Repair: results of the Everst II trial. Presented at: American College of Cardiology (ACC) Scientific Sessions; Atlanta, GA, USA. 14–16 March 2010.

51 Heart Transplant in Children and Adolescents

Heart transplantation, has been recently accepted as treatment of choice for children and adolescents with end stage heart disease. Selection of patients, follow-up and management of posttransplant patients as well as the surgical procedure and the immediate postoperative management are very important factors in their survival. Results from recent studies of long-term survival following pediatric heart transplantation is now excellent but limited long-term follow-up data is available as this operation has only been performed for about two decades. One year survival is now over 90% and 5 year survival is estimated to be close to 70% in major transplant centers around the world. Posttransplant coronary artery disease is mainly responsible for the decreased long-term survival. Complications of immunosuppression such as infections, lymphoprolifrative disorders and depressed renal function are still common but usually not life-threatening. Non-compliance with medication was observed amongst teenage recipients and can have lethal consequences. Despite this, it has been shown that heart transplantation can provide good quality of life and prolong survival in pediatric patients with end-stage heart disease.

A heart transplant is surgery done to remove a heart that is not working properly, in order to replace it with a healthy donor heart. A successful heart transplant in a child will extend the child's life and help him grow and develop more normally.

The first human heart transplant was done in 1967. At the Hospital for Sick Children, the first heart transplant was performed in 1990. The hospital now performs about 15 heart transplants each year, about 80% of Canada's paediatric heart transplants. At HSC, the survival for standard and moderate risk cases is 86% and 75% overall.

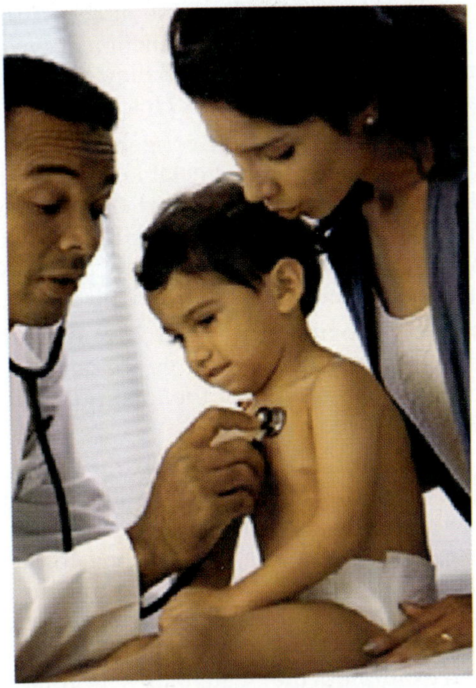

Fig. 51.1: *A young child being examined by a cardiac surgeon preoperatively for his medical fitness*

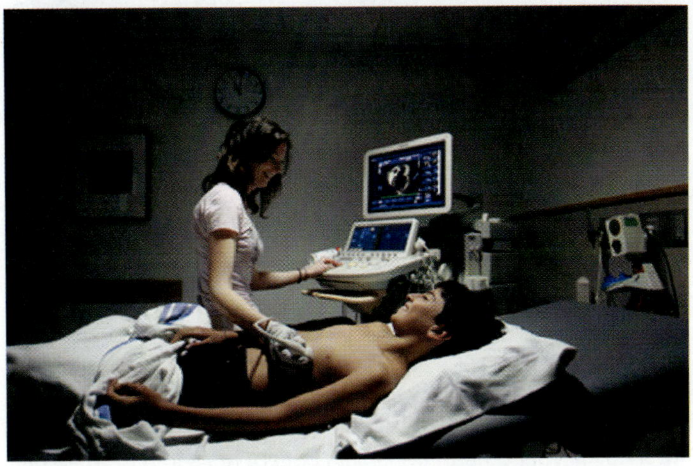

Fig. 51.2: *Teenager is being examined preoperatively with echoardiography for the degree of heart failure*

Table 51.1: *Description fo status levels in the united network of organ sharing list*

Status	*Description*
IA	Must be an inpatient Life expectancy < 7 days VAD related infection (including the pocket and the driveline) Extracorporeal membrane oxygenation (ECMO) Intraaortic balloon pump with inotropic criteria Continuous invasive hemodynamic monitoring with inotropic criteria Life-threatening arrhythmias Mechanical ventilation 30 days following medical stabilization after VAD implantation
IB	Inotrope dependent VAD not meeting criteria for IA status
II	Not inotrope dependent
VII	Inactive on list because of improved clinical status or short term contraindications to cardiac transplantation (e.g. active infection)

Inotrope criteria for status IA

1. Two or more inotropes, regardless of dose
2. Intravenous milrinone, at least 0.5 µg/kg/min by continuous infusion
3. Intravenous dobtuamine, at least 7.5 µg/kg/min by continuous infusion

Heart transplantation is not a cure. It is a very complex process that includes lots of medications, tests, procedures, and an intensive follow-up. As a parent, it can seem overwhelming. Just remember that you will have the ongoing support of the transplant team from start to finish. Team members will teach you what you need to know to help your child. The application of heart transplantation to infants and children has come of age. While many programs were outgrowths of adult heart transplant programs, most pediatric heart transplant programs have separate teams devoted to the care of infants and children. Most programs now have 5-year survival rates in excess of 70%. But, while an additional 5 years of life is important for all, the goal of pediatric heart transplantation is to provide as much of a normal life-span for these children as possible. This chapter describes the unique aspects of heart transplantation as applied to infants and children (Figs 51.9, 51.10 and 51.14).

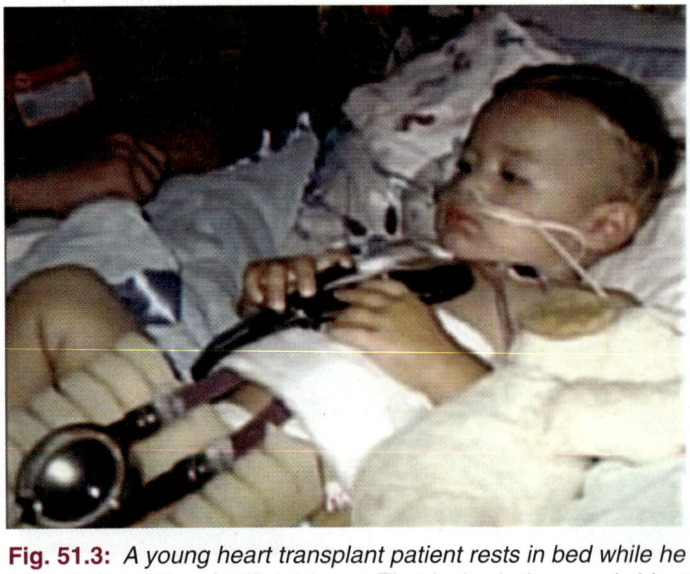

Fig. 51.3: *A young heart transplant patient rests in bed while he is kept alive with an artificial heart. The device is the round object in the lower part of the abdomen between two lower limbs*

Medical history: The first pediatric heart transplant was performed in 1968 when the heart of an anencephalic infant was transplanted into an 18-day-old infant with Ebstein anomaly. This neonate died 5 hours after the procedure. Older children occasionally underwent transplants during the 1970s and early 1980s. Routine successful cardiac transplantation began after the introduction of cyclosporine and with the pioneering efforts of Bailey and his team at Loma Linda University Children's Hospital in 1985.

Incidence: An estimated 10% of congenital heart disease cases have been deemed uncorrectable. One of the most common indications for infant heart transplantation is hypoplastic left heart syndrome (HLHS). This occurs in about 1 in 6,000 live births. Congenital cardiomyopathy occurs in approximately 1 in 10,000 live births.

Global burden: Worldwide, approximately 300–350 pediatric heart transplant procedures are performed each year, representing about 10% of the total number of heart transplants performed.

Etiology: The four etiologies leading to conditions that might require heart transplantation are errors in the formation of the heart, cardiac tumors, infections, and toxins (either endogenous or exogenous) leading to damage to the myocardium. Many of the congenital anomalies including congenital cardiomyopathy, now are known to have specific chromosomal abnormalities associated with them. A good example is the "Catch-22" syndrome, a 22q11 band deletion associated with DiGeorge syndrome and interrupted aortic arch.

Box 51.1: *Staff members of the transplant*

Transplant cardiologists
Cardiovascular surgeons
Clinical nurse specialists/nurse practitioners transplant nurses
Social workers
Psychiatrists
Clinical dieticians
Occupational therapists
Physiotherapists
Pharmacists
Adolescent medicine physicians
Discharge planners
Information coordinators
Cardiology, transplant and cardiovascular surgery fellows (physicians in training)
The donor heart

Box 51.2: *Indications for heart transplant surgery*

Conditions considered for pediatric heart transplantation include the following:

1. Cardiomyopathy (dilated, hypertrophic, restrictive)
2. Anatomically uncorrectable congenital heart disease (hypoplastic left heart syndrome, pulmonary atresia with intact ventricular septum plus sinusoids, congenitally corrected transposition of the great arteries with single ventricle and heart block, severely unbalanced atrio-ventricular septal defects)
3. Congenital heart disease at high risk for repair (severe Shone complex, interrupted aortic arch and severe subaortic stenosis, critical aortic stenosis with severe endocardial fibroelastosis, Ebstein anomaly in a symptomatic newborn)
4. Refractory heart failure after previous cardiac surgery
5. Unresectable symptomatic cardiac neoplasms

Age Factor

It is usually considered to suitable patients from infancy through to 18 years of age. In some cases, heart transplantation is an option prior to a baby being delivered if the heart disease is diagnosed before birth and there are no other problems with the baby.

Pathophysiology: The pathophysiology of conditions requiring heart transplantation is obviously as varied as the conditions themselves. Inherent in each condition, however, is the underlying principle of the inability of the pump to supply adequate perfusion for end-organ health and well being. Details of the pathophysiology of each condition should be obtained from the section in this text dedicated to that condition.

Care of Your Child while Waiting for a Donor Heart

You child's cardiologist will still be the main doctor caring for your child's heart problem while you wait for a donor heart. Your cardiac clinic nurse will know that your child is waiting for a heart transplant. While your child waits for a heart, you will see your transplant nurse from time to time. If your child's condition is more serious and she can't be cared for at home, she will be looked after in the hospital.

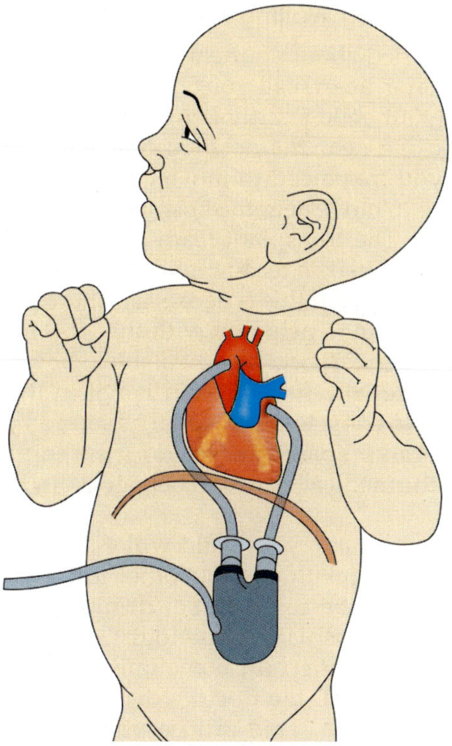

Fig. 51.4: *Diagrammatic representation of an artificial heart which has been fitted into the child just before heart transplantation*

There is no way of knowing how long your child may have to wait for a donor heart. Your child will be put on a waiting list and will get a donor heart when an appropriate one becomes available. The wait for a heart could be anywhere from days to months, depending on your child's size and blood type, and how sick your child is. This will all be explained to you in detail if your child gets listed for a heart transplant. Unfortunately, not many transplant organs are available. In Canada, about one in 4 people die while waiting for an organ transplant. There are only 1–4 donors for every 1 million people in Canada.

You and your family may find the time you spend waiting for a donor heart very frightening and difficult. This is particularly true if your child's condition gets worse. Your social worker will help you to plan for this stressful time (Box 51.2).

Depending on the severity of the condition, your child may need to stay in hospital while he waits for a heart. The transplant team will also help you make sure your child is in the best possible health at all times in case a heart becomes available. You will be alerted immediately when a suitable heart is available.

Keeping your child as healthy as possible before the heart transplant is very important. In particular, you need to make sure your child eats healthy foods and stays active. Your child's clinical dietician will help you choose the right foods to keep your child as healthy as possible before the heart transplant. Your child needs physical activity and exercise to keep the joints moving and the muscles strong. Your physiotherapist will help your child stay as active as possible before the transplant.

Emergency During Waiting for Transplant

If you are worried about your child's condition during the wait for a donor heart, call your cardiac clinic nurse. She will contact your child's cardiologist to confirm next steps. If you don't live near the hospital that will perform the transplant, you may need to move closer to the hospital. You will have to move near the hospital while you wait for a donor heart. The transplant team assesses each patient individually and makes recommendations about the need for family relocation. If this is necessary, there are multiple resources available to help you with this.

When a donor heart becomes available. The hospital will call you or page you. If your child is not in the hospital, you will need to come to the hospital as soon as you can so that the staff can prepare your child for surgery. Different members of the medical team will help get your child ready for surgery.

Once at the hospital, your child will get an IV, have his blood tested (along with possibly other tests), have a bath or shower, and not be able to eat or drink anything.

The surgeon, transplant cardiologist, anesthesiologist, and nurses will see your child. Sometimes, after you've been called to the hospital, the doctors decide that the donor heart is not suitable. This can be very disappointing, however it is more important that the donor heart be suitable. This is best for your child's health. If this should happen, your child's name will stay on the waiting list and the search for a suitable donor will continue.

The systems in place to match appropriate organs with appropriate recipients are very reliable. In extremely rare cases, there are reports in the media of patients who receive organs that aren't suitable for them. Safeguards are continually implemented and expanded to ensure this doesn't happen. Isolated incidents such as these should not cast doubt on the very dependable systems that are in place.

Evaluation of the Donor Heart Before Transplant?

A number of things are important in determining the suitability of a donor for your child including weight and the results of the heart tests on the organ donor. It doesn't matter if the donor is the same sex or ethnic background as the recipient. A team of surgeons at the donor hospital assesses the donor heart and surgically removes it for transfer back to the hospital. At the donor hospital—where the donor's heart was removed—the heart (also called the "graft") will be stopped with a fluid in a process called cardioplegia. It is then put in salt water and transported, in an ice cooler, to the hospital where the transplant patient is waiting (Fig. 51.1).

Clinical considerations in heart transplant patients: Infants with serious congenital heart disease generally present in the newborn period with varying degrees of cyanosis, tachypnea, tachycardia, dysrhythmias, poor perfusion, feeding intolerance, and other symptoms of heart failure. Symptoms of heart failure, either of rapid or slow onset, are associated with the cardiomyopathies. Children with tumors may present with congestive heart failure (CHF) or with syncope or cardiac arrest from arrhythmias. Specific presentations for each of the diagnoses can be found in the appropriate sections of this text. An increasing number of congenital lesions are diagnosable by fetal ultrasound. In the author's experience, almost half of all infants with hypoplastic left heart syndrome are diagnosed in utero.

High-risk children for corrective operation: Patients with potentially correctable congenital heart disease but at greatly increased operative risk also should be considered for transplantation. This decision is somewhat dependent on the surgical results at specific institutions. Lesions that should be considered include complex truncus arteriosus (with severe truncal valve insufficiency, interrupted aortic arch, or coronary artery anomalies), some severe forms of Shone complex, and complex interrupted aortic arch.

Contraindications in cardiac transplant surgery: Some anatomic considerations specifically referable to transplantation exist. The major anatomic contraindication is small pulmonary arteries that cannot be satisfactorily enlarged surgically. Other features that could preclude safe heart transplantation include subsets of anomalous pulmonary venous connection without a suitable pulmonary venous confluence for direct anastomosis to the donor left atrium. Few absolute contraindications to pediatric heart transplantation exist. Many children who are quite ill can make a remarkable recovery once a new heart restores adequate perfusion. The following, however, are considered incompatible with successful transplantation:

- Irreversible elevated pulmonary vascular resistance (> or = 5 Wood units M^2) (Table 51.2)

Table 51.2: *Modified recipient containdictions to heart transplantation*

Absolute contraindications
Severe irreversible pulmonary hypertension (>6 wood units)
Active systemic infection
Active systemic disease with poor prognosis
Active gastrointestinal bleeding
Probable contraindications
Irreversible renal and/or hepatic dysfunction
Hepatitis B positive serology
HIV positive serology
Active alcohol or drug abuse
Recent pulmonary infarction
Peripheral vascular or cerebrobascular disease
Psychosocial instability and lack of compliance
Potential contraindications
Hepatitis C positive serology
Chronic obstructive pulmonary disease
Renal insufficiency
Hepatic insufficiency
Peptic ulcer disease
Diverticular bowel disease
Active or recent malignancy
Diabetes mellitus
Excessive obesity

- Diffuse hypoplasia of right and left pulmonary arteries
- Total anomalous pulmonary venous connection without pulmonary venous confluence
- Ectopia cordis
- Active systemic infection
- Infection with HIV or chronic active hepatitis B or C
- Malignancy without cure or of recent onset
- Severe primary renal or hepatic dysfunction
- Multiorgan system failure
- Major central nervous system abnormality
- Severe dysmorphism
- Marked prematurity (<36 wk)
- Low birth weight (<2 kg)
- Positive drug screen
- Lack of family support.

Laboratory Studies

- ***Blood type:*** To be used to list for an appropriate organ
- ***Infection screening:*** CBC with differential, urine and blood cultures, cytomegalovirus (CMV) titer, hepatitis B surface antigen (HBsAg), HIV test, rapid plasma reagin (RPR) test, endotracheal tube (ETT) aspirate (if applicable)
- ***Assess renal and liver function:*** Electrolytes, BUN, creatinine and liver profile
- Assess pretransplant sensitization—panel reactive antibody.

Imaging studies: Head ultrasound, CT scan, MRI, EEG as appropriate to assess neurological status
- Chest X-ray (Fig. 51.6)
- Renal ultrasound.

Diagnostic Tests

1. Echocardiogram to assess anatomy and function (Fig. 51.2)
2. Cardiac catheterization.

May be needed to assess anatomy, rule out pulmonary venous drainage abnormalities, assess pulmonary artery adequacy, and assess pulmonary vascular resistance Recipients with elevated pulmonary vascular resistance (PVR) are at increased risk for acute right heart failure in the early posttransplant period (Fig. 51.8).

In the first few months of life, if the main and branch pulmonary arteries are of normal caliber and distribution, the elevated PVR of the newborn period usually rapidly normalizes shortly after transplantation. If there is pulmonary venous obstruction, pulmonary artery pressures may not normalize as quickly.

Estimation of pulmonary artery pressures may be possible by echocardiography but usually requires cardiac catheterization for a more formal analysis. Elevated PVR that is reactive (i.e. responds to vasodilator therapy) usually can be managed with oxygen and/or intravenous vasodilator therapy in the pretransplant period. This can lead to a decrease in the PVR, simplifying the posttransplant management. Elevated PVR that is fixed is an indicator of significant risk for acute graft failure.

Surgical Intervention

Donor operation: Attention to detail during the procurement of the donor organ and gentle handling of the donor organ is as important as the implantation of the organ. The donor operation must be tailored to the anatomic needs of the recipient. Recipient anomalies of pulmonary venous connection often require complete resection of the donor left atrium, dividing each donor pulmonary vein separately. In the case of anomalies of systemic venous return, extended removal of the superior vena cava, left innominate vein, and inferior vena cava may be required.

The pediatric cardioplegia solution usually is either the University of Wisconsin solution or Roe solution.

Preoperative assessment in a transplant patient: Meticulous care of the child awaiting transplant is essential to ensure the best possible outcome. For patients with ductal dependent physiology, the lowest dose possible of

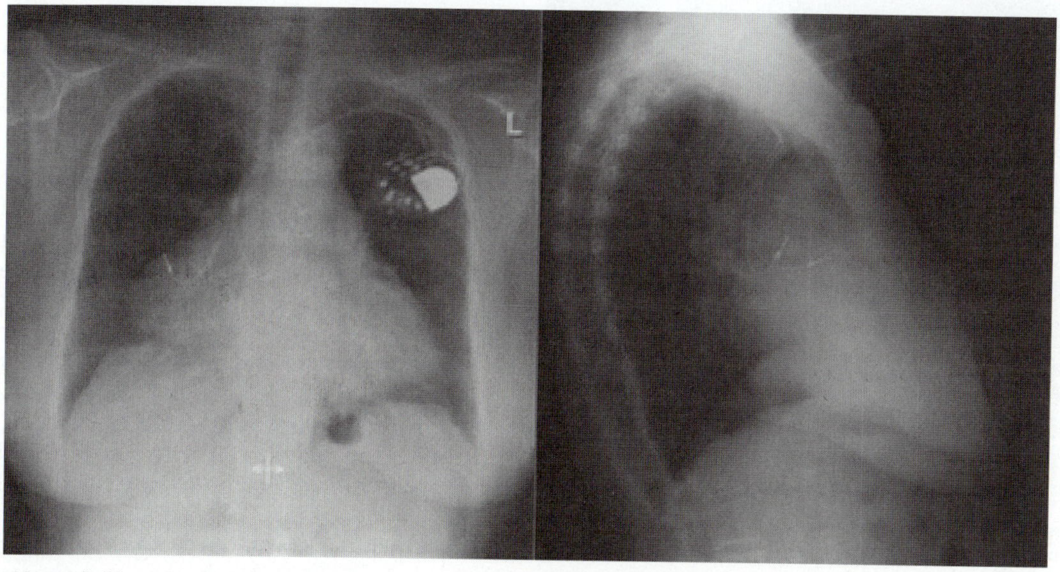

Fig. 51.5: *Chest X-ray (left) and lateral (right) after dual atrial pacemaker implantation with one screw-in lead into the right atrium of the donor graft and the second lead in the right atrium of the native heart*

prostaglandin (0.1–0.2 mcg/kg/min) should be used. The authors usually use a peripherally inserted central catheter (PICC) line, with a second heparin lock in place in the advent of sudden loss of the primary intravenous site. Oxygenation must be managed to balance the pulmonary and systemic blood flows. This may require adding nitrogen to the inspired gas mixture to render delivered oxygen at less than a fractional inspired oxygen (FiO_2) of 0.21. An important complication is a significantly restricted interatrial communication. Balloon atrial septostomy or surgical septectomy may be necessary. Among all children waiting for heart transplantation, the mortality prior to transplantation is approximately 15–20%. Mortality during the waiting period for infants with HLHS is significant when the infant has to wait longer than about 3 months, with infants only occasionally surviving until aged 6 months. In the group of less critically ill children [United Network for Organ Sharing (UNOS) status II], pretransplant mortality by 12 months is about 10%.

Intraoperative assessment: The operative method of transplantation in children with cardiomyopathy is the same as for adults. A median sternotomy is utilized to perform thymectomy and expose the recipient's native heart. If the donor heart is significantly larger than the native heart, the entire left pericardium anterior to the phrenic nerve is removed. Single venous and arterial cannulation generally is employed. A standard orthotopic technique utilizing biatrial or bicaval connection is used. Modifications for anatomy specific to congenital heart disease are as follows (Figs 51.9 and 51.10):

- For the infant with hypoplastic left heart syndrome, the ductus arteriosus is isolated and cannulated for arterial perfusion through a stab wound in the distal main pulmonary artery. All aortic arch vessels are isolated with loose tourniquets during the initial cooling phase in preparation for reconstruction. Implantation of the allograft is accomplished with systemic hypothermia, performing the atrial anastomoses under low-flow perfusion, with the pulmonary artery clamped and systemic perfusion maintained by means of the arterial cannula positioned in the ductus arteriosus. The aortic arch is then reconstructed under circulatory arrest with the arch vessel tourniquets tightened. The excision of ductal tissue at its entrance into the distal arch is important in providing secure aortic tissue for the anastomosis and to minimize the likelihood of a posttransplant stenosis in this area. The pulmonary artery anastomosis is completed while rewarming the patient.

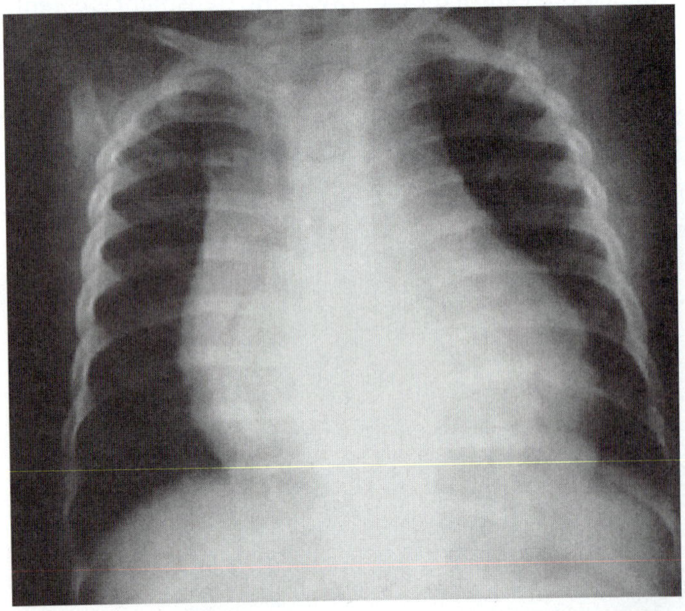

Fig. 51.6: *Skiagram chest PA view showing visceral situs solitus in levocardia. Enlarged cardiac silhouette with a cardiothoracic index of 0.70. Pulmonary network within normal limits in a child with end-stage heart failure*

Other complex congenital heart anomalies, such as transposition of the great arteries, often can be managed by direct anastomosis if sufficient lengths of donor arterial and venous connections are procured.

Postoperative evaluation: Management of the child who has undergone heart transplantation is similar to management for any pediatric cardiac surgery. Those details specifically referable to heart transplantation include the following (Figs 51.4 and 51.5):

- ***Prostaglandin therapy:*** For those patients on prostaglandin E (PGE) prior to transplantation, continuing for at least 1–2 days and then gradually weaning over 2–3 days to prevent rebound pulmonary hypertension is advisable.
- ***Pulmonary hypertension:*** The donor right ventricle is not tolerant of significant pulmonary hypertension and, for this reason, acute graft failure is one of the largest contributors to early mortality. Optimal therapy includes sedation, vasodilator therapy, alkalinization through hyperventilation, inotropic agents with minimal pulmonary vasoconstrictive effects, and inhaled nitric oxide when available.
- ***Pulmonary management:*** Many children receive donor organs that are larger than their native hearts. This leads to compression of lung parenchyma. Aggressive pulmonary toilet is indicated and close observation for respiratory compromise is required, especially after the initial extubation.

Perioperative immunosuppression: A number of protocols exist for immunosuppression in the perioperative and postoperative period. The following protocol is used at Loma Linda University Children's Hospital. Cyclosporine (CSA) is begun at 0.1 mg/kg/h IV when the donor is identified, stopped during surgery, and restarted after transplantation. This is switched to oral dosing when possible with a target trough CSA level of 250–300 ng/mL. Methylprednisolone is given IV at a dose of 20 mg/kg every 12 hours for 4 doses. Antithymocyte induction therapy (thymoglobulin) is given for recipients older than 30 days at a dose of 1.5 mg/kg/d once daily for the first 5 days. Azathioprine is started at 3 mg/kg/d IV or PO given once daily and adjusted downward as necessary to maintain a white blood cell count.

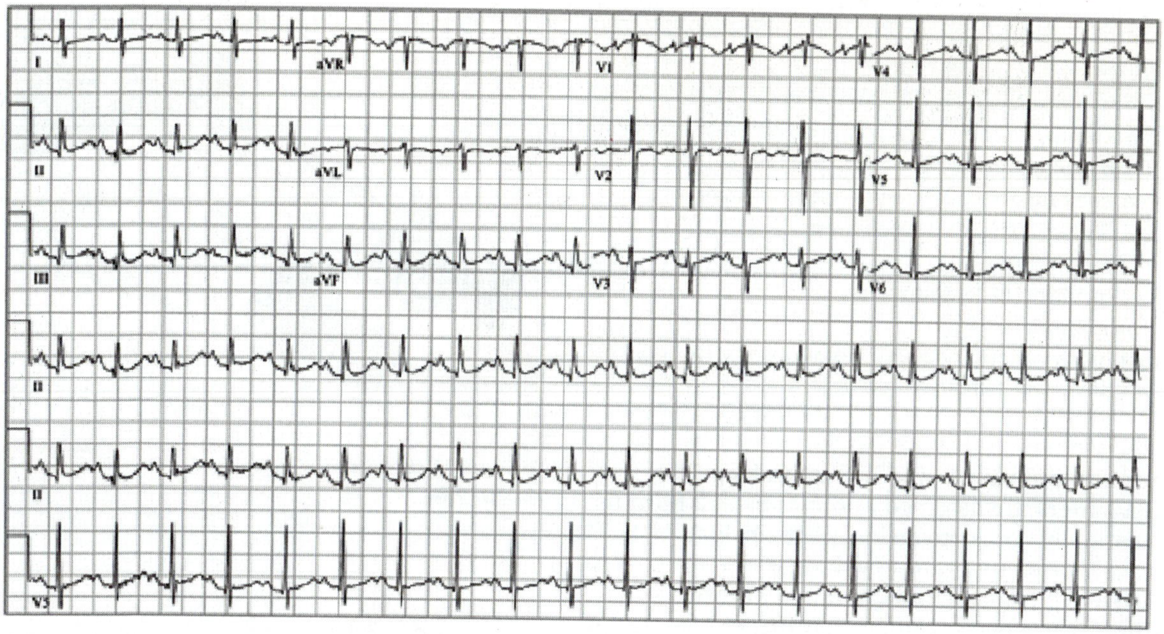

Fig. 51.7: *ECG shows sinus tachycardia, a prolonged QT interval, and a nonspecific T-wave abnormality. Cardiac transplant patients have a resting sinus tachycardia and a blunted chronotropic response to exercise due to a denervated sinus node as a result of transplantation. The QT interval is affected by autonomic tone. In the denervated transplanted heart, this is not unusual. Finally, a nonspecific T-wave abnormality is common in tachycardia and is not significant in the patient*

Adjunctive therapy includes intravenous immune globulin at a dose of 2 g/kg given over 24 hours beginning right after the transplant. Ranitidine is given while on methylprednisolone. Ganciclovir is given IV for 2 weeks for those recipients who are CMV positive or who receive a CMV positive donor. Aspirin at 3–5 mg/kg/d is given if the platelet count is chronically over 500 × 10/L.

Follow-up of transplant cases: Close outpatient follow-up is essential to ensure long-term success. The highest risk for complications occurs in the first few months after transplantation, and, for this reason, the child should remain near the transplant center for the initial follow-up. The outpatient-testing schedule at Loma Linda University Children's Hospital is as follows:

- Physician visits are twice weekly for 6 weeks, then less frequently as rejection free interval increases. Minimum visit frequency is monthly for the first year and every 3 months thereafter.
- **Echocardiogram/ECG** is obtained twice weekly for 4 weeks, then less often as the rejection free interval increases and should be performed at the same time as the routine physician visits thereafter. Full-study echocardiogram is obtained at 1 month, 3 months, and 12 months to evaluate the aortic arch in patients with arch reconstruction (Figs 51.7, 51.15–51.17, 51.21–52.23).
- **Chest X-ray** is taken monthly for 3 months, at 6 and 12 months, then annually (Figs 51.11 and 51.12).
- **Cyclosporine trough level** is assessed twice weekly for 2 weeks after discharge, weekly for 4 weeks, monthly for the first year, and then every 3 months thereafter. **Target CSA levels (with favorable rejection history)** are 250-300 ng/mL for 6 months, 200–250 ng/mL for 6–12 months, and then 125–150 ng/mL thereafter.
- **CBC with platelets** is obtained every 2 weeks for 2 months, then monthly for the first year and every 3 months thereafter.
- **Basic electrolytes** are obtained at the same time as the CBC for the first year with complete metabolic profile every 3 months.

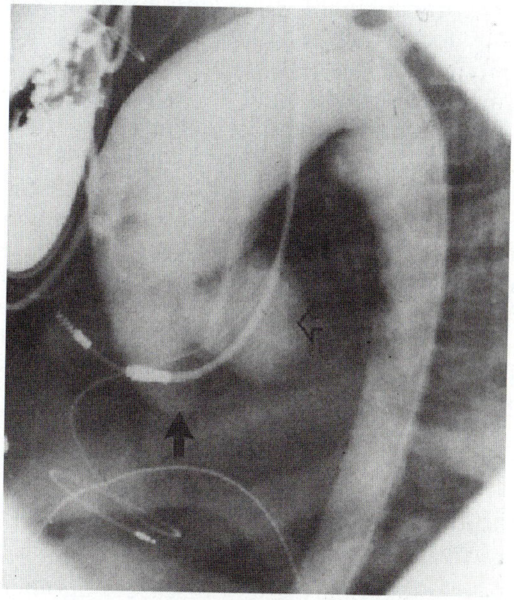

Fig. 51.8: *Lateral aortogram confirming false aneurysm posteriorly (open arrow). Note large ascending aorta and absence of distal aortic rupture after heart transplantation (closed arrow = native aortic root)*

Table 51.3: *Acute cardiac transplant rejection*

Acute cellular grade 2 or greater
Methylprednisolone 1,000 mg IV q.d. × 3 days
Prednisone 0.6 mg/kg tapering to 0.2 mg/kg over 3 weeks
Cellular recurrent grade 2 or greater
Methylprednisolone 500–1,000 mg IV q.d. × 3 days
Prednisone 0.6 mg/kg with 2 week taper
RATG or OKT3
Change cyclosporine to tacrolimus
Cellular, intractable
Total lymphoid irradiation 800 cGy total dose twice weekly (mantel and inverted Y distributions)

- **CMV immunoglobulin G (IgG) titer and Epstein-Barr virus (EBV) titers** are assessed at 6 months, 12 months, and then annually until conversion. (Antigen load by PCR may replace/supplement these values.)
- **HIV and HBsAg tests are obtained at 6 months.**
- **Developmental assessment is conducted at age 4 months and 18 months for infant recipients.**
- **Speech and language evaluation is conducted at age 3 years for infant recipients.**
- **Standard psychometric testing is conducted at age 5 years for those transplanted during infancy.**

Isotopic glomerular filtration rate (GFR) is assessed at 3 months, 12 months, and every year thereafter for those transplanted during infancy. Isotopic GFR is assessed every 2 years for those transplanted after the first year and for those children who are older than 2 years and whose most recent GFR is more than 100 mL/min/1.73 m^2.

- **Renal ultrasound is performed at 3 months, 12 months, and then every other year.**
- Metabolic exercise stress testing is started at age 6 years for those transplanted while younger than 6 years; test annually for all children older than 6 years.
- **Endomyocardial biopsy** is obtained annually for those who are newborn to aged 2 years at transplant; at 1 month, 3 months, 12 months, and annually thereafter for children aged 2–8 years at transplant; and prior to discharge, at 1 month, 2 months, 3 months, 6 months, 12 months, and annually thereafter for patients aged 9 years or older at transplant.

Coronary angiography is performed annually, starting at the first anniversary of transplant. (Consider intravascular ultrasound for children aged 6 years or older.) All routine vaccinations, except live virus vaccines [e.g. oral polio, varicella vaccine, measles-mumps-rubella (MMR)] should be given, starting as early as 6 weeks after transplantation (Fig. 51.19).

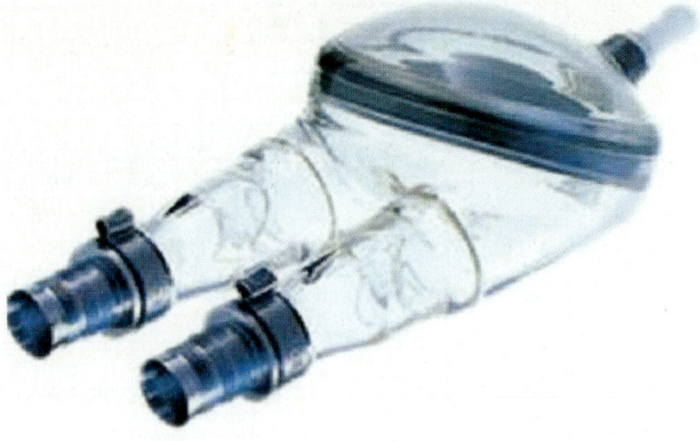

Fig. 51.9: *EXCOR pediatric blood pump 30 mL for children up to 66 pounds device stabilizes pediatric patients waiting for heart transplants*

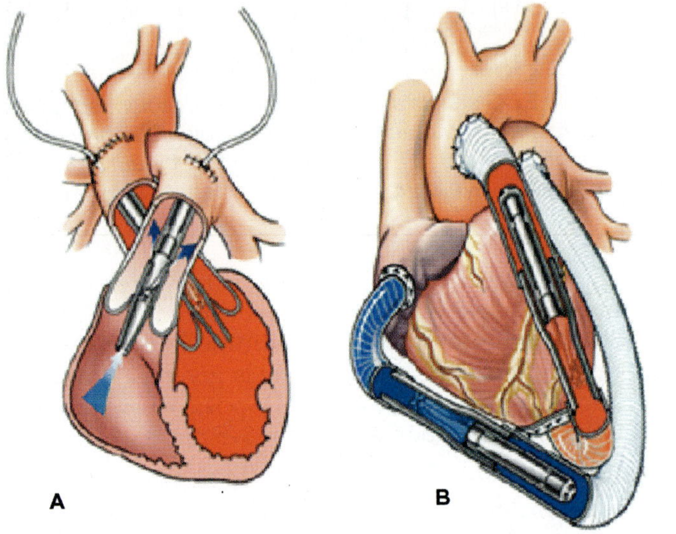

Fig. 51.10: *(A) Shows partial implantation of artificial (pedipump) providing support to the damaged left ventricle. (B) Shows completion of implantation in a newborn patient with end-stage cardiac failure*

Table 51.4: *Sample endomyocardial biopsy schedule*

Weeks after transplantation	*Biopsy frequency*
1–4	Weekly
5–12	Every 2 weeks
13–24	Monthly
25–52	Every 2 months
2 year	Every 3–4 months
3–4 year	Every 6 months
>4 years	Only if clinically indicated
After biopsy	2 weeks after initial biopsy acute rejection

Development of Coronary Atherosclerosis after Heart Transplant

Posttransplant coronary artery disease is another form of rejection also known as chronic vascular rejection or graft vasculopathy. The blood is supplied to the heart by little blood vessels called coronary arteries. After transplant, for reasons not fully understood, the coronary arteries can become narrow and thick. This is not the same kind of coronary artery disease you may have heard about in adult patients with heart disease or heart attacks. There are no good catheter lab or surgical options to treat posttransplant coronary artery disease. All patients after heart transplant undergo testing regularly to look for signs of coronary artery disease. Important things to help slow down or prevent coronary artery disease include a heart healthy diet, regular exercise, proper taking of all medications (for example, immunosuppression, blood pressure medications, cholesterol medications). Some children may require another heart transplant if the coronary artery disease becomes severe enough (Fig. 51.9).

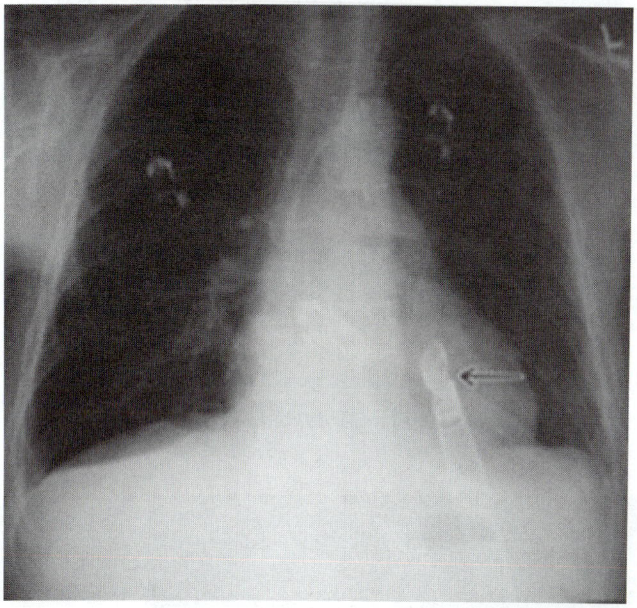

Fig. 51.11: *Frontal views of the chest show a thoratec left VAD (arrow)*

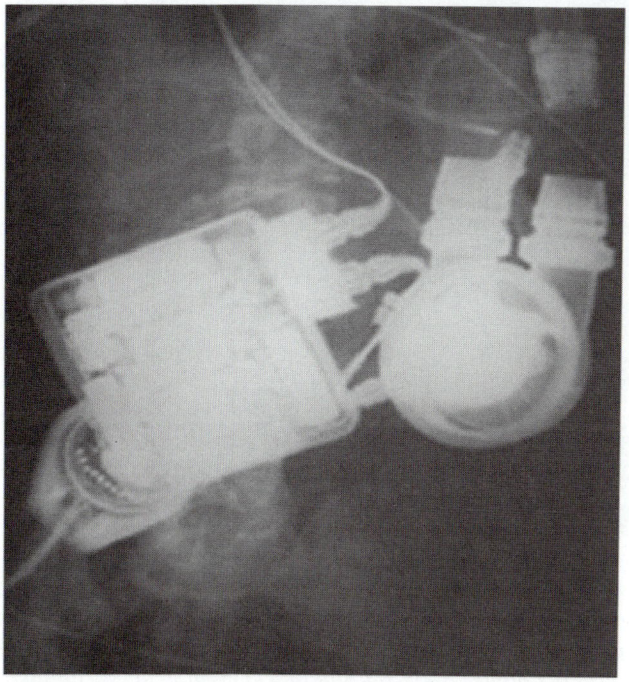

Fig. 51.12: *Abdominal image shows a heartmate VAD*

Risk of Infections after Transplant

Some parts of your child's immune system may be weaker because of the immunosuppressants she is taking for the new heart. Your child will get common illnesses, just like other children, that will not require any pecial treatment or precautions. However, certain infections may be more concerning in a patient who has had a transplant and require special monitoring or treatment including the chicken pox, and two specific viruses called cytomegalovirus (CMV) and Epstein-Barr virus (EBV). Information about this will be included in all of your posttransplant teaching and also provided to your family doctor or paediatrician after transplant (Table 51.6).

To prevent infection, you should keep your child away from crowded places for the first 3 months after the operation. This means that your child will not be able to school, the movies, restaurants, or swimming pools where there are large crowds. Your child will also need to stay away from other children or adults who have a cold, a cold sore, the flu, or diarrhea.

Lymphoproliferative Disease after Transplant

Posttransplant lymphoproliferative disorder (PTLD) is caused by an infection of the white blood cells in the body with Epstein Barr virus (EBV). This virus lives in your body once you have had it but, in most people, the immune system keeps it under control. Patients on immunosuppressant drugs may have a more difficult time controlling this virus in the body and it can cause the white blood cells to multiply out of control leading to varying stages of lymphoma, a type of cancer. Any post-heart transplant patient is susceptible to this, therefore, your child will be followed very regularly for the levels of EBV in the blood. She may require ultrasounds, X-rays, or other types of scans to look for tumours. If she does develop EBV, EBV disease, or any form of PTLD, she may require IV medications for many months to treat it. This can be administered at home. If the disease progresses, there may be a need for stronger forms of chemotherapy, but this is very rare.

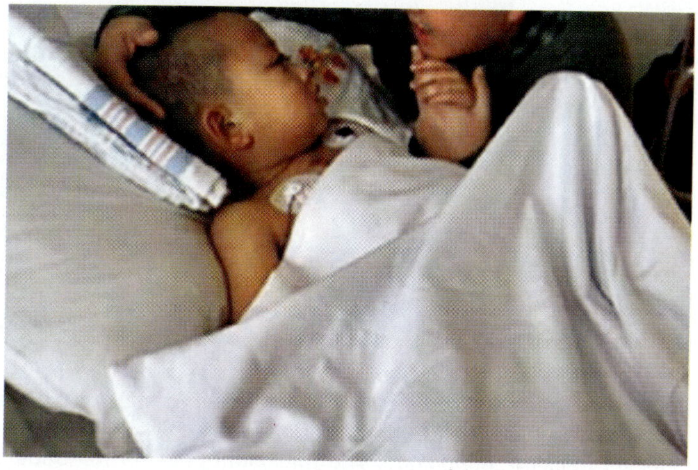

Fig. 51.13: *A 5-year-old child finally gets his permanent heart transplant after 7 months waiting with pediatric blood pump (pedipump)*

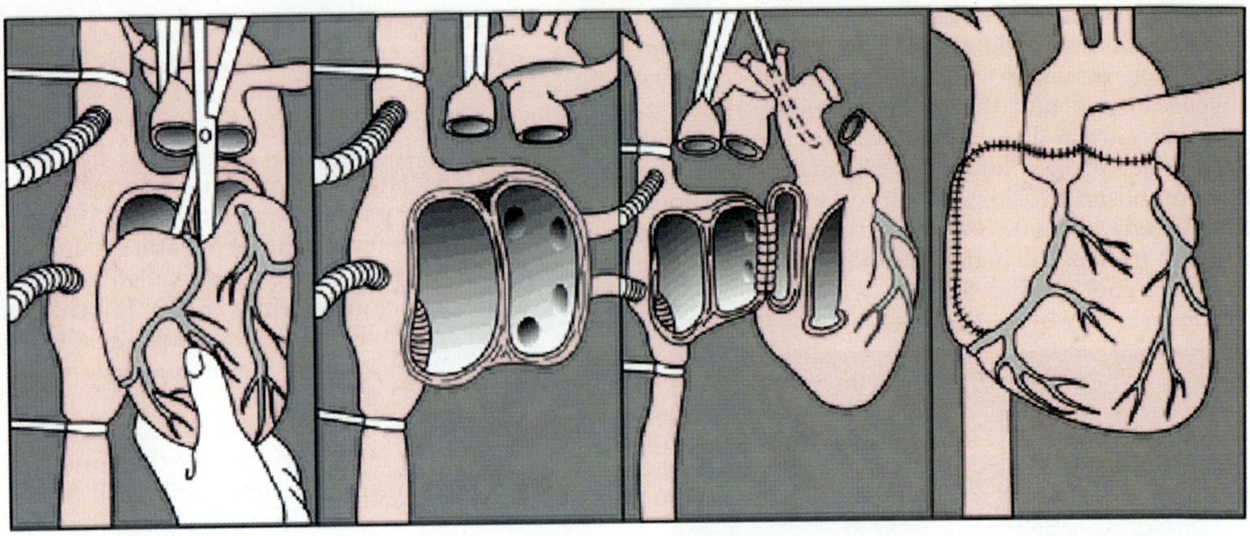

1. After the recipient is placed on cardiopulmonary bypass, the heart is removed
2. The posterior walls of the recipient's left and right atrial are left intact
3. The left atrium of donor heart is anastomosed to the recipient's residual posterior atrial walls, and the other atrial walls, the atrial septum, and the great vessels are joined
4. Postoperative result

Fig. 51.14: *Various surgical steps in the completion of heart transplantation*

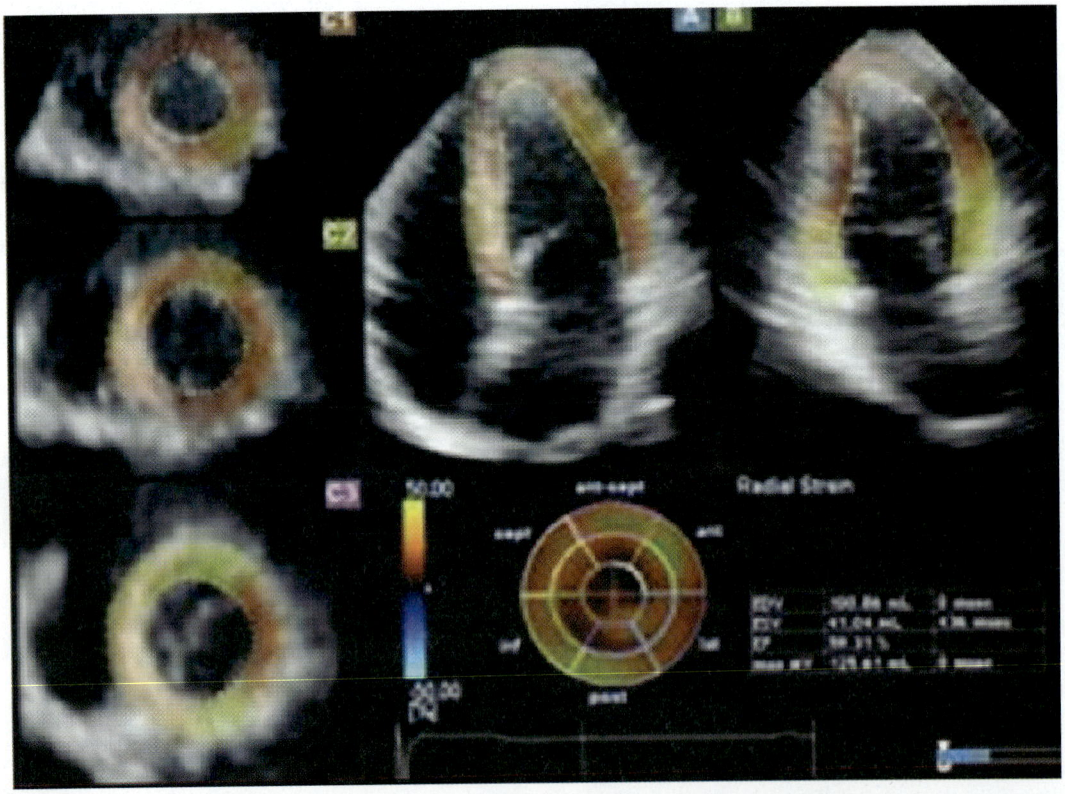

Fig. 51.15: *Analysis of myocardial deformation in heart transplant patients. Echocardiography has become vitally important for cardiac assessment of patients following heart transplant. This will investigate whether the contractile behaviour of the transplanted heart differs in general from that of healthy subjects. Myocardial deformation will therefore be evaluated using three dimensional speckle tracking technology. The transplant patients will undergo regular echocardiographic examinations as a part of outpatient follow-up examinations. The purpose of the study is to develop prognostic echocardiographic parameters in order to detect threatened rejection of the transplant earlier on*

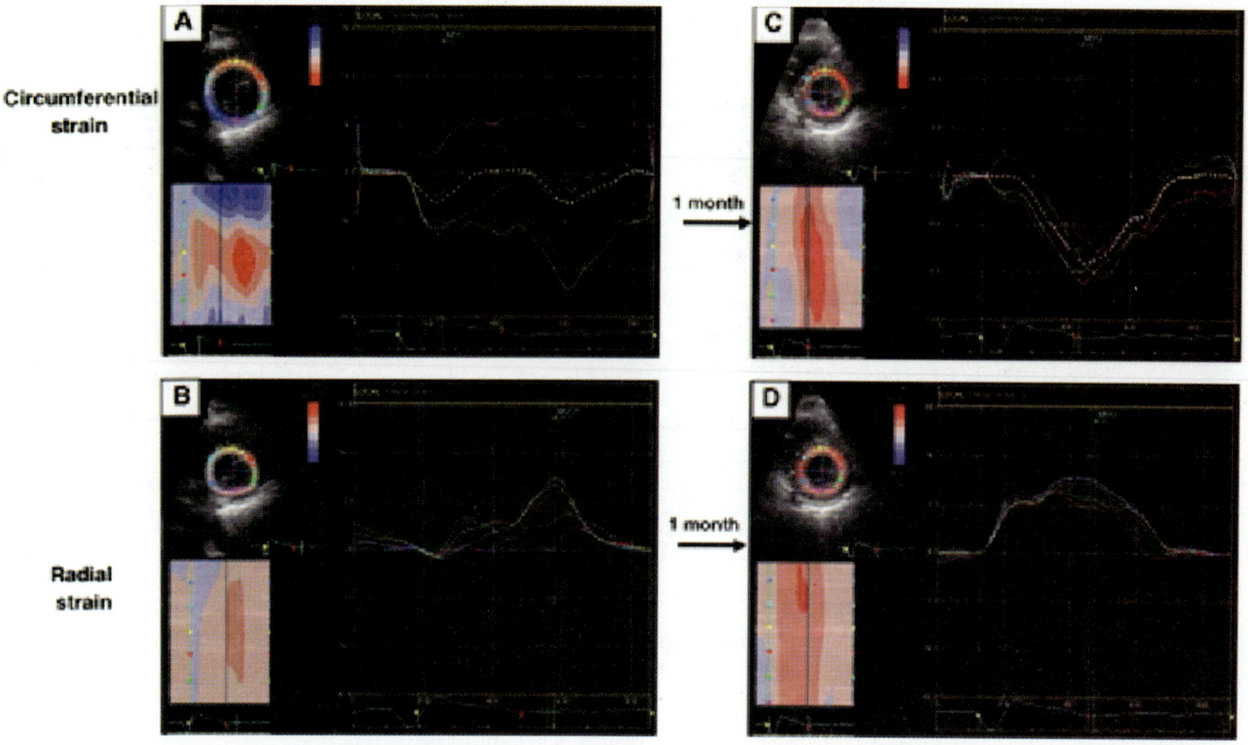

Fig. 51.16: *Strain and strain rate images in heart transplant recipients with focal stenoses of coronary arteries. (A and B): circumferential strain and strain rate in a patient with stenosis of the right coronary artery. (C and D): Longitudinal strain and strain rate in a patient with stenosis of the left anterior descending coronary artery. [Dandel et al. JHLT 2008;27(2):S95-96]*

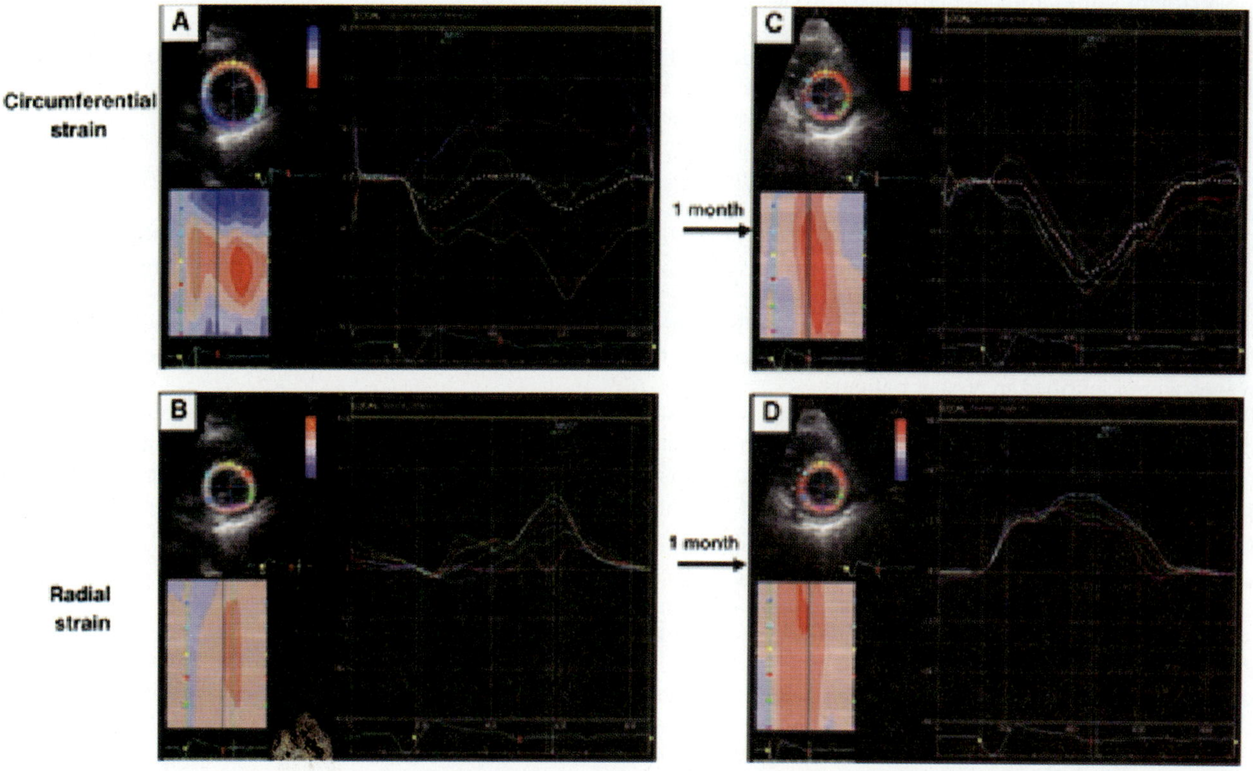

Fig. 51.17: *Time course of 2D-strain images recorded during reduction of the LVAD (Type Incor) rate in a patient with idiopathic dilated cardiomyopathy who showed relevant myocardial recovery during mechanical unloading. After LVAD implantation, the global strain values were low and regional strain curves showed important dyssynchrony (A and B). One month later global strain values were several times higher and regional strain curves indicated uniform circumferential shortening and radial thickening (C and D). (Dandel et al., 2007, oral abstract, AHA Scientific Sessions)*

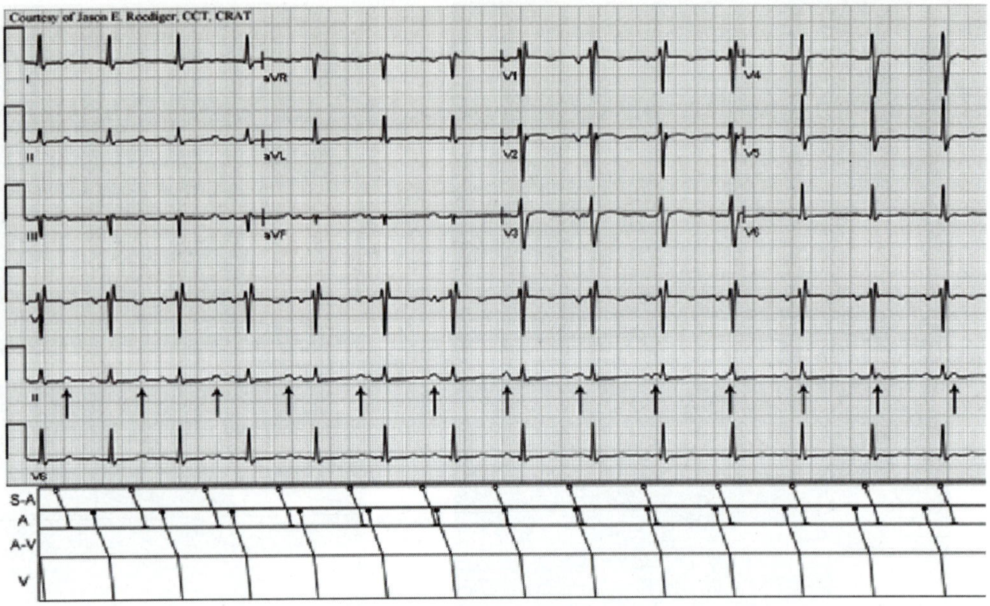

Fig. 51.18: *ECG shows orthotopic heart transplant. Recipient P-waves (arrows)*

Table 51.5: *ECG alternations in heart transplant patients*

General specifications

1. The recipient retains the posterior walls of his own atria.
2. The recipient's atria are vascularized by bronchial collateral vessels.
3. The transplanted heart is denervated and lacks autonomic neural control.
4. The EKG changes in these patients are mainly due to the remnant activity of the recipients atria, injury to the donor heart during the transplant procedure, and increased PVR in the recipient.
5. Atrial arrhythmias and ventricular conduction defects are common.
6. Role of the ECG in acute rejection is controversial.
7. MI may occur as a result of accelerated atherogenesis.

1. **Two sets of P waves (Fig. 51.18)**
   - The recipients native P waves are of a small amplitude donor P waves have normal amplitude and configuration
   - The suture line between the donor and the recipient atria blocks any interchange of the electrical impulses from the two sources. Atrial dissociation is present.
   - The donor P wave is conducted and stimulates the ventricles. The recipients atrial impulses are not conducted.
   - The rate of the denervated donor's heart is faster than that of the recipient's atrial remnant rate. In one series, two sets of P waves were identified in 86% of patients.
   - P waves of the recipient atrial remnants may not be seen because of their small amplitude or the presence of sinus node dysfunction or atrial fibrillation prior to the transplantation. May also lose the sinus node artery during surgery. Fib/flutter may be present in one set of atria while NSR is present in the other pair making interpretation difficult.
2. **RBBB (complete or incomplete):** Occurs in 83% of patients in Chou's experience, in 45% in another series.
3. **LAHB:** Occurs in about 25% of patients
4. **Bradyarrhythmias due to sinus node dysfunction**
   - Cause not explained by rejection or ischemic time during transplant
   - Subsidiary pacemakers may be unreliable in providing an escape rhythm and sudden death may occur.
   - Permanent pacemaker may be required.
   - PACs, PSVTs, afib and aflutter are seen postoperatively. Some investigators have felt that these episodes are associated with rejection episodes.
   - Presence of complex VEA is associated with accelerated atherosclerosis and early death.
5. **ST-segment and T-wave changes:** Some patients may develop diffuse ST-segment elevation followed by evolutionary changes of the ST segment and T wave changes consistent with acute pericarditis in the early postoperative period. as a rule these changes are transient
6. **ECG evidence of rejection:** Originally though that low voltage was indicative of rejection but this has been called into question.

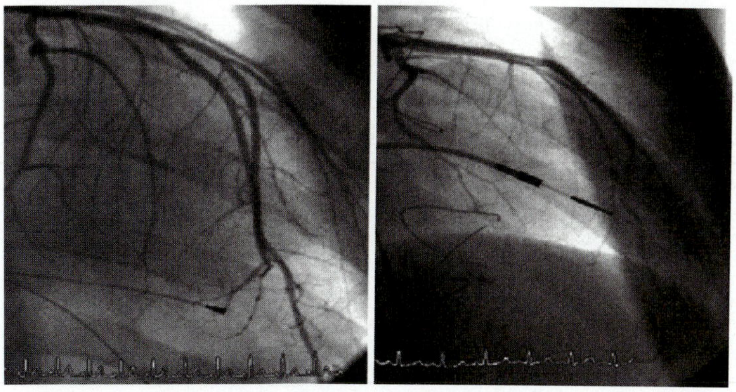

Fig. 51.19: *Angiographic studies from two patients. Left: a patient without signs of CAD. Right: signs of CAD with peripheral obliterations and B2 lesions with an intramyocardial pacemaker electrode (IMEG) in place*

Child's Diet after Heart Transplant

The immunosuppressant medicines may affect your child's appetite and weight after the operation, so a clinical dietician will help you and your child make sure that she eats healthy foods. Keeping a good weight will keep your child's new heart healthy.

It is important that your child eat foods that have little cholesterol and not too much salt. Foods with a lot of animal fat and cholesterol may make the chance of getting post-transplant coronary artery disease higher. Foods high in cholesterol can cause a thickening of the coronary arteries. Your child may also have high blood pressure after the transplant, so should not eat foods high in salt. The foods your child eats may change greatly after the operation. This is particularly true if, before the operation, your child had a restricted salt and fluid diet. After the transplant, your child should have lots of liquids to make sure that the medicines are well washed out through the kidneys.

Role of Exercise after Heart Transplant Surgery

After your child gets a new heart, she will be able to do lots of new things. A physiotherapist will work with you and your child so that she can get stronger and be able to exercise more. Your child will start doing exercises, called a physiotherapy program, in the hospital. Your child should continue to do this physiotherapy program after she goes home from the hospital (Fig. 51.20).

Appropriate Time of Discharge from the Hospital

Your child can go home when you, your child, and the heart transplant team believe the time is right. Often transplant patients start off on day passes, and then night passes, before they are completely discharged from the hospital. If you live more than a few hours away from the hospital, you'll need to find a place to stay close to the hospital for the first few weeks, and then a few months in the city.

Often getting your child ready to go home is a time filled with excitement and worry. After all, you will now be the main person caring for your child. You will be giving your child new medicines. You will also be arranging for all his regular medical needs, such as blood tests, heart biopsies, echocardiograms, electrocardiograms, and visits to the clinic. You may find this scary and wonder if you can deal with all this at home. This is very normal (Fig. 51.13).

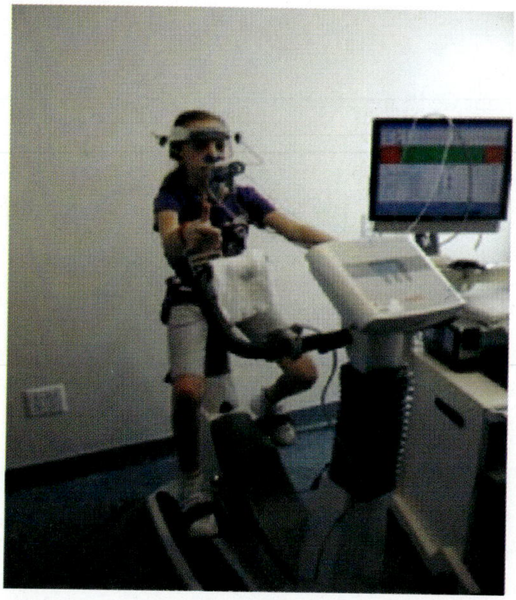

Fig. 51.20: *Young child with heart transplant is undergoing exercise stress test for knowing functional status of the heart*

To help with your child's care at home, the hospital may arrange for nurses to come to your home and check on your child. You'll also have help from a social worker and will come to clinic about twice a week for the first few weeks.

Prevention of Common Childhood Illnesses in a Transplant Patient

Brothers and sisters may get the common childhood conditions like coughs and colds, vomiting and diarrhea. Try to make sure that all members of your family wash their hands a lot. This is particularly important when you and your family change diapers and before making all meals and snacks.

For the first 3 months after the operation, let your child have only two visitors at a time. Make sure your child's friends do not visit when they have a fever, runny nose, cold, cough, vomiting, diarrhea, or rash. It is a good idea to ask all your visitors to wash their hands when they come to visit.

Make sure that all your pets have regular check-ups and have no fleas. Do not let your child touch your cat's litter box. That way your child should not get the germ called toxoplasmosis that cats sometimes have. Also, try to make sure that you and your child wash your hands after playing with cats and kittens.

Return of transplant child to his/her school or day **care**

In general, your child can return to school or day care 3 months after the transplant. Parents often go to the school before the child returns to talk to the child's teachers about what the child has been through. Members of the transplant team will send the school general information about having a student with a transplant and will be available to answer

Table 51.6: *Antimicrobial prophylaxis regimen postcardiac transplantation*

	Donor CMV negative	*Donor CMV positive*
Recipient CMB negative	No treatment	DHPG prophylaxis 34 days/cytovene/cytogam
Recipient CMB positive	DHPG prophylaxis 24 days	DHPG prophylaxis 24 days
DHPG (gancivlovir IV) 24 day regimen	5 mg/kg IV b.i.d. for 14 days 6 mg/kg IV q.d. for 10 days 5 mg/kg IV b.i.d. for 14 days 6 mg/kg IV b.i.d. for 20 days	
Cytovene (ganciclovir PO)		
1,000 mg PO TID for 6 weeks		
Cytogam (IgG gamma globulin)		
Within 72 hours posttransplant:	150 mg/kg	
Weeks 2, 4, 6, 8 posttransplant:	100 mg/kg	
Weeks 12 and 16 posttransplant:	50 mg/kg	
Pneumocystic carinii pneumonia prophylaxis		
Bactrim SS 1 table q.d. for life		
If bactrim allergic: pentamidine 300 mg nebulized Q month		
Aspergillus prophylaxis		
Amphotericin B aerosolized: 20 mg b.i.d. while hospitalized		

any questions that the school might have immunosuppressant drugs.

Complications in Heart Transplant Children (Figs 51.21–51.25)

The most significant causes of death after transplantation include early graft failure (either primary graft failure or secondary to pulmonary hypertension), allograft rejection, infection, allograft vasculopathy and malignancy.

Evaluation of an allograft rejection: The diagnosis of rejection is made based on clinical signs and symptoms, echocardiographic changes, and endomyocardial biopsy. Clinical clues to rejection include a decrease in the child's activity or feeding, low-grade fever, persistent resting tachycardia, ventricular ectopy, S_3 gallop, tachypnea/dyspnea, hepatic congestion, ileus, and other signs and/or symptoms of low cardiac output. Echocardiographic criteria for rejection are somewhat controversial, but include findings reflective of an increase in left ventricular mass, impairment of systolic and diastolic function, new pericardial effusion, and new mitral insufficiency. Endomyocardial biopsies are graded according to the criteria of the International Society for Heart and Lung Transplantation, with most centers only treating biopsies with a 3A (i.e. lymphocytic infiltration with myocyte degeneration) or greater histology.

Rejection is treated with bolus steroid therapy. The authors use methylprednisolone IV at a dose of 20 mg/kg/dose every 12 hours for 8 doses. For recurrent rejection or rejection accompanied by hemodynamic compromise, antithymocyte therapy is added. Various agents are available, such as orthoclone OKT3 (monoclonal mouse derived), antithymocyte gamma globulin (ATGAM) (polyclonal equine derived), and thymoglobulin (polyclonal rabbit derived). The authors use thymoglobulin at a dose of 1.5 mg/kg/dose given over 6 hours daily for 10 days. The target T-cell count (CD3 by flow cytometry) is 150/mL or less (Table 51.7).

Many options for adjusting immunosuppression protocols exist, depending on rejection history. Several programs now use tacrolimus and/or mycophenolic acid as primary immunosuppression therapy. These can also be used as

Table 51.7: *Stanford immunosuppressive regimen for cardiac transplantation*

Induction immunosupression	
Methylprednisolone	500 mg IV coming off bypass
Daclizumab	1 mg/kg coming off bypass (q2weeks for a total of 5 weeks)
Maintenance immunosuppression	
Sirolimus	2 mg per day 4 hours after Cyclosporine dose
Corticosteroids	Methylprednisolone 125 mg IV q8h for 3 doses postoperative
	Prednisone 1.0 mg/kg divided b.i.d. Days 1–14
	Prednisone Days 14 + taper to off as tolerated
Cyclosporine	25 mg p.o. b.i.d. postoperative day 1

"rescue" therapy for recalcitrant rejection. Total lymphoid irradiation also can be used for cases of rejection particularly difficult to treat.

- **Infection is an expected complication,** with a significant number of recipients experiencing one or more potentially serious infections in the first few months after transplantation. These infections in the early post-operative period usually are bacterial and include wound infections, pneumonia, bacteremia and urinary tract infections. CMV is a significant complication. *Pneumocystis carinii* occurs but is less frequent. Other opportunistic infections should be anticipated and aggressively treated when present.

Malignancy usually posttransplant ***lymphoproliferative disease associated with EBV infection, occurs in 2–10% of children.***

When the histology is low-grade (polymorphous hyperplasia), it usually responds to short-term cessation of immunosuppression. Higher-grade lymphomas also may respond to this therapy with chemotherapy reserved for rapidly progressive or persistent disease. A more recent development is the ability to use anti-CD20 monoclonal antibody (rituximab) to treat those tumors that express CD20.

- **Allograft vasculopathy** has emerged as the most important limiting factor for long-term survival. At 10 years after transplantation, as many as 20% of recipients will have developed significant allograft vasculopathy. Since the donor heart is denervated, children with graft vasculopathy rarely present with angina. They may have atypical angina such as shoulder or back pain, or, more frequently, abdominal pain. They also may present with syncope or sudden death. Significant vasculopathy that is diagnosed by coronary angiography probably is best treated with retransplantation (Figs 51.8 and 51.26).

Other modalities that have been useful in diagnosis are treadmill testing and dobutamine stress echocardiography. Data in adult heart transplantation suggest that calcium channel blockers and 3-hydroxy-3-methylglutaryl-coenzyme A reductase (HMG-CoA) inhibitors may help to prevent allograft vasculopathy, but data in children are lacking. Some transplant centers treat all children with these agents while others use them only in high-risk patients.

- Nephrotoxicity is the most import nonlethal complication. Hypertension, metabolic acidosis, and other metabolic abnormalities may be observed with varying frequency. Adjusting the calcineurin inhibitor to the lowest level possible helps ameliorate these problems. Minimizing steroid dosing also helps significantly with hypertension and with issues relating to growth and bone density.

Prognosis after Transplant Surgical Intervention

In the current era in experienced centers, expected 1-year survival is 80–90%, 2-year survival is 80–85%, and 5-year survival is approximately 70–80%. Mortality while waiting for a donor organ is additive to these survival figures. A survival advantage appears to exist for infants transplanted in the first month of life compared to infants transplanted during the remainder of the first year of life. This likely is related to immunologic and nonimmunologic factors.

The condition of the children who have survived beyond 10 years after transplant is good. Two-thirds of infant recipients who are older than 10 years are described as developmentally normal by their parents. More formal psychometric testing shows that infant heart transplant recipients score lower on IQ testing than normal controls, with about a 10-point decrement in standardized testing.

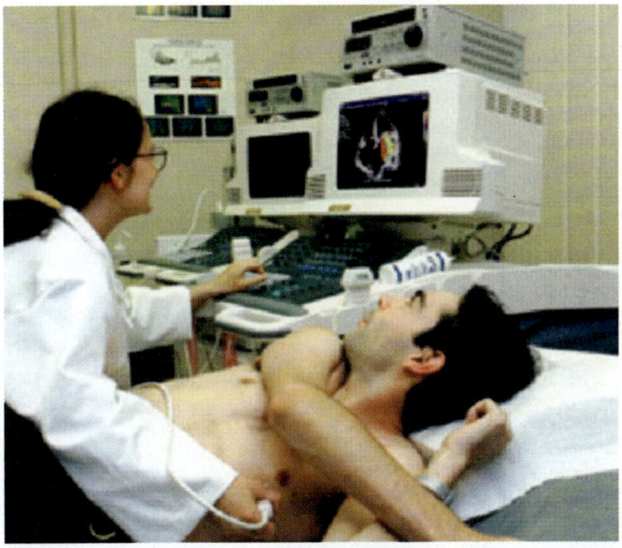

Fig. 51.21: *Teenager patient who received heart transplantation 6 months back is being investigated with strain and strain rate images for focal stenoses of coronary arteries. These patient are more prone to premature atherosclerosis and coronary artery disease*

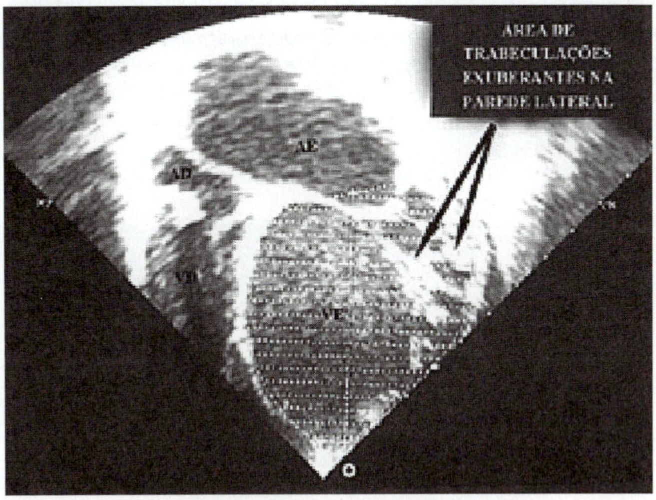

Fig. 51.22: *Echocardiogram showing dilatation of LV and LA cavities in dilated cardiomyopathy*

This is similar to infants undergoing other similar congenital heart surgery. In the absence of long-term higher-dose steroids, children grow appropriately after heart transplantation. Recent data indicate that they progress through puberty in a normal fashion. In the absence of repeated-graft rejection or graft vasculopathy, cardiac function and exercise tolerance are normal.

Rejection of the heart transplant: Rejection is the body's way of responding to something it thinks does not belong in the body. Some rejection is expected after the transplant. Most rejection events are mild and your child may not have any signs of the rejection. Rejection of your child's new heart could happen at any time, but happens most often during the first year after the heart transplant operation. There are different kinds of rejection. The most common type is called acute cellular rejection. There are more rare types of rejection that some patients are at higher risk of experiencing. If this is the case for your child, it will be explained to you by the transplant team.

Method of detection of rejection: A heart biopsy is one way to find out if your child's body is rejecting the new heart. It involves removing a small piece of heart muscle tissue for examination. Biopsies will be done regularly to check for rejection though less often if your child is a newborn or infant.

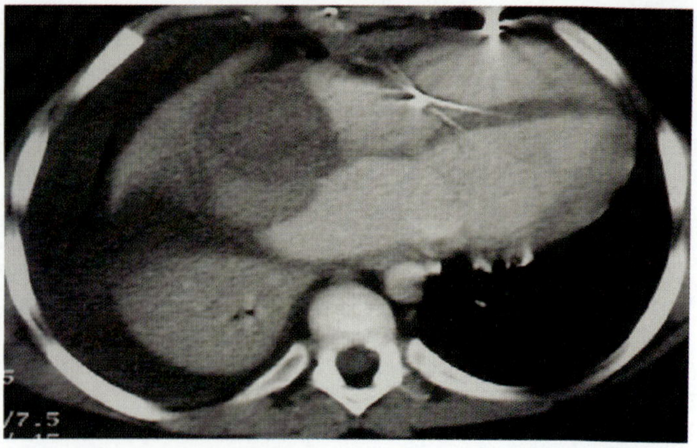

Fig. 51.24: *Axial CT scan with contrast through mid-chest region showing right pleural effusion and circular shadow adjacent to right atrium after heart transplantation*

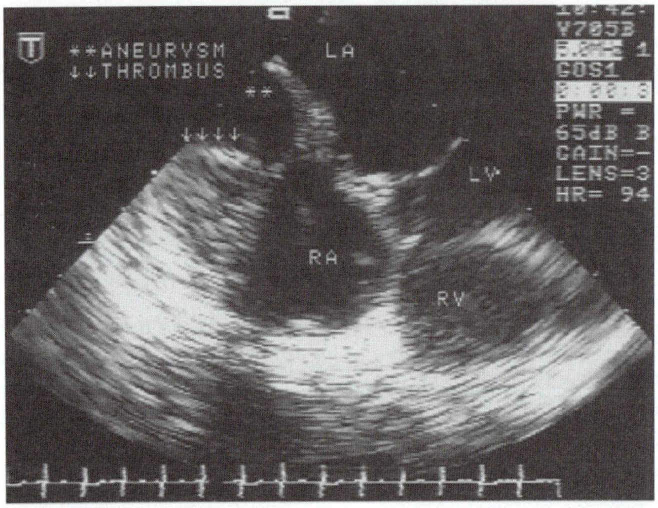

Fig. 51.23: *Transesophageal echocardiogram (four chamber view) showing large thrombus (arrowed) within aneurysm (asterisk) partly compressing the right atrium after heart transplantation (LA, left atrium; LV, left ventricle; RA, right atrium, RV, right ventricle)*

Immunosuppressive therapy: Immunosuppressant medications are the medications given to stop your child's body from rejecting the new heart. They are started in the operating room and your child will need to continue taking them for the rest of her life. The health of your child's new heart will depend on her taking these medications exactly as they are prescribed every day. Although these are critical for the health of your child's heart, they do have side effects which may need other medications to treat. All of these things will be explained and taught to you while your child is in the hospital. This will continue in the outpatient clinic visits (Table 51.8).

Type of immunosuppressant drugs used in heart transplant patients.

Your child will need to take immunosuppressants for the rest of his life. These drugs are used to prevent and treat rejection. There are three groups of immunosuppressants:

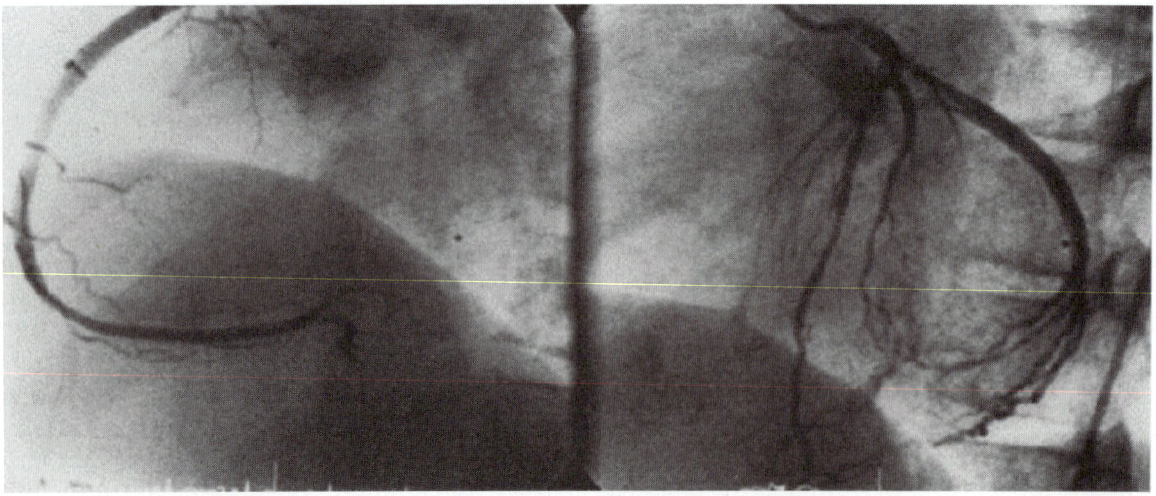

Fig. 51.25: *Selective right and left coronary angiograms showing graft dysfunction in a patient 5 years after transplant*

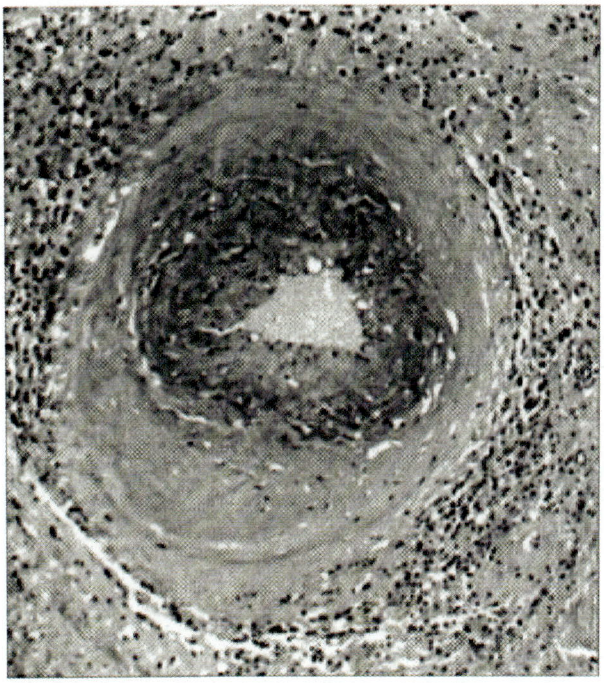

Fig. 51.26: *Postmortem histopathologic section of left anterior descending coronary artery from patient who died suddenly 8 years after heart transplantation. Note the extensive myointimal proliferation with obliteration of the coronary lumen. A mononuclear cell infiltrate is evident in the adventitia and a small number of lymphocytes infiltrate the vascular wall. Hematoxylin and Eosin, 20×*

cyclosporine or FK506 azathioprine or mycophenolate mofetil prednisone cyclosporine (Table 51.8).

Cyclosporine

Cyclosporine helps to prevent the body from rejecting the transplanted heart.

Cyclosporine is usually given twice a day, 12 hours apart at the same times each day. Blood levels of cyclosporine are checked to make sure your child is receiving the correct amount.

Food affects how the body absorbs cyclosporine. To maintain constant blood levels, your child must always take cyclosporine the same way—either always with food or always without food.

You may mix cyclosporine with water, juice or milk. Mixing improves the taste. Never use grapefruit juice or fruit juices containing grapefruit juice. It increases the amount of cyclosporine in the blood.

Do not use a styrofoam cup to mix the cyclosporine as some of the medication will be absorbed by the styrofoam. Cyclosporine will stick to rubber nipples. Do not put a soother or a bottle in an infant's mouth for at least 5 minutes after giving cyclosporine.

Cyclosporine is stored at room temperature. Do not store cyclosporine in direct sunlight or in the refrigerator. The shade of yellow of liquid cyclosporine may vary but it must be clear. Do not use if it is cloudy. Keep the foil on the cyclosporine capsules until just before you give them to your child.

If a cyclosporine dose is missed, give your child the missed dose soon as you remember. If it is almost time for the next dose, do not give the missed dose at all but give the regular dose as scheduled. Contact your clinical nurse specialist or transplant nurse if there has been more than 1 dose of cyclosporine missed or if your child is not taking her cyclosporine.

If your child throws up within 30 minutes of giving the cyclosporine dose, give your child the full dose again.

If your child throws up between 30 minutes and 1 hour of giving the cyclosporine dose, give your child half the dose.

If your child throws up more than 1 hour after giving the dose of cyclosporine, do not repeat the medication.

Most common side effects of cyclosporine increase in bodily and facial hair found mostly on eyebrows, arms and back bleeding, tender or overgrown gums high blood pressure shakiness in the hands and feet damage to the kidneys changes in the blood such as higher potassium levels and lower magnesium levels. If your child has diarrhea, this can affect the amount of cyclosporine absorbed. If your child has diarrhea or 6 watery bowel movements in 12 hours, contact your clinical nurse specialist or transplant nurse.

Several other medications may change the way cyclosporine works. Some raise the cyclosporine level in your child's blood and others lower the level. Always call your clinical nurse specialist or transplant nurse before using any new medications. If your child's paediatrician or family doctor orders a new medication for your child, you must ask the doctor to call us to make sure it is safe for your child to take that medication with cyclosporine.

If your child's paediatrician or family doctor orders a new medication or antibiotic for your child, you must ask the doctor to call the transplant clinic, or your child's clinical specialist nurse or transplant nurse, to make sure it is safe for your child to take that medication with cyclosporine. Your child should never take an antibiotic containing erythromycin while she is taking cyclosporine because the erythromycin causes the cyclosporine level to go very high.

FK506/Tacrolimus

FK506 helps to prevent the body from rejecting the transplanted heart. If your child has had several rejection episodes while taking cyclosporine or has problems with the cyclosporine side effects, your child will be switched to FK506. Cyclosporine and FK506 are never used at the same time.

FK506 is given twice a day, 12 hours apart at the same times each day. Blood levels of FK506 are checked to make sure your child is receiving the correct amount.

Food affects how the body absorbs FK506. To maintain constant blood levels, your child should always take FK506 the same way—either always with food or always without food.

FK506 is stored at room temperature. Do not store FK506 in direct sunlight or in the refrigerator.

If a FK506 dose is missed, give your child the missed dose soon as you remember. If it is almost time for the

Table 51.8: *Clinically used immunosuppresive agents*

Agent	*Mechanism of action*	*Toxicities*
Induction immunosuppression		
Antilymphocyte/antithymocyte	Deplete activated lymphocytes	Antibody response
Immunoglobulin	Deplete activated thymocytes	Allergic reaction
OKT3	Sequestration of CD3$^+$ T cells	Cytokine release syndrome
Interleukin-2	Inhibits T cell activation	None know
Receptor blocker		
Maintenance immunosuppression		
Glucocorticoids	Antiinflammatory	Cushingoid habitus Glucose intolerance Osteoporosis Cataracts Hypertension Hyperlipidemia Poor wound healing
Cyclosporine	Calcineurin inhibitor Inhibits T cell proliferation	Nephrotoxicity Neurotoxicity Hypertension Gingival hyperplasis Hyperlipidemia
Tacrolimus	Calcineurin inhibitor Inhibits T cell proliferation	Nephrotoxicity Neurotoxicity Hypertension Gingival hyperplasis Diabetes Alopecia
Azathioprine	Purine analogue Inhibits de novo and salvage purine synthesis pathways	Marrow toxicity Hepatotoxicity
Mycophenolate Mofetil	Inhibitis inosine monophosphate dehydrogenase: inhibits de novo purine synthesis	Hepatotoxicity Gastrointestinal distance
Rapamycin	Inhibits T cell activation? unknown mechanism	Hyperlipidemia Myelosuppression

next dose, do not give the missed dose at all but give the regular dose as scheduled. Contact your clinical nurse specialist or transplant. Nurse if there has been more than 1 dose of FK506 missed or if your child is not taking his/her FK506.

If your child throws up within 30 minutes of giving the FK506 dose, give your child the full dose again. If your child throws up between 30 minutes and 1 hour of giving the FK506 dose, give your child half the dose.

If your child throws up more than 1 hour after giving the dose of FK506 do not repeat the medication.

Side Effects of FK506? changes in the blood such as high blood sugar, high potassium levels and low magnesium levels shakiness in the hands and feet high blood pressure damage to the kidneys insomnia diarrhea or watery bowel movement.

If your child has diarrhea, this can affect the amount of FK506 absorbed. If your child has diarrhea or 6 watery bowel movements in 12 hours, contact your clinical nurse specialist or transplant nurse.

Several other medications may change the way FK506 works. Some raise the FK506 level in your child's blood and others lower the level. Always call your clinical nurse specialist or transplant nurse before using any new medications. If your child's paediatrician or family doctor orders a new medication or antibiotic for your child, you must ask the doctor to call the transplant clinic, or your child's clinical specialist nurse or transplant nurse, to make sure it is safe for your child to take that medication with FK506. Your child should never take an antibiotic containing erythromycin while she is taking FK506 because the erythromycin causes the FK506 level to go very high.

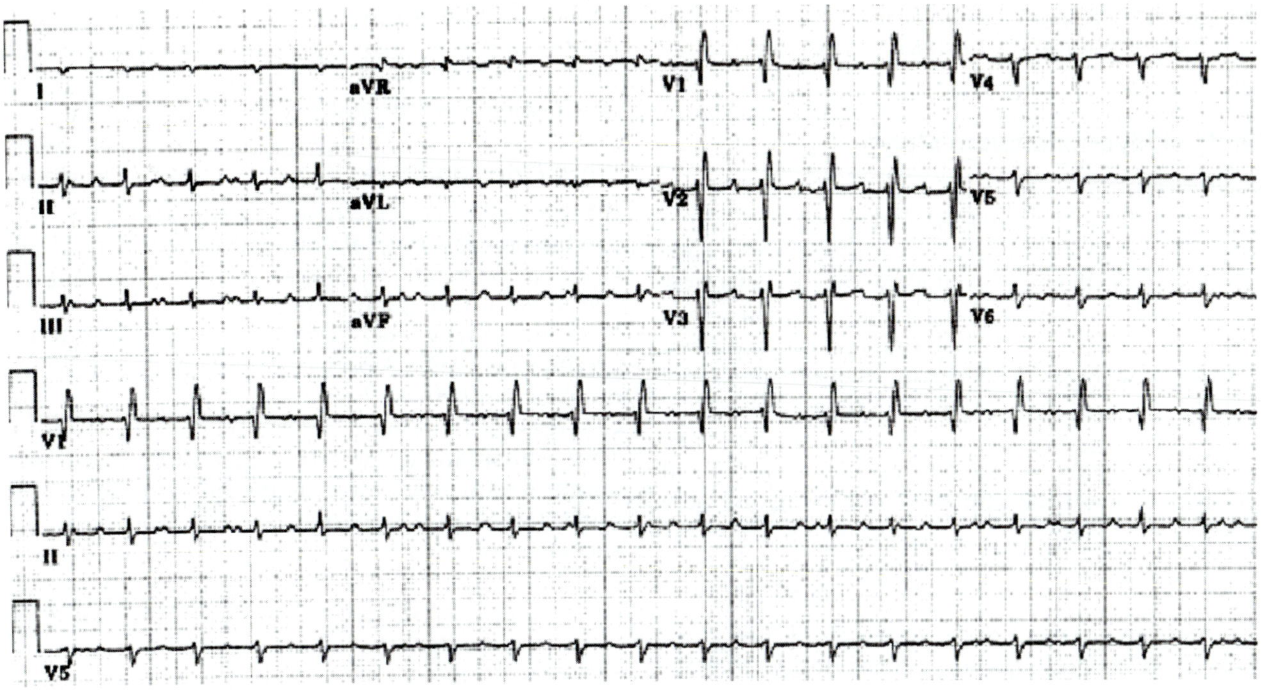

Fig. 51.27: *Twelve lead EKG shows accessory atrial activity (better seen in lead II at the end of the first complex in the middle between the second and the third complex and after the third complex) due to some of the original sinus node still remains in addition to the donor sinus node after a cardiac transplant. Because of a suture line in the right atrium the ectopic atrial rhythm rarely conducts to the AV node. Right-axis deviation and a rSR' which might suggest volume overload RVH also shown*

Azathioprine

Azathioprine helps to prevent the body from rejecting the transplanted heart.

- Azathioprine is given once a day in the morning.
- Azathioprine should always be given with food.
- Azathioprine pills are stored at room temperature.
- Azathioprine liquid is stored in the refrigerator.

If an azathioprine dose is missed, give your child the missed dose soon as you remember. Contact your clinical nurse specialist or transplant nurse if there has been more than 1 dose of azathioprine missed or if your child is not taking her azathioprine.

If your child throws up within 30 minutes of giving the azathioprine dose, give your child the full dose again.

If your child throws up between 30 minutes and 1 hour of giving the azathioprine dose, give your child half the dose.

If your child throws up more than 1 hour after giving the dose of azathioprine, do not repeat the medication.

Side Effects of Azathioprine

- Upset stomach
- Bruising
- Low white blood cell count in the blood.

If your child has diarrhea, this can affect the amount of azathioprine absorbed. If your child has diarrhea or 6 watery bowel movements in 12 hours, contact your clinical nurse specialist or transplant nurse. Several other medications may change the way azathioprine works. Always call your clinical nurse specialist or transplant nurse before using any new medications.

Mycophenolate Mofetil

Mycophenolate mofetil helps to prevent the body from rejecting the transplanted heart. If your child has had several rejection episodes while taking azathioprine, your child will be switched to mycophenolate mofetil. Azathioprine and mycophenolate mofetil are never used at the same time.

Mycophenolate mofetil is usually given twice a day, 12 hours apart at the same times each day. Food affects how the body absorbs mycophenolate mofetil. The most important thing is that your child should always take mycophenolate mofetil the same way each day—either always with food or always without food.

If your child has an upset stomach, your transplant cardiologist may tell you to give the mycophenolate 3–4 times a day in a lower dose. Never change the times you give the mycophenolate mofetil or the dose on your own. Mycophenolate mofetil is stored at room temperature. Keep mycophenolate mofetil in its package until your child needs a dose.

If a mycophenolate mofetil dose is missed, give your child the missed dose soon as you remember. If it is almost time for the next dose, do not give the missed dose at all but give the regular dose as scheduled. Contact your clinical nurse specialist or transplant nurse if there has been more than 1 dose of mycophenolate mofetil missed or if your child is not taking her mycophenolate mofetil.

If your child throws up less than 30 minutes after giving the mycophenolate mofetil dose, give your child the full dose again.

If your child throws up more than 30 minutes after giving the dose of mycophenolate mofetil do not repeat the medication.

Side Effects of Mycophenolate Mofetil

- Upset stomach
- Diarrhea or watery bowel movement
- Bruising.

If your child has diarrhea, contact your clinical nurse specialist or transplant nurse. Your child's diarrhea may mean that your child's dose of mycophenolate mofetil or the number of times you give it during the day may need to be changed.

Several other medications may change the way mychophenolate mofetil works. Always call your clinical nurse specialist or transplant nurse before using any new medications.

Prednisone

When children have a heart transplant, prednisone does two things: prednisone helps to prevent the body from rejecting the transplanted heart (Box 51.3).

Prednisone is also used to treat rejection after biopsy. If your child has a rejection, the transplant cardiologist will increase the dose of prednisone. Sometimes, the pill or liquid prednisone isn't strong enough to treat the rejection. Your child may need to have an intravenous form of prednisone called methylprednisolone.

Prednisone is given once a day in the morning. When prednisone is used to treat a 3A rejection, your child may need to take it twice a day for 4–5 days. Your clinical nurse specialist or transplant nurse will tell you exactly what to do if your child's prednisone dose changes and your child needs to take it more than once a day. Prednisone should always be given with food. It should never be given when your child's stomach is empty.

Prednisone pills are stored at room temperature. Prednisone liquid is stored in the refrigerator.

If a prednisone dose is missed, give your child the missed dose soon as you remember. Contact your clinical nurse specialist or transplant nurse if there has been more than 1 dose of prednisone missed or if your child is not taking her prednisone.

Box 51.3: *Side effects of prednisone*

Puffy cheeks
Weight gain
High blood pressure
Swelling of the hands and feet
Bruise easily
Hungry
Upset stomach
Mood changes
Higher amounts of sugar in your child's blood
Eye problems called cataracts
Weak bones

If your child throws up within 1 hour after giving the prednisone dose, give your child the full dose again.

If your child throws up after 1 hour after giving the prednisone dose, do not repeat the prednisone.

What One should do if your Child has Diarrhea?

If your child has diarrhea, this can affect the amount of prednisone absorbed. If your child has diarrhea or 6 watery bowel movements in 12 hours, contact your clinical nurse specialist or transplant nurse.

Several other medications may change the way prednisone works. Always call your clinical nurse specialist or transplant nurse before using any new medications. Changes in the dose of prednisone must only be done by your transplant doctor. If your child's paediatrician or family doctor wants to change the prednisone dose, you must call the transplant clinic, or your child's clinical specialist nurse or transplant nurse, immediately.

Controversies in Childhood Heart Transplant and Future Challenges

The oldest newborn recipient of a heart transplant reached age 15 years in 2000. Longer-term prognosis is unknown. Significant numbers of children are now entering the second decade after their transplantation and are generally in good health. The biggest challenge in the long-term is preventing or treating graft vasculopathy. Retransplantation, at some point in time, probably is inevitable for most, if not all, children who have undergone heart transplantation. If the vasculopathy is diagnosed in a timely manner, these children tolerate the second transplant well, with better survival rates than for the primary transplant. The role of calcium channel blockers, HMG-CoA reductase inhibitors, and newer immunosuppressive agents (e.g. mycophenolate, sirolimus) in the prevention of vasculopathy remains to be determined.

The most appropriate initial immunosuppression protocol is not known. Probably, a different protocol exists for nearly each transplant center. Clear data are difficult to obtain because of the small number of transplants performed each year and the need for centers to standardize practice across institutions. In addition, while early rejection and survival are important therapeutic end-points for research design, graft vasculopathy is the most important outcome measure. Vasculopathy does not become a significant issue for at least 5 years after transplantation. Much work remains to be done on this front.

Finally, donor supply is inadequate. Improved public and physician awareness of donor issues is the most important factor in increasing donor supply because many potential donors are not identified as such. Other more innovative and controversial sources of donors include resuscitation of asystolic donors and the use of xenografts.

BIBLIOGRAPHY

1. Armitage JM, Fricker FJ, del Nido P, et al: A decade (1982 to 1992) of pediatric cardiac transplantation and the impact of

FK 506 immunosuppression. J Thorac Cardiovasc Surg 1993 Mar; 105(3): 464–72.

2. Assaad A: Posttransplantation management of the newborn and the immunosuppressive role of prostaglandin E1. J Heart Lung Transplant 1993 Nov-Dec; 12(6 Pt 2): S191–4.
3. Bailey LL: Heart transplantation techniques in complex congenital heart disease. J Heart Lung Transplant 1993 Nov-Dec; 12(6 Pt 2): S168–75.
4. Bailey LL, Gundry SR, Razzouk AJ, et al: Bless the babies: one hundred fifteen late survivors of heart transplantation during the first year of life. The Loma Linda University Pediatric Heart Transplant Group. J Thorac Cardiovasc Surg 1993 May; 105(5): 805–14.
5. Bailey LL, Zuppan CW, Chinnock RE, et al: Graft vasculopathy among recipients of heart transplantation during the first 12 years of life. The Pediatric Heart Transplant Group. Transplant Proc 1995 Jun; 27(3): 1921–5.
6. Bauer J, Dapper F, Demirakca S, et al: Perioperative management of pulmonary hypertension after heart transplantation in childhood. J Heart Lung Transplant 1997 Dec; 16(12): 1238–47.
7. Baum D, Bernstein D, Starnes VA, et al: Pediatric heart transplantation at Stanford: results of a 15-year experience. Pediatrics 1991 Aug; 88(2): 203–14.
8. Baum M, Chinnock R, Ashwal S, et al: Growth and neurodevelopmental outcome of infants undergoing heart transplantation. J Heart Lung Transplant 1993 Nov-Dec; 12(6 Pt 2): S211–7.
9. Baum M, Freier MC, Freeman KR: Developmental outcomes and cognitive functioning in infant and child heart transplant recipients. Progress in Pediatric Cardiology 2000; 11: 159–163.
10. Berner M, Beghetti M, Spahr-Schopfer I, et al: Inhaled nitric oxide to test the vasodilator capacity of the pulmonary vascular bed in children with long-standing pulmonary hypertension and congenital heart disease. Am J Cardiol 1996 Mar 1; 77(7): 532–5.
11. Bork J, Chinnock R, Ogata K, Baum M: Infectious complications in infant heart transplantation. J Heart Lung Transplant 1993 Nov-Dec; 12(6 Pt 2): S199–202.
12. Boucek MM, Faro A, Novick RJ, et al: The Registry of the International Society of Heart and Lung Transplantation: Third Official Pediatric Report-1999. J Heart Lung Transplant 1999 Dec; 18(12): 1151–72.
13. Boucek MM, Mathis CM, Kanakriyeh MS, et al: Donor shortage: use of the dysfunctional donor heart. J Heart Lung Transplant 1993 Nov-Dec; 12(6 Pt 2): S186–90.
14. Boucek MM, Mathis CM, Boucek RJ Jr, et al: Prospective evaluation of echocardiography for primary rejection surveillance after infant heart transplantation: comparison with endomyocardial biopsy. J Heart Lung Transplant 1994 Jan-Feb; 13(1 Pt 1): 66–73.
15. Boucek RJ Jr, Naftel D, Boucek MM, et al: Induction immunotherapy in pediatric heart transplant recipients: a multicenter study. J Heart Lung Transplant 1999 May; 18(5): 460–9.
16. Burch M, Siddiqi SA, Celermajer DS, et al: Dilated cardiomyopathy in children: determinants of outcome. Br Heart J 1994 Sep; 72(3): 246–50.
17. Canter C, Naftel D, Caldwell R, et al: Survival and risk factors for death after cardiac transplantation in infants. A multi-institutional study. The Pediatric Heart Transplant Study. Circulation 1997 Jul 1; 96(1): 227–31.
18. Canter CE: Preoperative assessment and management of pediatric heart transplantation. Progress in Pediatric Cardiology 2000; 11: 91–97.
19. Cetta F, O'Leary PW, Seward JB, Driscoll DJ: Idiopathic restrictive cardiomyopathy in childhood: diagnostic features and clinical course. Mayo Clin Proc 1995 Jul; 70(7): 634–40.
20. Chartrand C, Guerin R, Kangah M, Stanley P: Pediatric heart transplantation: surgical considerations for congenital heart diseases. J Heart Transplant 1990 Nov-Dec; 9(6): 608–16.
21. Chen JM, Levin HR, Michler RE, et al: Reevaluating the significance of pulmonary hypertension before cardiac transplantation: determination of optimal thresholds and quantification of the effect of reversibility on perioperative mortality. J Thorac Cardiovasc Surg 1997 Oct; 114(4): 627–34.
22. Chiavarelli M, Gundry SR, Razzouk AJ, Bailey LL: Cardiac transplantation for infants with hypoplastic left-heart syndrome. JAMA 1993 Dec 22–29; 270(24): 2944–7.
23. Chinnock R, Baum M: Somatic growth in infant heart transplant recipients. Pediatr Transplant 1998 Feb; 2(1): 30–4.
24. Chinnock R, Emery J, Larsen R, et al: Methotrexate therapy for complex graft rejection in pediatric heart transplant recipients. The Pediatric Heart Transplant Team—Loma Linda. J Heart Lung Transplant 1995 Jul-Aug; 14(4): 726–33.
25. Chinnock RE, Baum MF, Larsen R, Bailey L: Rejection management and long-term surveillance of the pediatric heart transplant recipient: the Loma Linda experience. J Heart Lung Transplant 1993 Nov-Dec; 12(6 Pt 2): S255–64.
26. Chinnock RE: Pediatric heart transplantation at Loma Linda: 1985 to 1996. Clin Transpl 1996; 145–51.
27. Chinnock RE, Torres VI, Jutzy RV, et al: Cardiac pacemakers in pediatric heart transplant recipients: incidence, indications, and associated factors. Pediatric Heart Transplant Group- Loma Linda. Pacing Clin Electrophysiol 1996 Jan; 19(1): 26–30.
28. Chinnock RE, Cutler D, Baum M: Clinical outcome 10 years after infant heart transplantation. Progress in Pediatric Cardiology 2000; 11: 165–169.
29. del Rio MJ: Transplantation in complex congenital heart disease. Progress in Pediatric Cardiology 2000; 11: 107–113.
30. Denfield SW, Rosenthal G, Gajarski RJ, et al: Restrictive cardiomyopathies in childhood. Etiologies and natural history. Tex Heart Inst J 1997; 24(1): 38–44.
31. Dent CL, Canter CE, Hirsch R, Balzer DT: Transplant coronary artery disease in pediatric heart transplant recipients. J Heart Lung Transplant 2000 Mar; 19(3): 240–8.
32. Fricker FJ, Addonizio L, Bernstein D, et al: Heart transplantation in children: indications. Report of the Ad Hoc Subcommittee of the Pediatric Committee of the American Society of Transplantation (AST). Pediatr Transplant 1999 Nov; 3(4): 333–42.
33. Fritzsche SD, McCabe JL, Chinnock RE: Rare combined heart and kidney transplant in a pediatric patient: a case study. J Transpl Coord 1999 Sep; 9(3): 145–8.

34. Fukushima N, Gundry SR, Razzouk AJ, Bailey LL: Risk factors for graft failure associated with pulmonary hypertension after pediatric heart transplantation. J Thorac Cardiovasc Surg 1994 Apr; 107(4): 985–9.
35. Gajarski RJ, Towbin JA, Bricker JT, et al: Intermediate follow-up of pediatric heart transplant recipients with elevated pulmonary vascular resistance index. J Am Coll Cardiol 1994 Jun; 23(7): 1682–7.
36. Hirsch R, Huddleston CB, Mendeloff EN, et al: Infant and donor organ growth after heart transplantation in neonates with hypoplastic left heart syndrome. J Heart Lung Transplant 1996 Nov; 15(11): 1093–100.
37. Hsu DT, Garofano RP, Douglas JM, et al: Exercise performance after pediatric heart transplantation. Circulation 1993 Nov; 88(5 Pt 2): II238–42.
38. Jacobs ML, Blackstone EH, Bailey LL: Intermediate survival in neonates with aortic atresia: a multi-institutional study. The Congenital Heart Surgeons Society. J Thorac Cardiovasc Surg 1998 Sep; 116(3): 417–31.
39. Jenkins PC, Flanagan MF, Jenkins KJ, et al: Survival analysis and risk factors for mortality in transplantation and staged surgery for hypoplastic left heart syndrome. J Am Coll Cardiol 2000 Oct; 36(4): 1178–85.
40. Kawauchi M, Gundry SR, de Begona JA, et al: Prolonged preservation of human pediatric hearts for transplantation: correlation of ischemic time and subsequent function. J Heart Lung Transplant 1993 Jan-Feb; 12(1 Pt 1): 55–8.
41. Kirklin JK: Pediatric cardiac transplantation. Ann Thorac Surg 2000 May; 69(5): 1627–8.
42. Kuhn MA, Jutzy KR, Deming DD, et al: The medium-term findings in coronary arteries by intravascular ultrasound in infants and children after heart transplantation. J Am Coll Cardiol 2000 Jul; 36(1): 250–4.
43. Larsen RL, Applegate PM, Dyar DA, et al: Dobutamine stress echocardiography for assessing coronary artery disease after transplantation in children. J Am Coll Cardiol 1998 Aug; 32(2): 515–20.
44. Loker J, Darragh R, Ensing G, Caldwell R: Echocardiographic analysis of rejection in the infant heart transplant recipient. J Heart Lung Transplant 1994 Nov-Dec; 13(6): 1014–8.
45. Lynch BJ, Glauser TA, Canter C, Spray T: Neurologic complications of pediatric heart transplantation. Arch Pediatr Adolesc Med 1994 Sep; 148(9): 973–9.
46. Moran AM, Lipshultz SE, Rifai N, et al: Non-invasive assessment of rejection in pediatric transplant patients: serologic and echocardiographic prediction of biopsy-proven myocardial rejection. J Heart Lung Transplant 2000 Aug; 19(8): 756–64.
47. Morrow WR, Naftel D, Chinnock R, et al: Outcome of listing for heart transplantation in infants younger than six months: predictors of death and interval to transplantation. The Pediatric Heart Transplantation Study Group. J Heart Lung Transplant 1997 Dec; 16(12): 1255–66.
48. Morrow WR, Frazier E, Naftel DC: Survival after listing for cardiac transplantation in children. Progress in Pediatric Cardiology 2000; 11: 99–105.
49. Pahl E, Crawford SE, Swenson JM, et al: Dobutamine stress echocardiography: experience in pediatric heart transplant recipients. J Heart Lung Transplant 1999 Jul; 18(7): 725–32.
50. Pahl E, Zales VR, Fricker FJ, Addonizio LJ: Posttransplant coronary artery disease in children. A multicenter national survey. Circulation 1994 Nov; 90(5 Pt 2): II56–60.
51. Pahl E: Transplant coronary artery diseasein children. Progress in Pediatric Cardiology 2000; 11: 137–143.
52. Pietra BA, Boucek MM: Immunosuppression for pediatric cardiac transplantation in the modern era. Progress in Pediatric Cardiology 2000; 11: 115–129.
53. Razzouk AJ, Chinnock RE, Dearani JA, et al: Cardiac retransplantation for graft vasculopathy in children: should we continue to do it? Arch Surg 1998 Aug; 133(8): 881–5.

52 Practice of Yogic Exercises by Children and Adolescents in Reconditioning of Cardiovascular System

Influence of Yogic Exercises and Asanas in Health and Disease

Exercise has definite role to play in improving blood supply to the vital organs of the human body. This fact was not only known to yogacharyas but recently it has also been proved in animal experiments that exercise boosts brain power by building new brain cells in a brain region linked with memory and memory loss, US experts reported in their well-planed scientific study. Tests on mice showed they grew new brain cells in a brain region called the dentate gyrus, a part of the hippocampus that is known to be affected in the age-related memory decline that begins around age 30 years for most humans. Greg Quirk, a neurophysiologist from the Ponce School of Medicine in Puerto Rico, was quoted as saying.

Regular practice of yogic asanas also improves blood supply to the cardiovascular system thereby preventing many number of premature deaths due to fatal heart attacks. Problems of hypertension, ischemic heart diseases, dyslipidemia, dysmetabolic syndrome which are being frequently seen in daily practice if managed with yoga exercises as demonstrated in this chapter on both adolescents and in children would go in a long way in the prevention of these dreadly diseases. This chapter also illustrates a 3-year-old child in a attempt to perform some of the easy yogic exercises to create general awareness that such type of exercises can be practiced irregularly as her tender age.

Asanas Make you Strong and Healthy and Eradicate many Diseases such as

Bhastrika Pranayama develops lungs, destroys the germs of tuberculosis, augments lung-power and lung-capacity. Constipation is removed by the practice of **Bhujanga, Salabha and Dhanur Asanas.**

Dhanurasana is a combination of Bhujanga and **Salabha Asanas.**

Eating in moderation, plain living and high thinking help the Yogic student in attaining his goal quickly.

Fasting eliminates poison, purifies the system and invigorates the cells.

Garbhasana augments the digestive power, increases the appetite and removes many intestinal diseases.

Halasana makes the spine very supple and elastic.

Indriyas should be controlled by the practice of Pratyahara.

Japa of "Om" or "Hari Om" should go hand in hand with **Asanas and Pranayamas.**

Kumbhaka helps to attain longevity and awakens the Kundalini.

Lolasana strengthens the muscles of the arms and forearms.

Mind can be controlled by Vairagya, Abhyasa, Satsanga Vichara, eradication of Vasanas, destruction of egoism, Pranayama, meditation, and cultivation of virtues, such as mercy, complacency, self-denial, Santi and Santosha.

Pranayamas

Yoga Mudra removes the disorders of the abdomen and awakens Kundalini.

Zerosis is the disease of the eye owing to the deficiency of Vitamin "A". This is removed by the practice of mild Trataka and Sirshasana.

Padmasana

You must be able to sit in an Asana quite steady at a stretch for full 3 hours. Then only you will get mastery over the Asana (Asana Jaya). Without securing a steady Asana you cannot get on well in meditation. The more steady you are in your Asana, the more you will be able to concentrate and make your mind one-pointed. If you can be steady in the posture even for 1 hour, you will be able to acquire one-pointed mind and feel thereby infinite peace and atomic bliss inside. Four Asanas, viz., Padmasana, Siddhasana, Svastikasana and Sukhasana, are prescribed for meditative purposes. Rishis like Gheranda, Sandilya and others speak very highly of Padmasana. This is highly agreeable to householders. Spread a seat on the ground and take your seat facing North or East. Spread the legs forward. Take hold of your right foot and keep it on the left thigh and then place the left foot over the right thigh. Place the hands on the knees. You can make a finger-lock and keep the hands over the left ankle.

Nadi Suddhi can be Obtained by the Practice of Pranayama

Oordhva Padmasana checks wet-dreams and transmutes the sexual energy into Ojas.

Paschimottanasana removes fat, increases the gastric fire and eradicates diseases of the stomach.

Quetta earthquake is nothing when compared to the agitation caused in the mind by the turbulent senses.

Regularity in the practice of Asana and Pranayama is indispensably requisite for quick and solid progress.

Sirshasana is the king of all Asanas. It transmutes seminal energy into Ojas, develops memory and intellectual capacity, and removes a host of ailments.

Trataka helps concentration of the mind and removes diseases of the eyes.

Uddiyana Bandha imparts beautiful health, strength, vigour and vitality and removes the disorders of the alimentary system.

Vajrasana removes drowsiness, strengthens the spine, helps digestion and is very useful for meditation.

Winter is the best time for rigorous practice of Yoga.

Xerostomia (abnormal dryness of the mouth) can be removed by the practice of Sitali and Sitkari.

List of the Asanas

- Sukhasana-Easy Pose
- Padmasana-Lotus Pose
- Vajrasana-Hardy Pose
- Nata Vajrasana-Forward, bend Pose
- Vistrita Pad a Vajrasana-Hardy Pose with Parted Feet
- Supta Vajrasana-Horizontal Hardy Pose
- Gomukhasana-Cow, head Pose
- Ardha Matsyendrasana-Incomplete Matsyendra Pose
- Puma Matsyendrasana-Complete Matsyendra Pose
- Gorakshasanas-Goraksha Poses
- Goraksha Pose (Bhadrasana-Good Pose)
- Goraksha Pose
- Goraksha (Bhagasana-Vulvar Pose)
- Goraksha Pose (Guhyapadasana-Hidden Feet Pose)
- Vistrita Padasana-Lateral Stretched Legs Pose
- Janushirasana-Knee-Head Pose
- Veerya Stambhanasana-Semen Retention Pose
- Eka Pad a Shirasana-Foot-Head Pose
- Dvipada Shirasana-Feet-Head Pose
- Lolasana-Swing Pose
- Garbhasana-Foetus Pose
- Shirshasana-Head Stand Utthitapadasana-Raised Legs Pose
- Utthitapadashirasana-Raised Head and Legs pose
- Chakrasana-Wheel Pose
- Eka Pada Shalabhasana-Locust Pose
- Dvipada Shalabhasana-Locust Pose
- Urdhwa Sarvangasana-Shoulder Stand Pose
- Halasana-Plough Pose
- Matsyasana-Crocodile Pose
- Matsyasana-Crocodile Pose
- Bhujangasana-Serpent Pose
- Dhanurasana-Bow Pose
- Merusankarshasana-Spinal Traction Pose
- Pranayama-Yogic Breathing Shavasana
- Pose of Tranquillity

THE ASANAS

General Instructions

1. **Wake-up before sunrise:** This practice tones up the muscles of the eye as it protects the pupil of the eye against its sudden contraction which will inevitably result if the eye is opened in full daylight. Yoga always advices avoidance of sudden movements or jerks in all bodily activities. By rising before sunrise, you allow the pupil to take in the light gradually. As the sun rises, the pupil contracts slowly and gradually without its neuro, muscular structure contracting suddenly with a jerk. If, however, the nature of your work or routine forces upon you the need to sleep late, see that you wake-up in a room where sunlight, or even daylight, does not fall directly on your eyes when you wake-up, and where you can slowly and gradually get accustomed to light before they are subjected to the full impact of daylight.
   Another benefit of rising early is that you get a surplus of time in the morning which can protect you against jitters and nervousness arising out of rushing your morning activities to catch up with your office time. With a little more time at your disposal, you can go about your morning duties with a relaxed mind, a prerequisite to the practice of Yoga, and can easily extract your half-an-hour for the regular practice of Yoga. Thus, beginning your day with a cool and relaxed mind, instead of in a huff and a hurry, this tranquil beginning of the day may reflect beneficially on all your activities throughout the day. This little change in routine in getting up earlier may make all the difference to your career and your relationships with others.
2. **Ensure cleanliness of the bowels:** If your diet is correct, you observe punctuality and regularity with regard to the time of moving your bowels, you are not likely to suffer from constipation. Once the regular habits are formed, and the Yogic exercises are commenced, your chances of remaining free from constipation are considerably improved.
3. Your bowels must be clean at the time of practising the Asanas and Pranayama (Yogic exercises and breathing). Yoga is best practised on a clean bowel and an empty stomach. You are permittedto take a hot or cold bath before performing your exercises, if it suits your routine, but you can per form them even without taking a bath. You can have a hot bath anytime after

the exercise but you cannot take a cold bath within 15 minutes of completion of the Yogic exercises. Again, it is very desirable to have a bath daily but it is not absolutely essential in exceptionally cold climates. It may, however, be mentioned that both the hot and the cold baths are aphrodisiacs and are desirable from many angles-hygienic, tonic, aesthetic and, of course, aphrodisiac. You will start enjoying cold baths even in cold climates once you start your Yoga earnestly and regularly.

4. You can go through your exercises either in the morning or in the afternoon when the stomach is empty and the bowels clean. The duration of exercises should range from 15 to 45 minutes according to your capacity and the stage you have reached in the practice of your Asanas. Breakfast can be taken 30 minutes after completing the exercises but this period can be reduced to as little as 5 minutes, if you happen to be a very busy person. Remember that an empty bowel is a necessity before the exercises and not after them. If you want to give a demonstration of the Asanas before your friends, better choose an evening rather than a morning as the body is generally more flexible during the latter part of the day. If you perform your exercises in the evening, you are not to eat anything for at least 3 hours preceding the commencement of the exercises. This is to accommodate the needs of modern life. The classical Yogic demand is a 4-hour abstinence from food preceding the exercises.
5. If you practise prayer or meditation, it should usually be performed sitting in Sukhasana (Easy Pose) or Padmasana (Lotus Pose), before or after you do your pranayamic breathing exercises. If your prayers involve any rituals or visits to any shrines, better finish the Yogic exercises and breathing before commencing your religious practices. This will improve your concentration for prayer and meditation.
6. Both when practising Yoga and when not practising it, develop a habit of checking and rechecking your posture while standing or sitting and go on correcting the faulty posture, again and again, and day after day, until it becomes an unconscious habit with you. Sit and stand erect without sagging or hunching and without becoming stiff in your attempt at being erect. A large number of people associate erect posture with stiffness. This is unfortunate. The true posture is, both while standing or sitting, a *straight but relaxed* posture which you can easily develop through sustained practice of Yoga.
7. Begin with the practice of easier Asanas first. As the body acquires greater flexibility, add, gradually, to your practice comparatively more difficult Asanas. In trying to practise Asanas which are not easy for you to perform, stop at the stage when the pain becomes unpleasant. "Pleasant pain" is the boundary line up to which you can stretch your effort without restraining yourself. Remember that the most difficult pose is not necessarily the most beneficial pose. Should pain continue, consult a doctor immediately.
8. Relax your body with the following preliminary bending exercises before doing the Yogic ones:
   a. Stand erect with both your feet joined together, heel with heel and big toe with big toe. There should be no distance between the two big toes as is found in the stance adopted in modern exercises.
   b. Raise your arms as high as you can and bend your body backwards. Keep the legs steady and let the trunk go back as far as it can. Having reached the limit of your capacity to bend backward, start moving forward until your fingers touch the ground or the toes of your feet. Practise these bends ten times Breathe in when raising your hands from the ground and taking your body backward. Breathe out while bending forward. If you cannot cover one full backward movement in one inhalation and one full forward movement in one exhalation, stop in the process of bending, inhale or exhale your breath as needed, and resume the movement and the breathing where you left off.
   c. With your arms held against your waist on both sides, raise one leg as high up as you can and rotate it ten times, first clockwise and then anticlockwise. Bring the leg back into position and repeat the exercise with the other leg. In both cases, make your foot describe as large a circle during the rotation as possible. A photograph of Miss Lally has been included to show how high a leg can be raised for rotation if the body is well trained.
   d. Keeping your hands slightly away from your body, and standing erect with your feet slightly apart, rotate your pelvis, first clockwise and then anticlockwise, ten times in each case. You can place your hands on your waist as in (c) above to make it easier for you during the first few days or weeks of commencing the exercise.
   e. Similarly, holding the arms slightly away from your body with elbows partly relaxed, rotate your trunk first clockwise and then anticlockwise, ten times in each case. Here, too, you can place your hands on your waist as in (c) above to make the exercise easier.
   f. If short of time, reduce bends and rotations from ten each to five each, or even one each. Some of the Asanas, which the ancient Yogic texts have originally recommended for sublimation of the sex urge to promote celibacy among those involved in spiritual pursuits, will also prove to be excellent exercises for toning up the sex centres. The Asanas while contributing in varying degrees to general stability, strength, resilience, efficiency, flexibility and effective and satisfying functioning of all organs and tissues of the body, have a particular siant towards a rejuvenating, toning and sustaining effect on the sex centres (including the entire urogenital apparatus) of both men and women.

Sukhasana-Easy Pose Posture (Figs 52.1–52.5)

Sit on the ground. Fold your legs at the knees in such a way that one foot rests inside the knee, fold of the other leg

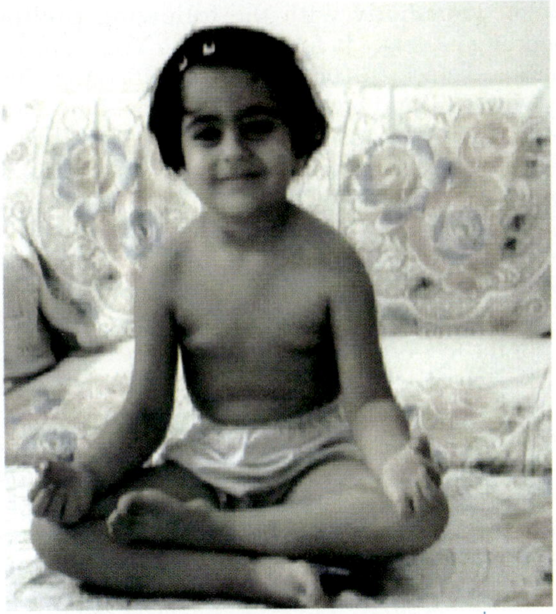

Fig. 52.1: *3-yrs-old girl performing lotus pose*

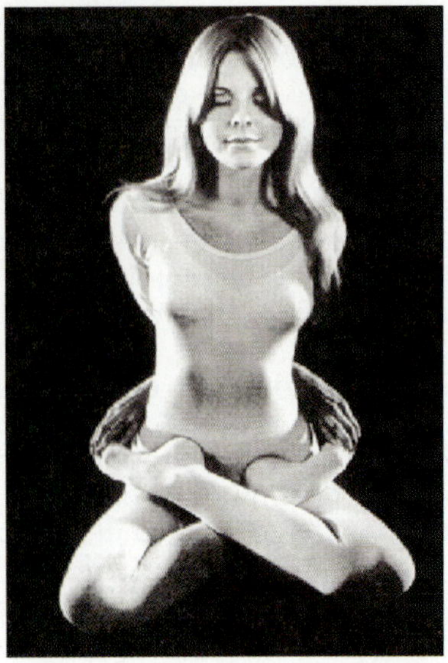

Fig. 52.3: *Full lotus posture*

and the other foot is on the ground beneath the knee, fold of the opposite leg, as shown in the plate.

Although the best pose for practising Yoga is **Padmasana (Lotus Pose)** which is described overleaf, the Sukhasana, being much easier, is widely practised by laymen in India at the time of meditation, worship and prayer. In the villages where people gather for a social chat or formal meetings or festive functions, or even in the houses where the only place to sit is on a carpet or a bare floor, Sukhasana is the pose generally adopted. Therefore, those of you who cannot perform Padmasana to begin with can use Sukhasana until you learn to sit comfortably in the Lotus Pose, and all the postures and Yogic breathing exercises which should be performed while sitting in the Lotus Pose can be practised in Sukhasana.

Benefits

The chief advantage of this posture is its availability to beginners in Yoga as a vehicle for Pranayama (Yogic breath culture) which has a direct bearing on reconditioning the nervous system and an indirect bearing on sexual performance. It is also a restful and tranquillizing pose which eliminates exhaustion and fatigue after strenuous games, drills or heavy manual labour. For relaxing the muscles of the body, including those related to the spine, Sukhasana is only bettered by Shavasana (Pose of Tranquillity) and Vajrasana (Hardy Pose).

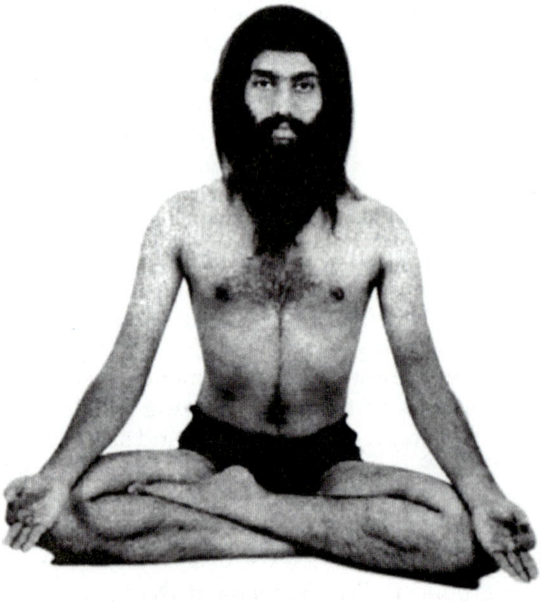

Fig. 52.2: *Lotus posture*

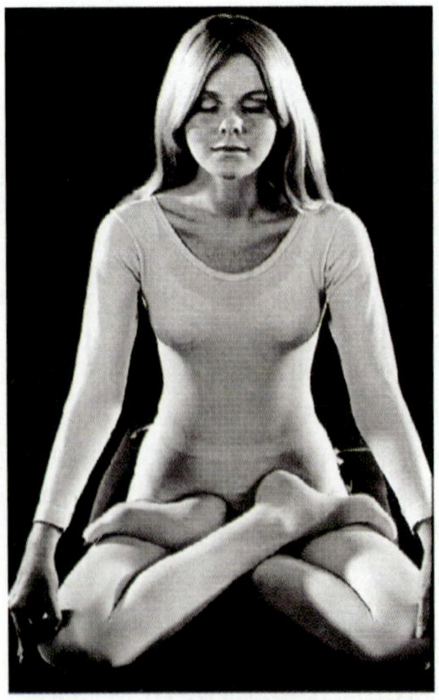

Fig. 52.4: *Sukhasana pose*

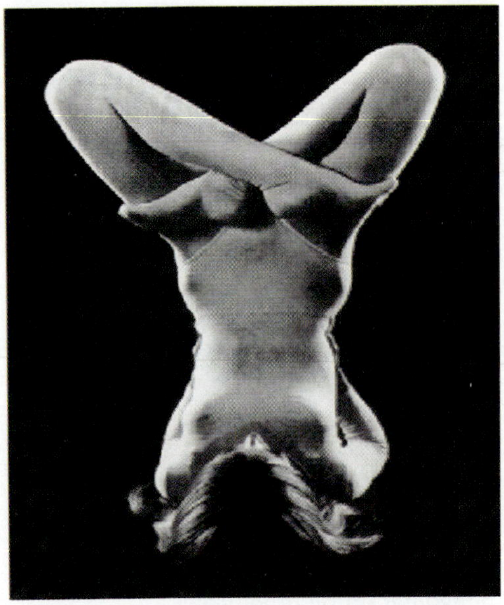

Fig. 52.5: *Lotus shoulder stand posture*

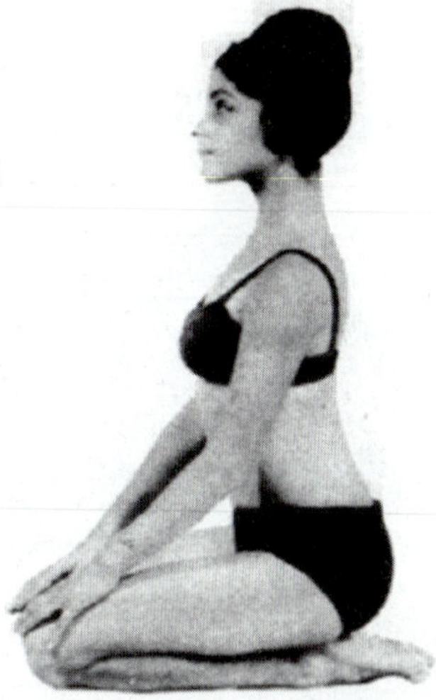

Fig. 52.6: *Vajrasna-hardy pose*

Vajrasana-Hardy Pose

Posture (Figs 52.6–52.11)

Kneel on the ground with your knees, ankles and big toes touching it. Then sit down on your heels. If you feel too much pressure from your weight on your feet you can move the heels outwards and then sit on them to distribute the weight over a larger portion of the soles. Place your hands on your knees, sit erect but relaxed.

Keep the eyes open and keep the breathing slow and deep. The chest should be expanded and abdomen drawn inwards.

Benefits

The great advantage of Vajrasana over all other postures is that it can be practised even by very advanced cases of heart disease. Also, unlike any other Asana except Vistrita Pada Vajrasana, it can be practised immediately after meals, however heavy.

Apart from its strengthening effect on the spine which I have dealt with in Yoga Against Spinal Pain, it improves the tone of the sexual organs in the male and the female. It is also supposed to be beneficial in cases of neuralgic headaches, sloth, stiffness, anger, anxiety, worry, cowardice, fear, hesitation, weakness and laxity of the sexual organs including the male and female gonads, thinness of semen and weak functioning of the kidneys. It effectively reduces flatulence and improves digestion. It prolongs youth and postpones old age. It contributes to self, confidence. The Yogis consider it a must for patients with heart disease. It is easy to perform and for patients of pronounced and discomforting flatulence it should be practised, in addition to regular morning exercises, after the two principal meals.

Important: No other variety of Vajrasana should be performed immediately after meals except this and *Vistrita Pada Vajrasana*.

Nata Vajrasana-Forward-Bend Hardy Pose

Posture (Fig. 52.17)

Sit down in Vajrasana (Hardy Pose) with both hands interlocked behind the back instead of being placed on the knees. Then bend your trunk slowly forward till your abdomen and chest comes into full contact with your thighs, and your chin and nose touch the ground infront of you. Hold this pose for 10 seconds or longer. Keep your eyes open. Take deep and slow breaths. Unlike the simple Vajrasana, Nata Vajrasana should not be performed immediately after meals. It must only be performed along with other Asanas on an empty stomach.

Benefits

As long as it is remembered that the Nata Vajrasana is not to be per, formed on a full stomach, the practice of this Asana confers all the benefits of the Vajrasana in a greater degree. In particular, its contribution to the flexibility of the spine and improvement of the tone of the sexual organs in both the sexes is more marked.

Vistrita Pada Vajrasana-Hardy Pose with Parted Feet Posture

Kneel down on the ground, spreading your feet as far apart as you can while keeping the knees together, so that you are sitting on the ground between your feet which are at a considerable distance from your body. Keep both your hands on your respective knees, sit erect but relaxed, keep the eyes open and continue slow and deep breathing.

Benefits (Fig. 52.18)

Like other Asanas which are practised by the Yogis for sublimation of the sex urge, this can also benefit the family man by toning up his sex centres.

Like the simple Vajrasana it can be practised after meals. It combines the benefits of the Vajrasana and the Gorakshasana poses as it is derived from both.

Supta Vajrasana-Horizontal Hardy Pose

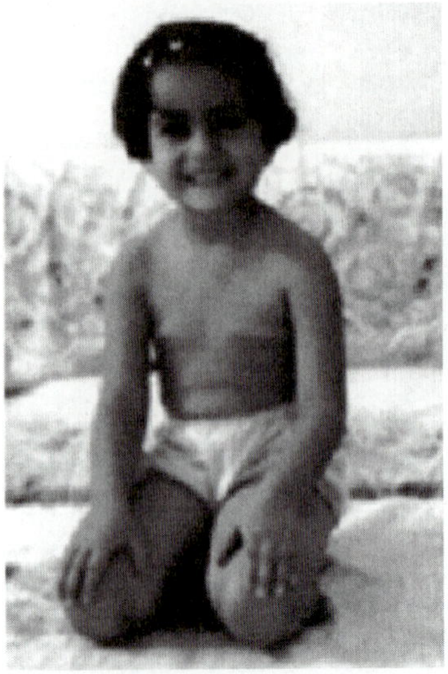

Fig. 52.7: *Vajrasna-hardy pose*

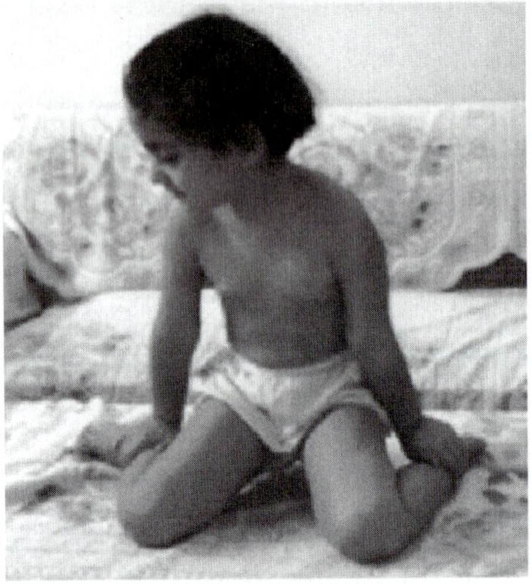

Fig. 52.8: *3-yrs-old girl showing an attempt to perform vajrasna-hardy pose*

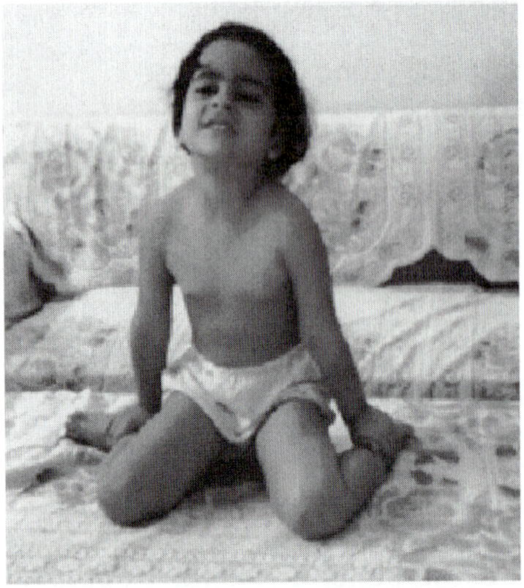

Fig. 52.9: *3-yrs-old girl making an attempt to perform Vistrita Pada Vajrasana-hardy pose with parted feet posture*

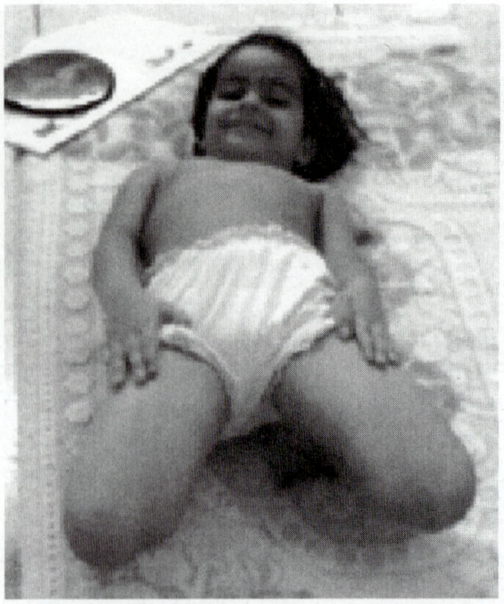

Fig. 52.10: *3-yrs-old girl making an attempt to perform Supta Vajarasna-horizontal Hardy (front view)*

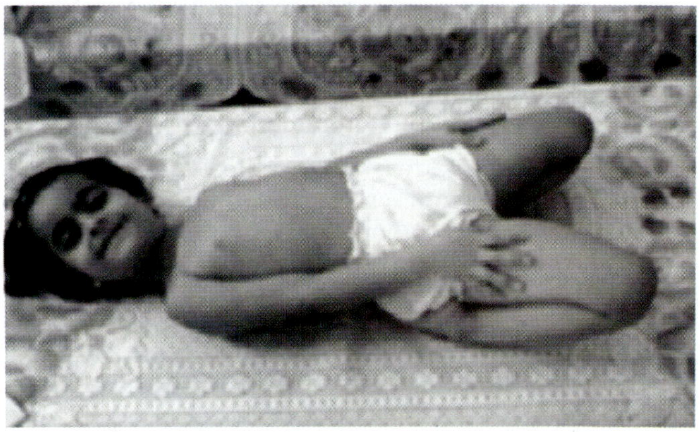

Fig. 52.11: *3-yrs-old girl making an attempt to perform Supta Vajarasna-horizontal Hardy (lateral view)*

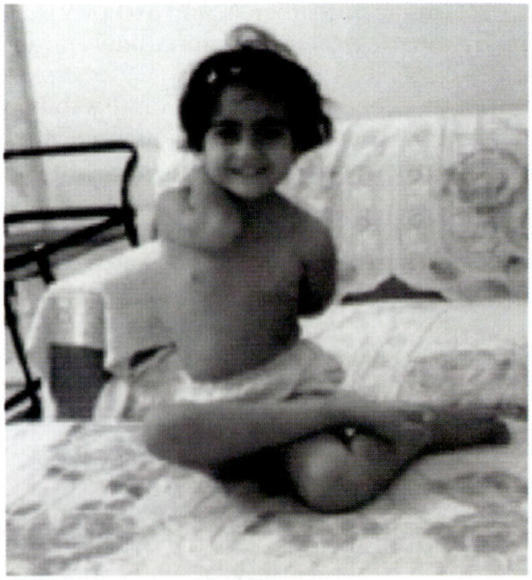

Fig. 52.12: *3-yrs-old girl making an attempt to perform Gomukh-asana-cow-head pose (front view)*

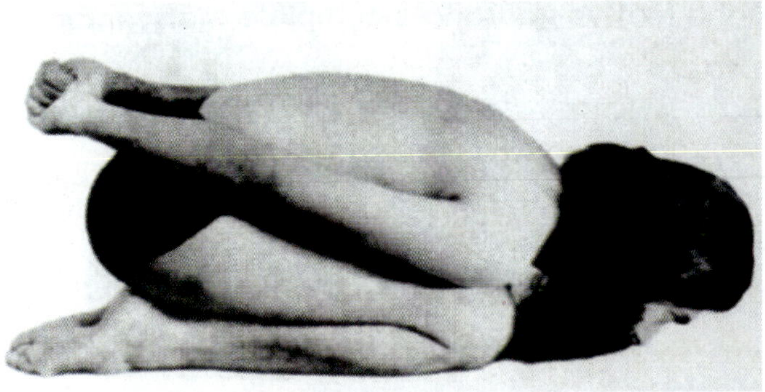

Fig. 52.13: *Nata Vajrasna*

Posture (Figs 52.13–52.15)

Kneel on the ground with the knees, ankles and big toes together as in Vajrasana (Hardy Pose). Then without shifting the position of the toes and the knees and only just separating the heels to make a place for your seat, bend slowly backwards till your head, shoulders and back touch the ground behind you. Keep both your hands on your thighs. The back should be in contact with the ground as much as possible. The eyes can be kept opened or closed. Continue deep breathing. Remain as relaxed as possible during the posture.

Important Pregnant Women should Avoid this Pose

Supta Vajrasana exercises the muscles and the blood vessels of the feet, knees, abdomen, ribs, throat and neck, mouth, eyes and the head and benefits all these parts. The exerciser experiences a stretching sensation along the whole length of the body. In spite of this, most of you would feel that the sensation of relaxation experienced while exhaling in this pose, and particularly at the end of exhalation, is even deeper and more soothing and tranquillizing than that experienced during the Shavasana (Tranquillity Pose) itself. The stretch on the inguinal muscles and blood vessels exercises a toning effect on the sex organs and the pelvic viscera. It also corrects certain defects of the spine, alleviates backache and tones up both the deep and the superficial muscles of the spine as well as its sex centres.

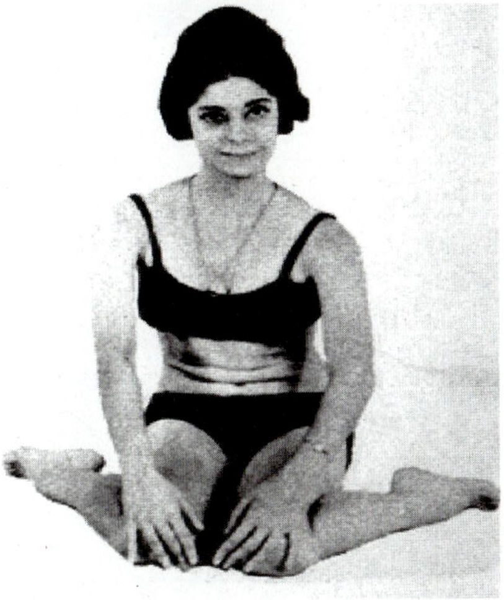

Fig. 52.14: *Hardy pose with parted feet posture*

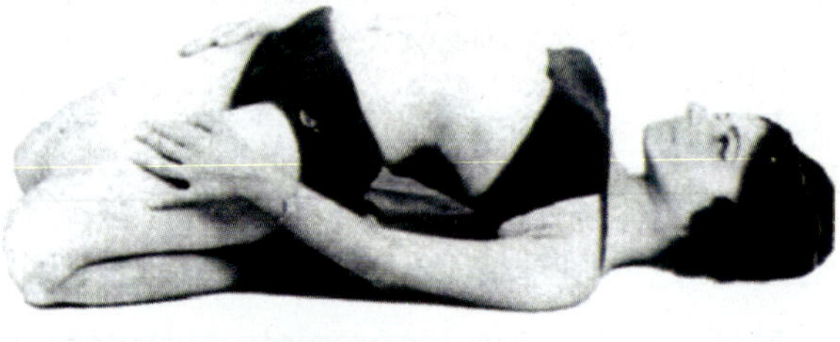

Fig. 52.15: *Supta Vajarasna-horizontal Hardy pose*

Gomukhasana-Cow-Head Pose
(Front and Back Views)

Posture (Fig. 52.16)

Sit on the ground with your right leg bent so that the centre of the rim of your heel is under the anus. The centre of gravity of the body should now be straight on the right heel on which the anus is resting. Now bend the left leg so as to bring the left heel as near the right hip as possible. In this posture, the left knee should be just above the right knee so that a straight line joining the two knees will fall perpendicular to the ground. Sitting in this posture, take your right hand behind your back so that your elbow bend is in contact with your head. Then take your left hand behind your back keeping the left elbow under your shoulder. Then lock both your hands together behind your back. The front aspect of the posture is shown in keep the eyes open, body straight and abdomen drawn inwards. Continue slow and deep breathing.

Benefits

This posture improves the circulation in the armpits and the sides. It also tones up the tissues of the feet, the knees and the waist. It improves the circulation and tones up the muscles, tendons and ligaments of the knees and the calves. The practice of this Asana, alternating the position of the arms and the legs so that both sides receive equal and balanced toning, improves the circulatory activity of both the lungs. It has been recommended for those suffering from tuberculosis of the lungs and it is beneficial to patients with asthma. It is very helpful in relieving backache, and can remove feelings of weakness and fatigue and of dislike for food. It also tends to reduce hyperacidity (heartburn).

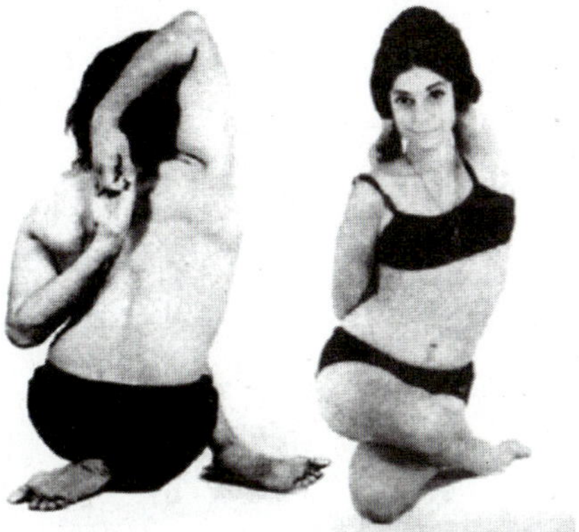

Fig. 52.16: *Gomukhasana-cow-head pose*

In particular, it effectively tones up the perineum, the prostate, the male and female genitalia and the rectal muscles. It prevents nocturnal emissions and in a number of cases has proved an effective cure for piles. It also relieves constipation. Its regular practice considerably counters the commonest of sex complaints-premature ejaculation-thereby improving sexual performance.

Ardha Matsyendrasana-Incomplete Matsyendra

Pose 1 (Front and Back Views)

Posture (Figs 52.17–52.19)

Matsyendra was the name of a great ancient Indian Yog whose habitual posture was named after him as Matsyendrasana. Here, the name of the posture is preceded by "Ardha" (Sanskrit for half or incomplete), for the beginner will find it difficult to perform the complete posture. To perform this incomplete posture, sit on the ground and spread the left leg in front of you at right angles to your trunk. Then place the right foot on the ground on the left side of your left knee as shown in the plate. Then pass your left arm round the right side of the left knee and hold your right foot with your left hand. Take your right hand behind your back, placing the back of your right hand on the extreme left of your waist. Continue deep breathing, expanding your chest as far as possible. Turn the head to your right as far as it can go so that the chin is in line with your shoulder. Keep the eyes open. Do not let the knee of the left leg rise from the ground. Try to press your abdomen with your right thigh while in this position.

Repeat the same in reverse by stretching the right leg and putting the left foot beside the right knee, and so on.

Benefits

This posture is usually prescribed for people with weak kidneys and lax urinary (bladder) muscles. It alleviates in the case of men and leucorrhoea due to mild inflammatory condition in the case of women. It tones up the entire urogenital apparatus, thereby considerably improving the sexual performance in both sexes. Leucorrhic discharge resulting from serious lesions like cancer abscesses, or venereal infections would, of course need medical treatment under expert guidance.

Ardha Matsyendrasana-Incomplete Matsyendra

Pose 2

Posture

The same as for incomplete Matsyendra Pose 1, except that the stretched leg is drawn in so that the heel touches the opposite hip.

Benefits

The same as from the previous pose.

Purna Matsyendrasana (Complete-Matsyendra Pose)

Posture

The complete Matsyendrasana is much more difficult than the incomplete poses described on the previous and can either be abandoned altogether or left until greater flexibility has been developed through practice of the previous Asanas.

Sit on the ground and place the left foot on the right thigh as you do in the Lotus Pose. The heel of the left foot is near the navel. Now, raise your right foot and place it beside the left knee as you did in the incomplete.

Pose I, the difference being that here the right leg is not stretched. See that the entire sole of your right foot by the side of the left knee is touching the ground and does not leave it. Then bring your left arm around the right knee and catch hold of the toes of the right foot with your left hand exactly as you did in the incomplete Matsyendra **Pose 2**. In the same manner, take your right arm behind your back and bring it to a position so that it touches the left heel, instead of just the waist as in the former posture. Turn the head to the right bringing the chin into line with the right shoulder. Repeat the Asana in reverse placing the right foot on the left thigh and changing the position of the limbs in the preceding posture.

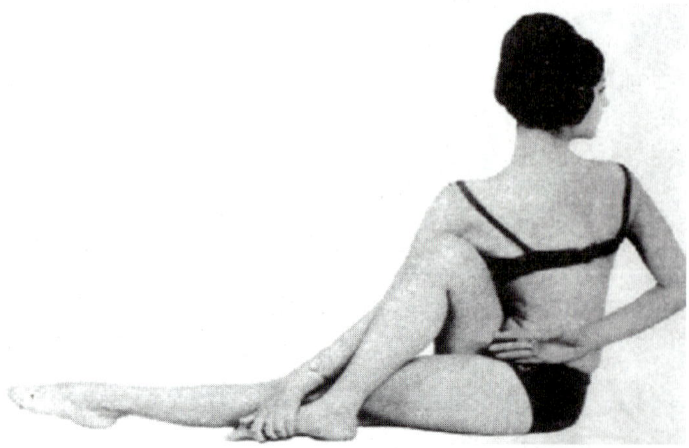

Fig. 52.17: *Ardhs Matsyendrasana-incomplete pose 1*

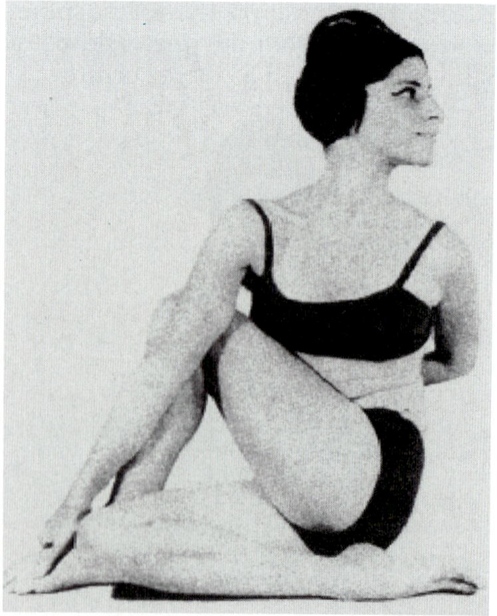

Fig. 52.18: *Ardha Matsyendrasana-incomplete pose 2*

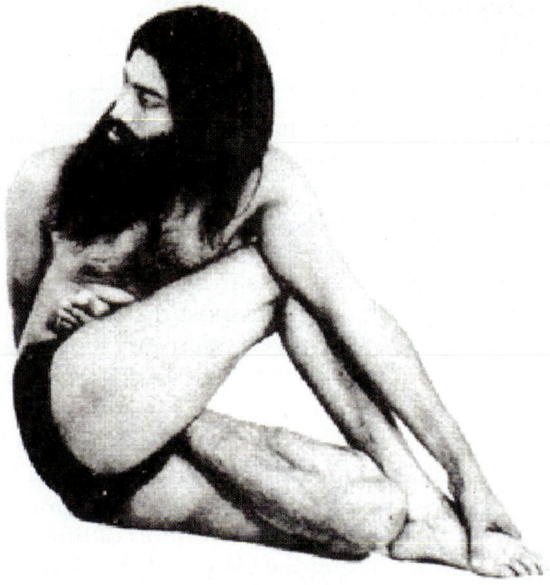

Fig. 52.19: *Purna Matsyendrasana-complete pose*

Benefits

This posture compresses the alimentary canal and almost all the viscen lying in the thorax, the abdomen, and the pelvis. It also twists the spine alternately on either side and stretches the muscles of the legs and the arms. When fully accomplished, the Matsyendra posture hardly leaves any portion of the body unexercised and unstimulated. Yogis prescribe it for disorders of the liver and the spleen particulady when they become chronic. It is very beneficial in chronic backache, toning up the nerves, and the deep as well as the superficial muscles of the spine. It improves the circulation of the entire body, increasing the efficiency of the spine and the spinal sex centre in particular. By maintaining deep breathing during this pose, the exerciser accelerates the blood circulation of all the glands and viscera from thyroid down to pelvis including the sex glands. It also improves digestion and assimilation of food and alleviates dyspepsia. Some Yogis go as far as to attribute anthelmintic properties to this posture-Le., destruction of worms found in the alimentary canal. How far it is effective in killing and expelling the worms is not possible to corroborate as no controlled experiments have been done, but there is no doubt that the practice of Matsyendra is very beneficial to the exerciser in search of sound health, sound sex life and longevity. It is a difficult pose and only through long practice and patience can average men and women master it. It is for this particular reason that I have offered a compromise in the form of the incomplete Matsyendrasana to enable the exerciser to gain some, if not all, the benefits of this posture.

Gorakshasanas-Goraksha Poses (Figs 52.20–52.40)

Goraksha Poses are named after one of the greatest and most "perfected" of Yogis and mystics of ancient and most "perfected" of Yogis and mystics of ancient India, Gqraksha or Gorakhanatha. There is no end to the stories and legends recounting the miracles and supernatural deeds performed by this yogi of yogis. It is appropriate that the postures should be associated with the name of one whose control over the sex urge was so complete that while he could perform the sex act at will at the highest level of efficiency, giving and deriving the maximum ecstasy, he could also totally sublimate the urge at will and switch off to complete detachment from sexual matters. Such mastery over the sex urge certainly lies within human potential but I do not expect anyone of you to approach Yoga with the dedication and persistent endeavour which is necessary to reach that state of development. Our aims are more modest and will be fully met by the practice of the series of Gorakshasanas that follow, or even the practice of one or two of them.

Goraksha Pose 1 (Bhadrasana-Good Pose)

Posture

Goraksha Pose 1 is referred to by some Yogis as Bhadrasana (Good Pose), a term which can also be applied to a type of Vajrasana (Hardy Pose). It is enough to remember this pose as Goraksha Pose 1.

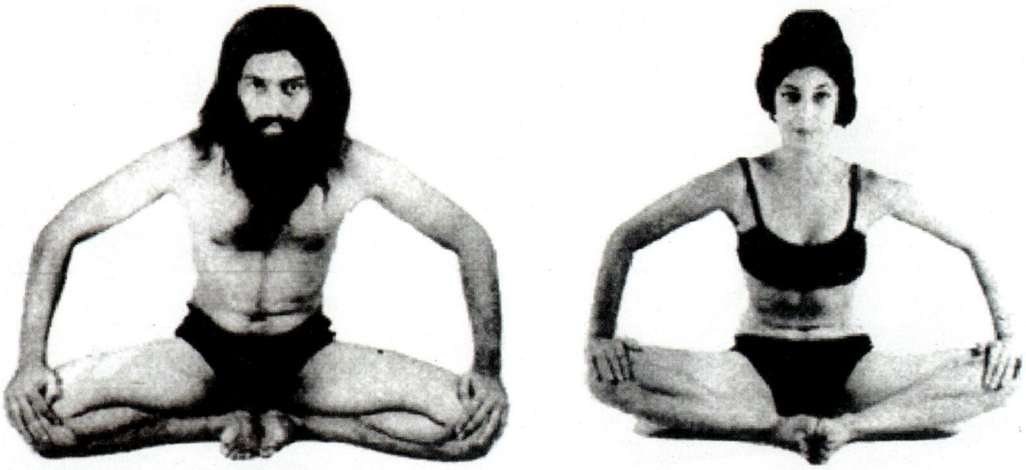

A B

Fig. 52.20A and B: *Goraksha pose 1*

Sit on the ground with your right knee pointing to your extreme right and the left knee pointing to your extreme left. In trying to do so, you will have to fold your legs inwards so that the calves are fully in contact with the thighs. Now, join the soles of your feet together so that from the heels to the toes they are in full contact. Keeping the knees in touch with the ground, or holding them as close to the ground as you can manage during the earlier stages of practice, draw in your joined feet close to your so that the heels of both the feet are touching the inner extremity of your thighs, or, better still, your perineum if you can draw the heels further inwards. Hold the pose with both your hands on your knees and your trunk as erect as possible, for a minimum of 10 seconds. Keep your eyes open and continue deep breathing.

Benefits

This posture tones up the nerves, the muscles and the circulatory system of the perineum and the genital organs of both men and women. Yogis believe that it improves the quality of the seminal fluid (which becomes thicker as a result of this exercise) and helps them sublimate their sex urge. However, they add that, since this posturetones up the sexual organs, a regular practitioner of this posture, if he happens to be a man of the world interested in legitimate progeny, will find this posture very effective in improving his sexual performance. It is believed that children whose parents performed this exercise regularly are strong, healthy and intelligent. This posture prevents and cures stiffness of body resulting from old age. Along with the whole series of Gorakshasanas it is said to lead to the removal of the stiffness of joints (particularly of the knees and ankles), oedema and swelling of the feet, premature ejaculation, lax erections and wet dreams. It strengthens the inguinal and hamstring muscles and affords prophylaxis to those with a tendency to hernia. It also strengthens the circulatory and neuromuscular system of the female urogenital organs and improves the chances of conception. A regular practice of this Asana is strongly recommended for both men and women.

Goraksha Pose 2

Posture

Sit in Goraksha Pose 1, and without moving the position of the joined feet place both hands on the ground in front of your knees. Raise your body on your hands and swing your hips forward and deposit them on your heels, so that you sit on your heels instead of on the ground with the inner side of your heels forming your seat. Having seated yourself on your feet, raise your hands from the ground and place them on your knees. Hold this posture for a minimum of 10 seconds. Keep your eyes open and continue deep breathing.

Benefits

The benefits of this posture are the same as those of Goraksha Pose 1 except that they are much more pronounced. Those of you who are short of time can select this posture from among the six Goraksha Poses for your regular practice as it is much superior to the earlier one and much easier than the next four poses in this category.

Goraksha Pose 3 (Bhagasana-Vulvar Pose)

Posture

Sit as in Goraksha Pose 1, and keeping the toes on the ground raise the heels upwards and outwards still keeping the soles joined together. In the completed pose, the feet will be supported on the ground by their toes only while the joined heels will be touching your pubic region. Some Yogis, in their writings, have named this pose "Bhagasana", a reference to the external appearance of the female genitals which is resembled by the ellipse formed by the hollows of the soles of the feet. It is enough for our purpose, however, to remember the pose.

GORAKSHA POSE 3

Benefits

The same as in Goraksha Pose 1.

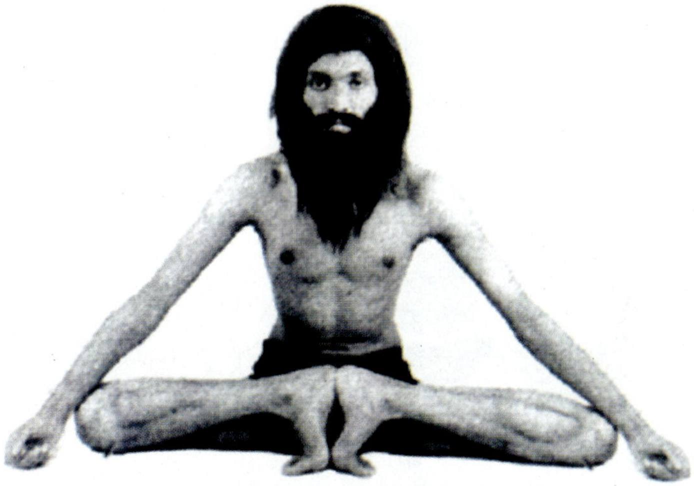

Fig. 52.21: *Goraksha pose 2*

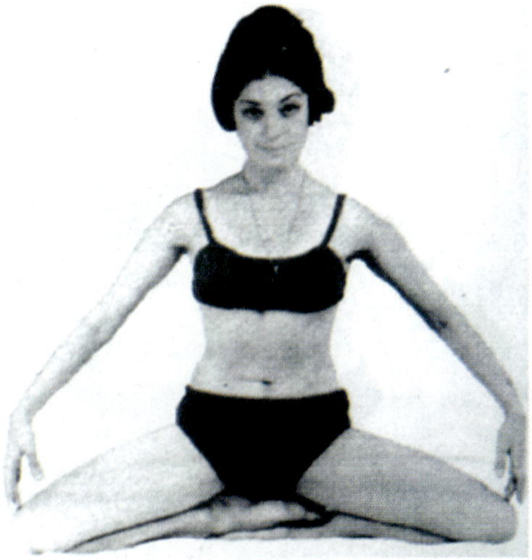

Fig. 52.22: *Goraksha pose 4*

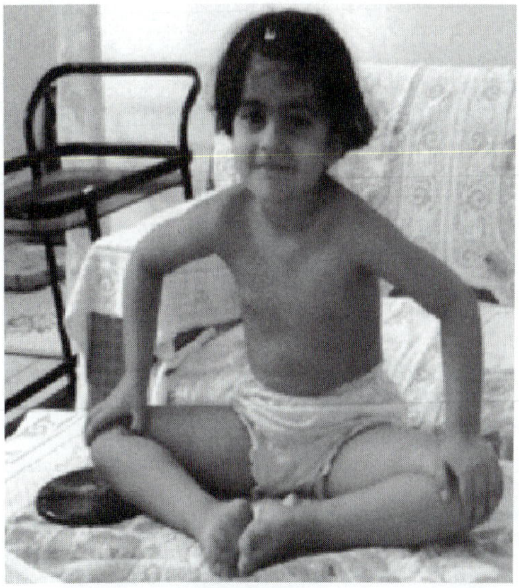

Fig. 52.23: *3-yrs-old girl attempting to perform Goraksha pose 2*

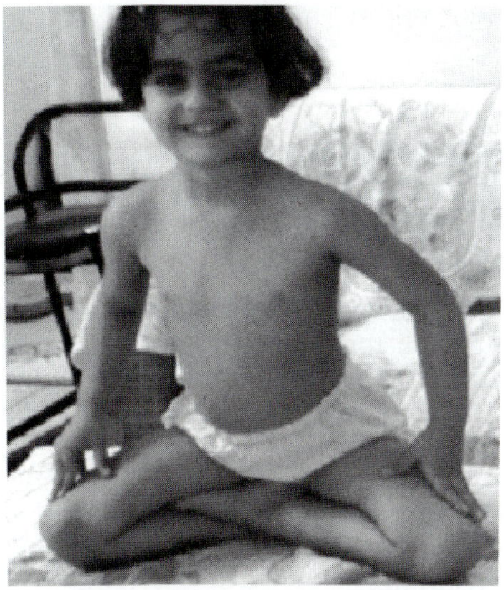

Fig. 52.24: *3-yrs-old girl attempting to perform Goraksha pose 4*

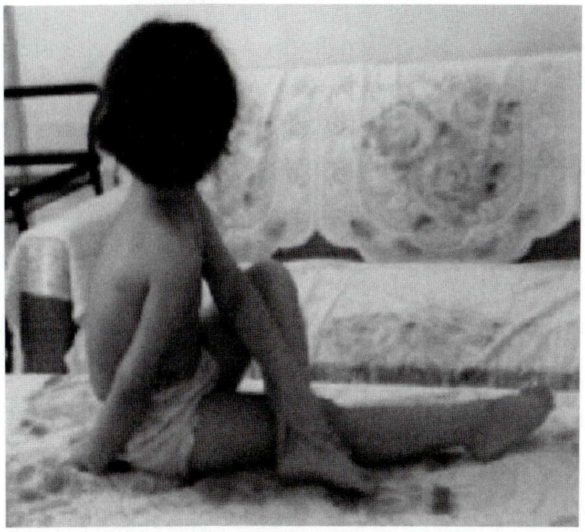

Fig. 52.25: *3-yrs-old girl attempting to perform Ardh Matsyendrasana-incomplete pose 2*

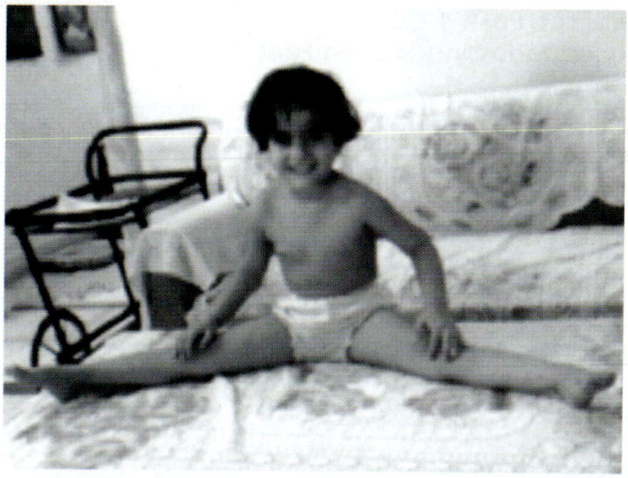

Fig. 52.26: *3-yrs-old girl attempting to perform Vistrita Padasana-lateral strech legs pose*

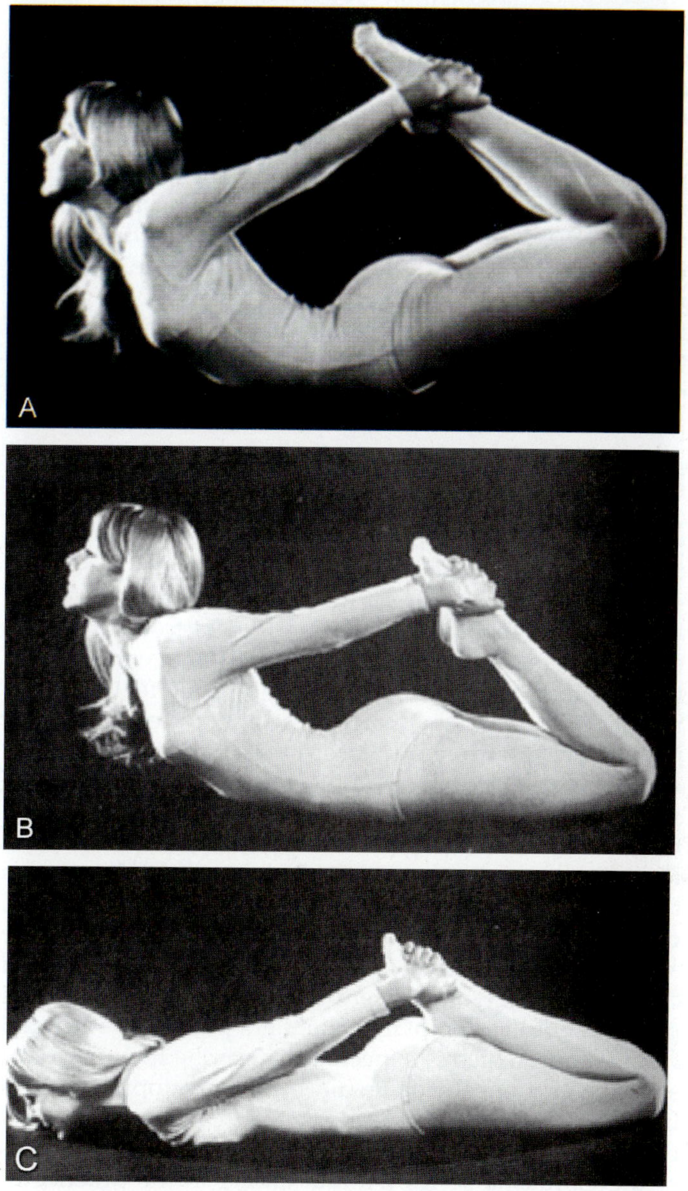

Fig. 52.27A to C: *Dhanurasana-Bow pose spine exercises*

Goraksha Pose 4 (Guhyapadasana-Hidden Feet Pose)

Posture

Sit down in Sukhasana, then placing your hands on the ground on both sides of your body raise your hips from the ground and draw both your feet under your hips, placing one foot on the, and sit down on your feet instead of on the ground. In this position, one foot will be on the ground with the other resting on it and the hips on top of the second foot. Then raise your hands from the ground and place them 011 your knees as you do in the Padmasana. Hold this pose wtlile you complete 10 Yogic breaths. Repeat the pose after changing the position of the feet so that the lower foot is placed on the upper in the second half of the exercise.

Benefits

Apart from strengthening the bones, muscles, arteries and nerves of the ankles and the feet, this Asana improves the circulation of the neuromuscular system serving the rectum, the perineum and the genitals. It strengthens the muscles and the nerves connected with the sex act. Consistent with the principle that flabby and weak sexual parts contribute to a greater craving for the sexual act, however ineffective they may be in performing it, the toning up of the sex centres by this. Asana enables the Yogi to practise celibacy effectively. At the same time, it greatly improves the functioning of the sex organs in the case of those who are not interested in celibacy. Thus, it is one of those Asanas which develop the individual's capacity to direct his libido either towards sublimation or towards sexual functioning at will.

Goraksha Pose 5

Posture (Fig. 52.28)

Sit in Goraksha Pose 3 as shown on the previous page. Then place your hands on the ground in front of you to then place your hands on the ground in front of you to enable you to raise your hips sufficiently above the ground to be able to turn the joined toes of your feet inwards underneath you so that you can sit on your feet with your joined heels pointing outwards in front of you. The inner sides of your feet are touching the ground and you are sitting on their outer edges. You will be able to understand the mechanics of this posture only if you keep Goraksha Pose 3 in your mind, and start turning your heels towards the ground in front of you and the toes inwards to go under your seat. This is a difficult posture and only those among you who are very keen to master all the poses and can afford to give sufficient time to the practice of the postute should attempt it. It could not possibly be omitted from a book which is expected to describe the important stages which constitute an aid to the development of an individual's sexual prowess but you can reap adequate benefits from the practice of the first and the second poses of the Goraksha series without taking to the practice of its more difficult postures.

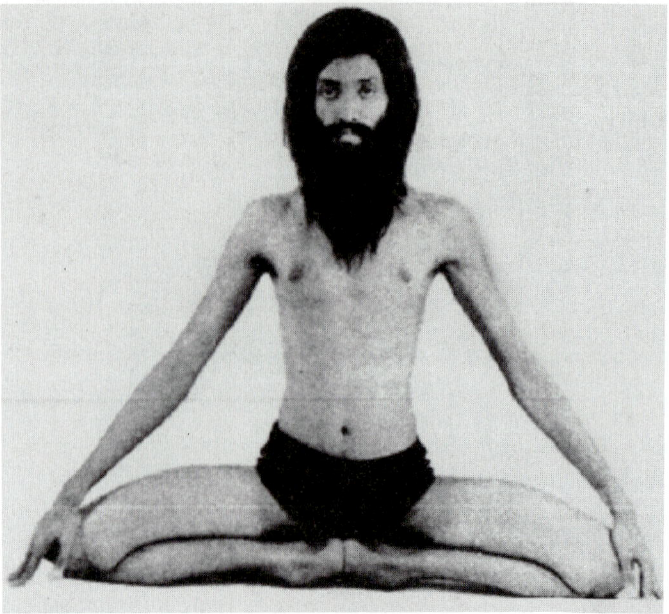

Fig. 52.28: *Goraksha pose 5*

Benefits

The same as in Goraksha Pose 2.

Goraksha Pose 6

Posture (Figs 52.29 and 52.30)

Sitting in Goraksha Pose 1, hold both your feet, which firmly on the ground on their outer edges with both your and bend your trunk forward without raising your hips from the ground till your nose and chin touch the ground. Hold yourself in this pose for 5–10 seconds or even less, to begin with. You can raise this period to 15–30 seconds when you have acquired adequate flexibility to practise this pose with comparative ease. Keep your eyes open and continue slow and deep breathing.

Benefits

The same as described in Goraksha Pose 5. It gives an added advantage of exercising your alimentary canal and stretching your spine, thereby improving the functioning of both these important areas.

Vistrita Padasana-Lateral Stretched Leg Pose

Posture (Fig. 52.31)

Sit down on the ground with both your legs stretched out to your right and your left respectively so that both the legs form one straight line. Keep your hands on your legs as shown in Plate 11. Keep the eyes open, body erect, legs straight and muscles relaxed to the greatest extent possible. Continue deep and slow breathing.

Benefits

This Asana improves the tone of the circulatory and neuromuscular systems of the entire pelvis including the organs of reproduction and elimination. It cures cramps of the

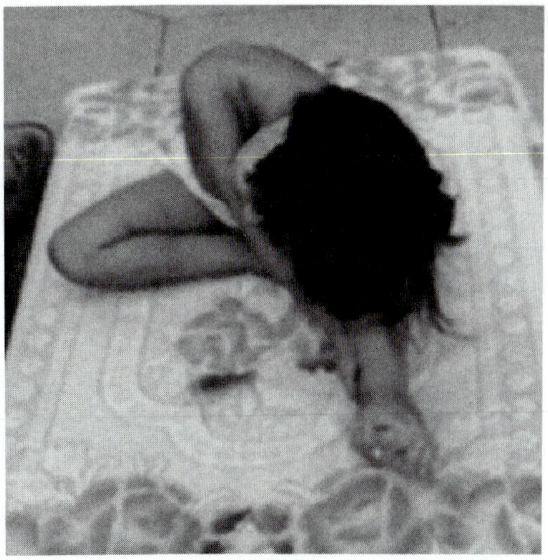

Fig. 52.29: *3-yrs-old girl attempting to perform Goraksha pose 6*

lower extremities and strengthens the muscles and the ligaments of the calves, the thighs and all the joints of the legs. It tends to increase the height if the exercise is done regularly and for a long time. It tones up the sex centres of the body both for purposes of sublimation of the sex urge in the case of the recluse and the ascetic and improvement of sexual efficiency in the case of the normal individual.

Janushirasana-Knee-Head Pose 1

Posture (Figs 52.32–52.35)

Sit down on the ground with your left leg stretched out straight before you and the right leg bent inwards at the knee so that the right heel is in touch with your body and if

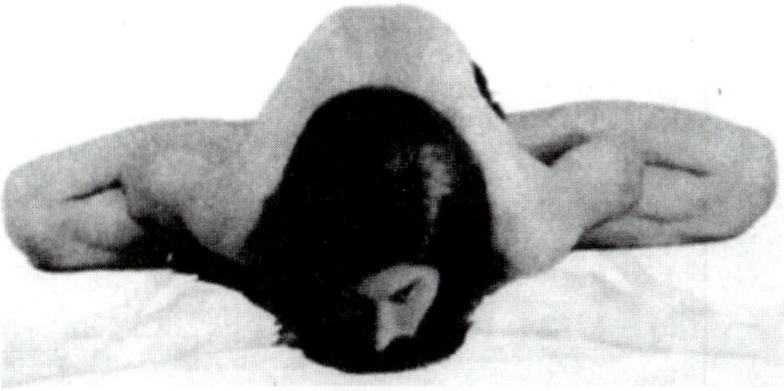

Fig. 52.30: *Goraksha pose 6 by an adolescent*

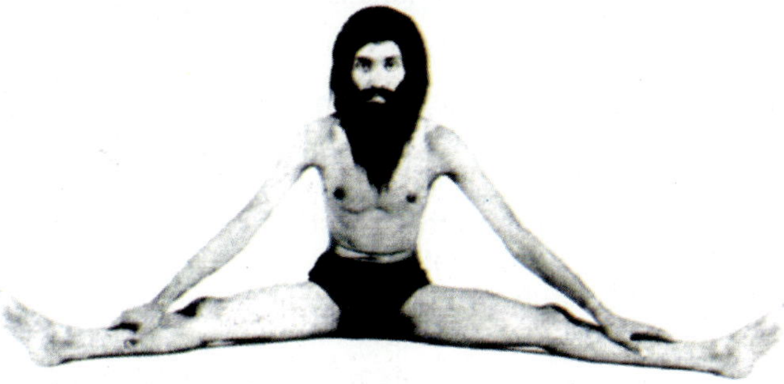

Fig. 52.31: *Vistrita Padasana-lateral strech legs pose*

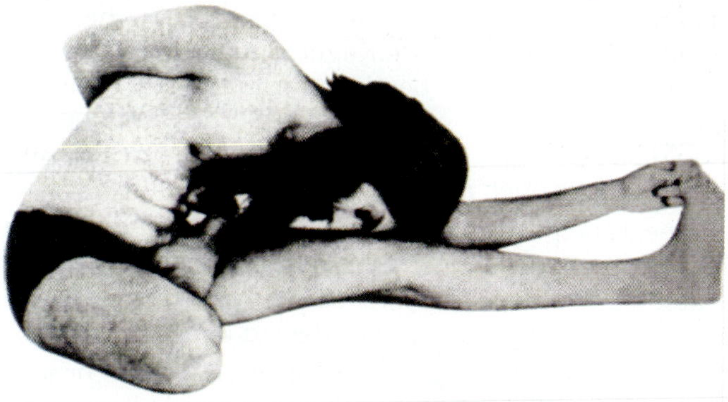

Fig. 52.32: *Janushirasana-knee-head pose 1*

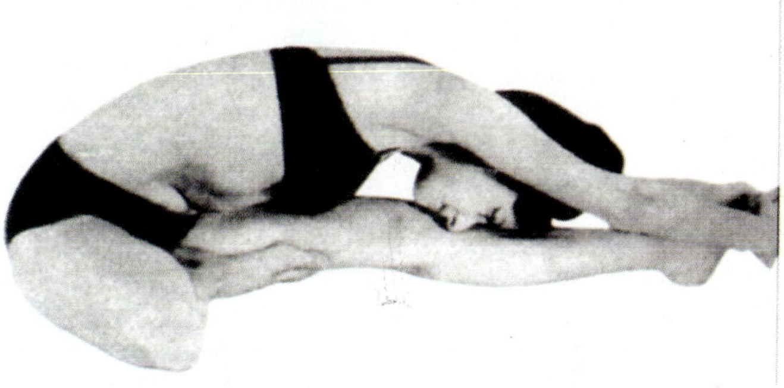

Fig. 52.33:*Janushirasana-knee-head pose 2*

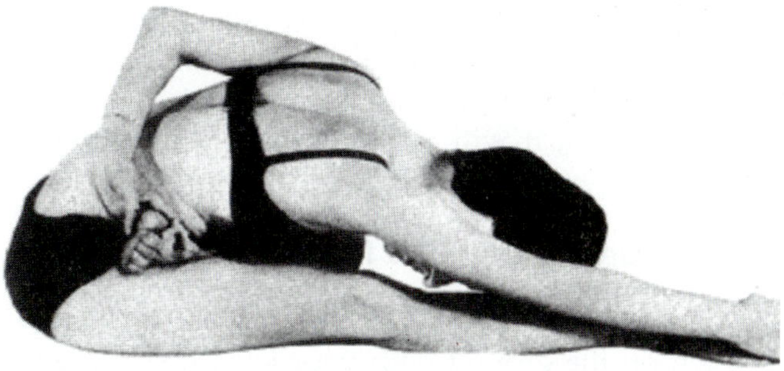

Fig. 52.34: *Janushirasana-knee-head pose 3*

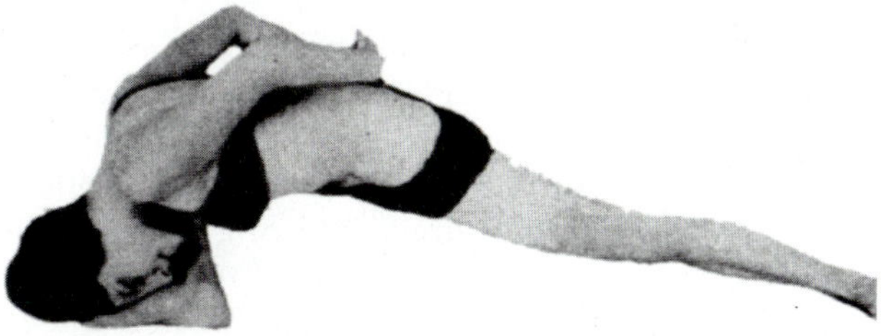

Fig. 52.35: *Janushirasana-knee-head pose 3*

possible touching your perineum. Then, bending forward, hold the big toe of your left foot with the thumb and two adjacent fingers of both hands. In this process, the left leg should be kept absolutely straight without permitting any bending of the left knee. Bend forward further to bring your forehead into contact with your knee. The right knee also should be kept in contact with the ground. The eyes can be kept closed or open and continue deep breathing.

Repeat the posture with the right leg stretched out and the left foot near the perineum, the rest of the posture remaining the same. The forehead in the latter posture will touch the right knee instead of the left knee.

Persons with bulging abdomens or stiff backs or joints will find it difficult to bring their foreheads into contact with their knees and they will find their knees rising from the ground to touch the forehead. Such a compromise is permissible for beginners. For the first few days, there is a possibility of the exerciser experiencing some pain in the parts exercised by this posture. This should not result in giving up the practice of this posture. The exercise should be continued in an imperfect manner, but regularly and daily.

Benefits

This exercise improves the circulation and tones up the neuromuscular system of the perineum and the gonads. Yogis prescribe it for spermatorrhoea, wet dreams and night emissions, defects in semen, and other sexual disorders. It also tones up the liver and the muscles and ligaments of the ribs and both sides of the trunk. It strengthens the urinary bladder and seminal vesicles. It is also prescribed for stones in the kidneys, urethra and bladder. It is often prescribed for women to tone up the muscles of the uterus, the fallopian tubes and to improve the functioning of the ovaries. Practised regularly by healthy couples, it will improve their sexual tone and performance.

Janushirasana-Knee-Head Pose 2

Posture

Sit down on the ground with your left leg stretched out infront of you and the right leg bent inwards at the knee so that the right heel is in touch with your left thigh.

Then hold your right ankle with your hands, raise your foot and place it on your left thigh instead of leaving it on the ground touching your perineum as was done in the previous pose, Janushirasana No. 1. The rest of the posture is exactly the same as Janushirasana No. i.e. the big toe of your left foot with both hands using the thumbs and two adjacent fingers and bend down to bring your forehead into contact with your left knee. Repeat the posture with the right leg stretched out and the left foot on the right thigh; the forehead in the reverse posture touching the right knee instead of the left knee.

Benefits

The same as in Janushirasana No.1.

Janushirasana-Knee-Head Pose 3

Posture

Sit down on the ground and stretch the right leg in front of you, bend the left leg inwards at the knee and place your left heel on the right thigh as in the reverse position of Janushirasana No. 2. Now bend forward and use only your right hand to hold the big toe of your right foot while your forehead touches the right knee and your left arm goes behind across your back to hold the big toe of your left foot which is resting on the right thigh.

Reverse the pose with the left leg stretched, the right foot on the left knee, the forehead on the left knee and left hand holding the big toe of the left leg, the right hand going behind across the back to hold the big toe of the right foot. Continue deep breathing as in the previous two poses.

Benefits

The benefits of the Janushirasana No. 3 are the same as from the previous two poses of this. Asana except that they are more pronounced. If you find it difficult to practise this pose, it can be abandoned in favour of the previous two Asanas which are quite adequate in conferring the benefits enumerated in Janushirasana No. 1.

Veerya Stambhanasana-Semen Retention Pose

Posture

Stand on the ground with one foot behind and one foot forward maintaining a distance of approximately one long stride between them. Then start bending the kame of the forward leg till the upper half of the leg is at right angles to the lower half and the latter is at right angles to the ground. While doing so, hold your hands behind your back and, keeping your back straight, bring your head down so that your nose touches the large toe of your leading foot. The leg behind should not be allowed to bend in this process. Hold yourself in this pose for half to one minute. Then rise slowly and disengage yourself from the pose. Repeat the posture reversing the position of the legs.

While disengaging from the pose, fill the lungs fully and then stand erect. The body should be kept immobile during the pose. The breath should be held in the lungs after full inhalation so that the chest remains a little thrown out and the abdomen drawn inwards. This posture is deemed to have been completed only after it has been done with both feet in the forward position. This Asana has also been called Padangushtha Nasa Sparshanasana.

Benefits

The benefits of this posture are similar to those of Bhadrasana and Gorakshasana. Yogic experts are unanimous in their praise of this. Asana as being very effective in toning up the sex centres. It is therefore practised both by the recluse for the effective sublimation of the sex urge and by the family man for the strengthening of the sex centres for better sexual performance. It promotes and prolongs youth and postpones and delays old age. It counters the effects of sexual excesses. It is supposed to cure borderline diabetes and to help bring the sugar levels in advanced diabetes towards the normal even when the drop in the level is not adequate.

Those of you who have a tendency to diabetes but have not started suffering from it yet, and also happen to have a sweet tooth, should perform it regularly. The pose also tends to control morbid, excessive sexual desires bordering on mania and helps counter the deleterious effects of sexual excesses. It is claimed that it cures mild glycosuria (sugar in the urine) resulting from excessive intake of food promoting tendency to diabetes. It is considered the best Asana for the cure of premature ejaculation and the thinness of seminal fluid. The regular practitioners of this Asana will notice that it thickens the consistency of the seminal fluid. It cures insomnia, anaemia, flatulence, abdominal pains, tendency to inguinal hernia. In general, it improves the tone of the entire body and is equally beneficial for the male and the female.

Eka Pada Shirasana-Foot-Head Pose

Posture (Figs 52.36 and 52.37)

Sit on the ground with the left leg stretched in front of you and lift your right foot with both your hands, bend your head and carry the foot over your head and place it on your neck. Then straighten your back and fold both your hands in front of your chest as is done in Indian salutation. Keep the head also erect. Continue normal deep breathing. Keep the eyes open. Don't relax the body in this pose. Repeat the same pose in reverse-lie, with the right leg stretched and the left foot on the neck, the rest of the pose remaining the same).

Benefits

Yogis prescribe this Asana for women who suffer from prolapse of the uterus, laxity of urogenital musculature and tendency to miscarriage and abortion. It is also prescribed, with good results, for piles. It tones up the male and female gonads and reduces minor swellings of the scrotum by improving the blood circulation. It reduces oedema in the extremities. It also tones up the respiratory tract and improves appetite. It improves the flexibility of the muscles of the legs, the back and the waist.

Dvipada Shirasana-Feet-Head Pose

Posture

Sit on the ground in the foot, head posture. Bend forward and lift the remaining foot off the ground with both your hands and bring it over your head to be placed on the back so that both feet are now behind your neck. Fold both your hands as you did in the previous posture. In a variant of this pose, place your palms on the ground either side of your body and, supporting your entire weight on your hands, raise yourself from the ground (as in the Swing Pose that follows next) without disturbing the position of your head and legs.

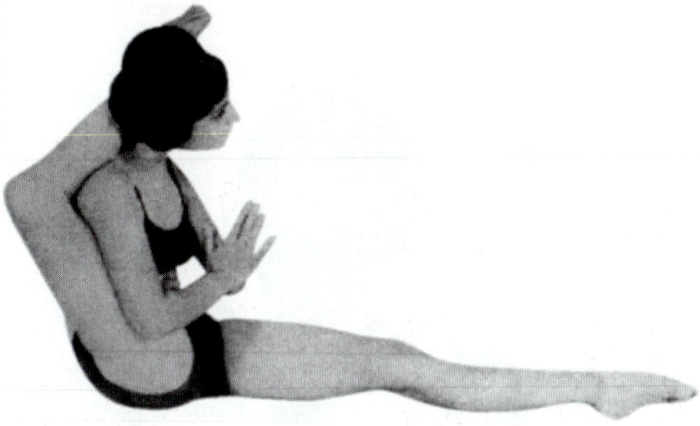

Fig. 52.36: *Eka Pada Shirasana (foot-head pose 1)*

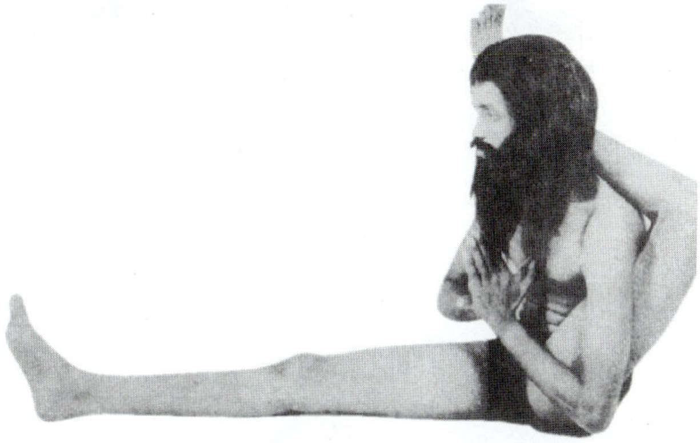

Fig. 52.37: *Eka Pada Shirasana (foot-head pose 2)*

Benefits

This posture confers the same benefits, in a greater degree, as those derived from the foot, head posture. It strengthens the spinal column and the shoulders. The calves and feet are strengthened. It improves the flexibility of the entire body and cures the stiffness of muscles in general. It improves physical efficiency and imparts great flexibility to the entire system. It also tones up the kidneys and promotes easier and more effective evacuation of the bladder and the bowels.

Loiasana-Swing Pose 1

Posture (Figs 52.40 and 52.41)

Sit in Padmasana (Lotus Pose), then place your palms on the ground on both sides of your body and, supporting your entire weight on your hands, raise the remaining part of the body from the ground keeping the Lotus Pose intact. Fill the lungs with a deep breath before lifting the body from the ground. Keeping the eyes open, take five deep breaths in this pose before gradually letting the body down to the ground, filling the lungs with a deep breath as you do so. Keep the abdomen contracted and the chest expanded during this exercise. Keep the body as steady as possible during the posture. If it is difficult to hold the body above the ground for the duration of five full deep breaths, you can terminate the pose earlier.

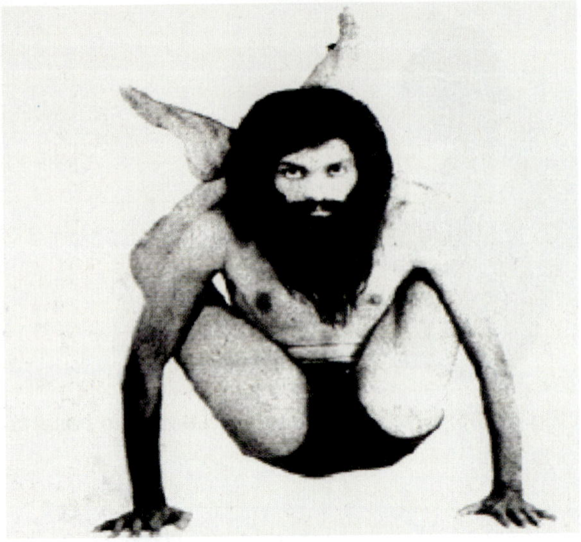

Fig. 52.38: *DviPada Shirasana (feet-head pose 1)*

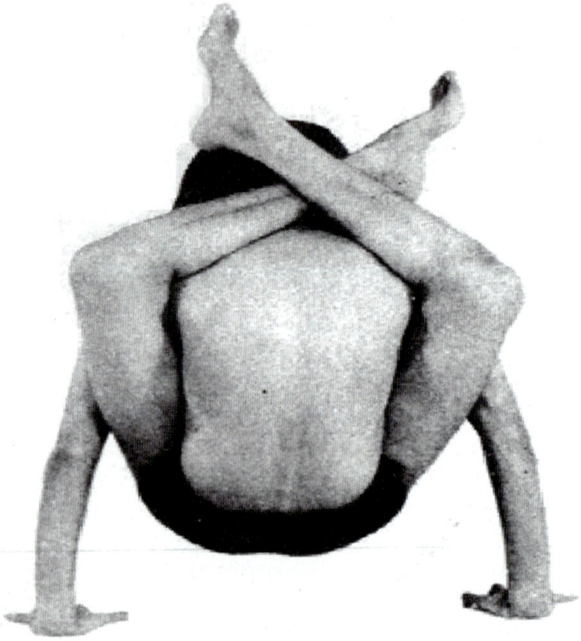

Fig. 52.39: *DviPada Shirasana (feet-head pose 2)*

Benefits

This posture strengthens the neuromuscular system of the fingers, the hands, the arms and the shoulders. It relieves constipation, flatulence, sperma, torrhoea andinvoluntary seminal discharges. It is also prescribed for excess of yawning, hiccups and lethargy.

Lolasana-Swing Pose 2

Posture

Another variety of Lolasana (Swing Pose) is raising the body still higher so that the knees rest against the arms above the elbows and the trunk is at right angles to the arms.

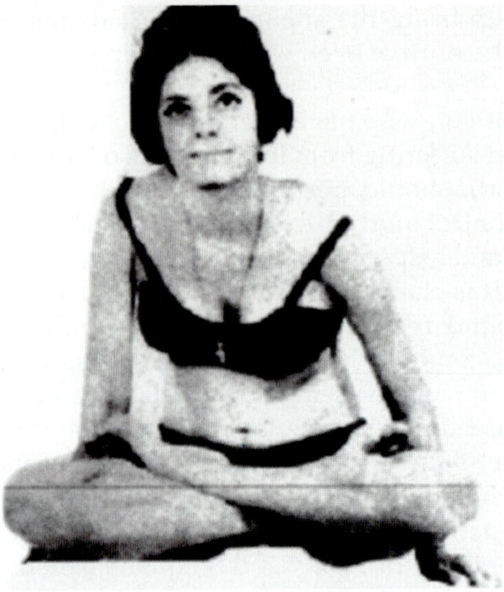

Fig. 52.40: *Lolasana-swing pose 1*

Benefits

The benefits are identical with those of the first variety of Loiasana.

Garbhasana-Foetus Pose

Posture (Fig. 52.42)

Sit on the ground with both hands resting on the ground infront of you with a distance of about one foot between them. Bring your right leg around the right arm so that the arm is placed between the inner side of the calf and the thigh touching the inner side of the knee joint. Similarly, the left arm should be embraced by the inner side of the left knee joint. Keeping the arms in position, bring in the right foot behind the left arm and the left foot behind the right arm. The position of the two feet now resembles, to some extent, that of the two feet in Padma, sana (Lotus Pose) except that now your arms are inside the respective folds

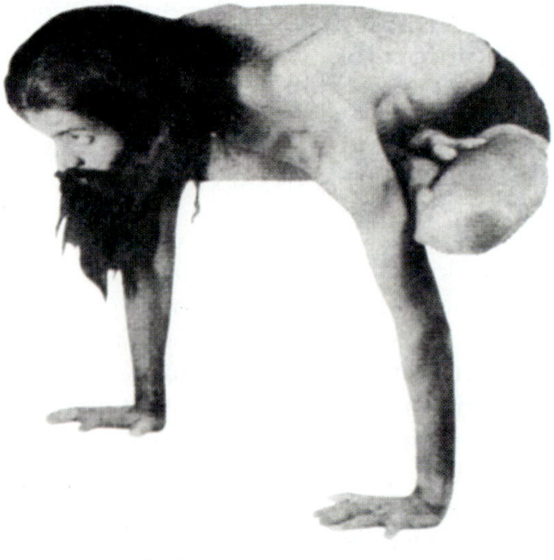

Fig. 52.41: *Lolasana-swing pose 2*

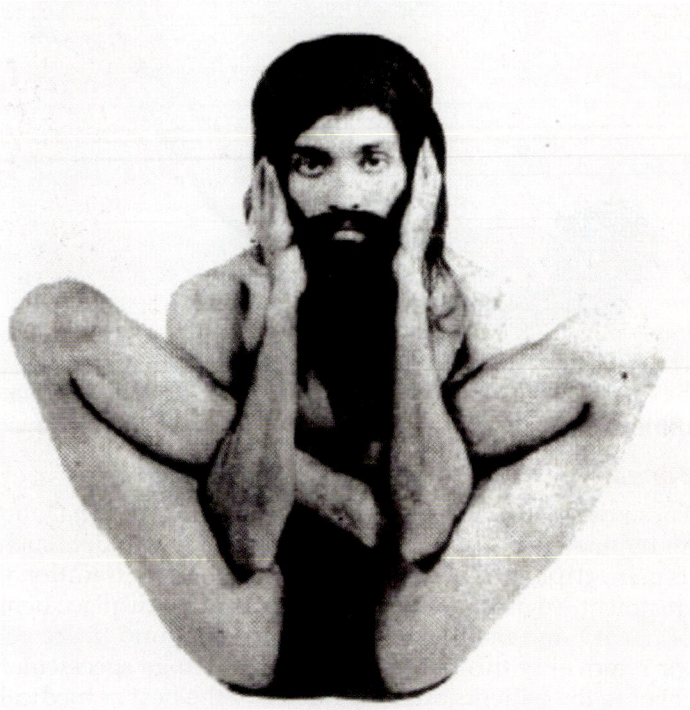

Fig. 52.42: *Garbhasana-foetus pose*

of your legs instead of outside them as in the Padmasana. Now raise your forearms and holding the lower portion of your calves in the inner folds of your elbows, raise your hands and place them on of your elbows, raise your hands and place them on both sides of your face. This will automatically raise your feet to the level of your abdomen against which they will be held by the folds of your elbows. Hold the pose from 5–15 seconds, keep the eyes open, contirfue to breathe comfortably, hold the body firmly during the pose, keep the head as straight as possible. If it is found difficult to hold the body in balance, through fear of toppling backwards, the Asana may be performed with the back supported against a wall. As confidence develops with the progress of the exercise, the support of the wall should be given up.

Benefits

This posture is named the Foetus Pose due to its partial resemblance to the position of the foetus in the womb. The Yogis also claim that this posture imparts the same softness and flexibility to the body as is possessed by the tissues of the foetus in the womb. It is supposed to confer a large number of benefits, the most surprising being relief in cases of granular pharyngitis and also of granulation on the back portion of the tongue. It is also prescribed for stomatitis, inflammatory conditions in general of the buccal cavity and the lips, pimples on the face, and poor complexion. It imparts considerable relief in cases of colitis. It tones up the organs of digestion and cures flatulence. It is also beneficial in cases of dysmenorrhoea. It tones up urogenital organs and cures impurities in urine. This is one of those postures which is freely prescribed for all, from childhood to ripe old age, and for both sexes.

Shirshasana-Head Stand

Posture (Fig. 52.43)

Spread a soft blanket or a thin foam, rubber mattress on the ground. Squat in the middle of the blanket. Interlocking the fingers of both hands in front of you with the palms facing towards you, bend slowly forward and place the interlocked hands on the ground in front of you keeping both palms open to support the back part of your head which you place on the ground. Then, gradually tilt your body upwards so that the weight of your body is borne by your head supported by the interlocked hands behind and the forearms in the front. The elbows and the head form a supporting triangle enabling you to stand straight on your head. Hold the pose for 1–2 minutes. Beginners may practise the pose for 15–30 seconds. Breathing should be normal.

If you cannot hold yourself erect whilst standing on your head, use the support of a wall. The benefit will be practically the same. Squat in front of the wall, place your hands on the ground (at a convenient distance from the wall) so that they form a triangle with your head when you place it on the ground against the wall (using a towel for protection). Using your hands to bear the weight of your body, raise your heels and legs, tilting them back, wards and upwards, so that they go up and touch the wall. Hold your body straight against the wall with the heels and the back of the head touching the wall. In this position, you cannot fall on any side as you have toe support of your hands at the front the sides and of the wall at your back.

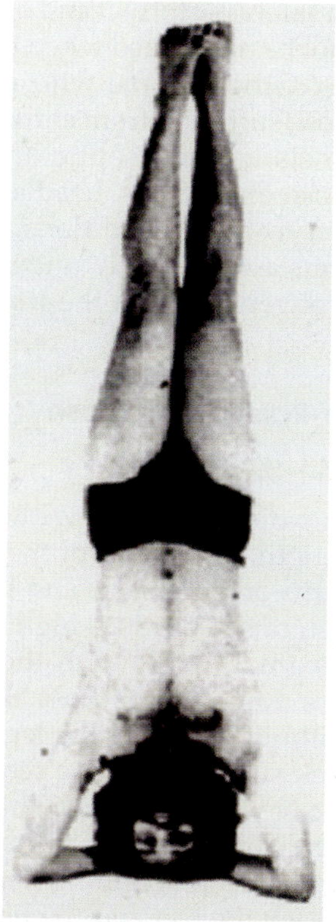

Fig. 52.43: *Shirshasana-head stand*

Benefits

The Head Stand has become popular in present, day Yoga in spite of the fact that no direct reference to it is to be found in any of the classical Yoga texts.

This pose improves the blood supply to the brain and the adjoining portion of the spinal cord. The practice of this Asana improves eye, sight, hearing and the sense of smell. It tones up the vocal cords and improves the voice. It promotes sound sleep. Normally, those who practise it can gain more benefit during a sleep session of 4 hours than others in 8 hours. The vascular system serving the brain and its nerves is exercised and strengthened by this posture and thereby feeding and serving the entire cerebral area with greater efficiency. It improves concentration and induces serenity and tranquillity. It tends to reduce funk and anxiety conditions and can therefore contribute to the cure of psychic sex disturbances. It is also supposed to make the greatest contribution of all the Asanas to intelligence and enthusiasm.

Important: Shirshasana should be immediately followed by Shavasana (Pose of Tranquillity) the duration of which should be equal to the duration of time given to Shirshasana. This is a must. The exerciser should not stand erect after the Shirshasana before completing the Shavasana which should follow it immediately. This Shavasana is normally practised at the end of all the exercises but in this case it should be done both after the Head Stand and as the last exercise of all. It is essential that the stomach should be empty when practising Shirshasana. People with a tendency to nose bleeds and high blood pressure should avoid it. However, people who have only a mildly high blood pressure can safely perform it and even derive benefit from it. It should not be performed when the body is heated by other exercises. Other people who should avoid the Head Stand are those suffering from chronic and advanced asthma, tuberculosis, cancer, septic and inflammatory diseases of ear, nose and throat, headaches, obesity and hyperacidity. Even in these conditions, this posture has been tried by enthusiasts, but only under the guidance of physicians fully conversant with the theory and practice of Yoga.

Utthitapadasana-Raised Legs Pose

Posture (Figs 52.44–52.46)

Lie on the ground on your back with the entire body stretched at full length. The palms of the hands should be touching your thighs on both sides and the feet should be held together. Then raise your legs high so that they form an angle of approximately 45° with the ground. This is Utthitapadasana or Raised Legs Pose this pose for 1–15 seconds. Then, without lowering the legs, raise the head, shoulders and back so that from the feet to the head the body forms a concave figure with the hips and the waist touching the ground Hold yourself in this position for half to 1 minute. Continue deep breathing. Finally, take a deep breath and bring back the feet and the head to the ground to terminate the pose.

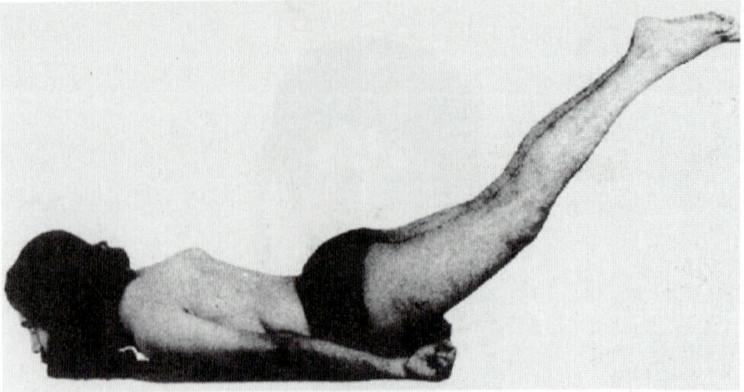

Fig. 52.44: *Utthitapadasana-raised leg pose*

Utthitapadashirasana-Raised Head and Legs Pose

Benefits

These two postures improve the tone of the intestinal and abdominal muscles. When certain intestinal disorders such as pain, griping, diarrhoea, etc. resist modern or traditional treatment, Yogis some times attribute them to "displacement of navel", and manipulation of the area around the navel for removal of this displacement often brings spectacular relief to the patients after the failure of the best of medical treatment. These postures counter the tendency to "displacement of navel" and disorders arising therefrom. They tone up the digestive apparatus and also exercise a beneficial effect on the blood vascular and neuromuscular systems of the pubic regions.

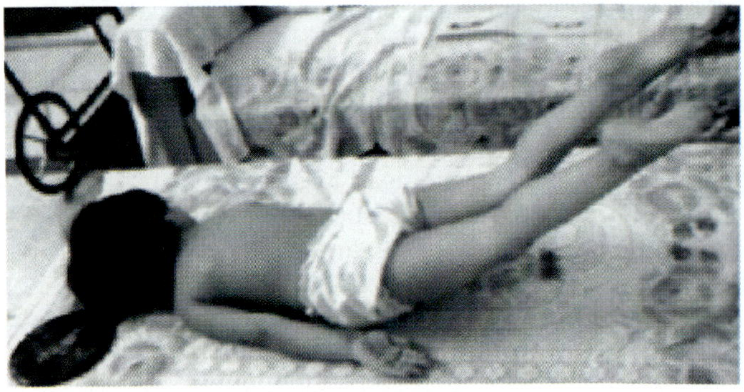

Fig. 52.45: *Utthitapadasana-raised leg pose (both legs, being helped by her mother) in a 3-yrs-old girl*

Chakrasana-Wheel Pose

Posture (Figs 52.47 and 52.48)

Lie down on your back, draw up the knees so that they point upwards while the heel of each foot touches the corresponding hip with the soles of the feet resting on the ground. Place your hands on either side of your head with the elbows pointing upwards and the palms and the fingers resting squarely on the ground. Then supporting the weight of your body on your hands and feet raise your hips and abdomen as high as you can so that the entire body describes an arch with only the hands and the feet touching the ground. Keep the body as still as possible. The hands and feet should hold the ground and remain firmly in

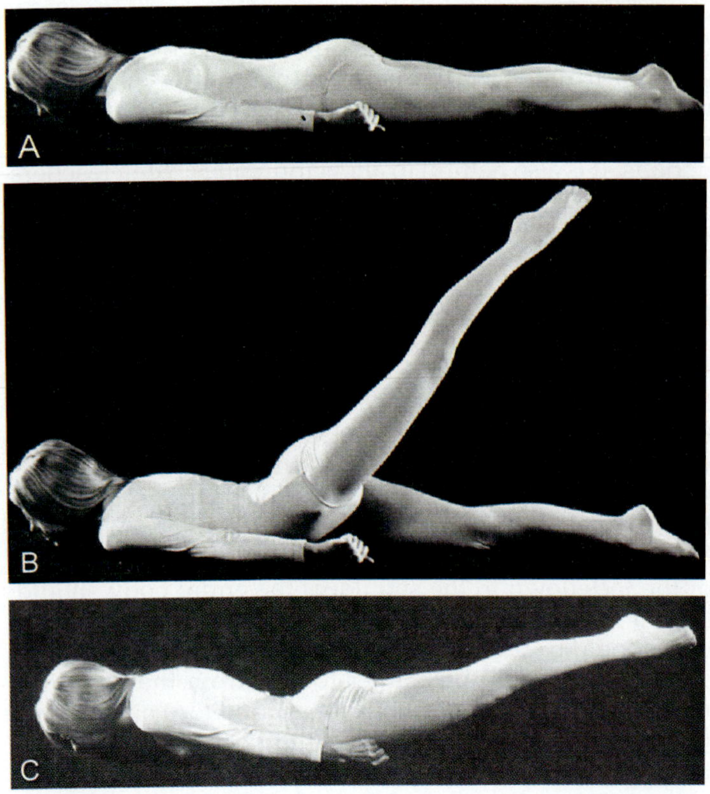

Fig. 52.46A to C: *Utthitapadashirasana-raised head and leg pose*

position. Raise the back as far up as possible so that the body imitates the shape of the rim of a wheel as much as possible. Take a deep breath before raising the body. Continue deep breathing during the posture. Fill the lungs again with air before slowly returning to the ground at the end of the exercise. After lying down on the ground, deep breathing should continue for a few seconds. The eyes may be open or closed.

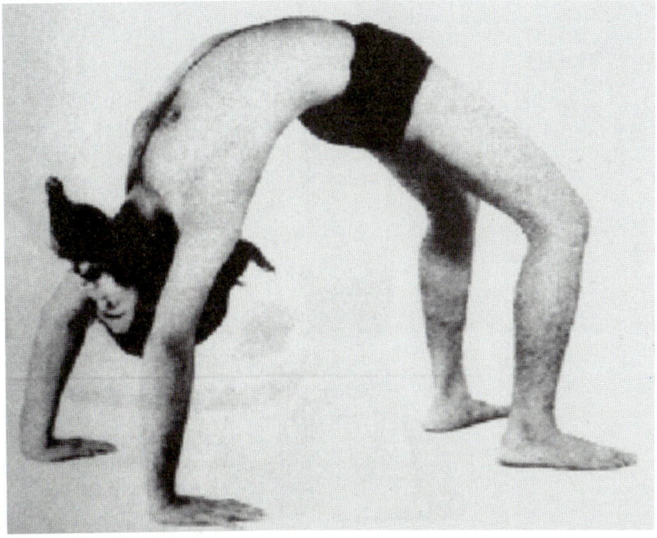

Fig. 52.47: *Chakarasana-wheel pose 1*

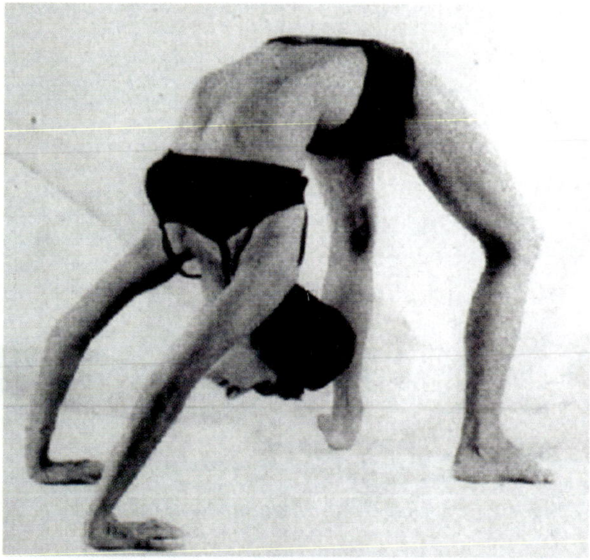

Fig. 52.48: *Chakarasana-wheel pose 2*

Benefits

This posture keeps the spine young and flexible even during old age. It helps the exerciser retain the flexibility and lightness of all the dorsal and ventral muscles. The Yogis prescribe this posture for improving the eyesight, and the richness and clarity of the voice. It is also claimed that it tones up the lymph glands and clears inflammatory conditions. It improves the texture and complexion of the skin. It tones up the sex centre in the spine. It also gives relief in cases of constipation, flatulence, nausea and asthma. It is claimed that it removes unpleasant sensations (pins and needles, burning, tenderness, pricking, general debility, rigidity, and anorexia, or lack of appetite). It tones up the nerves serving the organs of sight, hearing, smell and taste. It also improves the circulation of blood to the brain, thereby contributing to intelligence and alertness. It stretches and tones up the inguinal and pelvic muscles and vessels and tones up the pelvic organs.

Eka Pada Shalabhasana-Locust Pose

Posture (Figs 52.49 and 52.50)

Lie down flat and full length on your abdomen with both arms resting on the ground, close to your body. The chin should also be touching the ground. The upper surface of the stretched feet should also be in contact with the ground. Then take a deep breath and raise the left leg from the hip as far above the ground as you can, avoiding too much difficulty or distress. Then slowly exhale and take five deep breaths. Again fill your lungs with a deep breath and slowly bring down the leg to the original position on the ground. Repeat the entire process with the right leg. Do not bend your knees during the exercise and remember to keep the leg in a straight line with the body.

Benefits

The Locust Pose tones up the male gonads and the female pelvic viscera, thereby improving the general tone of the

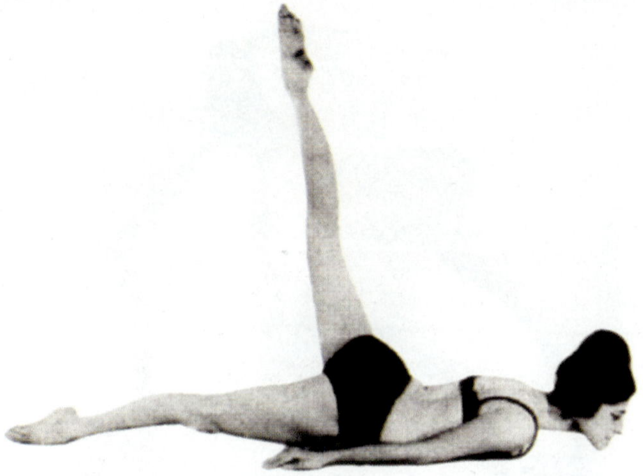

Fig. 52.49: *Eka Pada Shalabhasana-locust pose*

tissues connected with sexual and urogenital functions. It streamlines and dissolves fat from the knees, hips, waist and abdomen. It tones up the muscles of the dorsal, lumbar and sacral spine. It counters tendency to constipation and piles. It improves the circulation of the large intestines and removes flatulence. It also removes the aches and pains of the areas referred to above. Yoga teachers particularly recommend this posture for practice by women.

Dvipada Shalabhasana-Locust Pose

Posture

Lie down on the ground face downwards. The arms and hands should be on the ground, the entire length of the arm touching the body right up to the sides of the thighs. Fill the lungs with a deep breath, raise both the legs upwards as far as you can take them without experiencing too much discomfort or distress. Take three to five deep breaths in that position. Again fill the lungs with a deep breath and slowly bring the legs down till they rest on the ground. Do not bend the knees and throughout the exercise keep both the legs straight; the legs should not separate. The chin should remain in touch with the ground. The exerciser will not be able to raise the legs very far from the ground. Only through long practice will the requisite flexibility to practise the posture efficiently be acquired.

Benefits

This posture tones up the ligaments, tendons, muscles, and nerves of the lower back and the waist in general. It improves the circulation of the entire pelvic region, toning up all the organs and viscera of the area including the gonads. It tones up the entire urogenital apparatus. It reduces oedema of the ankles and feet. It is beneficial for women suffering from dysmenorrhoea and irregular periods. It is also helpful in alleviating piles. Yoga teachers also prescribe this Asana to patients for relie of painful urination, diabetes, and scanty urine as a further aid to the treatment they may be undergoing.

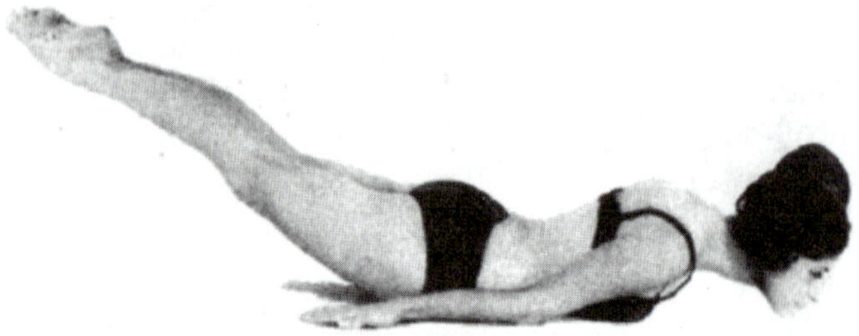

Fig. 52.50: *Dvipada Shalabhasana-locust pose*

Urdhwa Sarvangasana-Shoulder Stand Pose

Posture (Figs 52.51 and 52.52)

Lie on your back full length, legs together and arms touching your sides. Raise your legs and trunk so that entire weight of the raised legs and trunk is borne by the shoulders. The elbows should be resting on the ground with both hands and the forearms supporting the back to keep the body erect and in position for the posture. From the tip of the toes down to the shoulders the entire body should be in a straight line and at right angles to the ground. The chin should be pressing against the lower part of the neck. The elbows should be neither too far from the body nor too near it. Try to extend the feet and the toes upwards as much as possible. Do not bend the knees and keep still though relaxed. Fix your gaze on your toes. If this results in the eyes watering, close them and relax. Breathing during this posture should continue to be deep and slow. It may not be possible for obese people to perform this Asana to perfection. Probably, they will be able to raise only their legs and not the trunk. This should not discourage them. They should raise their legs as far as they can without feeling much discomfort and distress.

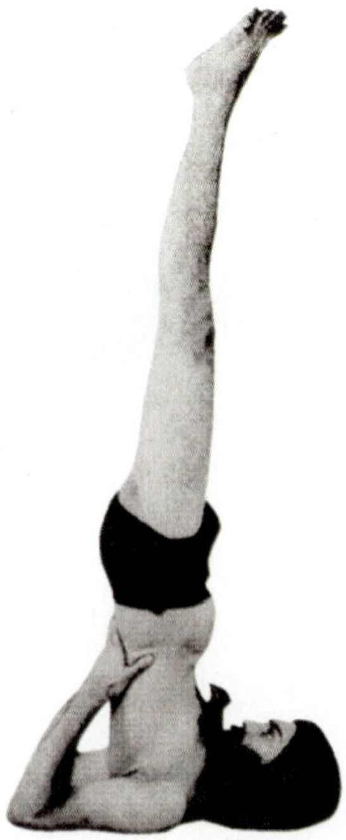

Fig. 52.51: *Urdhwa Sarvangasana-shoulder stand pose*

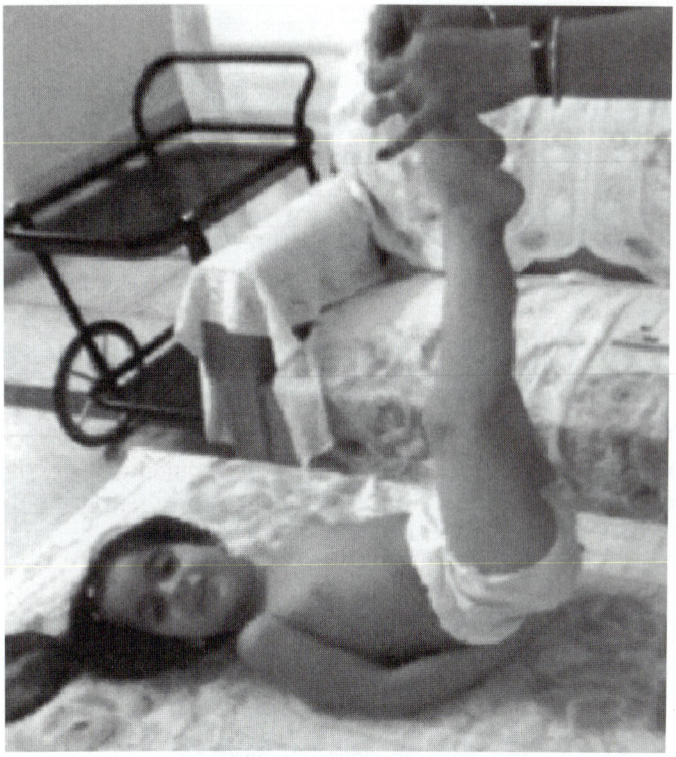

Fig. 52.52: *Urdhwa Sarvangasana-shoulder stand pose (helped by her mother)*

Benefits

The Yogic classification enumerates ten indriyas or organs of perception and action. The organs of sense are those of touch, taste, sight, hearing and smell. The organs of action are the hands and feet, the two excretory organs of urination and defecation and the organ of speech. This pose is considered to improve the action of all of them. It also improves the functioning of the cervical (neck) vessels and vocal cords and will improve a singer's voice. Experiments have confirmed that it improves the functioning of the liver and digestive system, and tones up the nerves and musculature of the head and the trunk. It is a prophylactic against many diseases. Yogis attach great importance to this posture as an aid to the awakening of the Kundalini, the mysterious power capable of leading the Sadhaka (Aspirant) to Absolute Perfection. But even for normal people, men and women alike, it is a highly beneficial posture conferring practically all the benefits that the head stand bestows without any of the possible harmful side effects.

Halasana-Plough Pose

Posture (Figs 52.53 and 52.54)

Lie down on the ground on your back, raise the legs upwards, then raise the back with the help of both hands until you attain the Urdhwa Sarvangasana. Then tilt your legs slowly until your toes touch the ground behind your head. Keep your legs straight and do not bend the knees stretch your arms behind your back so that they rest in the

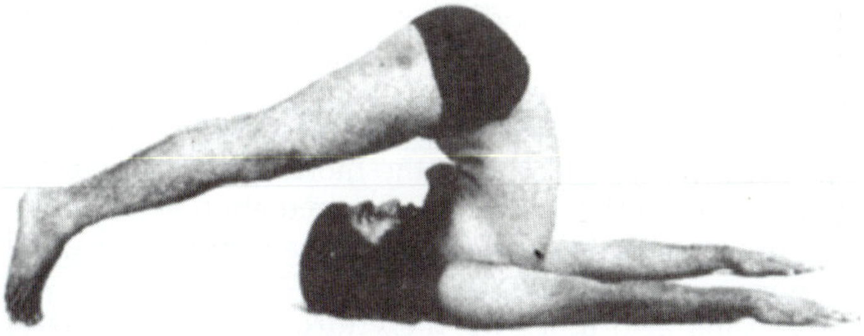

Fig. 52.53: *Halasana-plough pose 1*

opposite direction to the legs, lying parallel to each other with the palms touching the ground. The body now rests on the shoulders, neck and head, the pose resembling a plough. Keep the eyes open. If you cannot continue deep breathing in this posture you can breathe normally while holding this pose.

Benefits

This Asana is also known as Sarvangasana which literally means "all parts posture". It exercises and stretches the posterior muscles of the entire body. It improves the circulation and tone of the whole length of the spinal cord, and at the same time benefits the arms and legs. It tones up the thyroid gland. It imparts elasticity and pliability to the spinal cord, "oiling" the roots of the bilateral nerve branches of the spinal cord (32 pairs in all, serving the major part of the body). The stretching involved in this exercise enlarges the passages (vertebral foramina) through which the

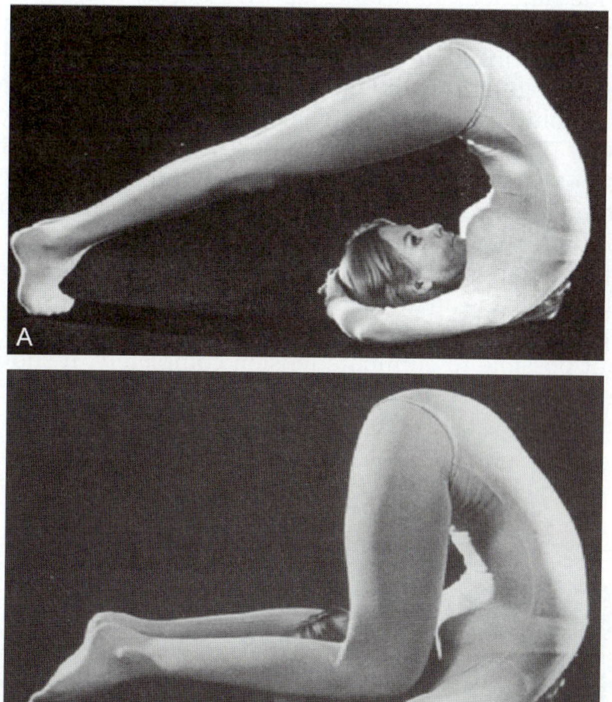

Fig. 52.54A and B: *Halasana-plough pose 2*

branches of the spinal cord pass out into the body, thereby raising considerably and sometimes spectacularly the efficiency and performance of the entire spinal nervous system and the areas served by it. Its regular practice improves the functioning of the thoracic and abdominal viscera in general. It improves the circulation of the brain, thereby contributing to intelligence, alertness and good memory.

Halasana also tones up the entire pelvic region and activates the gonadal secretions in the male and the female. It exercises the neuromusculo-circulatory systems and the tissues surrounding and adjoining the sex centres in the spipe, thereby substantially improving the sexual efficiency of the individual.

Matsyasana-Crocodile Pose 1

With Back and Head on Ground (Figs 52.55 and 52.56)

Posture: First, sit in the Lotus Pose (Padmasana), then gradually bend backwards until you are lying on your back with the legs still fixed in the Lotus posture. Flex your head backwards and arch your back by raising your chest and abdomen so that the entire body rests on the knees and the head. The head should be stretched backwards so that the highest point of the head is resting on the ground Breathe slowly and deeply, feeling relaxed.

Matsyasana-Crocodile Pose 2

(With Back and Head Stretched)

Benefits: This posture relieves constipation and tones up all the areas of the spine, including the sex centre. It is said to be particularly beneficial to women as it normalizes uterine functioning. It tones up the lungs and muscles of the chest. It improves the circulation of the throat and tends to reduce tonsils. It is said that those who practise this posture regularly maintain a strong and erect spine even during old age. Even if one has developed a slight stoop, regular practice of this posture will help to correct it. It is also said to help diabetics by improving their general metabolism. People suffering from spinal pain should practise it regularly. There is no harm in practising it in part if you are unable to achieve the perfect posture. Even while practising an imperfect posture, the exerciser should keep his mind and body free from tension and rigidity. If it is not possible to eliminate tension completely, it should be reduced to the minimum.

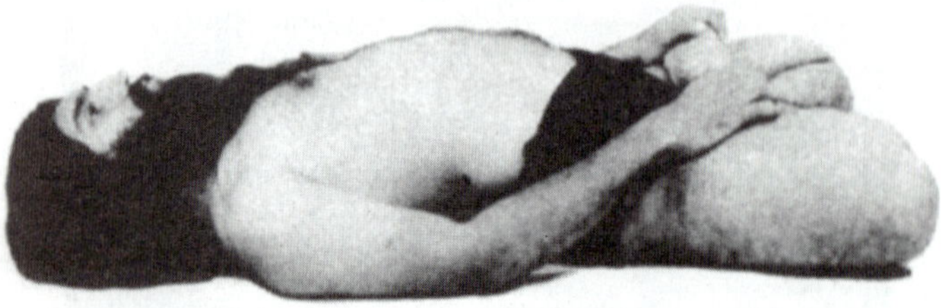

Fig. 52.55: *Matsyasana-crocodile pose 1 (with back and head on ground)*

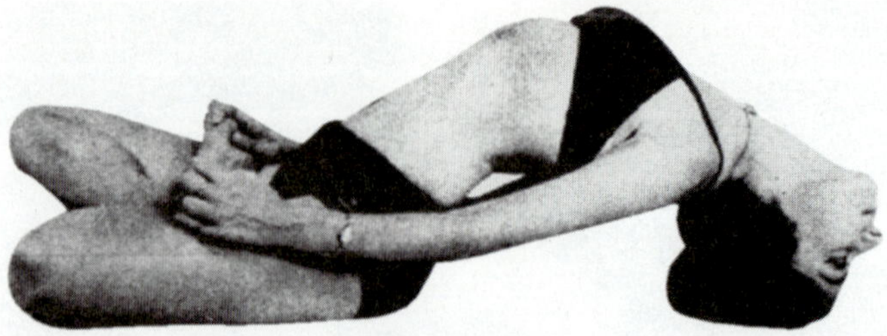

Fig. 52.56: *Matsyasana-crocodile pose 2 (with back and head stretched)*

Bhujangasana-Serpent Pose (Figs 52.60 and 52.61)

Posture

Down full length face downwards; then, placing both your hands on the ground alongside your shoulders, raise your

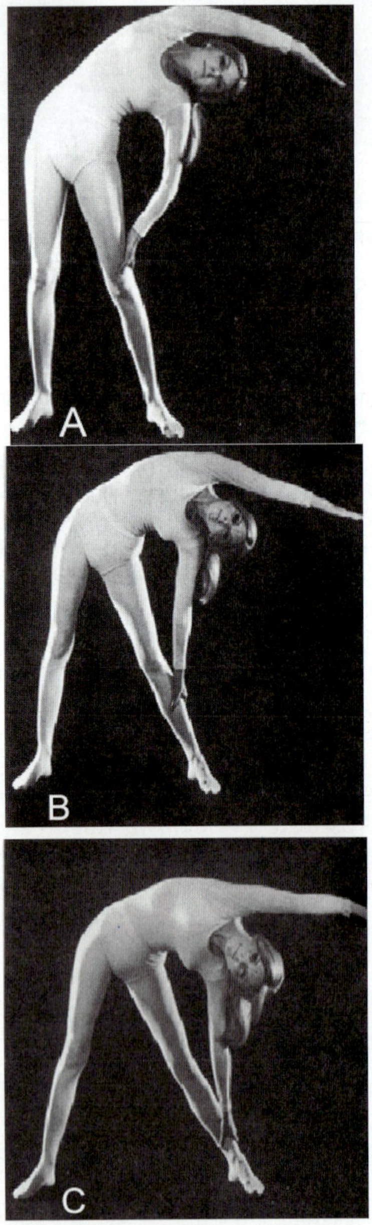

Fig. 52.57*(A-C)*: *Trinangle posture*

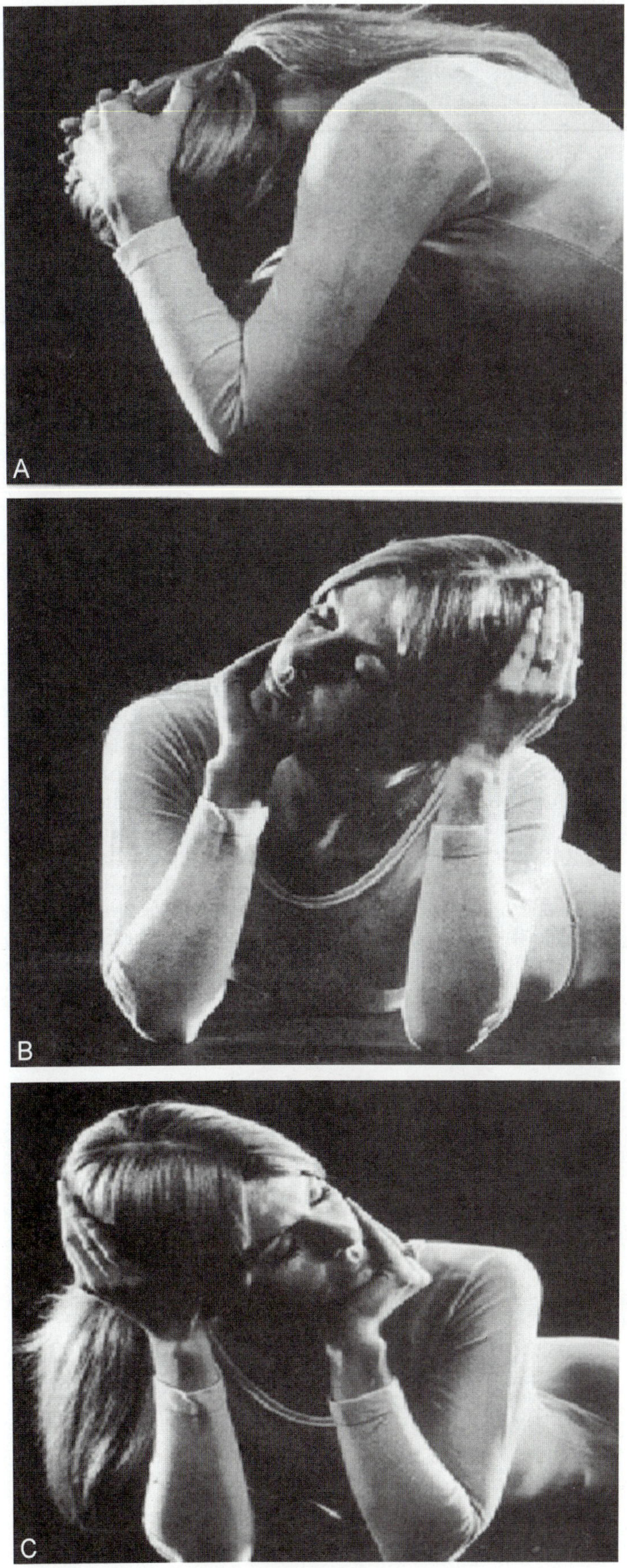

Fig. 52.58A to C: *Head twist*

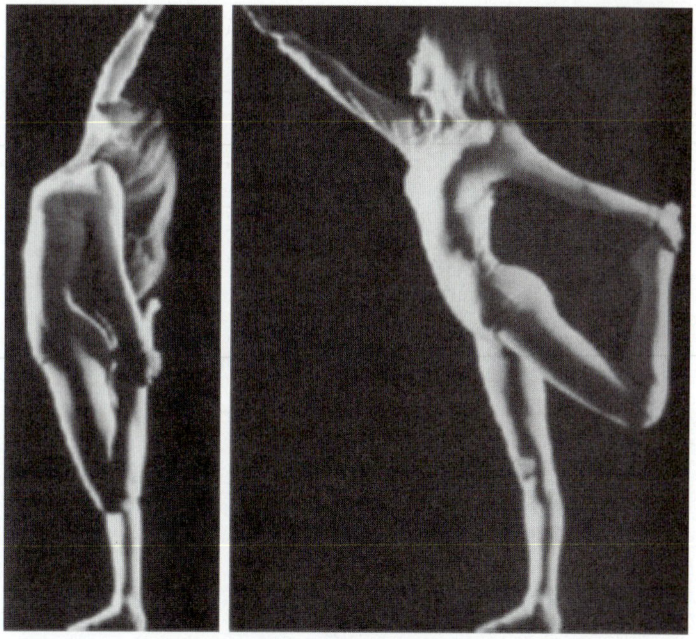

Fig. 52.59: *(Left to right) balance posture*

chest on your arms as high as you can with your head stretched backwards. The body from the waist down to the toes should remain in touch with the ground, the legs and the feet being held together. Breathe slowly and deeply.

Benefits

This is an excellent pose for reducing abdominal fat and relieving constipation and flatulence. Its contribution to relief from spinal pain is remarkable considering the simplicity of the pose. If practised patiently and diligently it helps the exerciser to get over spinal pain of long standing, even when caused by osteoarthritic changes in the spine. Its benefits affect the entire length of the vertebral column, including the cervical, the thoracic, the dorsal, and the sacral vertebrae, and the coccyx (these words denote the divisions of the spine into the neck, the upper back, the middle back, the lower back, and the tail bone respectively). It also tones up the muscles, tendons, and ligaments, the nerves and the blood vessels of the spinal region. Since this pose

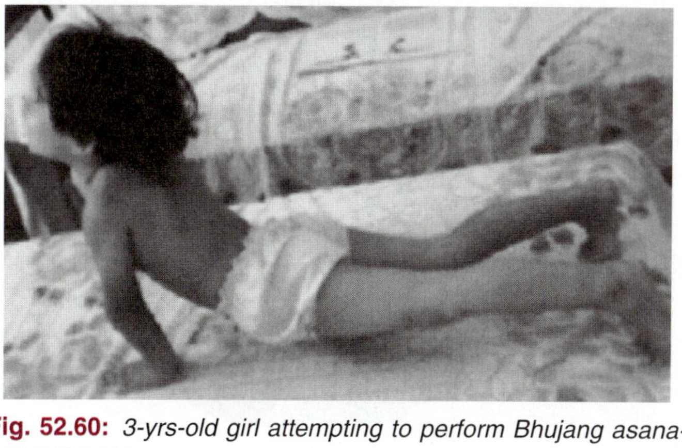

Fig. 52.60: *3-yrs-old girl attempting to perform Bhujang asana-serpent pose*

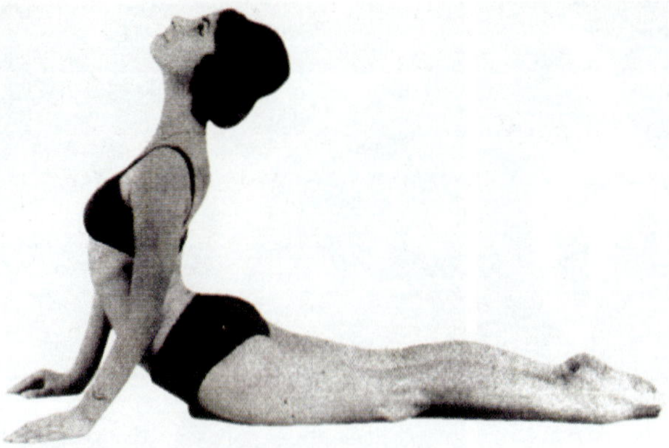

Fig. 52.61: *Bhujang asana-serpent pose*

exercises the spinal sex centre, it makes a substantial contribution to the effectiveness of the sexual performance of both men and women.

Dhanurasana-Bow Pose (Fig. 52.62)

Posture

Lie down on your chest and abdomen with your arms resting alongside your body. Throughout the exercise both the legs and the feet should remain joined together. Lift both the feet and legs upwards and backwards, bringing them towards your head until, with your arms raised behind you can hold both the ankles, the left ankle in the left hand and the right ankle in the right hand. The head should be held high. The chest also should be raised from the ground so that only the abdomen and the pelvis remain in contact with the ground. The pose should be held steady without any movement except that of the respiratory tract. Fill the lungs with air before raising the legs and the chest. At the completion of the pose continue normal breathing if deep breathing appears to be difficult. The feet may tend to come down towards the waist, but if you remain firm in your pose you can hold them steady. Keep the eyes open. Fill the lungs when returning to the ground to terminate the pose.

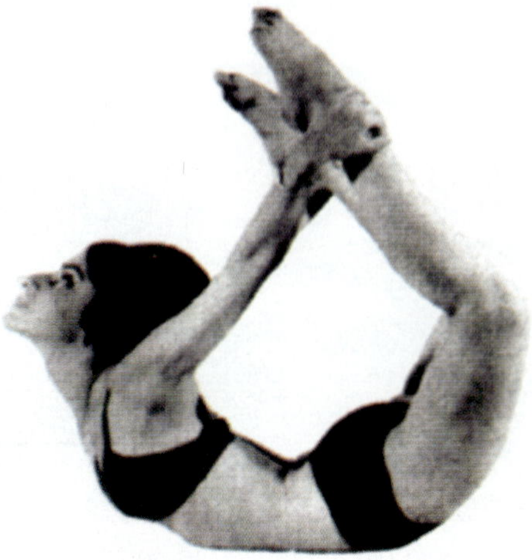

Fig. 52.62: *Dhanurasana-bow pose*

When you are accustomed to this posture learn to rock backwards and forwards (like a rocking chair).

Benefits: This posture exercises the entire body. It strengthens the deep and the superficial muscles of the entire spine, removing rigidity, stiffness, aches, pains, burning sensations, and tenderness of the spine and areas adjacent to it and served by the branches of the spinal cord. It also strengthens the spinal sex centre and both the male and female gonads, thereby improving the sexual performance. It tones up and develops the muscles of the chest. It improves the function of the liver, the kidneys, the bladder, the genital organs and other pelvic and abdominal viscera. It is a prophylactic against the formation of stones in the kidney and gall bladder. It relieves scanty, painful and burning urination. Practised regularly in middle age, it is believed to have a healthy effect on the prostate gland and to protect against enlargement or inflammation of this gland. It gives relief against piles, anorexia (dislike for food), flatulence, and halitosis (bad breath) when not caused by pyorrhoea. This Asana should not be performed by anyone suffering from a slipped disc.

Merusankarshasana-Spinal Traction Pose

Posture (Figs 52.63–52.67)

Lie down on a hard bed or table on your back with your body stretched full length but with the entire neck and head hanging beyond the edge of the bed, so that the full weight of the head is subjected to the gravitational pull of the earth without any support whatsoever. Relax' the entire body as much as you can so that the relaxed muscles of the neck do not interfere with the full force of gravity pulling the head downwards. In this way the maximum weight of the head will exert a tractional pullon the entire spine and tend to increase the intervertebral spaces. Lie thus for 5 minutes, then, retaining the same position, flex your feet, with heels firmly held against the surface of the bed, towards your

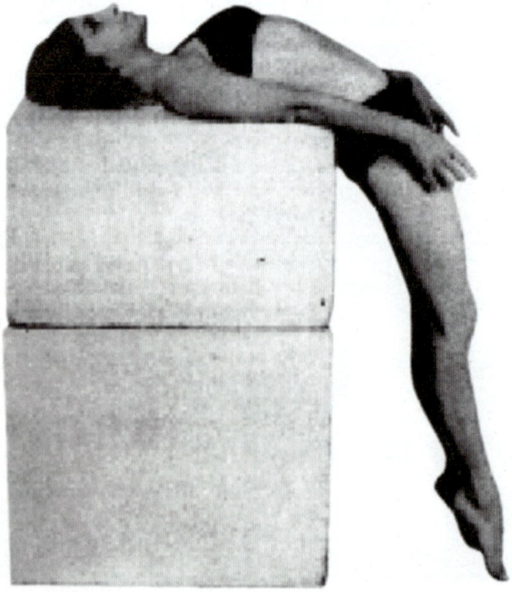

Fig. 52.63: *Merusankarsh asana-spinal traction pose*

face in aneffort to bring the toes of your feet into contact with your legs. This will exercise another strong pull on the back muscles of the body all along the line. Then slowly extend the feet in the opposite direction in an attempt to touch the surface of the bed with your toes. Of course, you can neither touch your legs nor the bed with your toes but try to cover fhe maximum distance in arching your feet on both sides. The movement should be slow and rhythmical and the pull in either direction the fullest you can manage. At the extreme end of the pull on either side hold the feet in position for 1 second. Repeat the exercise ten times. Keep the head hanging over the edge of the bed during this exercise.

During all this period both your arms should be spread out at right angles to your body and slipped slightly beyond the sides of the bed so that they, too, are unsupported. This will stretch the shoulders outwards. Even in this position, the arms should be so relaxed that their full gravitational pull downwards is not reduced by any tension of the muscles. This will exercise an outward pull on the muscles of the chest. The novice may feel the stretch of the chest muscles uncomfortable after a few seconds. If it becomes too uncomfortable, the arms should be taken back to the horizontal position until the sensation of discomfort in the chest muscles subsides. After five minutes of this exercise slide down so that the head now rests on the bed and the legs hang over the opposite end of the bed. This exercises an automatic stretch on the pelvis. After a few minutes slide your legs down so that your feet are on the floor and then sit up with the help of your hands in the bed. Keep sitting from half to 1 minute. This completes the exercise and you can then leave the bed.

Benefits

Orthopaedic surgeons usually treat spinal pains, sciatica, brachial neuralgia, pains in neck and shoulder blades, arising out of intervertebral pressure on spinal nerves, by subjecting the patients to traction by placing them in a horizontal position with their feet stretched outside the edge of the bed with weights tied to their ankles to exert a pull on the spine. Since the very concept of Yoga aims at using an individual's own body for meeting all its needs, the device of using the weight of the head in place of attaching extraneous weight to the feet not only fulfils this condition, but our experience has shown that its results

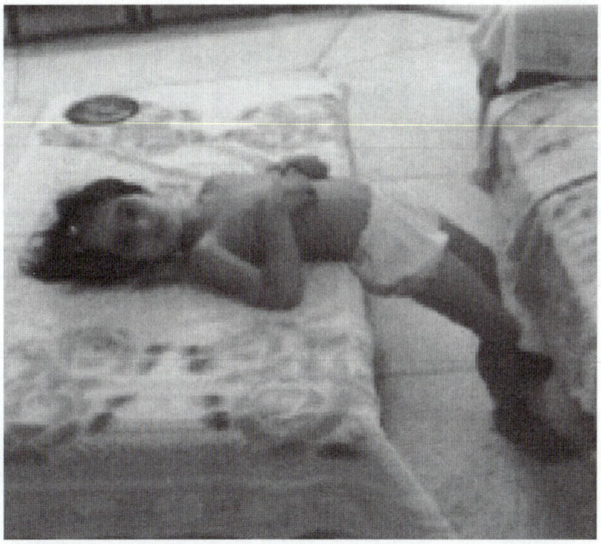

Fig. 52.64: *Merusankarsh asana-spinal traction pose in a 3-yrs-old girl*

are superior to those of the prevalent method of traction. The exercise brings about better and more speedy relief in all pains in which traction is indicated. This posture has not so far been mentioned by any books, ancient or modern, to my knowledge.

Pranayama-Yogic Breathing (Figs 52.68–52.70)

Pranayama should be performed after you have completed your routine of Asanas. Sit erect but relaxed in the Lotus Pose (Padmasana). If you do not feel comfortable and cannot relax in this pose, adopt the Easy Pose (Sukhasana). Sitting in this pose, complete a series of 25 unit yogic breaths in the following order:

Right nostril breathing: Close the left nostril with the little finger of your right hand and take 5 yogic breaths with your right nostril, i.e. inhale (Puraka), pause (Kumbhaka), exhale (Rechaka), and pause (Shunyaka). Repeat four more times.

Left nostril breathing: Now release the left nostril and close the right nostril with your right thumb. Take five 4, unit yogic breaths through your left nostril. Alternate breathing.

Inhale (Puraka) through the right nostril, keeping the left nostril closed with the little finger, pause (Kumbhaka), then

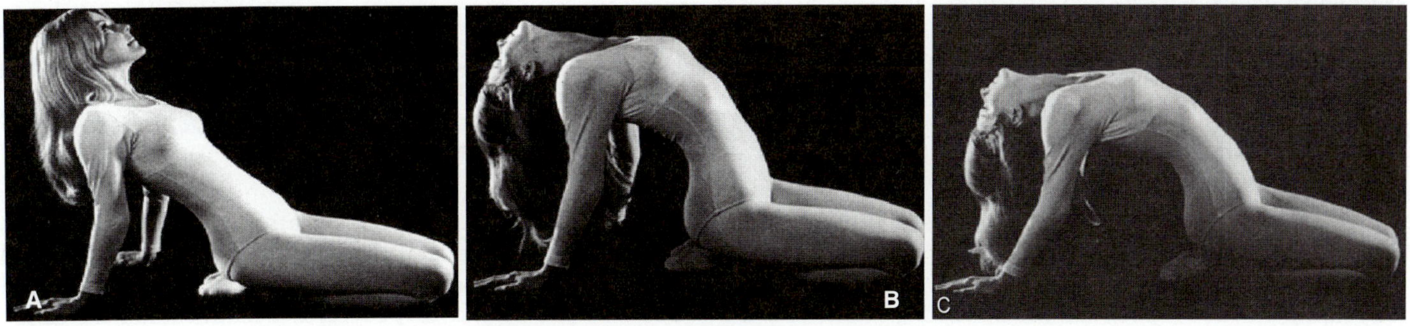

Fig. 52.65A to C: *Backward bend exercise*

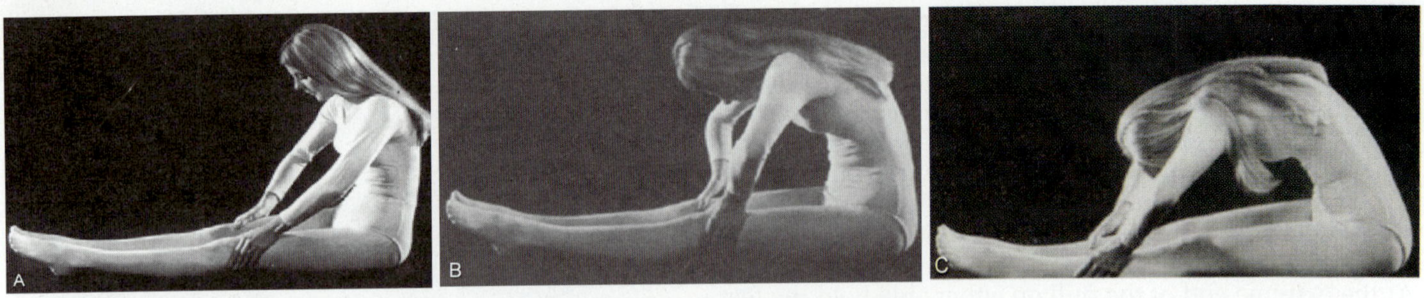

Fig. 52.66A to C: *Back stretch exercise*

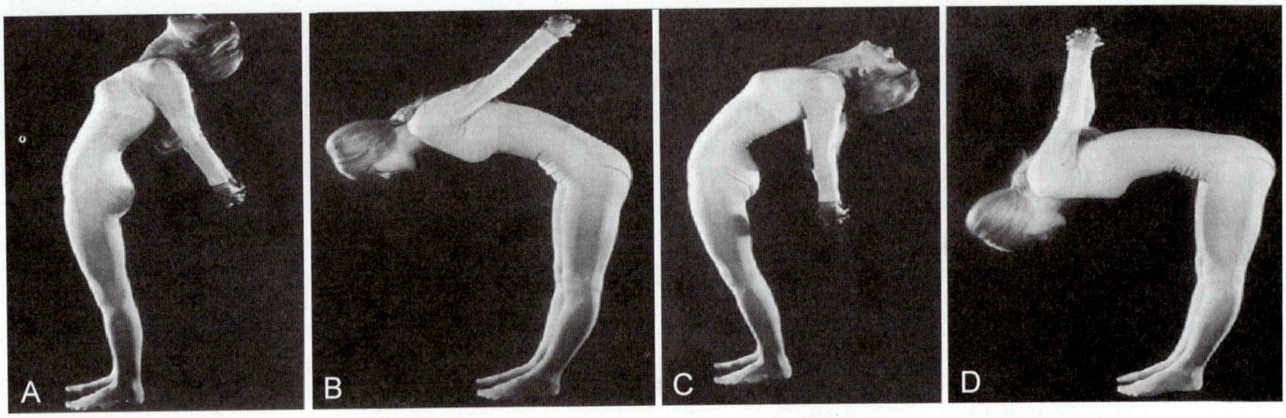

Fig. 52.67A to D: *Chest expansion exercise*

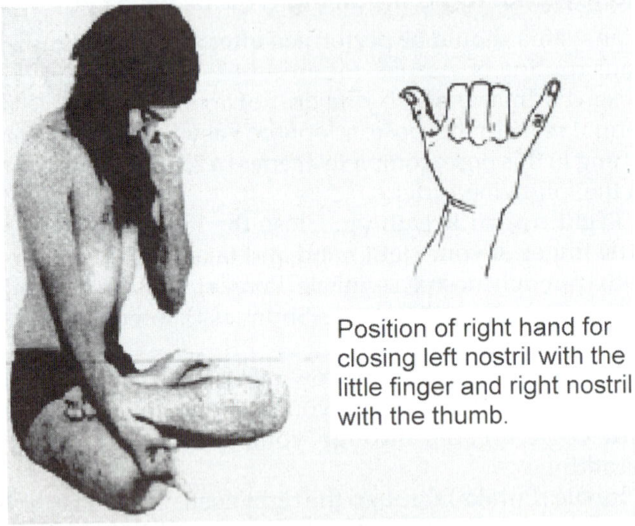

Fig. 52.68: *Young person performing Pranayama. In this exercise, the person positions the right hand for closing left nostril with little finger and right nostril with the thumb*

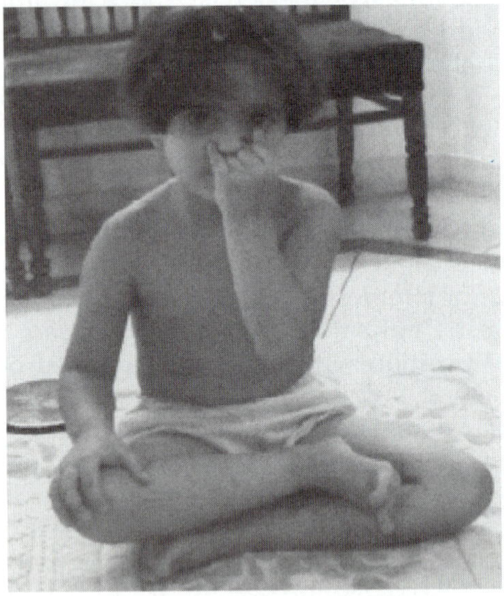

Fig. 52.69: *Alternate nostril breathing in a 3-yrs-old girl*

close the right nostril with the right thumb and exhale through the left nostril (Rechaka), and pause (Shunyaka). Repeat four more times.

Alternate Breathing 2

Repeat alternate breathing I in reverse. Simultaneous bilateral breathing: Take five full breaths with both nostrils open. While doing so, the backs of both your hands should be resting on your knees with the tips of the thumb and the index finger of each hand meeting together to form a circle between the two, the other three fingers of each hand remaining fully stretched.

Kapala, Bhati (Bellows Breathing)

The above, mentioned 25 pranayamic breaths should be followed by 10 quick deep breaths without any pauses between inhalations and exhalations or exhalations and inhalations. The posture for bellows breathing, so called because the sound of powerful breaths taken in quick succession resembles that of air being pushed out from

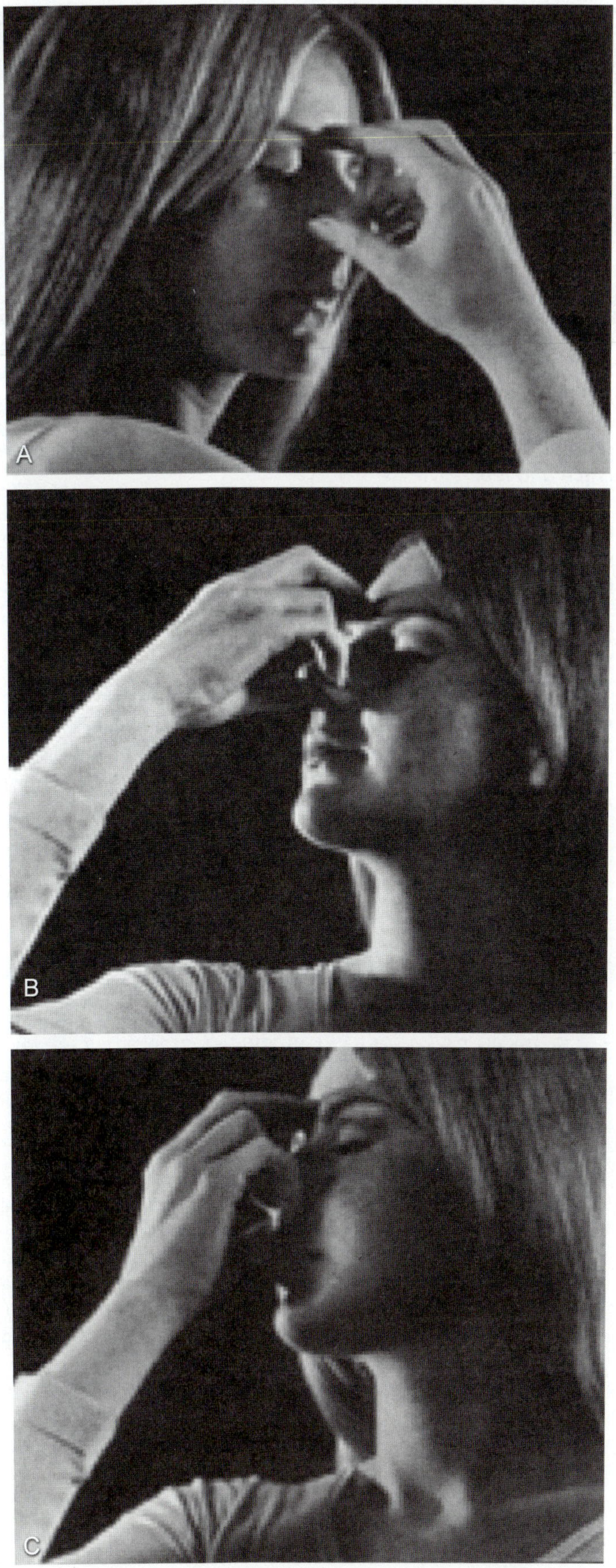

Fig. 52.70A to C: *Alternate nostril breathing*

bellows, has to be the same as for practising Pranayama, except that it is the palms of the hands that rest on the knees in the case of this type of breathing. Ordinarily; 10 such forceful and quick breaths suffice as an adequate exercise of the lungs and the nasal pas, sages for an average person. It is one of the most effective exercises to remove difficulty in breathing due to blocked nasal passages when the blocking does not result from polypi or tumours. The practice considerably enhances the efficiency of the respiratory system.

Shavasana-Pose of Tranquillity

Posture (Figs 52.71 and 52.72)

Lie down on your back with both arms lying close to your body. Relax yourself completely so that if someone raises your arm or leg, it falls down as if there were no life in it. No part of the body should make the slightest movement, and yet no tension should remain in any of the body. Detach yourself completely from the problems of your life arid if you have nothing better to concentrate upon, just give your entire attention to your breathing which should be deep, slow and easy.

At first glance, Shavasana appears to be the easiest of all Asanas to perform. A number of lazy people with blank

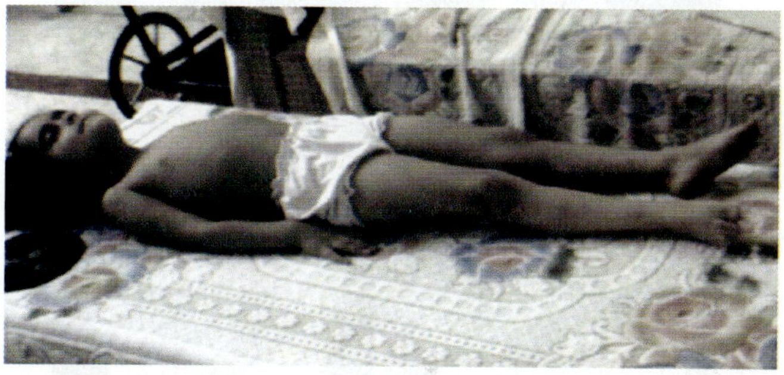

Fig. 52.71: *Shavasana-pose of tranquillity in a 3-yrs-old girl*

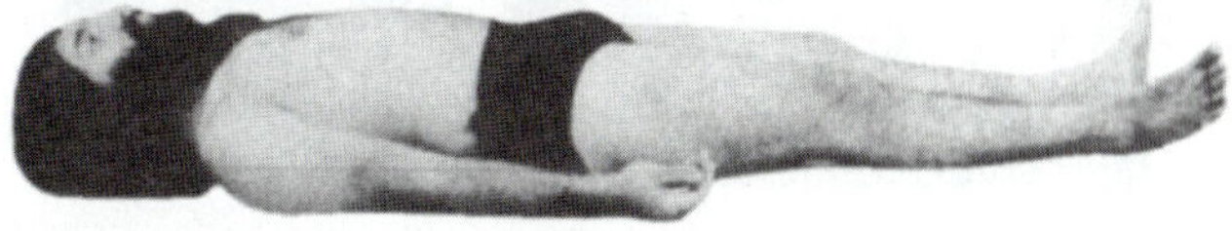

Fig. 52.72: *Shavasana-pose of tranquillity in adolescent*

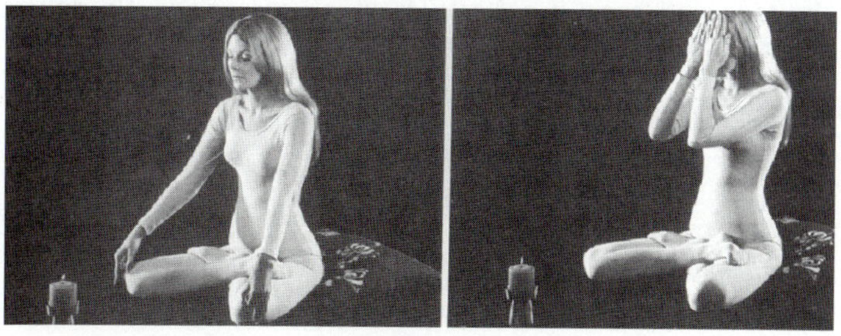

Fig. 52.73: *Candle concentration pose for turning the mind inward*

minds tend to perform it unconsciously. Yet, it is not so simple to achieve as it looks. In so far as one of the essential aspects of this, Asana is total detachment of the mind from the happenings round about, entailing a deliberate cultivation of total blankness of mind, it is one of the most difficult postures to perform completely. One must learn to perfect this pose not only physically but also mentally as it is not possible to get the best out of this pose without a completely coordinated relaxation of the mind and the body.

Benefits

This posture has been successfully utilized by eminent modern cardiologists in India to speed up the recovery of patients convalescing from heart diseases. It has been observed that patients practising Shavasana recover more quickly and completely. It also acts as a prophylactic against heart diseases in general. Practice of this posture helps to prevent the harmful effects on the body and mind of undue stress or anxiety, whether physical or mental. If one can achieve the right amount of detachment while relaxing in this pose, the feeling of relaxation will be far superior to that experienced from the use of tranquillizers and sedatives. It need hardly be pointed out that the role of a truly relaxed psychosomatic system in achieving a rewarding sexual gratification and performance is very important.

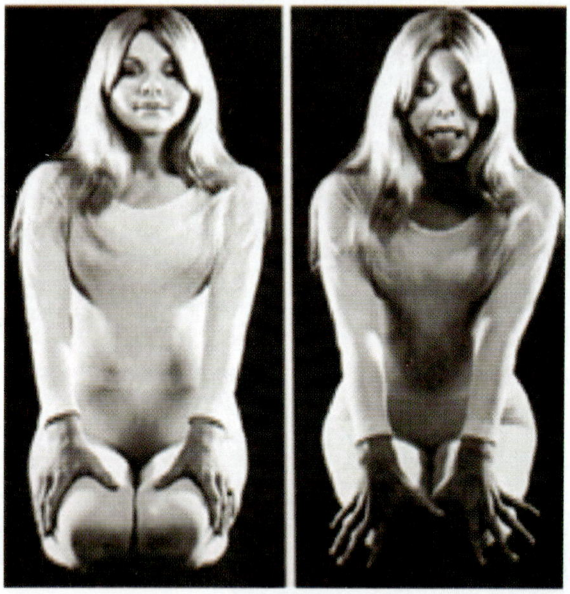

Fig. 52.74: *Loin pose for strengthening the muscles of the face and neck. Sit on heels hands rest on knees, slowly move trunk forward. Simultaneously widen eyes and extend tongue, fingers are spread far apart. You must feel a strong pull in all muscles of the face and neck; if not, you must intensify effort. Do not be reluctant to assume all the ferocity of a lion. Very slowly withdraw tongue. Relax eyes and fingers. Settle back into resting position and relax. Perform three times*

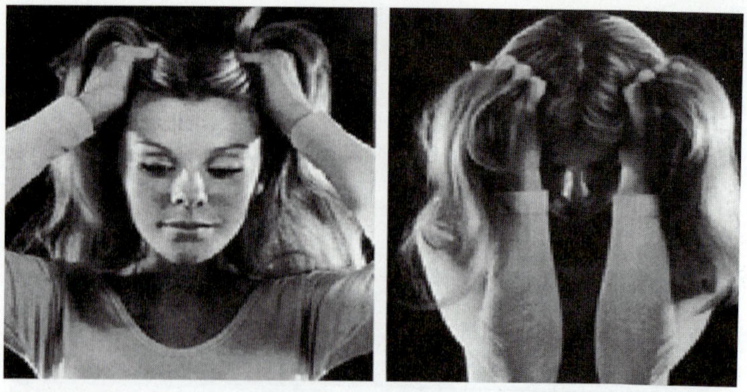

Fig. 52.75: *Scalp exercise for the healthy scalp. Sit in cross-legged posture. Grasp hair firmly at roots. Make scalp move as much as possible, first forward, then backward by pulling vigorously. Perform rhythmically and not too quickly 25 times without pause. Relax at conclusion of movements scalp should tingle and feel "alive"*

Strengthening the Muscles of the Face, Neck and Scalp (Figs 52.74 and 52.75)

Acknowledgment

The author is highly indebted to Pandit Shiv Sharma for utilizing some of photographs of yoga asanas from his book "Yoga and sex 1973".

BIBLIOGRAPHY

1. Monier-Williams, Sir Monier (1899). *A Sanskrit-English Dictionary*. Oxford Clarendon Press, p. 159.
2. Feuerstein, Georg (1996). The Shambhala Guide to Yoga. Shambhala Publications, Boston. p. 26.
3. "Patanjali Yoga sutras" by Swami Prabhavananda, published by the Sri Ramakrishna Math ISBN 81–7120–221–7 p. 111.
4. Verse 46, chapter II; for translation referred: "Patanjali Yoga Sutras" by Swami Prabhavananda, published by the Sri Ramakrishna Math ISBN 81–7120;221–7 p. 111.
5. Patanjali (± 300–200 B.C.) Yoga sutras, Book II:29.
6. Arya, Pandit Usharbudh (aka Swami Veda Bharati) (1977/1985). Philosophy of Hatha Yoga. Himalayan Institute Press, Pennsylvania.
7. Swami Prabhavananda (Translator), Christopher Isherwood (Translator), Patanjali (Author) (1996, 2nd ed.). Vedanta Press.
8. Vishnu-devananda, Swami (1959). The Complete Illustrated Book of Yoga.
9. Mittra, Dharma, (2003). Asanas: 608 Yoga Poses", ISBN 1–57731–402–6.

53 Telemedicine in Pediatric Cardiology

The newly developing field of telemedicine has the potential to benefit pediatric care by in creasing access to pediatric specialists and services. This report explores the current uses and limitations of telemedicine in pediatrics.

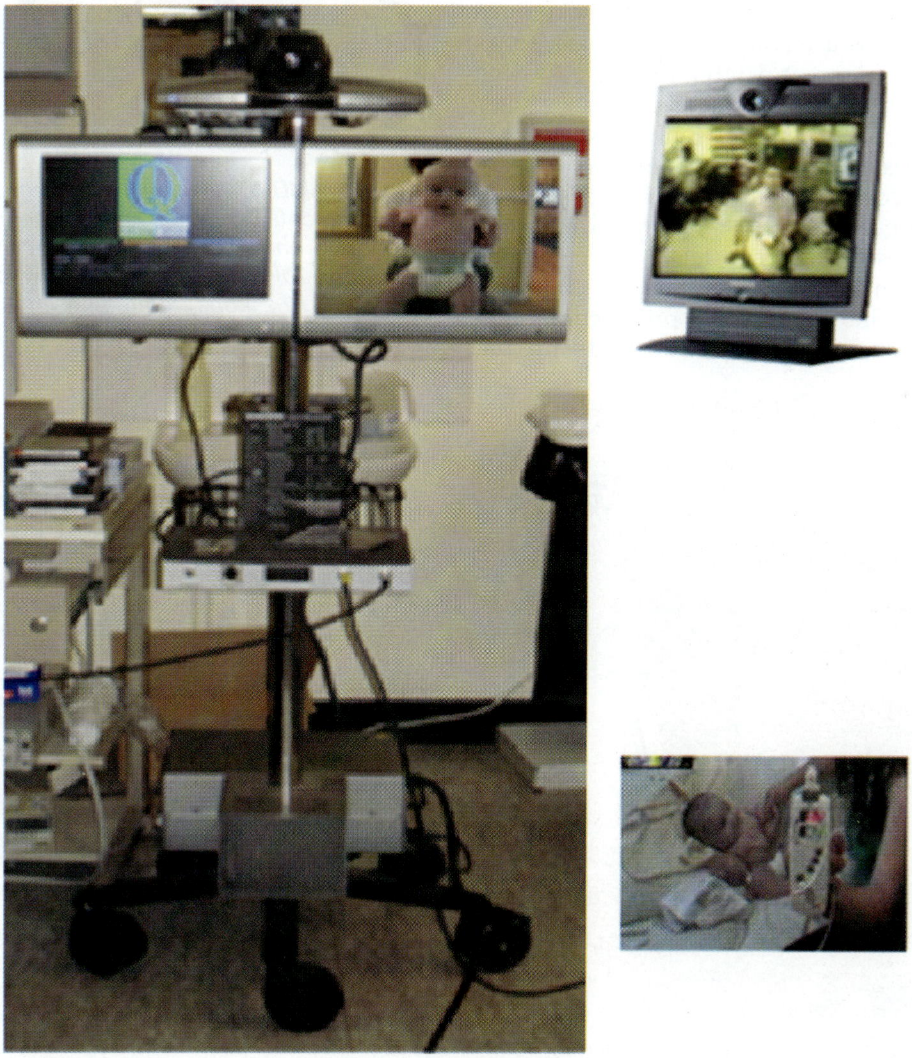

Fig. 53.1: *Telemedicine hardware needed for hospital-home videoconferencing. What the doctor sees and what the family sees*

Tele-echocardiography has the potential to bring real-time diagnoses to neonatal facilities without in-house pediatric cardiologists. Many neonates in rural areas, smaller cities, and community hospitals do not have immediate access to pediatric sonographers or echocardiogram interpretation by pediatric cardiologists. This can result in suboptimal echocardiogram quality, delay in initiation of medical intervention, unnecessary patient transport, and increased medical expenditures. Telemedicine has been used with increased frequency to improve efficiency of pediatric cardiology care in hospitals that are not served by pediatric cardiologists. Initial reports suggest that telecardiology is accurate, improves patient care, is cost-effective, enhances echocardiogram quality, and prevents unnecessary transports of neonates in locations that are not served by pediatric cardiologists (Fig. 53.1).

Echocardiography is often used to diagnose and exclude important cardiac diagnoses in children. Evolving telemedicine technology has the potential to improve access to echocardiography diagnoses in the intensive care unit, emergency room, and newborn nursery. The two primary modes of telemedicine practice are "store and forward" and "real-time" videoconferencing. A digital echocardiogram (often several one cardiac cycle loops) can be stored at one site and forwarded across a telemedicine network to a receiving station for review at a later time. Pediatric cardiologists often favor "real-time" telemedicine because of the ability to guide sonographers with limited experience in congenital heart disease. A complete telemedicine system requires a modified computer, a low- or high-speed connection, and telemedicine inputs. Several adult and pediatric clinical studies have shown telemedicine to be accurate, improve patient care, be cost-effective, enhance echocardiogram quality and sonographer proficiency, and promote practice expansion. Obstacles to widespread implementation of telemedicine include lack of standardization of telemedicine components, confusing legal issues and licensure requirements, and poor reimbursement.

Congenital Heart Diseases (Fig. 53.2)

Several telemedicine applications have become well established in paediatric cardiology but there is potential for improvement in and expansion of existing programmes and opportunities for new applications. This chapter shall discuss why telemedicine has an important role to play in paediatric cardiology, examine current applications from fetus to adult, including the evidence base and suggest what future steps may be taken to promote the use of telemedicine in paediatric cardiology. We shall also

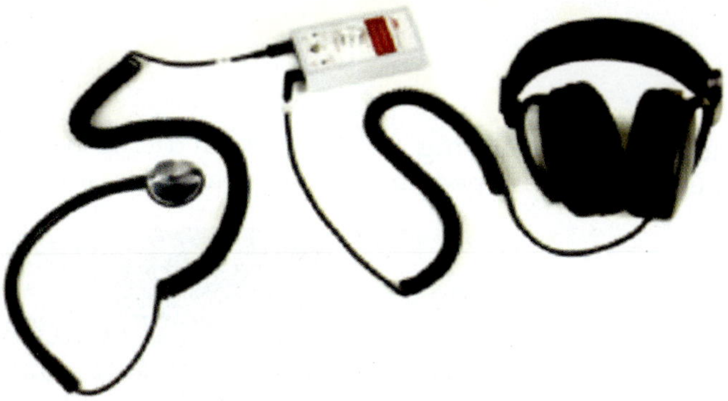

Fig. 53.3: *AMD-3700 telephonic stethoscope The AMD-3700 features low data bandwidth and high performance. Each module can operate on either transmit or receive mode auscultation bandwidth: 20Hz to 1,400Hz at low data communications bandwidth (19,2 kbps). Plugging chest piece automatically switches unit from send to receive mode*

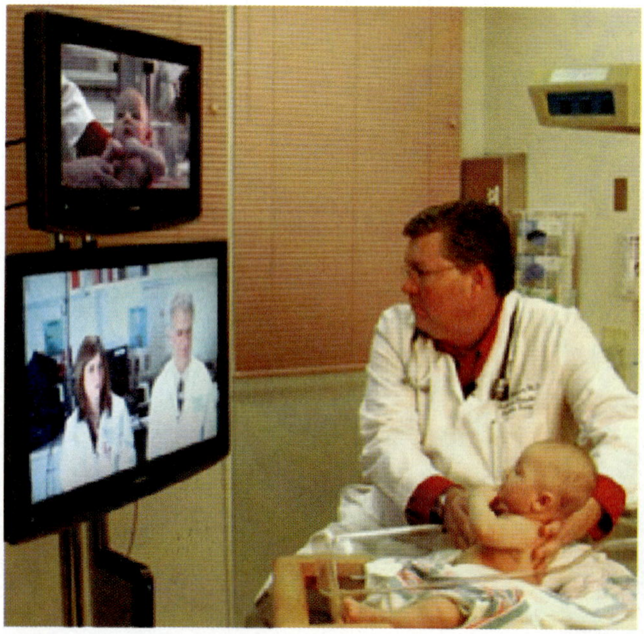

Fig. 53.2: *A telemedicine consultation for an infant with heart problem (top) and experts are advising accordingly (bottom)*

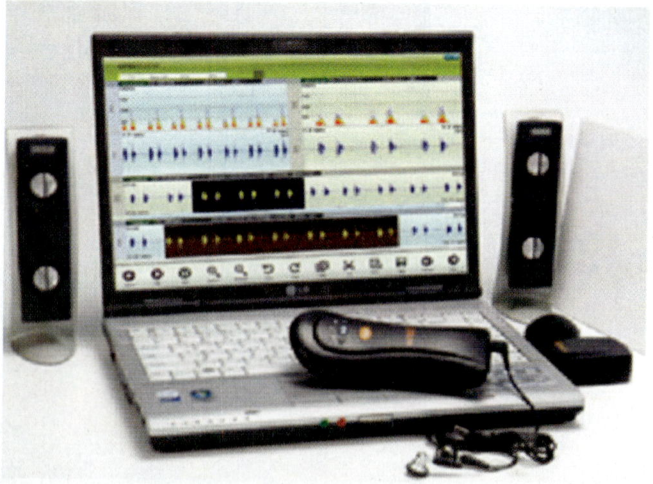

Fig. 53.4: *AMD-3130 E-scope stethoscope. The AMD-3130 E-scope stethoscope utilizes state of the art electronic technology to amplify heart, breath and Korotkoff sounds so they become much easier to hear. The sound is pure and clean. Compared to acoustic stethoscopes, murmurs and faint lows are much more distinguishable*

consider what equipment and personnel are necessary for successful telecardiology. However, before examining the role of telemedicine in paediatric cardiology, it is first important to understand what congenital heart disease is and how it presents to clinicians.

Why is Paediatric Cardiology Suited to Telemedicine

The single biggest reason why paediatric cardiology is suited to telemedicine is that it is a highly specialized field of medicine with a small cadre of professionals. Care is concentrated in a few regional centres. Therefore, large distances separate the patient and nonspecialist from expert advice. However CHD presents, it is unlikely that a nonspecialist will be confident in making a definitive diagnosis, counselling parents or instituting specific treatment without verification from a paediatric cardiologist. Fortunately, all forms of CHD can be diagnosed by a specialist using a combination of clinical examination including stethoscopy, ECG, chest X-ray and echocardigraphic images, i.e. on the analysis of data. These data are suitable for digitisation and electronic transmission and so used in telemedicine (Dowie et al., 2009). Babies with significant CHD may present to a hospital with on-site paediatric cardiology but considering only 13 hospitals in England and Wales have this facility compared with the 184 DGHs providing acute paediatric care, most will present to postnatal wards, neonatal units and emergency departments without on-site paediatric cardiology expertise (Workforce Review Team, 2009) (Figs 53.3–53.7).

Telemedicine can potentially support paediatricians faced with the predicament of a sick, cyanosed newborn baby with a suspected duct dependent CHD. Duct dependent lesions are a subgroup of severe CHD in which the circulation to either the lungs or body is dependent upon patency of the ductus arteriosus. This usually closes within the first 72 hours of life. In babies with duct dependent CHD, closure of the ductus arterious heralds the onset of severe symptoms. If not treated urgently duct dependent CHD is invariably fatal. The main differential diagnosis in this life-threatening scenario is persistent pulmonary hypertension of the newborn. The treatment of the two conditions is very different. Tele echocardiography interpreted by a paediatric cardiologist can offer timely diagnosis, institution of appropriate therapy and expedite or avoid transfer to a paediatric cardiology centre (Finley et al. 1997; Casey, 1999; Mulholland et al. 1999). Antenatal diagnosis of CHD is chiefly reliant upon an abnormality being suspected by a sonographer at a DGH, with very limited experience and knowledge of CHD during routine anomaly scanning.

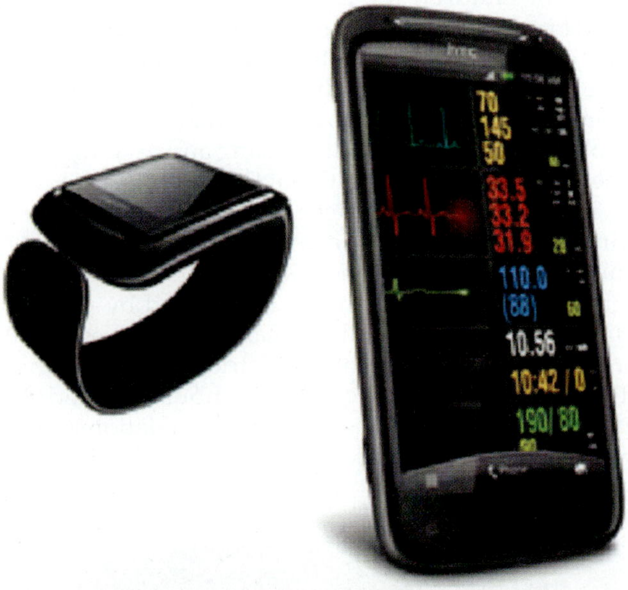

Fig. 53.5: *Wearable ECG monitor (wrist, wireless) CardioDefender is the first system to deliver mobile, real-time, beat-by-beat, and quantitative heart monitoring and automated reporting by combining patented analytical smartphone software with a Bluetooth device and electrodes*

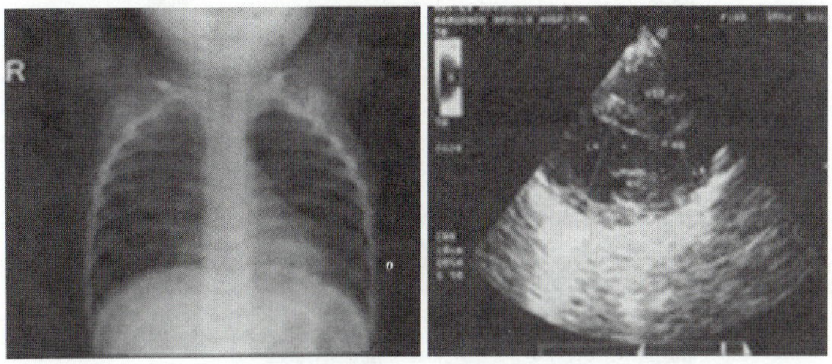

Fig. 53.6: *Chest X-ray and echocardiography as transmitted by internet*

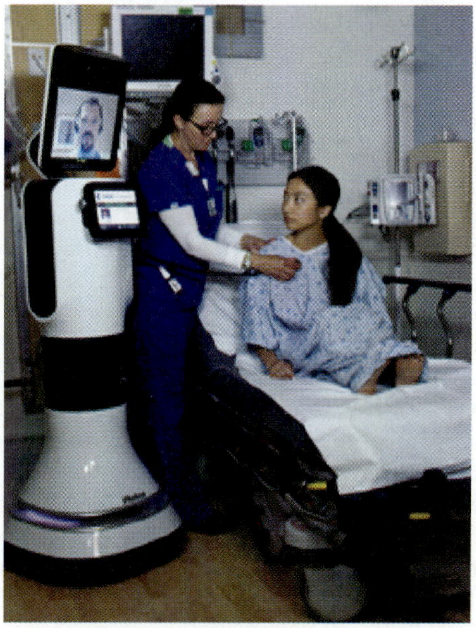

Fig. 53.7: *In touch health's specialty is remote-controlled robots for critical care, enabling people to be seen by doctors sooner than if they had to be in the same physical space as the physician. Getting a stroke victim, for example, to a specialist within 3 hours for diagnosis and treatment can make a huge difference to the patient. Similarly, specialists can provide care in intensive care units without having to physically be present which should lower health care costs and improve care*

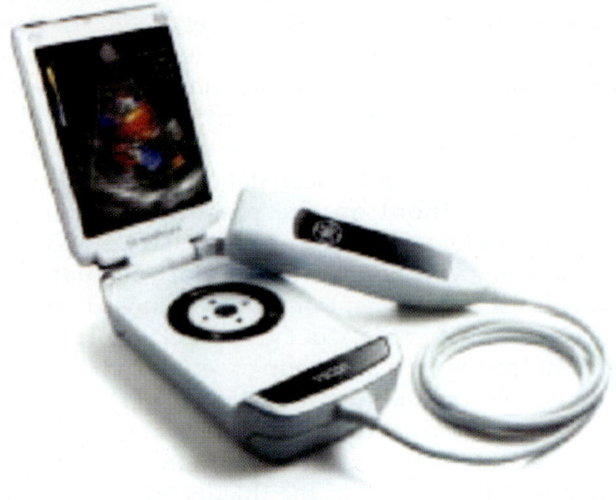

Fig. 53.8: *Echocardiography is a natural application for telemedicine, as handheld ultrasound devices and cloud-based transmission solutions make it possible to perform a test at a remote location and have consultation, in real-time, by an expert thousands of miles away. Telemedicine can eliminate the need for travel, reduce wait time for test results, and is cost effective*

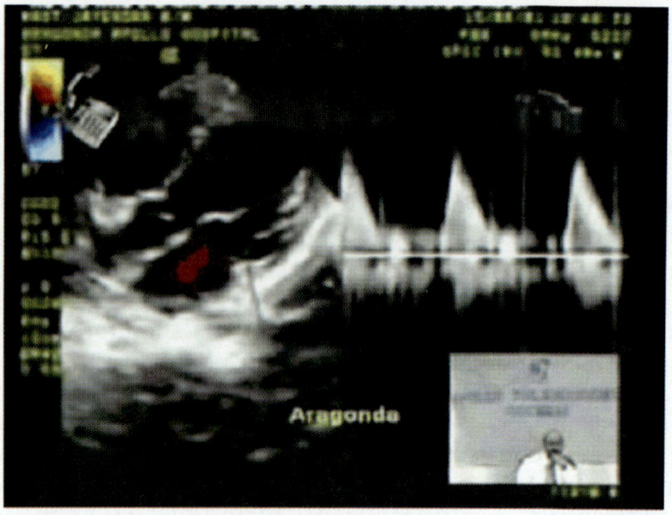

Fig. 53.9: *Specialist viewing transmitted live echocardiography from a remote centre*

Telemedicine may offer support to these radiographers. Telemedicine may also facilitate a rationalization of paediatric cardiology outreach clinics. Paediatric cardiologists hold outreach clinics at a number of DGHs within their region, travelling on a half day or full day once a month or once every 2 or 3 months. Lower thresholds for referring asymptomatic children with clear cut innocent murmurs for "a second opinion" have swollen outreach clinics (Dowie et al. 2009); (Dowie et al. 2009). Further pressures have been placed on service provision because of the need to comply with guidelines recommending screening of babies with various syndromes and family screening of certain inheritable conditions. Thus, the paediatric cardiologist may be away from the tertiary unit on average at least once a week. Whilst an excellent service is provided at the outreach clinic, it does not seem to be efficient from the tertiary unit's perspective (Qureshi, 2008). It is understood that most patient's first port of call will be their DGH. Therefore, it is important to foster confidence and competence in managing children with CHD. On the other hand, patients with a clinical problem requiring a paediatric cardiology opinion that cannot wait for the next out reach clinic, need transferred to the tertiary centre for a specialist opinion. A recent innovation has been the curriculum for paediatricians with special expertise in cardiology. Several posts have been appointed in DGHs throughout the UK (Royal College of Paediatrics and Child Health, 2009). The role of the paediatrician with special expertise in cardiology is to unload some of the outpatient work currently being done by the tertiary centres (e.g. evaluation of children with asymptomatic murmurs or chest pain), to be the link person for children with CHD followed up at that DGH and to be competent at performing 2D echocardiography. These paediatricians will need to be supported by the relevant tertiary centre. One of the key methods of providing this support could be via telemedicine links. Congenital cardiac surgery for children for England is currently provided across 11 centres. Each tertiary centre serves several DGHs staffed by paediatricians. A tertiary congenital cardiology service is provided by cardiac surgeons, specializing in congenital cardiac surgery, and paediatric cardiologists. The role of telemedicine in diagnosing and excluding CHD has been recognized at a national level in the UK. Various models of care have been debated leading to a number of recommendations including the establishment of telemedicine links between DGHs and the tertiary unit in order to have echocardiograms interpreted by paediatric cardiologists at all hours, all the year round (Qureshi, 2008). A proposed restructuring of paediatric cardiology services in the UK would reduce the number of paediatric cardiology surgical centres from 11 to 6 (National Health Service, Specialized Services, 2011). Several tertiary care

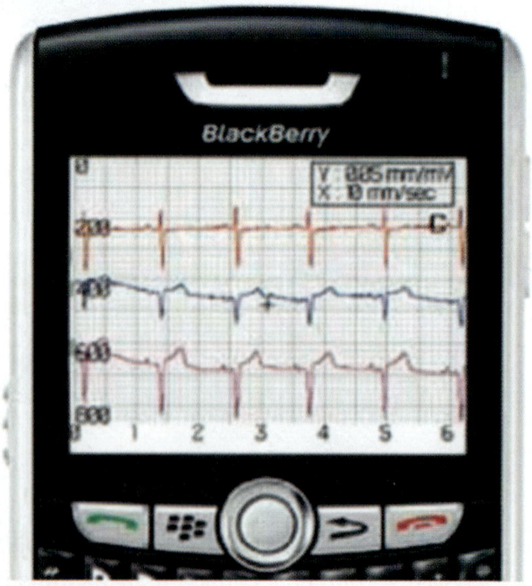

Fig. 53.10: *ECG record transmitted through mobile phone*

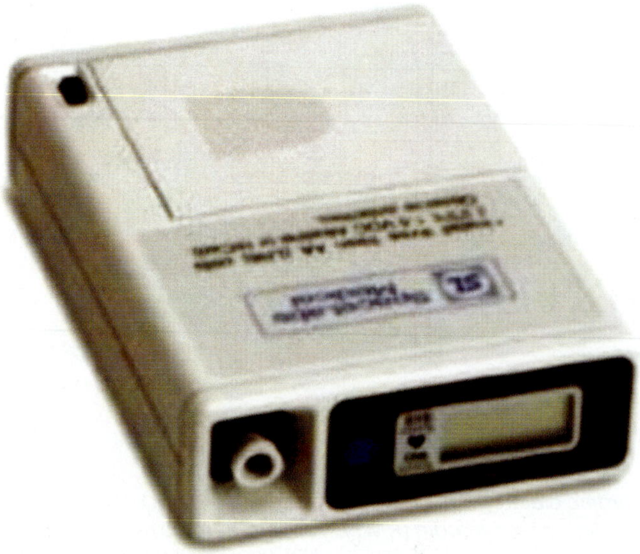

Fig. 53.11: *The features of ambulatory blood pressure monitoring recorder*

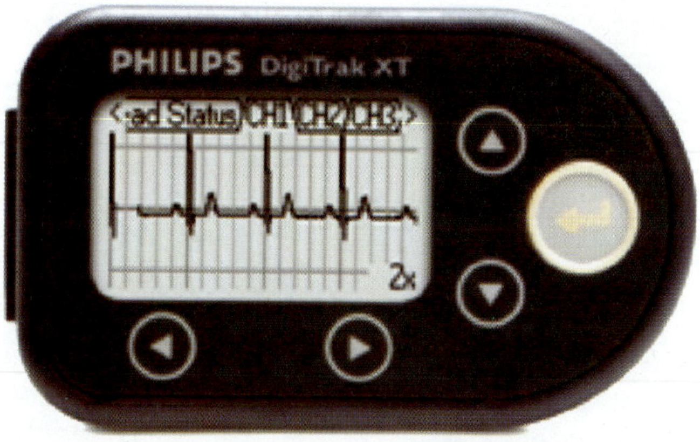

Fig. 53.12: *The features of cardiac event monitoring recorder*

centres will therefore need to significantly reorganize their working practices and become part of a large network of hospitals across a wide area. This development, which is likely to be adopted in other countries, is proposed in order to further centralise expertise and hopefully improve outcomes for patients. However, this may disadvantage paediatric cardiologists working in noncardiac centres and further isolate paediatricians in DGHs. The shared care of patients with CHD, between tertiary nonsurgical cardiac centres and the quaternary surgical centres, will necessitate excellent communication and case conferences. CHD case conferences are based around imaging data. It is easy to see that reliable telemedicine links between the various hospitals within this network will be essential.

In summary, congenital heart disease is potentially lethal. Its diagnosis is reliant upon interpretation of audio and visual data by a small number of experts, concentrated in a few tertiary units. Telemedicine seems to be the ideal tool to provide support to the nonspecialist thereby promoting access to specialist advice and improving patient care.

Common Diagnostic Difficulties for the Neonatologist

In terms of life or death of the patient, the defects that must be diagnosed are those causing cyanotic heart disease, major obstructive lesions of the left or right heart, and total anomalous pulmonary venous drainage (TAPVD). Cyanotic lesions such as transposition of the great arteries, pulmonary or tricuspid atresia, and other complex lesions with univentricular hearts do not usually present diagnostic difficulty if standard views can be obtained during the transmitted echocardiography. The diagnosis of TAPVD is the one likely to provide the most difficulty and is obviously a crucial one to make, particularly in babies where the differential diagnosis is persistent pulmonary hypertension. In our series, to date there has been only one patient with TAPVD. The correct diagnosis of supracardiac TAPVD was made with the transmitted scan, on which the pulmonary venous confluence and the ascending vein could be seen. The exclusion of a diagnosis of TAPVD requires a combination of imaging the pulmonary veins entering the left atrium and the demonstration of normal Doppler flow from them into left atrium. In the cases to date where a diagnosis of persistent pulmonary hypertension was being considered we have been able to satisfy ourselves that pulmonary venous drainage was normal (Figs 53.8–53.12).

For those with limited experience in echocardiography, obtaining good aortic arch views is one of the areas that causes most difficulty. The diagnosis of coarctation of aorta is essentially a clinical one, and if the femoral pulses are weak or absent in association with an arm-leg blood pressure gradient, the patient will require transfer to the regional centre for a definitive diagnosis.

The other common diagnostic dilemma for the neonatologist is in deciding whether the premature infant has a PDA, and, if there is one, how much is it contributing to the clinical condition of the patient? It is not practical to use a telemedicine link to confirm or exclude a PDA in all premature infants with this clinical problem. There is a case, however, for transmitting scans on ventilator dependent babies with chronic lung disease to determine whether a significant shunt through a PDA is exacerbating the problem. It is very useful in this situation to be able to answer the question by remote echocardiography and avoid transferring the ventilated patient.

Overview of Evidence Available in Paediatric Telecardiology (Figs 53.13–53.15)

There is a substantial body of research to support the feasibility of many applications of telecardiology in both paediatric and adult populations. There is much less good quality evidence demonstrating its clinical utility and cost-effectiveness. Most of the evidence is from small or uncontrolled studies. This is particularly difficult in paediatric cardiology because the numbers of patients involved are necessarily smaller than adult studies. However, there are larger scale randomized control trials in tele-homecare. There is now robust evidence advocating

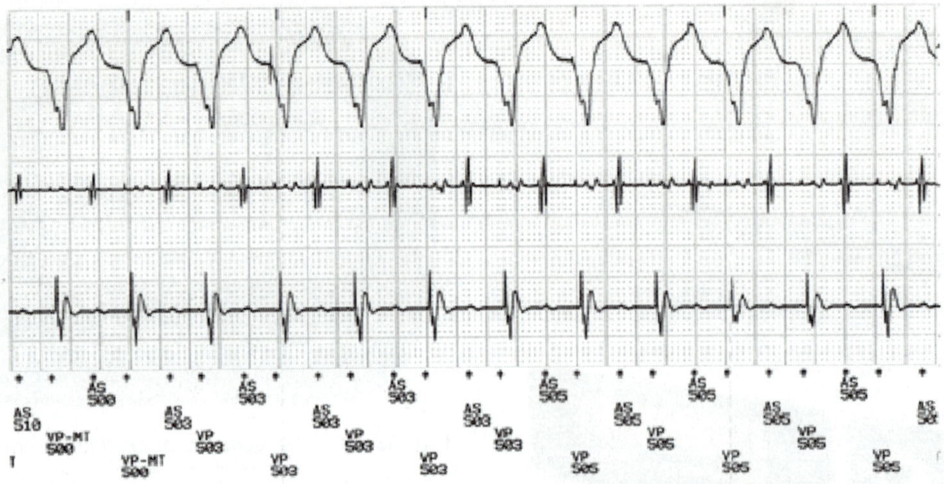

Fig. 53.13: *Telemetered ECG tracing with surface lead II (top) and intracardiac electrograms [atrial electrogram (center) and ventricular electrogram (lower)] and marker channel (bottom) showing pacemaker-mediated tachycardia (PMT). The intracardiac markers indicate that the retrograde P waves, labeled AS for atrial-sensed event, occur 280 milliseconds after the ventricular-paced beats, labeled VP*

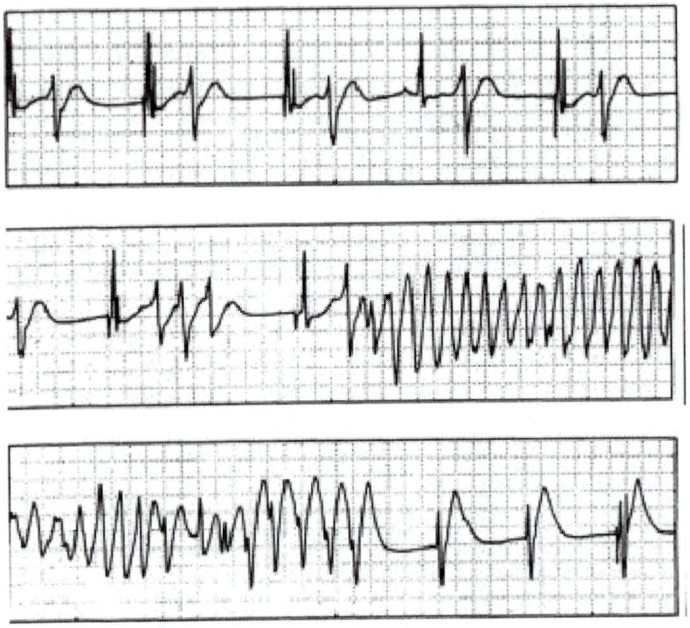

Fig. 53.14: *Continuous telemetry strip showing episode of TdP in a patient with a dual chamber pacemaker. The patient with sinus node dysfunction was started on quinidine and diltiazem in the hospital. The normally functioning pacemaker was programmed to the DDD mode with a lower rate of 50 beats per minute. She developed a junctional escape rhythm at around 50 bpm. Late-coupled ventricular bigeminy is followed by a three-beat run of ventricular tachycardia and then a 6-second run of TdP. The apparent ventricular undersensing is the result of "safety pacing" after sensing the ventricular electrogram in the nonphysiologic AV delay period after the atrial artifact. Torsades de pointes was suppressed by increasing the pacing rate*

a role for telemonitoring and structured telephone support for patients with chronic heart failure.

There is also evidence suggesting that remote monitoring of pacemakers and implantable cardiac defibrillators is reliable, safe, that it may improve patient satisfaction and reduce costs. Large randomizes control trials are ongoing which should hopefully clarify the role of remote monitoring in this patient group (Burri and Senouf, 2009).

Telemedicine Applied to Specific Cardiology Situations (Figs 53.13–53.15)

Telemedicine in fetal cardiology, there are a number of features of fetal cardiology that appear to make telemedicine an attractive proposition:

The clinical imperative

1. Fetal cardiology is a highly centralized subspeciality with even fewer specialists than paediatric cardiology.
2. Patients often travel large distances (up to 160 km in Northern Ireland) to attend a fetal cardiology clinic. The distance between home and the specialist centre is even greater in larger countries. In Quebec, 34% of mothers referred to a fetal cardiology service travel more than 100 km (Cloutier and Finley, 2004).

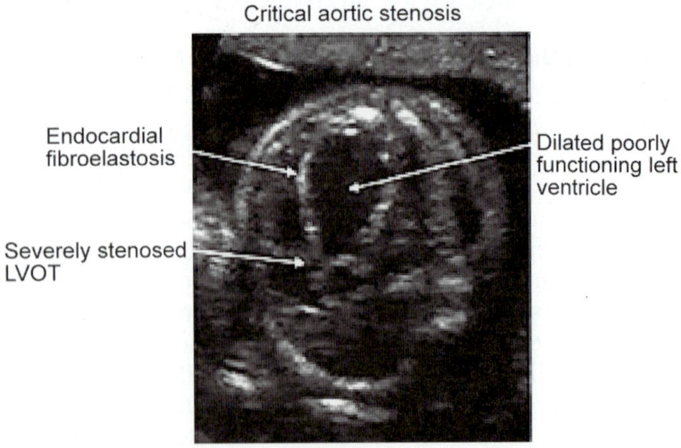

Fig. 53.15: *Example of severe congenital heart disease accurately diagnosed via tele-link in this study*

Table 53.1: *How congenital heart disease presents and the potential for telemedicine to support district general hospitals within a clinical network*

	Presentation	*Urgency*	*Potential for telemedicine*
Antenatal	Suspected CHD on routine anomally scan Risk factor for CHD	Nonurgent	Support sonographers Streamline antenatal screening
Neonate	Cyanosis Murmur Clinical shock Abnormal femoral pulses Risk factor for CHD	Usually an emergency	Immediate diagnosis or exclusion of CHD Institute potentially life-saving therapy Decide upon need for transfer
Infant and child	Hepatomegaly Abnormal femoral pulses Failure to thrive	Usually less urgent	Virtual clinics could help to recognize workload for peadiatric cardiologist

3. The summary of fetal cardiology literature demonstrates that timely, antennal diagnosis of CHD is important for improving outcomes for fetus and family by facilitating: parental counselling, elective delivery at an appropriate centre, parental choice in terms of termination and permitting fetal intervention in terms of pharmacotherapy for dysrhythmias and catheter intervention for severe complex lesions (Bonnet et al. 1999; Allan, 2000; Tworetzky et al. 2001; Gardiner, 2008).
4. The vast majority of fetuses with CHD are born from pregnancies without a recognisable antenatal risk factor. Obviously, formal evaluation by a fetal cardiologist cannot be offered to every single pregnancy. Therefore, in order to maximize antenatal detection of CHD, greater proficiency, from the non-specialist, is required at confirming normality and identifying pathology.

In the UK, the most practicable method of promoting antenatal detection of CHD is by improving cardiac evaluation during the routine anomaly scan. Previous studies have demonstrated the benefit and relative ease with which more detailed imaging of the heart may be incorporated into routine anomaly scanning (Stumpflen et al. 1996). However, such reports often reflect working practices immediately after the introduction of a training program. As the teaching study from Hunter et al demonstrated, there is a danger that if support from paediatric cardiology is not ongoing then the initial efficacy of training may diminish (Hunter et al. 2000). Telemedicine has the potential to facilitate earlier diagnosis of CHD by offering increased and quicker access to specialist opinion. Telemedicine may also support sonographers' education and training.

Fetal cardiology is predominantly a speciality of medical imaging as physical examination of the fetal cardiovascular system is obviously not possible and fetal catheter and surgical interventions are limited to a handful of centres worldwide. As is well documented, telemedicine lends itself to areas where medical imaging is crucial to diagnosis (Casey, 1999).

It may be suggested that performing fetal tele-echocardiography is much the same as tele-echocardiography in neonates but fetal echocardiography is significantly different from neonatal echocardiography:

1. The fetal heart is smaller and beats faster which may exacerbate motion artefact.
2. The fetus is surrounded by the mother so that ultrasound has to travel through more tissue impacting on image quality.
3. The fetus may move.
4. The fetus may be in a disadvantageous position e.g. back up. Experience of telemedicine in fetal cardiology is still in its infancy. The fetal cardiology telemedicine programs that are currently y active appear to have developed from centres with a major interest in telemedicine and fetal medicine. Whilst an acceptable bandwidth (384 kbps) has been established for neonatal tele-echocardiography. This is not the case with fetal tele-echocardiography. Therefore, research is required in this area.

Evidence for Fetal Telecardiology (Table 53.1)

a. Despite a potential role for telemedicine in fetal cardiology, there are very few studies investigating its potential. Only one study is reported to date that investigates the feasibility and acceptability of performing remote, real-time 2D fetal echocardiography. Sharma et al performed a study in two phases. Phase one was a laboratory study, investigating the effect of bandwidth on image quality and overall adequacy of scan. Sixty-four fetal echocardiograms were performed and randomly assigned to transmission across 128, 384 and 768 kbps and recorded on super VHS videotape for subsequent review. Six studies were excluded due to the presence of CHD. Of the 58 real-time studies interpreted, 15/58 were transmitted across 128 kbps, 21 across 384 kbps and 22 across 768 kbps. The image quality was felt to be significantly poorer at 128 kbps. At 128 kbps, the mean Likert score was 1.1/5 compared with 3.1/5 at 384 kbps ($p < 0.01$) and 3.4/5 at 768 kbps ($p < 0.01$). There was no significant difference in perceived image quality in transmission across 384 kbps compared with 768 kbps (p = 0.08). Similarly, there was no significant difference in the adequacy of studies transmitted across 384 kbps compared with 768 kbps. In this first phase, Sharma et al conclude that 384 kbps is an adequate bandwidth for the identification of normal heart structures.

In the second phase of the study, 34 fetal echocardiograms were successfully transmitted and interpreted in real-time. In four cases (11%), technical problems prevented transmission.

The fetal echocardiogram was performed by a fetal cardiac sonographer or a paediatric cardiology fellow with experience in fetal echocardiography. This was compared with a video recording of the study made at the transmitting site. Mothers were followed up with a face-to-face fetal echocardiogram if a concern was identified on the transmitted fetal echocardiogram. In order to evaluate patient satisfaction, a questionnaire was completed by all 34 expectant mothers and a control group of 195 patients referred from peripheral hospitals to the regional fetal cardiology clinic. There was no significant difference in the completeness of each study between the telefetal echocardiogram and the recorded fetal echocardiogram. CHD was identified correctly in two transmitted fetal echocardiograms with a third case of CHD being suspected but only confirmed on direct fetal echocardiography.

The satisfaction survey results were very positive. In all nine questions, the mean patient satisfaction score indicated high levels of satisfaction with the telemedicine consultation. In eight questions, there was no significant difference in patient satisfaction between the telemedicine and control groups. In addition, only 6% of patients stated that they felt uncomfortable talking to the doctor across the tele-link and only 3% felt it was difficult to ask questions. In this important study, the authors conclude that transmission of fetal echocardiograms across 384 kbps is feasible and adequate for the interpretation of screening fetal echocardiograms. Community acceptance of telemedicine screening and counselling is not adversely affected by a lack of direct personal contact with the specialist. Whilst this study is valuable there are some limitations. The majority of transmitted fetal echocardiograms were not followed up with a face-to-face fetal echocardiogram which is the gold standard. The proportion of fetuses with CHD was small in this cohort. Therefore, the diagnostic accuracy of the telemedicine process was not adequately assessed. The fetal echocardiograms were performed by an operator already skilled in fetal echocardiography. This may falsely enhance the adequacy and quality of the fetal echocardiogram being transmitted. It is suggested that most difficulties in interpreting echocardiograms transmitted via a tele-link are related to image acquisition rather than transmission (Cloutier, 2000). Eleven percent of studies were terminated due to technical difficulties.

A routine clinical service would be significantly limited if 11% of consultations were aborted due to technical difficulties. There are also reports of telemedicine facilitating 3D fetal echocardiography by spatiotemporal image correlation (STIC) and datasets transmitted across an ADSL link. STIC is a relatively new approach for clinical assessment of the fetal heart. It is an easy technique for acquiring data from the fetal heart (a single, automatic volume sweep) and produces a 4D cine sequence (Michailidis et al. 2001). A group from Chile conducted a similar study STIC transmitted across an ADSL connection with bandwidths of 300 and 600 kbps. In total, 50 scans were transmitted from two peripheral hospitals to the regional centre. On average complete fetal echocardiograms could be interpreted in 92% (Vinals et al. 2005). However, these isolated studies have not been followed up in the literature (Fig. 53.15).

In a study conducted in our own department we evaluated fetal echocardiography, performed by sonographers with little training in fetal cardiology, but guided by a fetalcardiologist and transmitted in real-time across ISDN 6. The remote consultation concluded with a video-conference in which the fetal cardiologist explained the diagnosis and answered any questions from the prospective parents. This fetal-telecardiology consultation was compared with the subsequent "face-to-face" fetal cardiology consultation at the regional centre. Sixty-eight fetal tele-echocardiograms were performed and followed up. The diagnostic accuracy was very high (ê – statistic = 0.89, sensitivity = 0.92, specificity = 0.98, ppv = 0.92, npv = 0.98). Sonographers were very positive regarding their involvement in the study and reported significantly improved levels of confidence in performing fetal echocardiography. A significant positive feature of real-time fetal tele-echocardioghraphy is the continued support provided to radiographers performing fetal anomaly scans in DGHs. Patients were very positive about the telemedicine process and were equally satisfied with the remote consultation as the face-to-face consultation. Patients were equally satisfied with each consultation but consistently replied that they would prefer to have the fetal cardiology consultation performed at the local hospital facilitated by a telelink rather by a face-to-face consultation at the regional centre.

Counselling parents during the study it was noted that the received fetal echocardiographic images were of poorer quality following an upgrade in the ultrasound scanner. This did not appear to affect diagnostic accuracy. With the superior imaging, this deterioration in received picture quality was probably due to excess data being transmitted down the 384 kbps connection with resulting package loss and pixellation. This problem would likely be reduced if a larger bandwidth was employed. Extensions to inter-hospital networks make this a realistic option. Alternatively SDSL links (2MBps) can be installed at much cheaper rates than corresponding ISDN bandwidths. The introduction of a remote fetal cardiology service would have attendant costs which are not offset by savings in interhospital transfers. However, the possible establishment of a "one-stop-shop" for "high-risk" pregnancies in which the routine fetal anomaly scan is followed by a remote fetal echocardiogram confidently identifying all relevant cardiac-structures (55% in this cohort) could potentially be cost neutral, relieve pressure on the regional unit and present time and cost savings to the patient. Ultimately, the aim of future work should be aimed towards the establishment of a regional fetal tele-echocardiography service.

Tele-Applications in Cardiology and Radiology in India (Fig. 53.6, Table 53.2)

A country like India , owing to it's vast geographical spread and the enormous population, requires tremendous resources and well-trained medical personnel so as to be able to deliver emergency medical care within a life-saving time frame in every nook and corner of the country. This may not always be possible given the fact that majority of the specialists are concentrated in urban areas with a significant paucity of trained specialists amongst the rural population. In a patient with a cardiac illness, the timing of medical intervention is crucial and dictates the outcome of treatment often proving to be the difference between life and death.

A typical example being the initiation of treatment early in a patient suffering a heart attack (golden hour), which can save life and have an important bearing on the quality of life post event (1) considering the fact that a significant proportion of the *Infant Mortality Rate* of 63.19 per 1,000 births (2) in our country could be attributed to the mortality associated with congenital heart defects, the burden posed by heart disease in the paediatric age group assumes enormous significance.

An estimated 48,000 to 1,28,000 babies are born every year with heart defects in India. This is based on the statistics that there are 16 million live births in India in a year and the incidence of heart disease in newborns is 8–12 per 1,000 live births. Only a bare 5% of these obtain medical attention and surgical care. Nearly 65% will die below 1 year of age and only 15% will survive beyond the age of 5 years. With at least 50,000 new cases of *Rheumatic fever* every year, it is estimated that there are currently more than 1 million patients with rheumatic heart disease in the country, which only adds to the disease burden. To compound these problems, there are less than 15 trained pediatric cardiologists in the country and less than 10 institutions in the country with the requisite infrastructure and manpower to offer surgical correction for neonates and infants with heart defects. There are, also, not more than 10 dedicated pediatric cardiothoracic surgeons.

The mismatch between the medical need and the availability of specialist care in our country is thus clearly evident. As mentioned earlier, this is because there is an estimated 620 million population living in the villages and the availability of specialist doctors there is inadequate. For

Table 53.2: *Potential measurements for heart failure monitoring*

Patient-report data
Signs and symptoms of congestion
Signs: Jugular venous distension, peripheral edema, pulmonary congestion/rales, pleural effusions, S3 gallop
Symptoms: Dyspnea on exertion, orthopnea, paroxysmal nocturnal dyspnea, fatigue, abdominal fullness, anorexia, nausea, vomiting
Daily weight
Sodium intake
Medication adherence/persistence
Laboratory data
• INR
• Natriuretic peptides (BNP and NT-proBNP)
• Other biomarkers
Directly recorded data
• Heart rate
• Blood pressure
• Atrial/ventricular arrhythmias
• Percentage pacing
• Pressure sensor data
• RV outflow
• Left atrial
• Pulmonary artery
• Device parameters
• Battery
• Alerts
• Leads
• Calculated/derived data
• Heart rate variability

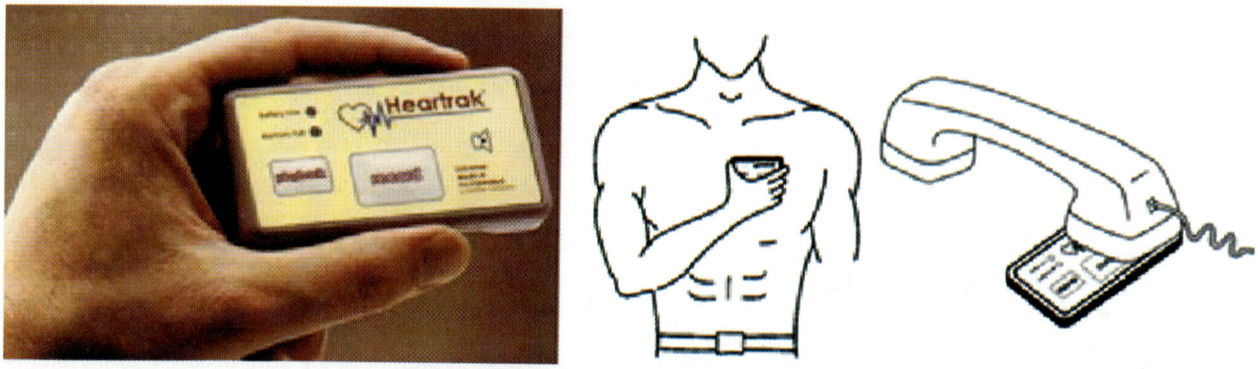

Fig. 53.16: *Left showing heartrak monitor, middle, shows patient placing the same over the heart area for record of ECG and right, shows a telephone through which the recorded information is transmitted*

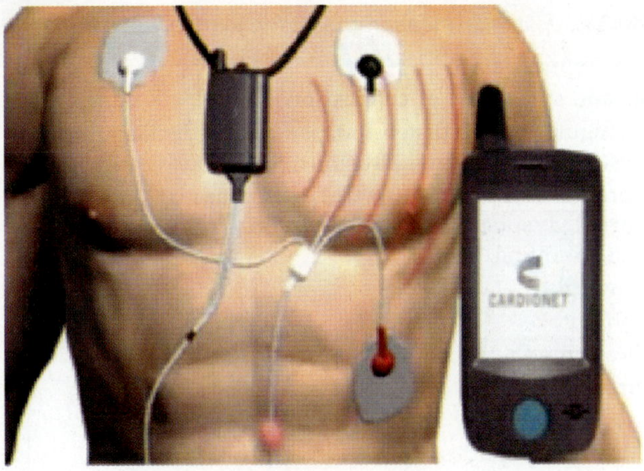

Fig. 53.17: *The sensor sends ECG information about every heart beat to a small portable monitor*

this reason, the rural population is known to be at twice the risk of death when compared to the urban population, for the same illness. Telemedicine can play a tremendous role in bridging the great divide between the patient and the medical specialist, especially in a country like India. By bringing together the patient and the specialist face to face and by its ability to allow the specialist to conduct an examination and view investigations both in report format and in real-time, telemedicine allows a comprehensive medical consultation in the initial stages of the disease presentation without requiring the patient to travel long distances.

Telecardiology in India (Fig. 53.18)

The basic requirement for telecardiac consultation is for a computer with a web camera, a modem and a standard telephone connection at the remote site with ISDN (Integrated Services Digital Network) or broadband capacity.

All aspects of a comprehensive cardiac consultation, such as

- A detailed history of the illness from the patient or the patient's attenders
- Visual general assessment of the patient's clinical status
- Auscultation of the patient's heart and lungs
- Reading the patient's ECG, chest X-ray and echocardiography
- Advising appropriate management including initiation of emergency life-saving treatment can be done to the

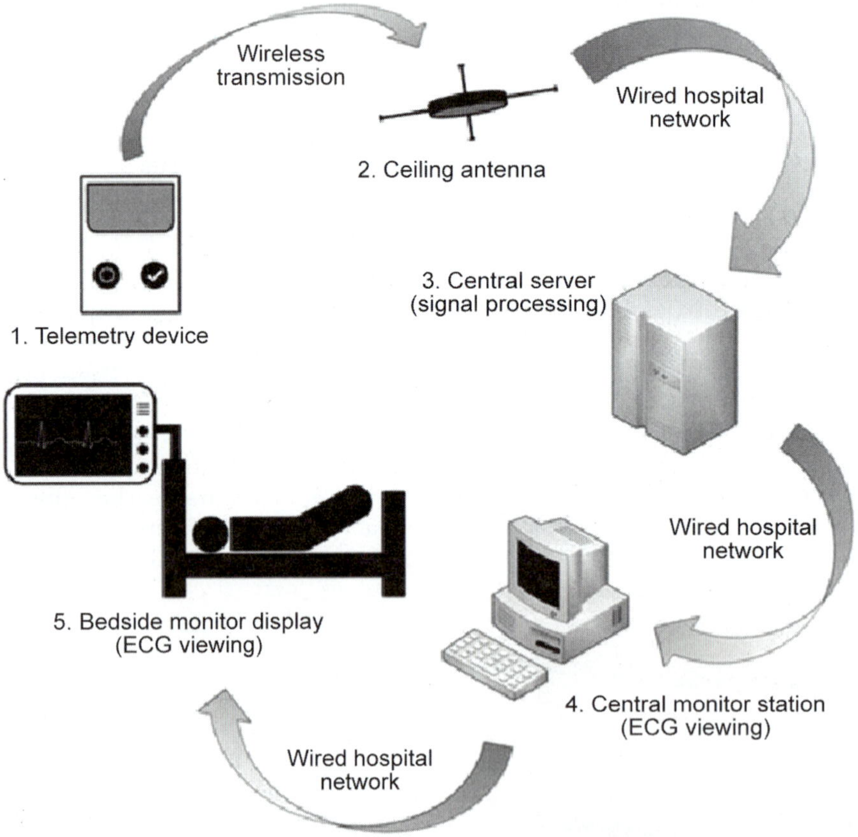

Fig. 53.18: *Illustration of configuration of a typical networked wireless telemetry system. This schematic is for illustrative purposes and does not represent the system of any single manufacturer. The patient's ECG signal is acquired with electrodes and lead wires connected to the telemetry device (1) and transmitted to ceiling antennae (2) via radio frequencies federally allocated to wireless medical telemetry services. The ECG is then transmitted directly over computer cables that link the ceiling antennae, central server (3), and central monitor station (4). The bedside monitor display typically receives the data from the central server or monitor station via a wired hospital network. There may be significant delays of up to several seconds from the time that a heart rhythm is experienced by the patient (step 1) to the time that the rhythm is displayed on the bedside monitor (step 5)*

satisfaction of the clinician and the patient through teleconferencing.

Auscultatory findings play a crucial part in diagnosing cardiac ailments, especially in those with congenital heart disease. Recent technological aids such as electronic stethoscope makes it possible for the clinician to hear the patients' heart sounds for himself across many miles and come to an accurate clinical diagnosis. This eliminates the risk of error associated with having to rely on the attending persons clinical auscultation. Even a narrow bandwidth (analog) telephonic stethoscope has been proven to be effective in distinguishing accurately between an innocent and a pathological murmur. The clinical diagnosis, thus arrived at, can then be confirmed by reviewing investigations such as electrocardiogram (ECG), chest X-ray, echocardiogram, treadmill test, angiocardiography, cardiac CT scan, cardiac MRI scan, ambulatory ECG monitoring, pacemaker evaluation, and relevant blood tests. Most of these test results are reviewed using a ***store and forward*** technique from the remote site, where the tests are initially performed, captured and stored in the computer which is then forwarded as still frames to the specialist for review. Transtelephonic ECG provides the means of transmitting an electrocardiogram recorded in a patient with rhythm disorders or a myocardial infarction, enabling immediate initiation of treatment. Having connectivity between an ultrasound (echocardiography) equipment and the computer, enables the transmission of streaming video pictures of the heart scan in real time to the specialist. This is particularly useful in situations where a child is brought in with a complex cardiac lesion. The primary doctor or technician may not be skilled to perform a detailed scan of the heart of the child and interpret them accurately, and in such cases the specialist is required to view the test ***live*** to be able to make an accurate diagnosis. Telemedicine can be effectively used to transmit fetal echocardiography images as identifying fetal cardiac anomalies early on in gestation prepares the parents and the attending doctor towards care immediate post-partum thus greatly enhancing the outcome of management for that baby. As not many are trained to identify cardiac anomalies in early pregnancy, a technician could be directed by the clinical specialist at the referral center to show the required views to enable a diagnosis of fetal cardiac problem.

Chest X-ray and Echocardiography as Transmitted by Internet (Fig. 53.6)

The practice of diagnosing complex congenital heart defects by transmission over an ISDN line is well established. However, in our experience, it was found that broadband or VSAT connectivity was superior to ISDN connectivity in that it enhanced the quality of the transmitted images as well as ensured an uninterrupted transmission, especially when transmitting streaming images such as online echocardiography. This is crucial for ensuring accuracy of the diagnosis, particularly in the case of a complex congenital cardiac anomaly. There are previous studies corroborating the accuracy of a diagnosis by telemedicine as compared to one by personal clinical examination.

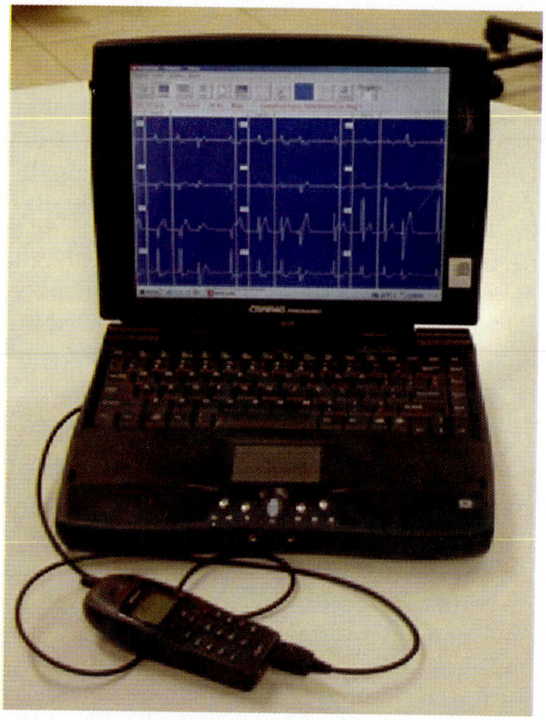

Fig. 53.19: *Remote computer connected to a mobile phone of the digital tele-ECG system. The PC anywhere 32 is the telecommunication software, which is installed in the host and the remote computers, a system that allows data transmission via phone for remote analysis*

Specialist Viewing Transmitted Live Echocardiography from a Remote Centre

In acute cardiac events, telecardiology provides the means by which the specialist is able to guide the primary doctor or the paramedical personnel at the scene to undertake measures which would help save the life of the cardiac patient based on the history provided, and the investigation findings. An extremely important aspect of telecardiology is that it achieves shared care of the patient by the primary physician and the specialist and also in the process entrains the primary physician in the ways of specialist management for the specific condition. Telemedicine can also be effectively utilized to propagate the knowledge of the specialist to primary care physicians and the public through teleconferencing continuing medical education (CME) programs.

Applications in Radiology

Images in radiology are predominantly plain X-ray pictures, ultrasound scan images and images of CT scans, MRI scans, cine angiography, etc. These images can be digitally scanned and stored in an archival server in DICOM (digital imaging and communications in medicine) format even if they are previously in non-DICOM format. Subsequently, the images can be stored in the web server in either compressed or noncompressed form and be available for acquisition either within the institution through internet or worldwide through internet. It is important to adhere to the DICOM-ACR-NEMA-3 standard for storing images and also important not to alter or edit the image during acquisition. Telemedicine plays a crucial role of networking whereby technicians in rural settings can acquire radiological images and transmit to a central hub where it can be reported on by a qualified radiologist and the report sent back to the primary physician in the rural center within a matter of minutes. Complicated imaging procedures or ultrasound-guided procedures can be undertaken confidently in remote settings while being guided by a specialist from elsewhere be it within the country or from abroad.

Specifications for Setting Up a Telemedicine Unit

The World Health Organization defines telemedicine as "The delivery of health care services, where distance is a critical factor, by all healthcare professionals using information and communication technologies for the exchange of valid information for diagnosis, treatment and prevention of disease and injuries, research and evaluation, and for the continuing education of healthcare providers, all in the interests of advancing the health of individuals and their communities".

Required Infrastructure

An **air-conditioned, sound-proof room** with electrical outlets for connecting various equipments and a very good earthing pit.

Recommendation

Five 15 amps Sockets for UPS, five 5 amps socket for other diagnostic equipments, UPS of atleast 3 KVA capacity.

Curtains/walls preferably light blue or gray in colour to give good contrast for video conferencing.

Video Conferencing Hardware (Fig. 53.1, 53.2 and 53.7)

A **television** preferably with 29" screen. Alternatively, if Tele CMEs (Continuing Medical Education) are planned a LCD projection on to a big screen.

A video conferencing system—these can be:

1. Stand-alone code based system **(recommended)**
2. PC based using PC add-on card codec
3. PC based with in-camera codec
4. PC based web camera and software only codec.

IT Hardware

A computer with printer and a scanner (capable of scanning X-ray films also or alternatively a X-ray digitizer).

Data such as images and video pictures that are NOT in digital format require to be converted to digital format for transmission. This is done using **"codec"** units. (short for coder/decoder).

Compression softwares help transmit large files in shorter time. Digital Imaging and Communications in Medicine (DICOM) compression is the recommended standard for transmitting medical images.

Connectivity Hardware

It can be either terrestrial or satellite based.

- Terrestrial communication can be through analog modems, DSL modems, ISDN and broadband.
- Satellite communication is usually through Very Small Aperture Terminals (VSATs). It provides much better image transfer quality than terrestrial mode of communication as well as instantaneous global coverage.

Medical Hardware

Various instrumentation that can be connected to the video-conferencing unit to directly relay data from the patient are: Digital 12 lead ECG, electronic stethescope, digital microscope, digital blood pressure monitor, skin camera, doppler ultrasound and echocardiography equipment, etc. Stored images such as X-rays, ultrasound images, CT/MRI images or pathology slide images can be scanned into a computer and transmitted. Moving video images of echocardiography can be transmitted by connecting the video player/DVD player to the video-conferencing system (Figs 53.1–53.5, 53.7–53.12, 53.16–53.17).

Recommendations in Telemedicine

Accessibility to telemedicine centers can be enhanced if such models as the one in this study are developed on a larger scale networking the entire length and breadth of the country. This could be done with government and private sector partnership nurturing the way to establishment of a platform for dispensing uniform healthcare to one and all in the country despite the geographical restrictions.

Risk vs Benefit in Telecardiology

The earlier diagnosis and initiation of appropriate treatment that can be achieved using telemedicine links should reduce morbidity and mortality but as yet there are no published controlled trials measuring this benefit. A further significant benefit is that unnecessary transfers are avoided. In our series of 63 cases, the need for transfer to obtain a diagnosis was avoided in 47. There are therefore potentially significant financial savings for the referring hospital.

For the paediatric cardiologist the concern about participating in diagnosis by telemedicine is that a serious lesion may be missed and false reassurance given. The medicolegal aspects of patient responsibility after remote consultation in this way are still unclear. In our series of 61 transmitted studies using ISDN2, there were four errors in diagnosis: three small ventricular septal defects and one moderate pulmonary valvar stenosis were not detected. Twenty eight major lesions were accurately diagnosed. In the series reported by Finlay et al, patients in whom a diagnosis was made by using their telemedicine link had follow-up echocardiography by "paediatric cardiology echocardiography staff".

No significant diagnostic discrepancies were found. Sobczyk et al reported their experience of remote diagnosis in 47 patients from prerecorded images transmitted transtelephonically studies were normal. Lesions accurately diagnosed included persistent ductus arteriosus (PDA) (n = 8), ventricular septal defect (n = 6), and ventricular septal defect with interrupted aortic arch (n = 1). They reported an inappropriate clinical decision causing delay in transfer of a patient with a PDA requiring ligation due to an inconclusive transmitted study.

The available evidence thus suggests that remote echocardiography can be used to diagnose or exclude major lesions with accuracy. The diagnosis made on the transmitted scan should not, however, be considered the definitive cardiac consultation. This is not an issue for patients transferred to the regional centre on the basis of the remote consultation as they will all have a "hands on" consultation and echocardiography. I would advocate that babies considered to be normal or to have minor lesions on the transmitted scan should also electively have a follow-up direct consultation by a paediatric cardiologist.

Conclusion

It is likely that with further improvements in, and increasing availability of the equipment necessary to transmit good quality echocardiographic images, an increasing number of telemedicine links will be established from neonatal units to paediatric cardiology centres. It is not appropriate or necessary to apply this technology to the assessment of the child where an urgent clinical decision does not need to be made such as the evaluation of a murmur. Telemedicine links should be used to diagnose or exclude significant neonatal CHD and that over the next few years paediatric cardiologists will find that providing remote diagnosis in this way could become an increasingly important part of their workload.

BIBLIOGRAPHY

1. Boersma E, Maas AC, Deckers JW, Simoons ML. Early thrombolytic treatment in acute myocardial infarction: reappraisal of the golden hour. Lancet 1996 Nov 9;348(9037): 1312–3.
2. The world fact book 2001, CIA publication, Office of public affairs.
3. Belmont JM, Mattioli LF. Accuracy of analog telephonic stethoscopy for paediatric telecardiology. Pediatrics. 2003 Oct;112(4):780–6.
4. Fisher JB, Alboliras ET, Berdusis K, Webb CL: Rapid identification of serious congenital heart disease using real-time transtelephonic transmission of echocardiograms. Am Heart J 1996;131(6):1225–27.
5. Randolph GR, Hagler DJ, Khandheria BK, Lunn ER, Cook WJ, Seward JB, O'Leary PW: Remote telemedical interpretation of neonatal echocardiograms: Impact on clinical management in a primary care setting. J Amer Coll Cardiol 1999;34(1):241–245.
6. Stevenson JG. Evolution of echocardiography in neonatal diagnosis. Acta Paediatr Suppl. 1995;410:8–14.
7. Du ZD, Roguin N, Barak M. Clinical and echocardiographic evaluation of neonates with heart murmurs. Acta Paediatr. 1997;86:752–756.
8. Hurwitz RA, Caldwell RL. Should pediatric echocardiograms be performed in adult laboratories? Pediatrics. 1998;102(2).
9. Afset JE, Lunde P, Rasmussen K. Accuracy of routine echocardiographic measurements made by an inexperienced examiner through teleinstruction. J Telemed Telecare. 1996;2:148–154.
10. Casey F, Brown D, Corrigan N, et al. Value of a low-cost telemedicine link in the remote echocardiographic diagnosis of congenital heart defects. J Telemed Telecare. 1998;4(suppl 1):46–48.
11. Casey F, Brown D, Craig BG, Rogers J, Mulholland HC. Diagnosis of neonatal congenital heart defects by remote consultation using a lowcost telemedicine link. J Telemed Telecare. 1996;2:165–169.
12. Finley JP, Sharratt GP, Nanton MA, et al. Pediatric echocardiography by telemedicine—nine years' experience. J Telemed Telecare. 1997;3:200–204.
13. Fisher JB, Alboliras ET, Berdusis K, Webb CL. Rapid identification of congenital heart disease by transmission of echocardiograms. Am Heart J. 1996;131:1225–1227.
14. Hassol A, Irvin C, Gaumer G, Puskin D, Mintzer C, Grigsby J. Rural applications of telemedicine. Telemed J. 1997;3:215–225.
15. Randolph GR, Hagler DJ, Khandheria BK, et al. Remote telemedical interpretation of neonatal echocardiograms: impact on clinical management in a primary care setting. J Am Coll Cardiol. 1999;34:241–245.
16. Sable C, Roca T, Gold J, Gutierrez A, Gulotta E, Culpepper W. Live transmission of neonatal echocardiograms from underserved areas: accuracy, patient care, and cost. Telemed J. 1999;5:339–347.
17. Sobczyk WS, Solinger RE, Rees AH, Elbl F. Transtelephonic echocardiography: successful use in a tertiary pediatric referral center. J Pediatr. 1993;122:S84–S88.
18. Colton T. Statistics in Medicine. Boston, MA: Little, Brown and Company; 1974:237–250.
19. Finley JP, Human DG, Nanton MA, et al. Echocardiography by telephone—evaluation of pediatric disease at a distance. Am J Cardiol. 1989;63:1475–1477.
20. Trippi JA, Kopp G, Lee KS, et al. The feasibility of dobutamine stress echocardiography in the emergency department with telemedicine interpretation. J Am Soc Echocardiogr. 1996;9:113–118.
21. Trippi JA, Lee KS, Kopp G, Nelson D, Kovacs R. Emergency echocardiography telemedicine: an efficient method to provide 24-hour consultative echocardiography. J Am Coll Cardiol. 1996;27:1748–1752.
22. Trippi JA, Lee KS, Kopp G, Nelson DR, Yee KG, Cordell WH. Dobutamine stress tele-echocardiography for evaluation of emergency department patients with chest pain. J Am Coll Cardiol. 1997;30:627–632.
23. Houston A, McLeod K, Richens T, et al. Assessment of the quality of neonatal echocardiographic images transmitted by ISDN telephone lines. Heart. 1999;82:222–225.
24. Rendina MC, Downs SM, Carasco N, Loonsk J, Bose CL. Effect of telemedicine on health outcomes in 87 infants requiring neonatal intensive care. Telemed J. 1998;4:345–351.
25. Rendina MC, Long WA, deBliek R. Effect size and experimental power analysis in a pediatric cardiology telemedicine system. J Telemed Telecare. 1997;3(suppl 1):56–57.
26. Sable C. Telecardiology: potential impact on acute care. Crit Care Med. 2001;29:N159–N165.

27. Scholz TD, Kienzle MG. Optimizing utilization of pediatric echocardiography and implications for telemedicine. Am J Cardiol. 1999;83: 1645–1648.
28. Thomas JD, Main ML. Digital echocardiographic laboratory: where do we stand? J Am Soc Echocardiogr. 1998;11:978–983.
29. Egan EA, Eitzman DV. Umbilical vessel catheterization. Am J Dis Child. 1971;121:213–218.
30. Ades A, Sable C, Cummings, Martin G. Echocardiographic assessmentof umbilical venous catheter placement. Pediatr Res. 2000;47:383A.
31. Dunn PM. Localization of the umbilical catheter by post-mortem measurement. Arch Dis Child. 1966;41:69–7527. Burdussis K. Tele-echocardiography and telecardiology. Telemed Today. 1999;7:25–26, 35–36.
32. Jenkins KJ, Newburger JW, Lock JE, Davis RB, Coffman GA, Iezzoni LI. In-hospital mortality for surgical repair of congenital heart defects: preliminary observations of variation by hospital caseload. Pediatrics. 1995;95:323–330.
33. Millman DS, Kiesel AB. Telecardiology: legal issues and new developments. Telemed Today. 1999;7:27–29.
34. States where Medicaid reimbursement of services utilizing telemedicine is available, June 27, 2000, Health Care Financing Administration.

54 Newer Innovations in the Field of Cardiology

NEWER INNOVATIONS IN CARDIAC PACING

The world's first leadless pacemaker, by Indian-origin scientist. The world's first leadless pacemaker, developed by an Indian-origin scientist Vivek Reddy, has shown promising results after 1 year of human trials on 32 patients who received the pacemaker.

"This is the first time we have seen 1 year follow-up data for this innovative, wireless cardiac pacing technology. Our results show the leadless pacemaker is comparable to traditional pacemakers", said Reddy, director of arrhythmia services at the Mount Sinai Hospital here.

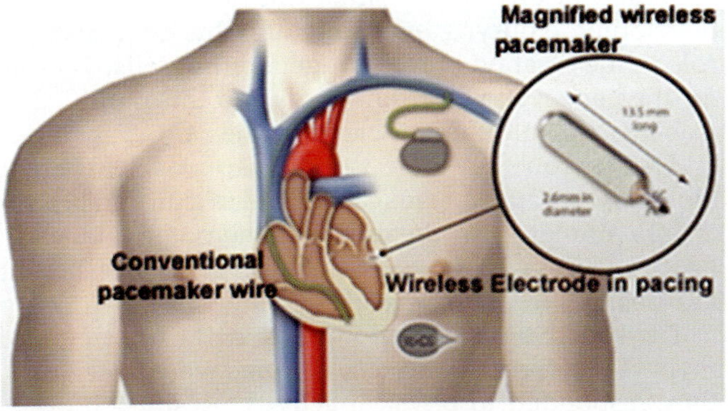

Fig. 54.1: *Leadless pacemaker. EBR systems, a start-up out of Sunnyvale California, and Cambridge Consultants, the technology design and development firm, have developed a leadless pacemaker system for patients with advanced heart failure. The wireless cardiac stimulation system (WiCS) comprises two units, an implantable electrode and an external control unit. The electrode incorporates an ultrasonic, wireless receiver and delivers an electrical stimulus to the heart based on triggering signals from the external control unit. In its current iteration the WiCS system is designed to work with conventional pacemakers/ defibrillators pacing the right ventricle of patients requiring biventricular pacing. The WiCS external control unit senses the pacing stimulus delivered to the right ventricle and initiates a burst of stimulus from the electrode implanted in the left ventricle. According to the company, the wireless left ventricular pacing approach removes the need for complex surgery and the complications often associated with the coronary sinus leads used to pace the left ventricle*

The findings further support the promising performance and safety of this minimally-invasive, nonsurgical pacing device.

The leads-free pacemaker is implanted by a cardiac electrophysiologist directly inside the heart during a catheter-guided procedure through the groin via the femoral artery. The device, resembling a small, metal silver tube, is only a few centimeters in length, making it less than 10% the size of a traditional pacemaker.

The follow-up study evaluated 32 patients with a slowed heartbeat (bradycardia) who successfully received St. Jude Medical's "Nanostim" leadless pacemaker at two hospitals in Prague and one in Amsterdam. "There was no experience of infections or failure to sense, pace or communicate with the pacemaker", Reddy noted. The leadless cardiac pacemaker is placed directly inside a patient's heart without surgery during a catheter-guided procedure through the groin via the femoral vein.

The device, resembling a tiny, silver tube and smaller than a triple-A battery, is only a few centimetres in length, making it less than 10% the size of a traditional pacemaker.

It works by closely monitoring the heart's electrical rhythms and if the heart beat is too slow it provides electrical stimulation therapy to regulate it.

"More long-term follow-up of these 'leadless' study patients will further our understanding of the potential advantages, benefits, and complication risks of leadless pacemaker technology, along with additional ongoing, larger trials," Reddy said.

More than 4 million patients globally have a pacemaker, and 700,000 new patients receive one each year. Reddy presented the 1 year "leadless" study data findings at "Heart Rhythm 2014," the Heart Rhythm Society's 35th annual scientific sessions in San Francisco city in the US May 9.

Biological Pacemaker Created with Gene Therapy

What is a biological pacemaker?

The sinoatrial node is the primary biological pacemaker in the heart and a potential template for any biological pacemaker to be fabricated. All channels and transporters necessary to generate the heartbeat in mammals are present in the sinoatrial node myocyte membrane and in other pacemaker tissues of the conducting system and myocardium. The sinoatrial node has the following characteristics:

1. It is a specialized tissue well-integrated electrically and structurally into the cardiac substrate, whose pacemaker current is optimally suited to initiate the cardiac impulse.
2. Its operation is determined by interactions among ion channels and pumps to initiate phase 4 depolarization and carry membrane potential towards the threshold voltage at which action potentials are elicited.
3. It initiates an impulse whose rhythm tends to be regular while the rate varies in nearly instantaneous response to the physiological and emotional demands of the body. The modulatory checks and balances on rate and rhythm are largely the province of the sympathetic (excitatory) and parasympathetic (inhibitory) nervous systems.

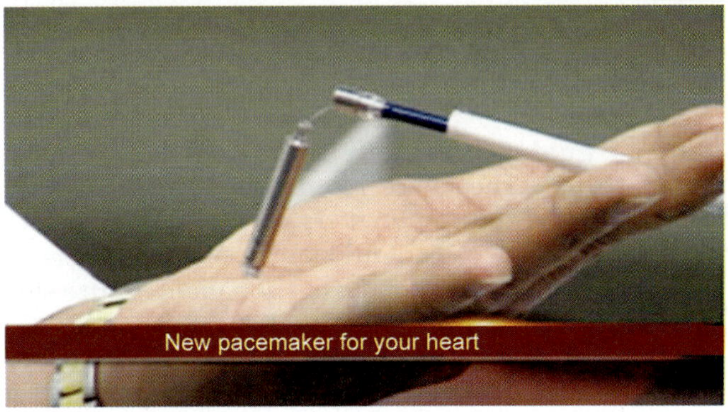

Fig. 54.2: *Tiny leadless pacemaker less than 10% the size of a traditional pacemaker*

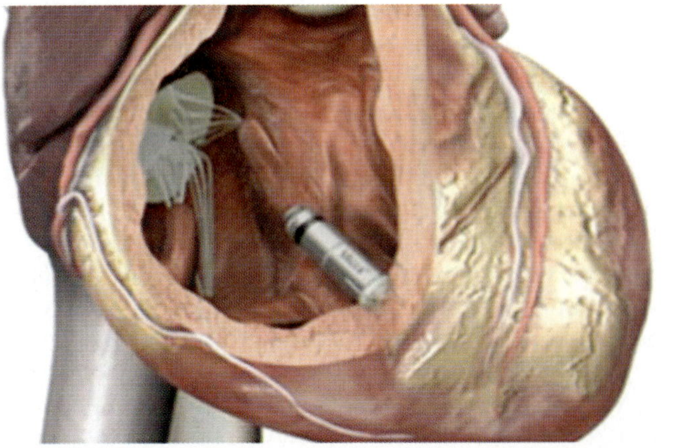

Fig. 54.3: *Leadless pacemake implanted by Dr Vivek Reddy, MD, launches international leadless II clinical research trial testing a miniature-sized, leadless pacemaker placed inside the heart without surgery*

4. The propagation of its impulse maximizes efficiency of cardiac contraction and output.

A biological pacemaker was created in the hearts of pigs using gene therapy. Specifically, heart cells called cardiomyocytes were converted into pacemaker cells that could be used to control the rate of heartbeats. If this research effort achieves its goal, it could mean that humans who need pacemakers would not need to have a mechanical device implanted but would only need to have cells in their heart transformed to provide the electrical pulses needed to make the heart pump.

In a normal, healthy heart, cells signal the heart muscle to contract and pump the blood throughout the circulatory system. In an unhealthy heart, this function can be slowed or the heartbeats can become irregular. A mechanical pacemaker is then sometimes implanted to make the heartbeats regular. A conventional mechanical pacemaker must be implanted under the skin with surgery. It controls the rate of heartbeats by emitting electrical pulses to the muscles of the heart. Infection, however, is often a complication with conventional pacemakers.

Gene therapy is a procedure where genes (or segments of DNA) are inserted into a cell and the cell then takes up the gene and incorporates it into its own genome. Any cells that are reproduced from the original cell will contain the inserted gene as well. *The gene that was transferred into the cardiomyocyte cells was TBX18, which stands for embryonic transcription factor T-box 18.* The TBX18 gene is known to play a role in heart development. The gene TBX18 is activated briefly in the sinoatrial node of the hearts of developing embryos, and therefore, this gene may play a role in the creation of rhythm-generating cells. The carrier for the gene was a modified virus and this modified virus was injected into the muscle of the heart.

The reason this gene therapy approach to create a biological pacemaker was carried out in a pig is a pig's heart is very similar to a human heart. The potential use of pig hearts in human heart transplants has been a consideration in research efforts for a while.

During the research experiment, after the cardiomyocytes were transformed, the pigs were tested on how they responded to physical activity. Results showed the heart rates increased when the pigs exercised and slowed when the pigs rested, which confirmed the biological pacemaker was working.

The creation of a biological pacemaker will circumvent the problems of conventional, mechanical pacemakers. It is unknown, however, what potential complications there might be with biological pacemakers in which cells are "reprogrammed" with gene therapy. Since this procedure involves the insertion of a foreign virus into cells, the immune system may respond and try to destroy the cells. This would mean the biological pacemaker would be short-lived.

Eugenio Cingolani, MD, the director of the Institute's Cardiogenetics-Familial Arrhythmia Clinic who worked with Dr Marbán on the biological pacemaker research team, said that in the future pacemaker cells also could help infants born with congenital heart block.

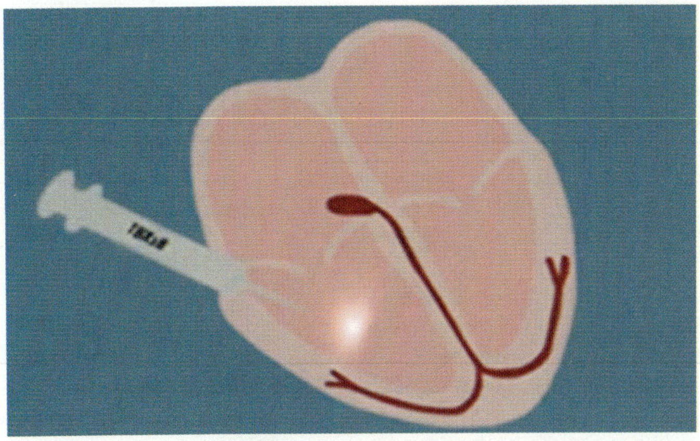

Fig. 54.4: *Gene therapy is a procedure where genes (or segments of DNA) are inserted into a cell and the cell then takes up the gene and incorporates it into its own genome*

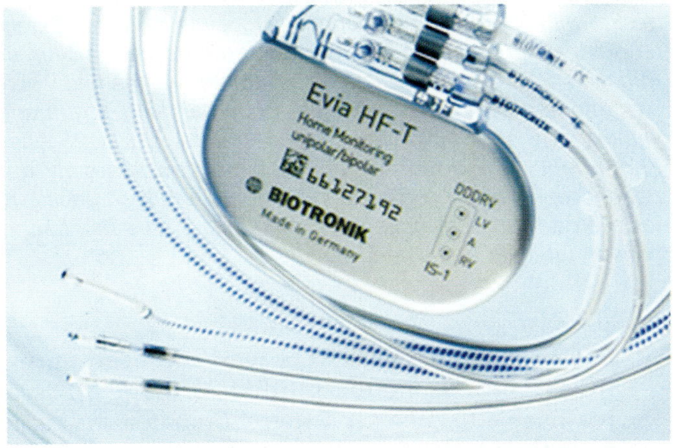

Fig. 54.5: *BIOTRONIK's Evia HF-T, world´s first MR conditional CRT-P system. Main features of this device are "world´s first MR conditional CRT-P system." Wide choice of MR conditional leads for RA, RV and LV application with excellent; handling and optimal electrical performance. "Capture control (RA, RV and LV) and 6 multiselect LV pacing polarities as part of a range of solutions for continuous, effective biventricular pacing without complications." Closed loop stimulation (CLS) to optimize individual rate regulation for patient with chronotropic incompetence (CI). CI is a common comorbidity present in 70% of the advanced HF patients 1. CLS is the most physiological rate adapting system and is the only sensor to react on both physical and mental stress. "Timely intervention using BIOTRONIK Home Monitoring. The results of the COMPAS study show a median gain of 122 days for medical intervention through early detection of clinically relevant events in pacemaker patients 2." Clinical trend data with Heart Failure Monitor offer a daily updated view on the patients HF status and the effectiveness of the CRT therapy*

"Babies still in the womb cannot have a pacemaker, but we hope to work with fetal medicine specialists to create a life-saving catheter-based treatment for infants diagnosed with congenital heart block", noted Dr Cingolani. "It is possible that one day we might be able to save lives by replacing hardware with an injection of genes."

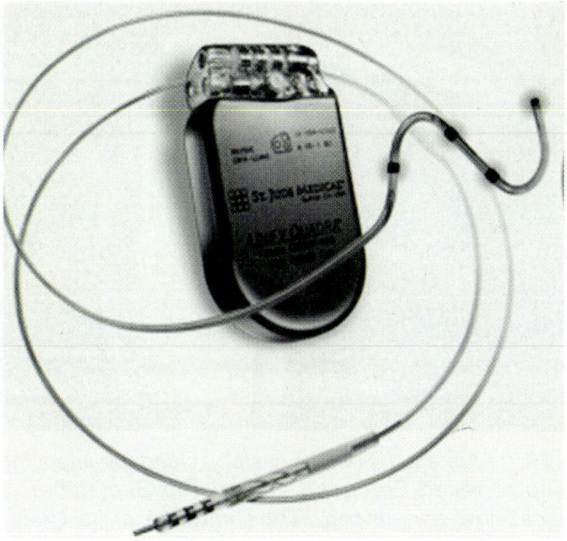

Fig. 54.6: *The energencardiac resynchronization therapy defibrillator (CRT-D) and implantable cardioverter defibrillator (ICD) is used to treat heart failure and sudden cardiac death. The system is designed to simplify and reduce the time needed for the implant procedure by combining three separate lead terminals into one integrated connector and reducing the number of connections and set screws needed in the device header. In addition, some patients will receive a remote monitoring system where an at-home communicator will allow physicians to monitor the patient's device, as well as vital signs such as blood pressure and weight, in order to better*

2014 AHA/ACC Guideline for the Management of Patients With Non-ST-Elevation Acute Coronary Syndromes: A Report of the American College of Cardiology/American Heart Association Task Force on Practice Guidelines

The following are 10 points to remember about this guideline from the American College of Cardiology/ American Heart Association on the management of patients with non-ST-elevation acute coronary syndromes (NSTE-ACS):

1. Patients with suspected ACS should be risk stratified based on the likelihood of ACS and adverse outcome(s) to decide on the need for hospitalization and assist in the selection of treatment options.
2. In patients with chest pain or other symptoms suggestive of ACS, a 12-lead electrocardiogram (ECG) should be performed and evaluated for ischemic changes within 10 minutes of the patient's arrival at an emergency facility.
3. Cardiac-specific troponin (troponin I or T with a contemporary assay) levels should be measured at presentation and 3–6 hours after symptom onset in all patients who present with symptoms consistent with ACS to identify a rising and/or falling pattern.
4. Oral beta-blocker therapy should be initiated within the first 24 hours in patients who do not have any of the following: (1) signs of heart failure, (2) evidence of low-output state, (3) increased risk for cardiogenic

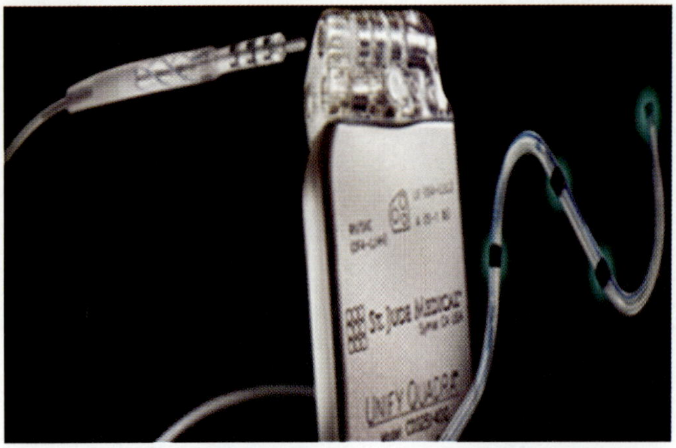

Fig. 54.7: *Quadripolar pacing system. Quadripolar pacing system having received European approval in September, St. Jude Medical now announced FDA clearance of its Unify Quadra cardiac resynchronization therapy defibrillator (CRT-D) and the matching quartet left ventricular quadripolar pacing lead. The lead features four electrodes and the CRT-D is able to take advantage of them by providing up to ten different pacing configurations. Because the electrodes cover a greater area, precise placement of the lead is less critical as adjustments of the electrical signal can be made via software. Like many other implantable devices from St. Jude, the Unify Quadra can wirelessly interface with the Merlin.net system for reporting both on the health of the patient and the status of the device. The quartet lead - used as part of the Unify Quadra system-features four electrodes spaced over 4.7 centimeters, enabling up to 10 pacing configurations. Multiple pacing configurations allow the physician to implant the lead in the most stable position without making trade-offs in electrical performance. This includes pacing closer to the base of the left ventricle, which recent studies associate with better patient outcomes and which may be more difficult with traditional bipolar leads. The quadripolar pacing electrodes also provide physicians more options to optimize CRT performance, such as pacing around scar tissue in the heart and avoiding the most common pacing complications. The many benefits conferred from the quartet lead's unconventional pacing have been demonstrated by implanters around the world and reported in a number of published studies*

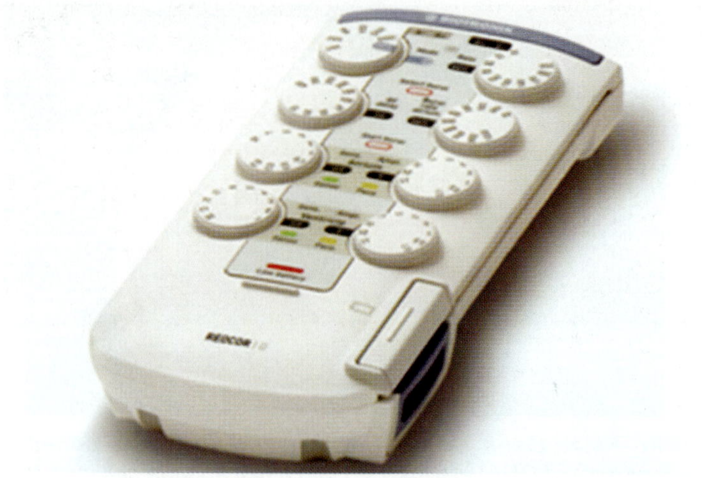

Fig. 54.8: *BIOTRONIK's reocor external pacemaker. Biotronik's reocor external pacemaker, that is available in two models for dual- and single-chamber pacing. "Reocor combines intuitive design with unprecedented longevity for simplified use. Extended longevity increases reliability and reduces costs over time" Function dials display selectable parameter values and visualize programmed settings at a glance. Easy handling is guaranteed without any specific training requirements. Up to 25 days of permanent pacing therapy and backup power supply during battery replacement. High pacing outputs and high pacing rates for a broad range of patients. Continuous status monitoring for patient safety at any time*

shock, or (4) other contraindications to beta-blockade (e.g. PR interval >0.24 second, second- or third-degree heart block without a cardiac pacemaker, active asthma, or reactive airway disease).

5. High-intensity statin therapy should be initiated or continued in all patients with NSTE-ACS and no contraindications to its use.
6. A P2Y12 inhibitor (either clopidogrel or ticagrelor) in addition to aspirin should be administered for up to 12 months to all patients with NSTE-ACS without contraindications who are treated with either an early invasive or ischemia-guided strategy. P2Y12 inhibitor therapy (clopidogrel, prasugrel or ticagrelor) continued for at least 12 months is indicated in postpercutaneous coronary intervention (PCI) patients treated with coronary stents. It is reasonable to use ticagrelor in preference to clopidogrel for P2Y12 treatment in patients with NSTE-ACS who undergo an early invasive or ischemia-guided strategy. It is also reasonable to choose prasugrel (initiated during PCI) over clopidogrel for P2Y12 treatment in patients with NSTE-ACS who undergo PCI whoare not at high risk of bleeding complications.
7. In patients with NSTE-ACS, anticoagulation, in addition to antiplatelet therapy, is recommended for all patients irrespective of initial treatment strategy. In patients with NSTE-ACS, anticoagulant therapy should be discontinued after PCI unless there is a compelling reason to continue such therapy.
8. An urgent/immediate invasive strategy (diagnostic angiography with intent to perform revascularization if appropriate based on coronary anatomy) is indicated in patients with NSTE-ACS who have refractory angina or hemodynamic or electrical instability (without serious comorbidities or contraindications to such procedures). An early invasive strategy (diagnostic angiography with intent to perform revascularization if appropriate based on coronary anatomy) is indicated in initially stabilized patients with NSTE-ACS (without serious comorbidities or contraindications to such procedures) who have an elevated risk for clinical events. An early invasive strategy (i.e. diagnostic angiography with intent to perform revascularization) is not recommended in patients with extensive comorbidities (e.g. hepatic, renal, pulmonary failure, cancer), in whom the risks of revascularization and

comorbid conditions are likely to outweigh the benefits of revascularization and those with acute chest pain and a low likelihood of ACS who are troponin-negative, especially women.

9. All eligible patients with NSTE-ACS should be referred to a comprehensive cardiovascular rehabilitation program either before hospital discharge or during the first outpatient visit.
10. An evidence-based plan of care (e.g. guideline-directed medical treatment) that promotes medication adherence, timely follow-up with the healthcare team, appropriate dietary and physical activities, and compliance with interventions for secondary prevention should be provided to patients with NSTE-ACS. In addition to detailed instructions for daily exercise, patients should be given specific instruction on activities (e.g. lifting, climbing stairs, yard work, and household activities) that are permissible and those to avoid. Specific mention should be made of resumption of driving, return to work, and sexual activity.

Optical Coherence Tomography

Optical coherence tomography (OCT) is a high-resolution imaging technique that offers microscopic visualization of coronary plaques. The clear and detailed images of OCT generate an intense interest in adopting this technique for both clinical and research purposes. Recent studies have shown that OCT is useful for the assessment of coronary atherosclerotic plaques, in particular the assessment of plaque rupture, erosion, and intracoronary thrombus in patients with acute coronary syndrome. In addition, OCT may enable identifying thin-cap fibroatheroma, the proliferation of vasa vasorum, and the distribution of macrophages surrounding vulnerable plaques. With its ability to view atherosclerotic lesions in vivo with such high resolution, OCT provides cardiologists with the tool they need to better understand the thrombosis-prone vulnerable plaques and acute coronary syndromes.

Future Perspectives of OCT

Recently, a second-generation OCT technology, named frequency-domain OCT, has been developed. This new technology will solve the current time-domain OCT limitations by imaging at much higher frame rates with slightly deeper penetration depth and greater scan area. In combination with a short, nonocclusive flush and rapid spiral pullback, the higher frame rates generated by frequency-domain OCT enable imaging of the three dimensional microstructure of longer segments of coronary arteries. In addition, frequency-domain OCT facilitates the acquisition of spectroscopic and polarization data for tissue characterization. The development of frequency-domain

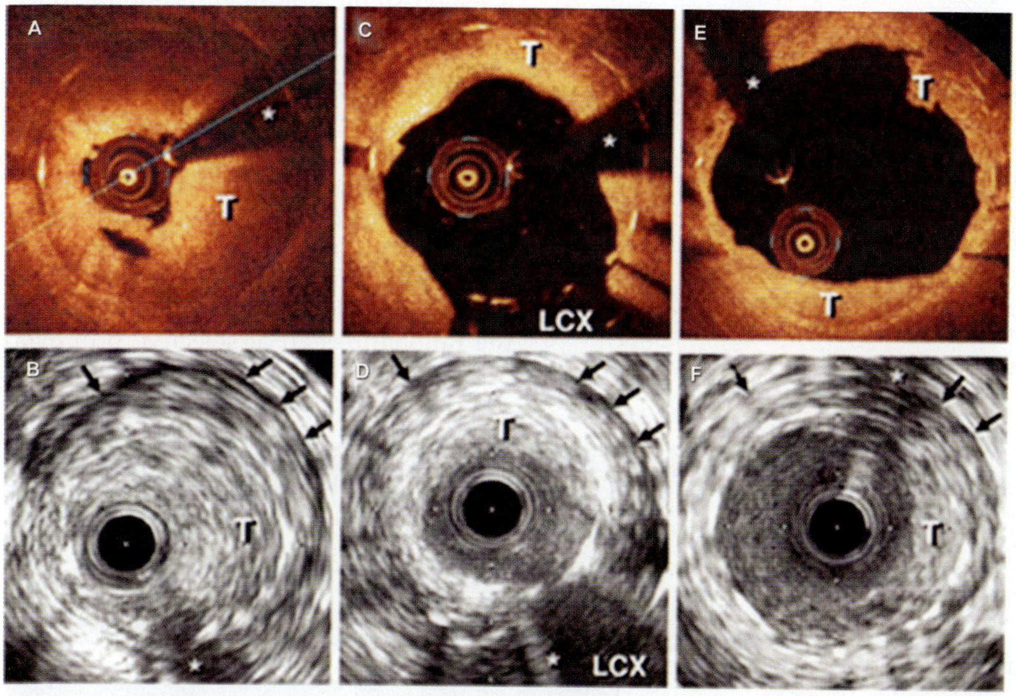

Fig. 54.9: *OCT (top) and IVUS (bottom) findings at the time of LST. (A) An obstructive thrombus (T) is visualized by OCT in the midsegment of the stent. Notice a tiny residual lumen and significant shadowing of the stent struts (mainly from 10 to 6 o'clock). (B) IVUS findings at the same position showing an occlusive thrombus (T). Stent struts and the external elastic lamina (black arrows) can be clearly visualized. (C) OCT findings at the origin of the left circumflex coronary artery (LCX) revealing significant lining thrombus (T) opposite to the flow divider. (D) IVUS findings at the same location. Please notice again the blurred interface between lumen and thrombus but a nice delineation of the outer vessel wall (black arrows). (E) OCT findings after intervention at the midpart of the stent. A better expansion of the stent with adequate lumen was visualized but also significant residual thrombus (T). (F) Postintervention IVUS findings at the same location. *Wire artifact. Note that a larger field of view is always displayed in the IVUS images to allow visualization of the entire vessel. OCT indicates optical coherence tomography; IVUS, intravascular ultrasound; LST, late stent thrombosis.*

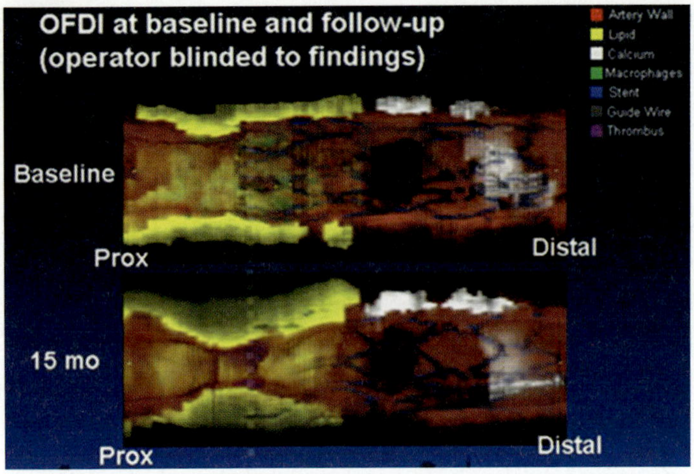

Fig. 54.10: *Optical frequency domain imaging (OFDI) represents an advance over optical coherence tomography for evaluating plaque deposits in coronary arteries, offering faster image acquisition and wider fields-of-view. A blinded study at Waxman's institution used OFDI to study the history of vulnerable plaque over 15 months. Above, restenosis, thrombus, and progression of calcification can be seen compared to baseline image poststenting. Images courtesy of Dr. Guillermo Tearney, Ph.D., and Dr. Sergio Waxman*

OCT would allow easy and precise identification of vulnerable plaque in daily clinical practice.

Positron Emission Tomography

Positron emission tomography (PET) is a powerful, quantitative imaging modality that has been used for decades to noninvasively investigate cardiovascular biology and physiology. Due to limited availability, methodologic complexity, and high costs, it has long been seen as a research tool and as a reference method for validation of other diagnostic approaches.

This perception, fortunately, has changed significantly within recent years. Increasing diversity of therapeutic options for coronary artery disease, and increasing specificity of novel therapies for certain biologic pathways, has resulted in a clinical need for more accurate and specific diagnostic techniques. At the same time, the number of PET centers continues to grow, stimulated by PET's success in oncology. Methodologic advances as well as improved radiotracer availability have further contributed to more widespread use. Evidence for diagnostic and prognostic usefulness of myocardial perfusion and viability assessment by PET is increasing. Some studies suggest overall cost-effectiveness of the technique despite higher costs of a single study, because unnecessary follow-up procedures can be avoided. The advent of hybrid PET-computed tomography (CT), which enables integration of PET-derived biologic information with multislice CT-derived morphologic information, and the key role of PET in the development and translation of novel molecular-targeted imaging compounds, have further contributed to more widespread acceptance. Today, PET promises to play a leading diagnostic role on the pathway toward a future of high-powered, comprehensive, personalized, cardiovascular medicine. This review summarizes the state-of-the-art in current imaging methodology and clinical application, and outlines novel developments and future directions. While the basic principles of PET are similar to those of SPECT, PET systems are generally more sensitive than SPECT systems, have better spatial resolution and provide the possibility of more accurate attenuation correction. The consequence of these advantages with PET is the possibility for quantification of tracer concentration in absolute units.

Genetic Aspects of Cardiovascular Diseases

Despite high contribution of factors such as hypercholesterolemia, systemic hypertension, smoking, and diabetes in development of coronary artery disease (CAD), evidence from family studies show that genetic factors also contribute significantly to the predisposition to CAD. Knowledge of genetic risk factors will help define the mechanisms of the disease and could ultimately assist in the rational design of selective prophylaxis or therapy. Many single genes have been identified as the basis for different cardiovascular diseases. However, unlike other

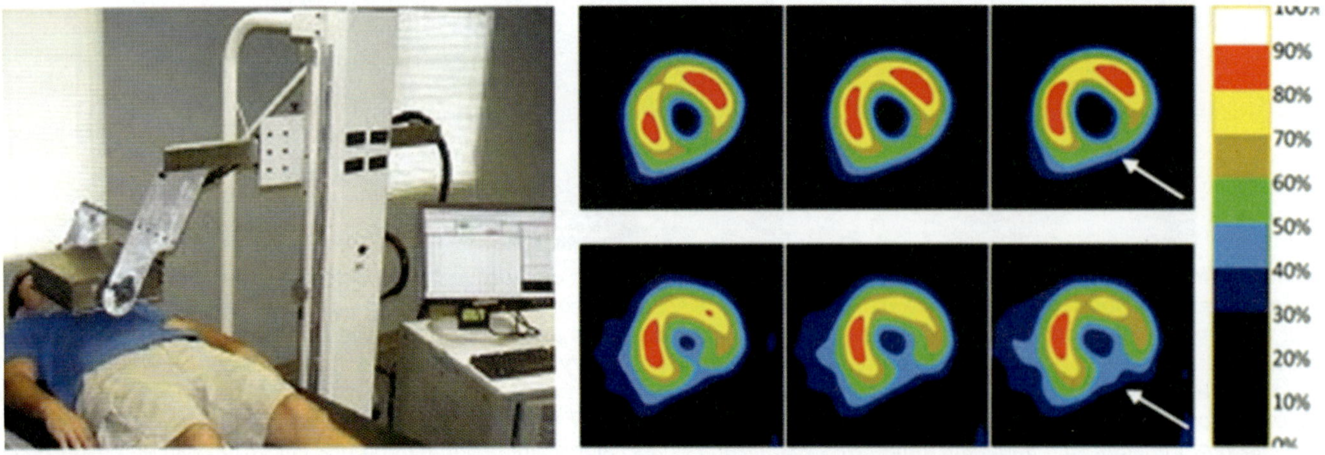

Fig. 54.11: *The images in the top row were obtained from a conventional cardiac SPECT system and the images in the bottom row were obtained from the mobile system*

genetic disorders, cardiovascular diseases are not solely due to a single gene mutation/polymorphism. The major genetic causes for cardiovascular diseases are:

i. Chromosomal disorders and single gene disorders (8%)
ii. Environmental teratogens (2%)
iii. Multifactorial disorders, which means both genetic and environmental factors interact (90%). Hence, it is important to bear in mind that in cardiovascular diseases one has to study multiple genes focusing on different aspects like lipids, blood coagulation, circulation as well as gene environment interactions.

Stem Cell Pioneers Honoured with Nobel

Winners of this year's (2007) Nobel prize for medicine are Mario Capecchi, Oliver Smithies and Martin Evans US citizens who won the 2007 Nobel Prize in medicine for ground breaking stem cell discoveries that led to a technology known as gene targeting. This gene targeting technology helps in undertsanding gene disease releationship. The three scientists modified the DNA of mice in so called "knockout" experiments that have advanced the understanding of the relationship between genes and human ailments, including cystic fibrosis, cancer and high blood pressure. "We're on the cusp of having a much better understanding of the relationship between genes and disease and how, when genes go wrong, they cause disease", said Steve Brown, director of the Medical Research Council at the Mammalian Genetics Unit in London. The citation from the Nobel award committee said the trio had discovered "principles for introducing specific gene modification in mice by the use of embryonic stem cells." They used "knockout mice" animals whose genetic code has been altered in the laboratory to either turn on or off certain genes that mice and humans share. Although gene targeting uses embryonic stem cells from mice, the research is very different from how stem cells would be used to treat disease in humans. In people, stem cells would be prodded to become replacement tissue like nerve cells for transplant into patients. Capecchi, 70, did work that "shed light on the cause of several human inborn malformations", the prize citation said, while Evans, 66, applied gene targeting to develop mouse models for human diseases. Smithies, 82, also used gene targeting to develop mouse models for inherited diseases such as cystic fibrosis and the blood disease thalassemia, and other diseases such as hypertension and atherosclerosis AP.

Long before "Human Genome Project" was even conceived, clinical studies showed that cardiovascular diseases are associated with strong genetic components with different types of inheritance. After the completion of "Human Genome Project", by proper linkage analysis of various families with different kinds of hereditary cardiovascular disorders it is now possible to localize and amplify such genes. If its function is unknown then from gene library of different animals it is possible to find out whether similar genes in animals are known with identified function. Other technical advances in biological sciences and in information technology with powerful software programme allow us to study the precise location of the abnormal gene in the members of the affected family. Once the location of the abnormal gene is known, that gene can be amplified by using information from genome project. These oligonucleotides on a PCR reaction can amplify the target area a million times. Apart from possible therapeutic developments, once the abnormalities in the gene leading to disease in the family is identified, it may be possible to assign the risk to the other members of the family who have not yet developed the disease or to offer prenatal diagnosis.

The implications of the human genome for medicine and in particular, cardiovascular diseases are unparalleled partly because the information targeted to the inter workings of mankind is enormous. The genomic sequences contain the actual blueprint that determines all of our actions as well as the inherent biological functions. We know for example that 80% of all the deaths in the world today are due to 20 diseases. It is estimated that about 200 to 300 genes are responsible for susceptibility to these diseases which are amenable to vaccines and other preventive therapies. It is expected that most of these genes will be identified within next 5–10 years. The human genome sequence will facilitate markedly our search for genes responsible for diseases and various physiological functions. At present, however, only 1,000 genes have been identified to be responsible for human diseases. The remaining 39,000 genes, all of which have either a physiological or pathological function, are yet to be identified and their appropriate function determined. The genes and genomes of over 50 organisms have been identified such as haemophylus in fluenza and *Treponema palidum* which provide novel targets for antibiotics and vaccines. It has been recognised that the cloning of certain growth factors can be directed to selectively modulate cardiac myocyte growth and to inhibit unwarranted growth of fibroblasts.

DNA was established in the 1940s to be responsible for passing on inherited characteristics as opposed to the previously held hypothesis of protein. The DNA is contained in 23 pairs of chromosomes enclosed in the nucleus and collectively referred to as the genome. These chromosomes are paired with the homologous chromosomes in the case of 22 pairs referred to as autosomes. The remaining two chromosomes are the sex chromosomes, which in the female consist of two X chromosomes, and in the male an X and a Y chromosome. The two homologous chromosomes of each pair carry the same set of genes with one inherited from each parent, but

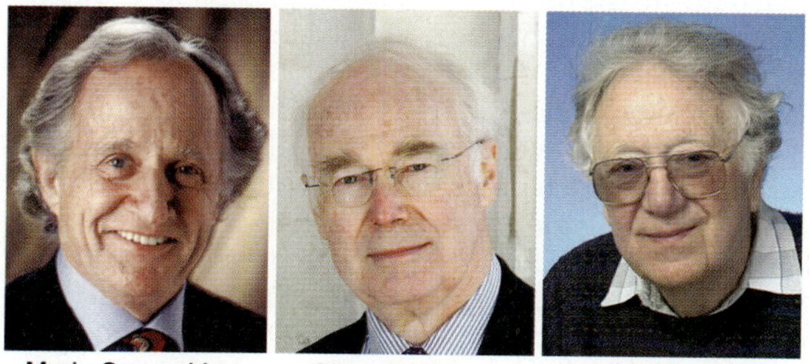

Mario Capecchi Oliver Smithies Martin Evans

despite their homology and potential identical function, there are minor differences in the DNA sequence which mayor may not alter the function of the corresponding gene. A chromosome consists of a single long linear molecule of DNA. DNA has a three-dimensional structure which consists of two helical strands coiled around a common axis forming a double helix. Each strand of DNA is composed of four different monomers called nucleotides or bases. The two strands of DNA each coiled in a helix, antiparallel to each other, are held together by hydrogen bonds formed between the bases. A nucleotide consists of a phosphate group linked by a phosphodiester bond to a pentose sugar, which in turn is linked to an organic base. In DNA, the pentose sugar is deoxyribose and in RNA is ribose. DNA consists of 4 bases, adenine (A), guanine (G), thymine In, cytosine (C) as does RNA except that thymine is replaced by uracil (U). The DNA sequence of a chromosome is always read from left to right with the proximal sequence (left) referred to as the 5' end, the distal sequence (right), the 3' end. The two strands of DNA of each chromosome are held together by hydrogen bonds between the organic bases in a precise and obligatory format. The base adenine (A) on one strand can only pair with T on the other strand and does so through two hydrogen bonds and G can only pair with C through three hydrogen bonds. Complementary base pairing between two strands of DNA contributes to the stability of the double helix and is a unique feature of DNA. Breaking down of these bonds, referred to as'denaturation of the DNA molecule' can be induced through several mechanisms such as increased temperature with the helix separating into two single strands. Restoration of the lower temperature induces the two strands to come together (reanneal) in the same precise order as prior to separation. This precise order is maintained by the complementary base pairs whereby A only pairs with T and C with G. This feature of DNA to denature and reanneal is the basis of practically all DNA diagnostic tests.

Human Genome Organisation and Matrix

The 46 chromosomes are compacted to occupy less than 10% of the volume of the cell. An average cell has a diameter of about 0.0015 cm, yet the chromosomes, if joined together head and tail would average about 3 metres. The combination of DNA with the protein around which it is attached for compaction is referred,to as chromatin. The most abundant protein binding to the DNA is a family of histones which are rich in lysine, a positively charged amino acid that binds to the negatively charged phosphate groups in the DNA. Recently it has been learned that the chromatin structure of DNA is a major determinant of whether a particular gene will undergo transcription. The chromatin structure of DNA is very compact with tight binding between histones which prevents transcription, acetylation-deacetylation of histone proteins is now recognised as fundamental to the regulation of gene expression. Histone acetyltransferases (HAC) acetylate the lysine groups on the histones, which displace binding to the DNA resulting in relaxation of the nucleosomes and increased transcription of the gene. Histone deacetylation (HDAC) antagonises this action and represses transcription through compaction of chromatin. There are at least 16 known HDACs in humans. Class II HDACs are known to repress transcription of MEF II, one of the pivotal transcription factors in cardiac development. Thus, chromatin compaction and decompaction, although recently explored mechanisms, determine whether a gene will be transcribed and expressed into its functional unit, namely, the protein.

Genes are referred to as the units of heredity and are responsible for passing on the various characteristics that distinguish each individual. Genes are distinct sequences which have a start and stop site varying in size from 10,000 to 2 million base pairs (bp). The average estimate of the human gene is about 20,000 bp. Genes are distinct units of heredity with each of their transcripts, messanger RNA (mRNA) encoding for a single polypeptide. They do not directly participate in function but participate through their intermediary Mrna code for a polypeptide which is determined by the sequence of its amino acids. The linear sequence of the amino acids in the polypeptide corresponds to the linearity of the codons (triplet of bases) in the gene. Each codon encodes for a specific amino acid and determines its position in the polypeptide. The human genome has about 40,000 genes which is only about 2% of the human DNA. About 1/3rd of the DNA is transcribed into mRNA but most of it is spliced out in the processing of the mature mRNA before it exits the nucleus to serve as a polypeptide template. The mature mRNA is derived from DNA sequences referred to as exons (exiting the nucleus) while the intervening DNA sequences spliced out of the mRNA are referred to as introns (remaining in the nucleus). The overall structure of a gene consists of three parts. The middle portion consists of those sequences which ultimately end up in the mRNA to serve as a template to code for the protein and is referred to as the protein coding portion. The two ends referred to as the 5' (left) and the 3' (right) contain important sequences to which proteins that determine transcription of the gene are bound. The 5' end contains sequences specific for transcription factors which bind to determine whether a gene will be transcribed. The 3′ end has a sequence which stabilises the mRNA and is essential for the over all function of the mature mRNA. There are three kinds of proteins that regulate transcription: (1) promoters, which increase transcription; (2) enhancers that enhance transcription and (3) silencers which repress transcription. All of these proteins primarily bind to the 5′ end of the gene and regulate its overall function. Thus, a gene has coding sequences interspersed with noncoding sequences and represents the entire genomic DNA sequence required for synthesis of a functional polypeptide.

Human Genome Project

The Human Genome Project (HGP) was initiated in 1990 to be completed in 2005. The overall goal of the HGP was to obtain a physical map of the Human Genome, namely, to determine the sequence of all the bases in each chromosome. This was the first international project devoted to understanding the biology of the human being.

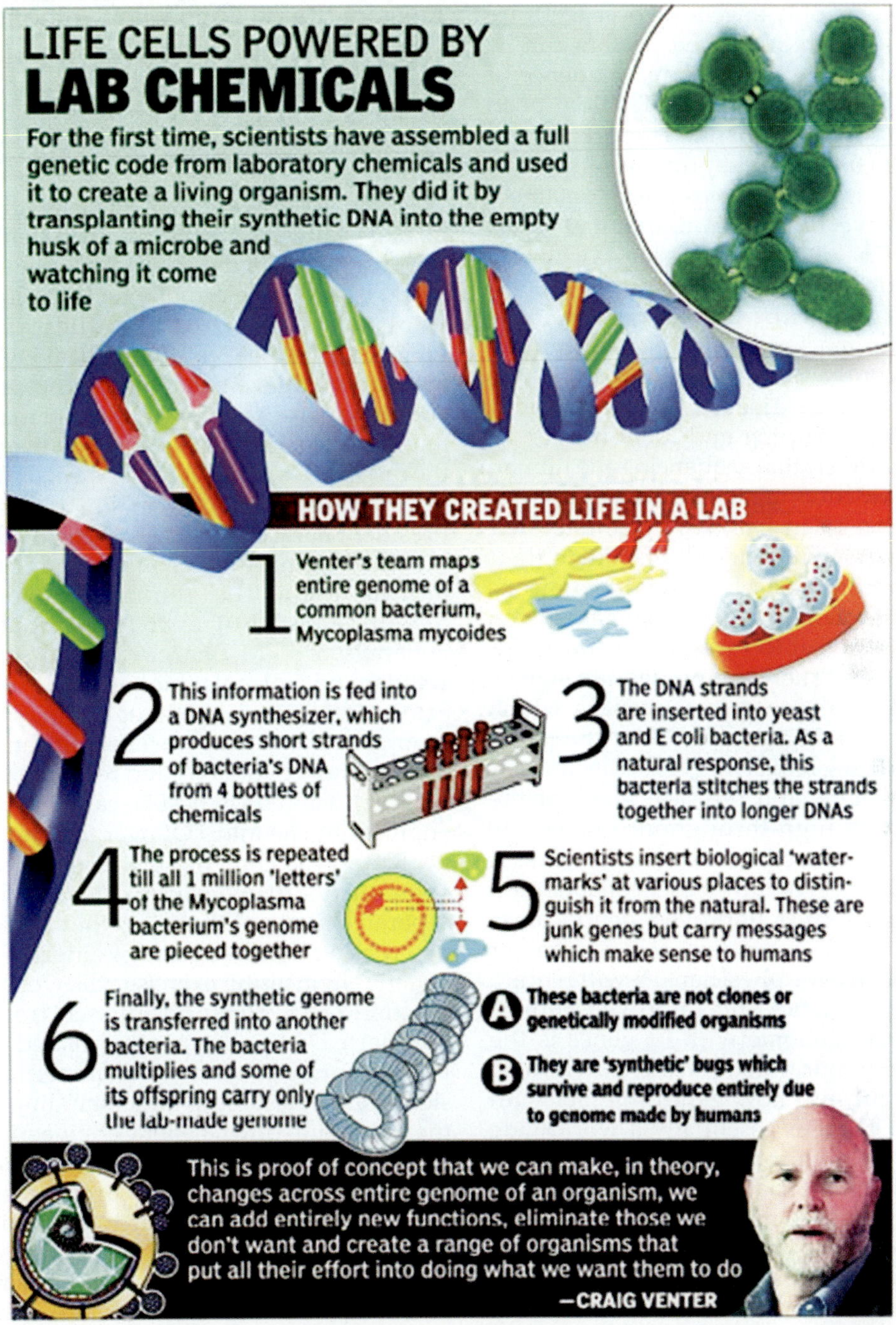

Fig. 54.12: *Laboratory techniques in the creation of artificial life by J Craig Venter and his associates.*

A rough draft covering about 90% of the human sequences is available. In the meantime, HGP also developed genetic maps based on short DNA sequences of known chromosomal location distributed throughout the human genome to be used as signposts or markers for the mapping and identification of genes.

Chromosomal markers to map the human genome were available prior to HGP but were limited in their distribution and provided minimal information. A new set of DNA markers were developed from the repeat microsatellite sequences. These markers are repeats of di-, tri-, or tetranucleotides referred to as short tandem repeat polymorphisms (STRPs). Genetic maps are now available with thousands of markers that span the human genome at less than 1 million bp intervals. These genetic markers made possible the widespread application of genetic linkage analysis. This is a computerised technique utilised in families with familial disease, to map the chromosomal location (locus) of the responsible gene and has led to identification of several genes responsible for inherited cardiovascular disease. The HGP also spurred the movement to identify a genetic map based on markers that are expressed sequences. These were referred to as Expressed Sequence Tags (ESTs) and are unique genomic sequences which are present only in genes. These ESTs are short sequences of two or three hundred bp that can be used as a probe to identify the full genomic sequence of the gene. Hundreds of thousands of ESTs have been sequenced and entered into GenBank. These ESTs are cloned in vectors such as bacteria and provide a library of human ESTs from which multiple copies can be obtained. Many of these ESTs have now been mapped to their chromosomal location. The ultimate aim is to have an EST accurately annotated to a chromosomal position at least every 100,000 bp throughout the human genome. The development of genetic markers spanning the human genome and more recently the generation of ESTs as candidate genes for human disease have markedly accelerated chromosomal mapping and identification of genes It must not be assumed that sequencing the human genome is analogous to identifying the human genes. The human genomic sequences will markedly facilitate their human genomic sequences will markedly facilitate their identification, but do not in themselves provide a means to identify the genes. One cannot identify the genes even when it were visually possible to observe the DNA sequence of a chromosome. There are no definite signals to indicate the 2 percent of genomic sequences which comprise the genes. Identifying most or all of the genes responsible for a human being remains a goal of the future.is conceivable with the genetic and physical maps of the human genome and with high throughput nucleotide sequencing it could be achieved in the next 5 years. It remains a major effort and will require closer collaboration of the physician with the scientist. Improved identification of phenotypes due to single gene disorders is a major opportunity and a challenge for physicians. It will require increased awareness of genetics and improved clinical observations. The human genome with its genes is the blueprint for human biological activities and will also provide immense insight into how genes interact with environmental stimuli. There is essentially a worldwide interest in the human genome scientifically, culturally, racially, medically and commercially. It is predicted that within 5 to 10 years personalised medicine will be a reality with the type of drug and its dose determined by the individual's genetic profile. The commercial spin off and utilisation is already evident from the large role played by biotechnology in our everyday commercial world. In conjunction with the initiation of the human genome project, computerised gene bank (GenBank) accessible at HTTP://www.ncuv.nhm.nih.gov was established by the National Centre for Biotechnology Information (NCBI) and is part of the International Nucleotide Sequence Database Collaboration alongwith its two partners, the European Molecular Biology Laboratory (EMBL) nucleotide database and the European Bioinformatics Institute and the DNA Databank of Japan. It is available without any cost to physicians and scientists throughout the world. It contains billions of DNA sequences from over 40,000 species and expands every day. The availability of these databases has markedly facilitated research in human molecular genetics and biology to the extent that it is now a necessary resource.

Artificial Life on Earth with Synthetic Gene

J. Craig Venter, PhD, from t he Institute for Genomic Research in Maryland.is regarded as one of leading scientists of the 21st century for his invaluable contributions in genomic research and is one of the most frequently cited scientists.

A day after genome pioneer J Craig Venter announced he had created synthetic life, the scientific world was agog over the merits and demerits of Craigs seemingly dramatic work. Is the future actually here The jury is still out. Arthur Caplan, professor of bioethics at the University of Pennsylvania told Nature medical journal that Venter and his teams achievement undermines a fundamental belief about the nature of life that is likely to prove as momentous to our view of ourselves and our place in the Universe as the discoveries of Galileo, Copernicus, Darwinand Einstein. The US governments reaction was more guarded with President Barack Obama announcing that the White House bioethics committee would submit a report within six months about the genuine concerns raised by this development. But even back home, Indias premier geneticist Dr PM Bhargava, who set up the Centre for cellular and molecular biology (CCMB) in Hyderabad, was categorical that venter, though a fine scientist, had this time around overstated his works significance.Venters team took a cell, removed its DNA and replaced it with a host of other material. This can at best be called a massive bit of genetic engineering, he told TOI over telephone from Hyderabad. Dr Bhargavas contention was simple: A cell has several components. If we can take each of those components separately and put them together to create life, that would be creating synthetic life. Venters experiment is just a genetic engineering exercise. His words find an echo in the reaction of Dr Steen Rasmussen from the University of Southern Denmark. In a published statement, he said, Implementing a synthetic genome in a modern cell is a significant milestone in understanding life today. However, the radical top down genetic engineering that Venters team has done, does not quite constitute a synthetic cell by my definition. Bottom-up researchers, like myself, aim to assemble life including hardware and the programme as simply as possible, even if the result is different from what we think of as life. Constructing life using different material and blueprints will teach us more about the nature of life than reproducing life as we know it. The stand of the non-governmental organizations was clear as well. A statement released by the Friends of the Earth, an environmental group in the US, denounced the synthetic genome as dangerous new technology, saying that Mr Venter should stop all further research until sufficient regulations are in place. Some NGOs felt that even the environmental uses of synthetic cells (it is hoped the bacteria, for instance, can be used to neutralize greenhouse gases) were exaggerated. BBC quoted Dr Helen Wallace from Genewatch UK, an organization that monitors developments in genetic technologies,as saying, If you release new organisms into the environment,you can do more harm than good.

We dont know how these organisms will behave in the environment.

The synthetic genome also raised some philosophical points. Mark Bedau, a professor at Reed College in Oregon, said: It (the new prosthetic genome) will revitalize perennial questions about the significance of life what is it, why it is important and what role humans should have in its future.

Scientists Find way to Increase Length of Human Telomeres—Life Map of Humans

The shortening of human telomeres—caps that protect our chromosomes from deterioration—has been associated with aging and disease.

Now, researchers from the Stanford University School of Medicine, CA, say they have found a way to lengthen these telomeres, potentially opening the door to new treatments for many age-related and genetic conditions. Researchers say they have found a way to lengthen human telomeres - the protective caps at the end of chromosomes. The research team, led by John Ramunas, PhD, and Eduard Yakubov, PhD, publish their findings in The FASEB Journal. Chromosomes are thread-like structures situated at the end of DNA strands that contain all our genetic information. Telomeres protect our chromosomes from becoming damaged during cell division. However, telomeres become shorter with each cell division and can reach a point where they are no longer able protectthe chromosomes, leaving them open to deterioration. This leads to aging and disease development. Studying human cells in the laboratory is important for finding new ways to treat such diseases, but the team says the shortening of telomeres makes this challenging; it only allows researchers to monitor cells over a few divisions before they die.But now, Ramunas, Yakubov and their team say they have found a way to extend the length of telomeres, which could increase the number of human cells available for studying.

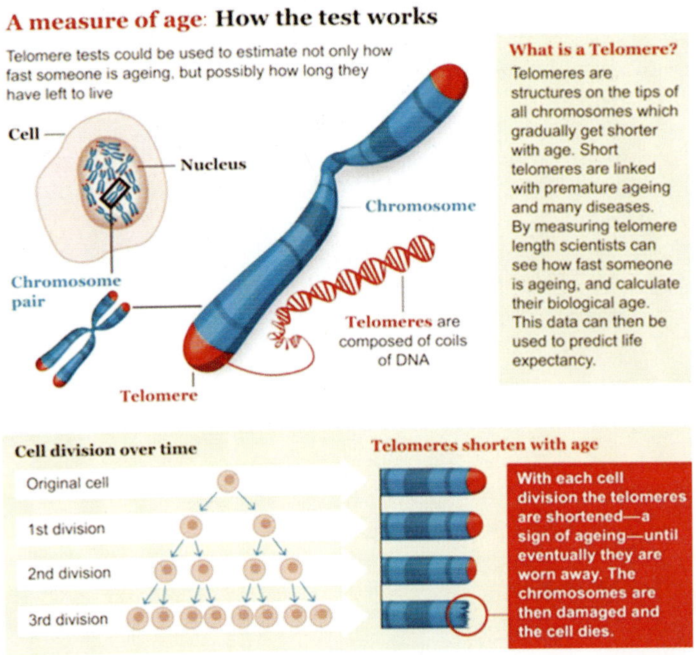

Fig. 54.13: *Cell containing chromosomes, blown up picture of chromosome with telomere in the shape of cap at the ends of each chromosome. How ageing affects the length of telomere in human beings (right bottom)*

New method increased telomere length by up to 10% To increase telomere length, the team used a modified type of ribonucleic acid (RNA) that contained the coding sequence of TERT. TERT is the active component of telomerase - an enzyme expressed by stem cells that maintains the health of telomeres as they are passed to the next generation. Though stem cells express TERT, the researchers note that most other cell types do not. In their study, the researchers explain that introducing as few as three applications of the modified RNA (called modified TERT mRNA) to human cells over a few days increased telomere length by up to 10%. Young humans possess telomeres that are around 8,000–10,000 nucleotides long, the team notes, but the modified TERT-encoding RNA increased telomere length by around 1,000 nucleotides. What is more, the researchers say that human skin cells treated with modified TERT mRNA divided around 28 more times than those that remained untreated, while treated human muscle cells divided around three more times. Ramunas says the team was pleasantly surprised to find that modified TERT mRNA effectively increased telomere length. "Previous attempts to deliver mRNA-encoding TERT caused an immune response against telomerase, which could be deleterious," he adds."In contrast, our technique is nonimmunogenic. Existing transient methods of extending telomeres act slowly, whereas our method acts over just a few days to reverse telomere shortening that occurs over more than a decade of normal aging. This suggests that a treatment using our method could be brief and infrequent."

Findings may lead to new treatments for genetic, age-related disorders.

The researchers say their new technique could lead to new treatments for age-related diseases and genetic conditions that are associated with telomere shortening, such as Duchenne muscular dystrophy—an inherited neuromuscular condition estimated to affect 1 in 3,600 male infants in the US.

Study co-author Helen Blau adds: "Now, we have found a way to lengthen human telomeres by as much as 1,000 nucleotides, turning back the internal clock in these cells by the equivalent of many years of human life. This greatly increases the number of cells available for studies such as drug testing or disease modeling.One day it may be possible to target muscle stem cells in a patient with Duchenne muscular dystrophy, for example, to extend their telomeres. There are also implications for treating conditions of aging, such as diabetes and heart disease. This has really opened the doors to consider all types of potential uses of this therapy". The researchers now plan to investigate how modified TERT mRNA affects other types of human cells. In June last year, Medical News Today reported on a study led by the University of California-San Francisco, in which researchers claim—contrary to other studies—longer telomeres are associated with an increased risk of brain cancer.

Appendix

Cardiovascular Drug Therapy and Current Innovations in Cardiology

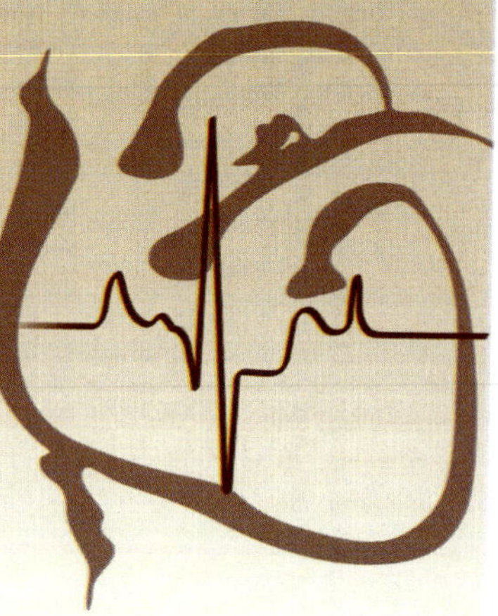

Advances in cardiology, surgical techniques, postoperative care, and medications have improved the chances of long-term survival of the neonatal and pediatric patient with complex congenital cardiac anomalies. Rather than undergoing palliative repair, these children are now frequently taken to the operating room for complete repair. As complete repair becomes the norm, collaborative management and a thorough understanding of the pre- and postoperative medications used become essential to the care of these patients. The nurse's ability to understand preop, postop, and management medications is enhanced by an understanding of the principles of cardiac anatomy and physiology, as well as developmental changes in cardiac function. All of these are reviewed. In addition, since the safe and effective administration of these drugs depends on the pediatric intensive care unit (PICU) and neonatal intensive care unit (NICU) nurse's thorough knowledge of these medications and their effects on the cardiovascular system, a brief review of these medications is presented. While new technology and techniques are improving survival rates for children with congenital heart anomalies, it is the postoperative care that these children receive that enhances the patient's survival even more.

Antihypertensive Drugs

Drug category: **Diuretics**
Cause diuresis, which decreases plasma volume and edema, thereby decreasing cardiac output and blood pressure.

Drug: Hydrochlorothiazide (esidrix, hydroDIURIL, microzide).

Description: Inhibits reabsorption of sodium in distal tubules, causing increased excretion of sodium, water, potassium and hydrogen ions.

Adult dose: 25–100 mg PO qd; not to exceed 200 mg/kg/d.

Pediatric dose: < 6 months: 2–3 mg/kg/d PO divided bid, > 6 months: 2 mg/kg/d PO divided bid.

Contraindications: Documented hypersensitivity; anuria; renal decompensation.

Interactions: May decrease effects of anticoagulants, antigout agents, and sulfonylureas; may increase toxicity of allopurinol, anesthetics, antineoplastics, calcium salts, loop diuretics, lithium, diazoxide, digitalis, amphotericin B, and nondepolarizing muscle relaxants.

Table 1: *Presents normal hemodynamics and oxygen consumption in children*

Age (weight/BSA)	*Cardiac output (mL/min)*	*Heart rate*	*Stroke volume (mL)*	*Oxygen consumption (mL/min*	
					mL/min/m
Newborn (3.2 kg/0.2 m)	700–800	145	5	36–54	180–270
6 months (8 kg/0/42 m)	1000–1600	120	10	70–100	167–238
1 year (10 kg/0/5 m)	1300–1500	115	13	85–110	170–220
2 years (13 kg/0.59 m)	1500–2000	115	18	91–123	154–211
4 years (17 kg/0.71 m)	2300–2375	105	27	110–150	155–211
5 years (19 kg/0.77 m)	2500–3000	95	31	115–170	149–221
8 years (28 kg/0.96 m)	3400–3600	83	42	150–208	156–200
10 years (35 kg/1.1 m)	3800–4000	75	50	190–250	122–227
15 years (50 kg/1.4 m)	5000–6000	70	85	300–400	120–200

Table 2: *Drug therapy in children*

Medication	*Indication for use*	*Dosing*	*Onset*	*Side-effects*	*Half-life*	*Metabolism*	*Contraindications*
Dopamine	Pre- and postoperatively to increase cardiac output, blood pressure, and urine output. Volume depletion should be corrected prior to starting dopamine	Renal and mesentetric vasodilation: 2–5 mcg/kg/min (beta) effect: 5–10 mcg/kg/min Vasoconstriction and pressor (alpha) effect. >10 mcg/kg/min IV infusion	Within 5 mins	Tachydysthythmias, vasocontriction, gangrene of the extremities, anginal pain and palpitations	2 mins	Metabolized in the plasma kidney and liver	Hypersensitivity to sulfiters, phechromocytoma or ventricular fibrilation. Care must be given to ensure that extravasation does not occur. Extravasation causes severe tissue necrosis. In the event of extravasation, phentolamine should be instilled locally
Dobutamine	Pre-and postoperatively to increase cardiac output and to manage short-term cardiac decompensation. Volume depletion should be corrected prior to starting dobutamine	2–20 mcg/kg/min IV infusion. Transient hypotension may occur when starting this medication	1–10 mins	Ectopic heart beats, increased heart rate chest pain, headche, nausea and vomiting dyspnea, and in higher doses, ventricular dysrhythmias	2 mins	Metabolized in the tissues and liver	Hypersensitivity to sulfiltes and idiopathic hypertophic subaortic stenosis
Epinephrine	Pre- and postoperatively to increase cardiac output and blood pressure. Care must be taken when using this drug. The benefits of increased cardiac output and blood pressure must be weighed against the effects of increased consumption of myocardial oxygen, tachycardia, and decreased renal blood flow	0.1 to 1 mcg/kg/min IV infusion	5 mins	Pallor, tachycardia hypertension, increased myocardial oxygen consumption, anxiety, headache, dilated pupils, nausea, acute urinary retention, weakness, tremor, and decreased renal blood flow	3 mins	Metabolized in the liver and tissues	Hypersensitivity to epinephrine, cardiac dysrhythmias, and angle-closure glaucoma
Mllrinone amrinone	Postoperatively to treat low cardiac output syndrome and congestive heart failure. Both drugs increase cardiac output and stroke volume, decrease intracardiac filling pressure, and decrease systemic vascular resistance without changing heart rate or myocardial oxygen consumption. Milrinone has fewer side effects.	Loading dose: 50 mcg/kg IV over at least 10 mins Maintenance infusion: 0.2 to 1 mcg/kg	5–15 mins	Headache, ventricular dysthythmias, hypotension, and chest pain	1–5 hours	Excretion by the kidneys	Severe pulmonary or aortic obstructive disease and hypersensitivity to milrinone
Digoxin	Most frequently used in chronic heart failure, its primary use is to increase the force of contraction in the myocardium thus increasing cardiac output. May be given IV or PO	Digitalizing: 30–50 mcg/kg IV (Q 8 hrs: 1/2, 1/4. 1/4) Maintenance: 2–12 mcg/kg/day must be individualized according to age	5–30 mins	Sinus bradycardia, A-V and S-A block, ventricular dyrhythmias lethargy, confusion, nausea, vomiting, feeding intolerance, blurred vision	18–36 hours	Excretion by kidneys, removed by dialysis, dose must be adjusted for renal failure patients (follow levels closely)	Hypersensitivity to digoxin, ventricular fibrilation, A-V block, idiopathic hypertrophic subaortic stenosis, or constrictive pericarditis

(Contd...)

Table 2: *Drug therapy in children (Contd...)*

Medication	*Indication for use*	*Dosing*	*Onset*	*Side-effects*	*Half-life*	*Metabolism*	*Contraindications*
Nitroglycerin	Postoperatively to dilate the coronary arteries, improving oxygenation of the myocardial tissues. As a venous dilator, nitroglycerine reduces left ventricular diastolic pressure and systemic vascular resistance, reducing myocardial oxygen demand	Initial dose: 0.25–0.5 micrograms/kg/min via infusion. May titrate by 0.5 to 1 microgram/kg/min every 3–5 min to a maximum dose of 5–10 mcg/min Caution: when mixing nitroglycarin, the maximum concentration is 400 micrograms/mL, it must be diluted in glass, and special non-polyviryl chloride tubing must be used	1–2 min	Severe hypotension, headache, dizziness, reflex tachycardia, nausea, and vomiting	1–4 min	Extensively during first-pass and excreted in the urine	Hypersensitivity to nitroglycerin, organic nitrates, glucoma, severe anemia, increased ICP, pericardial tamponae, constrictive pericarditis and hypotension
Nitroprusside	Indicated preoperatively and postoperatively for hypertensive crisis. Nitroprusside, a peripheral vasodilator, increases cardiac output by decressing afterload and systemic vascular resistance	Starting dose: 0.3 to 0.5 micrograms/kg/min IV infusion, titrating to effect to a maximum of 8 of 10 micrograms/kg/min. Nitroprusside must be protected from light (light greatly increases decomposition) D_5W should be used for dilution	Within 2 min	Profound hypotension, metabolic acidosis, increased ICP, thyroid suspression, and CNS toxicity. Cyanide and thiocyanate toxicity may occur if nitroprusside is used for greater than 4 days, if the infusion is > 4 micrograms/kg/min or in the presence of renal dysfunction. Monitor thiocyanate and cyanide levels keeping	Less than 10 min	Metabolized in the liver and excreted in the urine	Hypersensitivity to nitropresside and decreased cerebral perfusion
Lidocaine	A class IB antiarrhythmic indicated pre- and post operatively for ventricular dysrthythmias. Lidocaine suppresses automaticity of conduction tissues by increasing the electrical threshold of the ventricles	Loading: 1 mg/kg IV, may be repeated in 10–15 min times 2 doses, followed by a continuous infusion of 10–50 mcg/kg/min Lower loading doses: 0.5 mg/kg IV and lower infusion rates may be required in patients with CHF or hepatic disease.	45–50 sec after single IV bolus dose	Bradycardia, hypoten sion, heart block, lethargy, coma, agitation slurred speech, seizures, hallucinations, nausea, vomiting, muscle twiching, blurred vision, respiratory depression or arrest	Biphasic ranging from 7 min to 3.2 hours	Metabolized in the liver and excreted in the urine	Hypersensitivity to lidocaine Adams-strokes syndrome, or severe degree of S-A or A-V or ventricular heart block without a pacemaker

(Contd...)

Table 2: *Drug therapy in children (Contd...)*

Medication	*Indication for use*	*Dosing*	*Onset*	*Side-effects*	*Half-life*	*Metabolism*	*Contraindications*
Amiodarone	A class III antiarrhythmic indicated postoperatively for life-threatening ventricular dysthythmias and junctional ectopic tachycardia (JET). Amiodarone decreases A-V and S-A node conduction and prolongs the refractory period.	Loading: 5 milligram/kg IV over 1 hour followed by a maintance infusion of 0.3 to 1 milligram/kg/hr Aminodarone must be mixed with D_5W and in a glass bottle	Within hours of the loading dose	Worsening A-V block, bradycardia, hypotension. With long-term use hypothyroidism, liver toxicity	Extremely long 5 days	Metabolized in the liver and is excreted in the biliary tract and urine	Hypersensitivity to amiodarone, sinus bradycaria, second and third degree A-V block and cardiogenic shock. Many drug inter-actions; amiodarone is a very potent inhibitor of P450 liver enzymes
Precainamide	A class 1A antiarrhythmic indicated postoperatively for SVT, ventricular tachycardias, and atrial tachycardia. Procainamide inhibits the sodium pump decreases myocardial excitability and conduction velocity and depresses myocardial contractility.	*Loading:* 5–15 milligram/kg IV over 5 min to a maximum dose of 100 milligrams followed by a maintenance infusion of 20–80 microgram/kg/min to a maximum dose of 2 gm/24 hrs	10–30 min	Prolongation of the QT interval (stop infusion if QT increases by 50% of premedication length), hypotension, A-V block, confusion, tachycardia, nausea, and vomiting. Long-term side effects systemic lupus	1.7 hours	Metabolized in the liver and excreted in the urine	Complete heart block, A-V block, long QT interval, hypersensitivity to procainamide, and torsades de pointe
Furosemide	A loop diuretic indicated postoperatively to reduce preload, and in patients with postperfusion syndrome. Postperfusion syndrome is a systemic inflammatory response to cardiopulmonary bypass. This syndrome manifests itselft, in part, as renal insufficiency. Renal insuffciency (oliguria and fluid retention) affects 5% to 30% of all children after pediatric cardiac surgeries with the aid of cardiopulmonary bypass. Furosemide as either a continuous drip or intermittent boluses can be given. The study indicates that a constant infusion yields comparable urine output at a lower dose of furosemide while decreasing the fluctuations in urinary output and the need for volume replacement.	IV infusions: 0.05 mg/kg/hrs thrated to clinical effect. intermittent IV: 1–2 mg/kg/dose every 6–12 hrs	IV 5 min PO: 30–60 min	Hypotension, dizziness, utcaria, electrolyte imbalances, potential ototoxicity with high doses, and jaundice	Normal renal function 30 min, with renal failure 9 hrs	Metabolized by the liver and 80% excreted in the urine	Indomethacin decreases effect

(Contd...)

Table 2: *Drug therapy in children (Contd...)*

Medication	*Indication for use*	*Dosing*	*Onset*	*Side-effects*	*Half-life*	*Metabolism*	*Contraindications*
Bumetanide	A loop diuretic is indicated postoperatively to reduce preload	0.015–0.1 mg/kg/dose given every 6–24 hrs IV	Within a few min when given IV	Hypotension, chest pain dizziness, rash, hyperglycemia, electrolyte imbalance, elevated liver enzymes, ototoxicity and elevated serum creatinine	Ranges from 1 hr to 2-1/2 hrs	Partially metabolized in the liver and excreted in the urine	Hypersensitivity to bumetanide and anuria or increasing azotemia
Ethacrynic acid	A loop diuretic is indicated postoperatively to reduce preload	1 mg/kg/dose given once. If necessary may be repeated every 8–12 hrs	5 min when given IV	Hypotension, chest pain, dizziness, rash, hyperglycemia, electrolyte imbalance, elevated liver enzymes, ototoxicity, and elevated serum creatinine	Range from 1 hr to 2½ hrs	Partially metabolized in the liver and excreted in the urine	Hypersensitivity to bumetanide and anuria or increasing azotemia
Ethacrynic acid	A loophdiuretic is indicated postoperatively to reduce preload	1 mg/kg/dose given once. If necessary may be repeated every 8–12 hrs	5 min when given IV	Hypotension, electrolyte imbalance, rash, hyperglycemia, abdominal pain, and renal injury	2 hrs if given IV	Metabolized in the liver and excreted in the bile and urine	Hypersensitivity to etacrynic acid, hypotension, hyponatremic dehydration, metabolic alkalosis with hypokalemia and anuria
Spironolactone	A potassium-sparing diuretic acting on the distal collecting duct of the nephron This drug is indicated for treatment of CHF. May be used in conjunction with lasix and digoxin	1–3 mg/kg/day, given once a day or divided into two doses given every 12 hours	1–3 hrs	Dysrhythmias, lethargy confusion, ataxia, rash electrolyte imbalance, dehydration, and decreased renal function		Metabolized in the liver and excreted in the urine and biliary tracts	If given with potassium supplements may increase potassium serum levels. Spironolactone, when given with potassium supplements, may potentiate inotropic affect of digoxin while decreasing digoxin clearance.
Calcium Chloride Calcium Gluconate	Often indicated in the postoperative cardiovascular patient to increase contractility of the myocardium. when choosing which calcium supplement to use, attention must be paid to the strength of the supplement and the purpose for using it. For example, calcium chloride has three times more elemental calcium than calcium gluconate. Since the body will be able to utilize the calcium from calcium chloride much more	Calcium chloride: 10 to 20 mg/kg/IV dose Calcium gluconate: 50–100 mg/min IV infusion		Vasodilation hypotension bradycardia, dysrhythmias ventricular fibrilation, syncope, headache, confusion, lethargy, coma constipation, nausea, vomiting and elevated serum amylase. Ionized calcium (amount of calcium) available for use) levels should be used instead of serum calcium (total amount of calcium in body) levels when monitoring calcium supplementation			Hypercalcemia, renal calculi ventricular fibrilation

(Contd...)

Table 2: *Drug therapy in children*

Medication	*Indication for use*	*Dosing*	*Onset*	*Side-effects*	*Half-life*	*Metabolism*	*Contraindications*
	Quickly, calcium chloride is used during emergent situations. Calcium gluconate releases the calcium more slowly and is utilized, via infusion, for long-term correction.						
Esmolol	A beta-blocker indicated postoperatively for the treatment of systemic hypertension, right or left-sided outflow tract obstruction, and is a class II antiarrhythmic	200–500 mcg/kg/ IV over 1–2 min followed by a maintenance infusion of 50–250 mcg/kg/min	1– 2 min after loading dose	Heart failure, bradycardia, hypotension, nausea, and vomiting	3–5 min	Metabolized in the blood and excreted in the urine	Bradycardia, heart block, uncompensated heart failure, cardiogenic shock, and hypersensitivity to esmolol or any other beta-blocker
Indomethacin	A nonsteroidal antiinflammatory drug (NSAID) that inhibits the production of prostaglandin. It is indicated for pharmacological closure of a patent ductus arteriosus.	0.2 mg/kg intravenously if the ductus does not dose with the initial dose, two additional doses may be given. The amount and timing of those closes are determined by postnatal age, urine output, clinical assessment, and/or echocardiography. A second series of indomethacin may be necessary in some neonates to assure ductal closure		Transient renal dysfunction (decreased urine output, decreased urine sodium and chloride excretion, free water clearance, hyponatremia, transient hypoglycemia, decreased platelet aggregation and increased risk of hemorrhage, necrotizing enterocolitis, and gastric perforation. These side effects will usually disipate 72 hrs after the last dose of indomethacin	Ranges from 15–50 hrs and is partially dependent on postnatal age	Metabolized in the liver and excreted in the urine and feces	Bleeding, necrotizing enterocolitis, platelet count < 50,000 and impaired renal function Use with caution in patients with diabetes mellitus and/or insipidis as symptoms may become exaggerated. Contraindicated with recent MI, uncorrected adrenal insufficiency, thyrotoxicosis and hypersensitivity to liothyronine
Liothyronine (continued)	On the heart, increased systemic vascular resistance, and an association with increased morbidity in the postoperative period						
Prostaglandin E_1	An endogenous fatty acid indicated preoperatively to the ductus arteriosus. This is vitally important with ductal dependent lesions such as severe coarctation of the aorta, critical pulmonary stenosis, and transposition of the great arteries	0.05 mcg/kg/min may be doubled every 15–30 minutes up to a maximum dose of 0.2 mcg/kg min until desired effect is obtained. The infusion may be decreased to the lowest effective close once ductal pattency is achieved	Relatively short with immediate effects	Apnea, hypotension seizures, flushing and elevated temperature		Metabolized rapidly in the pulmonary circulation and excreted by the kidneys	

Pregnancy: C-fetal risk revealed in studies in animals but not established or not studied in humans; may use if benefits outweigh risk to fetus.

Precautions: Caution in renal and hepatic disease, gout, diabetes mellitus, and lupus erythematosus.

Drug: Spironolactone (Aldactone).

Description: Used for management of hypertension. May block effects of aldosterone on arteriolar smooth muscles.

Adult dose: 25–200 mg/d PO qd or divided bid.

Pediatric dose: 1.5–3.5 mg/kg/d PO in divided doses q6–24h.

Contraindications: Documented hypersensitivity; anuria; renal failure; hyperkalemia.

Interactions: May decrease effect of anticoagulants; potassium and potassium-sparing diuretics may increase toxicity of spironolactone.

Pregnancy: D-fetal risk shown in humans; use only if benefits outweigh risk to fetus.

Precautions: Caution in renal and hepatic impairment.

Drug: Amiloride (Midamor)

Description: l-carbonyl-guanidine unrelated chemically to other known antikaliuretic or diuretic agents. Potassium-conserving (antikaliuretic) drug that, compared with thiazide diuretics, possesses weak natriuretic, diuretic, and antihypertensive activity.

Adult dose: 5–20 mg PO qd.

Pediatric dose: Not established.

Contraindications: Documented hypersensitivity; elevated serum potassium levels > 5.5 mEq/L; impaired renal function, acute or chronic renal insufficiency, and evidence of diabetic nephropathy.

Interactions: Concomitant therapy with potassium supplementation may increase serum potassium levels (if concomitant use indicated because of demonstrated hypokalemia, use caution and monitor serum potassium frequently); lithium generally should not be administered with diuretics because may reduce renal clearance and increase risk of lithium toxicity; administration of nonsteroidal antiinflammatory agents can reduce diuretic, natriuretic, and antihypertensive effects of loop, potassium-sparing, and thiazide diuretics (when used concomitantly, observe patient closely to determine if desired effect of diuretic achieved); indomethacin and potassium-sparing diuretics including amiloride, may be associated with increased serum potassium levels, so consider potential effects on potassium kinetics and renal function.

Pregnancy: B-fetal risk not confirmed in studies in humans but has been shown in some studies in animals.

Precautions: Potassium retention associated with use of an antikaliuretic agent accentuated in presence of renal impairment and may result in rapid development of hyperkalemia; monitor serum potassium level; mild hyperkalemia usually not associated with abnormal ECG findings; monitor electrolytes closely if evidence of renal functional impairment present, BUN > 30 mg/100 mL, or serum creatinine levels >1.5 mg/100 mL.

Drug: Furosemide (lasix)

Description: Increases excretion of water by interfering with chloride-binding cotransport system, which, in turn, inhibits sodium and chloride reabsorption in ascending loop of Henle and distal renal tubule. Dose must be individualized to patient. Depending on response, administer at increments of 20–40 mg no sooner than 6–8 h after previous dose until desired diuresis occurs. When treating infants, titrate with 1-mg/kg per dose increments until satisfactory effect achieved.

Adult dose: 20–80 mg/d PO/IV/IM; titrate up to 600 mg/d for severe edematous states.

Pediatric dose: 1–2 mg/kg/dose PO; not to exceed 6 mg/kg/dose; not to administer more often than q6h Alternatively, 1 mg/kg IV/IM slowly under close supervision; not to exceed 6 mg/kg.

Contraindications: Documented hypersensitivity; hepatic coma; anuria; state of severe electrolyte depletion.

Interactions: Metformin decreases furosemide concentrations; furosemide interferes with hypoglycemic effect of antidiabetic agents and antagonizes muscle-relaxing effect of tubocurarine; auditory toxicity appears to be increased with coadministration of aminoglycosides and furosemide; hearing loss of varying degrees may occur; anticoagulant activity of warfarin may be enhanced when taken concurrently with this medication; increased plasma lithium levels and toxicity possible when taken concurrently.

Pregnancy: C-fetal risk revealed in studies in animals but not established or not studied in humans; may use if benefits outweigh risk to fetus.

Precautions: Perform frequent serum electrolyte, CO_2, glucose, creatinine, uric acid, calcium, and BUN determinations during first few mo of therapy and periodically thereafter.

Drug: Alpha1-adrenergic blockers

Selectively block postsynaptic alpha1-adrenergic receptors. Dilate arterioles and veins, thus lowering blood pressure.

Drug: Prazosin (Minipress), Terazosin (Hytrin)

Description: Prazosin treats prostatic hypertrophy. Improves urine flow rates by relaxing smooth muscle, which is caused by blocking alpha1-adrenoceptors in bladder neck and prostate. When increasing dose, administer first dose of each increment at bedtime to reduce syncopal episodes. Although doses > 20 mg/d usually do not increase efficacy, some patients may benefit from as much as 40 mg/d. Terazosin decreases arterial tone by allowing peripheral postsynaptic blockade. Has minimal alpha2 effect.

Adult dose: Prazosin: 1 mg PO bid/tid initial; 6–15 mg/d PO bid/tid maintenance. Terazosin: 1 mg PO hs; increase slowly to effect; not to exceed 20 mg/d.

Pediatric dose: Prazosin: not established; suggested dose is 0.5-7 mg PO tidTerazosin: not established.

Contraindications: Documented hypersensitivity.

Interactions: Acute postural hypotensive reaction from beta-blockers may worsen; indomethacin may decrease antihypertensive activity; verapamil may increase serum levels and may increase patient's sensitivity to drug-induced postural hypotension; may decrease anti-hypertensive effects of clonidine.

Pregnancy: C-fetal risk revealed in studies in animals but not established or not studied in humans; may use if benefits outweigh risk to fetus.

Precautions: Caution in renal impairment; may cause marked hypotension following first dose and coadministration with beta-blockers.

Drug: Beta-adrenergic blocking agents

Used to treat hypertension as initial agents or in combination with other drugs (e.g., thiazides).

Drug: Atenolol (tenormin), metoprolol (lopressor, toprol XL), propranolol (inderal), nebivolol (bystolic).

Description: Atenolol and metoprolol selectively block beta1-receptors with little or no effect on beta2 types. Propranolol is a class II antiarrhythmic, nonselective, beta-adrenergic receptor blocker with membrane-stabilizing activity that decreases automaticity of contractions. Nebivolol actions depend on metabolic factors and dose. In extensive metabolizers (majority of the population) and doses ≤10 mg, preferentially elicits beta1 selective inhibition whereas in poor metabolizers and at higher doses, inhibits both beta1- and beta2-receptors.

Adult dose: Atenolol: 50 mg PO qd; increase to 100 mg/d, if necessary. Metoprolol: 100 mg/d PO qd or divided bid/tid initial; increase at 1-wk intervals prn to a total of 450 mg/d if necessary. Propranolol: 40–80 mg PO bid initial; increase to 160–320 mg/d (may require up to 640 mg/d). Nebivolol: 5 PO qd initially if further blood pressure. reduction required after 2 wk, may increase dose at 2 wk intervals, not to exceed 40 mg/d; decrease initial dose to 2.5 mg/d for CrCl <30 mL/min and moderate hepatic impairment.

Pediatric dose: Atenolol: 1–2 mg/kg/dose PO qd Metoprolol: 1–5 mg/kg/d PO divided bid. Propranolol: 0.5 mg/kg/d PO divided bid/qid; increase gradually q3–7d; range is 2–4 mg/kg/d divided bid; not to exceed 2 mg/kg/d. Nebivolol: not established.

Contraindications: Documented hypersensitivity; congestive heart failure; pulmonary edema; cardiogenic shock; AV conduction abnormalities; heart block (without a pacemaker).

Interactions: Coadministration with aluminum salts, barbiturates, calcium salts, cholestyramine, NSAIDs, penicillins, and rifampin may decrease effects; haloperidol, hydralazine, loop diuretics, and MAOIs may increase toxicity; coadministration with myocardial depressants, AV conduction inhibitors (e.g. verapamil, diltiazem), or antiarrhythmic agents (e.g. disopyramide) may increase risk for bradycardia; if coadministered with clonidine, discontinue nebivolol several days before gradually tapering clonidine

Pregnancy: C-fetal risk revealed in studies in animals but not established or not studied in humans; may use if benefits outweigh risk to fetus.

Precautions: Beta-adrenergic blockade may reduce signs and symptoms of acute hypoglycemia and may decrease clinical signs of hyperthyroidism; abrupt withdrawal may exacerbate symptoms of hyperthyroidism including thyroid storm; monitor patient closely and withdraw drug slowly during IV administration, carefully monitor blood pressure, heart rate and ECG.

Drug: Alpha/beta-adrenergic blocking agents

Block alpha-, beta1-, and beta2-adrenergic receptor sites, thus decreasing blood pressure.

Drug: Labetalol (normodyne, trandate), carvedilol (coreg).

Description: Nonselective beta- and alpha-adrenergic blockers. Do not appear to have intrinsic sympathomimetic activity. May reduce cardiac output and decrease peripheral vascular resistance. Use in aortic dissection not advisable when titratable drugs, such as esmolol and nitroprusside, available.

Adult dose: Labetalol: 20–30 mg IV over 2 min followed by 40–80 mg at 10-min intervals; not to exceed 300 mg/dose. Carvedilol: 6.25 mg PO bid; maintain for 1–2 wk if tolerated and increase to 12.5 mg bid to maximum 25 mg bid.

Pediatric dose: Labetalol: not established; suggested dose is 0.4-1 mg/kg/h; not to exceed 3 mg/kg/h. Carvedilol: not established.

Contraindications: Documented hypersensitivity; cardiogenic shock; pulmonary edema; bradycardia; AV block; uncompensated congestive heart failure; reactive airway disease; severe bradycardia.

Interactions: Labetalol decreases effect of diuretics and increases toxicity of methotrexate, lithium and salicylates; may diminish reflex tachycardia resulting from nitroglycerin use without interfering with hypotensive effects; cimetidine may increase labetalol and carvedilol blood levels; glutethimide may decrease labetalol effects by inducing microsomal enzymes; rifampin, barbiturates, cholestyramine, colestipol, NSAIDs, salicylates, and penicillins may decrease carvedilol effects; carvedilol may increase effects of antidiabetic agents, digoxin, and calcium channel blockers; concurrent administration with clonidine may increase blood pressure and decrease heart rate; carvedilol may decrease effect of sulfonylureas; fluoxetine, paroxetine, and propafenone may increase carvedilol levels

Pregnancy: C-fetal risk revealed in studies in animals but not established or not studied in humans; may use if benefits outweigh risk to fetus.

Precautions: Caution in impaired hepatic function; discontinue therapy if signs of liver dysfunction present; in elderly patients, a lower response rate and higher incidence of toxicity may be observed; caution in congestive heart failure being treated with digitalis, diuretics, or ACE inhibitors (AV conduction may be slowed); caution in peripheral vascular disease, hyperthyroidism, and diabetes mellitus.

Drug category: Peripheral vasodilators
Relax blood vessels to improve blood flow, thus decreasing blood pressure.

Drug: Hydralazine (apresoline), minoxidil (rogaine loniten)

Description: Hydralazine decreases systemic resistance through direct vasodilation of arterioles. Minoxidil relaxes arteriolar smooth muscle, causing vasodilation, which, in turn, may reduce blood pressure.

Adult dose: Hydralazine: 10–20 mg/dose IV/IM q 4–6h prn initial; increase to 40 mg/dose if necessary; change to PO as soon as possible. Minoxidil: 5 mg PO qd; increase gradually q3d; 10–40 mg/d PO qd or divided bid maintenance; not to exceed 100 mg/d.

Pediatric dose: Not established.

Contraindications: Documented hypersensitivity; mitral valve, rheumatic heart disease (hydralazine); pheochromocytoma (minoxidil).

Interactions: MAOIs and beta-blockers may increase hydralazine toxicity; pharmacologic effects of hydralazine may be decreased by indomethacin; concurrent use of minoxidil with guanethidine, diuretics, or hypotensive agents may result in additive hypotension.

Pregnancy: C-fetal risk revealed in studies in animals but not established or not studied in humans; may use if benefits outweigh risk to fetus.

Precautions: Hydralazine has been implicated in MI; minoxidil may exacerbate angina pectoris; caution in pulmonary hypertension, congestive heart failure, coronary artery disease, and significant renal failure.

Drug category: Calcium channel blockers
May be a more effective class of medication for black patients.

Drug: Diltiazem (cardizem, dilacor), verapamil (calan, covera-HS), nifedipine (adalat).

Description: During depolarization, inhibits calcium ion from entering slow channels or voltage-sensitive areas of vascular smooth muscle and myocardium.

Adult dose: Diltiazem: cardizem SR: 60–120 mg PO bid. Cardizem CD: 180–240 mg PO qd.

Hypertension: 180–240 mg PO qd. Angina: 120 mg/d PO; titrate slowly over 7–14 d up to 480 mg/d prn; not to exceed 540 mg/d. Verapamil: 240–480 mg/d PO divided tid/qid. Nifedipine: 10–30 mg IR cap PO tid; not to exceed 120–180 mg/d 30–60 mg SR tab PO qd; not to exceed 90–120 mg/d.

Pediatric dose: Diltiazem: not established. Verapamil: Not established. Nifedipine: 0.25–0.5 mg/kg/dose PO tid/qid prn.

Contraindications: Documented hypersensitivity; severe CHF; sick sinus syndrome; second- or third-degree AV block; hypotension (<90 mmHg systolic).

Interactions: May increase carbamazepine, digoxin, cyclosporine, and theophylline levels; when administered with amiodarone, may cause bradycardia and a decrease in cardiac output; when administered with beta-blockers, may increase cardiac depression; cimetidine may increase levels.

Pregnancy: C-fetal risk revealed in studies in animals but not established or not studied in humans; may use if benefits outweigh risk to fetus.

Precautions: Caution in impaired renal or hepatic function; may increase LFTs, and hepatic injury may occur; nifedipine may cause lower extremity edema.

Drug category: Angiotensin-converting enzyme (ACE) inhibitors
Competitive inhibitors of ACE. Reduces angiotensin II levels, thus decreasing aldosterone secretion.

Drug: Captopril (capoten), enalapril (vasotec), lisinopril (zestril), ramipril (altace).

Description: Prevents conversion of angiotensin I to angiotensin II, a potent vasoconstrictor, resulting in lower aldosterone secretion.

Adult dose: Captopril: 12.5–25 mg PO bid/tid; may increase by 12.5–25 mg/dose at 1- to 2-wk intervals up to 50 mg tid. Enalapril: 2.5–5 mg/d PO (increase as necessary); range is 10–40 mg/d PO in 1–2 divided doses 1.25 mg/dose IV over 5 min q6h. Lisinopril: 10 mg/d PO; increase 5–10 mg/d at 1- to 2-wk intervals; not to exceed 40 mg. Ramipril: 2.5–5 mg PO qd; not to exceed 20 mg/d.

Pediatric dose: Captopril: 6.25–12.5 mg/dose PO q 12–24 h; not to exceed 6 mg/kg/d. Enalapril: not established. Lisinopril: not established. Ramipril: not established.

Contraindications: Documented hypersensitivity; history of angioedema.

Interactions: NSAIDs may reduce hypotensive effects; ACE inhibitors may increase digoxin, lithium, and allopurinol levels; rifampin decreases levels; probenecid may increase levels; hypotensive effects of ACE inhibitors may be enhanced when administered concurrently with diuretics.

Pregnancy: C-fetal risk revealed in studies in animals but not established or not studied in humans; may use if benefits outweigh risk to fetus.

Precautions: Category D in second and third trimester of pregnancy; caution in renal impairment, valvular stenosis, or severe congestive heart failure.

Drug category: Angiotensin II receptor antagonists. For patients unable to tolerate ACE inhibitors.

Drug: Losartan (cozaar), valsartan (diovan).

Description: Nonpeptide angiotensin II receptor antagonists that block vasoconstrictor and aldosterone-secreting effects of angiotensin II. May induce more complete inhibition of renin-angiotensin system than ACE inhibitors, do not affect response to bradykinin, and are less likely to be associated with cough and angioedema.

Adult dose: Losartan: 25–100 mg PO qd/bid. Valsartan: 80 mg/d PO; may increase to 160 mg/d if needed.

Pediatric dose: Not established.

Contraindications: Documented hypersensitivity.

Interactions: Ketoconazole, troleandomycin, sulfaphenazole, and phenobarbital may decrease effects; cimetidine may increase effects.

Pregnancy: C-fetal risk revealed in studies in animals but not established or not studied in humans; may use if benefits outweigh risk to fetus.

Precautions: Category D in second and third trimester of pregnancy; caution in unilateral or bilateral renal artery stenosis, severe hepatic insufficiency, biliary cirrhosis or obstruction, primary hyperaldosteronism, and hyperkalemia.

Drug: Eprosartan (teveten), olmesartan (benicar).

Description: Angiotensin receptor antagonist that binds to AT1 angiotensin II receptor, blocking vasoconstrictor and aldosterone-secreting effects of angiotensin II. May induce a more complete inhibition of renin-angiotensin system than ACE inhibitors and do not affect response to bradykinin and, thus, is less likely to be associated with cough and angioedema. For patients unable to tolerate ACE inhibitors.

Adult dose: Eprosartan (teveten): 400–800 mg PO qd or divided bid. Olmesartan (benicar): 20 mg PO qd initially; may increase to 40 mg/d after 2 wk if further BP reduction required. Note: lower dose in volume- or salt-depleted patients.

Pediatric dose: Not established.

Contraindications: Documented hypersensitivity; bilateral renal artery stenosis and preexisting renal insufficiency; significant aortic/mitral stenosis.

Interactions: May increase toxicity of lithium; may decrease angiotensin II antagonist efficacy; may increase risk of hyperkalemia if taken concurrently with potassium supplements.

Pregnancy: C-fetal risk revealed in studies in animals but not established or not studied in humans; may use if benefits outweigh risk to fetus.

Precautions: Pregnancy category D in second and third trimester of pregnancy; avoid use or use lower dose in patients who are volume depleted (correct volume depletion first); renal deterioration can occur with initiation of therapy; caution in unilateral renal artery stenosis and preexisting renal insufficiency; caution in aortic/mitral stenosis.

Drug category: Aldosterone antagonists

Compete with aldosterone receptor sites, reducing blood pressure and sodium reabsorption.

Drug: Eplerenone (INSPRA).

Description: Selectively blocks aldosterone at the mineralocorticoid receptors in epithelial (e.g. kidney) and nonepithelial (e.g. heart, blood vessels, brain) tissues, thus decreasing blood pressure and sodium reabsorption.

Adult dose: 50 mg PO qd; may increase dose after 4 wk, not to exceed 100 mg/d.

Pediatric dose: Not established.

Contraindications: Documented hypersensitivity; hyperkalemia or coadministration with drugs causing increased potassium; type 2 diabetes with microalbuminuria; moderate-to-severe renal insufficiency [i.e. CrCl < 50 mL/min or serum creatinine >2 mg/dL (males) or > 1.8 mg/dL (females)].

Interactions: CYP450 3A4 substrate; potent CYP3A4 inhibitors (e.g. ketoconazole) increase serum levels about fivefold, less potent CYP3A4 inhibitors (e.g. erythromycin, saquinavir, verapamil, fluconazole) increase serum levels about twofold; grapefruit juice increases serum levels about 25%; coadministration with potassium supplements, salt substitutes, or drugs known to increase serum potassium (e.g. amiloride, spironolactone, triamterene, ACE inhibitors, angiotensin II inhibitors) increases risk of hyperkalemia.

Pregnancy: B-fetal risk not confirmed in studies in humans but has been shown in some studies in animals.

Precautions: May cause hyperkalemia, headache, or dizziness; caution with hepatic insufficiency.

Drug category: Alpha-adrenergic agonists.

Stimulate presynaptic alpha2-adrenergic receptors in the brain stem which reduces sympathetic nervous activity.

Drug: Methyldopa (aldomet).

Description: Stimulates central alpha-adrenergic receptors by a false transmitter, resulting in decreased sympathetic outflow. This results in inhibition of vasoconstriction.

Adult dose: 250 mg PO bid/tid; increase q2d prn; not to exceed 3 g/d.

Pediatric dose: 10 mg/kg/d PO divided bid/qid; increase q2d prn to maximum 65 mg/kg/d; not to exceed 3 g/d.

Contraindications: Documented hypersensitivity; acute liver disease.

Interactions: Effects may decrease with concurrent administration of barbiturates and tricyclic antidepressants; increase in blood pressure may occur with coadministration of iron supplements, MAOIs, sympathomimetics, phenothiazines and beta-blockers.

Pregnancy: C-fetal risk revealed in studies in animals but not established or not studied in humans; may use if benefits outweigh risk to fetus.

Precautions: Caution in previous history of liver disease; hemolytic anemia and liver disease may occur; reduce dose in renal disease.

Table 3: *Medications for pediatric resuscitation and arrhythmias*

Medication	*Dose*	*Remarks*
Adenosine	0.1 mg/kg (maximum 6 mg) Repeat: 0.2 mg/kg (maximum 12 mg)	Monitor ECG Rapid IV/IO bolus
Amiodarone	5 mg/kg IV/IO; repeat up to 15 mg/kg Maximum: 300 mg	Monitor ECG and blood pressure Adjust administration rate to urgency (give more slowly when perfusing rhythm present) Use caution when administering with other drugs that prolong QT (consider expert consultation)
Atropine	0.02 mg/kg IV/IO 0.03 mg/kg ET* Repeat once if needed Minimum dose: 0.1 mg Maximum single dose Child 0.5 mg Adolescent 1 mg	Higher doses may be used with organophosphate poisoning
Calcium chloride (10%)	20 mg/kg IV/IO (0.2 mL/kg)	Slowly
Epinephrine	0.01 mg/kg (0.1 mL/kg 1:10,000) IV/IO 0.1 mg/kg (0.1/kg 1:1,000) ET* Maximum dose: 1 mg IV/IO; 10 mg ET	Adult dose: 5–10 mL
Glucose	0.5–1 g/kg IV/IO	D10W: 5–10 mL/kg D25W: 2–4 mL/kg D50W: 1–2 mL/kg
Lidocaine	Bolus: 1 mg/kg IV/IO Maximum dose: 100 mg Infusion: 20–50 1/4 g/kg per minute ET*: 2–3 mg	
Magnesium sulfate	25–50 mg/kg IV/IO over 10–20 min faster in torsades Maximum dose: 2 g	
Naloxone	< 5 y or 20 kg: 0.1 mg/kg IV/IO/ET* 5 y or > 20 kg: 2 mg IV/IO/ET*	Use lower doses to reverse respiratory depression associated with therapeutic opioid use (1–15 1/4 g/kg)
Procainamide	15 mg/kg IV/IO over 30–60 min Adult dose: 20 mg/min IV infusion upto total maximum dose 17 mg/kg	Monitor ECG and blood pressure Use caution when administering with other drugs that prolong QT (consider expert consultation)
Sodium bicarbonate	1 mEq/kg per dose IV/IO slowly	After adequate ventilation

IV indicates intravenous; IO intraosseous; and ET, via endotracheal tube.
*Flush with 5 mL of normal saline and follow with 5 ventilations.

Drug: Clonidine (catapres)

Description: Stimulates alpha2-adrenoreceptors in brain stem, activating an inhibitory neuron, which, in turn, results in reduced sympathetic outflow. These effects result in a decrease in vasomotor tone and heart rate.

Adult dose: 0.1 mg PO bid initial; 0.2–1.2 mg/d divided bid/qid maintenance; not to exceed 1.2 mg/d.

Pediatric dose: Not established.

Contraindications: Documented hypersensitivity.

Interactions: Tricyclic antidepressants inhibit hypotensive effects of clonidine; coadministration of clonidine with beta-blockers may potentiate bradycardia; tricyclic antidepressants may enhance hypertensive response associated with abrupt clonidine withdrawal; hypotensive effects of clonidine are enhanced by narcotic analgesics.

Pregnancy: C-fetal risk revealed in studies in animals but not established or not studied in humans; may use if benefits outweigh risk to fetus.

Precautions: Caution in cerebrovascular disease, coronary insufficiency, sinus node dysfunction and renal impairment.

Drug category: Renin inhibitor

Newest class of antihypertensive drugs. Acts by disrupting the renin-angiotensin-aldosterone system feedback loop.

Drug: Aliskiren (tekturna)

Description: Direct renin inhibitor. Decreases plasma renin activity and inhibits conversion of angiotensinogen to angiotensin I (as a result, also decreasing angiotensin II) and, thereby, disrupts the renin-angiotensin-aldosterone system (RAAS) feedback loop. Indicated for hypertension as monotherapy or in combination with other antihypertensive drugs.

Adult dose: 150 mg PO qd initially; if needed, may increase to 300 mg/d.

Pediatric dose: <18 years: not established.

Contraindications: Documented hypersensitivity.

Interactions: Coadministration with irbesartan decreases C_{max} by 50%; coadministration with atorvastatin increases C_{max} and AUC by 50%; ketoconazole increases plasma levels by about 80%; does not inhibit CYP450 isoenzymes or induce CYP3A4; coadministration with furosemide decreases furosemide C_{max} and AUC by 30% and 50%, respectively; high-fat meals substantially decrease absorption; use with maximal dose of ACE inhibitors has not been studied.

Pregnancy: D-fetal risk shown in humans; use only if benefits outweigh risk to fetus.

Precautions: Discontinue use in pregnancy as soon as possible because use of drugs affecting the renin-angiotensin system during second and third trimesters has been associated with fetal and neonatal injury including hypotension, neonatal skull hypoplasia, anuria, renal failure, and fetal death; may cause angioedema; dose-related GI adverse effects may occur.

Drug category: Anticoagulants

Unfractionated IV heparin and fractionated low molecular weight SC heparins are the two choices for initial anticoagulation therapy. Warfarin therapy may be initiated after 1–3 days of effective heparinization.

Drug: Heparin.

Description: Usually administered as CIV infusion for the treatment of acute thrombosis. For prevention of thrombosis, unfractionated heparin is administered SC.

Adult dose: Initial dose: 80 U/kg IV bolus. Maintenance: 18 U/kg/h CIV infusion (See discussion under introduction to medications section regarding target aPTT and dose monitoring).

Pediatric dose: Administer as in adults.

Contraindications: Documented hypersensitivity; subacute bacterial endocarditis; active bleeding; history of heparin-induced thrombocytopenia; relative contraindications include recent surgery (especially ocular and neurosurgical procedures) and hereditary bleeding disorders.

Interactions: Digoxin, nicotine, tetracycline, and antihistamines may decrease effects; NSAIDs, aspirin, dextran, dipyridamole, and hydroxychloroquine may increase heparin toxicity.

Pregnancy: B-fetal risk not confirmed in studies in humans but has been shown in some studies in animals.

Precautions: Bleeding is most frequent complication; occurrence of thrombocytopenia during heparin therapy may indicate onset of heparin immune reaction, termed heparin-induced thrombocytopenia (HIT); syndrome can be life-threatening and can be associated with new-onset paradoxical arterial or venous thrombosis; elevations of liver enzymes have been observed during heparin therapy; heparin is not indicated for IM injection; IM medications should be administered by alternate route; in neonates, preservative-free heparin is recommended to avoid possible toxicity (gasping syndrome) by benzyl alcohol, which is used as preservative; caution in severe hypotension and shock.

Drug: Enoxaparin (lovenox).

Description: Enhances inhibition of factor Xa and thrombin by increasing antithrombin III activity. In addition, preferentially increases inhibition of factor Xa. Average duration of treatment is 7–14 d.

Adult dose: Treatment of established DVT with or without PE: 1 mg/kg SC q12h can be administered in the hospital or in an outpatient setting under supervision. Alternatively, 1.5 mg/kg SC once qd, administered at same time qd is approved for in-hospital treatment of DVT without symptomatic PE. Prevention of DVT: 30 mg SC q12h or 40 mg qd. These two regimens differ by indication, i.e. hip replacement versus knee surgery, and in use as extended prophylaxis; in acutely ill patients at high risk for DVT/PE, a dose of 40 mg SC once qd has reported efficacy.

Pediatric dose: Not established. Suggested dose: 0.75 mg/kg/dose SC bid for <2 mo; 0.5 mg/kg/dose SC bid if > 2 mo.

Contraindications: Documented hypersensitivity; major bleeding; thrombocytopenia.

Interactions: Platelet inhibitors or oral anticoagulants (e.g. dipyridamole, salicylates, aspirin, NSAIDs, sulfinpyrazone, ticlopidine) may increase risk of bleeding.

Pregnancy: B-fetal risk not confirmed in studies in humans but has been shown in some studies in animals.

Precautions: LMWH is cleared by renal mechanisms; LMWHs should be used with caution, if at all, in patients with renal impairment (i.e. CrCl <30 mL/min); if thromboembolic event occurs despite LMWH prophylaxis, discontinue drug and initiate alternate therapy; elevation of hepatic transaminases may occur but is reversible; heparin-associated thrombocytopenia may occur with fractionated LMWHs; 1 mg of protamine sulfate reverses effect of approximately 1 mg of enoxaparin if significant bleeding complications develop; however, protamine sulfate provides incomplete reversal of the anti-Xa effect of LMWHs including Lovenox. LMWHs are safe and effective in preventing or treating thrombosis during pregnancy; prophylactic regimens are preferred in patients with no history of thrombosis; guidelines for the use of LMWHs in pregnancy are still formative; some authors recommend monitoring LMWH blood levels to maintain trough anti-Xa activity of 0.15–0.2 U/mL and 2 h postinjection peak levels of 0.4–0.6 U/mL; levels are checked monthly during pregnancy; most women may require dosage increase at 20.5 wk gestation (SD 8.2 wk); in women with prosthetic valves, heparin use during pregnancy presents additional challenges and extreme caution with close monitoring is needed; reports exist of thrombosis of cardiac valves while on usual doses of LMWH; this is an evolving field and clinical trials are required to determine optimal dosage and safety in this setting; recommended to continue treatment with LMWH for 4–6 wk postpartum. Cases of epidural hematoma have been described following epidural/spinal anesthesia and concomitant LMWH heparin administration; these events occurred with prophylactic doses of LMWH; risk of hematoma is increased by indwelling catheters, concomitant NSAID use, and traumatic or repeated epidural or spinal puncture; current guidelines suggest LMWH therapy be started 24 h after epidural anesthesia; epidural catheter removal should be: (1) > 2 h before first dose of LMWH or (2) no less than 12 h after the last dose of LMWH.

Drug: Dalteparin (fragmin)

Description: Enhances inhibition of factor Xa and thrombin by increasing antithrombin III activity. In addition, preferentially increases inhibition of factor Xa. Average duration of treatment is 7–14 d.

Adult dose: 2,500–5,000 U SC qd for prevention of DVT; current recommended dose in patients undergoing abdominal surgery is 2,500 U SC qd.

Pediatric dose: Not established.

Contraindications: Documented hypersensitivity; major bleeding; thrombocytopenia.

Interactions: Platelet inhibitors or oral anticoagulants, such as dipyridamole, salicylates, aspirin, NSAIDs, sulfinpyrazone and ticlopidine, may increase risk of bleeding.

Pregnancy: C-fetal risk revealed in studies in animals but not established or not studied in humans; may use if benefits outweigh risk to fetus.

Precautions: LMWH is cleared by renal mechanisms; LMWHs should be used with caution, if at all, in patients with renal impairment (i.e. CrCl <30 mL/min); if thromboembolic event occurs despite LMWH prophylaxis, discontinue drug and initiate alternate therapy; elevation of hepatic transaminases may occur but is reversible; heparin-associated thrombocytopenia may occur with fractionated LMWHs; 1 mg of protamine sulfate reverses effect of approximately 1 mg of enoxaparin if significant bleeding complications develop; however, protamine sulfate provides incomplete reversal of the anti-Xa effect of LMWHs including Fragmin. Cases of epidural hematoma have been described following epidural/spinal anesthesia and concomitant LMWH administration; these events occurred with prophylactic doses of LMWH; the risk of hematoma is increased by indwelling catheters, concomitant NSAID use, and traumatic or repeated epidural or spinal puncture; current guidelines suggest LMWH therapy be started 24 h after epidural anesthesia; epidural catheter removal should be (1) >2 h before the first dose of LMWH or (2) no less than 12 h after the last dose LMWH.

Drug: Fondaparinux sodium (arixtra).

Description: Only synthetic compound in this class of LMW heparins. This compound is a novel pentasaccharide capable of inhibiting factor Xa via the action of antithrombin (AT) but devoid of anti-factor IIa (thrombin) activity. Interestingly, this compound does not appear to cross-react with HIT antibodies. Approved for use in hip fracture surgery, knee replacement surgery, and hip replacement surgery. Only FDA-approved anticoagulant drug for hip fracture surgery. Also used and approved for extended prophylactic dosing for 21 d following hip fracture surgery.

Adult dose: Symptomatic DVT and acute symptomatic PE:<50 kg BW: 5 mg SC qd for 5 d50–100 kg BW: 7.5 mg SC qd for 5 d>100 kg BW: 10 mg SC qd for 5d. Treatment should be continued until therapeutic oral anticoagulant effect is established (INR 2-3) with at least two determinations. For prophylaxis of VTE: 2.5 mg SC qd; initial dose recommended to be given 6–8 h following surgery, after hemostasis established; administration <6 h after surgery associated with increased risk of major bleeding.

Pediatric dose: Not established.

Contraindications: Documented hypersensitivity; seriously impaired kidney function or patients who weigh <110 lb; patients given spinal anesthesia or spinal puncture; major bleeding; thrombocytopenia.

Interactions: None reported; increased risk of bleeding possible with concurrent administration of platelet inhibitors, oral anticoagulants, or thrombolytic agents.

Pregnancy: C-Fetal risk revealed in studies in animals but not established or not studied in humans; may use if benefits outweigh risk to fetus.

Precautions: When spinal anesthesia or spinal puncture used, blood clot in spine may develop, which can result in long-term or permanent paralysis (holding 2 doses prior to LP or surgery is recommended); major bleeding risk increased when initiated before 6 h following surgery; elimination decreased in elderly persons and in those with renal impairment. Use caution in patients with severe renal impairment (i.e. CrCl <30 mL/min); if thromboembolic event occurs despite LMWH prophylaxis, discontinue drug and initiate alternate therapy; elevation of hepatic transaminases may occur but is reversible; no known antidote exists for this drug. Protamine sulfate does not appear to reverse effect of this compound; if significant bleeding complications develop; some authors have recommended the use of recombinant factor VIIa as a means of hemostasis. Cases of epidural hematoma have been described following epidural/spinal anesthesia and concomitant LMWH administration; these events occurred with prophylactic doses of LMWH; risk of hematoma is increased by indwelling catheters, concomitant NSAID use, and traumatic or repeated epidural or spinal puncture; current guidelines suggest LMWH therapy be started 24 h after epidural anesthesia; epidural catheter removal should be (1) >2 h before first dose of LMWH or (2) no less than 12 h after last dose of LMWH.

Drug: Tinzaparin (innohep).

Description: Enhances inhibition of factor Xa and thrombin by increasing antithrombin III activity. In addition, preferentially increases inhibition of factor Xa. Average duration of treatment is 7–14 d.

Adult dose: 175 U/kg SC qd, at same time qd, for treatment of DVT/PE.

Pediatric dose: Not established; adult dose suggested.

Contraindications: Documented hypersensitivity; major bleeding; thrombocytopenia.

Interactions: Platelet inhibitors or oral anticoagulants, such as dipyridamole, salicylates, aspirin, NSAIDs, sulfinpyrazone, and ticlopidine, may increase risk of bleeding.

Pregnancy: B-fetal risk not confirmed in studies in humans but has been shown in some studies in animals.

Precautions: LMWH is cleared by renal mechanisms; LMWHs should be used with caution, if at all, in patients with renal impairment (i.e. CrCl <30 mL/min); if thromboembolic event occurs despite LMWH prophylaxis, discontinue drug and initiate alternate therapy; elevation of hepatic transaminases may occur but is reversible; heparin-associated thrombocytopenia may occur with fractionated LMWHs; 1 mg of protamine sulfate reverses effect of approximately 1 mg of enoxaparin if significant bleeding complications develop; however, protamine sulfate provides incomplete reversal of anti-Xa effect of LMWHs including Lovenox. Cases of epidural hematoma have been described following epidural/spinal anesthesia and concomitant LMWH administration; these events occurred with prophylactic doses of LMWH; the risk of hematoma is increased by indwelling catheters, concomitant NSAID use, and traumatic or repeated epidural or spinal puncture; current guidelines suggest LMWH therapy be started 24 h after epidural anesthesia; epidural catheter removal should be (1) >2 h before the first dose of LMWH or (2) no less than 12 h after the last dose of LMWH.

Drug: Warfarin (coumadin).

Description: Oral anticoagulant that antagonizes action of vitamin K in normal synthesis of clotting factors II, VII, IX, and X. Safe and effective for long-term oral management of thrombotic disorders. See articles on deep venous thrombosis or pulmonary embolism (discussed in Treatment section) for additional details on dosing and monitoring of warfarin. Therapy is initiated without a loading dose at a dose range of 5–10 mg qd for 70 kg adult. Monitor PT/INR daily during initiation of therapy to measure anticoagulation effect. After initial 5–10 d and stabilization of warfarin dose, measure PT/INR 2–3 times qwk for 2–4 wk, then monthly thereafter.

Adult dose: 5–10 mg PO qd; adjust dose according to desired INR.

Pediatric dose: 0.05–0.34 mg/kg/d PO qd; adjust dose according to desired INR.

Contraindications: Documented hypersensitivity; severe liver or kidney disease; open wounds or GI ulcers.

Interactions: Drugs that may decrease anticoagulant effects include griseofulvin, carbamazepine, glutethimide, estrogens, nafcillin, phenytoin, rifampin, barbiturates, cholestyramine, colestipol, vitamin K, spironolactone, oral contraceptives, and sucralfate; medications that may increase anticoagulant effects include oral antibiotics, phenylbutazone, salicylates, sulfonamides, chloral hydrate, clofibrate, diazoxide, anabolic steroids, ketoconazole, ethacrynic acid, miconazole, nalidixic acid, sulfonylureas, allopurinol, chloramphenicol, cimetidine, disulfiram, metronidazole, phenylbutazone, phenytoin, propoxyphene, sulfonamides, gemfibrozil, acetaminophen, and sulindac.

Pregnancy: D-fetal risk shown in humans; use only if benefits outweigh risk to fetus.

Precautions: Contraindicated in first trimester; warfarin skin necrosis (see Medical/Legal Pitfalls); do not switch brands after achieving therapeutic response; caution in active tuberculosis or diabetes; patients with protein C or S deficiency are at risk of developing skin necrosis.

Drug category: Antiplatelet agents—these agents prevent formation of thrombi associated with MI and inhibit platelet function by blocking aggregation. Antiplatelet therapy has been shown to reduce mortality by reducing the risk of fatal MIs, fatal strokes and vascular death. Pooled data from over 2,000 patients revealed reduction of death or MI from 11.8% to 6% with aspirin in cases of unstable angina. A recent randomized clinical trial involving 12,562 patients showed a reduction of cardiovascular death, MI, or stroke from 11.4% to 9.3% by adding clopidogrel to aspirin therapy.

Drug: Aspirin (anacin, bayer buffered aspirin, ecotrin)—administer as soon as possible. Inhibits cyclo-oxygenase, which produces thromboxane A2, a potent platelet activator. Early administration has been shown to reduce mortality.

Adult dose: 160–324 mg PO qd.

Pediatric dose: Not established.

Contraindications: Documented hypersensitivity; liver damage; hypoprothrombinemia; vitamin K deficiency; bleeding disorders; asthma; patients <16 y with influenza (because of association of aspirin with Reye syndrome).

Interactions: Effects may decrease with antacids and urinary alkalinizers; corticosteroids decrease salicylate serum levels; additive hypoprothrombinemic effects and increased bleeding time may occur with coadministration of anticoagulants; may antagonize uricosuric effects of probenecid and increase toxicity of phenytoin and valproic acid; doses > 2 g/d may potentiate glucose-lowering effect of sulfonylurea drugs.

Pregnancy: D-unsafe in pregnancy.

Precautions: May cause transient decrease in renal function and aggravate chronic renal disease; avoid use in patients with severe anemia, those with history of blood coagulation defects, or those taking anticoagulants.

Drug: Clopidogrel (plavix)—selectively inhibits adenosine diphosphate (ADP) binding to platelet receptor and subsequent ADP-mediated activation of glycoprotein llb/llla complex, thereby inhibiting platelet aggregation.

This agent is used as an alternative to aspirin or in addition to aspirin after coronary stenting (CAPRIE Steering Committee, 1996 #158). The recently concluded randomized clinical trial clopidogrel in unstable angina to prevent recurrent events (CURE) showed an absolute risk reduction in cardiac death, MI, or stroke of 2.1% (11.4% down to 9.3% at 1-y) at the cost of increased major bleeding by 1.0% (3.7% versus 2.7%).

Adult dose: CURE protocol for unstable angina patients within 24 h of symptom onset: 300 mg loading dose PO followed by 75 mg PO qd for 3–12 mo (mean = 9 mo) in conjunction with aspirin 75–325 mg/d PO.

Pediatric dose: Not established.

Contraindications: Documented hypersensitivity; active pathological bleeding, such as peptic ulcer, or intracranial hemorrhage.

Interactions: Coadministration with naproxen is associated with increased occult GI blood loss; clopidogrel prolongs bleeding time; safety of coadministration with warfarin not established.

Pregnancy: C-safety for use during pregnancy has not been established.

Precautions: Caution in patients at increased risk of bleeding from trauma, surgery, or other pathological conditions; caution in patients with lesions with propensity to bleed (e.g. ulcers).

Drug category: HMG-CoA reductase inhibitors used to treat hypercholesterolemia. Highly efficacious and very well tolerated.

Drug: Atorvastatin (lipitor) can provide up to 60% reduction in LDL-C. Inhibits 3-hydroxy-3-methylglutaryl coenzyme A (HMG-CoA reductase), which in turn inhibits cholesterol synthesis and increases cholesterol metabolism. The half-life of atorvastatin and active metabolites is longer than that of all the other statins (i.e. approximately 48 h compared to 3–4 h). The myocardial ischemia reduction with aggressive cholesterol lowering (MIRACL) randomized clinical trial randomized 3,086 patients with unstable angina to high-dose atorvastatin versus placebo. Therapy resulted in a reduction in the primary end-point (i.e., death, MI, resuscitated cardiac arrest, severe recurrent symptomatic ischemia) from 17.4% to 14.8% (P = .048) within a relatively short period of 4 mo. The benefit was mostly for recurrent symptomatic ischemia with objective evidence and requiring emergency rehospitalization (8.4% down to 6.2%, P = .02).

Adult dose: 10 mg PO qd in the evening; titrate to a maximum 80 mg/d prn. MIRACL protocol: 80 mg PO qd commenced within 1–4 d after admission for unstable angina, continue for at least 16 wk.

Pediatric dose: Not established.

Contraindications: Documented hypersensitivity; significant hepatic impairment; pregnancy; breastfeeding.

Interactions: Toxicity increases when coadministered with triazole antifungals, CNS depressants, macrolide antibiotics, and mibefradil; atorvastatin increases the action of anticoagulants and levothyroxine.

Pregnancy: Contraindicated in pregnancy.

Precautions: Thirty-one cases of rhabdomyolysis (out of 1.33 million total prescriptions) were reported in Canada, resulting in 1 death associated with concomitant use of gemfibrozil, a fibric acid derivative; concomitant use with nicotinic acid (niacin) also advised. Stop drug use or decrease doses for elevations of transaminases more than 3 times the upper limit of the reference range; elevations generally resolve upon withdrawal of drug; if symptoms of myopathy and rhabdomyolysis occur, stop the drug and obtain a CKDo not exceed daily dose; caution in patients receiving drugs that prolong QRS or Q-T interval; monitor transaminase levels before treatment, at 6 wk and 12 wk, then q6mo.

Drug category: Glycoprotein IIb/IIIa receptor antagonists Up to 80,000 copies of these integrins on the platelet cell surface serve as ligands for fibrinogen cross-linkage, the final common pathway for platelet aggregation and thrombus formation, even under arterial shear stress conditions. To date, more than 40,000 patients have been enrolled in randomized clinical trials evaluating glycoprotein IIb/IIIa antagonists in ACS. These trials have shown 30 day relative risk reductions of 22–56% in composite end-points, with beneficial trends in each of the component outcomes, largely in association with percutaneous coronary intervention.

Drug: Tirofiban (aggrastat)—nonpeptide antagonist of platelet GP IIb/IIIa receptor that reversibly prevents von Willebrand factor, fibrinogen, and other adhesion ligands from binding to the GP IIb/IIIa receptor, thereby inhibiting platelet aggregation. Effects persist over the duration of maintenance infusion and are reversed after stopping the infusion. Approved by the FDA for use in combination with heparin for patients with ACS who are being managed medically and for those undergoing PCI. Dose should be halved in patients with severe renal insufficiency (CrCl <30 mL/min).

Adult dose: 0.4 mcg/kg/min IV for 30 min, followed by 0.1 mcg/kg/min for up to 72 h. If CrCl <30 mL/min, then reduce dose by 50%.

Pediatric dose: Not established.

Contraindications: Documented hypersensitivity; severe hypertension (systolic BP >200 mmHg); active internal bleeding; history of intracranial hemorrhage, intracranial neoplasm, arteriovenous malformation, or aneurysm; acute pericarditis; bleeding diathesis; trauma or stroke within previous 30 d; platelet count <100,000/mm^3; history of thrombocytopenia following exposure to this product; serum creatinine >2 mg/dL (for 180 mcg/kg bolus and 2 mcg/kg/min infusion) or > 4 mg/dL (for 135 mcg/kg bolus and 0.5 mcg/kg/min infusion); history of bleeding diathesis within 30 d; intracranial hemorrhage; history of hemorrhagic stroke; severe hypertension (systolic BP >200 mmHg or diastolic BP >110 mmHg); major surgical procedure within past mo.

Interactions: Possible increased risk of bleeding with coadministration of heparin or aspirin; closely monitor when using concurrently with drugs that affect hemostasis (e.g., warfarin)

Pregnancy: B-usually safe but benefits must outweigh the risks.

Precautions: Bleeding events are the most common complications encountered during therapy with eptifibatide; caution with platelet count <150,000/mm^3 and hemorrhagic retinopathy; prior to treatment, monitor platelet counts, serum creatinine, hemoglobin, hematocrit, and PT/aPTT within 6 h after loading infusion and at least daily thereafter (more frequently if evidence of significant decline); because these agents inhibit platelet aggregation, caution when using concurrently with drugs that affect hemostasis (e.g. thrombolytics, ticlopidine, NSAIDs, warfarin, dipyridamole, clopidogrel); measure ACT and maintain aPTT 50–70 seconds unless a PCI needs to be performed; maintain ACT 300–350 seconds during PCI; if platelet count decreases to <100,000/mm^3, perform additional platelet counts to exclude pseudothrombocytopenia; if thrombocytopenia is confirmed, discontinue GP IIb/IIIa inhibitors and heparin and appropriately monitor and treat the condition; to monitor unfractionated heparin, monitor aPTT 6 h after beginning heparin infusion; adjust to maintain aPTT higher than 2 times baseline.

Drug: Eptifibatide (integrilin)—cyclic heptapeptide antagonist of the platelet GP IIb/IIIa receptor that reversibly prevents von Willebrand factor, fibrinogen, and other adhesion ligands from binding to the GP IIb/IIIa receptor, thereby inhibiting platelet aggregation. Effects persist over duration of maintenance infusion and are reversed when infusion ends. Approved by the FDA for use in combination with heparin for patients with ACS, patients who are being managed medically, and for those undergoing PCI.

Adult dose: Unstable angina: 180 mcg/kg IV bolus, followed by continuous infusion of 2 mcg/kg/min for up to 72 h. Undergoing PCI: additional 180 mcg/kg IV bolus 10 min after the first bolus. For patients with serum Cr >2 mg/dL: Lower dose to 135 mcg/kg bolus and 0.5 mcg/kg/min infusion.

Pediatric dose: Not established.

Contraindications: Documented hypersensitivity; severe hypertension (systolic BP >200 mmHg); active internal bleeding; history of intracranial hemorrhage, intracranial neoplasm, arteriovenous malformation or aneurysm, acute pericarditis, or bleeding diathesis; trauma or stroke within previous 30 d; platelet count <100,000/mm^3; history of thrombocytopenia following prior exposure to this product; serum Cr >4 mg/dL.

Interactions: Possible increased risk of bleeding with coadministration of heparin, warfarin, or aspirin; closely monitor when using other drugs that affect hemostasis.

Pregnancy: B-usually safe but benefits must outweigh the risks.

Precautions: Bleeding events are the most common complications encountered during therapy with eptifibatide; caution in platelet count <150,000/mm^3 and hemorrhagic retinopathy; because agent inhibits platelet aggregation, caution when using concurrently with drugs that affect hemostasis (e.g. thrombolytics, ticlopidine, NSAIDs, warfarin, dipyridamole, clopidogrel); measure ACT and maintain aPTT 50-70 seconds unless a PCI needs to be performed; maintain ACT 250-350 seconds during a PCI; if platelets decrease to <100,000/mm^3, perform additional platelet counts to exclude possibility of pseudothrombocytopenia; if thrombocytopenia is confirmed, discontinue GP IIb/IIIa inhibitors and heparin and appropriately monitor and treat the condition; monitor aPTT 6 h after start of heparin infusion and at least daily thereafter.

Drug category: Platelet aggregation inhibitors inhibit platelet aggregation.

Drug: Abciximab (ReoPro)—chimeric human-murine monoclonal antibody approved for use in elective/urgent/emergent PCI. Binds to receptor with high affinity and reduces platelet aggregation by 80% for up to 48 h following infusion. The recently concluded GUSTO-4 randomized clinical trial did not show any benefit for abciximab in medically treated patients who do not undergo PCI. In fact, longer duration of abciximab use was associated with a negative trend in event rates. On the other hand, in the context of PCI, it has been shown to be superior to tirofiban.

Adult dose: 0.25 mg/kg IV bolus, followed by 10 mcg/min IV for 12 h after PCI.

Pediatric dose: Not established.

Contraindications: Documented hypersensitivity; severe hypertension (systolic BP >200 mmHg); active internal bleeding; history of intracranial hemorrhage, intracranial neoplasm, arteriovenous malformation or aneurysm, acute pericarditis, or bleeding diathesis; trauma or stroke within previous 30 d; platelet count <100,000/mm^3; history of thrombocytopenia following prior exposure to this product.

Interactions: Possible increased risk of bleeding with coadministration with heparin, warfarin, or aspirin; closely monitor when using other drugs that affect hemostasis.

Pregnancy: B-usually safe but benefits must outweigh the risks. Bleeding events are the most common complications encountered during therapy with abciximab; caution in platelet count <150,000/mm^3 and hemorrhagic retinopathy; because agent inhibits platelet aggregation, caution when using concurrently with drugs that affect hemostasis (e.g. thrombolytics, ticlopidine, NSAIDs, warfarin, dipyridamole, clopidogrel); measure ACT and maintain aPTT 50–70 seconds unless a PCI needs to be performed; maintain ACT 250–350 seconds during a PCI; if platelets decrease to <100,000/mm^3, perform additional platelet counts to exclude possibility of pseudothrombocytopenia; if thrombocytopenia is confirmed, discontinue GP IIb/IIIa inhibitors and heparin and appropriately monitor and treat condition; monitor aPTT 6 h after start of heparin infusion and at least daily thereafter; abciximab is associated with an incidence of thrombocytopenia in approximately 2% of patients.

Drug category: Beta-adrenergic blocking agents—limit heart rate and reduce blood pressure to decrease myocardial oxygen demand, oppose effects of elevated catecholamines, and produce antiarrhythmic properties. Clinical trials of beta-adrenoreceptor blockers in cases of unstable angina have shown decreases in ischemic symptoms and in occurrence of MIs. In vitro studies have shown inhibition of platelet aggregation with this drug class. Infrequent situations in which beta-blocker therapy should be avoided in patients with unstable angina include nonischemic exacerbation of heart failure, cocaine-induced coronary vasoconstriction, and vasospastic angina.

Drug: Metoprolol (lopressor, toprol XL)—selective beta1-adrenergic receptor blocker that decreases automaticity of contractions. During IV administration, carefully monitor blood pressure, heart rate and ECG.

Adult dose: 5 mg IV slow infusion q5min up to 3 times until resolution of angina or titrate to reduce heart rate to 50–70 bpm.

Pediatric dose: Not established.

Contraindications: Documented hypersensitivity; uncompensated congestive heart failure; bradycardia; asthma; cardiogenic shock; AV conduction abnormalities.

Interactions: Aluminum salts, barbiturates, NSAIDs, penicillins, calcium salts, cholestyramine, and rifampin may decrease bioavailability and plasma levels of metoprolol, possibly resulting in decreased pharmacologic effects; toxicity of metoprolol may increase with coadministration of sparfloxacin, phenothiazines, astemizole, calcium channel blockers, quinidine, flecainide and contraceptives; may increase toxicity of digoxin, flecainide, clonidine, epinephrine, nifedipine, prazosin, verapamil, and lidocaine.

Pregnancy: B-usually safe but benefits must outweigh the risks.

Precautions: Beta-adrenergic blockade may reduce signs and symptoms of acute hypoglycemia and may decrease clinical signs of hyperthyroidism; abrupt withdrawal may exacerbate symptoms of hyperthyroidism including thyroid storm; closely monitor patient and slowly withdraw the drug; caution in patients taking other negative chronotropes or inotropes (e.g. verapamil).

Drug: Esmolol (brevibloc)—shown to reduce episodes of chest pain and clinical cardiac events compared to placebo. The very short half-life (8 min) allows a large degree of dosing flexibility, such that cardiovascular benefits are comparable to PO propranolol, yet adverse effects can be managed promptly. It is particularly useful for patients at risk for complications with beta-blockade (e.g. reactive airway disease or COPD, severe bradycardia, or poor left ventricular function).

Adult dose: 0.05 mg/kg/min IV over 1 min initially; 0.1 mg/kg/min IV maintenance; titrate in increments of 0.05 mg/kg/min q10–15 min until resolution of angina, until heart rate of 50–70 bpm is attained, or until maximum dose of 0.2 mg/kg/min is reached.

Pediatric dose: Not established.

Contraindications: Documented hypersensitivity; uncompensated congestive heart failure; bradycardia; asthma; cardiogenic shock; AV conduction abnormalities.

Interactions: Aluminum salts, barbiturates, NSAIDs, penicillins, calcium salts, cholestyramine, and rifampin may decrease bioavailability and plasma levels of metoprolol, possibly resulting in decreased pharmacologic effects; toxicity of metoprolol may increase with coadministration of sparfloxacin, phenothiazines, astemizole, calcium channel blockers, quinidine, flecainide and contraceptives; metoprolol may increase toxicity of digoxin, flecainide, clonidine, epinephrine, nifedipine, prazosin, verapamil and lidocaine.

Pregnancy: C-safety for use during pregnancy has not been established.

Precautions: Beta-adrenergic blockade may mask signs and symptoms of acute hypoglycemia and may decrease clinical signs of hyperthyroidism; abrupt withdrawal may exacerbate symptoms of hyperthyroidism including thyroid storm; closely monitor patient and slowly withdraw the drug; during IV administration, carefully monitor blood pressure, heart rate and ECG.

Drug: Propranolol (inderal)—nonselective beta-blocker that is lipophilic (penetrates CNS). Although generally short-acting agent, long-acting preparations are also available.

Adult dose: IR: 40–160 mg PO bid; SR: 60–320 mg PO qd.

Pediatric dose: Not established.

Contraindications: Documented hypersensitivity; history of bronchospasm; uncompensated congestive heart failure; bradycardia; cardiogenic shock; AV conduction abnormalities.

Interactions: Coadministration with aluminum salts, barbiturates, NSAIDs, penicillins, calcium salts, cholestyramine, and rifampin may decrease propranolol effects; calcium channel blockers, cimetidine, loop diuretics, and MAOIs may increase toxicity of propranolol; toxicity of hydralazine, haloperidol, benzodiazepines, and phenothiazines may increase with propranolol.

Pregnancy: C-safety for use during pregnancy has not been established.

Precautions: Beta-adrenergic blockade may hide signs of acute hypoglycemia and hyperthyroidism; abrupt withdrawal may exacerbate symptoms of hyperthyroidism, including thyroid storm; slowly withdraw drug and closely monitor patient; adverse effects include bronchial constriction, Raynaud phenomenon, hypotension, decreased libido, impotence, lethargy, depression, and decreased HDL; caution in Wolff-Parkinson-White syndrome and renal or hepatic dysfunction.

Drug: Nadolol (corgard)—competitively blocks beta-1 and beta-2 receptors. Does not exhibit membrane stabilizing activity or intrinsic sympathomimetic activity.

Adult dose: 40 mg/d PO initially; gradually increase dose by 40–80 mg increments at 3–7 d intervals up to 160–240 mg/d.

Pediatric dose: Not established.

Contraindications: Documented hypersensitivity; congestive heart failure; pulmonary edema; cardiogenic shock; AV conduction abnormalities; heart block (without a pacemaker).

Interactions: Coadministration with aluminum salts, barbiturates, calcium salts, cholestyramine, NSAIDs, penicillins, and rifampin may decrease effects; haloperidol, hydralazine, loop diuretics, and MAOIs may increase toxicity of nadolol.

Pregnancy: C-safety for use during pregnancy has not been established.

Precautions: Beta-adrenergic blockade may reduce symptoms of acute hypoglycemia and mask signs of hyperthyroidism; abrupt withdrawal may exacerbate symptoms of hyperthyroidism and cause thyroid storm; closely monitor patients and slowly withdraw drug; during an IV, carefully monitor BP, heart rate and ECG.

Drug category: Antithrombotic agents—thrombin, the end product of the coagulation mechanism, initiates transformation of fibrinogen to a fibrin clot and activates platelets. Its antagonist, antithrombin III, is the major endogenous inhibitor of the coagulation cascade and is the essential cofactor for heparin.

Drug: Heparin (hep-lock)—catalyzes the effect of antithrombin III on coagulative proteinases (e.g. factors II, XII, XI, IX, and X; tissue factor VIIa). Prevents reaccumulation of clot after endogenous fibrinolysis. Meta-analysis shows modest benefit (when compared to aspirin alone) and slight increase in bleeding. Reactivation of unstable angina after discontinuation of heparin has been documented among subjects not receiving concomitant aspirin therapy. When unfractionated heparin is used, the aPTT should not be checked until 6 h after initial heparin bolus.

Table 4: *Treatment of hypercyanotic spells in tetralogy of Fallot*

Knee to chest position
Supplemental oxygen
Morphine sulfate (0.1 mg/kg 1 m or SC)
If not responding to above:
Obtain IV access
Repeat morphine sulfate if agitated
IV fluid bolus 00 mL/kg
Phenylephrine infusion 0.5–5.0 (~kg/min fitrate to effect)
$NaHCO_3$ (1 mEq/kg IV)
Propraolol (0.5–0.10 mg/kg IV maximum dose 1 mg)
If remains criticat:
Consider general anethesia and paralytic agent.
Urgent consultation with cardiothoracic surgery is needed for

Adult dose: 80 U/kg IV bolus, followed by infusion of 18 U/kg/h; titrate to maintain aPTT 1.5-2.5 times control; decrease initial bolus dose to 50 U/kg IV when used in conjunction with GP IIb/IIIa antagonist.

Pediatric dose: Not established.

Contraindications: Documented hypersensitivity; subacute bacterial endocarditis; active bleeding; history of heparin-induced thrombocytopenia.

Interactions: Digoxin, nicotine, tetracycline, and antihistamines may decrease effects; NSAIDs, aspirin, dextran, dipyridamole, and hydroxychloroquine may increase heparin toxicity.

Pregnancy: B-usually safe but benefits must outweigh the risks.

Precautions: Most important risk with unfractionated heparin is ineffectiveness because of insufficient dose; may cause hemorrhagic complications; if significant bleeding complications develop, 15 mg protamine sulphate (infused over 3 min) usually reverses anticoagulant effect; can trigger immune thrombotic thrombocytopenia 1–2 wk after beginning of treatment; heparin-associated thrombocytopenia is serious, causes widespread thrombosis refractory to treatment, and can be fatal if not recognized quickly and managed appropriately; some preparations contain benzyl alcohol as a preservative, which can be associated with fetal toxicity (gasping syndrome) when used in large amounts; use of preservative-free heparin is recommended in neonates; caution in shock or severe hypotension.

Drug: Enoxaparin (lovenox) or dalteparin (fragmin)—enoxaparin: only LMWH now approved by the FDA both for treatment and for prophylaxis of deep venous thrombosis and pulmonary embolism. LMWH has been widely used in pregnancy, although clinical trials are not yet available to demonstrate that it is as safe as unfractionated heparin. Except in overdoses, checking PT or aPTT is not useful because aPTT does not correlate with the anticoagulant effect of fractionated LMWH. Dalteparin: LMWH with many similarities to enoxaparin but with a different dosing schedule. Except in overdoses, checking PT or aPTT is not useful because aPTT does not correlate with the anticoagulant effect of fractionated LMWH. Approved for deep venous thrombosis and pulmonary embolism prophylaxis for patients undergoing orthopedic and abdominal surgery.

Adult dose: Enoxaparin: 1 mg/kg SC q12h or 1.5 mg/kg SC qd. Prophylaxis against DVT: 30 mg SC q12h. Dalteparin: 120 IU/kg SC q12h; not to exceed 10,000 IU for at least 5 d or until revascularization is performed (FRISC-2 regimen).

Pediatric dose: Not established.

Contraindications: Documented hypersensitivity; major bleeding; thrombocytopenia.

Interactions: Platelet inhibitors or PO anticoagulants (e.g. dipyridamole, salicylates, aspirin, NSAIDs, sulfinpyrazone, ticlopidine) may increase risk of bleeding.

Pregnancy: B-usually safe but benefits must outweigh the risks.

Precautions: If thromboembolic event occurs despite LMWH prophylaxis, discontinue drug and initiate alternate therapy; elevation of hepatic transaminases may occur but is reversible; heparin-associated thrombocytopenia may occur with fractionated LMWHs; 1 mg of protamine sulfate reverses effect of approximately 1 mg of enoxaparin if significant bleeding complications develop; if necessary, 1 mg of protamine can neutralize 100 U dalteparin.

Drug category: Thrombin inhibitors—lepirudin and bivalirudin are direct thrombin inhibitors. Advantages over heparin are efficacy against clot-bound thrombin, resistance to inactivation by platelet factor 4 and thrombospondin, and nondependence on antithrombin III pathways. Data to date suggest only a modest reduction in adverse events at the cost of increased nonmajor bleeding complications. GUSTO IIB investigators compared recombinant hirudin and heparin in 12,142 patients, a third of whom had ST elevation MI. The hirudin group had a 9% relative risk reduction in 30-d death or MI rates (8.9% vs 9.8%), but more moderate bleeding events occurred (8.8% vs 7.7%).

OASIS-2 was an international randomized clinical trial that involved 10,141 patients. Patients were randomized between heparin (aPTT maintained between 60 and 100 seconds) or lepirudin, which is recombinant hirudin (0.4 mg/kg bolus followed by 0.15 mg/kg/h 72-h IV infusion). Unlike for GP IIb/IIIa antagonists, no evidence indicates attenuation of myocardial necrosis (based on CK or troponin measurements). Approved by the FDA in patients with heparin-induced thrombocytopenia and associated thrombotic disease. Goal is 1.5-2.5 times the control aPTT values. Dose needs to be adjusted for patients with renal impairment. Bivalirudin (angiomax) is a thrombin inhibitor used for anticoagulation in patients with unstable angina undergoing PTCA.

Drug: Bivalirudin (angiomax) used for anticoagulation in patients with unstable angina undergoing PTCA. Synthetic analogue of recombinant hirudin. Inhibits thrombin. Potential advantages over conventional heparin therapy include more predictable and precise levels of anticoagulation, activity against clot-bound thrombin, absence of natural inhibitors (e.g. platelet factor 4, heparinase), and continued efficacy following clearance from plasma (due to binding to thrombin).

Adult dose: 1 mg/kg IV bolus initially; followed by 2.5 mg/kg/h IV for 4 h; may administer additional IV infusion at 0.2 mg/kg/h (not to exceed 20 h); administer with 300–325 mg/d aspirin.

Pediatric dose: Not established.

Contraindications: Documented hypersensitivity; cerebral aneurysm; intracranial hemorrhage; general uncontrollable hemorrhage; active major bleeding.

Interactions: Coadministration with antiplatelets (other than aspirin) or other anticoagulants not fully evaluated (use caution)

Pregnancy: B-usually safe but benefits must outweigh the risks.

Precautions: Adjust dose in renal impairment; caution in recent surgery, trauma, or GI ulceration; bleeding may occur; may cause back pain, nausea, headache and hypotension.

Drug: Lepirudin (refludan)—recombinant hirudin derived from yeast cells. Highly specific direct inhibitor of thrombin. Natural hirudin is produced in trace amounts as a family of highly homologous isopolypeptides by the leech *Hirudo medicinalis.* Biosynthetic lepirudin is identical to natural hirudin except for substitution of leucine for isoleucine at the *N*-terminal end of the molecule and the absence of a sulfate group on the tyrosine at position 63. Activity of lepirudin is measured in a chromogenic assay. One antithrombin unit (ATU) is the amount of lepirudin that neutralizes one unit of World Health Organization preparation 89/588 of thrombin. Specific activity of lepirudin is >16,000 ATU/mg. Mode of action is independent of antithrombin III. Platelet factor 4 does not inhibit lepirudin. One molecule of lepirudin binds to one molecule of thrombin and thereby blocks the thrombogenic activity of thrombin. As a result, all thrombin-dependent coagulation assays are affected (e.g. aPTT values increase in a dose-dependent fashion).Goal is 1.5-2.5 times the control aPTT values. Dose needs to be adjusted for patients with renal impairment.

Adult dose: 0.4 mg/kg IV bolus over 15–20 seconds, followed by continuous infusion of 0.15 mg/kg/h.

Pediatric dose: Not established.

Contraindications: Documented hypersensitivity; major bleeding; thrombocytopenia.

Interactions: Intracranial bleeding may be life-threatening following concomitant fibrinolytic therapy.

Pregnancy: B-usually safe but benefits must outweigh the risks.

Precautions: Associated with increased need for transfusion (vs unfractionated heparin) and slightly increased risk of intracranial hemorrhage; no specific antidote.

Drug category: Vasodilators—relieve chest discomfort by improving myocardial oxygen supply, which in turn dilates epicardial and collateral vessels, improving blood supply to the ischemic myocardium. Opposes coronary artery spasm, which augments coronary blood flow and reduces cardiac work by decreasing preload and afterload. Effective in the management of symptoms in acute MI but may reduce mortality only slightly. Nitroglycerin can be administered sublingually by tablet or spray, topically, or IV. In acute MI, topical administration is a less desirable route because of unpredictable absorption and onset of clinical effects.

Drug: Nitroglycerin (minitran, nitrogard, nitrol, nitrolingual, nitrostat, nitro-dur)—causes relaxation of vascular smooth muscle by stimulating intracellular cyclic guanosine monophosphate production. Whether administered topically, SL, PO, or IV, nitrates ameliorate several pathways of unstable angina and reduce the incidence of symptomatic ischemia. Nitrates lower systemic arterial pressure and decrease venous return to the heart, both of which reduce myocardial wall stress. Similarly, nitrates are excellent coronary vasodilators. Other possible beneficial effects include transient inhibition of platelet aggregation, increase in coronary collateral blood flow, and a favorable redistribution of regional flow. Of note, induction of heparin resistance has been reported.

Adult dose: 400 mcg SL tab or spray q5min, repeated up to 3 times; if symptoms persist, infuse IV at a rate of 5–10 mcg/min; titrate dose to a 10% reduction in mean arterial pressure.

Pediatric dose: Not established.

Contraindications: Documented hypersensitivity; severe anemia; shock; postural hypotension; head trauma; closed-angle glaucoma; cerebral hemorrhage; known right ventricular infarct.

Interactions: Aspirin may increase nitrate serum concentrations; marked symptomatic orthostatic hypotension may occur with coadministration of calcium channel blockers (dose adjustment of either agent may be necessary).

Pregnancy: C-safety for use during pregnancy has not been established.

Precautions: Caution in CAD and low systolic blood; limiting adverse effects include hypotension (>30% reduction in mean arterial pressure or systolic BP < 90).

Treatment and Prevention of GAS

Treatment and prevention of GAS pharyngitis outlined here are based on the current recommendations of the Committee on Infectious Disease (American Academy of Pediatrics). Medical therapy is directed toward elimination of GAS pharyngitis (if still present), suppression of inflammation from the autoimmune response, and supportive treatment of CHF. Attempts are being made to produce vaccines against GAS infection, but the vaccines will not be available for years.

Antibiotics for endocarditis prophylaxis are administered to patients with certain cardiac conditions, such as carditis caused by rheumatic fever before procedures that may cause bacteremia are performed. For more information:

Drug category: Antibiotics—the roles for antibiotics are to (1) initially treat GAS pharyngitis, (2) prevent recurrent streptococcal pharyngitis, RF, and RHD, and (3) provide prophylaxis against bacterial endocarditis.

Drug: Penicillin VK (Beepen-VK, Pen.Vee K, V-Cillin K, Veetids)—DOC for treatment of GAS pharyngitis. Although ampicillin or amoxicillin may be used instead, they have no microbiologic advantage. Do not use tetracyclines and sulfonamides to treat GAS pharyngitis. For recurrent GAS pharyngitis, a second 10-d course of same antibiotic may be repeated. Alternate drugs include narrow-spectrum cephalosporins, amoxicillin-clavulanate, dicloxacillin, erythromycin, or other macrolides.

Adult dose: 500 mg PO bid/tid for 10 d.

Pediatric dose: Children: 250 mg (400,000 U) PO bid/tid for 10 d. Adolescents: administer as in adults.

Contraindications: Documented hypersensitivity.

Interactions: Probenecid may increase effectiveness by decreasing clearance; tetracyclines are bacteriostatic, causing decrease in effectiveness of penicillins when administered concurrently.

Pregnancy: B-usually safe but benefits must outweigh the risks.

Precautions: Renal impairment, anaphylaxis, thrombocytopenia.

Drug: Benzathine (Bicillin L-A)/procaine penicillin (Crysticillin A.S., Wycillin) used when PO administration of penicillin is not feasible or dependable. IM therapy with penicillin is painful, but discomfort may be minimized if penicillin G is brought to room temperature before injection or combination of benzathine penicillin G and procaine penicillin G is used. Initial course of antibiotics administered to eradicate streptococcal infection also serves as first course of prophylaxis. An injection of benzathine penicillin G IM q4wk is recommended regimen for secondary prevention for most United States patients. Administer same dosage q3wk in areas where RF is endemic, in patients with residual carditis, and in high-risk patients.

Adult dose: Eradication: 1.2 million U of benzathine penicillin G or a combination of 900,000 U of benzathine penicillin G with 300,000 U of procaine penicillin G IM as a single dose. Secondary prevention: administer eradication dose q3wk (in high-risk areas, high-risk patients) or q4wk (for most areas in United States).

Pediatric dose: Eradication <60 lb: 600,000 U of benzathine penicillin G IM as a single dose. Secondary prevention: Administer eradication dose q3wk (in high-risk areas, high-risk patients) or q4wk (for most areas in United States)

Contraindications: Documented hypersensitivity.

Interactions: Increases risk of bleeding when administered concurrently with warfarin; ethacrynic acid, aspirin, indomethacin, and furosemide may compete with penicillin G for renal tubular secretion, increasing penicillin serum concentrations.

Pregnancy: B-usually safe but benefits must outweigh the risks.

Precautions: Never use IV route to administer penicillin G procaine; impaired renal function; anaphylaxis; thrombocytopenia.

Drug: Erythromycin (EES, E-Mycin, Eryc, Ery-Tab, Erythrocin)—used for patients who are allergic to penicillin. Other options include clarithromycin, azithromycin, or a narrow-spectrum cephalosporin (i.e., cephalexin). As many as 15% of penicillin-allergic patients also are allergic to cephalosporins.

Adult dose: 250 mg erythromycin stearate/base (or 400 mg ethylsuccinate) q6h PO 1 h ac for 10 d.

Pediatric dose: 20-40 mg (as base, estolate, or stearate)/kg/d PO divided bid/qid for 10 d; not to exceed 1 g/dAlternatively, 40 mg (as ethylsuccinate)/kg/d PO divided bid/qid for 10 d.

Contraindications: Documented hypersensitivity; with terfenadine (off US market) or astemizole (use in combination with erythromycin may cause prolongation of QT interval, with increased risk of ventricular arrhythmias and sudden death).

Interactions: Coadministration may increase toxicity of theophylline, digoxin, carbamazepine and cyclosporine; may potentiate anticoagulant effects of warfarin; coadministration with lovastatin and simvastatin increases risk of rhabdomyolysis.

Pregnancy: B-Usually safe but benefits must outweigh the risks.

Precautions: Caution in liver disease; estolate formulation may cause cholestatic jaundice; GI adverse effects are common (administer doses pc); discontinue use if nausea, vomiting, malaise, abdominal colic, or fever occurs.

Drug: Clarithromycin (biaxin)—alternate antibiotic for treating GAS pharyngitis in patients allergic to penicillin.

Adult dose: 250–500 mg PO bid for 10 d.

Pediatric dose: 7.5 mg/kg PO bid for 10 d.

Contraindications: Documented hypersensitivity; coadministration of pimozide; patients taking terfenadine (off US market); patients with long QT syndrome.

Interactions: CYP450 1A2 and 3A4 inhibitor; toxicity increases with coadministration of fluconazole and pimozide; clarithromycin effects decrease and GI adverse effects may increase with coadministration of rifabutin or rifampin; may increase toxicity of anticoagulants, cyclosporine, tacrolimus, digoxin, omeprazole, carbamazepine, ergot alkaloids, triazolam, and HMG CoA-reductase inhibitors; plasma levels of certain benzodiazepines may increase, prolonging CNS depression; arrhythmias and increase in QTc intervals occur with disopyramide; coadministration with omeprazole may increase plasma levels of both agents.

Pregnancy: C-safety for use during pregnancy has not been established.

Precautions: Coadministration with ranitidine or bismuth citrate is not recommended with CrCl <25 mL/min; administer one half dose or increase dosing interval if CrCl <30 mL/min; diarrhea may be sign of pseudomembranous colitis; superinfections may occur with prolonged or repeated antibiotic therapies.

Drug: Azithromycin (zithromax)—alternate antibiotic for treating GAS pharyngitis in patients allergic to penicillin.

Adult dose: 12 mg/kg (not to exceed 500 mg) PO qd for 5 d.

Pediatric dose: Administer as in adults.

Contraindications: Documented hypersensitivity; hepatic impairment; do not administer with pimozide.

Interactions: May increase toxicity of theophylline, warfarin, and digoxin; effects are reduced with coadministration of aluminum and/or magnesium antacids; nephrotoxicity and neurotoxicity may occur when coadministered with cyclosporine.

Pregnancy: B-usually safe but benefits must outweigh the risks.

Precautions: May increase hepatic enzymes and cholestatic jaundice; caution in patients with impaired hepatic function, prolonged QT intervals, or pneumonia; caution in patients who are hospitalized, geriatric, or debilitated.

Drug: Cephalexin (keflex, biocef, keftab)—alternate antibiotic for treating GAS pharyngitis in patients allergic to penicillin.

Adult dose: 250–500 mg PO qid for 10 d.

Pediatric dose: 25–50 mg/kg/d PO divided qid for 10 d.

Contraindications: Documented hypersensitivity.

Interactions: Coadministration with aminoglycosides increases nephrotoxic potential.

Pregnancy: B-Usually safe but benefits must outweigh the risks.

*Precautions:*Adjust dose in renal impairment.

Drug: Amoxicillin (amoxil, biomox, trimox)—DOC used for bacterial endocarditis prophylaxis. Administered as single PO dose 1 h before dental work or surgery.

Adult dose: 2 g PO once as a single dose.

Pediatric dose: 50 mg/kg PO once as a single dose.

Contraindications: Documented hypersensitivity.

Interactions: None significant for prophylaxis.

Pregnancy: B-usually safe but benefits must outweigh the risks.

Precautions: Adjust dose in renal impairment.

Drug category: Antiinflammatory agents—manifestations of acute RF (including carditis) typically respond rapidly to therapy with anti-inflammatory agents. Aspirin, in anti-inflammatory doses, is DOC. Prednisone is added when evidence of worsening carditis and heart failure exists.

Drug: Aspirin (anacin, ascriptin, bayer aspirin)—begin administration immediately after diagnosis of RF. Initiation of therapy may mask manifestations of disease.

Adult dose: 4–8 g/d PO divided q4-6h; maintain aspirin levels in 20-25 mg/dL range until all symptoms have resolved and APRs have returned to normal.

Pediatric dose: 80–100 mg/kg/d PO divided q4–6h; maintain aspirin levels in 20–25 mg/dL range until all symptoms have resolved and APRs have returned to normal.

Contraindications: Documented hypersensitivity; liver damage; hypoprothrombinemia, vitamin K deficiency; bleeding disorders; asthma.

Interactions: Effects may decrease with antacids and urinary alkalinizers; corticosteroids decrease salicylate serum levels; additive hypoprothrombinemic effects and increased bleeding time may occur with coadministration of anticoagulants; may antagonize uricosuric effects of probenecid and increase toxicity of phenytoin and valproic acid; doses > 2 g/d may potentiate glucose-lowering effect of sulfonylurea drugs.

Pregnancy: D-unsafe in pregnancy.

Precautions: Risk of salicylate intoxication and poisoning; watch for hyperventilation with prolonged expiratory phase with respiratory alkalosis and metabolic acidosis; risk of tinnitus, GI discomfort, and ulceration; when taken during pregnancy, increased risk of pulmonary hypertension exists in fetus in neonatal period.

Drug: Prednisone (deltasone, orasone) if moderate-to-severe carditis is present as indicated by cardiomegaly, CHF, or third-degree heart block, use 2 mg/kg/d PO prednisone in addition to or in lieu of salicylate therapy. Continue prednisone for 2–4 wk depending on severity of carditis and taper during last week of therapy. Discontinuing prednisone therapy after 2 wk while adding or maintaining salicylates for additional 2–4 wk may minimize adverse effects.

Adult dose: 2 mg/kg/d PO for 2–4 wk.

Pediatric dose: Administer as in adults.

Contraindications: Documented hypersensitivity; viral infection; peptic ulcer disease; hepatic dysfunction; connective tissue infections; fungal or tubercular skin infections; GI disease.

Interactions: Coadministration with estrogens may decrease prednisone clearance; concurrent use with digoxin may cause digitalis toxicity secondary to hypokalemia; phenobarbital, phenytoin, and rifampin may increase metabolism of glucocorticoids (consider increasing maintenance dose); monitor for hypokalemia with coadministration of diuretics.

Pregnancy: C-safety for use during pregnancy has not been established.

Precautions: Abrupt discontinuation of glucocorticoids may cause adrenal crisis; hyperglycemia, edema, osteonecrosis, myopathy, peptic ulcer disease, hypokalemia, osteoporosis, euphoria, psychosis, myasthenia gravis, growth suppression, and infections may occur with glucocorticoid use.

Drug category: **Therapy for congestive heart failure**—heart failure in RHD probably is related in part to severe insufficiency of the mitral and aortic valves and in part to pancarditis. Therapy traditionally has consisted of an inotropic agent (digitalis) in combination with diuretics (furosemide, spironolactone) and afterload reduction (captopril).

Drug: Digoxin (lanoxin, lanoxicaps)—inotropic agent widely used in past. Its efficacy in CHF is under review. Potential for toxicity is present. Therapeutic levels and clinical effects are observed more quickly if loading doses of digitalis are administered before routine maintenance doses. Acts directly on cardiac muscle, increasing myocardial systolic contractions. Indirect actions result in increased carotid sinus nerve activity and enhanced sympathetic withdrawal for any given increase in mean arterial pressure. Therapeutic digoxin levels are present at trough levels of 1.5–2 ng/mL.

Adult dose: Total digitalizing dose (TDD) to be administered over 24 h; first dose is one half the TDD; second dose is one-fourth the TDD, given 8 h later; third dose is one-fourth the TDD, given 8 h after the second. TDD: 0.75–1.5 mg PO. Maintenance dose: 0.125–0.5 mg PO qd.

Pediatric dose: TDD to be administered over 24 h; first dose is one half the TDD; second dose is one-fourth the TDD, given 8 h later; third dose is one-fourth the TDD, given 8 h after the second TDD: preterm infant: 20–30 mcg/kg PO, Term infant: 25–35 mcg/kg PO. 1 month to 2 years:

Table 5: *Medications to maintain cardiac output and for postresuscitation stabilization*

Medication	*Dose range*	*Comment*
Inamrinone	0.75–1 mg/kg IV/IO over 5 minutes; may repeat × 2 then: 2–20 µg/kg per minute	Inodilator
Dobutamine	2–20 mg/kg per minute IV/IO	Inotrope; vasodilator
Dopamine	2–20 mg/kg per minute IV/IO	Inotrope; chronotrope; renal and splanchnic vasodilator in low doses; pressor in high doses
Epinephrine	0.1–1 mg/kg per minute IV/IO	Inotrope; chronotrope; vasodilator in low doses; pressor in higher doses
Milrinone	50–75 µg/kg IV/IO over 10–60 min then 0.5–0.75 µg/kg per minute	Indilator
Norepinephrine	0.1–2 µg/kg per minute	Inotrope; vasopressor
Sodium nitroprusside	1–8 µg/kg per minute	Vasodilator; prepare only in D5W

IV, intravenous; IO, intraosseous

Alternative formula for calculating an infusion:

Infusion rate (mL/h) - [weight (kg) × dose (µg/kg/min) × 60 (min/h)]/concentration µg/mL.

Table 6: *Meanings of terms used in pediatric cardiology*

Adrenergic: Activating the sympathetic nervous system
Afterload: The resistance against which the myocardium must eject
Agonist: Acting positively toward an action
Alpha: Vasoconstriction
Antagonist: Opposite in action
Beta1: Increasing contractility, heart rate
Beta2: Vasodilation and bronchodilation
Cardiac output: (Heart rate) × (Stroke volume)
Cholinergic: Activating the parasympathetic nervous system
Chronotropic: Affecting heart rate
Contractility: The intrinsic ability of the myocardial fibers to contract
Dopaminergic: Renal perfusion
Half-life: The time required for 50% of a dose to be excreted, used to determine intervals for dosing
Heart rate: The rate of ventricular contraction
Inotropic: Affecting contractility
Preload: The amount of blood distending the ventricles prior to contraction
Stroke volume: Determined by preload, afterload, and contracility

35–60 mcg/kg. PO_2-5 years: 30–40 mcg/kg PO. 5–10 years: 20–35 mcg/kg PO>10 years: Administer as in adults. Maintenance dose: preterm infant: 5–7.5 mcg/kg/d PO divided bid. Term infant: 6–10 mcg/kg/d PO divided bid 1 month to 2 years: 10–15 mcg/kg/d PO divided bid 2–5 years: 7.5–10 mcg/kg/d PO divided bid 5–10 years: 5–10 mcg/kg/d PO divided bid > 10 years: Administer as in adults.

Contraindications: Documented hypersensitivity; beri beri heart disease; idiopathic hypertrophic subaortic stenosis; constrictive pericarditis; carotid sinus syndrome.

Interactions: Medications that may increase digoxin levels include alprazolam, benzodiazepines, bepridil, captopril, cyclosporine, propafenone, propantheline, quinidine, diltiazem, aminoglycosides, PO amiodarone, anticholinergics, diphenoxylate, erythromycin, felodipine, flecainide, hydroxychloroquine, itraconazole, nifedipine, omeprazole, quinine, ibuprofen, indomethacin, esmolol, tetracycline, tolbutamide, and verapamil. Medications that may decrease serum digoxin levels include aminoglutethimide, antihistamines, cholestyramine, neomycin, penicillamine, aminoglycosides, PO colestipol, hydantoins, hypoglycemic agents, antineoplastic treatment combinations (e.g. carmustine, bleomycin, methotrexate, cytarabine, doxorubicin, cyclophosphamide, vincristine, procarbazine), aluminum or magnesium antacids, rifampin, sucralfate, sulfasalazine, barbiturates, kaolin/pectin, and aminosalicylic acid.

Pregnancy: C-safety for use during pregnancy has not been established.

Precautions: Hypokalemia may reduce positive inotropic effect of digitalis; IV calcium may produce arrhythmias in patients receiving digitalis; hypercalcemia predisposes patient to digitalis toxicity, and hypocalcemia can make digoxin ineffective until serum calcium levels are normal; magnesium replacement therapy must be instituted in patients with hypomagnesemia to prevent digitalis toxicity; patients diagnosed with incomplete AV block may progress to complete block when treated with digoxin; caution in hypothyroidism, hypoxia, and acute myocarditis; initiate digoxin only after checking electrolytes and correcting abnormalities in serum potassium.

Drug: Captopril (capoten)—systemic afterload reduction may be helpful in improving cardiac output, particularly in setting of mitral and aortic valve insufficiency. Some patients have unusually large hypotensive response. Use small starting dose, particularly with hypovolemia.

Adult dose: Starting dose: 6.25–12.5 mg PO tid. Typical dose: 50–100 mg PO tid.

Pediatric dose: Starting dose: 0.1–0.5 mg/kg/d PO divided tid; typically 1–2 mg/kg/d PO divided tid.

Contraindications: Documented hypersensitivity; renal impairment.

Interactions: NSAIDs may reduce hypotensive effects of captopril; ACE inhibitors may increase digoxin, lithium, and allopurinol levels; rifampin decreases captopril levels; probenecid may increase captopril levels; hypotensive effects of ACE inhibitors may be enhanced when administered concurrently with diuretics.

Pregnancy: C-safety for use during pregnancy has not been established.

Precautions: Pregnancy category D in second and third trimesters; caution in renal impairment, valvular stenosis, or severe CHF.

Drug: Furosemide (lasix)—diuretics frequently are used in conjunction with inotropic agents for patients with CHF. When used aggressively, may result in hypokalemia and hypovolemia. Risk of hearing loss in premature infants. Increases excretion of water by interfering with chloride-binding cotransport system, which, in turn, inhibits sodium and chloride reabsorption in ascending loop of Henle and distal renal tubule.

Adult dose: 20–40 mg PO/IV/IM bid/tid.

Pediatric dose: 1–2 mg/kg/dose PO/IV/IM qd/tid.

Contraindications: Documented hypersensitivity; hepatic coma; anuria; state of severe electrolyte depletion.

Interactions Metformin decreases furosemide concentrations; furosemide interferes with hypoglycemic effect of antidiabetic agents and antagonizes muscle-relaxing effect of tubocurarine; auditory toxicity appears to be increased with coadministration of aminoglycosides and furosemide; hearing loss of varying degrees may occur; anticoagulant activity of warfarin may be enhanced with concurrent administration; increased plasma lithium levels and toxicity are possible with concurrent administration.

Pregnancy: C-safety for use during pregnancy has not been established.

Precautions: Obtain frequent serum electrolyte, carbon dioxide, glucose, creatinine, uric acid, calcium, and BUN determinations during first few months of therapy and periodically thereafter.

Drug: Spironolactone (aldactone) used in conjunction with furosemide as potassium-sparing diuretic. Competes with aldosterone for receptor sites in distal renal tubules, increasing water excretion while retaining potassium and hydrogen ions.

Adult dose: 100 mg PO divided qd/bid.

Pediatric dose: 2–4 mg/kg/d PO divided bid.

Contraindications: Documented hypersensitivity; anuria; renal failure; hyperkalemia.

Interactions: May decrease effect of anticoagulants; potassium and potassium-sparing diuretics may increase toxicity of spironolactone.

Pregnancy: D-unsafe in pregnancy.

Precautions: Caution in renal and hepatic impairment mmHg or severe headache.

BIBLIOGRAPHY

1. Bailey JM, Miller BE, Lu, W, Tosone, SR, Kanter, KR, & Tam, VK (1999). The pharmacokinetics of milrinone in pediatric patients after cardiac surgery. Anesthesiology, 90, 1012–1018.
2. Bell SG. (1998). Neonatal cardiovascular pharmacology. Neonatal Network, 17, 7–15.
3. Berg RA, & Padbury JF. (1997). Sulphoconjugation and renal excretion contribute to the interpatient variation of exogenous catecholamine clearance in critically ill children. Critical Care Medicine, 25, 1247–1251.
4. Bindler RM, & Howry, LB (1997). Pediatric drugs and nursing implications (2nd ed.). Upper Saddle River, NJ: Pearson Education.
5. Chowdhury C, Parnell VA, Ojamaa K, Boxer R., Cooper, R., & Klein, I. (1999). Usefulness of triodothyronine (T3) treatment after surgery for complex congenital heart disease in infants and children. The American Journal of Cardiology, 84, 1107–1109.
6. Fineman JR, & Soifer SJ (1998). The fetal and neonatal circulations. In AC Chang, FL Hanley, G Wernovsky, & C.L. Wessel (Eds.), Pediatric cardiac intensive care (pp. 17–20). Baltimore: Williams & Wilkins.
7. Hazinski MF (1999). Cardiovascular disorders. The manual of pediatric critical care (pp. 112, 284–288). St. Louis: Mosby.
8. Kohr LM, & Sims SL (1998). Alterations of cardiovascular function in children. Pathophysiology: The biologic basis for disease in adults and children (3rd ed.) (pp. 1093–1101). St. Louis: Mosby.
9. McCance KL (1998). Structure and function of the cardiovascular and lymphatic systems. Pathophysiology: The biologic basis for disease in adults and children (3rd ed.) (pp. 968–988). St. Louis: Mosby.
10. Noerr, B. (1999). Pointers in practical pharmacology: Spironolactone. Neonatal Network, 18, 43–46.
11. Rosen DA (1996). Effects of T3 to treat postoperative cardiac failure in congenital cardiac surgery patients. Critical Care Medicine, 24 (1), A121.
12. Taketomo CK, Hodding, JH, & Kraus, CK (2000). Pediatric dosage handbook (7th ed.). Hudson, OH: Lexi-Comp, Inc.

Index

A

D

E

F

G

H

I

J

K

L

Q

R

S

Reader's Notes

Reader's Notes